T0331121

Clinical Exercise Pathophysiology for Physical Therapy

Examination, Testing, and Exercise Prescription for Movement-Related Disorders

Clinical Exercise Pathophysiology for Physical Therapy

Examination, Testing, and Exercise Prescription for Movement-Related Disorders

Editor

Debra Coglianese, PT, DPT, OCS, ATC
Clinical Specialist
Mercy Rehab & Wellness Center at Havertown
Havertown, Pennsylvania
Mentor for Professional Development and Portfolios
Rehabilitation Services
Mercy Fitzgerald Hospital
Darby, Pennsylvania

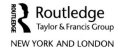
Routledge
Taylor & Francis Group

NEW YORK AND LONDON

Clinical Exercise Pathophysiology for Physical Therapy: Examination, Testing, and Exercise Prescription for Movement-Related Disorders includes ancillary materials specifically available for faculty use. Included are PowerPoint Slides. Please visit http://www.routledge.com/9781617116452 to obtain access.

First published 2015 by SLACK Incorporated

Published 2024 by Routledge
605 Third Avenue, New York, NY 10158

and by Routledge
4 Park Square, Milton Park, Abingdon, Oxon OX14 4RN

Routledge is an imprint of the Taylor & Francis Group, an informa business

Library of Congress Cataloging-in-Publication Data

Clinical exercise pathophysiology for physical therapy : examination, testing, and exercise prescription for movement-related disorders / [edited by] Debra Coglianese.
        p. ; cm.
Includes bibliographical references and index.
ISBN 978-1-61711-645-2 (hardback : alk. paper)
I. Coglianese, Debra, - editor.
[DNLM: 1. Exercise--physiology--Case Reports. 2. Physical Therapy Modalities--Case Reports. WB 460]
RM725
615.8'2--dc23
                        2014011379

ISBN: 9781617116452 (hbk)
ISBN: 9781003523048 (ebk)

DOI: 10.4324/9781003523048

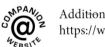

Additional resources can be found at
https://www.routledge.com/9781617116452

CONTENTS

Clinical Exercise Pathophysiology for Physical Therapy: Examination, Testing, and Exercise Prescription for Movement-Related Disorders includes ancillary materials specifically available for faculty use. Included are PowerPoint Slides. Please visit http:// www.routledge.com/9781617116452 to obtain access.

CONTRIBUTING AUTHORS

Joanell A. Bohmert, PT, DPT, MS (Case Study 2-1)
Physical Therapist
Anoka-Hennepin Independent School District No. 11
Anoka, Minnesota

Lisa Brown, PT, DPT, NCS (Chapter 12)
Clinical Assistant Professor
Boston University
Sargent College of Health and Rehabilitation Science
Boston, Massachusetts

Cheryl L. Brunelle, PT, MS, CCS, CLT (Chapter 7, Case Study 7-1)
Clinical Specialist, Physical Therapy Services
Massachusetts General Hospital
Boston, Massachusetts

LeeAnne Carrothers, PT, PhD (Chapter 4, Chapter 5)
Program Director, Physical Therapist Assistant Program
Term Assistant Professor
University of Alaska Anchorage
Anchorage, Alaska

David Chapman, PT, PhD (Chapter 2)
Associate Professor
Physical Therapy Program
St. Catherine University
Minneapolis, Minnesota

Debra Coglianese, PT, DPT, OCS, ATC (Chapter 10, Case Study 10-1)
Clinical Specialist
Mercy Rehab & Wellness Center at Havertown
Havertown, Pennsylvania
Mentor for Professional Development and Portfolios
Rehabilitation Services
Mercy Fitzgerald Hospital
Darby, Pennsylvania

Kathleen Coultes, PT, PCS (Case Study 2-2)
Pediatric Clinical Specialist
Rehabilitation Services
Mercy Fitzgerald Hospital
Darby, Pennsylvania

Vanina Dal Bello-Haas, PT, PhD (Case Study 12-2)
Associate Professor
Assistant Dean, Physiotherapy Program
School of Rehabilitation Science
McMaster University
Hamilton, Ontario, Canada

Skye Donovan, PT, PhD, OCS (Chapter 5)
Associate Professor
Department of Physical Therapy
Marymount University
Arlington, Virginia

Susan L. Edmond, PT, DSc, OCS (Chapter 11, Case Study 11-1)
Professor
School of Health Related Professions
Department of Movement Sciences
Rutgers, The State University of New Jersey
Newark, New Jersey

Nancy Gage, PT, DPT (Case Study 13-2)
Director Rehabilitation Services
Beth Israel Deaconess Hospital-Plymouth
Plymouth, Massachusetts

Paul D. Gaspar, PT, DPT, CCS (Case Study 7-1)
Founder/President
Gaspar Doctors of Physical Therapy, APC
Carlsbad, California

Melanie A. Gillar, PT, DPT, MA (Chapter 13, Case Study 13-1, Case Study 13-2)
Owner/President
Gillar Physical Therapy
New York, New York

Scot Irwin, PT, DPT, CCS (Chapter 6, Case Study 6-1)
Deceased

Laura Klassen, DipPT, BPT, MSc (Case Study 12-1)
Clinical Associate
Bourassa & Associates Rehabilitation Centre
Adjunct Professor
School of Physical Therapy
University of Saskatchewan
Saskatoon, Saskatchewan, Canada

Kerri Lang, PT, DPT (Case Study 4-1)
Physical Therapist
Advantage Sports Medicine
Stoneham, Massachusetts

Daniel Malone, PT, PhD, CCS (Chapter 1, Chapter 6)
Assistant Professor
Physical Therapy Program
Department of Physical Medicine and Rehabilitation
University of Colorado Denver
Aurora, Colorado

Mary Jane Myslinski, PT, EdD (Case Study 5-2)
Associate Professor
Doctoral Program in Physical Therapy
School of Health Related Professions
Rutgers, The State University of New Jersey
Newark, New Jersey

Lola Sicard Rosenbaum, PT, DPT, MHS (Case Study 5-1)
Physical Therapist
Cantrell Center for Physical Therapy
Warner Robins, Georgia

Brian D. Roy, PT, DPT, MS, CCS (Chapter 9, Case Study 9-1)
Cardiovascular and Pulmonary Clinical Specialist
Acute Therapies
University of Vermont Medical Center
Adjunct Faculty
The University of Vermont
Burlington, Vermont

Robert M. Snow, PT, DPT, OCS, ATC (Case Study 7-1)
CEO
Gaspar Doctors of Physical Therapy, APC
Carlsbad, California

Alison L. Squadrito, PT, DPT, GCS, CEEAA (Chapter 3, Case Study 3-1)
Clinical Specialist
Physical Therapy Services
Massachusetts General Hospital
Boston, Massachusetts

Jane L. Wetzel, PT, PhD (Chapter 8, Case Study 8-1, Chapter 9)
Associate Professor
Department of Physical Therapy
College of Health and Human Services
Youngstown State University
Youngstown, Ohio

About the Editor

Debra Coglianese, PT, DPT, OCS, ATC is a clinical specialist with the Mercy Health System, with over three decades' experience. She holds her Doctor of Physical Therapy from the MGH Institute of Health Professions and her MS in physical therapy from the University of Southern California. After initially practicing in a thoracic surgery ICU, Dr. Coglianese focused on treating musculoskeletal patients in outpatient settings and is specialty board certified in orthopedics. She has lectured nationally, taught for four years as a section leader for the Comprehensive Case course for entry-level DPT students at MGH Institute of Health Professions, and frequently supervised students in clinical training. Prior to her current practice in Pennsylvania, she practiced with the University of Michigan Health System, Massachusetts General Hospital, and Beth Israel Deaconess Medical Center. Still earlier, she served as a physical therapist assistant at the Idaho State School and Hospital and then as an athletic trainer at the College of Idaho. Dr. Coglianese has previously been published in the *Journal of Orthopaedic & Sports Physical Therapy* and as a regular abstractor and book reviewer for the *Journal of Physical Therapy*. She continues to be certified as an athletic trainer.

DEDICATION

For teachers and mentors who lit the way,
colleagues with whom we share the path,
and future physical therapists yet to begin the journey.

FOREWORD

Dr. Scot Irwin, PT, DPT, CCS had a unique perspective on the practice of physical therapy (PT). While most PT practitioners consider the multiple facets of human movement response to pathology from a biomechanical or motor function perspective, Scot consistently focused on the scientific principles of oxygen uptake and delivery as crucial factors in human performance. This perspective, possibly borne of an undergraduate degree in exercise physiology followed by two graduate degrees in PT, led him into a relatively new practice area in the mid-1970s—cardiac rehabilitation.

During the 1960s and early 1970s, conventional wisdom in medical practice managed an individual's post-cardiac event with rest to preserve the injured myocardial tissue from experiencing further damage. Exercise in a general form was discouraged, and prescribed exercise for these "at risk" patients was not yet recognized as a therapeutic intervention. The recognition and physiologic description of deconditioning, or the "deleterious effects of bed rest" on normal individuals, had only begun to evolve in the late 1960s,[1] so the application of these concepts to patient populations was not yet common.

It was into this evolving intersection of basic science knowledge and clinical practice protocols that Scot began developing his career as a "cardiopulmonary physical therapist." He joined several PT colleagues to form Specialized Cardiac Outpatient Rehabilitation (SCOR), a PT practice focused on diagnostic exercise testing and training of individuals with history and risk of coronary artery disease (CAD). They were at the forefront of the cardiac rehabilitation trend, and by the late 1970s, they had collected substantial population data. Scot and his partners presented and published their findings on the safety and efficacy of exercise testing and training patients with CAD at their angina threshold—a whole new way of managing patients by documenting their pathophysiologic response to activity, identifying abnormalities, and then using the information to safely prescribe exercise for effective rehabilitation.[2]

Scot and his colleagues were not simply advancing clinical practice and disseminating their work through publication, they were teaching these cutting-edge concepts in academic and continuing education settings nationally. Their fundamental message relied heavily on the background science of exercise physiology, the human movement science database from PT, and descriptive and experimental research in the current literature. As a result, the suggested reading list for the courses they taught required the participants to either purchase multiple textbooks, spend days in a medical library, or both. To remedy that inefficient situation, Scot partnered with another colleague to develop the first and definitive text on the physical therapist's management of individuals with cardiovascular and pulmonary disorders. *Cardiopulmonary Physical Therapy* by Irwin and Tecklin was first published in 1985, and in its fourth edition,[3] it remains one of the most comprehensive and well-referenced texts on the subject.

As practical a clinical reference as that text has been, it addressed only "half of the problem" from Scot's perspective. Despite his seemingly narrow cardiopulmonary clinical practice specialty, Scot's very early practice experiences with broad rehabilitation populations, including those with amputation, spinal cord injury, or other neuromusculoskeletal disorders, produced a clinician who always addressed the entire patient. His physiologic mindset and physical therapist's clinical perspective on functional human movement combined to produce patient evaluations that considered both the cellular and systemic aspects of human movement as carefully as the functional or task performance. The diagnostic exercise testing Scot performed was intended to measure the oxygen cost of an activity such as ambulation simultaneously with the gait abnormality. Similarly, biomechanical analysis of workload could be measured with the physiologic cost of movement. From his vantage point, accurate evaluation of human movement to diagnose limitations required assessment of performance elements from the cellular to the person level.[4]

Scot fundamentally believed that a broad pathophysiologic perspective is truly essential for all professionals managing humans and their desire to move. He recognized there was a large gap between the science of exercise in normal human movement and the science of exercise associated with prevention or remediation of human movement abnormalities. In the mid-1990s, Scot set out to rectify that gap by locating clinical scientists who practiced PT by considering the cellular through systemic physiologic principles governing human motion. The clinicians, researchers, and academicians he approached spanned the spectrum of neurologic, orthopedic, cardiovascular-pulmonary, pediatric, and geriatric specialties. He challenged them to reflect on the scientific basis of their practice and attempt to describe the primary texts that served as their reference points. Individually and collectively, they could easily cite anatomic and physiologic references for the normal resting state or exercise physiology references for the same. Similarly, all could name favorite general or focused pathology texts. None could cite a single exercise text focusing on the pathophysiologic response to increased workload across systems.

As a result, Scot set out to remediate the situation by creating a text for that "missing link" in the exercise science scope. Preliminary research demonstrated that the essential science existed and was being well-used by PT practitioners who accessed it one article at a time, mostly focusing on their clinical specialty. However, there was no summary compilation of the information to be accessed by PT practitioners and students alike. Additionally, there were other health practitioners who could similarly benefit from understanding the demarcation between normal and abnormal response to increased oxygen demand or workload across systems.

This book was subsequently started as a project more than a decade ago. Its production was stalled by Scot's early and untimely death mid-production. However, the information that has been assembled here is a testament to the importance of the work. Many of these authors are members of the originally assembled group, and they have persevered to fulfill promises made as the need for the dissemination of this information has not diminished. Some of the newer authors were taught by Scot and have become knowledgeable, authoritatively informed, professional resources in their own right. They too believe in the value of this assembled evidence. Collectively, we remain grateful for the vision and leadership Dr. Scot Irwin, PT, DPT, CCS demonstrated over the full trajectory of his career. I believe this work honors his memory and fulfills his expectation.

References

1. Saltin B, Blomqvist G, Mitchell JH, Johnson RL Jr, Wildenthal K, Chapman CB. Response to exercise after bed rest and after training. *Circulation.* 1968;38(5 Suppl):1-78.
2. Blessey R, et al. Therapeutic effects and safety of exercising coronary patients at their angina threshold. *Med Sci Sports Exer.* 1979;11:110 (abstract).
3. Irwin S, Tecklin J. *Cardiopulmonary Physical Therapy.* 4th ed. St Louis, MO: Mosby; 2004.
4. Hislop HJ. Tenth Mary McMillan lecture. The not-so impossible dream. *Phys Ther.* 1975;55(10):1069-1080.

Cynthia Coffin-Zadai, DPT, MS, FAPTA
Professor Emerita
MGH Institute of Health Professions Charlestown Navy Yard
Boston, Massachusetts

PREFACE

To effectively examine, test, and treat patients with exercise, physical therapists need to understand how physiology from the cellular to systems level provides the basis for normal responses to exercise. But that is not enough. Knowledge about pathophysiology—the changes that lead to abnormal responses to exercise in different patient populations—is also essential.

Other texts cover normal exercise physiology well. Information about abnormal responses to exercise, however, has to be gathered from a variety of sources for different patient populations. Examination and testing information can be found in articles and texts for some specific patient populations, but for not all. In addition, a smattering of case studies can be found in the literature. Until now, though, no text has compiled all of this information together for physical therapists.

Clinical Exercise Pathophysiology for Physical Therapy: Examination, Testing and Exercise Prescription for Movement-Related Disorders shows why, and offers examples of how, to treat patients with exercise, offering comprehensive information from the research literature as well as original patient cases. Its coverage is broad, ranging from a cellular metabolism review to the discharge summary—with all of the connections in between.

To ensure that this exceptional sweep of information would not overwhelm the reader, the talented authors contributing to this book have created chapters that follow a consistent format. That alone is a remarkable feat for a text with different contributors. Further, the authors have distilled and refined the content for clarity to further assist the reader.

This book's chapters are arranged into 3 distinct sections: Foundations of Physiological Responses; Pathophysiology of Deconditioning and Physiology of Training; and Pathophysiological Considerations and Clinical Practice.

In Section I, the first chapter, "Cardiovascular and Pulmonary System," begins with a review of cellular metabolic pathways as the basis for why a delivery system in the form of the cardiovascular and pulmonary system even exists. The chapter presents the structure and physiology for each component of this essential system. The chapter then discusses the normal physiological responses of the components to show how the system responds as a whole during an exercise session. The next 2 chapters in Section 1 show the normal physiology in developing and aging systems, respectively. These 2 chapters have been placed early in this text rather than toward the end because it is not a pathology to be young or old. Along with presenting the normal physiology associated with development and aging, however, these chapters do identify the pathophysiology that can occur simultaneously with each phase of life.

Section II of this book provides chapters exploring the changes that occur from decreased, and then increased, physiological demands. A clarification needs to be made at the outset about the dual routes to a deconditioned status. Is it deconditioning when a high-performance athlete follows a much lighter-than-usual workout for several weeks, or is deconditioning what occurs when a person who has been functioning adequately with daily activities experiences a drop in activity level? Chapter 4, entitled "Fatigue and Deconditioning," offers the true physiologic definition of a deconditioned status that applies to both situations. In the groundbreaking collection of information that makes up that chapter, however, the emphasis is on the latter scenario. Chapter 5, "Principles of Training and Exercise Prescription," summarizes the training information many readers will recognize from previous exposure to exercise physiology content. Here again, though, the focus of the chapter is to highlight the principles for patient—not athlete—applications.

In Section III of this book, the chapters present the physiology and pathophysiology for defined patient populations consistent with the *American Physical Therapy Association* (APTA) *Guide to Physical Therapy Practice*. For clarity, the chapters in Section 3 follow a consistent organizational structure. Each chapter begins with a presentation of the basic physiology principles appropriate for the systems involved. This information then serves as the foundation to link to the pathophysiology that occurs in the defined patient population. The pathophysiology content then spans the components to be included, or considered, in therapists' examination, testing, evaluation, and treatment of these patients. It is worth repeating that these chapters have the same structure: basic physiology, pathophysiology, and the impact on clinical practice.

The order of chapter topics reflects, as does this text as a whole, a view of patients through a cardiovascular and pulmonary system lens. As such, chapters on cardiovascular and pump dysfunctions, peripheral vascular disorders, ventilatory pump dysfunctions, and gas exchange disorders appear first in Section 3. Next, the musculoskeletal system is introduced with chapters on localized, and then systemic, musculoskeletal disorders. Similarly, the neuromuscular system is introduced and associated disorders presented in the next chapter. The text concludes with a chapter that considers multi-system disorders.

Throughout this book, all of the chapters except the first are followed by at least one patient case. The cases serve to illustrate how understanding the content in each chapter informs physical therapy examination, testing, and treatment. Just as the chapters follow a consistent structure, so do the patient cases. The patient/client management model from the *Guide* defines the structure. Three exciting upgrades from the *Guide* enhance the cases in this book.

First, the *Guide* recommends a list of pathology, impairments, functional limitations, and disability in the diagnosis portion of the evaluation. Although there are plans to upgrade the *Guide* language to be consistent with that identified in the *International Classification of Function, Disability and Health* (ICF), the APTA had yet to make this upgrade at the time this book was submitted for publication. To better reflect the profession's acceptance of ICF language, and prepare physical therapists for anticipated changes in the *Guide*, the ICF model of disablement has been inserted into the patient case presentations in this text.

Second, special attention has been paid in the patient cases to the writing of the exercise prescriptions. The *Guide* does mention that physical therapists prescribe exercise as a therapeutic intervention. The APTA has more recently highlighted exercise and physical activity prescription as a component of the tasks physical therapists perform as the health service delivery providers of choice. The patient cases in this book, therefore, model taking exercise prescription to a higher level. Any exercise recommended in a patient case here is accompanied by an exercise prescription that contains a specified mode, intensity, duration, and frequency, along with a description of the intervention.

Finally, the third innovative upgrade distinguishes the patient cases in this book and enhances their educational value. A defined format for writing a case report exists that renders the case suitable for publication, or poster presentation, but might not be the best form for teaching. For one thing, when students are asked to write cases about "average" patients encountered in clinical affiliations, the defined format for the journal and posters focuses on novel cases. For another, this format, or one that presents bulleted facts following the *Guide* structure, does not allow an "in the moment" identification of the critical thinking involved during a patient encounter. It can be useful to know more about what a patient's therapist is thinking, moment by moment. We think these limitations have now been solved with the introduction here of a "Clinician Comments" feature that emphasizes critical thinking and moves beyond the "just the facts" structure of case presentations.

Highlighted "Clinician Comments" appear throughout each patient case in this book to point out the critical thinking considerations. The reporting of information from the patient case is periodically interspersed with "Clinician Comments" that allow the case author to step outside the traditional narration of the case, so to speak, to summarize what is now known about the patient or what additional information needs to be gathered or clarified. The evidence to support the interpretation of the case facts also appears in these comments, as well as the decisions being made by the physical therapist as the case unfolds. Once the critical thinking required for this portion of the case is completed, the highlighted "Clinician Comments" section ends and the case reporting resumes. Various "Clinician Comments" are inserted into the cases to explain the decision making about matters such as the selection of the tests and measures to be used, the practice pattern chosen, and the mode of exercise selected, to list a few examples. Further, "Clinician Comments" are included to bring forward chapter content to aid in patient management.

Clinical Exercise Pathophysiology for Physical Therapy will be an effective resource tool for physical therapists at many levels. Entry-level Doctor of Physical Therapy (DPT) students will be well-guided by the scope and depth of content in this book when used as the primary text for a clinical exercise pathophysiology course. Advanced master's students will find the extensive pathophysiology content to be an exemplary supplement to any clinical research inquiry.

The extensive patient cases illustrate not only the application of physiological and pathophysiological principles for patient management, but the critical thinking employed as well. The information in the cases will inform future clinical practice for students at all levels. In addition, entry-level and transitional DPT students will find the format used for patient cases to be an invaluable model as they prepare their own patient cases in comprehensive case classes.

Constant retooling is required to maintain competency in physical therapy. Knowledge of the various physical therapy practice areas can only enhance the skills of the experienced and well-rounded practitioner. For this reason, all physical therapists who desire a single reference to update their knowledge base will find this text useful. The content provides a clear delineation of the physiology, pathophysiology, and research evidence that supports therapeutic exercise intervention across the scope of physical therapy practice.

Debra Coglianese, PT, DPT, OCS, ATC

ACKNOWLEDGMENTS

When much is owed to the contributions of many, it can be difficult to know where to start. Let me begin with the talented chapter and case authors whose work built this text. I cannot possibly express adequate gratitude for the countless hours and expertise each put into their respective chapters and cases. Although their previous experience with published writing varied, all approached the writing assignments with fresh eyes and infectious enthusiasm. We needed that spirit to keep up resolve when the exhausting "breaking trail" nature of the writing proved daunting at times.

Some of the authors have been with this project from the beginning. That meant that they accepted the assignment of periodic rewriting of their work to provide updated evidence and references as the project spread out over years. As challenging as it can be to write a chapter or case the first time, the task of rewriting can seem a punishment for being prompt with the first deadline. Other authors, brought on board late in the project, delivered on short writing deadlines so that the entire project would not have to be subjected to another updating. Heroes, all.

It was not just the incredible expertise that the authors brought to their work. They were, to a person, a pleasure to work with. Countless times I benefited from individual and collective goodwill. No group could have been more supportive. I will always be grateful for the experience of working with them. It has been a privilege to promote their work to successful publication.

Initially, I was asked to join this project to provide support to a few authors working to finish chapters. Cyndi Coffin-Zadai appealed to my regard for Scot Irwin to help her complete the project he had started. It was not a tough sell. She did not know it at the time, but, to paraphrase the line from the movie, *Jerry Maguire*, the project "had me" at the idea of incorporating "Clinician Comments" into the book's patient cases.

After taking a comprehensive case course in the transitional Doctor of Physical Therapy (DPT) program at the MGH Institute of Health Professions (IHP) and serving as adjunct faculty for 4 years in the same course for entry-level DPT students, I knew that patient cases were my interest. Specifically, I had hoped to identify the process of writing a case in a manner that would be accessible for all physical therapists who wanted to write one. I tabled my how-to book idea to help with this project and, in the process, gained an insight into case writing that I might not have discovered on my own. Cyndi's brilliant creation of the "Clinician Comments" tool was key to the effective educational form the cases have taken in this book. Once again, the profession owes her much appreciation for coming up with a solution to a perplexing situation. I am grateful to her for the opportunity to be involved with this project. I am appreciative of her confidence in me to ultimately carry on as the editor when the demand for her extensive professional skills spread her time too thinly to allow her to continue.

There will be those who may question a text that views patients from a cardiovascular and pulmonary perspective being edited by a physical therapist with a predominant expertise in orthopedics. It is a reasonable question and one I have considered also. However, as I look back over my career thus far, the influence of cardiovascular and pulmonary concerns for patients has always appeared as a broadening correction to my focus in rehabilitation of athletes and patients with musculoskeletal disorders.

During the first year as a physical therapy assistant student, a serendipitous opportunity led me to Bob Moore and the training room at San Diego State University. Once we had the athletes ready for practice and out of the training room in the late afternoon, I was equally curious about the participants in the cardiac rehab group who gathered in the area outside the training room. During my second year, John Iames arranged a class field trip to Rancho Los Amigos. There I was oriented to, and then observed, cardiac stress testing by Scot Irwin and cardiac rehab by Ray Blessey. While providing athletic training services at a youth John Wooden Basketball Camp, I spent a week of mornings talking with Coach Wooden during the time he cooled down from his own cardiac rehab walking program. Events such as these leave an impression.

Even with subsequent moves to other parts of the country, the trend of pursuing musculoskeletal rehabilitation with an awareness of cardiovascular/pulmonary concerns continued to be reinforced by the professionals from whom I had the good fortune to learn. My practice in Idaho as a physical therapist assistant and then athletic trainer benefited from the knowledge I gained from Sheri Robison, Ron Pfeiffer, Ross Vaughn, and Bob Murray. As an entry-level master's physical therapy student at the University of Southern California, exposure to the wisdom of Joan Walker, Ray Blessey, and Cyndi Coffin-Zadai was invaluable. In Michigan, as a member of the chest team in my first year of practice as a physical therapist, I was fortunate to learn from Peg Clough, and later from Steve Goldstein, Jim Goulet, and Pete Loubert.

A move to Massachusetts provided the truly amazing opportunity to work with the extraordinarily talented physical therapists at Massachusetts General Hospital, Beth Israel Deaconess Medical Center, and Mount Auburn Hospital. Do you think a physical therapist would be allowed to ignore cardiovascular and pulmonary considerations in orthopedic patients when working in a department headed by Cyndi Coffin-Zadai? Of course not.

I am grateful to have had the opportunity to meet and learn from the gifted clinicians, teachers, and researchers named above. To the countless others, including patients, who have influenced my patient care, I give thanks.

This project benefited from the generous assistance of many. Ellen Abramowitz, the medical librarian at Mercy Fitzgerald Hospital, was an incredible resource herself in tracking down elusive references. Megan Fennell provided much development expertise to the manuscript. I am grateful to Mike Johnson for stepping in to make an introduction for me when it became clear that Dan Malone held the solution for the first chapter. I owe Dan Malone more pies than I could possibly provide. Not only did Dan contribute a wonderful chapter and update a second one, he also provided invaluable advice at various points in the manuscript construction. Dan, in turn, made an introduction for me to Brien Cummings, the Acquisitions Editor at SLACK Incorporated.

I appreciate Brien for his wonderful encouragement when he was first shown this manuscript. He deftly steered the project through all the required steps for approval. His unfailing optimism is a gift to all who have the opportunity to work with him. Thank you, Brien, for all you did to ensure that our manuscript would become a book we can hold in our hands.

Many thanks as well to the members of the SLACK team whose dynamic work launched the project to new heights. Brien and his assistant, Katherine Rola, each stepped outside their usual job duties and offered assistance with the permission process. John Bond, Chief Content Officer at SLACK, championed our project and adjusted the budget to allow the project to move forward. Special thanks to April Billick, the Managing Editor, for lining up such great talent for the book's production. The artists at SLACK induced smiles all around the country when the authors saw the masterful cover design for the first time. An equally beautiful interior design by Jean-Marc Yee will greet and guide readers. The new illustrations will further enhance the readers' experience. Also, April found us Dani Malady, Senior Project Editor. Working with Dani has been a joy. She managed us more gently than one would expect for a project this size. Thank you, Dani, for your diligent attention to detail—the book is better for it.

I am grateful to the continued team effort for the published book. Tony Schiavo competently stepped in to fill big shoes when Brien Cummings accepted broader duties at SLACK. The book is in good hands with Michelle Gatt, SLACK Incorporated's Marketing Communications Director; Trevor Hirsh for the marketing campaign; and Jim Clark, who will promote the book in his duties as SLACK's sales representative for physical therapy.

Cyndi gave me Laurie Hack's contact information when I moved from Boston to Pennsylvania. Little did I know that Laurie, my first physical therapy contact in Pennsylvania, would be such an amazing source of wisdom and lovely friendship. My colleagues in Havertown, Pennsylvania—Linda Price, Nathalie Wilson, and Janet Buckley—were so nice to me during this project. No colleagues have had to witness more editorial hand-wringing than them, yet they consistently provided encouraging responses in return. There is not enough chocolate in the world to repay them for their kindness.

With the ease of social media, I am fairly certain that my children, on more than one occasion, sent text warnings to each other such as, "Unless you want an earful, don't ask Mom about the book." I would like to thank Patrick, John, and Anne—and now my lovely daughter-in-law, Erin—for their patience when birthdays, holidays, and general home life seemed to be given a backseat constantly to this project—not to mention all the space taken up at home with piles.

To my amazing husband, Cary Coglianese, I owe much. From my time studying in physical therapy school to the extra hours I continue to need to complete documentation at work, he has been wonderfully supportive of my career. Countless times during this project, I benefited from Cary's well-informed advice. I am especially appreciative that he understood my desire to see the authors' work published despite the never-ending quest it seemed at times. Through it all, he bore every bit of angst to which he was exposed with good cheer. Thank you.

DC
2014

SECTION I

FOUNDATIONS OF
PHYSIOLOGICAL RESPONSES

1

Cardiovascular and Pulmonary System

Daniel Malone, PT, PhD, CCS

CHAPTER OBJECTIVES

- Identify the central and peripheral cardiovascular responses that occur during an acute exercise session.
- Identify the pulmonary responses during an acute exercise session and relate these responses to the homeostasis of oxygen (O_2) and carbon dioxide (CO_2) concentrations within the blood.
- Discuss the interrelationships between the cardiac, vascular and pulmonary systems as it relates to human movement and exercise training.
- List abnormal exercise responses using the concepts of normal exercise physiology as a guideline to prevent untoward patient responses during a physical therapy session.

CHAPTER OUTLINE

- Mortality and Survivorship
- Interdependence of Systems
- Cellular Metabolism
  - Adenosine Triphosphate
    - Resynthesis of Adenosine Triphosphate
  - Cellular Respiration
  - One-Celled to Multi-Celled Organisms: Development of Transport Systems
- Cardiovascular and Pulmonary Systems
  - Overview
  - The Cardiovascular System
    - Overview

- Cardiac Component
  - Cardiac Pump
  - Cardiac Muscle
  - Generation of Heart Rate: The Cardiac Conduction System
  - Neurohumoral Control: Autonomic Innervation of the Heart
  - The Cardiac Cycle
  - Common Cardiac Reflexes
    - Frank-Starling Mechanism
    - Bainbridge Reflex
    - Baroreceptor Reflex
    - Force-Frequency Relationship (Bowditch Effect)
- Vasculature Component
  - Structure and Network
  - Neurohumoral Control of Blood Flow
  - Blood Flow
  - Blood Pressure
- Pulmonary Component
  - Overview
  - Ventilatory Pump
    - Structure
    - Properties
    - Ventilation
    - Control of Ventilation
    - Ventilation Volumes and Flow

Coglianese D, ed. *Clinical Exercise Pathophysiology for Physical Therapy: Examination, Testing, and Exercise Prescription for Movement-Related Disorders (pp 3-26).*
© 2015 Taylor & Francis Group.

- Gas Exchange
  - Perfusion
    - Blood Flow to Lungs
    - Properties of Perfusion
    - Ventilation to Perfusion Ratio
  - Properties of Gas Exchange, Including Surface Area
  - Gas Partial Pressures
- Blood
  - Oxygen in Blood/Oxygen Delivery
  - Hemoglobin Saturation Curve
- Exercise Physiology: Tying It All Together
  - Overview
  - Maximal Oxygen Consumption and Metabolic Equivalents
  - Energy Utilization
  - Normal Response to Increasing Loads
    - The Cardiovascular Responses
      - Cardiac Output and Stroke Volume
      - Heart Rate
      - Blood Pressure
    - Pulmonary Responses
      - Overview
      - Minute Ventilation (Respiratory Rate × Tidal Volume
      - Gas Exchange
- Summary
- References

Mrs. Mason is a 73-year-old female who was referred to outpatient physical therapy for evaluation and treatment of a left-sided pelvic fracture sustained 10 weeks prior when she fell in her doctor's waiting room. She reported pain in her left groin, left buttock, and anterior left thigh with standing transfers and stair climbing. Her chief complaint is that it takes her twice as long to bathe and dress herself because she gets severely short of breath. Her past medical history is significant for pulmonary sarcoidosis, myocardial infarction, hypertension, osteopenia, and a significant leg length difference.

Is she a candidate for physical therapy? If so, how do we identify which of the possible underlying pathologies is affecting her breathing, thus her functional status, most? Is there evidence in the literature to support exercise training for this patient? Are there long-term benefits if she begins an exercise program? Should she be referred to another health care practitioner before initiating physical therapy?

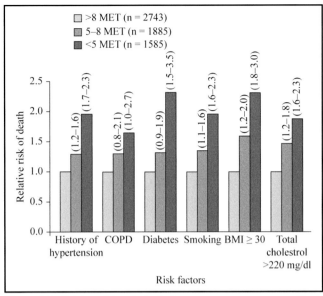

Figure 1-1. Relative risks of death from any cause among subjects with various risk factors who achieved an exercise capacity of less than 5 metabolic equivalents (MET) or 5 to 8 MET, as compared with subjects whose exercise capacity was more than 8 MET. Numbers in parentheses are 95% confidence intervals for the relative risks. BMI, body mass index. (Reprinted with permission from Myers J, Prakash M, Froelicher V, Do D, Partington S, Atwood JE. Exercise capacity and mortality among men referred for exercise testing. *N Engl J Med.* 2002;346(11):793-801.)

The patient's case history may appear straightforward initially. She will primarily be viewed as an orthopedic patient, but the subjective comments add complexity and question this treatment approach. The physical therapist (PT) starts the examination process not knowing where the patient sits on a continuum of activity tolerance. Knowing the fundamentals of normal exercise physiology will allow the PT to compare and contrast this patient's physiologic and symptomatic responses to the normal or expected responses. Through the examination and evaluation process, the PT must determine the potential causes of the patient's limited exercise capacity in order to design the most efficacious and safe treatment plan as well as determine the patient's prognosis for attaining anticipated goals and expected outcomes.

MORTALITY AND SURVIVORSHIP

A common physical therapy goal is to improve the patient's activity tolerance, and this is most often accomplished by exercise training. Research has shown that physical activity is associated with a marked decrease in cardiovascular and all-cause mortality in men and women.[1-3] Physically fit patients have excellent prognoses even if they have significant heart disease, risk factors for heart disease, and other comorbid conditions (Figure 1-1).[4-7] Additionally, improvements in exercise capacity, even modest advances in physical fitness, are associated with a significantly lowered risk of death.[3,8] It is imperative, therefore, that an attempt be made to improve the exercise tolerance of patients.

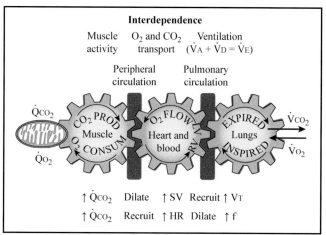

Figure 1-2. The gas transport mechanisms coupling cellular (internal) respiration of muscle to pulmonary (external) respiration by way of the cardiovascular system. The movement system relies on each of these linked systems during activities of daily living and exercise. (Reprinted with permission from Wasserman K, Hansen JE, Sue DY, et al. *Principles of Exercise Testing and Interpretation.* 3rd ed. Philadelphia, PA: Lippincott Williams & Wilkins; 1999.)

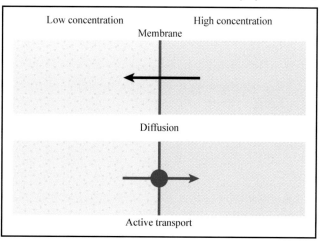

Figure 1-3. Direction of net solute flux crossing a membrane by diffusion (high to low concentration) and active transport (low to high concentration with energy expenditure). (Reprinted with permission from Vander A, Sherman J, Luciano D. *Human Physiology: The Mechanism of Body Function.* 7th ed. New York, NY: McGraw-Hill; 1999:118. Copyright The McGraw-Hill Companies, Inc.)

INTERDEPENDENCE OF SYSTEMS

The challenge is to carefully assess the patient's status and begin exercise, being aware of a desired outcome but equally mindful of the patient's ability and potential risks for an untoward event. These clinical decisions are guided by an understanding of cellular metabolism, properties of organ and system function, and the overarching interdependence of the involved body systems. This overarching interdependency of systems has been conceptualized by Wasserman et al (Figure 1-2).[9] The muscular, cardiovascular, pulmonary, and bioenergetic systems are represented as gears depicting how alterations in one system lead to changes in the others. This model highlights the functional interdependence of the physiological components that are responsible for energy production, waste elimination, and O_2 delivery and transport.

Viewing the Wasserman schematic starting on the left, the model shows the link between internal cellular respiration at the mitochondria level and external respiration of the lungs by way of the circulation. As the human body begins to move, energy derived from O_2 is used to fuel muscle contraction and results in the production of a waste product, CO_2. If additional O_2 is not provided, energy production slows and activity will stop. If waste products increase without adequate removal, activity will stop. Providing transport of O_2 as well as providing waste removal from the working muscle is the role of the cardiovascular and pulmonary systems.

It is necessary that the practicing PT and PT assistant (PTA) have an understanding of the basic physiologic mechanisms underlying normal functioning of the human body. This understanding of normal physiology and exercise physiology allows the clinician to compare and contrast physiologic responses and fully appreciate the pathophysiology of disease and the negative impact on the movement system.

CELLULAR METABOLISM

All biological systems share common cellular process in their quest to function and survive. These common features include the following:

- Exchange of essential materials between the internal environment of a cell and its external environment
- Production of energy from organic compounds
- Synthesis of complex proteins
- Replication of the cell itself
- Detection of, and response to, signals in the external environment

A single-celled organism low in essential nutrients can obtain nutrients from the relatively more abundant supply in the external environment. Simple diffusion allows nutrients to pass through the cell's membrane down a concentration gradient from the external environment into the cell. Waste products from the cell will follow the reverse path and diffuse from a higher concentration within the cell to a lower concentration in the external environment. Fluid movement across semipermeable cell membranes by osmosis is similarly driven by equalizing concentrations on either side of the cell membrane. However, cells cannot rely on simple diffusion for the movement of all nutrients and waste products. Movement of nutrients or fluids against concentration gradients requires active transport by the cell (Figure 1-3). Active transport, as well as other common cellular functions,

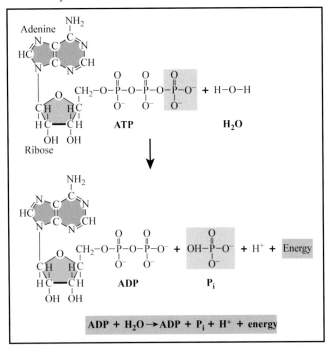

Figure 1-4. Chemical structure of ATP. Its breakdown to ADP and P_i is accompanied by the release of energy that is used to fuel cellular processes. (Adapted from Widmaier EP, Hershel R, Strang KT. *Vander, Sherman & Luciano's Human Physiology: The Mechanism of Body Function.* 9th ed. New York, NY: McGraw-Hill; 2004:46.)

requires a ready supply of energy to allow prolonged cellular function and survival.

Adenosine Triphosphate

The basic unit of fuel used by cells is adenosine triphosphate (ATP). ATP is a complex molecule made up of adenosine and 3 phosphate groups. The usefulness of ATP lies in the energy released when the high-energy bond holding the third phosphate is broken, forming adenosine diphosphate (ADP), inorganic phosphate (P_i): ATP $\rightarrow$ ADP + P_i + energy (Figure 1-4). This energy is used by the cell to perform work such as active transport and protein synthesis. Unfortunately, cells have limited ATP stores. When cellular energy demands exceed the available free ATP molecules, these energy stores need to be replaced to maintain ongoing cellular activity.

Resynthesis of Adenosine Triphosphate

ATP is created and restored by sequences of enzyme-mediated reactions known as *metabolic pathways*. For example, in skeletal muscle, there are limited stores of a high-energy phosphate compound, phosphocreatine (PC), which can be used to immediately resynthesize ATP from ADP and inorganic phosphates (ADP + PC $\rightarrow$ ATP + C). Use of PC preserves the levels of ATP during short-duration, quick bursts of muscle activity.

For longer duration activity, ATP is resynthesized by oxidation. At rest or with submaximal activities, the optimal restoration of ATP occurs via oxidation in the mitochondria, leaving CO_2 and water (H_2O) as the waste products

(Figure 1-5). A cell that needs to resynthesize ATP rapidly requires the ability to quickly obtain greater quantities of O_2. This requirement partially explains the evolutionary development of complex organizational structures of the cardiovascular and pulmonary systems as well as the internal structure of the mitochondria.

The synthesis of ATP in the presence of O_2 relies on metabolic pathways that can utilize carbohydrates, lipids, and proteins. Though not immediate sources of energy, oxidative pathways lead to increased ATP production compared to anaerobic pathways (Figure 1-6). Oxidative pathways limit the accumulation of lactic acid because its chemical precursor, pyruvic acid, is metabolized in the presence of O_2. The body's use of oxidative pathways in muscle work delays the onset of muscle fatigue (see Figure 1-6).

For shorter duration activity, ATP can be resynthesized without O_2 by nonoxidative, or anaerobic, metabolic pathways to give the muscles another immediate source of energy. Anaerobic pathways are useful for short-duration activity because ATP production is limited and the accumulation of the metabolic byproduct, lactic acid, leads to muscular fatigue. Nonoxidative pathways use only glucose or its storage form, glycogen.

Cellular Respiration

As stated previously, cellular respiration is the use of O_2 to resynthesize ATP and results in the production of CO_2. The rate of cellular respiration reflects the extent of the metabolic work being performed by the cell. When the amount of O_2 used by the cell (QO_2) is proportional to the CO_2 produced (QCO_2), the cell is functioning in a steady-state condition. The cell remains in steady state as long as respiration remains balanced with waste removal.

One-Celled to Multi-Celled Organisms: Development of Transport Systems

In single-celled organisms, a cell membrane separates the internal environment of the cell from the external environment of H_2O, O_2, and organic molecules. Needed O_2 diffuses across the cell membrane and the produced H_2O and CO_2 diffuse out to the external environment. The limits of simple diffusion, however, dictate the distance that molecules can cover, thereby dictating the size and complexity of cells (Figure 1-7).

As single-cell organisms evolved into multi-cell organisms, cells and organelles would no longer be exposed to the external environment. As multi-cell organisms evolved with differentiation of cells into specialized tissues and organs, transport mechanisms also evolved. These transport systems carried essential nutrients and wastes to and from the external environment to each cell. Over time, through exoskeletons, gills, and primitive hearts and lungs, transport mechanisms evolved into cardiovascular and pulmonary organ systems of increasing complexity.

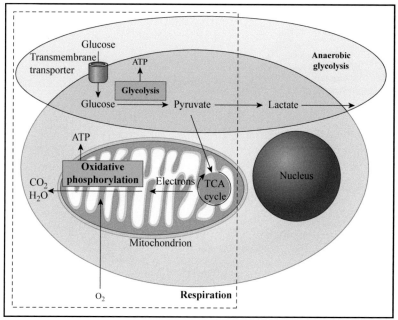

Figure 1-5. Simplified schema of glycolysis and oxidative phosphorylation in a cell. Anaerobic glycolysis results in forming 2 ATP from each glucose molecule while aerobic respiration yields 38 ATP highlighting the efficiency of aerobic metabolism. (Reprinted by permission from MacMillan Publishers Ltd: Sitkovsky M, Lukashev D. Regulation of immune cells by local-tissue oxygen tension: HIF1 alpha and adenosine receptors. *Nat Rev Immunol.* 2005;5:712-721. Copyright 2005.)

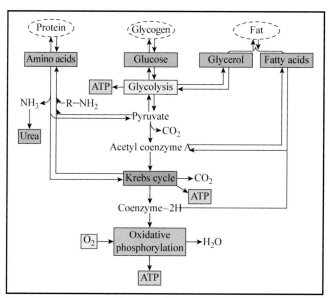

Figure 1-6. Interrelations between the pathways for the metabolism of carbohydrate, fat, and protein. (Adapted from Widmaier EP, Hershel R, Strang KT. *Vander, Sherman & Luciano's Human Physiology: The Mechanism of Body Function.* 9th ed. New York, NY: McGraw-Hill; 2004:104.)

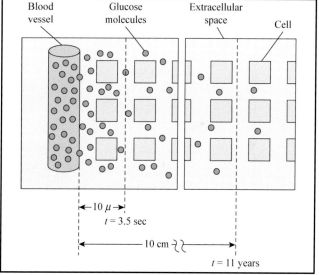

Figure 1-7. The time required for diffusion to raise the concentration of glucose at a point 10 μ (about one cell diameter) away from a blood vessel to 90% of the blood glucose concentration is about 3.5 sec, while it will take more than 11 years for the glucose to reach that same concentration at a point 10 cm away (3.9 in). (Reprinted with permission from Vander A, Sherman J, Luciano D. *Human Physiology: The Mechanism of Body Function.* 7th ed. New York, NY: McGraw-Hill; 1999:44. Copyright The McGraw-Hill Companies, Inc.)

CARDIOVASCULAR AND PULMONARY SYSTEMS

Overview

In its simplest description, the pulmonary system extracts air from the external environment and the cardiovascular system delivers O_2 to the internal environment of cells for metabolism. The transport of air and blood occurs by 2 distinct mechanisms: diffusion and bulk flow. Diffusion defines the movement of particles through random motion from regions of higher concentration to regions of lower concentration. Bulk flow defines the movement of substances under the influence of pressure.[10,11]

Bulk flow of air occurs through the activity of the ventilatory pump of the lungs while bulk flow of blood occurs through activity of the cardiac pump. Bulk flow of air and blood must be continuous. In the transition from the cardiac pump or ventilatory pump to the tubes of the vascular and bronchial tree, flow is ultimately dependent on the amount of pressure generated by the pump and limited by the resistance

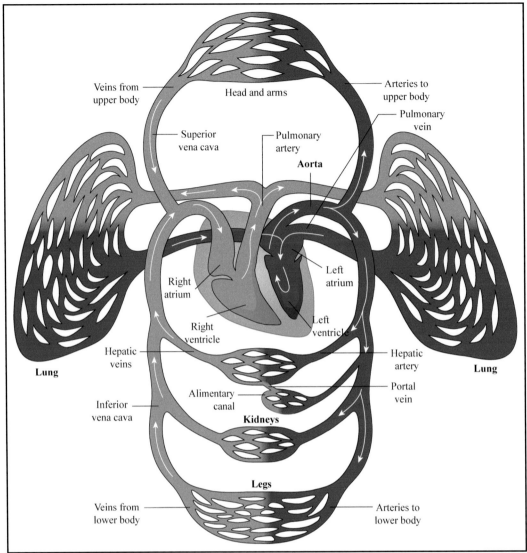

Figure 1-8. Schematic view of the cardiovascular system indicating the heart and the pulmonary and systemic vascular circuits. Red shading depicts oxygen-rich arterial blood; blue shading denotes deoxygenated venous blood. The situation reverses in the pulmonary circuit; oxygenated blood returns to the heart in the right and left pulmonary veins.

of the tubes. Diffusion occurs across capillary membranes at the alveolar-capillary membrane of the lung, and the capillary networks of skeletal muscle and other organ systems.

The energy requirements of repetitively contracting skeletal muscle cells exceed the energy that can be supplied by the cell's stored ATP. The efficient transport of O_2 to exercising muscle and removal of CO_2 and other metabolic acids is integral to improving activity tolerance at the muscle level. Fortunately, the O_2 transport system is able to adjust to the varied demands of each individual.

The Cardiovascular System

Overview

Distilled down to its basic elements, the human cardiovascular system is a circuit of tubes with 2 interspersed pumps whose primary purpose is to deliver adequate amounts of O_2 and remove wastes from the body (Figure 1-8). The right

heart pumps to the lungs and is referred to as the *pulmonary circuit*, while the left heart is the systemic circuit pumping to the remainder of the body.

Cardiac Component

Cardiac Pump

Though sitting side-by-side and joined by the intraventricular septum, the 4-chambered human heart can be viewed as a 2-sided pump of similar structure—each side with a primer pump (the atrium) and a more powerful pump (the ventricle; Figure 1-9A). The 2 pumps often referred to as the *right* and *left heart* are aligned in a series occupying different locations in the vascular circuit. In brief, deoxygenated blood from the peripheral circulation fills the right atrium (RA), which guides and pumps the blood through the tricuspid valve to the right ventricle (RV). The RV pumps the blood through the pulmonary valve to the lungs via the main pulmonary artery. The main pulmonary artery divides into the right

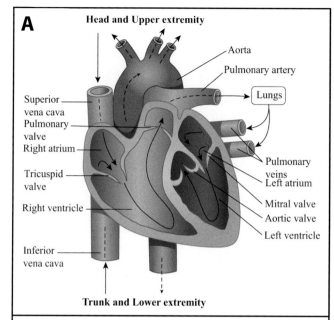

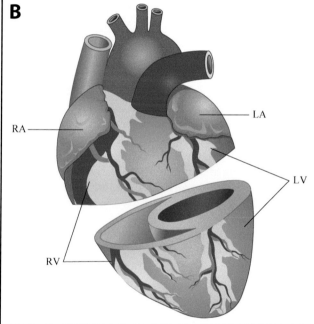

Figure 1-9. (A) Structure of the heart and course of blood flow through the heart chambers. (B) The anatomical relationship of the RV to the LV, showing the thicker globular shape of the LV and the half-moon shape of the RV as it drapes around the LV. (Adapted from Hall J. *Guyton and Hall Textbook of Medical Physiology.* 12th ed. Philadelphia, PA: Saunders; 2010:101, 289.)

BODY AREA	BLOOD VOLUME	
	mL	*Percentage*
Heart	360	7.2
Lungs		
Arteries	130	2.6
Capillaries	110	2.2
Veins	200	4.0
Systemic		
Aorta, large arteries	300	6.0
Small arteries	400	8.0
Capillaries	300	6.0
Small veins	2300	46.0
Large veins	900	18.0
Total	5000	100.0

TABLE 1-1. ABSOLUTE AND PERCENTAGE DISTRIBUTION OF TOTAL BLOOD VOLUME IN THE PULMONARY AND SYSTEMIC VASCULAR CIRCUITS OF A TYPICAL ADULT MALE AT REST

Reprinted with permission from McArdle WD, Katch FI, Katch VL. *Exercise Physiology: Nutrition, Energy and Human Performance.* 7th ed. Philadelphia, PA: Lippincott, Williams & Wilkins; 2010:305.

Although each ventricle contracts and propels an equal volume of blood, the distribution of the blood volume and pressures developed are markedly different (Table 1-1). These differences are reflected in the structure of the RV and LV. The pulmonary circuit is a low-pressure, high-capacity system that receives the entire cardiac output (CO) while maintaining pressures that are usually 20% to 25% of the systemic circulation. The RV has a thicker myocardium than the atria but is approximately one-third the thickness of the LV. The thicker LV myocardium is related to the higher afterload, the resistance to ventricular ejection, within the systemic circuit compared to the afterload of the pulmonary circuit.

Cardiac Muscle

The heart is composed of connective tissue and cardiac muscle, an involuntary striated muscle tissue. Cardiac muscle is 1 of the 3 major types of muscle, the others being skeletal muscle and smooth muscle. Though all 3 muscle types share monofilament sliding for contraction, their morphology and activation patterns differ (Figure 1-10). Cardiac muscle is multinucleated, differing from skeletal muscle but having a striated arrangement of the filaments similar to skeletal muscle promoting forceful contractions. Cardiac muscle cells (myocytes) are connected via intercalated discs that couple the cells both mechanically and electrically. This conductivity defines the ability of the myocytes to transmit impulses rapidly to successive cells, allowing the heart to contract as a unit, a functional syncytium. The interconnectedness of the

and left pulmonary arteries, supplying blood via the pulmonary circulation to each lung. The blood is oxygenated at the alveolar-capillary interface surrounding the alveoli and then returns to the left atrium (LA) via the pulmonary veins. The LA pumps the oxygenated blood through the mitral valve into the left ventricle (LV), which, in turn, pumps the oxygenated blood through the aortic valve into the aorta to be distributed to the rest of the body. The continuous pumping of the heart ensures that blood continues moving through the circulatory system by bulk flow.

Figure 1-10. Structure of the 3 different types of muscle fibers. (A) Skeletal muscle consists of long, parallel multinucleated fibers that provide rapid, forceful contraction. (B) Cardiac muscle fibers are irregular, branched fibers connected by intercalated discs with a central nuclei; contraction is a variable rhythm. (C) Smooth muscle fibers are spindle shaped with a single central nucleus and contraction is slow, sustained, or rhythmic in nature.

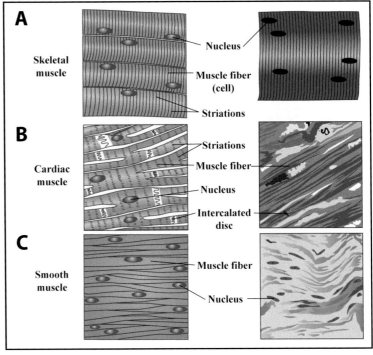

cardiac muscle filaments—different from skeletal muscle but similar to smooth muscle—leads to a sequential contraction of a muscle sheet when one muscle fiber is stimulated (ie, "all or none" phenomenon).

All 3 muscle types will contract with nerve stimulation, but cardiac and smooth muscle can be directly stimulated by circulating hormones, while only cardiac muscle can generate its own stimulus for rhythmic contraction. This unique property of cardiac muscle, termed *automaticity*, refers to the ability of a cardiac myocyte to discharge an electrical current without stimulation from the nervous system. The pacemaker cells of the sinoatrial (SA) node, atrioventricular (AV) node, and Purkinje system highlight this property, but other regions of the myocardium can initiate electrical impulses and take over pacemaker function as seen in various heart dysrhythmias (eg, atrial fibrillation/flutter).

The walls of the heart are made up of 3 layers: an inner layer (endocardium), an outer protective layer (epicardium), and muscular middle layer (myocardium; Figure 1-11). The innermost layer, the endocardium, is a thin layer of endothelial cells supported by underlying connective tissue that repeatedly folds on itself to form the valves of the heart and is continuous with the innermost layer of the large blood vessels (tunica intima). The conduction pathways are found beneath the endocardium in the subendocardial layer.[12] The middle layer, the myocardium, is the contractile layer of the heart and is composed primarily of cardiac muscle fibers. The outer layer, the epicardium, is a thin membrane that encases the myocardium and is the root of the great vessels. The epicardium turns back on itself to form a sac that surrounds the heart (the pericardium).[13,14]

Generation of Heart Rate: The Cardiac Conduction System

The average resting adult heart contracts 72 beats per minute (bpm). The contraction is generated by the specialized cardiac muscle fibers of the SA node located in the muscle wall of the RA. The electrical signal from the SA node travels throughout the muscle sheet of the RA and LA. It then travels to the AV node, located at midline just above the junction of the atria and ventricles. While the atria contract, the transmitted electrical signal is slightly delayed in the AV node before traveling along the bundle of fibers (AV bundle). The delay in the signal at the AV node allows the atria to contract and complete ventricular filling before the ventricles contract and eject the blood out of the heart.[15,16] The signal then travels along the 2 large bundle branches of the Purkinje system that transmit the electrical stimulus for contraction to the ventricles (Figure 1-12).

The SA node, known as the *pacemaker of the heart*, generally sets the rate of heart contraction. Its rate (72 bpm) overrides the self-generating rate of the AV node (40 to 60 bpm) and the Purkinje system (15 to 40 bpm). However, the heart rate (HR) can be stimulated to increase with a stretch of the heart muscle walls due to an increased arrival of blood volume to the heart (see the Bainbridge Reflex section on p 13) as well as by hormone and autonomic nervous system (ANS) input.

Neurohumoral Control: Autonomic Innervation of the Heart

The heart and vascular systems receive neurologic input from the ANS. Specifically, the heart is innervated by cranial nerve X (the vagus nerve) and sympathetic fibers arise

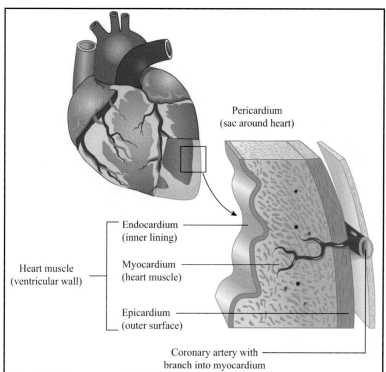

Figure 1-11. Layers of the heart wall from innermost (the endocardium), through the middle layer (the myocardium), to the exterior (the epicardium). The epicardium is continuous with the visceral or serous pericardium that lubricates and reduces friction during contraction. The outermost covering, the parietal or fibrous pericardium, is a dense fibrous sac that limits its distension and retains the heart in its anatomic position.

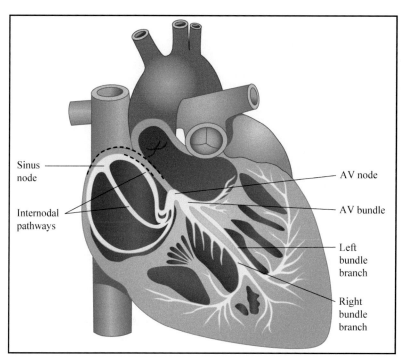

Figure 1-12. Sinus node and the Purkinje system of the heart, also showing the AV node, atrial internodal pathways, and ventricular bundle branches. (Adapted from Hall J. *Guyton and Hall Textbook of Medical Physiology.* 12th ed. Philadelphia, PA: Saunders; 2010.)

from the sympathetic chain ganglia from the thoracolumbar region of the spinal cord (levels T1 to L2; Figure 1-13). The medulla, located in the brainstem, is the primary site in the brain for regulating sympathetic and vagal outflow to the heart and blood vessels. The sympathetic nervous system (SNS) uses norepinephrine (NE) and the parasympathetic nervous system uses acetylcholine as neurotransmitters. Sympathetic and parasympathetic effects on heart function are mediated by beta-adrenoceptors and muscarinic receptors, respectively (Table 1-2).[10,17] Sympathetic stimulation with release of NE increases HR (positive chronotropy), increases the strength of ventricular contraction (positive inotropy), and increases the velocity of the action potential throughout the conduction system (positive dromotropy), whereas parasympathetic stimulation with release of acetylcholine has opposite effects (eg, negative chronotropy). The adrenal glands located superior to the kidneys are also stimulated by the SNS and will release epinephrine (EPI) into the circulation. Although this response is delayed, EPI has similar effects on heart and vascular function as NE.

Figure 1-13. The ANS showing distribution of sympathetic and parasympathetic nerve fibers to the myocardium. (Adapted from McArdle WD, Katch FI, Katch VL. *Exercise Physiology: Nutrition, Energy and Human Performance.* 7th ed. Philadelphia, PA: Lippincott, Williams & Wilkins; 2010:330.)

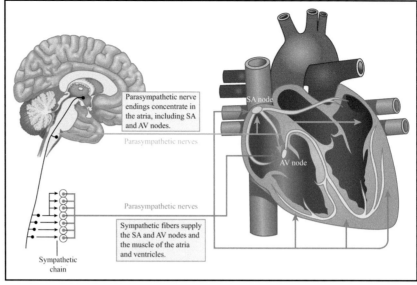

TABLE 1-2. AUTONOMIC NERVOUS SYSTEM INFLUENCES ON CARDIOVASCULAR SYSTEM			
NEUROTRANSMITTER	**RECEPTOR TYPE**	**LOCATION**	**RESPONSE**
Parasympathetic nervous system Cholinergic: acetylcholine	Muscarinic	Airway smooth muscle (bronchi/bronchioles)	Contraction
		Vasculature of genitalia	Dilation
		SA node; AV node Atria	Decreased rate (– chronotropy), conductive velocity (– dromotropy), and force of contraction (– inotropy)
SNS Adrenergic: NE/EPI	Alpha1	Vascular smooth muscle	Contraction
	Beta1	SA node and AV node Atria and ventricle	Increased rate (+ chronotropy), conductive velocity (+ dromotropy), and force of contraction (+ inotropy)
	Beta2	Airway smooth muscle (bronchi/bronchioles)	Dilation
		Skeletal muscle and hepatic vascular smooth muscle	Dilation

The Cardiac Cycle

The cardiac cycle defines the combined electrical and mechanical forces acting within the heart to complete one heartbeat. It includes a phase of contraction (systole) and a phase of relaxation or filling (diastole). Systole begins with the contraction of the ventricle resulting from electrical stimulation by the pacemaker of the heart transmitted through the conduction system. The amount of blood ejected from the heart with each ventricular contraction is called the *stroke volume* (SV). The amount of blood ejected from the ventricles per minute defines the CO. At rest, the adult heart pumps about 5 to 8 liters of blood each minute. This volume of blood (the CO) is the product of the SV. The rate of heart contractions per minute (the HR) is expressed as bpm. CO is represented by the equation CO = SV × HR. SV and ultimately CO are influenced by multiple factors, including the end-diastolic volume (EDV), ventricular contractility, afterload, and HR.[18]

The EDV is the maximal filling volume in the ventricle prior to ejection. The EDV in the normal adult averages 120 mL, representing the ventricular preload. The SV mathematically is expressed as the difference between the EDV and the end-systolic volume (ESV) volume of blood remaining in the heart at the end of ejection (SV = EDV – ESV). The ejection fraction (EF) is the fraction of blood pumped out of the ventricles with each heartbeat and compares the filling volume of the ventricle to the volume ejected with each beat. EF is SV divided by EDV where: EF = EDV – ESV/EDV or SV/EDV. Normal EF is approximately 55% to 70% and is widely considered an index of contractility.[19] Since the

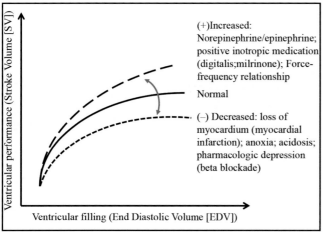

Figure 1-14. Diagram showing the major factors that influence cardiac contractility. These factors will elevate (+) or depress (−) left ventricular performance at any given level of ventricular filling (ie, EDV). (Adapted from Braunwald E, Ross J, Sonnenblick H. Mechanisms of contraction of the normal and failing heart. *N Engl J Med.* 1967;277:1012-1022.)

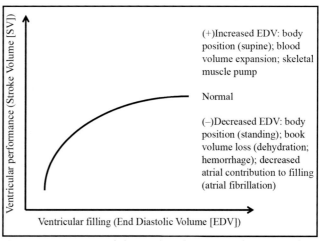

Figure 1-15. Diagram of the Frank-Starling curve. This curve relates ventricular filling (EDV) to ventricular performance. Factors that increase EDV will stretch the myocardium and increase ventricular performance leading, to enhanced SV. Factors that reduce EDV decrease ventricular performance and SV. (Adapted from Braunwald E, Ross J, Sonnenblick H. Mechanisms of contraction of the normal and failing heart. *N Engl J Med.* 1967;277:1012-1022.)

cardiovascular system is a closed pressure and closed volume system, the heart can eject only what enters it during diastole. It is evident that the SV is highly dependent on the EDV. Changes in the EDV will directly change the SV as described by the Frank-Starling mechanism (see the Common Cardiac Reflexes section next).

Afterload is the resistance to ejection and is defined as the force against which the ventricle must contract to eject blood.[10] Afterload will directly affect the SV. For example, an increase in afterload (eg, increased aortic pressure as seen in hypertension and aortic valve stenosis) will increase the resistance to ejection and may decrease SV. Conversely, a decrease in afterload (eg, anti-hypertension medications; aortic valve replacement) enhances SV. It is important to note, however, that the SV in a normal, nondiseased ventricle is not strongly influenced by afterload. In contrast, the SV of hearts that are failing is very sensitive to changes in afterload.[17]

Contractility, or inotropy, is often defined as the strength of ventricular contraction and refers to the ventricular performance at a given preload and afterload. The heart can increase its SV with reductions in afterload or increases in preload. The heart, however, can also modify its contractile performance for any given EDV or afterload. For example, consider the "fight or flight response." Activation of the SNS will increase the calcium released in the myocardium, which increases the force of ventricular contractions independent of the EDV (Figure 1-14). Conversely, a decrease in inotropy as seen in heart failure reduces SV and limits CO.

Common Cardiac Reflexes

Frank-Starling Mechanism

The Frank-Starling mechanism or Starling's Law of the Heart is mechanically similar to the length-tension relationship defining skeletal muscular contraction. The heart can change its force of contraction and therefore its SV in response to changes in venous return. Increased venous

return augments the EDV, leading to an increased stretch of the cardiac myocytes prior to contraction. Myocyte stretching increases the sarcomere length, optimizing actin and myosin overlap and resulting in enhanced force production and, therefore, an increased SV. Reducing EDV will have a reverse response. This mechanism enables the heart to eject the additional venous return that accompanies exercise even though the filling time is reduced, thereby increasing SV and CO during activity (Figure 1-15).

Bainbridge Reflex

The Bainbridge reflex is also called the *RA stretch reflex.* This reflex occurs when an increased blood volume reaches the RA and stretches the wall of the RA. The RA contains stretch receptors that respond by a reflex arc increasing HR. As the increased right ventricular output reaches the left heart, the left ventricular EDV is increased, which increases the CO (see Frank-Starling Mechanism section).

Baroreceptor Reflex

The baroreceptor reflex is mediated by stretch receptors in the walls of the aortic arch and carotid sinus. These mechanoreceptors are called *baroreceptors* because they respond to changes in pressure, and the role of the arterial baroreflex is to prevent excessive fluctuations of arterial blood pressure (BP). For example, as BP decreases, which may be seen in conditions such as dehydration and heart failure, these receptors respond by inducing a sympathetic reflex that increases HR and contractility and promotes vasoconstriction in the periphery. These factors will increase CO and total peripheral resistance (TPR), leading to an increased BP. Failure of this reflex may lead to orthostatic hypotension, the sudden fall in BP upon standing—a potential manifestation of prolonged immobility and bed rest. Baroreceptor reflex failure, although infrequent, can be manifested as wide changes in BP and HR.[20,21]

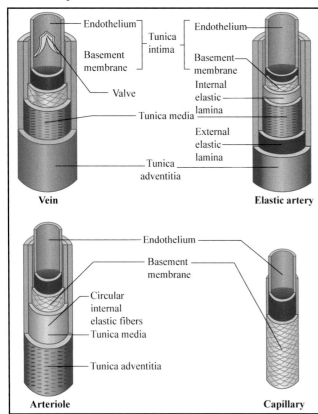

Figure 1-16. Schematic highlighting the structure of arteries, veins, and capillaries. Lining the interior of all blood vessels is a continuous endothelial cell layer. The arteries, arterioles, and veins have additional smooth muscle that spirals around the blood vessels. The aorta and other large arteries contain large amounts of elastic tissue. (Adapted from Carroll RG. *Integrated Physiology.* Philadelphia, PA: Mosby Elsevier; 2007.)

Force-Frequency Relationship (Bowditch Effect)

The "treppe" or Bowditch effect defines the positive relationship between ventricular force production and frequency of stimulation. An increased frequency of stimulation leads to an increased force of contraction of the heart. In other words, an increasing HR increases cardiac contractility. This is an important reflex when we consider exercise or stress responses. As the HR accelerates, the duration of diastolic filling decreases; however, the reduced filling time is normally compensated by an enhanced ventricular contractility. It should also be noted that the Bowditch effect does not apply to patients with severe heart failure, which may contribute to poor exercise performance.[22,23]

Vasculature Component

Structure and Network

All vessels larger than the capillaries consist of 3 distinct layers: the tunica intima, the media, and the adventitia (Figure 1-16). The innermost layer (the tunica intima) consists of a smooth layer of endothelial cells, isolated smooth muscle cells, and loose connective tissue. The endothelium promotes smooth laminar blood flow and is selectively permeable to many different molecules (eg, low-density lipoprotein cholesterol). Additionally, the endothelium secretes and responds to a variety of vasoactive substances that influence

TABLE 1-3. VASOACTIVE INFLUENCES ON PERIPHERAL ARTERIES AND VEINS

VASODILATION	VASOCONSTRICTION
Nitric oxide	Adrenergic stimulation (NE/EPI)
Adenosine	
Bradykinin	Endothelin
Low oxygen concentration	Angiotensin II
High CO_2 concentration	Aldosterone
Decreased blood pH (ie, acidosis)	

the contraction or relaxation of the smooth muscle within blood vessels. The middle layer (the media) consists of multiple layers of smooth muscle cells and elastic tissue. The media is the site of vasoconstriction/dilation through chemical, mechanical, and neurologic stimuli (see Tables 1-2 and 1-3). The outer layer (the adventitia) consists of collagen and loose connective tissues providing a supportive structure to the vessel as well as containing nerves and small blood vessels, the vasa vasorum that provides nutrients to the vessels themselves.[14]

The blood vessels provide the conduit for the distribution and return of blood and waste products to their appropriate destinations. Under normal circumstances, the resistances throughout the vascular system adjust to regulate the pressure and flow through the various organ systems, resulting in increased or reduced flow to match metabolic needs. Structurally, the pulmonary circulation and the systemic vasculature continually branch into vessels of progressively smaller diameters (the arteries, arterioles, and capillaries) to form parallel circuits that provide nutrient-rich blood to the organ systems of the body. This change in the tube structure reduces vascular resistance and aids diffusion of necessary respiratory gases and nutrients down their respective concentration gradients. Blood returns to the heart from the capillaries passing through vessels of progressively larger diameters called *venules* and *veins*.

Neurohumoral Control of Blood Flow

Blood flow is the movement of blood through the vessels. It is pulsatile in the large arteries and diminishes in amplitude as it approaches the capillaries. The blood vessels actively control the flow and distribution of blood throughout the body by smooth muscle vasoconstriction or dilation that results from the influences of vasoactive substances, hormones, and neurologic input.

The blood vessels are innervated by SNS within the tunica adventitia and mediated by alpha-adrenergic receptors. Activation of vascular sympathetic nerves causes vasoconstriction of the arteries and veins.[17] Interestingly, capillaries are not innervated and the capacitance vessels (the veins) are more responsive to sympathetic stimulation than the resistance vessels (arterioles).[22] Venous constriction reduces blood storage in the venous system, increasing venous return to the heart during periods of stress and exercise. Parasympathetic fibers are only found associated with blood vessels in certain organs such as salivary glands, gastrointestinal glands, and erectile tissue of the genitalia. The release of acetylcholine from these parasympathetic nerves has a direct vasodilatory action.[17]

Blood Flow

Blood flow relies on ventricular ejection to provide a driving pressure that must overcome vascular resistance. The flow in arteries is the result of SV, as well as the elastic recoil of the large arteries. Venous blood flow is nonpulsatile and results from several factors, including residual arterial pressure, pressure fluctuations due to respiratory movements, and muscle compression of the veins aided by one-way valves. Blood flow (Q) is directly proportional to the pressure differences across the vasculature ($\Delta P = P_1 - P_2$ [ΔP = upstream pressure – downstream pressure]) and inversely proportional to the resistance (R) within the vessels. Quantitatively, this is expressed as $Q = \Delta P/R$ (Figure 1-17).[19]

Blood flow can be viewed across the entire circulatory system, where the pressure difference is left ventricular pressure minus right atrial pressure, or across a single capillary bed, where the pressure gradient is defined by the arterial pressure minus venous pressure. The greater the pressure difference (ie, ΔP), the greater the blood flow. Opposing blood flow is the vascular resistances. Again, this can be viewed across the entire circulatory system, where the sum of all vascular resistances is the TPR, or it can be viewed across a single capillary bed, where vascular resistance is defined by the resistances in the artery and arterioles supplying the capillary.

The 3 primary factors that determine the resistance to blood flow within a vessel include vessel diameter or radius (r), vessel length (L), and blood viscosity (η). The relationship between these factors is described by Poiseuille's equation, where resistance (R) is: $R \sim \eta \times L/r^4$. A 2-fold decrease in radius (ie, vasoconstriction) increases resistance 16-fold ($24 = 2 \times 2 \times 2 \times 2$), but a 2-fold increase in vessel length or blood viscosity (eg, increased hematocrit; polycythemia) will increase resistance only 2-fold. The most important factor impacting vascular resistance quantitatively and physiologically is vessel radius and vessel radius changes because of contraction and relaxation of the vascular smooth muscle within the tunica media of the blood vessel.

Considering the equation $Q = \Delta P/R$, the concept of autoregulation is explained. Autoregulation is the intrinsic ability of an organ to maintain a constant blood flow despite changes in arterial perfusion pressure. The ability to autoregulate is intrinsic to the small arteries and arterioles and is most readily identified in the cerebral and renal vascular systems but is also believed to occur in skeletal muscle, termed the *myogenic reflex*. For example, if arterial perfusion pressure would decrease to exercising muscle, vasodilation of the arteries and arterioles will reduce vascular resistance, allowing adequate blood flow to be maintained to the muscle.[19] If the vasculature did not dilate, muscle perfusion and O_2

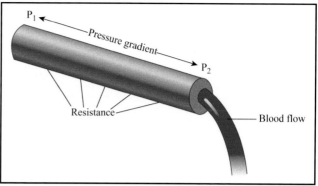

Figure 1-17. Interrelationships of pressure, resistance, and blood flow. (Adapted from Hall J. *Guyton and Hall Textbook of Medical Physiology.* 12th ed. Philadelphia, PA: Saunders; 2010.)

delivery would be impaired, ATP would fail to be produced, and muscle fatigue would necessitate stopping the exercise session.

Blood Pressure

BP is defined by the CO of the heart and the TPR of the vascular system: $BP = CO \times TPR$. Since the CO from the LV and RV is similar, the differences in pressures that need to be generated by the right and left sides of the heart are explained by the differences in the peripheral resistances. On the right, the resistance of only the pulmonary circulatory system needs to be countered, while the LV needs to generate pressure to overcome the resistances of multiple vascular systems, including the skeletal, hepatic, renal, cerebral, and the heart muscle itself, to name just a few.

BP is the pressure exerted by circulating blood upon the walls of blood vessels. During each heartbeat, BP varies between a maximum (systolic) and a minimum (diastolic) pressure. It should be remembered that systolic and diastolic arterial BPs are not static but undergo natural variations from one heartbeat to another, and measurements will reflect this variation. The mean arterial pressure (MAP) is the average pressure over a cardiac cycle and is determined by the CO, systemic vascular resistance (SVR), and central venous pressure (CVP): $MAP:MAP = (CO \times SVR) + CVP$. Clinically, MAP can be estimated by adding the diastolic BP to the pulse pressure ($PP = SBP - DBP$) in the following equation: $MAP \sim DP + 1/3$ (PP) (Figure 1-18).

The PP fluctuates because of the pulsatile nature of the cardiac cycle and is directly proportional to SV and inversely proportional to the compliance (ability to expand) of the aorta. For example, a widened PP would be seen during exercise because of an increased SV, or it could be seen in atherosclerosis of the aorta because of stiffening of this usually highly elastic artery. A narrowed PP may signify a poor SV as seen in heart failure.

MAP is an important variable to consider because it reflects the perfusion pressure of the organ systems of the body, and it is generally accepted that a MAP greater than 60 mm Hg is necessary to maintain sufficient blood flow to meet an organ's metabolic needs. If the MAP falls

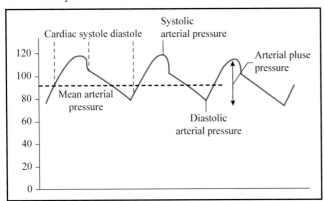

Figure 1-18. The arterial pressure waveform highlighting SBP, DBP, MAP and PP in relation to the cardiac cycle. (Reprinted with permission from Carroll RG. *Integrated Physiology.* Philadelphia, PA: Mosby Elsevier; 2007.)

significantly below 55 mm Hg for an extended time, the organ will not have sufficient blood flow, resulting in ischemia and organ dysfunction.

BP drops most rapidly along the small arteries and arterioles and continues to decrease as the blood moves through the capillaries and back to the heart through the veins. The pressure drop in the arterioles is due to increased vascular resistance in this region of the circulatory system. It is the alterations in vascular contraction and relaxation of the arterioles that regulates organ blood flow and primarily dictates the arterial BP.[24]

Pulmonary Component

Overview

A simple way to conceptualize the respiratory system is to divide the system into the gas-exchanging organ and the musculoskeletal ventilatory pump. The gas-exchanging organ is composed of the lung tissue and airways that conduct airflow from the external environment to the alveoli and the specialized interface between inspired air and the circulation—the alveolar-capillary membrane. Additionally, the gas-exchanging organ includes the pulmonary and bronchial circulations.[25] The musculoskeletal pump consists of the thoracic rib cage, cervical and thoracic spine, and upper pelvic area and the muscles of respiration. The bony structures allow for the origin and insertion of the respiratory muscles and also provide protection and support of the lung tissue. The muscles of ventilation alter the configuration of the thoracic cage by contracting and relaxing in synchrony, creating the pressure fluctuations that result in inspiration and expiration. These 2 systems (the gas-exchanging organ and musculoskeletal pump) must work in concert to maintain adequate O_2 supply and CO_2 removal, allowing metabolic processes to continue.

Ventilatory Pump

Structure

The ventilatory pump creates a vacuum, a lower intrathoracic pressure that draws air down a pressure gradient, from the external environment and into the lungs. The respiratory muscles develop force to overcome the resistances of the airways, lung tissue, and chest wall to create the negative intrathoracic pressure.[26] The forces produced by the musculoskeletal pump may be considered the "work of breathing" (WOB).

The primary muscle of inspiration, the diaphragm, accounts for approximately 60% of quiet breathing, and this dome-shaped muscle separates the abdomen from the thoracic cavity. The diaphragm consists of 2 separate halves (ie, right and left) with 3 distinct portions.[27,28] The costal diaphragm fans out to originate within the inner surfaces of the costal cartilages and adjacent portions of the lower 6 ribs; the xiphoid portion attaches on the posterior surface of the xiphoid process; and the crural diaphragm inserts into a central tendon that attaches to the lumbar vertebrae.[29] The phrenic nerve, originating from cervical nerve roots C3 to C5, innervates the diaphragm, activating the muscle.

Properties

Contraction of the diaphragm pulls the central tendon downward, combining with the rib cage attachments promoting thoracic expansion in both the lateral and vertical plane. The accessory muscles of inspiration (the sternocleidomastoid, erector spinae, trapezius, and scalenes) activate during tasks that require increased ventilation, allowing greater elevation of the rib cage. Expiration is normally a passive process. The inspiratory muscles relax, allowing the rib cage and the diaphragm to return to their resting positions. This combines with the elastic recoil of the lungs and airways, resulting in a reduced thoracic volume and higher intrathoracic pressures compared to the environment.[10]

Exceptions to the passive nature of expiration are forced expirations such as coughing, sneezing, and exercise as well as expiration for patients with increased airway resistance (eg, chronic obstructive pulmonary disease [COPD]). Forced exhalation combines the activities of the abdominals, the primary expiratory muscles, with the postural back, cervical, and pelvic muscles to contribute to force development.[27]

Ventilation

Air enters through the mouth and nose and travels via the trachea through the repeatedly branching conducting airways to the sites of gas exchange. The airflow divides at the level of the 2 mainstem bronchi to enter the right and left lungs. The right lung divides into 3 lobes: the middle, upper, and lower. The left lung is divided into 2 lobes: the upper and lower. Part of the left upper lobe, the lingula, is considered anatomically similar to the right middle lobe. The left lung is slightly smaller than the right because of the space occupied in the left thorax by the heart. Air moves from large bronchi to smaller branches (the bronchioles) to reach the air-filled sacks (the alveoli). The tree-like branching structure of the airways, branching upwards of 28 times, greatly increases the surface area for gas exchange (Figure 1-19). The conducting airways extend from the oral and nasal pharynx to the 17th generation of branching bronchi (the terminal bronchioles). The transitional zone consists of respiratory bronchioles, alveolar ducts, and the alveolar sacs, and is the site of gas exchange. Gas exchange occurs by diffusion through the cell membranes of the alveoli and the capillaries of the cardiovascular system.

Control of Ventilation

Breathing is largely regulated by the respiratory center in the medulla of the brainstem. The breathing rhythm is driven by neurons originating in the inspiratory area of the respiratory center.[11,30] Changes in ventilation rate and breathing pattern can occur with a variety of stimuli, including blood gases. Central and peripheral chemoreceptors will detect the changing amounts of O_2, CO_2, and pH in the blood and will stimulate an adaptive change in respiratory rate (RR).[30,31] Additional factors that alter the breathing pattern include stimuli from the cerebral cortex (eg, breath holding, volitional hyperventilation, phonation), hypothalamus and limbic systems (eg, emotional states), and irritant and pain receptors within the lung and muscle spindle receptors of the chest wall and extremities.[10,11,29] For example, at the onset of increased activity, skeletal muscle can provide input that will lead to an increase in ventilatory pump force and frequency.[32]

Ventilation Volumes and Flow

At rest, the volume of air that enters the lungs in 1 minute in the average adult is 4 to 8 liters. This volume of air (the minute ventilation [VE]) is determined by the volume of air that is inspired in one normal resting breath (the tidal volume [VT]) and the number of breaths in 1 minute (the RR). VE, therefore, can be represented by the equation $VE = VT \times RR$. An average RR of 10 to 16 breaths per minute with an average VT at rest of 500 mL yields the average adult VE noted previously.

Since ventilation is the volume of inspired gas that enters and leaves the lungs but not all of the inspired volume participates in gas exchange, the VT and VE can be further divided. The VT consists of air that reaches the alveoli (alveolar ventilation [VA]) and the volume of air in the conducting zones at the level of the mouth to the terminal bronchioles, termed *anatomic dead space* (VD), or the volume of air that does not contribute to gas exchange. VE, therefore, consists of both alveolar ventilation and dead space ventilation and can be represented by the following equation: $VT = VA + VD$.

On average, dead space volume is approximately one-third of the resting VT and is usually in the range of 150 mL.[11] Hypothetically, if the VT was the same as the VD volume, minimal gas exchange would occur since the inspired volume of air would not reach the level of the alveoli. A vital task of the musculoskeletal pump is to provide VT breaths that exceed the VD.

Ventilation is influenced by multiple factors, including lung and chest wall compliance, and the frictional forces within the airways. Airway friction or airway resistance is affected by the geometry of the airways (bronchodilation versus bronchoconstriction; see discussion of Poiseuille's equation on p 15) and velocity and type of airflow (laminar versus turbulent, slow versus rapid breathing frequency). Turbulent

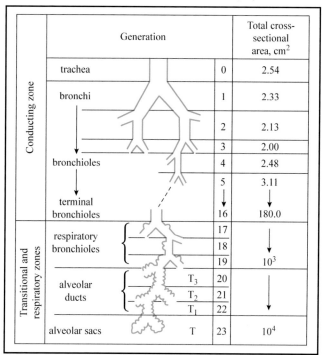

Generation		Total cross-sectional area, cm^2
trachea	0	2.54
bronchi	1	2.33
	2	2.13
	3	2.00
bronchioles	4	2.48
	5	3.11
terminal bronchioles	16	180.0
respiratory bronchioles	17	
	18	
	19	10^3
alveolar ducts T_3	20	
T_2	21	
T_1	22	
alveolar sacs T	23	10^4

(Left margin labels: *Conducting zone*; *Transitional and respiratory zones*)

Figure 1-19. The conducting and respiratory zones of the respiratory system. Note the increased cross-sectional area with each airway generation and airway branching. (Reprinted with permission from Levitzky M. *Pulmonary Physiology*. 8th ed. New York, NY: McGraw-Hill; 2013. Copyright The McGraw-Hill Companies, Inc.)

airflow occurs primarily in the larger airways (eg, trachea to the fourth or fifth generation of bronchi), requiring an increased driving pressure (an increased WOB) to maintain flow down the tracheobronchial tree. Compliance defines the ease of lung and chest wall expansion. Compliance is the ability of the lung or chest wall to change volume relative to an applied change in pressure and is defined by the equation $C = \Delta V / \Delta P$. As compliance decreases, expansion is resisted and greater force is required by the musculoskeletal pump to promote a volume change. Lung compliance is influenced by the fluid content of pulmonary tissues and the structural components of the lung parenchyma. For example, pulmonary edema and fibrosis of the lung will decrease lung compliance, leading to an increased demand on the musculoskeletal pump and increasing the WOB. The musculoskeletal pump will also be influenced by the structural make-up of the soft tissues and the mechanical alignment of the rib cage. Chest wall compliance would be reduced by fibrosis of the costovertebral joints (eg, ankylosing spondylitis) or a horizontal rib alignment (eg, COPD), resulting in an increased WOB.

Ventilation is influenced by many factors and will not be uniform throughout the lung. For example, the lung is often compared to the childhood toy, the Slinky (Figure 1-20). The alveoli in the upper part of the upright lung (the apex) are more expanded because of the weight of the dependent portion of the lung (the base). These alveoli will be stiffer and have a lower lung compliance compared to the smaller alveoli at the base. Therefore, as the individual breathes,

Figure 1-20. Diagram of the "Slinky" analogy of the lung, where the apical alveoli are larger and more distended compared with alveoli at the base at resting volume (ie, functional residual capacity). (Adapted from Grippi MA. *Pulmonary Pathophysiology*. Philadelphia, PA: Lippincott Co.; 1995, and Leff AR, Schumacker PT. *Respiratory Physiology: Basics and Application*. Philadelphia, PA: W.B. Saunders Company; 1993.)

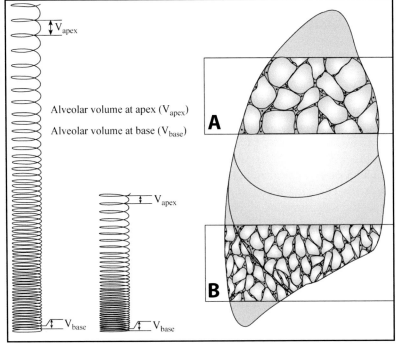

Alveolar volume at apex (V_{apex})

Alveolar volume at base (V_{base})

the majority of the VT will take the path of least resistance and airflow will be directed to the base of the lung. Disease processes can lead to regional alterations in lung compliance that can result in regional changes in ventilation. Consider the patient with right lower lobe pneumonia. In this case, inflammation and hypersecretion of mucus lead to lung consolidation and decrease lung compliance in the right lower lobe. Airflow will be restricted to this region and redistributed to the higher compliant middle and upper lobes.

Gas Exchange

Perfusion

Blood Flow to Lungs

Blood flow to the lungs occurs via 2 separate circulations: the pulmonary circulation and the bronchial circulation. The bronchial circulation arises from the aorta or from intercostal arteries and supplies oxygenated blood to the conducting airways, pulmonary vessels, nerves, interstitium, and pleura. The pulmonary circulation is responsible for bringing the systemic venous blood into contact with the alveoli, allowing gas exchange. Additionally, the pulmonary circulation filters the blood, serves as a blood reservoir, provides nutrients to the lungs, and metabolizes many blood-borne chemicals.

Properties of Perfusion

The pulmonary circulation is a high-capacity, low-resistance circuit allowing pulmonary BP to remain low even though the lung receives the entire CO. Anatomically, blood enters the pulmonary circulation at the main pulmonary artery after being ejected from the RV. Just as the airways repeatedly divide into smaller but more numerous units, the pulmonary circulation follows a similar tree-like pattern of branching until forming the alveolar-capillary membrane and then converging into the pulmonary venous system,

which carries oxygenated blood to the LA via the pulmonary veins. Just as ventilation is not uniform, lung perfusion is heterogeneous. CO, gravity, and the pulmonary vascular resistance (PVR) affect blood flow, creating regional differences that are classically defined as 3 separate "Zones of West":

1. Zone 1 defines the upper one-third of the lung

2. Zone 2 defines the middle

3. Zone 3 defines the lower one-third

Recall that the alveoli in the apex are more distended compared with alveoli in the basilar portions of the lung. The pressure from these air-filled alveoli compresses the capillaries, leading to an increase in the PVR. The increased PVR combined with the resistive force of gravity will limit blood flow to the apical regions. The result is relatively greater ventilation (V) compared to perfusion (Q), V > Q, and this is termed *dead space physiology*. The alveoli in the lower one-third of the lung have greater compliance and will receive the majority of the ventilation. However, gravity and a decreased PVR will preferentially allow greater blood flow at the base of the lung. Even though more airflow goes to the base compared to the apex (approximately 3 times more air), blood flow is much greater in the base (approximately 10 times greater), resulting in perfusion exceeding ventilation (Q > V). When Q > V, this is termed *shunt physiology*.

Ventilation to Perfusion Ratio

The V/Q ratio defines the relationship between airflow and blood flow, and the physiologic coupling of these 2 factors determines the gas-exchanging function of the lung. Regions of low V/Q (ie, shunt physiology) result in decreased partial pressure of O_2 in arterial blood (PaO_2) and elevated arterial concentrations of CO_2 ($PaCO_2$). The concentrations of the respiratory gases in the blood in a low V/Q state

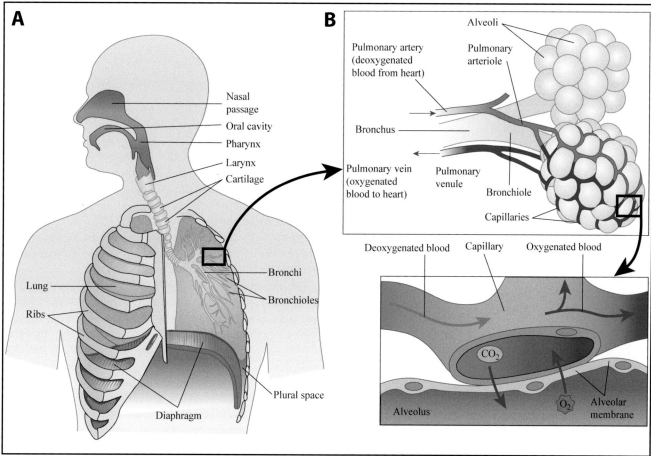

Figure 1-21. (A) Major pulmonary structures within the thoracic cavity. (B) General overview of the ventilatory system showing the respiratory passages, alveoli, pulmonary circulation, and gas exchange function in an alveolus. (Adapted from McArdle WD, Katch FI, Katch VL. *Exercise Physiology: Nutrition, Energy and Human Performance.* 7th ed. Philadelphia, PA: Lippincott, Williams & Wilkins; 2010:254.)

resemble venous blood even though the blood has passed through the pulmonary circulation. It is as if the blood exited the RV, bypassed the lungs, and entered the LV (ie, a right-to-left shunt). Shunt refers to the entry of blood into the systemic arterial system without going through ventilated areas of lung. This mismatch between ventilation and perfusion is a common cause of hypoxemia in adult patients.[31,33] To compensate for V/Q mismatch, the pulmonary vasculature is sensitive to low O_2 and high CO_2 tensions as seen in poorly ventilated lung regions. The vasculature will adapt by "shunting" blood to better ventilated areas of the lungs for gas exchange by the process of hypoxic vasoconstriction.[25] Increased PVR in poorly ventilated regions enhances blood flow to normally ventilated regions. Blood flow will take the path of least resistance, and this adaptive mechanism optimizes V/Q matching. This may become pathologic when there is extensive tissue destruction of the lung or alterations of the pulmonary vascular bed leading to increased PVR, pulmonary hypertension, and right heart failure. Regions of high V/Q are termed *dead space* and result in reduced $PaCO_2$ and insignificant changes in PaO_2 (eg, hyperventilation). An example of ventilation exceeding perfusion would be a patient with a pulmonary embolism restricting pulmonary blood flow.

Properties of Gas Exchange, Including Surface Area

The alveolar-capillary junction plays a critical role in gas exchange. The lungs and the cardiovascular system directly connect when the pulmonary arteries branch into single-cell walled capillaries that surround the alveoli of the lungs (Figure 1-21). The O_2 requirements for all of the other cells in the body, and CO_2 removal, rely on the successful diffusion of respiratory gases across the cell membranes at this juncture.

Diffusion within the lung is defined by the Fick equation (Fick's Law of Diffusion): $V = d\,A \times (P_1 - P_2)/T$. This equation states that the diffusion of a volume of gas (V) is directly proportional to the gas constant (d), the surface area available for gas exchange (A), and the difference of the partial pressures of the specific gas across the alveolar capillary membrane ($P_1 - P_2$). Diffusion is inversely proportional to the tissue thickness across the alveolar capillary membrane (T). The diffusion constant (d) represents the solubility of the gas within the membrane. The respiratory gases are highly soluble in lipids and therefore pass through cell membranes easily.[11] CO_2 is approximately 20 times more soluble than O_2 and will more readily diffuse in the lung.

The adult lung contains approximately 300 million alveoli, creating a large surface area (A) for gas exchange (approximately 100 m^2 or the area of 2 tennis courts).[10] The alveolar capillary membrane (T) is thin and in some places less than 0.5 μm (10^{-6} meters; one-millionth of a meter), which aides in diffusion of respiratory of O_2 and CO_2.[10,14] For comparison, a single strand of human hair usually has a diameter of 20 to 180 μm while red blood cells (RBCs) are approximately 8 μm in diameter.[14]

With consideration of Fick's equation, it is easy to understand how various lung pathologies affect gas exchange. For example, the thickness of the alveolar-capillary junction (T) may be increased with pulmonary edema or pulmonary fibrosis, reducing gas diffusion. The surface area (A) could be reduced when alveoli are destroyed, as seen in emphysema. If a patient has a gas-exchange defect and is provided supplemental O_2, the inhaled O_2 increases the partial pressure gradient ($\uparrow \Delta P$) for this gas across the alveolar-capillary membrane, increasing diffusion of O_2 from the alveoli into the bloodstream (see Chapter 9).

Gas Partial Pressures

At standard temperature and pressure, the composition of atmospheric air is 21% O_2 (a fraction of inspired O_2 [FiO_2] = 0.21) and 79% nitrogen (FiN_2 = 0.79). At sea level, 1 atmosphere of pressure is 760 mm Hg. The partial pressure of O_2 (PO_2) in air is equal to its portion in the mixture, thus 21% of 760 mm Hg. Therefore, the PO_2 in atmospheric air, inhaled into the lungs, would be 160 mm Hg. However, as we breathe, the air is humidified and warmed as it passes through the mouth, nose, and conducting airways. Saturating the dry atmospheric air with water vapor effectively lowers the PO_2 to 149.13 mm Hg, or just more than 19.5%.[11] Additionally, inspired air will mix with air already in the tracheobronchial tree, further reducing the concentration of O_2 and raising the concentration of CO_2. The PO_2 becomes 104 mm Hg, or 13.6%. This pressure of O_2 becomes the driving force for the diffusion of O_2 across the alveolar capillary membrane (see ΔP—Fick's Law of Diffusion).

O_2 diffusing from the alveoli into capillaries follows a pressure gradient. The relatively higher concentration of O_2 in the alveoli (~100 mm Hg) contrasts with the lower O_2 concentration in the venous blood (40 mm Hg) arriving from the pulmonary arteries and arterioles into the pulmonary capillaries. The net rate of O_2 diffusion through the cell membranes of the alveoli and blood capillaries is proportional to the concentration difference on either side ($P_1 - P_2 = \Delta P$ or 100 mm Hg – 40 mm Hg = 60 mm Hg). The PO_2 in the capillary blood rises rapidly and quickly combines with hemoglobin of the RBCs. Under normal circumstances, the total transit time of an RBC within a pulmonary capillary is approximately 0.75 seconds. However, when an RBC is about one-third of the way through the capillary, PaO_2 equilibrates and matches that of the alveoli. O_2 tensions equilibrate in approximately 0.25 seconds, and hemoglobin will fully saturate with O_2. As long as there is normal perfusion through the pulmonary circulation and the alveolar capillary membrane is not altered, gas exchange will continue normally. This defines the perfusion limit for gas exchange in the normal lung.

Blood

Oxygen in Blood/Oxygen Delivery

The erythrocyte or RBCs' primary functions are the delivery of O_2 to tissues, the uptake of cellular metabolic byproducts (specifically CO_2 and H+), and maintenance of acid-base balance. A single RBC contains 4 hemoglobin molecules and can carry 4 molecules of O_2 when fully saturated, for a total O_2 content of approximately 20 mL/dL of blood. RBCs last 120 days in the bloodstream and are removed by macrophages in the liver and spleen.[14] Only 3% of the O_2 in the pulmonary capillaries remains dissolved in the blood. The remaining molecules, the majority at 97%, are loosely bound to hemoglobin molecules within RBCs.

The number of RBCs and the volume of blood that is RBCs will vary with age and gender. The numbers of RBCs are carefully regulated by the body to ensure there is an adequate supply to deliver O_2 to the cells of the body. Hypoxia, low O_2 tensions in the blood due to pulmonary disease, heart failure, or altitude, may upregulate RBC production in response to the production of the hormone erythropoietin from the kidneys. RBC production is also regulated to avoid an excessive concentration that would increase blood viscosity, thereby increasing resistance and impeding blood flow.

Hemoglobin Saturation Curve

The oxyhemoglobin dissociation curve defines how our RBCs acquire and release O_2. Specifically, the oxyhemoglobin dissociation curve relates O_2 saturation (SpO_2) measurable by pulse oximetry on the "X" axis and PaO_2 on the "Y" axis. The sigmoid shape of the curve relates to the reversible binding properties of hemoglobin itself (Figure 1-22). For example, consider the saturation of hemoglobin at a PaO_2 of 60 mm Hg. Hemoglobin's affinity for O_2 increases as successive molecules of O_2 bind and more molecules of O_2 bind as the PaO_2 increases. Each RBC can carry 4 O_2 molecules, and as this limit is approached, hemoglobin is fully saturated and additional binding cannot occur, regardless of an increase in PaO_2, and the curve plateaus. This process occurs in the lung.

Consider the shape of the curve as O_2 partial pressure decreases below 50 mm Hg. This is the process that occurs in peripheral tissues such as exercising skeletal muscle. In this steep area of the curve, O_2 is unloaded to peripheral tissue as the hemoglobin's affinity diminishes and O_2 is released into the surrounding plasma. The O_2 molecules will diffuse into the skeletal muscle and will ultimately be available for metabolic pathways to create ATP.

Complicating the understanding of the oxyhemoglobin dissociation curve is the fact that hemoglobin-O_2 binding can be affected by several factors, and this is represented by the curve shifting to the left or right. A rightward shift occurs in states of lower pH (acidosis), high CO_2, fever, and increased 2,3-diphosphoglycerate (DPG). 2,3-DPG is a substance created during glycolysis in RBCs during periods of inadequate O_2 availability such as hypoxemia and inadequate O_2 delivery such as heart disease, and facilitates hemoglobin's release of O_2. A rightward shift defines a reduced affinity of hemoglobin for O_2. In other words, hemoglobin will release the O_2 it is carrying and hemoglobin's saturation will be reduced for a given PaO_2 compared to normal.[10,11,34]

Consider the case of exercising muscle. This muscle will need greater O_2 to maintain energy production. As a result of exercise, heat is produced, CO_2 and lactic acid are released, and this will promote hemoglobin release of O_2, making it available for ATP production within the exercising muscle. Pathologically, a rightward shift may accompany many disease processes such as respiratory failure in COPD, reducing binding of O_2 and hemoglobin, which will decrease the delivery of O_2 to peripheral tissues.

Conversely, a leftward shift defines an increased affinity of hemoglobin for O_2; hemoglobin holds onto O_2, limiting its availability for metabolic processes. This occurs in states where pH is higher (alkalosis), and when CO_2 and 2,3-DPG are reduced, as is seen in the resting state or pathologically during sepsis (see Chapter 9).

EXERCISE PHYSIOLOGY: TYING IT ALL TOGETHER

Overview

The transition from rest to exercise involves the coordinated functioning of the cardiovascular, respiratory, musculoskeletal, neurologic systems, and bioenergetic systems. Successful completion of any exercise or activity is based on adequate O_2 transport and waste removal (see Figure 1-2). Ultimately, the movement system is limited by the weakest link in this "interdependent" chain, and this weakest link or combination of impairments will be the cause of activity intolerance and functional limitations.

Maximal Oxygen Consumption and Metabolic Equivalents

The maximal capacity to transport and utilize O_2 during exercise is considered the "gold standard" measurement of cardiorespiratory fitness. This measurement, VO_2 maximum (also called maximal O_2 consumption, maximum O_2 uptake, or aerobic capacity), implies that an individual's physiological limit has been reached. Conceptually, VO_{2max} is defined by O_2 delivery and O_2 extraction ($VO_2 = O_2$ delivery × O_2 extraction). Mathematically, this is represented by Fick's equation: $VO_2 = CO \times (A-V)\ O_2$ difference. O_2 delivery is a function of the CO (HR × SV) while O_2 extraction is a function of the arterial-venous O_2 difference, or the ability of peripheral tissues to extract O_2 and create ATP by aerobic metabolism.

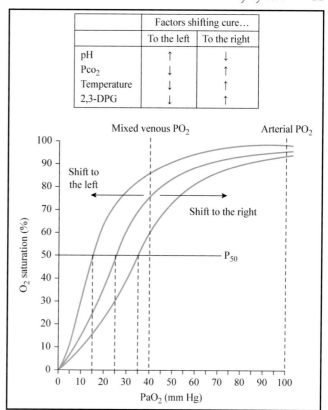

Figure 1-22. Hemoglobin affinity for O_2 can be altered. The hemoglobin affinity for O_2 is decreased by factors that occur during exercise: a decrease in pH, an increase in PCO_2, or an increase in temperature. Prolonged hypoxia generates 2,3-DPG, which also decreases hemoglobin affinity for O_2. Each of these changes allows a greater proportion of the bound O_2 to dissociate from hemoglobin and be delivered to the tissues. The decrease hemoglobin affinity for O_2 is called a shift to the right of the oxyhemoglobin dissociation curve, or an increase in P50, the PO_2 at which 50% of the hemoglobin is saturated with O_2. (Reprinted with permission from Carroll RG. *Integrated Physiology*. Philadelphia, PA: Mosby Elsevier; 2007.)

Accurately measuring VO_{2max} involves a physical effort sufficient in duration and intensity to overload the aerobic energy system. This typically involves a graded exercise test performed on either a treadmill or a cycle ergometer. Testing requires an exercise intensity that is progressively increased while measuring vital signs including HR and rhythm (ie, electrocardiogram), BP, RR, VTs, VE, pulse oximetry, as well O_2 and CO_2 concentration of the inhaled and exhaled air.[35,36] VO_{2max} is achieved when O_2 consumption plateaus and the HR and BP fail to increase despite an increase in workload. The point during exercise where CO_2 production rises disproportionately to O_2 consumed ($VCO_2 > VO_2$) or lactate accumulates in the blood are termed the *ventilatory* or *lactate threshold*, respectively. The lactate threshold may also be referred to as the onset of blood lactate accumulation.[32] Technically, this is a challenging test to perform and requires a highly motivated subject. Few patients will achieve true maximum, however, and the highest achieved workload is termed *peak*. VO_{2max} is expressed either as an absolute rate in liters of O_2 per minute (L/min), or it can be normalized to the patient's body weight in milliliters of O_2 per kilogram (mL/kg/min).

TABLE 1-4. ACTIVITIES OF DAILY LIVING AND METABOLIC EQUIVALENTS

ACTIVITY	METHOD	METS	AVERAGE HR RESPONSE (ELEVATED FROM RESTING HR)
Toileting	Bed pan Commode Urinal (in bed) Urinal (standing)	1.0 to 2.0	5 to 15 bpm
Bathing	Bed bath Tub bath Shower	2.0 to 3.0	10 to 20 bpm
Walking (flat surface)	2 mph	2.0 to 2.5	5 to 15 bpm
	2.5 mph	2.5 to 2.9	5 to 15 bpm
	3 mph	3.0 to 3.3	5 to 15 bpm
Stair climbing (1 flight = 12 steps)	Down 1 flight of stairs	2.5	10 bpm
	Up 1 flight of stairs	4.0	10 to 25 bpm
	Down 1 flight of stairs carrying objects (25 to 49 pounds)	5.0	15 to 30 bpm
Upper body exercise (while standing)	Upper extremity	2.0 to 2.2	10 to 20 bpm
Leg calisthenics		2.5 to 4.5	15 to 25 bpm

Adapted from Ainsworth BE, Haskell WL, Herrmann SD, et al. 2011 Compendium of Physical Activities: a second update of codes and MET values. *Med Sci Sports Exerc.* 2011;43(8):1575-1581; and National Cancer Institute. Metabolic equivalent (MET) values for activities in American time use survey (ATUS). *Applied Research Cancer Control and Population Sciences.* http://appliedresearch.cancer.gov/atus-met/met.php. Accessed August 6, 2014.

Another method to express patients' aerobic capacity is the metabolic equivalent (MET). The measured O_2 consumption of a 70-kg man at rest is approximately 3.5 mL/kg/min, and this value is used as the standard unit for setting the resting energy expenditure, or 1 MET. Therefore, any physical activity can be viewed as a multiple of this unit. For example, most activities of daily living require an energy expenditure of approximately 1.5 to 4 METs, moderate work and typical sexual activities require an energy expenditure of approximately 3 to 6 METs, and heavy work or high-level sport activities require an energy expenditure of 5 to 15 METs (Table 1-4).[37] Since exercise testing will reveal the highest achievable workload and vital sign responses to progressive activity, clinicians can use this information to determine if a patient can safely participate and complete various activities. For example, if a patient had a peak achieved O_2 consumption of 35 mL/kg/min (10 METs), it would be risky for him to return to work as a firefighter since this job requires an estimated energy expenditure of 12 METs.

Measurements during exercise testing assume a steady-state condition. Steady state occurs when the amounts of O_2 and CO_2 exchanged in cellular respiration is in balance, and this is balanced by the inspired O_2 (VO_2) and expired CO_2 (VCO_2) from the lungs. A steady state assumes the amounts of inspired VO_2 and expired VCO_2 measured at the mouth accurately reflect the extent of cellular work at a particular level of exercise.[35] The ratio of VCO_2/VO_2 is called the *respiratory exchange ratio* (RER) or is sometimes referred to as the *respiratory quotient* (RQ) if measured at the tissue level. Although related, the RER and RQ are not completely interchangeable.[36] Normally, blood and gas transport systems are keeping pace with tissue metabolism and the RER can be used as an index of metabolic events or RQ. Additionally, the ratio of VO_2 to VCO_2 will reflect the energy substrate used to create ATP. For example, an RQ of 1.0 indicates metabolism of primarily carbohydrates, whereas an RER < 1.0 indicates a mixture of carbohydrates and fat (RER ~ 0.7) or protein (RER ~ 0.8). RER greater than 1.0 could be caused by CO_2 derived from lactic acid or by hyperventilation, and this value is used to determine whether the patient has achieved the anaerobic threshold.[35,36,38]

Energy Utilization

Energy utilization will depend on the exercise duration and intensity. Short-duration, high-intensity exercise primarily utilizes anaerobic metabolic pathways. For example, exercise lasting less than 10 seconds primarily relies on the ATP-PC system, between 10 seconds to 1 minute will rely on ATP created from glycolysis, and longer than 45 seconds will utilize a combination of anaerobic (ATP-PC; glycolysis) and aerobic systems. Longer-duration activities, especially submaximal exercises at moderate intensity, will use ATP generated from aerobic metabolism. However, as exercise intensity increases toward maximum as in an incremental or graded exercise test, there is increased reliance on anaerobic pathways. This switch is identified by the rise in lactic acid in the plasma as well as increased VE with increased CO_2 elimination (RER > 1.0, where $VCO_2 > VO_2$). The switch from aerobic to more anaerobic metabolism is termed the *anaerobic threshold*, *lactate* or *ventilatory threshold* or the *onset of blood lactic acidosis*.[11,13] During endurance tasks, anaerobic metabolism is triggered when the preferable aerobic system can no longer match the demand for ATP production and fatigue and the cessation of activity will soon occur.

Normal Response to Increasing Loads

The Cardiovascular Responses

The cardiovascular changes associated with exercise will increase O_2 delivery to working muscle, allowing aerobic metabolism to continue. Consider the case of running on a treadmill or a patient performing gait training. At the start of the therapy session, the patient's HR increases. This initial increase in HR is due to inhibition of tonic parasympathetic tone. Vagus nerve activity is reduced, acetylcholine levels decline, and the heart is released from this negative chronotropic influence and HR begins to accelerate. As workload increases, sympathetic activity increases. NE and later EPI are released and combine with the beta1-type receptors, leading to an increased HR and increased cardiac contractility, while stimulation of the alpha1 receptors promotes vasoconstriction of the peripheral vasculature, increasing peripheral resistance (see Table 1-2). The increased HR and contractility will promote an increased SV and CO, thus increasing O_2 delivery, and the increased CO and TPR will increase BP.[35,36] TPR will later decrease as exercise continues because of local mediators as described next.

Cardiac Output and Stroke Volume

CO increases in direct proportion to work rate and results from both an increase in HR and SV (Figure 1-23). As noted previously, SV is influenced by the changes in contractility, afterload, HR, and preload.[39] SNS activation will enhance contractility and HR, increasing CO. Vasoconstriction of nonworking vasculature, most notably the splanchnic circulation (vasculature of the abdominal viscera—mesenteric, splenic and hepatic circulations), combined with ongoing muscle contraction and the increased rate and depth of breathing will support venous return and increase the EDV (see Bainbridge reflex and Frank-Starling mechanism on p 13), leading to elevations in SV and, consequently, the CO. SV, however, will plateau in the untrained or moderately trained at approximately 40% to 60% of VO_{2max}.[40,41] During progressive exercise, SV will increase by as much as 50%, with the greatest change occurring earlier in the exercise

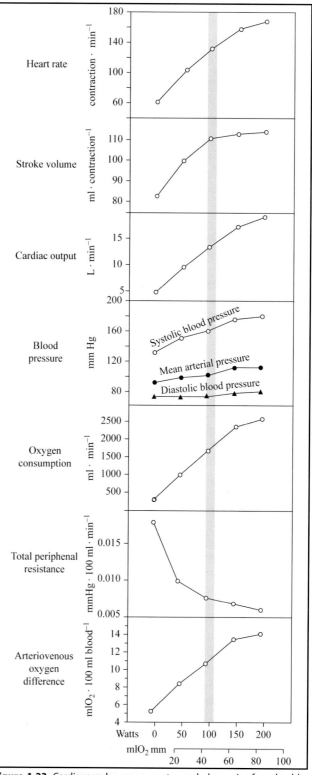

Figure 1-23. Cardiovascular responses to graded exercise for a healthy sedentary individual. Values are plotted against specific work rates and percentage of VO_{2max}. The shaded area represents the lactate threshold. (Reprinted with permission from *ACSM's Resource Manual for Guidelines for Exercise Testing and Prescription*. 2nd ed. Malvern, PA: Lea & Febiger; 1993.)

session.[42] This implies that the increase in CO at higher workloads is due primarily to increases in HR. Maximal CO tends to decrease in both men and women after 30 years of age, but the age-related decline in CO is still uncertain.[41,43] Challenging this traditional view of SV changes with increasing exercise intensity is recent evidence demonstrating that SV may progressively increase throughout the exercise session. However, this finding requires further research as it appears SV may be influenced by multiple factors, including training status, age, mode of training, and gender.[44-46]

Heart Rate

HR increases nearly linearly with increasing workload but plateaus as exercise approaches maximum, as noted in Figure 1-23. The HR acceleration will increase the CO, especially at higher workloads, and is primarily due to SNS stimulation of the beta adrenergic receptors, but cardiac reflexes (eg, Bainbridge reflex) also contribute to the rise in HR. Maximal HR declines in a linear fashion in men and women after 30 years of age.[47,48] It should also be noted that peak HR is reduced in many, but not all, patients with different cardiovascular and/or pulmonary diseases (either because of the disease itself or because of medications used to treat the disease), and therapists should modify their expectations while patients perform therapeutic interventions.[33] Common equations to determine the age-predicted maximal HR include $220 - age$ and $208 - (age \times 0.7)$. Both give similar values for people younger than 40 years. However, the first equation appears to underestimate the maximal HR in older people and variability of 10 to 15 bpm within an age group is expected.[35,48] Determining the HR reserve (HRR) is clinically important since it provides information regarding an individual's potential reserve capacity and may allow the clinician to set exercise parameters. HRR is calculated by subtracting the resting and measured or age-predicted maximum HR ($HRR = HR_{max} - HR_{rest}$).

Another concept related to the exercise HR response is the HR recovery following exercise. HR recovery refers to the early deceleration of the HR following an exercise session and is believed to be associated with vagal tone reactivation.[36] HR recovery has generated interest in recent years because studies have demonstrated that the longer the HR remains elevated following an exercise test, there is increased cardiovascular risk of death.[49,50] Vagal reactivation is an important cardiac deceleration mechanism after exercise; it is accelerated in well-trained athletes but may be blunted in deconditioned and/or "medically ill" patients.[51] The reasons why patients are at increased risk is poorly understood and is still under investigation.

Blood Pressure

BP, as previously noted, is dependent on CO and TPR. As the working muscle continues to contract, waste products build and the local mediators cause intense vasodilation (see Table 1-3). The vasodilation overrides the sympathetic-derived vasoconstriction and lowers TPR (see Figure 1-23). Although generalized vasoconstriction occurs, local vasorelaxation reduces peripheral resistance and diverts blood flow from low-demand visceral areas to the skeletal muscles.[52] Remember that blood flow is inversely proportional to vascular resistance ($Q = P/R$) and blood flow will increase

to working muscle as the resistance falls. Enhanced blood flow ensures O_2 delivery and CO_2 removal, supporting the metabolic demands of the muscle. The observed increase in BP results from marked increases in CO that counteracts the decrease in TPR. As a result of the increase in CO, systolic and MAP increase with a progressive increase in workload. Systolic BP will continue to rise until maximal workload with little change in diastolic BP (+10 to 15 mm Hg; see Figure 1-23). Exercise-induced hypotension is an abnormal finding, and the clinician should terminate the exercise session if this is observed. Knowing that BP relies on CO and TPR, it is not surprising that abnormal BP responses are due to alterations in CO such as aortic valve or other outflow obstruction, impaired LV function, global severe myocardial ischemia, and/or alterations in TPR, most notably an exaggerated peripheral vasodilation.[36,52] Each factor increases the risk for an exercise-related untoward event, and the clinician should immediately stop the exercise and evaluate the patient. Exercise-induced hypotension, as a general rule, is associated with a poor prognosis and should raise emergent consideration of significant cardiac disease.[36]

Conversely, an excessive rise in BP is often seen in patients with known resting hypertension, but an abnormal rise with exercise in the face of normal resting BP is also indicative of abnormal BP control.[35] It is also important to consider the site of BP measurements. For measurements taken in the lower extremities, the diastolic pressure in the legs is usually similar to that in the arms, while the systolic pressure may be 20 to 30 mm Hg higher in normal individuals.[53]

Pulmonary Responses

Overview

Exercise increases the metabolism of the working muscles, leading to increased O_2 consumption, CO_2, and lactic acid production. The respiratory system, in combination with the cardiovascular system, responds to these demands by increasing the volume of O_2 supplied to the exercising tissues and increasing the removal of CO_2 and hydrogen ions (H+) from the body. Although the lungs and heart are coupled in gas exchange, they differ with regard to physiologic reserve during maximal exercise. Under normal circumstances, the respiratory system has a larger reserve capacity and normally exceeds the demands of maximal exercise. For example, VE can increase 20 times in healthy subjects to meet the needs of O_2 uptake and CO_2 removal. Exercising subjects will usually reach maximum O_2 consumption (VO_{2max}) when pulmonary ventilation is 60% to 70% of maximal breathing capacity, reflecting a 30% to 40% breathing reserve.[40] This highlights that maximal exercise is normally limited by restricted O_2 delivery from the cardiovascular system and not limited by a lack of pulmonary reserve.

Minute Ventilation (Respiratory Rate × Tidal Volume)

During exercise, the increase in depth and rate of breathing are early signs for the clinician to observe (Figure 1-24). The stimulus to increase ventilation results from feedback loops emerging from the respiratory centers in the brainstem and volitional activity from the motor cortex, and through feedback from the proprioceptors in the muscles and joints of the working muscles.[11,13,31] Bronchial dilation due to SNS stimulation of beta2 adrenergic receptors within the airways leads to reduced airway resistance, promoting increased airflow (see Poiseuille's equation on p 15 and Table 1-2). During prolonged and/or intense exercise, CO_2 production and H+ from lactic acid will stimulate the central and peripheral chemoreceptors associated with respiratory control, further increasing the rate and depth of breathing. The increases in VT and RR increase VE, specifically alveolar ventilation. The initial increase in ventilation is due to an increase in VT greater than RR. However, with increasing exercise intensity (typically 70% to 80% of peak exercise), increases in RR predominate due to greater resistive and elastic loads on the lung with large VTs (> 75% of vital capacity).[31,35] Considering that the normal RR is 10 breaths per minute, RR can increase 1- to 3-fold (25 to 45 breaths/minute) in most adult subjects, but in athletes, it may be increased by 6- to 7-fold (60 to 70 breaths/minute).[35]

Gas Exchange

Efficient pulmonary gas exchange function is important for a normal exercise response. The increases in CO in combination with increased pulmonary ventilation will lead to improved matching of ventilation and perfusion. The increased pulmonary perfusion due to the enhanced CO, especially of apical lung units, will decrease dead space, and increases in alveolar ventilation in basilar regions will reduce shunting, thereby optimizing gas exchange. Normally, oxygenation is well-maintained during an exercise session. However, a decrease of > 5% in the pulse oximeter estimate of arterial saturation during exercise is suggestive of abnormal exercise-induced hypoxemia likely due to a V/Q mismatch, most notably Q > V (ie, shunt physiology).[36] True arterial desaturation of 5% to 10% from baseline can occur in extremely fit healthy individuals but is uncommon in the general population. In fit individuals, desaturation occurs during sustained high-intensity exercise because of a diffusion limitation resulting from rapid pulmonary vascular transit time associated with very high COs. In these instances, the O_2 tensions between the alveoli and the blood do not equilibrate, the RBCs do not fully saturate with O_2, and the pulse oximeter values decline.[33,36]

Summary

This chapter introduced the integrative functions of the cardiovascular and pulmonary systems. The interaction of these systems aids the increased metabolic needs of the body during the stress of exercise. The clinician has a special challenge to carefully monitor and assess a patient's exercise responses and compare those responses to the expected "normal" outcomes. The ultimate goal is to improve the patient's activity tolerance in the most safe and efficacious manner.

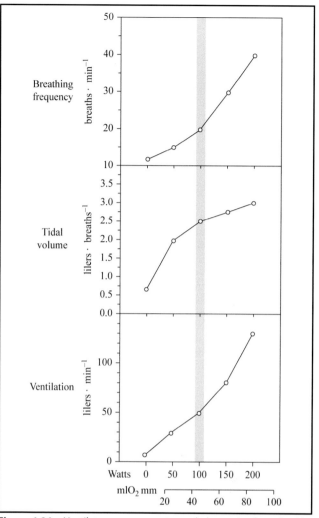

Figure 1-24. Ventilatory responses to graded exercise for a healthy sedentary individual. Values are plotted against specific work rates and percentage of VO_{2max}. The shaded area represents the lactate threshold. (Reprinted with permission from *ACSM's Resource Manual for Guidelines for Exercise Testing and Prescription.* 2nd ed. Malvern, PA: Lea & Febiger; 1993.)

References

1. Snader CE, Marwick TH, Pashkow FJ, et al. Importance of estimated functional capacity as a predictor of all-cause mortality among patients referred for exercise thallium single-photon emission computed tomography: report of 3,400 patients from a single center. *J Am Coll Cardiol.* 1997;30:641-648.

2. Gulati M, Pandey DK, Arnsdorf MF, et al. Exercise capacity and the risk of death in women: the St James Women Take Heart Project. *Circulation.* 2003;108:1554-1559.

3. Blair SN, Kohl HW 3rd, Barlow CE, Paffenbarger RS Jr, Gibbons LW, Macera CA. Changes in physical fitness and all-cause mortality: a prospective study of healthy and unhealthy men. *JAMA.* 1995;273:1093-1098.

4. Weiner DA, Ryan TJ, McCabe CH, et al. The role of exercise testing in identifying patients with improved survival after coronary artery bypass surgery. *J Am Coll Cardiol.* 1986;8:741-748.

5. Bourque JM, Holland BH, Watson DD, Beller GA. Achieving an exercise workload of > or = 10 metabolic equivalents predicts a very low risk of inducible ischemia: does myocardial perfusion imaging have a role? *J Am Coll Cardiol.* 2009;54(6):538-545.

6. Myers J, Prakash M, Froelicher V, Do D, Partington S, Atwood JE. Exercise capacity and mortality among men referred for exercise testing. *N Engl J Med.* 2002;346(11):793-801.

7. Berry JD, Willis B, Gupta S, et al. Lifetime risks for cardiovascular disease mortality by cardiorespiratory fitness levels measured at ages 45, 55, and 65 years in men. The Cooper Center Longitudinal Study. *J Am Coll Cardiol.* 2011;57:1604-1610.

8. Erikssen G, Liestøl K, Bjørnholt J, Thaulow E, Sandvik L, Erikssen J. Changes in physical fitness and changes in mortality. *Lancet.* 1998;352(9130):759-762.

9. Wasserman K, Hansen JE, Sue DY, et al. *Principles of Exercise Testing and Interpretation.* 2nd ed. Malvern, PA: Lea & Febiger; 1994.

10. Rhoades RA, Tanner GA. *Medical Physiology.* Baltimore, MD: Lippincott Williams & Wilkins; 1995.

11. Guyton AC, Hall JE. *Textbook of Medical Physiology.* Philadelphia, PA: W.B. Saunders Company; 2000.

12. Kierszenbaum AL. *Histology and Cell Biology: An Introduction to Pathology.* St Louis, MO: Mosby Inc; 2002.

13. Powers SK, Howley ET. *Exercise Physiology: Theory and Application to Fitness and Performance.* Dubuque, IA: Brown & Benchmark Publishers; 1997.

14. Kerr J. *Functional Histology.* 2nd ed. Chatswood, NSW: Mosby Elsevier Australia; 2010.

15. Hillegass EA. Electrocardiography. In: Hillegass EA, Sadowsky HS. *Essentials of Cardiopulmonary Physical Therapy.* 2nd ed. Philadelphia: WB Saunders Company; 2001.

16. Berne RM, Levy MN. Electrical activity of the heart. In: *Cardiovascular Physiology.* 8th ed. St Louis, MO: Mosby Inc; 2001.

17. Klabunde RE. *Cardiovascular Physiology Concepts.* Philadelphia, PA: Lippincott Williams & Wilkins; 2005.

18. Gleim GW, Coplan NL, Nicholas JA. Acute cardiovascular response to exercise. *Bull N Y Acad Med.* 1986;62(3):211-218.

19. Berne RM, Levy MN. Hemodynamics. In: *Cardiovascular Physiology.* 8th ed. St Louis, MO: Mosby Inc; 2001.

20. Ketch T, Biaggoioni I, Robertson RM, Robertson D. Four faces of baroreflex failure: hypertensive crisis, volatile hypertension, orthostatic tachycardia, and malignant vagotonia. *Circulation.* 2002;105:2518-2523.

21. AAJ Smit, Halliwill JR, Low P, Wieling W. Pathophysiological basis of orthostatic hypotension in autonomic failure. *J Physiol.* 1999;519(Pt 1):1-10.

22. Schmidt U, Hajjar RJ, Gwathmey JK. The force-interval relationship in human myocardium. *J Cardiac Failure.* 1995;4:311-321.

23. Erdmann E. Pathophysiology of heart failure. *Heart.* 1998;79(Suppl 2):S3-S5.

24. Berne RM, Levy MN. The peripheral circulation and its control. In: *Cardiovascular Physiology.* 8th ed. St Louis, MO: Mosby Inc; 2001.

25. West JB. *Respiratory Physiology: The Essentials.* 3rd ed. Baltimore, MD: Williams & Wilkins; 1985.

26. Crystal RG, West JB, eds. *The Lung: Scientific Foundations.* New York, NY: Raven Press Ltd.; 1991.

27. Mead J, Loring SH. Analysis of volume displacement and length changes of the diaphragm during breathing. *J Appl Physiol Respir Environ Exerc Physiol.* 1982;53:750-755.

28. Polkey MI, Moxham J. Clinical aspects of respiratory muscle dysfunction in the critically ill. *Chest.* 2001;119:926-939.

29. Hollinshead WH, Rosse C. *Textbook of Anatomy.* 4th ed. Philadelphia, PA: Harper & Row; 1985.

30. Remmers JE, Lahiri S. Regulating the ventilatory pump: A splendid control system prone to fail during sleep. *Am J Respir Crit Care Med.* 1998;157:S95-S100.

31. Grippi MA. *Pulmonary Pathophysiology.* Philadelphia, PA: J.B. Lippincott Co.; 1995.

32. McArdle WD, Katch FI, Katch VL. *Exercise Physiology: Energy, Nutrition and Human Performance.* 5th ed. Philadelphia, PA: Lippincott Williams & Wilkins; 2001.

33. Hopkins SR. Exercise induced arterial hypoxemia: the role of ventilation-perfusion inequality and pulmonary diffusion limitation. *Adv Exp Med Biol.* 2006;588:17-30.

34. Klocke RA. Oxygen transport and 2,3-diphosphoglycerate (DPG). *Chest.* 1972;62:79S-85S.

35. American Thoracic Society and the American College of Chest Physicians. ATS/ACCP statement on cardiopulmonary exercise testing. *Am J Respir Crit Care Med.* 2003;167:211-277.

36. Balady GJ, Arena R, Sietsema K, et al. Clinician's Guide to cardiopulmonary exercise testing in adults: a scientific statement from the American Heart Association. *Circulation.* 2010;122(2):191-225.

37. Squires RW, Gau GT, Miller TD, Allison TG, Lavie CJ. Cardiovascular rehabilitation: status, 1990. *Mayo Clin Proc.* 1990;65:731-755.

38. Milani RV, Lavie CJ, Mehra MR. Cardiopulmonary exercise testing: how do we differentiate the cause of dyspnea? *Circulation.* 2004;110:e27-e31.

39. Gleim GW, Coplan NL, Nicholas JA. Acute cardiovascular response to exercise. *Bull N Y Acad Med.* 1986;62(3):211-218.

40. Gerstenblith G, Renlund DG, Lakatta EG. Cardiovascular response to exercise in younger and older men. *Fed Proc.* 1987;46(5):1834-1839.

41. Powers SK, Howley ET. *Exercise Physiology: Theory and Application to Fitness and Performance.* Dubuque, IA: Brown & Benchmark Publishers. Times Mirrow Higher Education Group; 1997.

42. Petrof BJ, Grippi MA. Exercise physiology. In: Grippi MA. *Pulmonary Pathophysiology.* Philadelphia, PA: J.B. Lippincott Co.; 1995.

43. McGuire DK, Levine BD, Williamson JW, et al. A 30-year follow-up of the Dallas Bedrest and Training Study: I. Effect of age on the cardiovascular response to exercise. *Circulation.* 2001;104(12):1350-1357.

44. Zhou B, Conlee RK, Jensen R, Fellingham GW, George JD, Fisher AG. Stroke volume does not plateau during graded exercise in elite male distance runners. *Med Sci Sports Exerc.* 2001;33(11):1849-1854.

45. Vella CA, Robergs RA. A review of the stroke volume response to upright exercise in healthy subjects. *Br J Sports Med.* 2005;39:190-195.

46. McLaren PF, Nurhayati Y, Boutcher SH. Stroke volume response to cycle ergometry in trained and untrained older men. *Eur J Appl Physiol Occup Physiol.* 1997;75(6):537-542.

47. Kostis JB, Moreyra AE, Amendo MT, Di Pietro J, Cosgrove N, Kuo PT. The effect of age on heart rate in subjects free of heart disease. Studies by ambulatory electrocardiography and maximal exercise stress test. *Circulation.* 1982;65:141-145.

48. Tanaka H, Monahan KD, Seals DR. Age-predicted maximal heart rate revisited. *J Am Coll Cardiol.* 2001;37:153-156.

49. Imai K, Sato H, Hori M, et al. Vagally mediated heart rate recovery after exercise is accelerated in athletes but blunted in patients with chronic heart failure. *J Am Coll Cardiol.* 1994;24:1529-1535.

50. Cole CR, Blackstone EH, Pashkow FJ, Snader CE, Lauer MS. Heart-rate recovery immediately after exercise as a predictor of mortality. *N Engl J Med.* 1999;341:1351-1357.

51. Fletcher GF, Balady GJ, Amsterdam EA, et al. Exercise standards for testing and training: a statement for healthcare professionals from the American Heart Association. *Circulation.* 2001;104:1694-1740.

52. Le VV, Mitiku T, Sungar G, Myers J, Froelicher V. The blood pressure response to dynamic exercise testing: a systematic review. *Prog Cardiovasc Dis.* 2008;51(2):135-160.

53. Perloff D, Grim C, Flack J, et al. Human blood pressure determination by sphygmomanometry. *Circulation.* 1993;88:2460-2470.

2

Developing Systems
Birth to Adolescence

David Chapman, PT, PhD

CHAPTER OBJECTIVES

- List the mature tissues and anatomical structures that arise from the ectoderm, mesoderm, and endoderm.
- Outline the developmental changes that occur in the musculoskeletal system during the germinal, embryonic, and fetal periods of prenatal development.
- Describe typical development of the cardiovascular/pulmonary system during prenatal development, infancy, childhood, and adolescence.
- Explain the age-related changes that occur in motor control during infancy, childhood, and adolescence.
- Outline the impact that training has on the development of aerobic endurance and muscular strength during childhood and adolescence.
- Explain the protective role the nervous systems plays when children and adolescents participate in training programs.
- Identify the age-related changes in the cardiovascular/pulmonary system to consider during the physical therapy examination process.

CHAPTER OUTLINE

- Overview of Embryogenesis and Prenatal Development
  - Prenatal Nervous System Development
  - Prenatal Musculoskeletal System Development
    - Prenatal Skeletal Development
      - Intramembranous Ossification
      - Endochondral Ossification
    - Prenatal Muscle Development
  - Prenatal Cardiovascular Development
    - Prenatal Heart Development
    - Prenatal Circulatory System Development
  - Prenatal Lung Development
  - Development of the Endocrine System
  - Neuromotor Development and Motor Control
    - Neurological Changes in Neuromotor Development and Control
    - Development of Motor Milestones
    - Development of Fundamental Motor Skills
  - Summary: Using this Information to Guide the Physical Therapy Examination
- Development of Systems That Influence Aerobic Capacity During Infancy, Childhood, and Adolescence
  - Heart Development During Infancy, Childhood, and Adolescence
  - Circulatory System Development During Infancy, Childhood, and Adolescence
  - Lung Development During Infancy, Childhood, and Adolescence
  - Support System/Structures
  - Developmental Changes in Aerobic Capacity and Endurance Training
  - Summary: Using this Information to Guide the Physical Therapy Examination

Coglianese D, ed. *Clinical Exercise Pathophysiology for Physical Therapy: Examination, Testing, and Exercise Prescription for Movement-Related Disorders* (pp 27-93).
© 2015 Taylor & Francis Group.

Physical therapists (PTs) who treat or work with pediatric patients usually begin an episode of care by completing an in-depth history and thorough systems review with the child and his or her parent or caregiver. These essential first steps enable the PT to establish a productive working relationship with the child and parent/caregiver as well as develop an understanding of the reason(s) for this episode of care. The results of this initial interview and systems review can be used by the PT to guide the examination process and procedures that will be implemented with this particular child and his or her family.

Ideally, the PT will recognize that each child develops holistically in real time and that clinical observations of how a child moves and functions are a reflection of the complex interactions of his or her multiple systems at that point in development. For example, when an infant leaves the compact and supportive environment of the womb at birth, she "comes with" certain characteristics and faces multiple developmental tasks. Her joints are used to being flexed, she has relatively weak muscles, and her head is quite large in relation to her body. In addition, she has a nervous system that will continue to develop for nearly 2 decades, lungs that need to mature, and virtually no experience with gravity. And yet, during the first year of life, she will learn to suck and chew for nutrition, bond with her parents and other caregivers, as well as coordinate her musculoskeletal system as she prepares to walk and manipulate objects with her hands.

Then, during childhood, as her nervous system matures and her muscles gain strength, she will learn to explore her environment physically as she develops a variety of complex neuromotor skills, such as running, hopping, skipping, and galloping. Simultaneously, she will develop the cognitive skills needed to solve basic problems and begin to reason abstractly. Her development of oral and written language skills will enable her to interact with and understand the world around her and the people in it. As her social skills expand, her ability to comprehend nonverbal communication and the emotional aspects of relationships will continue to grow, as will her need to be independent at home and school.

With the arrival of adolescence and the changes associated with puberty, she will develop secondary sexual characteristics and experience changes in her body composition that boys will not. In fact, certain physical abilities will begin to plateau as she reaches physical maturity. Alternatively, her male counterparts will continue to develop increasingly higher levels of muscle performance and aerobic capacity as they grow and develop. Adolescents of both genders will continue to develop and refine their cognitive, language, and social skills as they seek to develop their own identity and sense of purpose in the world.

The behaviors we observe during infancy, childhood, and adolescence reflect the developmental status of multiple body systems and structures. Our "everyday" observations of these traits, however, may mask the underlying complexity of the developmental trajectories for each of these systems. For instance, why do infants have higher heart rates (HRs), but lower blood pressure (BP) values compared to children and adolescents? What changes occur within an infant or child's system(s) that allow him or her to demonstrate improved neuromotor control over time? Why are prepubescent girls and boys able to increase their muscle strength in the absence of androgens and without showing any hypertrophy of their muscle tissues? Why do boys show a positive relationship between their growth spurt and improvements in muscle performance and aerobic capacity while girls do not? Answers to these questions can be established by examining the influence typical development of selected body systems has on observable traits, such as aerobic capacity and muscle performance. This type of knowledge will enable us, as PTs, to provide effective examinations, evaluations, and interventions with infants, children, and adolescents who may present in the clinic for known or suspected impairments in one or more of these body structures and functions.

In light of the PT's need to interpret a child's movement patterns and accurately predict how he or she will respond to prescribed therapeutic exercises, the purposes of this chapter are to (1) describe typical development of the cardiovascular-pulmonary musculoskeletal, neurological, integument, and endocrine systems during prenatal development, infancy, childhood, and adolescence and (2) review the developmental changes that occur in aerobic capacity, muscle performance, and neuromotor development/motor control during infancy, childhood, and adolescence. Suggestions regarding how this information can be used to guide the physical therapy examination and evaluation process for infants, children, and adolescents will also be offered.

The chapter begins with an overview of embryogenesis and prenatal development. This information is followed by a review of the endocrine system and neuromotor development/control. A comprehensive review of how the subsystems that support aerobic capacity and muscle performance typically develop will then be offered. This section will also include a review of how these traits respond to training. How this knowledge can be used to guide the physical therapy examination and evaluation process for infants, children, and adolescents will be presented next. Finally, 2 patient cases will be offered as a means to integrate how the development of these various systems affect typical and atypical responses to exercise during infancy, childhood, and adolescence.

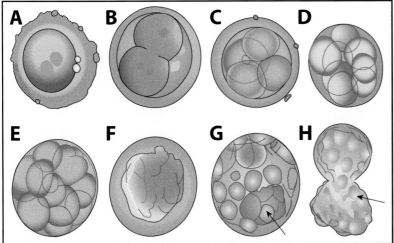

Figure 2-1. Human development begins with cleavage of the fertilized egg. (A) The fertilized egg at day 0 with 2 pronuclei and the polar bodies. (B) A 2-cell embryo at day 1 after fertilization. (C) A 4-cell embryo at day 2. (D) The 8-cell embryo at day 3. (E) The 16-cell stage later in day 3, followed by the phenomenon of compaction, whereby the embryo is now termed a *morula*. (F) Day 4. (G) The formation of the blastocyst at day 5, with the inner cell mass indicated by the arrow. (H) Finally, the embryo (arrow) hatches from the zona pellucida. (Adapted from Ogilvie CM, Braude PR, Scriven PN. Preimplantation diagnosis—an overview. *J Histochem Cytochem.* 2005;53:255-260.)

OVERVIEW OF EMBRYOGENESIS AND PRENATAL DEVELOPMENT

Embryology commonly refers to the study of prenatal development but literally means the study of embryos.[1] Examining the developmental changes that occur during gestation allows therapists to acquire knowledge regarding how life begins as well as typical and atypical development of the anatomical structures and function(s) we treat in patients. Perhaps more importantly, it provides us with the knowledge needed to answer the questions that parents and caregivers often express regarding, "How did this happen?" and "What can we do about it now?"[1]

A typical human pregnancy lasts approximately 280 days, or 40 weeks, and consists of 3 trimesters that encompass 3 periods of prenatal development. The first trimester is the most critical trimester and includes the germinal and embryonic periods of gestation as well as the first month of the fetal period. This is when all systems, organs, appendages, and sense organs develop. It is known as the most critical trimester because the embryo/fetus is the most vulnerable to the potentially negative effects of drugs, viruses, nutritional deficits, and the impact of radiation.[2] The germinal period lasts approximately 2 weeks from conception to full implantation in the uterine wall. This is followed by the embryonic period, which begins at the end of the second week of gestation and continues through the eighth week of prenatal development. The fetal period begins with the onset of the ninth week of gestation and continues until the baby is born.

Human development begins when an egg or ovum is fertilized by a sperm cell and is defined as change over time (Figure 2-1).[1,3] Thus, the developmental age of the zygote, embryo, and developing fetus can be calculated from the day of conception, which is assumed to be approximately 14 days after the first day of the mother's last normal menstrual period (LNMP). Alternatively, gestational age is calculated from the first day of the mother's LNMP. This approach usually over estimates developmental age by about 2 weeks

since the mother's LNMP began approximately 14 days prior to conception. Here, we will use developmental age when referring to the age of the embryo or fetus during prenatal development.

Cell division begins approximately 30 hours after conception.[1,2] At this point, the zygote begins to travel through the fallopian tube on its week-long journey to the womb. During this time, the zygote becomes a *morula*—a raspberry like structure—that consists of 16 identical cells. Note, cell differentiation has yet to begin (see Figure 2-1E).[1,2]

Cell differentiation begins near the end of the first week of gestation with the zygote developing into a blastocyst (see Figure 2-1G).[1,2] The blastocyst consists of an outer cell layer known as the *trophoblast* and an inner cell layer called the *embryoblast*. The trophoblast becomes the placenta, which will attach to the uterine wall, and the embryoblast becomes the embryo. Full implantation into the uterine wall generally occurs by the tenth day following fertilization.[2]

The next phase of gestation is known as the *embryonic period*.[1,2] As mentioned earlier, it begins at the end of week 2 and continues through the eighth week of gestation. During this time, the blastocyst undergoes rapid cell differentiation, known as *gastrulation*, and change that includes development of multiple body systems and organs, including the head, vertebrae, arm and leg buds, a heart that beats, internal organs such as the liver and kidneys, and sense organs (eg, eyes and ears).

Gastrulation continues throughout the embryonic period. Specifically, development of the 3 germ layers known as the *ectoderm*, *mesoderm*, and *endoderm* takes place during weeks 2 and 3 of embryonic development as is illustrated in Figure 2-2. These 3 layers of tissue are known as *germ layers* because all other tissues arise or germinate from them. Each will continue to undergo cell differentiation as well as further growth and development during the embryonic period. As we will see, each layer contributes to the development of more specialized structures and systems that will support the development of neuromotor control, aerobic capacity, and muscle performance during infancy, childhood, and adolescence.

Figure 2-2. A cross-sectional view of an embryonic diagram at 16 days of gestation showing the endoderm, mesoderm, and ectoderm. (Adapted from Moore KL, Persaud TVN. *Before We Are Born: Essentials of Embryology and Birth Defects.* 7th ed. W.B. Saunders Company; 2007.)

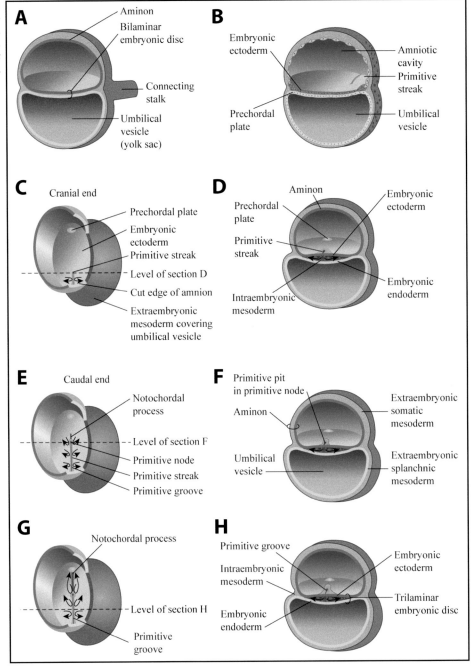

The ectoderm forms the dorsal or posterior layer of the embryo.[1,2] Cells from the ectoderm develop into the neural tube, spinal cord, brain, sensory organs, and epidermal portion of the integumentary system.[1,2] The spinal cord, brain, and sensory organs provide structures and systems that support typical development of neuromotor control as well as influence muscle performance and aerobic capacity during infancy, childhood, and adolescence. Prenatal development of the brain and spinal cord is presented next.

Prenatal Nervous System Development

The brain and spinal cord begin to develop during the third week of gestation when thickening mesenchyme cells within the ectoderm give rise to the neural plate.[1,2] The neural plate develops thickened neural folds superiorly and a longitudinal groove surrounded by neural folds inferiorly.[2] Cells in the thickened neural folds located at the superior end of the neural plate then fuse to form the prosencephalon, or forebrain; the mesencephalon, or midbrain; and the rhombencephalon, or hindbrain. A complete discussion of brain development, which continues well into the second decade of life, is beyond the scope of this chapter. However, Table 2-1 identifies the relationship between these primitive brain structures and the corresponding area or region of the mature brain.[2]

The neural folds that surround the longitudinal groove also fuse to form the neural tube (Figure 2-3). At this point

TABLE 2-1. THE RELATIONSHIP BETWEEN EMBRYONIC AND MATURE BRAIN STRUCTURES

PRIMARY BRAIN VESICLES	SECONDARY BRAIN VESICLES	AREA OF THE MATURE BRAIN
Hindbrain	Myelencephalon	Medulla
	Metencephalon	Pons and cerebellum
Midbrain	Mesencephalon	Midbrain
Forebrain	Diencephalon	Thalamus, epithalamus, hypothalamus, subthalamus
	Telencephalon	Cerebral hemispheres: cortex, medullary center, corpus striatum, and olfactory system

Adapted with permission from Moore KL. *Essentials of Human Embryology.* Burlington, Ontario: B.C. Decker Inc; 1988.

in development, cells deep within the neural tube begin to divide and produce neuroblasts and glioblasts.[1,2] Neuroblasts develop into nerve cells, while glioblasts become neuroglial or supporting cells. In addition, select cells from the neural folds cluster to form the neural crest. These cells eventually give rise to dorsal root ganglia, autonomic nervous system ganglia, some cranial nerve ganglia, and peripheral nerve sheaths.[1,2] Simultaneously, a shallow groove known as the *sulcus limitans* develops along the midline of the neural tube. This developmental process results in 2 groups of nerve cells. One is located dorsally to the sulcus limitans and is known as the alar plate. The second is recognized as the basal plate and is ventral to the sulcus limitans. Nerve cells that develop from the alar plate are predominantly sensory or afferent neurons. These cells lead to the formation of the dorsal or posterior horn of the gray matter within the spinal cord and function to receive sensory information from the periphery. Nerve cells that come from the basal plate become organized in the ventral or anterior horn of the gray matter and are typically motor or efferent neurons. These cells eventually provide the motor signals needed for skeletal muscles to function.

During the first 12 weeks of prenatal development, the spinal cord is essentially the same length as the vertebral column. This enables the nerve roots to exit directly through the corresponding intervertebral foramen. Later in prenatal development and after birth, the vertebral column grows faster in length than the spinal cord itself and the caudal or inferior end of the spinal cord degenerates. These 2 processes coupled with the fact that the cranial end of the spinal cord is attached to the brain cause the caudal end of the spinal cord to ascend within the vertebral canal. Eventually, the conus medullaris, or tapered end of the spinal cord, resides at the end of the third lumbar vertebrae in newborn infants. These events and structures are represented in Figure 2-4.[1]

The middle germ layer, or mesoderm, is the origin of the muscles, bones, cartilage, tendons, and ligaments; dermal layer of the integumentary system; and the circulatory system.[1,2] As we will observe, the circulatory system plays a vital role in the development of aerobic capacity throughout infancy, childhood, and adolescence. The connective tissues listed previously will be reviewed next as they contribute to

the development of neuromotor control and muscle performance in the developing infant, child, and adolescent.

Prenatal Musculoskeletal System Development

Prenatal Skeletal Development

Skeletal development also begins during the third week of gestation via gastrulation, when mesenchymal cells condense to form fibrous membrane and hyaline cartilage templates for later skeletal development.[1,2] Initially, somites—a series of paired block cells—form from the mesoderm approximately 22 days after gestation. The ventral or anterior segment of each pair of somites develops into the cartilage and bone of the vertebral columns and ribs. The posterior or dorsal portion gives rise to the dermis of the back and to the skeletal muscles of the body and limbs. Figure 2-5 illustrates somites at 22 days of gestation.[2]

The embryo consists of fibrous membranes and hyaline cartilage until approximately 6 to 7 weeks of gestation. Cartilaginous upper limb buds begin to form during week 4 of gestation, with the lower limb buds appearing 1 to 2 days later (Figure 2-6A).[1,2] The digits of the hands and feet develop during weeks 6 and 7 of prenatal development (Figure 2-6B).[1,2] By the end of the seventh week of gestation, all 206 bones have been "set down" as cartilage. Synovial joints then develop during weeks 8 and 9 of gestation. Osteogenesis/ossification begins during this same time period and will continue throughout life.

There are 2 types of human osteogenesis/ossification. Intramembranous (IM) ossification leads to the formation of flat bones including the skull, a portion of the mandible, and the clavicles. Endochondral (EC) ossification results in the long and short bones of the upper (UE) and lower extremities (LE) as well as the vertebrae (irregular bones). Days 24 to 36 of embryonic development are especially critical for healthy bone development. It is during this time—weeks 4 through 7—that the embryo is most sensitive to teratogens and/or genetic mutations that may affect typical bone development.

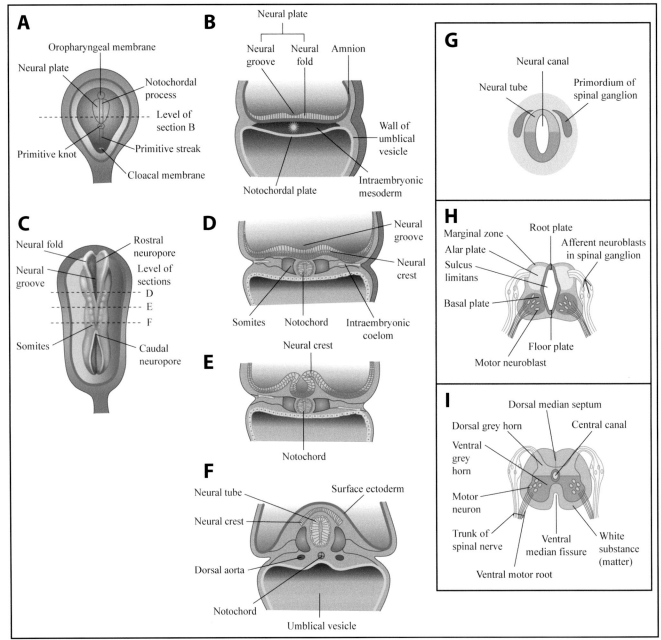

Figure 2-3. The neural plate and its folding to form the neural tube. (A) Dorsal view of an embryo at approximately 18 days, exposed by removing the amnion. (B) Transverse section of the embryo, showing the neural plate and early development of the neural groove and neural folds. (C) Dorsal view of an embryo at approximately 22 days. The neural folds have fused opposite the fourth to sixth somites, but are spread apart at both ends. (D) to (F) Transverse sections of this embryo at the levels shown in (C), showing the formation of the neural tube and its detachment from the surface ectoderm. Note that some neuroectodermal cells are not included in the neural tube but remain between it and the surface ectoderm as the neural crest. (G) to (I) Development of the spinal cord. (G) Transverse section of the neural tube of an embryo at approximately 23 days. (H) and (C) Similar sections in 6- and 9-week embryos, respectively. (D) Section of the wall of the neural tube shown in (G). (I) Section of the wall of the developing spinal cord, showing its 3 zones. In (G) to (I), note that the neural canal of the neural tube is converted into the central canal of the spinal cord. (Adapted from Boron WF. *Medical Physiology, Updated Edition.* St. Louis, MO: Saunders; 2005.)

Intramembranous Ossification

IM ossification means that bony tissue develops within flat membranes. This process begins after connective tissue has formed sheets of mesenchymal cells, where the flat bones will be located. These cells are highly vascularized and differentiate into osteoblasts. Osteoblasts "lay down" spongy bone cells that get trapped in a hard matrix. They are known as *osteocytes* and provide the basis for compact bone development that is typically observed in the skull, mandible, and clavicles. Over time, more and more osteoblasts are formed from sheets of connective tissue and become layers of osteocytes that build up at the edge of spongy bone. Osteocytes continue to lay down more hard matrix that becomes compact over time and enables flat bones to develop to an appropriate level of thickness. IM ossification is illustrated in Figure 2-7.

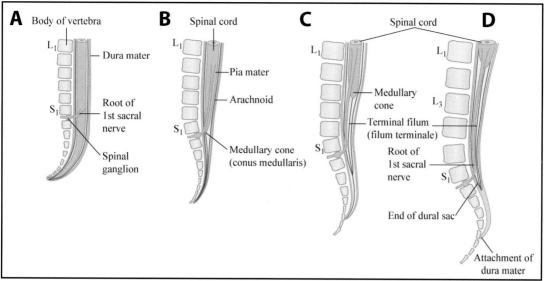

Figure 2-4. Spinal cord development (A) at 8 weeks of gestation, (B) at 24 weeks of gestation, (C) at the time of delivery, and (D) in an adult. Note the relationship of the vertebra with the spinal cord itself, including the conus medullaris, and how the spinal cord tapers throughout development. (Adapted from Moore KL, Persaud TVN. *Before We Are Born: Essentials of Embryology and Birth Defects.* 7th ed. W.B. Saunders Company; 2007.)

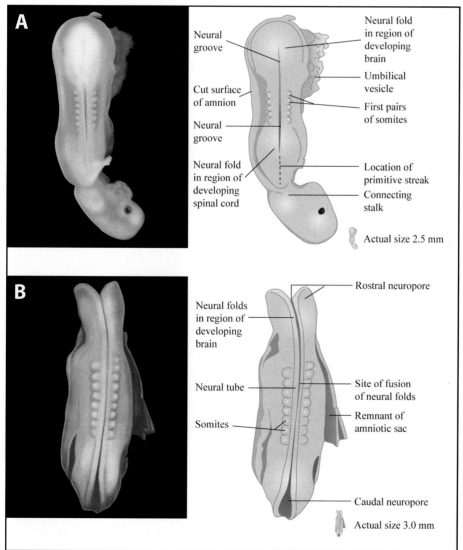

Figure 2-5. (A) A microphotograph of a 22-day-old embryo from the dorsal view that illustrates 5 paired somites with a corresponding drawing of the same-aged embryo in (B). Note these are the first pairs of somites that will give rise to the dermis of the back and the skeletal muscles of the body and limbs. (Adapted from Moore KL, Persaud TVN. *Before We Are Born: Essentials of Embryology and Birth Defects.* 7th ed. W.B. Saunders Company; 2007.)

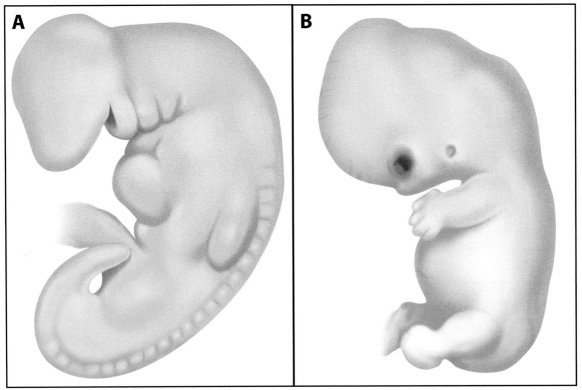

Figure 2-6. (A) A 4-week-old embryo showing UE and LE limb buds. (B) A 6- to 7-week-old embryo displaying the early development of the UEs and LEs, including the hands and feet. (Adapted from Moore KL, Persaud TVN. *The Developing Human: Clinically Oriented Embryology.* 7th ed. Philadelphia, PA: Saunders; 2003.)

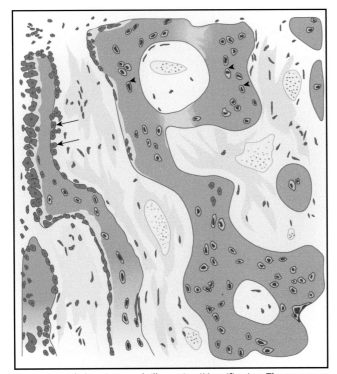

Figure 2-7. A light micrograph illustrating IM ossification. The arrows on the left side of the micrograph point out the trabeculae of bone that is being formed by osteoblasts lining their surface. The arrowheads in the upper middle portion of the micrograph are pointing out the osteocytes that are being trapped in the lacune. (Adapted from Gartner LP, Hiatt JL. *Color Textbook of Histology.* 2nd ed. Philadelphia, PA: Saunders; 2001.)

Endochondral Ossification

EC ossification occurs when bony tissue replaces a hyaline cartilage model (Figure 2-8). Chondrocytes within the cartilage begin to die off and a layer of periosteum forms on the outside of the cartilaginous model. The periosteum provides the osteoblasts needed for bony tissue to develop. Chondrocytes die first in the middle of the diaphysis, which is the primary ossification center and is where spongy bone develops. The next set of chondrocytes to die are found in the secondary ossification centers known as the *epiphyses*. The epiphyses are typically located near the end of long bones and are also known as the *growth plate*. While osteoblasts make hard extracellular matrix, the periosteum produces osteoblasts that get "laid down" as compact bone along the edges of the long, short, and irregular bones. Note that cartilage near the epiphyses is retained and functions as articular cartilage within the synovial joints.

Prenatal joint development begins during the sixth week of gestation and is complete 2 weeks later.[1,2] Synovial joints form when interzonal mesenchyme cells that are located between the long bones differentiate to form the joint capsule and ligaments in the peripheral areas of the developing joint (Figure 2-9). Centrally, these cells disappear, which leads to the development of the joint space.[2] These cells also form the synovial membrane that lines the joint capsule and articular surfaces. Fibrous joints develop as the interzonal mesenchyme cells differentiate into the dense fibrous cartilage that exists between the developing bones, such as the suture joints

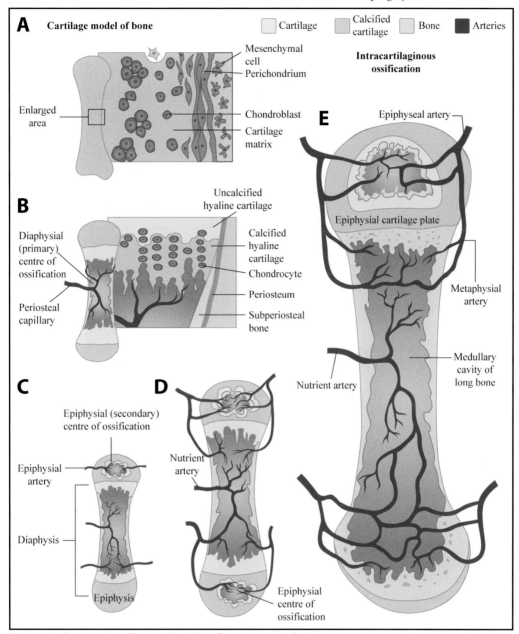

Figure 2-8. Drawings that illustrate the EC ossification process that begins at approximately 5 weeks of gestation. (Adapted from Moore KL, Persaud TVN. *Before We Are Born: Essentials of Embryology and Birth Defects.* 7th ed. W.B. Saunders Company; 2007.)

in the skull.[2] The hyaline cartilage of the costochondral joints and the fibrocartilage of the pubic symphysis develop in the same manner. That is, the interzonal mesenchyme cells differentiate into hyaline cartilage and fibrocartilage. By the end of the eighth week of gestation, the developing joints resemble those of an adult.[2]

Prenatal Muscle Development

Prenatal skeletal muscle development begins during the fourth week of gestation. Most skeletal muscle tissue develops before birth from embryonic mesoderm with the exception of the dilator and sphincter papillae muscles of the iris.[1,2] These muscles develop from the ectoderm. In general, mesenchymal cells migrate from myotome regions of the somites located on the posterior aspect of the embryo and become myoblasts (Figure 2-10). These fibers fuse to form multinucleated muscle fibers. Soon after, myofibrils appear in the cytoplasm of the developing muscle cells. This process is followed by the development of cross striations that leads to the formation of striated muscle fibers. From the anterolateral body walls of the embryo, mesenchyme cells from the somatic layer of the mesoderm give rise to striated muscle fibers for the body walls and limbs.

The ventral or anterior layer of the embryo is composed of the endoderm, which gives rise to the endocrine system, gut, liver, pancreas, respiratory system, gastrointestinal tract, and genitourinary system. The respiratory system along with the circulatory system that develops from the mesoderm

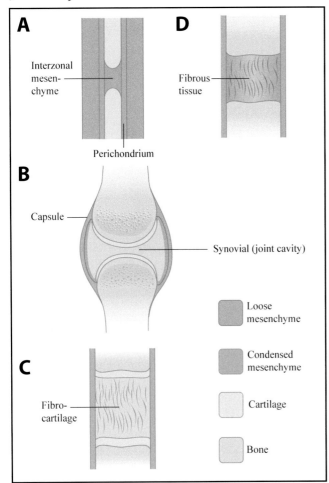

Figure 2-9. Schematic drawings of synovial joints and fibrous joints. (Adapted from Moore KL, Persaud TVN. *Before We Are Born: Essentials of Embryology and Birth Defects.* 7th ed. W.B. Saunders Company; 2007.)

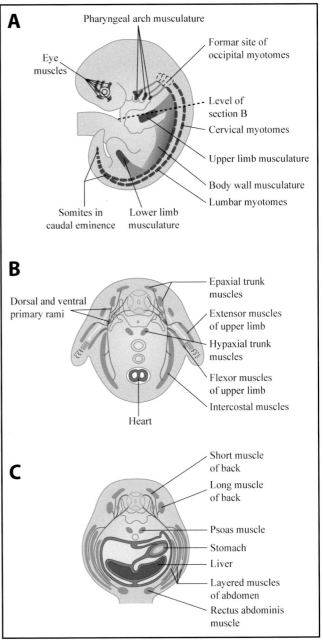

Figure 2-10. Drawings illustrating early prenatal muscular development at approximately 41 days of gestation. Note the myotomes in (A) as well as the transverse section of the developing embryo in (B) and (C), respectively. The embryo represented in drawing (C) is now 7 weeks old. (Adapted from Moore KL, Persaud TVN. *Before We Are Born: Essentials of Embryology and Birth Defects.* 7th ed. W.B. Saunders Company; 2007.)

play key roles in the development of aerobic capacity, while the endocrine system heavily influences the development of muscle performance and aerobic capacity during puberty. The prenatal development of circulatory and respiratory system components will be presented next.

Prenatal Cardiovascular Development

Prenatal Heart Development

The heart is the central pump that supplies blood to the pulmonary or venous blood transport loop and the peripheral or arterial blood transport loop. Heart development begins with the appearance of cardiogenic cords of cells that are located in the cardiogenic area of the fetus (Figure 2-11).[1,2] These consist of mesenchymal cells that become canalized and form a primitive tube. This original structure develops into a thin-walled, 2-tube structure by the end of the third week of gestation. This primitive heart begins to beat at approximately 22 days of gestation and connects to blood vessels in the embryo, connective stalk, chorion, and yolk sac to form a primitive cardiovascular system. Then, through a series of constrictions and dilations, the sinus

venosus, primitive atrium, primitive ventricle, bulbus cordis, and truncus arteriosus are formed.[1]

The sinus venosus is located in the caudal region of the primitive heart. Initially, it functions to receive blood that is returning to the heart from the common cardinal veins, vitelline veins, and umbilical vein and later is incorporated into the right atrium. The truncus arteriosus dilates to form the aortic sac, which eventually develops into the aortic arches. The primitive ventricle becomes the left ventricle while the bulbus cordis develops into the right ventricle.[2]

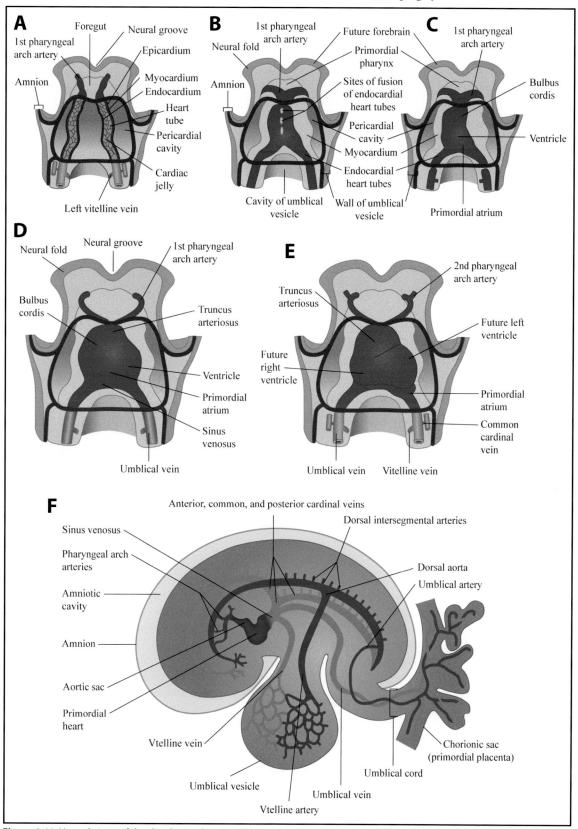

Figure 2-11. Ventral views of the developing heart and the pericardial region (22 to 35 days). The ventral pericardial wall has been removed to show (A) the developing myocardium and fusion of the 2 heart tubes to form (B) a single heart tube. (C) Fusion begins at the cranial ends of the tubes and extends caudally until a single tubular heart is formed. (D) As the heart elongates, it bends on itself, forming (E) an S-shaped heart. (F) The embryonic cardiovascular system (at approximately 26 days), showing vessels on the left side only. The umbilical vein carries well-oxygenated blood and nutrients from the chorion (the embryonic part of the placenta) to the embryo. The umbilical arteries carry poorly oxygenated blood and waste products from the embryo to the chorion. (Adapted from Moore KL, Persaud TVN. *Before We Are Born: Essentials of Embryology and Birth Defects.* 7th ed. W.B. Saunders Company; 2007.)

Figure 2-12. Schematic drawings of the developing heart from 28 days of gestation through 8 weeks (56 days) of prenatal development. Note the plane cutting through the heart in drawing (A) that is the basis for drawings (B) through (E). Drawing (E) represents a typical 4-chambered heart at 56 days of gestation. (F) Sonogram of a second trimester fetus showing the 4 chambers of the heart. Note the septum secundum (arrow) and the descending aorta. (Adapted from Moore KL, Persaud TVN. *Before We Are Born: Essentials of Embryology and Birth Defects.* 7th ed. W.B. Saunders Company; 2007.)

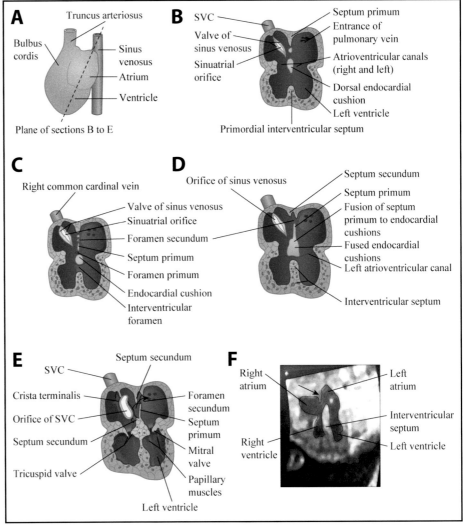

During days 22 to 24, the primitive heart begins to bend to the right and folds back on itself (see Figure 2-11B) to create a left- and right-sided double-chambered pump for each of the 2 circulatory loops mentioned previously.[1,2] During weeks 4 and 5, the primitive heart divides into the typical 4-chambered heart with 2 atria and 2 ventricles. The formation of the atrioventricular pumping chambers is complete by 8 weeks of gestation (Figure 2-12).[1,2]

Prenatal Circulatory System Development

The circulatory/vascular system begins to develop during the third week of gestation in the extra-embryonic mesoderm of the yolk sac, connecting stalk, and chorion.[1,2] Blood vessels begin to appear when groups of mesenchymal cells, known as *angioblasts*, located in the yolk sac form "blood islands." Cavities then form within these islands. Next, mesenchymal cells begin to arrange themselves around these cavities to form the endothelium of the primitive blood vessels. These primitive vessels begin to fuse and form a networks of vessels within the wall of the yolk sac. This process is also repeated in the connecting stalk and chorion as well as within the embryo itself. All of these vessels extend into adjacent areas and fuse with other vessels. The blood vessels

in the embryo join those in the yolk sac, connecting stalk and chorion to form a primitive vascular system. In particular, the cardinal veins return blood from the embryo while the vitelline veins return blood from the yolk sac, and the umbilical veins return oxygenated blood from the placenta (see Figure 2-11F).[1,2]

Prenatally, a majority of fetal blood moves from the right atrium through the foramen ovale—a small opening located between the right and left atria—into the left atrium to the left ventricle and then to the body via the aorta.[1] A small amount of fetal blood also flows from the right atrium to the right ventricle through the ductus arteriosus, located in the pulmonary trunk that connects to the aorta.[1] This allows a portion of the fetal blood supply to flow out to the body. The ductus arteriosus is a small opening that connects the right ventricle with the arterial circulation. These openings provide for intrauterine circulation of the arterialized placenta blood directly through the heart and into the arterial tree, essentially bypassing the lungs (Figure 2-13A). In neonatal circulation, the lungs are now involved because of closure of the foramen ovale and ductus arteriosus shortly after birth (Figure 2-13B).

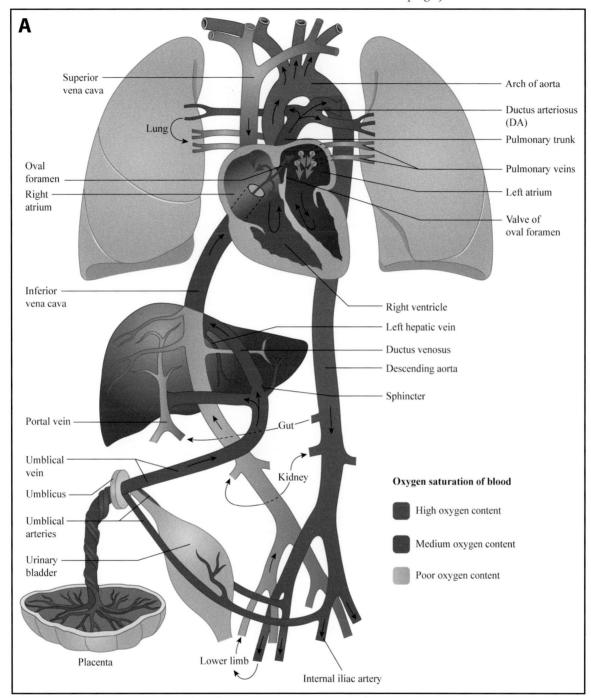

Figure 2-13. (A) Prenatal and (B) neonatal circulation. It is important to note the foramen ovale and the ductus arteriosus. Both contribute to the observation that intrauterine circulation bypasses the lungs completely. Note that both the foramen ovale and ductus arteriosus are now closed in the neonate, which allows the infant to circulate blood between the heart, body, and lungs for typical perfusion of all body tissues. (Adapted from Moore KL, Persaud TVN. *Before We Are Born: Essentials of Embryology and Birth Defects.* 7th ed. W.B. Saunders Company; 2007.) *(continued)*

Prenatal Lung Development

Development of the lungs begins at approximately 4 weeks of gestation via the primitive endoderm and mesoderm tissues mentioned previously. Endoderm from the pharynx develops into the epithelial lining with the mesoderm surrounding the lung buds, developing into smooth muscle, connective tissue, and cartilage. At the end of the laryngotracheal tube, a single lung bud develops during week 4 of gestation. A tracheoesophageal septum develops that divides the single lung bud into 2 lung buds (Figure 2-14). Figure 2-15 highlights the development of the bronchial buds, bronchi, and lungs between 28 and 56 days of gestation. By 16 weeks of gestation, the bronchi, bronchioles, and terminal bronchioles develop (Figure 2-16). The respiratory bronchioles and alveolar ducts develop next, with a large

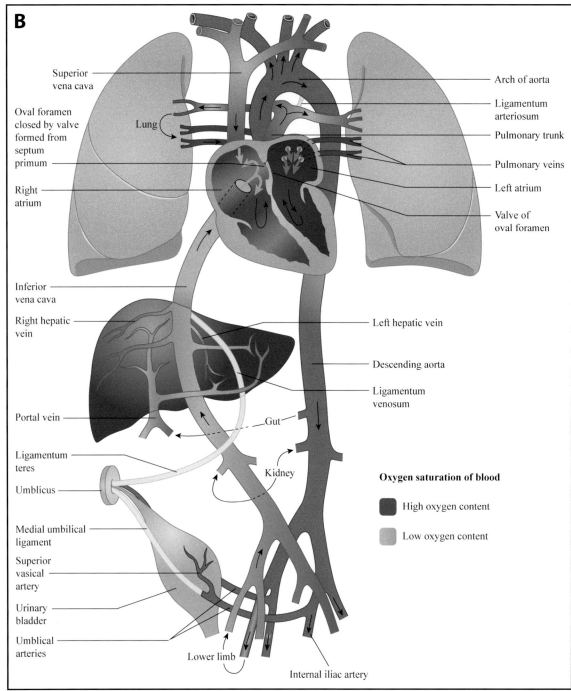

Figure 2-13 (continued). (A) Prenatal and (B) neonatal circulation. It is important to note the foramen ovale and the ductus arteriosus. Both contribute to the observation that intrauterine circulation bypasses the lungs completely. Note that both the foramen ovale and ductus arteriosus are now closed in the neonate, which allows the infant to circulate blood between the heart, body, and lungs for typical perfusion of all body tissues. (Adapted from Moore KL, Persaud TVN. *Before We Are Born: Essentials of Embryology and Birth Defects.* 7th ed. W.B. Saunders Company; 2007.)

number in place by week 24 of gestation. From 24 weeks of gestation until birth, terminal respiratory units continue to form alveoli. The alveolar sacculi are the last to develop, with only one-third of alveoli developed at birth. Surfactant also begins to be produced at approximately 24 weeks of gestation. By weeks 26 to 28, there are enough vascularized terminal sacs developed and appropriate levels of surfactant for the fetus to survive if he or she is born at this point in development. However, it normally takes 36 weeks of gestation for the prenatal lungs to develop fully. Approximately 75% of infants born between 26 and 28 weeks of gestation will experience respiratory distress syndrome due to a lack of surfactant. Thus, it is important to recognize that the number of vascularized terminal sacs multiplies rapidly during the last few weeks of fetal life and that the number of alveoli will continue to increase following birth.

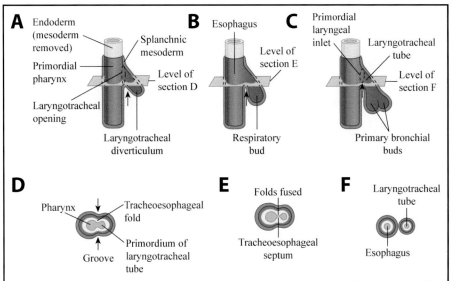

Figure 2-14. Early development of the upper and lower respiratory system during the fourth and fifth weeks of gestation. Note the tracheal bud in drawing (B) and how it then divides into the primary bronchial buds in (C). (Adapted from Moore KL, Persaud TVN. *Before We Are Born: Essentials of Embryology and Birth Defects.* 7th ed. W.B. Saunders Company; 2007.)

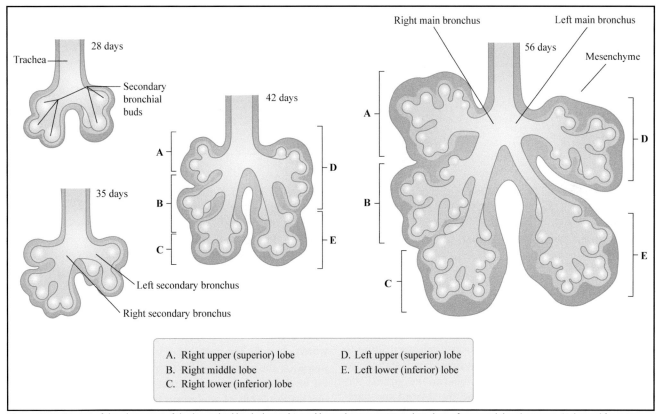

Figure 2-15. Stages of development of the bronchial buds, bronchi, and lungs between 28 and 56 days of prenatal development. (Adapted from Moore KL, Persaud TVN. *Before We Are Born: Essentials of Embryology and Birth Defects.* 7th ed. W.B. Saunders Company; 2007.)

The final segment of prenatal development is the fetal period. The fetal period, as noted previously, begins during the ninth week of gestation and continues until the infant is delivered. During this period, the brain cells begin to mature. The fetus also begins to demonstrate early neuromuscular system function as is evidenced by his or her ability to kick legs, curl toes and fingers, as well as squint with his or her eyes.[4] In addition, the heartbeat is stronger than earlier in development with a typical range of 120 to 160 beats per minute (bpm) during the last trimester of pregnancy.[5] The integument becomes coarser during the final trimester, while the fetus grows by approximately 8 inches in length and gains nearly 6 pounds on average during the final 3 months of gestation.[2]

Underlying many of the changes observed in the development of aerobic capacity and muscle performance during infancy, childhood, and adolescence are the all-encompassing influences of the endocrine system, as well as changes

Figure 2-16. An illustration of the histological development of the terminal bronchioles, saccules, and alveoli between 6 weeks of gestation and 8 years of age. (Adapted from Moore KL, Persaud TVN. *Before We Are Born: Essentials of Embryology and Birth Defects.* 7th ed. W.B. Saunders Company; 2007.)

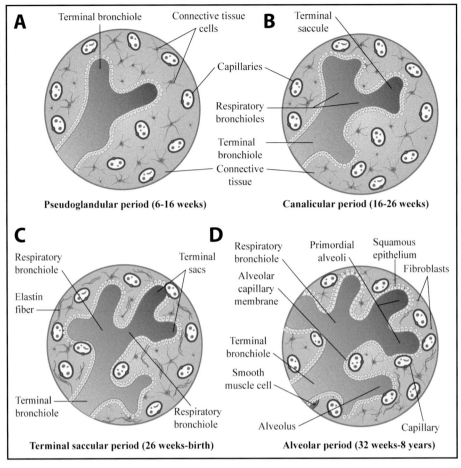

in the child's level of neuromotor development and motor control. Because both of these systems have fundamental effects on the development of aerobic capacity and muscle performance for typically developing infants, children, and adolescents, they will be reviewed next.

Development of the Endocrine System

The endocrine system begins to develop approximately 24 days after fertilization when the thyroid gland begins to form from the endoderm.[1] All 3 germ layers contribute to the development of the endocrine system. For instance, the pituitary gland develops from the ectoderm, the adrenal cortex develops from the mesoderm, and the thyroid and parathyroid originates in the endoderm. The testes in boys and ovaries in girls develop from the mesoderm, mesenchyme cells, and primordial germ cells.[1]

Figure 2-17 illustrates the endocrine system, which consists of ductless glands that are located throughout the body.[6] The primary tasks of the endocrine system are to integrate the various metabolic activities needed to sustain life; influence growth and development of the body, including the development of secondary sexual characteristics; and regulate internal body functions in light of environmental and activity-based demands. They accomplish these primary tasks by secreting hormones (ie, chemical messengers that are circulated throughout the body via the bloodstream).

These chemical messengers influence or target very specific tissues while selectively bypassing most body structures. For example, in females, the ovaries secrete progesterone and estrogen. Progesterone functions to support pregnancy, minimize inflammation within the body, and assists the thyroid in promoting bone growth, while estrogen influences the development of secondary sexual characteristics in women, including the percentage of body fat in females, the rate of growth in height in girls, and bone formation in children of both genders. In addition, estrogen alters serotonin activity, which changes the perception of pain during the follicular phase of the menstrual cycle when estrogen is at its lowest level during the menstrual cycle.[6] This may change the motivation levels of adolescent females when they are training. Alternatively, the testes in boys impact the development of their secondary sexual characteristics and enhance the development of muscle mass, strength, height, and bone density during puberty. Testosterone has also been linked to an increase in aggressive behaviors in mature males, which may change their levels of motivation when they train to enhance their aerobic capacity and muscle performance. In addition, the thyroid secretes thyroxine, which functions to stimulate oxygen (O_2) and energy consumption that influences the child's metabolic rate at rest and during activity. Finally, the pituitary gland secretes growth hormone (GH), which influences the growth of the body and body tissues throughout infancy, childhood, and adolescence.

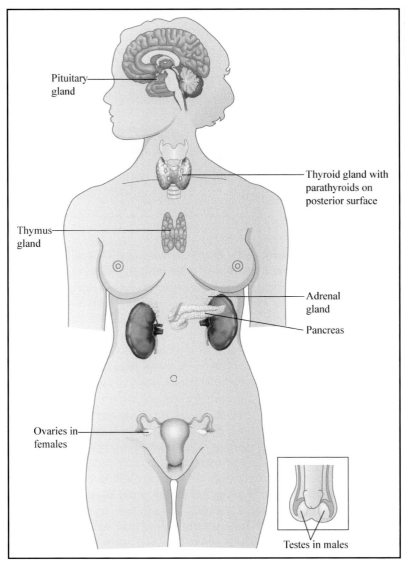

Figure 2-17. A schematic drawing of the endocrine system. (Adapted from LaFleur Brooks M. *Exploring Medical Language: A Student-Directed Approach.* 7th ed. St. Louis, MO: Mosby; 2009.)

Although a complete discussion of endocrine system development and function is beyond the scope of this chapter, it is important to recognize the comprehensive integrating role and influence these hormones play throughout life in the ongoing development of aerobic capacity and muscle performance. As we will see, the development of aerobic capacity and muscle performance are significantly influenced by the effects of the endocrine system.[6]

Neuromotor Development and Motor Control

The neuromotor skills demonstrated by the infants, children, and adolescents that we examine in the clinic reflect the developmental status and cooperative interactions of their multiple subsystems (eg, muscles, nervous, and vestibular systems) in a given environment as they attempt to meet the demands of a specific task.[7-13] These "snapshot" views of their neuromotor development afford us with the opportunity to compare their current level of performance with age-related norms, gain insight into their ability to coordinate their movements, develop preliminary hypotheses regarding how efficiently they move, and determine which of their many subsystems may be preventing them from moving in a more functional or adaptive manner.

By definition, motor development means changes in motor behavior over the lifespan and the process(es) that underlie these changes.[3] The development of motor skills at every age is the result of the interaction of the individual mover, the task(s), and the environment(s) in which he or she is placed.[13] Motor control has been defined as an area of study that attempts to understand the neural, physical, and behavioral aspects of movement.[14] Motor learning is frequently thought to be synonymous with *motor development* and *motor control* but has been defined as an area of study that focuses on the acquisition of skilled movements as a result of practice.[14] Given these definitions and the purposes of this chapter, our focus here will be on neuromotor development, motor control, and the developmental processes, including those within the nervous system, that influence these 2 characteristics.

Figure 2-18. An illustration of an unmyelinated and myelinated nerve fiber. (Adapted from Purves D, Augustine GJ, Fitzpatrick D, et al, eds. *Neuroscience.* 4th ed. Sunderland, MA: Sinauer Associates Inc; 2008.)

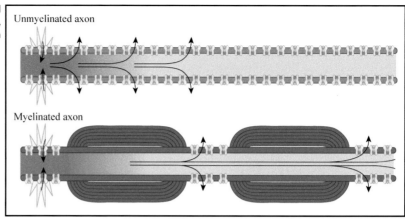

Neurological Changes in Neuromotor Development and Control

As mentioned in the embryogenesis and prenatal development section of this chapter, nervous system development begins during the third week of gestation and may not be complete, depending on the child, until sometime during the third decade of life. This is because there are multiple developmental processes within the nervous system itself that literally continue throughout life. Here, however, we are concerned only with those changes that occur during infancy, childhood, and adolescence. Thus, concepts such as neural migration, myelination, and neuroplasticity as they affect the child's developing levels of motor development and control will be reviewed next.

Neural migration occurs in both the peripheral (PNS) and central nervous systems (CNS). Neural migration within the embryo and developing child involves chemical processes at the cellular and extra-cellular levels and physical relocation of various types of neurons and their developing axons. For example, motor neurons are able to move into close proximity with each other as well as their "target" tissue(s), in this case muscle fibers, because of peptide hormones, cell surface ligands and receptors, extracellular matrix molecules, existing axons within the CNS, and radial glial cells.[15] This allows them to interact in an appropriate manner during development and facilitates the physical relationship needed between neurons and their targeted receptors for the child to display typical levels of neuromotor development and control. This physical proximity is assumed to be particularly important because it enables the developing nervous system to organize itself in a manner that is consistent with the neural map(s) needed to generate functional and adaptive motor behaviors over time.[15] For example, when infants spontaneously generate leg movements that involve flexion and extension of their legs at the hip and knee, they strengthen the muscles used to move their legs at those joints, the efferent neural signals that result in leg kicks, and the afferent fibers that send sensory information back to their brain and cerebellum about the consequences of those movements.[10,11] This is an example of how the developing infant relies on experience to "learn" how to move and control his or her body.

Myelination is the formation of myelin sheaths around the axons by glial cells (Figure 2-18).[15] Myelin is a fatty insulating material that consists of select lipids and proteins that function to insulate the nerve fibers and enhance nerve conduction velocities in the PNS and CNS. Schwann cells accomplish this task in the PNS while oligodendrocytes do so in the CNS. Myelination begins about 24 weeks after conception in the spinal cord and moves to the primitive hind-, fore-, and midbrain and the periphery during prenatal development. Following delivery, there is an intense period of central and peripheral myelination that occurs early in the infant's life and continues through adolescence. In fact, magnetic resonance images of 111 living children and adolescents indicate that myelination of the nerve fibers that support motor functions continues through late childhood and into adolescence.[16] Functionally, this neural maturation process explains, in part, why children and adolescents are able to refine their motor skills and learn to move more efficiently throughout childhood and adolescence. As we will observe, the ability to move more efficiently over time influences a child's ability to improve his or her aerobic capacity and muscle performance.

Neuroplasticity is the brain's ability to organize itself during development or reorganize itself as a consequence of a brain injury through the formation of new neural connections that result from novel experiences.[17] During development, as the brain grows and neurons mature, they send out multiple axons and dendrites that increase the number of synaptic connections within the brain. (Note: Axons send out neural signals and dendrites receive information back from the periphery.) This process increases the number of synapses within the brain from approximately 2500 at birth to nearly 15,000 by age 2 or 3.[18] Because of genetics and as a result of evolutionary development of the human brain, new information coming into the brain via the sensory receptors "finds" its way to the correct area of the brain. For example, information that excites nerve cells within the eye gets sent to the primary visual area in the occipital lobe of the brain and not to another area of the brain, such as the motor cortex. In this way, neural connections between neurons in the eye and the primary visual area of the brain are strengthened. If a child is born without vision and the ability to see, then these connections would not be strengthened over time. Instead, they would become weakened and eventually die out. This process is known as *synaptic pruning*.[17] During development, synapses can be selectively strengthened or weakened depending on the experiences the child is provided. This suggests that the child and his or her developing nervous system will benefit from a variety of movement experiences throughout infancy, childhood, and adolescence. Multiple movement experiences will optimize his or her ability to strengthen the neural connections that will support a relatively rich and diverse movement repertoire during these developmental periods.

Development of Motor Milestones

To be able to interpret the motor performance of an infant, child, or adolescent, the examining PT must be knowledgeable about when in development most children demonstrate particular motor skills, like rolling over, pulling to a stand, and walking. During the first year of life, developing infants typically learn to perform a number of gross and fine motor skills.[19] These are summarized in Table 2-2.

Development of Fundamental Motor Skills

Throughout childhood, the developing child will then learn to walk, run, and perform a number of other fundamental locomotor and object control skills.[20] These skills will be refined during childhood depending on the child's movement experiences and will enable him or her to successfully participate in recreational and sport activities of his or her choice during late childhood and throughout adolescence (Table 2-3). Recreational sport and athletic experiences will allow the child to continue to refine his or her movement repertoire as well as strengthen the neural connections that support his or her well-developed set of movement skills.

Summary: Using This Information to Guide the Physical Therapy Examination

During the initial physical therapy examination, the PT should keep in mind that how the child moves reflects the developmental status of his or her neuromuscular and musculoskeletal systems as well as the integrity of his or her nervous system and the impact of his or her previous movement experiences. While it is important to be mindful of when selected motor milestones are typically achieved, there is a great deal of variability as to when a given child demonstrates a particular skill. As a result, it is equally important to recognize that each child develops at his or her own rate. Thus, it becomes our responsibility to facilitate that process in light of the child's strengths and weaknesses.

TABLE 2-2. DEVELOPMENTAL MOTOR MILESTONES DURING THE FIRST YEAR OF DEVELOPMENT

AVERAGE AGE IN MONTHS	AGE RANGE IN MONTHS	MOTOR MILESTONE
0.1		Lateral head movements
0.8	0.3 to 3.0	Arm and leg thrusts in play
1.6	0.7 to 4.0	Head erect and steady
1.8	0.7 to 5.0	Turns from side to back
2.3	1.0 to 5.0	Sits with slight support
4.4	2.0 to 7.0	Turns from back to side
4.9	4.0 to 8.0	Partial thumb opposition
5.3	4.0 to 8.0	Sits alone momentarily
5.4	4.0 to 8.0	Unilateral reaching
6.4	4.0 to 10.0	Rolls from back to front
6.6	5.0 to 9.0	Sits alone steadily
6.9	5.0 to 9.0	Complete thumb opposition
7.4	6.0 to 10.0	Partial finger prehension
8.1	5.0 to 12.0	Pulls to a stand
8.6	6.0 to 12.0	Stand by furniture
8.8	6.0 to 12.0	Stepping movements
9.6	7.0 to 12.0	Walks with help
11.0	9.0 to 16.0	Stand alone
11.7	9.0 to 17.0	Walks alone
14.6	11.0 to 20.0	Walks backward
16.1	12.0 to 23.0	Walks up stairs with help
16.4	13.0 to 23.0	Walks down stairs with help
23.4	17.0 to 30.0	Jumps off floor, both feet
24.8	19.0 to 30.0+	Jumps from bottom step

In the presence of a known or suspected functional limitation or participation restriction, the PT needs to uncover during examination which system(s) is/are preventing the child from moving more effectively. This will allow the PT to design intervention strategies that will minimize the level of impairment of the involved system(s), expand the child's movement repertoire, and take advantage of the intrinsic plasticity that exists in all of his or her developing systems.

TABLE 2-3. DEVELOPMENT OF FUNDAMENTAL LOCOMOTOR AND OBJECT CONTROL SKILLS	
LOCOMOTOR SKILLS	AGE IN YEARS WHEN CHILDREN DEMONSTRATE MATURE FORM OF SKILL
Running	5
Hopping	8
Skipping	7
Galloping	8
Side slide	5
Horizontal jump	9
Leap	8
OBJECT CONTROL SKILLS	
Two-hand strike	8
Overhand throw	8
Kick	10
Catch	7
Bouncing ball	7

Adapted from Ulrich DA. *Test of Gross Motor Development 2.* Austin, TX: PRO-Ed Publishers; 2000.

DEVELOPMENT OF SYSTEMS THAT INFLUENCE AEROBIC CAPACITY DURING INFANCY, CHILDHOOD, AND ADOLESCENCE

The cardiovascular system is the first organ system to reach a functional state and includes the heart, veins, and arteries, which are all connected in a continuous loop system.[1,2] The pulmonary system includes the lungs and musculoskeletal structures that support these organs and participate in their physiologic function. The skeletal system, which provides specific structural support to the cardiovascular and pulmonary systems, includes the vertebral column, ribs, and sternum, collectively known as the *thorax.* The muscular system contributing to physiologic function includes the primary and accessory muscles of respiration/ventilation as well as the muscles that provide for stabilization of this system. These include the diaphragm, intercostal muscles, sternocleidomastoid, scalenes, serratus anterior, pectoralis major, pectoralis minor, trapezius, erector spinae, and abdominal wall (rectus, obliques, transverses) muscles. The pulmonary system structures that participate in ventilation and gas delivery include the nose, pharynx, larynx, trachea, bronchi, bronchioles, and terminal units or respiratory bronchioles and alveoli.

The aerobic capacity of infants, children, and adolescents reflects the developmental status of and changes in the heart, circulatory system, and lungs. As will be shown, each system affects the relative efficiency of aerobic capacity at rest and during exercise throughout these developmental periods. In addition, these systems also influence how children and adolescents respond to endurance training.

Heart Development During Infancy, Childhood, and Adolescence

At birth, a typically developing infant is born with an intact, fully functional heart. It is, however, considerably smaller than it will be later in childhood and adolescence. As a result, an infant's heart is able to pump less blood per beat when compared to the amount of blood pumped per beat by a child, adolescent, or adult. The amount of blood pumped per beat is known as stroke volume (SV) and depends on the size of the left ventricle and myocardial contractility.[21] Myocardial contractility does not change over time or with growth.[21] Thus, SV is the primary factory that affects cardiac output (CO) throughout life. CO generally increases during development and is the amount of blood pumped by the heart in 1 minute. It is the product of HR multiplied by SV. In equation format it appears like: $CO = HR \times SV$.

A newborn infant's HR is generally higher at rest and during activity when compared to a child, adolescent, or adult. This is because an infant's heart and left ventricle are relatively small compared to his or her basal metabolic needs and the energy he or she needs to grow. In fact, a newborn infant's average resting HR is 120 bpm.[22] This figure can reach as high as 190 bpm when the infant is crying and generally will be higher if the infant is ill, especially if he or she has a fever and/or is fighting an infection.[22]

Following birth, the heart continues to grow in size throughout infancy, childhood, and adolescence parallel to the individual's body growth and development until maturity is reached. This results in a larger left ventricle, which results in an increase in SV and CO, and ensures adequate perfusion of the body throughout development.

As children get older, their HRs at rest and with activity decrease. For example, at 2 years of age, the average resting HR has dropped to 110 bpm because of the increased size of the heart/left ventricle and a corresponding increase in SV and CO compared to a newborn infant.[22] Throughout childhood and adolescence, resting HR values continue to decline so that an average 10 year old's resting HR is 90 bpm.[22] By age 14, the typical resting HR for females is 85 bpm and for males is 80 bpm.[22] By age 16, the average resting HR has dropped to 80 bpm for females and 75 bpm for males.[22]

The resting HR values observed during childhood and adolescence parallel the increase in SV and CO experienced by these individuals. Typically, developing children have an average SV of 3 to 4 mL per ventricular contraction compared to 40 to 60 mL per ventricular contraction for adolescents.[23] Although SV is generally greater in boys than in girls, this 10-fold increase in SV for both genders directly facilitates the observed lower resting HR and corresponding higher CO values in children and adolescents compared to infants and newborns.[23] Alternatively, maximum HR values for children and adolescents have been reported to range from 195 to 215 bpm and then begin to decrease by 0.7 to 0.8 bpm every year after maturity has been reached.[21] The resting HR, SV, and CO values during infancy, childhood, and adolescence are presented in Table 2-4.

Circulatory System Development During Infancy, Childhood, and Adolescence

At birth, the lungs expand, which allows for a rapid increase in blood flow to and from the lungs. Typically, the foramen ovale and ductus arteriosus close when the umbilical cord is cut because circulation to the placenta is terminated, which causes a change in blood flow and an increase in BP within the chambers of the heart. This results in the reflex closure of the ductus arteriosus and foramen ovale.[1] This phenomenon is presented in Figure 2-19.

If the foramen ovale does not close spontaneously, O_2-rich blood will leak from the left atrium into the right atrium instead of moving to the left ventricle and then out to the aorta and body. Minor atrial septal defects (ASDs) will present without symptoms, but larger ASDs will need to be repaired surgically. In a similar manner, if the ductus arteriosus remains patent or open, some blood that should flow through the body will go to the lungs. This may lead to heart failure and/or cardiac infections. Infants with this condition are usually treated with medications, while older children and adults have their ASDs repaired surgically. These conditions are illustrated in Figure 2-19.

Following delivery, infants and children have hypokinetic circulation.[24] This means that their CO is less when compared with adults. This is primarily because infants and children have smaller left ventricles and hearts than adults, so their SV—the amount of blood pumped per beat—is less than adults. Thus, as noted earlier, when compared to adults, infants and children will have higher/faster HRs at rest and at a given level of work. In addition, infants and children have lower levels of hemoglobin in their blood compared to adults. For example, the total hemoglobin concentration in adults is approximately 22% greater than in typical 11- and 12-year-old children.[25] This suggests that they have a decreased ability to carry O_2 in their blood. Fortunately, their lower hemoglobin levels are offset by an enhanced ability to extract O_2 when compared with adults.[26,27] Hemoglobin concentrations plateau in females during adolescence but continue to rise in males throughout adolescence, which suggests that

AGE	HEART RATE	RESPIRA-TION RATE	BLOOD PRESSURE
Newborn	120	30 to 40	60 to 90/20 to 60
1 year	120	20 to 40	74 to 100/50 to 70
2 years	110	25 to 32	80 to 112/50 to 80
4 years	100	23 to 30	82 to 110/50 to 78
6 years	100	21 to 26	84 to 120/54 to 80
8 years	90	20 to 26	84 to 120/54 to 80
10 years	90	20 to 26	84 to 120/54 to 80
12 years			
Female	90	18 to 22	84 to 120/54 to 80
Male	85	18 to 22	84 to 120/54 to 80
14 years			
Female	85	18 to 22	94 to 120/62 to 80
Male	80	18 to 22	94 to 120/62 to 80
16 years			
Female	80	16-20	94 to 120/62 to 80
Male	75	16-20	94 to 120/62 to 80
18 years			
Female	75	12 to 20	90 to 120/60 to 80
Male	70	12 to 20	90 to 120/60 to 80

TABLE 2-4. NORMAL VALUES FOR HEART RATE, STROKE VOLUME, CARDIAC OUTPUT, AND BLOOD PRESSURE DURING DEVELOPMENT

males will have an easier time delivering O_2 to their working muscles.[21]

BP is the amount of pressure exerted by the blood on the walls of the blood vessels.[24] It is influenced by an individual's HR, volume of blood, resistance to blood flow due to the radius and length of the blood vessels, and the viscosity of the blood itself.[21] Resting systolic, diastolic, and systemic BP values all rise during infancy, childhood, and adolescence. For instance, a healthy full-term newborn infant's average BP is on average 60 to 90/20 to 60. By age 10, it will rise to 84 to 120/54 to 80 and will be 94 to 120/62 to 80 for the average 15 year old.[21] (These values are summarized in Table 2-4.) This trend reflects the increase in SV children and adolescents demonstrate as well as changes in peripheral resistance that are likely due to changes in sympathetic innervation, blood viscosity, arteriolar radius, and blood vessels that continue to lengthen as the child grows and develops into maturity.[21]

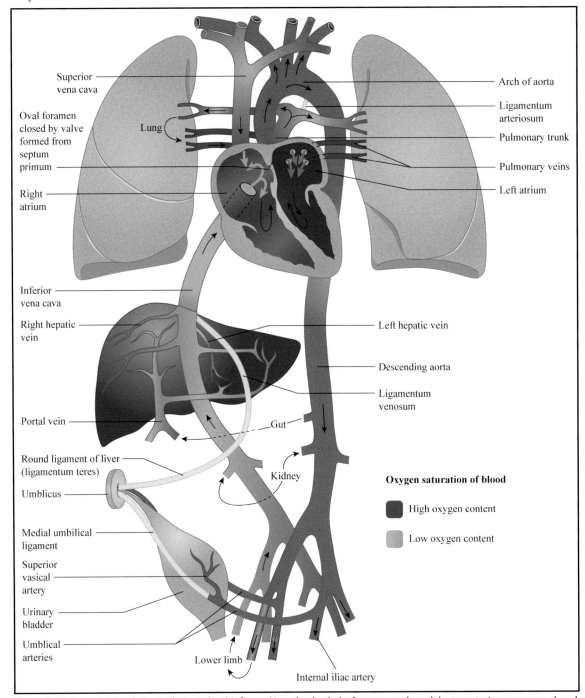

Figure 2-19. Neonatal circulation is illustrated in this figure. Note that both the foramen ovale and ductus arteriosus are now closed, which allows the infant to circulate blood between the heart, body, and lungs for typical perfusion of all body tissues. (Adapted from Moore KL, Persaud TVN. *The Developing Human: Clinically Oriented Embryology.* 7th ed. Philadelphia, PA: Saunders; 2003.)

Lung Development During Infancy, Childhood, and Adolescence

Lung development, similar to heart development and function, improves as the child and his or her lungs get bigger during infancy, childhood, and adolescence. Initially, the lungs develop as an organ that participates in the production and drainage of the amniotic fluid that also fills the developing air spaces. Just prior to birth, the existing alveoli are collapsed and the lungs are filled with amniotic fluid. Then, during the birthing process, the amniotic fluid is expressed from the lungs in 3 ways as they convert to managing gas exchange and supplying the O_2 transport system. Fifty percent is reabsorbed by the lymph system, and 25% is pressed out as the infant's thorax is significantly compressed as it passes through the birth canal. Of course, this does not take place if the baby is born via caesarian section; the remaining 25% is absorbed into the circulatory system through the capillaries.[28] This complex system for expressing fluid is essential for the conversion to successful gas exchange in the neonate as the high surface tension in the relatively wet alveoli causes them to continually collapse.

The 2 physiologic mechanisms that combat alveolar collapse are the filling of the alveoli with air and the production of surfactant by type II alveolar cells. At birth, the neonate has a low arterial pH and low partial pressure of arterial O_2 that will both drive the respiratory rate and increase ventilatory pump action to result in a higher level of ventilation. Simultaneously, the stretch of alveoli enhances the production of surfactant to lower intra-alveolar surface tension. Consequently, the inhalation of air and the reduction in alveolar surface tension by surfactant results in gradually more and more alveoli unfolding to participate in gas exchange.

During the first 6 months of life, there is a rapid increase in the number of alveoli, with the process continuing until the baby is approximately 18 months old. A significant increase in the size of the alveoli and an increase in the number of alveoli continue through adolescence.[1,2]

Support System/Structures

The function of the cardiovascular/pulmonary system is interdependent with the musculoskeletal system. Development of ventilatory pump, gas exchange, and cardiovascular pump functional capacity depends not only on the growth and development of the heart and lungs, but also on the musculoskeletal system's increasing structural strength and endurance capacity as this will impact the ability of the child to perform work against gravity.

The thorax as a structure has been biomechanically described as having 3 degrees of movement freedom that allow it to expand in 3 dimensions: anteroposterior, superoinferior, and transverse or lateral.[29] Expansion and compression of the chest wall boundaries or surfaces may be assisted or resisted by the forces of gravity, strength of supporting muscles, or a support surface. Figure 2-20 shows the 3 chest wall motions.

At birth, all of the infant's systems have been influenced by the limited space available in the womb. The anterior chest wall is shortened and the connective tissues are short and tight because of the forward flexed position of the fetus in the womb. The thorax is triangular-shaped at birth, taking up only one-third of the trunk. The ribs are positioned horizontally with limited intercostal space and there is sternal instability primarily because the skeletal tissue is composed entirely of cartilage. The lack of skeletal rigidity is what allows for the compression of the thorax as it passes through the birth canal and the minimal resistance or load the ventilatory muscles face to perform the work of breathing.[29]

The work of breathing in the infant is accomplished primarily through the piston action of the diaphragm.[30] The diaphragm works by contracting against the load of the abdominal contents to displace the fluid volume and create the negative inspiratory pressure for inhalation.

Infants at birth are obligatory nose breathers, so the resistance of the upper airways has to be overcome. This immature

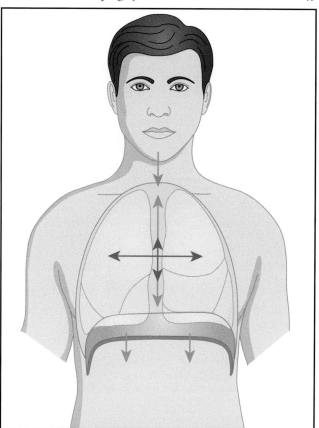

Figure 2-20. Chest wall motions. (Adapted from Massery M. Multisystem clinical implications of impaired breathing mechanics and postural control. In: Frownfelter D, Dean E, eds. *Cardiovascular and Pulmonary Physical Therapy: Evidence to Practice.* 4th ed. St. Louis, MO: Elsevier-Mosby; 2006.)

breathing pattern is essential to allow for ventilation during feeding. The intercostal muscles are also immature and are unable to produce force for movement of the ribs. The lungs have formed with large bronchi and few alveoli. As a result, they have limited vital capacity (VC) and their breathing is shallow and rapid. The typical respiration rate for newborns and infants up to 6 months of age is 30 to 40 breaths per minute, while infants between 6 and 12 months of age breathe between 20 and 40 times per minute.[24] As infants begin to move against gravity and change positions, they strengthen the muscles of respiration, which facilitates migration of the ribs in a downward direction. Increased extensor activity relative to their flexed in utero position facilitates the "opening up" of the anterior chest wall.

Between 6 and 12 months of age, the infant transitions to moving against gravity while in an upright position. The general muscle strength increases that occur during this time allow for a downward pull and expansion of the ribs from the abdominals, diaphragm, and intercostals muscles. Head control is gained, resulting in elongation of the neck. The thorax becomes more rectangular in shape and takes up one-half of the trunk cavity.[30] Intra-abdominal pressure increases as the diaphragm achieves a more optimal position supported by the abdominal viscera and downward pull of the ribs by the abdominals. The intercostals muscles stabilize

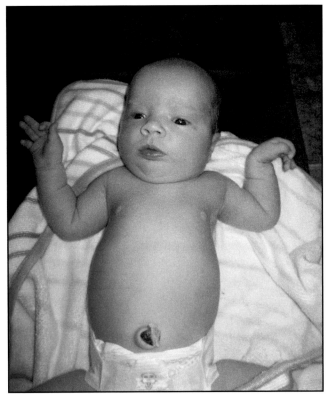

Figure 2-21. Chest wall shape at birth.

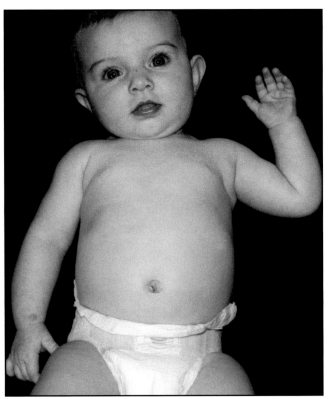

Figure 2-22. Chest wall shape at 6 months.

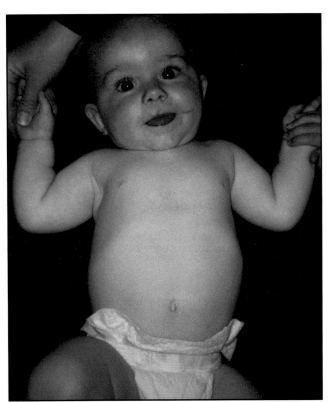

Figure 2-23. Chest wall shape at 12 months.

age. Further changes occur with growth spurts through bone growth and lengthening of muscles. The rib cage continues to rotate downward and does not fully ossify until the mid-20s.[31] Figures 2-21 to 2-23 depict the shape of the chest at birth, 6 months, and 12 months of age, respectively.

During childhood and early adolescence, there is a marked increase in total lung capacity. Starting at age 5 years, total lung capacity is estimated to be approximately 1400 cm³. By age 14 years, total lung capacity will triple to nearly 4500 cm³. This increase in total lung capacity parallels the child's growth in stature and is positively correlated with the height and weight of the child.[32] This increase in lung capacity results in a slowing of respiration from an average of 24 breaths per minute at age 6 years to 13 breaths per minute on average at age 17 years.[33] Note that this phenomenon parallels what we observed with heart development; that is, as the child grows and develops, his or her left ventricle increases in size, enabling the heart to pump more blood per beat and minute, which allows his or her HR to slow. Thus, as children get older and bigger, they tend to show decreased rates of respiration as well as slower HRs.

Although breathing rates decline during childhood and adolescence, tidal volume (VT) and VC both increase during these same periods of development. VT is the amount of air that is moved into and out of the lungs during normal inspiration and expiration.[21] VC is the greatest amount of air that can be expelled in one single maximum expiratory effort.[21] Both increase with lung growth and body size. VC per kilogram (kg) of body weight has been found to be greater in

the chest wall, allowing for changes in the dimensions of the chest during inhalation and exhalation. The general shape of the thorax and chest cavity are established by 12 months of boys than girls.[34] Research has shown that VC per kg to be 2.5 L for 11-year-old boys and 2.19 L for 11-year-old girls when mass and height are controlled.[34]

It is important to note that VT at rest decreases with respect to mass and surface area during childhood. For example, 6- to 8-year-old girls demonstrate VTs of 321 mL/m^2 of body surface compared to 297 mL/m^2 for 8- to 12-year-old females and 242 mL/m^2 for 12- to 17-year-old females, respectively.[35] This suggests that the percentage of VC used for VT decreases (ie, breathing becomes more efficient as children develop and mature). This is thought to be the result of improved lung compliance and reduced airway resistance demonstrated by late childhood.[21]

Resting minute ventilation (VE) also decreases during childhood but is consistently higher in children than adults at all activity levels. VE is the volume of air inhaled or exhaled in 1 minute and reflects both the rate or frequency of breaths taken and VT expressed relative to body size.[21] In equation format, it appears as: VE = VT × respiration rate

Typically, developing 10-year-old children show VE values of 200 mL·kg^{-1}·min^{-1} while typical 16-year-old adolescents have VE values of 158 mL·kg^{-1}·min^{-1}.[21] As such, it makes logical sense that resting VE would decrease as a result of the decreases observed during childhood for respiration rate and VT.

Maximal VE (VE$_{max}$) reflects maximal metabolic activity and the influence of excessive carbon dioxide (CO_2) produced during activity and the need to modulate metabolic waste products, such as lactate, during peak levels of activity.[36] Unfortunately, no normative values exist for VE$_{max}$ in children.[21] In spite of this gap in our knowledge, it is thought that VE increases during maximal exercise because of the observed increase in total lung capacity throughout childhood. It is important for PTs to keep in mind that VE$_{max}$ reflects the metabolic rate of the exercising child or adolescent and is influenced by cellular level metabolic processes, like lactate production and levels of CO_2 in the blood.

To summarize, as a child gets older, he or she typically experiences an increase in size that parallels the growth he or she experiences in his or her heart, circulatory system, and lungs. These changes enable the child's heart to pump more blood per beat and beat less often at rest and with activity; levels of circulating hemoglobin increase and the child breathes more efficiently as he or she grows and develops. With these thoughts in mind, we can now focus on the developmental changes in aerobic capacity demonstrated during childhood and adolescence.

Developmental Changes in Aerobic Capacity and Endurance Training

Aerobic capacity is the amount of physiologic work that a person can perform as measured by how much O_2 he or she consumes during activity.[37] This ability is influenced by a person's age, gender, genetics, experiences, social factors such as economic status, and the relative condition of his or her cardiovascular system. During infancy, childhood, and adolescence, aerobic capacity is also affected by developmental changes in the heart, circulatory system, and lungs as reviewed earlier. Thus, the development of aerobic capacity is a dynamic trait that needs to be thoughtfully considered by the PT.

Aerobic capacity is often associated with the concept of physical fitness. Physical fitness consists of motor fitness and health-related fitness.[38] Motor fitness focuses on the skills and abilities needed to participate and compete in athletics. Health-related fitness includes having enough energy to complete activities of daily living (ADL) in an appropriate manner and maintaining a low level of risk for prematurely developing diseases related to being inactive (eg, hypertension, coronary artery disease, and obesity).[39] Four basic components of health-related fitness have been identified.[40] These include cardiorespiratory endurance (ie, aerobic capacity), muscular strength and endurance, flexibility, and body composition. Muscle strength and endurance will be addressed later in the muscle performance section of this chapter. Developmental changes in aerobic capacity at rest and with exercise during infancy, childhood, and adolescence as influenced by development of the heart, circulatory system, and lungs will be presented next. The focus here is on aerobic activity rather than anaerobic activity.

Aerobic fitness is usually measured by maximum O_2 consumption (VO$_{2max}$), which equals the amount of O_2 consumed in mL or L per minute. VO$_{2max}$ expressed in L/min is an absolute measure of O_2 consumed. It can be normalized to body weight (mL/min/kg) by dividing the absolute measure by the child's weight in kg.[21] Either measure represents the highest rate that O_2 can be delivered and used by working skeletal muscle.[21] Functionally, it can be thought of as the time it takes to walk, run, or bike a given distance.[21] VO$_{2max}$ is influenced by multiple factors and generally improves throughout childhood and adolescence.[21]

The factors that influence the development of VO$_{2max}$ include SV, skeletal muscle mass (lean body mass), percentage of body fat, oxidative enzymatic activity within skeletal muscle cells, the level of hemoglobin in the blood, endurance training, and nervous system activity.[21] VO$_{2max}$ is approximately 200 mL·kg^{-1}·min^{-1} greater for boys than for girls throughout childhood, but both genders demonstrate improved VO$_{2max}$ values as they grow and their SV improves over time. For instance, a typical 6-year-old boy will demonstrate a VO$_{2max}$ of 1.2 L/min^{-1} and by age 12 years, and this will rise to 2.7 L/min^{-1}.[41-43] This trend continues to approximately 16 years of age for boys, but only age 14 years for typically developing girls.[41-43] Girls actually experience a plateau or decline in VO$_{2max}$ beginning at the time of puberty, and by age 16 years, their VO$_{2max}$ will be 32% lower than boys their age.[41-43]

SV has been found to be sensitive to endurance training in prepubescent children. Mobert et al reported a 20% increase in SV from 55 to 66 mL for twelve 13- to 14-year-old boys who completed 7 months of an aerobic training program.[44]

Obert et al reported similar results for 10 girls and 9 boys who were 10 years old after they finished a 13-week aerobic training program.[45] These researchers documented a 15% increase in SV for the boys and an 11% increase in SV for the girls who participated in this study.

Skeletal muscle mass and percentage of body fat have a positive and negative effect on VO_{2max} depending on the gender of the child. Boys show an 11% increase in skeletal muscle mass, from 42% to 53%, as a percentage of their body weight during puberty because of the influence of testosterone.[26] Females experience only a 1% increase in skeletal muscle mass as a percentage of their body weight during puberty.[26] Thus, they will have nearly the same amount of skeletal muscle mass as a percentage of their body weight by the end of puberty as they did at the beginning of puberty. They will, however, experience a significant increase in body fat as a percentage of their total body weight. A typical female gains nearly twice as much body fat during puberty compared to a typical boy.[26] This trend reflects gender differences that began prior to birth (eg, newborn baby boys average 11% body fat, while infant girls are born with 14% body fat) and are observed during childhood, then accelerate throughout adolescence.[21] Ultimately, when a female reaches maturity, she will, on average, have twice the amount of body fat as a percentage of her total body weight that a boy has when he reaches maturity.[26] This is due to an increase in the number and size of her fat cells. Functionally, it means that her cardiovascular system has become relatively less efficient during puberty, especially when compared to a boy her age.

Oxidative enzymatic activity within skeletal muscle cells appears to limit the development of and absolute values at maturity for VO_{2max} for adults and children.[21] This is because cellular-level aerobic enzyme function decreases at rest as body mass increases.[21] Currently, it is assumed that this "rule" also applies to when children and adults are working at peak levels of activity. Unfortunately, it is not known whether oxidative enzymatic activity in children improves with training, nor is it clear why this mechanism functions in this manner.

Hemoglobin levels range from 11.5 to 15.5 grams/deciliter (g/dL) in boys and girls prior to puberty and cannot be used to explain the gender differences observed in VO_{2max} in prepubescent children.[22,44] However, as noted previously, adults have approximately 22% greater levels of hemoglobin in their blood compared to children.[25] These differences occur during puberty as boys' hemoglobin levels rise to 14 to 18 g/dL, while girls experience a smaller increase to 12 to 16 g/dL on average.[22] As result, this difference explains, in part, the greater VO_{2max} values observed in adults compared with children and why adolescent boys begin to show increased VO_{2max} values when compared with girls their age.

Endurance training is the next factor to consider as we explore the developmental changes observed in VO_{2max} during childhood and adolescence. Fifteen well-designed studies that employed appropriate control groups and sufficient training protocols with adequate levels of frequency, duration, and intensity with nontrained boys and girls have been completed.[44-58] These studies examined the impact of endurance training on VO_{2max}, resting HR, ventricular size, plasma volume, and VE in prepubescent children.

Improvements in VO_{2max} ranged from 0% to 10% across the 15 studies, with an average improvement of 5.8%. Two experiments specifically examined gender differences in VO_{2max} after completing a 12- or 13-week training program but did not reveal any gender differences for this trait.[46,47] Two additional studies reported that 11-year-old girls had greater gains in VO_{2max} than boys of the same age after they completed an endurance training program.[46,48] These authors suggested that the observed post-training gender differences were due to the fact that the girls had lower pretraining VO_{2max} values than did the boys.

Resting HR and vascular resistance to blood flow were consistently observed to be lower after these children completed the required endurance training program.[49] Concurrently, left ventricle size (volume) and plasma volume were found to be improved as a result of participating in an aerobic training program.[49]

The length of the training program (duration) did not show a significant overall impact on any of the variables measured in this set of studies. However, the 3 longest programs showed the greatest gains in VO_{2max}. These program were run for 15, 28, and 72 weeks and obtained VO_{2max} increases of 10.3%, 12.2%, and 18.9%, respectively.[44,50,51]

Collectively, these studies suggest that VO_{2max} and the traits related to VO_{2max} can be improved in prepubescent children. However, the training program must last for a sufficient period of time, be frequent enough, and require the children to work at high enough levels of intensity to obtain these benefits. They also show, but do not explain, why children's gains in VO_{2max} with training are 15% to 30% less than those enjoyed by adults who complete similar types of programs, nor do they address how the nervous system affects the development of VO_{2max} in children and adolescents.[21]

The nervous system may affect the development of VO_{2max} in children and adolescents in several ways. The brain exerts a protective influence on exercising children by sending neural signals to the child that lets him or her know that he or she is feeling uncomfortable, nauseated, light headed, and/or is experiencing excessive leg fatigue.[21] The perception of these "fatigue signals" may function to prevent myocardial ischemia and cardiogenic shock when the child exercises at maximum levels of intensity.[21] The autonomic nervous system also influences aerobic capacity by controlling regional blood flow, perspiration rates, bronchodilation, and myocardial contractility. Beyond these protective mechanisms, it is not clear if these neural activities limit the development of VO_{2max} or simply function to keep the exercising child safe.[21]

Summary: Using This Information to Guide the Physical Therapy Examination

Health-related fitness is influenced by multiple factors, including aerobic capacity, which is frequently associated with physical fitness. Typically, as the child grows and develops, components of his or her cardiovascular and pulmonary systems also grow to ensure adequate perfusion of his or her body tissues at rest and during activity. It is important for the examining PT to realize that none of these systems will be mature until the child has completed puberty and reaches a mature physical state. Until that time, the child's HR, respiration rate, and VE will usually get lower as he or she develops. Simultaneously, BP, SV, CO, VT, and VC will all increase over time. To complete a thorough systems review during the initial physical therapy examination and subsequent treatment sessions, it is imperative that the examining PT be aware of the normal values for HR, BP, and respiration rate. This knowledge will allow the PT to rule in or rule out any impairment that may exist in one or more of these functions.

It is also important for the involved PT to recognize that, prior to puberty, boys and girls have similar levels of aerobic capacity and respond to aerobic training programs in a comparable manner with the exception that girls often show greater gains in VO_{2max} after completing an endurance training program when compared with boys of the same age. During puberty, the aerobic capacity of girls plateaus, while the ability of boys to deliver and use O_2 during activity improves. Children of all ages and both genders experience less improvement in VO_{2max} as a result of participating in endurance training programs than adults. In spite of the limited impact endurance training programs have on VO_{2max} in children, they do result in lower HRs, less vascular resistance, and greater SVs and plasma levels after an endurance training program has been completed. Thus, aerobic training programs that are of sufficient frequency, duration, and intensity are considered to be beneficial to most children. Finally, the treating PT must keep in mind the protective role the nervous system plays in letting the child know when she is becoming fatigued, feeling nauseated, light-headed, or otherwise uncomfortable. This is nature's way of letting her know is it time to take a break.

DEVELOPMENT OF MUSCLE PERFORMANCE SYSTEMS DURING INFANCY, CHILDHOOD, AND ADOLESCENCE

Muscle performance reflects the developmental status of an individual's muscular strength, endurance, and power as well as the influence of his or her nervous system on these types of traits.[38] Strength refers to a person's ability to generate maximal contractile force. Muscular endurance depends, in part, on muscular strength and is the ability of the muscle(s) to perform work when work is equal to force multiplied by distance. The equation for work is: work = force × distance.

For example, if a child moves a 5-pound dumbbell 2 feet, he or she would have performed 10 pounds-feet of work. In equation form, this would appear as: work = 5 pounds × 2 feet = 10 pounds-feet.

Muscular power is the ability to generate maximal muscular force in a specified time. In an equation, muscular power presents as Power = (force × distance)/time; with power being defined as the amount of work completed per unit of time. In the previous example, if a child moves the 5-pound dumbbell 2 feet in 1 second, he or she would have completed 10 pounds-feet per second of work. Likewise, if a child moves the 5-pound dumbbell 2 feet in 0.5 seconds, he or she would have generated 20 pounds-feet per second of work. In equation format, these examples would look like the following:

- Power = (5 pounds × 2 feet)/1 second = 10 pounds-feet/second
- Power = (5 pounds × 2 feet)/0.5 seconds = 20 pounds-feet/second

As a result, muscular power increases when velocity increases or time decreases. Because muscular endurance and power are dependent on muscular strength, strength will be the focus of the information presented here.

Development of Muscle Tissue

The number of muscle fibers that each child possesses is established at or shortly after birth. Following birth, muscle tissue enlarges in size because of an increase in the diameter of individual muscle cells secondary to more myofilaments within each fiber and an increase in the protein content with the muscle fibers themselves.[59] The skeletal muscle mass of all children, under the influence of GH and insulin-like growth factor I (IGF-I), increases linearly with age until puberty. This is because GH and IGF-I promote the development of muscle mass and greater levels of strength by promoting muscle protein synthesis during childhood.[59-61] Prepubescent boys tend to demonstrate relatively larger muscles than girls of the same age.[21] During puberty, boys experience a marked increase in muscle mass (11%), while girls show only a 1% gain in muscle mass during this same time period.[21] It has been observed that boys experience this marked increase in muscle mass and strength approximately 1 year after their peak change in height.[59-61] Unfortunately, there are no data that describe this type of effect in females.[21]

Development of Bony Tissue

There is a gradual increase in bone density throughout childhood for children of both genders prior to puberty.[62-67] During puberty, bone density increases from 17% to 70% in

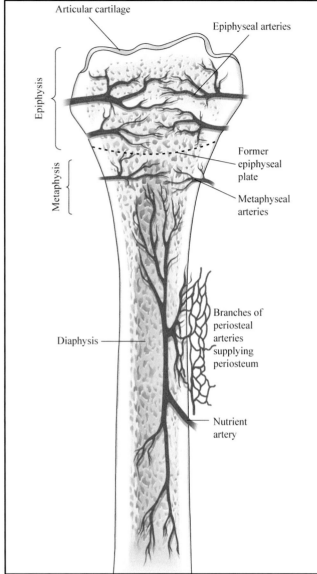

Figure 2-24. A schematic drawing of a mature long bone. (Adapted from Whiting WC, Zernicke RF. *Biomechanics of Musculoskeletal Injury.* Champaign, IL: Human Kinetics; 1998.)

girls.[68] These influences may shape when in development the long bones stop growing for boys and girls. Skeletal development is also shaped by movement and the forces exerted on the bones during movement as well as injuries that may occur in or near the growth plates located at the end of the long bones.[69] A schematic drawing of a mature long bone is presented in Figure 2-24.

Developmental Changes in Muscle Performance and Strength Training

Little is known about the development of strength prior to age 6 years, but cross-sectional and longitudinal studies of muscle strength show that children of both genders safely demonstrate, with no injuries, an increase in isometric and isokinetic strength when they are trained on weight machines, free weights, calisthenics, and sport-specific activities.[70-73] These studies examined the effects of strength training in prepubescent boys and girls and showed that children demonstrated a 30% to 40% increase in strength following an 8- to 12-week training program without a concomitant hypertrophy of muscle tissue.[70-73] The authors of these studies have suggested that the increases in strength demonstrated by prepubescent children with training may be due to learning effects as well as developmental changes in motor unit firing, motor unit recruitment, nerve conduction velocity, modulation in CNS inhibition, and/or an increase in the contractile forces of skeletal muscle. Each of these influences will be examined next.

A motor unit consists of one motor neuron in the anterior horn of the spinal cord and its axons that synapse with a number of muscle fibers. The number of muscle fibers innervated by one motor neuron, depending on the area of the body involved, may range from 3 to 2000 fibers.[21] Note that motor units fire on an all-or-nothing principle. As a result, the increase in strength observed in children in the absence of muscle hypertrophy may be due to an increase in the frequency of firing by a given motor unit and/or recruitment of more motor units during the execution of a given task. In other words, a given motor unit may fire more often and/or a child may be able to selectively recruit more motor units while performing a particular task. Both would enable the child to demonstrate more strength without an increase in the muscle fibers themselves.

A second neurological influence on strength development in childhood is nerve conduction velocity. Research has shown that motor nerve and sensory nerve conduction velocities increase between birth and 4 to 5 years of age.[71-73] Adults demonstrate nerve conduction velocities that are 2 times faster than neonates.[73] However, these researchers noted that nerve conduction velocities are similar between 4 to 5 year olds and adults.[71-73] Other researchers have found that nerve conduction velocities continue to increase until age 20 years.[73] As a result, it is possible then that the increases in strength shown by adolescents may also be due to neurological factors in addition to the influence of testosterone

girls and 11% to 75% in boys, depending on the source.[62-67] Researchers doubt the accuracy of these values because of variations caused by the dual energy X-ray absorptiometry method of measurement that was employed in each of these studies. There is, however, general consensus that there is a large gain in bone density during adolescence. Several studies suggest that peak bone density development occurs between the ages of 16 and 26 years for females and 16 and 25 years for males.[62-67]

Several factors influence skeletal development throughout childhood and adolescence. For example, hormonal factors influence how fast and how much the long bones grow. In particular, testosterone, thyroxin, and GH stimulate cell differentiation of the cartilage within the growth plate of long bones.[68] Simultaneously, estrogen acts to suppress growth of the cartilage but stimulates bone growth both in boys and in males. Corticospinal tract conduction velocities (motor nerve conduction velocities) have also been found to increase between children aged 6 to 9 years and young adults between 22 and 26 years old.[74] Collectively, these lines of research show that increases in strength can be due, in part, to neurological factors into early adulthood.

The final neurological factor to consider is the role of the CNS in the development of strength during childhood and adolescence. The CNS influences the development of strength via cognitive, autonomic, and reflexive processes. In particular, the CNS sends signals from the brain through the spinal cord that affect the relative contractile force demonstrated by the child as he or she exercises.[21] At a conscious level, the CNS can also influence the child or adolescent's level of motivation when performing a given task. Subconsciously, the CNS modulates the child's HR and BP at rest and during activity. In addition, the autonomic portion of the CNS affects how the child or adolescent may perform because of its influences on how efficiently he or she loses heat during exercise via perspiration and controls regional blood flow to the muscles, internal organs, integument, and bronchodilation that may or may not enhance the child's ability to exercise at a given level of intensity during exercise.

For clinicians, it is perhaps most important to realize that the CNS exerts a powerful protective influence on the exercising child and/or adolescent. The relative threshold of this central inhibitory function may change during childhood, but it will always exert this protective function.[21] It is through this mechanism that the child will sense that he or she is becoming fatigued and that it is time to stop working. This may limit the development of strength but will prevent damage to exercising muscles.[21] Evidence of this effect is observable in the clinic and occurs when the child reports feeling nauseated, light headed, or uncomfortable, and/or reports, "I need to stop."

Currently, it is not clear whether the contractile properties of skeletal muscle cells change during development. Although this may change during childhood, it is more likely that individual muscle fiber architecture improves during childhood and adolescence.[21] This suggests that the angle of pennation (ie, the angle of the muscle fibers themselves) in relation to the direction of the insertion of the muscle tendon into the bone may facilitate the increase in strength observed in children. If this relationship improves during childhood and adolescence, then it would enable the child to show greater strength without showing an increase in the size of the muscle fiber under study.

Summary: Using This Information to Guide the Physical Therapy Examination

Muscle performance consists of strength, endurance, and power. Because muscular endurance and power are dependent on strength, it is most appropriate for practicing PTs to focus on the development of strength rather than muscular endurance or power during childhood and adolescence. In general, muscle mass and strength improves linearly throughout childhood because of the effects of GH and IGI-I. During puberty, boys naturally experience a greater gain in muscle mass and strength than girls do during this period of development. Concurrently, females will experience a marked increase in their percentage of body fat, which implies from a movement perspective that their systems will become relatively less efficient as they mature during puberty.

Bone density also increases linearly for boys and girls during childhood. Throughout adolescence, bone density continues to increase for boys and girls because of the influence of several hormones. Skeletal development is also sensitive to movement and the forces that are exerted on the bones as the child and adolescent moves.

Little is known about how children younger than age 6 years respond to strength training programs, but the literature clearly documents that prepubescent children of both genders can safely increase their isometric and isokinetic strength when they complete training programs that involve free weights, weight machines, calisthenics, and sport activities under supervision. These gains are due primarily to neurological factors, so the treating PT needs to recognize that, prior to adolescence, children may gain strength without an observable increase in the size of their muscles. With training, of course, adolescent boys and girls will continue to demonstrate increases in muscle size and strength, but it is essential that the involved PT recognize that the skeleton is usually immature prior to and during adolescence, which suggests that children and skeletally immature adolescents should not perform one-repetition maximum lifts.

Finally, as we observed in the development of aerobic capacity, the involved PT needs to be aware that the nervous system exerts a protective role in the development of muscle strength. As such, intensity levels that cause the child to feel nauseated, light headed, or unduly fatigued should be avoided.

INTEGUMENTARY SYSTEM DEVELOPMENT

The integumentary system includes the skin and its appendages, such as hair, glands, and fingernails and toenails, as well as the mammary glands and teeth. Because of space constraints, only the skin will be examined in detail here. The epidermis develops from the ectoderm of the fetus and the dermis arises from the mesoderm.[1,2] Initially, the epidermis consists of only one layer of ectodermal cells. By week 7 of gestation, a second layer has formed so that the fetus is covered by a superficial layer of dermal tissue known as *periderm* and a deeper layer called the *basal layer*. During the remainder of gestation, the periderm is continuously sloughed off. These cells become mixed with hair and sebaceous gland secretions to form vernix caseosa.[1,2] Vernix caseosa is a greasy, whitish material that is thought to protect the skin of the fetus while surrounded by the amniotic fluid in utero. The basal layer serves as a germinal layer that leads to the development of the mature epidermis.[1,2]

In the absence of significant scar tissue, the skin will not biomechanically limit an infant or child's movement or ability to exercise. It may, however, affect how a child responds to exercise if the skin's ability to generate perspiration is impaired and limits the child's ability to lose body heat.

SUMMARY

The purposes of this chapter were to describe typical development of the cardiovascular-pulmonary, musculoskeletal, neurological, integument, and endocrine systems from conception through adolescence and review the developmental changes that occur in aerobic capacity, muscle performance, and neuromotor development/motor control during infancy, childhood, and adolescence. To achieve these purposes, the literature was reviewed in each of these areas with regard to the PT's need to be able to understand a child's movement patterns and then correctly predict how he or she will respond to therapeutic interventions.

Our review of embryology and prenatal development revealed that the first trimester is the most critical or sensitive period for typical development of all body organs, systems, and structures. This area of study provides us with the foundation needed to understand the beginning of development and how tissues become specialized very early in life and enable us to address many of the questions and concerns that are often raised by parents and other caregivers.

The information presented about neuromotor development and motor control during infancy, childhood, and adolescence reinforces the idea that each child possesses a great deal of intrinsic plasticity relative to how and when he or she develops new motor skills. This suggests that, in the presence of impairment, each child and treating PT have many options and choices to make regarding how to best design treatment programs that will minimize the impact of the child's impairment(s), take advantage of his or her intact systems, and optimize his or her ability to move in multiple environments.

Developmental changes in a child's aerobic capacity and his or her heart, lungs, and circulatory system before and with training were examined and showed that, throughout childhood and adolescence, a child experiences growth in these organs and systems that parallel his or her physical growth to ensure adequate perfusion of his or her tissues at rest and during exercise. During adolescence, boys will continue to show improvements in VO_{2max}, but girls will not. Normative values were presented to enhance the PTs' ability to conduct a thorough review of the systems that influence aerobic capacity. Endurance training programs that are of sufficient frequency, intensity, and duration result in only modest improvements in VO_{2max} but positively affect several

important cardiovascular functions in prepubescent children. The nervous system plays an important and sometimes protective role in influencing the development of aerobic capacity of children and adolescents.

Muscle performance includes strength, muscular endurance, and power. An examination of the developmental changes that children and adolescents experience in muscle and bony development as well as how they respond to resistance training indicates that prepubescent children usually experience linear growth of their muscle mass and strength. They may safely participate in resistance training programs that are designed to improve their isometric and isokinetic strength with multiple types of equipment. They should not, however, complete any activities that require a one-repetition maximum effort. During adolescence, boys demonstrate marked increases in their muscle mass and strength with and without training, but girls do not show similar gains as they mature during puberty.

It is recommended that the evaluating and treating PT recognize the important role a thorough systems review plays in conducting an effective physical therapy examination for children and adolescents. This necessary first step provides the basis for completing a comprehensive examination of the child or adolescent that will reveal his or her individual strengths and weaknesses and current levels of development. Then, an effective and efficient treatment program can be implemented.

REFERENCES

1. Moore KL, Persaud TVN. *The Developing Human: Clinically Oriented Embryology.* 7th ed. Philadelphia, PA: Saunders; 2003.
2. Moore KL. *Essentials of Human Embryology.* Burlington, Ontario: B.C. Decker Inc; 1988.
3. Clarke J, Whitall J. What is motor development? The lessons of history. *Quest.* 1989;41:182-202.
4. Turner JS, Helms DB. *Lifespan Development.* 5th ed. Fort Worth, TX: Harcourt Brace College Publishers; 1995.
5. Fetal heart & heartbeat facts. *Fetal Sure.* www.fetalsure.com/fetal-heart.html. Accessed September 12, 2011.
6. Crouch JE. *Functional Human Anatomy.* 4th ed. Philadelphia, PA: Lea & Febiger; 1985.
7. Thelen E. Developmental origins of motor coordination: leg movements in human infants. *Dev Psychobio.* 1986;18:1-22.
8. Thelen E, Smith L. *A Dynamic Systems Approach to the Development of Cognition and Action.* Cambridge, MA: MIT Press; 1994.
9. Thelen E, Ulrich BD. Hidden skills: a dynamic systems analysis of treadmill stepping during the first year. *Monogr Soc Res Child Dev.* 1991;56(1):1-98.
10. Chapman D. Context effects on the ability of young infants with myelomeningocele to generate complex patterned leg movements. *Proceedings of the 3rd International 'Come to Your Senses Conference.'* Toronto, Canada: Mukibaum Press; 2009.
11. Chapman D. Context effects on the spontaneous leg movements of infants with spina bifida. *J Ped Phys Ther.* 2002;14(2):62-73.
12. Kamm K, Thelen E, Jensen JL. A dynamical systems approach to motor development. *Phys Ther.* 1990;70:763-775.
13. Newell K. Constraints on the development of coordination. In: Wade MG, Whiting HTA, eds. *Motor Development in Children: Aspects of Coordination and Control.* Amsterdam: Martin Nijhoff; 1986:341-361.

14. Schmidt R, Lee TD. *Motor Control and Learning: A Behavioral Approach.* Champaign, IL: Human Kinetics, 1999.

15. Purves D, Augustine GJ, Fitzpatrick D, et al. *Neuroscience.* 4th ed. Sunderland, MA: Sinauer Associates Inc; 2008.

16. Paus T, Zijdenbos A, Worsley K, et al. Structural maturation of neural pathways in children and adolescents: in vivo study. *Science.* 1999;283:1908-1911.

17. Chudler EC, ed. *Brain Plasticity: What Is It? Learning and Memory.* http://faculty.washington.edu/chudler/plast.html. Accessed November 9, 2011.

18. Gopnick A, Meltzoff A, Kuhl P. *The Scientist Crib: What Early Learning Tells Us About the Mind.* New York, NY: HarperCollins Publishers; 1999.

19. Bayley N. *Bayley Scales of Infant and Toddler Development.* 3rd ed. San Antonio, TX: Pearson; 2005.

20. Ulrich DA. *Test of Gross Motor Development 2.* Austin, TX: PRO-Ed Publishers; 2000.

21. Rowland TW. *Children's Exercise Physiology.* 2nd ed. Champaign, IL: Human Kinetics; 2005.

22. Jarvis C. *Physical Examination and Health Assessment.* Philadelphia, PA: W.B. Saunders Company; 1996.

23. Bar-Or O. *Pediatric Sports Medicine for the Practitioner.* New York: Springer-Verlag; 1983.

24. Bar-Or O, Shephard RJ, Allen CL. Cardiac output in 10- to 13-year-old boys and girls during submaximal exercise. *J Appl Physiol.* 1971;30:219-223.

25. Krahenbuhl GS, Skinner JS, Kohrt WM. Developmental aspects of maximal aerobic power in children. *Exerc Sport Sci Rev.* 1985;13:503-538.

26. Malina R, Bouchard C. *Growth, Maturation, and Physical Activity.* Champaign, IL: Human Kinetics; 1991.

27. Shephard RJ. *Physical Activity and Growth.* Chicago, IL: Year Book Medical; 1982.

28. Chinoy MR. Lung growth and development. *Front Biosci.* 2003;8:d392-d415.

29. **Massery M.** Multisystem clinical implications of impaired breathing mechanics and postural control. In: Frownfelter D, Dean E, eds. *Cardiovascular and Pulmonary Physical Therapy: Evidence to Practice.* 5th ed. St. Louis, MO: Elsevier-Mosby; 2012.

30. Campbell S, Palisano RJ, Orlin MN. *Physical Therapy for Children.* 4th ed. Phildelphia, PA: Elsevier; 2010.

31. Williams PL, Warwick R, eds. *Gray's Anatomy.* 36th ed. Philadelphia, PA: W.B. Saunders Company; 1980.

32. Lyons HA, Tanner TW. Total lung volume and its subdivisions in children: normal standards. *J Appl Physiol.* 1962;17:601-604.

33. Robinson S. Experimental studies of physical fitness in relation to age. *Arbeitsphysiologie.* 1938;10:318-323.

34. Armstrong N, Kirby BJ, McManus AM, Welsman JR. Prepubescents' ventilatory responses to exercise with reference to sex and body size. *Chest.* 1997;112:1554-1560.

35. Cassels DE, Morse M. *Cardiopulmonary Data for Children and Young Adults.* Springfield, IL: Charles C Thomas; 1962:52-57.

36. Morse M, Schultz FW, Cassels DE. Relation of age to physiological responses of the older boy (10-17 years) to exercise. *J Appl Physiol.* 1949;1:683-709.

37. *Mosby's Medical Dictionary.* 8th ed. Philadelphia, PA: Elsevier; 2009.

38. Stout J. Physical fitness during childhood and adolescence. In: Campbell S, Vander Linden DW, Palisano RJ, eds. *Physical Therapy for Children.* 3rd ed. Philadelphia, PA: Elsevier; 2006.

39. Pate RR. A new definition of youth fitness. *Phys Sportsmed.* 1983;11:77-83.

40. Pate RR, Shephard RJ. Characteristics of physical fitness in youth. In: Gisolfi CV, Lamb DR, eds. *Perspectives in Exercise Science and Sports Medicine. Vol. 2: Youth, Exercise, and Sport.* Indianapolis, IN: Benchmark Press; 1989:1-45.

41. Armstrong N, Welsman J. Assessment and interpretation of aerobic fitness in children and adolescents. *Exerc Sport Sci Rev.* 1994;22:435-475.

42. Armstrong N, Welsman J. Development of aerobic fitness. *Pediatr Exerc Sci.* 2000;12:128-149.

43. Mácek M, Vávra J, Novosadová I. Prolonged exercise in prepubertal boys: I. Cardiovascular and metabolic adjustment. *Eur J Appl Physiol.* 1976;35:291-298.

44. Mobert J, Koch G, Humplik O, Oyen EM. Cardiovascular adjustment to supine and seated postures: effect of physical training. In: Oseid S, Carlsen KH, eds. *Children and Exercise.* XIII. Champaign, IL: Human Kinetics; 1989:165-182.

45. Obert P, Mandigout S, Nottin S, Vinet A, N'Guyen D, Lecoq AM. Cardiovascular responses to endurance training in children: effect of gender. *Eur J Clin Invest.* 2003;33:199-208.

46. Mandigout SA, Melin A, Lecoq AM, Courteix D, Obert P. Effect of gender in response to an aerobic training programme in prepubertal children. *Acta Paediatr.* 2001;90:9-15.

47. Rowland TW, Boyajian A. Aerobic response to endurance training in children. *Pediatrics.* 1995;96:654-658.

48. Tolfrey K, Campbell IG, Batterham AM. Aerobic trainability of purepubertal boys and girls. *Pediatr Exerc Sci.* 1998;10:248-263.

49. Eriksson BO, Koch G. Effect of physical training on hemodynamic response during submaximal and maximal exercise in 11-13-year old boys. *Acta Physiol Scand.* 1973;87:27-39.

50. Williford HN, Blessing DL, Duey WJ. Exercise training in black adolescents: changes in blood lipids and VO_{2max}. *Ethnicity Dis.* 1996;6:279-285.

51. Yoshizawa SH, Honda H, Nakamura N, Itoh K, Watanbe N. Effects of an 18-month endurance run training program on maximal aerobic power in 4- to 6-year-old girls. *Pediatr Exerc Sci.* 1997;9:33-43.

52. Eliakim A, Scheet T, Allmendinger N, Brasel JA, Cooper DM. Training, muscle volume, and energy expenditure in nonobese American girls. *J Appl Physiol.* 2001;90:35-44.

53. Ignico AA, Mahon AD. The effects of physical fitness programs on low-fit children. *Res Q Exerc Sport.* 1995;66: 85-90.

54. McManus AN, Armstrong N, Williams CA. Effect of training on the anaerobic power and anaerobic performance of prepubertal girls. *Acta Paediatr.* 1997;86:456-459.

55. Rowland TW, Martel L, Vanderburgh P, Manos T, Charkoudian N. The influence of short-term aerobic training on blood lipids in healthy 10-12 year old children. *Int J Sports Med.* 1996;17:487-492.

56. Shore S, Shephard RJ. Immune responses to exercise and training: a comparison of children and young adults. *Pediatr Exerc Sci.* 1998;10:210-226.

57. Welsman JR, Armstrong N, Withers S. Responses of young girls to two modes of aerobic training. *Br J Sports Med.* 1997;21:139-142.

58. Williams CA, Armstrong N, Powell J. Aerobic responses of prepubertal boys to two modes of aerobic training. *Br J Sports Med.* 2000;34:268-173.

59. Rowland TW. Effect of prolonged inactivity on aerobic fitness in children. *J Sports Med Phys Fitness.* 1994;34:147-155.

60. Rowland TW, Blum JW. Cardiac dynamics during upright cycle exercise in boys. *Am J Hum Biol.* 2000;12:749-757.

61. Payne VG, Morrow JR. The effect of physical training on prepubescent VO_2 max: a meta-analysis. *Res Q.* 1993;64:305-313.

62. Jones DA, Round JM. Strength and muscle growth. In: Armstrong N, van Mechelen W, eds. *Paediatric Exercise Science and Medicine.* Oxford University Press; 2000:133-142.

63. Blimkie CJR, Sale DG. Strength development and trainability during childhood. In: Van Praagh E, ed. *Paediatric Anaerobic Performance.* Champaign, IL: Human Kinetics; 1998:193-224.

64. Froberg K, Lammert O. Development of muscle strength during childhood. In: Bar-Or O, ed. *The Child and Adolescent Athlete.* Oxford: Blackwell Science; 1996:42-53.

65. Guesens P, Cantator F, Nijis J, Proesmans W, Emma F, Dequeker J. Heterogeneity of growth of bone in children at the spine, radius, and total skeleton. *Growth Dev Aging.* 1991;55:249-256.

66. Bonjour JF, Theintz G, Buch B, Slosman D, Rizzoli R. Critical years and stages of puberty for spinal and femoral bone mass accumulation during adolescence. *J Clin Endocrin Soc.* 1991;73:555-563.

67. Southard RN, Morris JD, Mahan JG, Hayes JR, Torch MA, Sommer A. Bone mass in healthy children: Measurement with quantitative DXA. *Radiology.* 1991;179:735-738.

68. Gordon CL, Halton JM, Atkinson SA, Webber CE. The contributions of growth and puberty to peak bone mass. *Growth Dev Aging.* 1991;55:257-262.

69. Glastre C, Braillon P, David L, Cochat P, Meunier PJ, Delmas PD. Measurement of bone mineral content of the lumbar spine by dual energy X-ray absorptiometry in normal children: correlations with growth parameters. *J Clin Endocrinol Metab.* 1990;70:1330-1333.

70. Gilanz V, Gibbons DT, Carlson M. Peak trabecular vertebral density: a comparison of adolescent and adult females. *Calcif Tissue Int.* 1988;43:260-262

71. Whiting WC, Zernicke RF. *Biomechanics of Musculoskeletal Injury.* Champaign, IL: Human Kinetics; 1998.

72. Carter DR, Fyhrie CB, Whalen RT. Trabecular bone density and loading history: regulation of connective tissue biology by mechanical energy. *J Biomech.* 1987;20:785-794.

73. Payne VG, Morrow JR, Johnson L, Dalton SN. Resistance training in children and youth: a meta-analysis. *Res Q Exerc Sport.* 1997;68:80-88.

74. Cronin JB, McNair PJ, Marshall RN. Is velocity-specific training important in improving functional performance? *J Sports Med Phys Fitness.* 2002;42:267-273.

CASE 2-1

Joanell A. Bohmert, PT, DPT, MS

EXAMINATION

History

Current Condition/Chief Complaint

Jill, a 15-year-old female with cerebral palsy (CP), was referred to physical therapy for an evaluation as part of her comprehensive 3-year reevaluation for special education services. She was a general education ninth-grader at her local public high school.

Clinician Comment *CP is a nonprogressive neurological condition that results from an insult to the CNS in utero, at birth, or within the first 2 years that results in a movement disorder.[1] Cognition, learning ability, vision, and hearing may also be affected. The term CP covers a wide array of symptoms that have been classified by area of body affected, type of movement disorder, or functional movement abilities.*

While the pathology in the CNS does not progress, it has ongoing impact on development, growth, and movement. CP affects motor coordination, postural control, and the use of muscles in a smooth, efficient manner. The ability of the muscle to relax, extend, or contract easily and smoothly may also be affected. Spasticity may be present and may interfere or assist with movement and posture.[2]

Federal legislation mandates free and appropriate education for all children. The Individuals with Disabilities Education Act established the criteria and requirements that individual states must follow when providing educational services to students with identified special needs.[3] A student may receive special education services if he or she meets state education eligibility criteria, requires specialized instruction, or demonstrates an educational need. These services support the student to be successful in general education. Physical therapy is a related service available to special education students to aid them in being successful in their educational setting. For example, physical therapy is available to a special education student who needs help to access and move in his or her current, and future, educational settings. By age 16 years, schools must address any needs the student may have in the areas of transition, training, education, employment, independent living skills, and community participation.[4]

Social History/Environment

Jill lived with her mother, stepfather, and 2 brothers aged 5 and 9 years in a 3-bedroom split-entry home. Her mother worked at a law office as an administrative assistant. Her stepfather was a department store manager. Her father lived 2 hours away and worked in construction. Jill would spend holidays and 1 month in the summer with her father.

Jill was a ninth-grade student at her neighborhood high school. To accommodate the large number of students, the school building was large and multilevel with elevators. She used a manual wheelchair for her primary mobility. She was, however, able to walk for short, in-room distances by holding onto objects or with the assistance of a classmate or teacher. Jill had an Individual Education Plan (IEP) that listed accommodations and program modifications that she needed while at school. The accommodations included the following:

- A table/desk close to the classroom exit door
- Shortened or modified assignments
- Copy of teacher's notes
- Extra set of textbooks to keep at home
- Early release from classes to avoid congestion in hallways
- A locker on the end of a row
- Assistance for getting lunch and carrying a tray
- Use of handicapped-accessible bathroom with rails and large enough to accommodate her wheelchair
- Special transportation
- An evacuation plan

Jill was reported to be a good self-advocate by informing her teachers of her abilities and needs.

Clinician Comment *Transition to high school is a major event. Students typically move from a smaller middle school to a larger high school. In Jill's case, she went from a single-level middle school with 1240 students to a large, multilevel high school with 2870 students.*

The physical environment at home, school, and in the community may be a challenge for Jill when using her wheelchair or when walking. The environment can aid or hinder movement. She also needed to be aware of how the environment changed when people were added and it became highly variable and unpredictable. An open hallway was easy to wheel through when empty but quite challenging when filled with students going in multiple directions or just standing still, talking, and passing time. Jill also needed to be aware of routes to exit her home or school for emergency evacuation as the designated route may not be accessible to her.

Social/Health Habits

Jill and her family were very active in school and community activities. Jill enjoyed going out with friends, shopping, movies, and reading. The family had a family membership to a community health club. She enjoyed using the pool at the health club. She hadn't used the weight machines because she didn't think she could get on and off or lift the weights.

Clinician Comment *Jill enjoyed going out in the community and participating in activities with her brothers and friends. Membership at the community health club allowed her to incorporate fitness into her weekly routine.*

Medical/Surgical History

Jill was diagnosed with CP, spastic diplegia, as an infant. Jill was born at 28 weeks weighing 2 pounds, 6 ounces. She had delays in gross and fine motor skills, while language and cognition followed appropriate developmental milestones. Jill had multiple orthopedic surgeries to correct the alignment of her legs. Jill's spasticity had been managed with Botox injections to specific leg muscles at various times throughout her childhood. Jill reported that the injections were not successful, so she had an intrathecal baclofen pump (ITBP) implanted 4 years prior. Jill reported she felt her legs were "looser" and it was easier to move since she had received the pump.

Her most recent orthopedic surgery was a single-event multilevel surgery (SEMLS) 2 years prior and included bilateral proximal femoral derotation osteotomy, bilateral distal femoral extension osteotomies, bilateral patellar tendon advancements, right distal tibial derotation osteotomy, and bilateral Vulpius Achilles tendon lengthening. Her hardware from this surgery was to be removed in the upcoming summer. She had solid ankle-foot orthoses (AFOs) following surgery to assist in maintaining length of her Achilles tendons.

Clinician Comment *Spasticity is a symptom of an upper motor neuron insult that presents as muscle hyperactivity to a velocity-dependent passive stretch.[2,5,6] It can interfere with the ability of the muscles to function appropriately and may affect range of motion (ROM) and movement.[7] It can also provide tension in the muscle that allows the performance of functional activities.[2,8] Spasticity has been viewed as a major contributor to the difficulties with movement and function in children with CP and is frequently managed with pharmacological agents, surgery, orthotics, and therapy.[2,8-10]*

Botox, or botulinum toxin, is a medication that provides a chemical denervation of the motor unit within a specific muscle, decreasing its ability to contract.[2] It is administered through injection into the muscle at the motor unit endplate, causing inhibition of acetylcholine release at the synaptic cleft.[11] It has been used in children with CP to decrease muscle tightness and improve movement by decreasing the ability of the muscle to contract. There has been debate about spasticity and how it actually affects movement, which has resulted in reconsideration of Botox as an appropriate method of improving function.[2,7,9,10]

An ITBP is an implanted device that provides baclofen medication directly into the intrathecal space of the spinal column.[8,12] It provides a more general impact on overall limb or trunk spasticity and is removable if it is not effective for the individual.[2] The ITBP is about the size and shape of a hockey puck that is inserted through an incision over the lateral aspect of the abdomen. It is secured in place under the skin, over the abdominal muscles. A catheter is attached to the pump and runs internally to the spine. Through a small incision along the spine, the tip of the catheter is inserted into the intrathecal space of the spinal column. The vertebral level at which the catheter is inserted is dependent on the functional effect that is desired. For example, placement at T10 or lower will affect the legs more than the arms, while placement at C5 to T2 will affect the arms more than the legs.[8,12]

Orthopedic surgeries are used to correct alignment issues that may be present because of imbalance in muscle tension, flexibility, and decreased strength. The purpose of SEMLS of the LEs is to decrease crouch and prevent future complications of crouch including arthritis, pain, contractures, and loss of walking ability as an adult.[13,14]

A proximal femoral derotation osteotomy is performed to correct excessive femoral anteversion that leads to hip internal rotation and subluxation. It involves removing a wedge of bone of the proximal femur then rotating the bone to the desired angle of alignment. The new bone location is secured with pins, screws, and/or plates.

A distal femoral extension osteotomy is performed to increase knee extension lost because of excessive crouch when standing and walking.[14] It involves removing a wedge of the distal femur from the anterior surface then realigning bone and securing it in place with screws and plates.

A patellar tendon advancement is performed to correct for an over-lengthened patella tendon as a result of a crouched stance/gait.[14] If the epiphyseal plate is still present, only the tendon is moved. If it is closed, then a wedge of bone with the tendon attached is cut out of the proximal tibia and moved lower and reattached with plates, screws, wire, or sutures.

The Vulpius Achilles tendon lengthening is performed to lengthen the Achilles tendon and correct pull on the calcaneous.[13,15] It is performed through a longitudinal incision over the Achilles tendon, which is then cut to allow lengthening.

Reported Functional Status

Jill reported that she was fairly independent getting dressed at home but needed help getting her shoes on over her AFOs. She did her own hair and makeup. She was independent with bathing, including getting in and out of tub with the use of a bath chair outside of the tub to assist her transfer. She was able to do simple cooking. She had concerns about using the stove and oven because her impaired balance might compromise her safety handling hot items. Jill reported she needed some assistance with dressing at school, such as getting her coat on and changing for physical education. At home, she walked up stairs using the wall and hand railing, but she would often scoot down on her seat as she felt safer and it was faster.

Jill reported she used her wheelchair at school because she did not think she could walk safely in the congested hallways. She left class early, which helped her avoid crowds. Jill reported she would like to be more independent in her mobility and daily routine. She wanted to be able to be more active in her community. She especially wanted to go to her friends' houses. This was difficult because it required transporting her wheelchair, and her friends' homes might not be accessible. Jill wanted to improve her ability and confidence with walking.

Clinician Comment *Students with CP who were walkers in elementary and middle school frequently transition to using a wheelchair as they age as the amount of energy needed to walk greater distances in shorter periods is too high. It is also challenging to use a wheelchair in the halls and a walker in the classroom as it is difficult to transport a walker while wheeling. Staff could transport a walker; however, this is not reality in future settings or in current community settings. Jill needed to bring one or the other. It would be appropriate to explore other assistive*

devices such as forearm crutches, walking sticks, or various canes as these could be easily attached to the wheelchair.

Jill would like to be more independent. She would like to be able to do more with her friends but has difficulty getting into their vans or trucks. She also would like to be able to walk up and down stairs instead of scooting on her seat. At school, she would like to be able to change into shorts and a T-shirt for physical education.

Medications

Jill had an ITBP implanted 4 years ago. Her baclofen dosage was monitored at her medical facility. She had an increased dose before bed to aid in sleeping and a smaller dose throughout her day. She did not take any other medications.

Clinician Comment *ITBPs are used to deliver a specific dosage of baclofen directly into the intrathecal space of the spinal column. The pump holds a reserve of medication, in this case baclofen, which is released based on the programming of the pump. The pump is refilled using a transdermal needle puncture.[12] How frequent the pump needs to be refilled is dependent on the dosage and the size of the pump. Baclofen is used to decrease muscle tone. It can be taken orally; however, it is more effective when delivered directly into the spinal fluid. Baclofen, acting prior to the synapse, inhibits and suppresses the excitatory neurotransmitters at the synaptic junction.[16] When the desired outcome is to have more effect on the legs, the catheter is commonly placed between T8 and T12. While this level will affect the legs, it will also affect the activity of the abdominals, which may make it difficult to gain strength to stabilize the core for weight shifting through the pelvis. Adjusting dosage and delivery times to allow more activity for strengthening and use of muscles may be beneficial. Reviews on use of ITBPs in children and adolescents with spasticity who can walk indicate that it may improve their ability to move, but it does not change their level of functional walking.[2,8,17] Possible loss of function needs to be considered if the individual is using her spasticity to stand or transfer.*

Other Clinical Tests

Additional educational testing took place as part of this comprehensive educational evaluation. Cognition and academic status were assessed by the school psychologist; communication by the speech and language pathologist; impact of disability on education by the special education teacher for students with physical and health disabilities; and motor skill development and abilities by the adapted physical education teacher. Jill qualified for special education under the category of Physically Impaired. She also qualified for adapted physical education.

Clinician Comment *Jill had a diagnosis that was known to affect movement and ability to participate in home, school, work, and community activities. She had a supportive family and school program and was interested in becoming more independent. She reported decreased strength and endurance and safety concerns.*

Next, in the examination portion of the evaluation, was the systems review. The limited examination of the systems review aided in the identification of indicated tests and measures as the examination moved forward as well as establishing that there were no contraindications for Jill to be seen in physical therapy. As Jill had a diagnosis that was known to affect her systems, it was expected that her results would vary from typical.

Systems Review

Cardiovascular/Pulmonary

HR (resting): 94 bpm
Respiration rate: 24 bpm
BP: 100/70 mm Hg
Edema: no edema present

Clinician Comment *Jill demonstrated vital signs within the normal range for typical adolescents when at rest. CP frequently results in difficulty moving in an efficient manner, so it was important to measure Jill's response to activity and exercise to determine not only how she responded to movement, but also how quickly she recovered.*

Integumentary

Skin Integrity

Jill had mild acne on her face. She wore bilateral solid-ankle AFOs. Her skin was calloused over the medial malleolus, bilaterally, especially on the right. She reported no problems with skin breakdown from sitting. She relieved pressure by getting out of her wheelchair or doing wheelchair pushups.

Presence of Scar Formation

Jill had well-healed incision scars bilaterally on hips, thighs, knees, and over her Achilles tendons from previous orthopedic and soft tissue surgeries. Also, she had a well-healed incision scar on her right lower abdomen and posterior spine from placement of the intrathecal pump and catheter.

Clinician Comment *Use of orthotics and assistive devices can result in pressure on bony prominences, which can affect alignment and position of feet, legs, and body. Changes as a result of growth are often seen first in the fit of orthotics, so they should be monitored on a regular basis. Pressure-relieving strategies need to be used throughout the day.*

Musculoskeletal

Gross Symmetry/Posture

Jill's standing posture was asymmetrical with shoulders rounded forward, increased lumbar lordosis, and internally rotated and flexed hips and knees. Her sitting posture in the wheelchair was asymmetrical. She sat with her trunk leaning to the left with rounded back and shoulder girdle posture and her pelvis rotated forward on the left, causing the left knee to be further forward than the right.

Gross Range of Motion

Limitations in gross active shoulder, hip, and knee motions.

Gross Strength

Limitations noted in extremities and trunk.

Height/Weight

61 inches; 108 pounds

Clinician Comment *It is common to have asymmetry and postural deviations with CP. Changes in posture may be due to multiple factors, including decreased strength, limited ROM, contractures, and difficulty with movement.*

Neuromuscular

Balance

With her AFOs, Jill was unable to stand still in one place, requiring stepping to avoid falling. She tended to weave and used increased trunk movements to maintain her balance. She reported falling whenever she was bumped while in class or tripped herself.

Locomotion

She was able to wheel her manual wheelchair independently for distance. She walked in classrooms using the wall or objects for balance. Observed lateral sway when walking in class with or without hand support.

Transfers

Reported independent from wheelchair to/from walker, desk, and toilet.

Transitions

Movements were slow and deliberate. Jill had difficulty ascending and descending stairs and needed to use the handrail going up or down. She had difficulty with eccentric control and sustaining postures when moving. This was seen when she was descending stairs and when she lowered herself to sit in her wheelchair or desk.

Clinician Comment *Observation of movement provided valuable information that helped to decide what needed further testing. Jill demonstrated ability to move independently using natural supports. While this type of movement may be considered functional for CP, it was not performed with the speed or efficiency of her peers.*

Communication, Affect, Cognition, Language, and Learning Style

Jill reported she got As and Bs in her classes. English was her first language. She preferred demonstration and picture diagrams for learning movement. She reported that she learned better by listening and discussing in classes. Jill was alert and oriented to person, place, time, and situation. She demonstrated selective attention typical for her age. Interested in becoming more active and fit, she was motivated to improve her movement.

Clinician Comment *Jill demonstrated characteristics that were consistent with a diagnosis of CP spastic diplegia. While her resting vitals were within an acceptable range, it needed to be known how she responded to activity. Testing of her aerobic capacity and endurance was needed. Since children with CP tend to grow at a slower rate, it was important to have baseline measurements for height and weight as well as other anthropometric measures to document rate of change. Her ROM was limited actively and her posture suggested potential contractures.*

Individuals with CP have difficulty moving as part of their condition; it was important, therefore, to determine what was interfering with her movement and mobility independence. Her muscle performance was decreased as demonstrated in posture and gait deviations and difficulty with balance. Her motor function needed further examination looking at how she planned and varied movement.

Fit and functional use of her wheelchair and assistive device needed to be evaluated. The integumentary screen identified a number of scars; however, all were healed and did not require further examination. Her orthotics did need further examination to assess their fit in relation to her growth as well as the impact on her function.

Jill was 15 years old and in high school, so areas of transition needed to be assessed to further address her functioning in self-care and home management, as well as work and leisure integration. Environmental, home, and work barriers as they limit or aid function needed to be assessed.

Tests and Measures

Aerobic Capacity/Endurance

Energy Expenditure Index (EEI): Jill was asked to walk independently at a fast pace for 2 minutes. She was able to walk the entire time but would periodically veer toward the wall, touching it to maintain her balance. The following measures were recorded:

	HEART RATE (BPM)	OXYGEN SATURATION %
Starting	103	98
Stopping, after 2 minutes	188	100
MINUTES OF RECOVERY		
1	132	96
2	110	97
3	107	97
4	106	97
5	103	96

EEI in Heartbeats/Meter

Wheeling regular pace	0.168
Wheeling at fast pace	0.334
Walking independently at regular pace	1.24
Walking independently at fast pace	1.80

Clinician Comment *The EEI measures the amount of energy used over a 2-minute walk or run. It is easy to use in a school setting and is based on change in HR over distance walked per minute (walking HR – resting HR/ distance in meters/minute).[18-20] The result is a ratio that provides the heart bpm walked. Resting HR was measured after sitting for 5 minutes. Walking HR was the HR taken immediately upon stopping the walk. Rate of recovery can also be measured by tracking HR each minute for 5 minutes after stopping. O$_2$ saturation may also be measured when a pulse oximeter is used. A measurement wheel is used to measure distance walked; an advantage of this instrument is you can follow the path walked by the student rather than just a straight line.*

In typically developing adolescents, 0.4 bpm is common for walking at a preferred pace, while running is 0.7 bpm.[18,20] Jill's EEI demonstrated she was very efficient when wheeling on a flat, smooth indoor surface. When walking, however, her energy use spiked, indicating she was using a lot of energy to walk, even when walking at her preferred rate. She walked farther in her first minute compared to the second, indicating she had little reserves from which to draw. The EEI requires walking for only 2 minutes, which is too short of a time period for Jill to get to most of her classes. In addition to improving her aerobic capacity and endurance, Jill needed a method to conserve her energy to allow optimal academic performance throughout her school day. Whether to use the wheelchair or to walk still needed to be determined.

Anthropometric Characteristics

Body Fat Composition

SKINFOLD CALIPER MEASUREMENT		
Side (Dominant)	*Area*	*Measurement (mm)*
Right	Tricep	16
Right	Bicep	6
Right	Subscapular	12
Right	Suprailiac	16
Total mm measured		50
% body fat		26.5

Body Fat Percentage

Body fat handheld analyzer	27.4%
Skinfold measurement	26.5%
Height/weight formula (kg/m²)	20.43%

Clinician Comment *Body composition may be measured in many ways. For body fat, it has become popular to use an impedance device such as a handheld analyzer or a scale as it is easy to administer and takes age, weight, height, and gender into consideration. Another method is the use of a skinfold caliper in which the skin in 4 specific locations (tricep, bicep, subscapular, suprailiac) is pinched and measured with the specifically designed caliper. The last method is to calculate the body mass index (BMI) using height and weight. There are a variety of formulas that attempt to take age, gender, and muscle mass into account; however, this calculation may overestimate or underestimate the actual percentage of body fat. While none of these methods are totally accurate, they are easily available and easy to use in the clinic or school setting and give an estimation of body fat. Because of the impact of the endocrine system on body composition at puberty, it is important to use a scale that differentiates males and females.*

Body Measurements/Circumference

AREA MEASURED	MEASUREMENT (INCHES) *All measurements are circumference except height and weight*		
		LEFT	RIGHT
Height	61		
Weight	108 pounds		
Shoulders	34		
Chest (under arms)	32		
Bicep (flexed)		9⁷/₈	10¹/₄
Forearm (wrist flexed)		9	9⁵/₈
Waist	28		
Hips	34⁷/₈		
Thigh (midpoint)		17³/₈	17³/₄
Thigh (widest point)		18⁷/₈	19¹/₈
Calf (widest when flexed)		11³/₈	11³/₈

Clinician Comment *Body circumference is measured using a standard flexible tape measure. The purpose of measurement is to evaluate how interventions affect changes in body dimensions. Body circumference is frequently used to monitor weight loss as it more accurately measures change than weighing. The comparison is against self and not other adolescents as there are no standardized measures. Circumference measurements are often motivated as they show the student how his or her body has changed with exercise that may be attributed to weight loss and/or muscle gain. It is important to take height and weight measurements at the same time as circumference since changes in circumference may also be from growth or weight gain/loss.*

Overall, Jill appeared healthy with weight appropriate for height. It was noted that the widest part of calf was just below her knee joint and stopped on top of where her AFO ended. Her lower leg was very flat under the area covered by the AFO. Her feet also appeared flat with little muscle development and definition.

Jill demonstrated body dimensions for her right arm and leg (her dominant side) that were slightly larger on the left. Lack of lower leg and foot muscular development is typical when AFOs, especially solid ankle, are worn. An AFO is designed to restrict unwanted movement and may, therefore, limit muscle development. It can impose a "forced disuse" of the lower leg, ankle, and foot. The gastrocnemius, being a 2-joint muscle, will develop above the brace but is limited in how much it can develop because of the constraint of the brace around the leg and the limited (or no) motion at the ankle. For development of ankle and foot muscles, the ankle needs to be allowed to move. Consideration needs to be given to the benefits and limitations of orthotics in relation to the development of strength while maintaining appropriate alignment.

Range of Motion (Including Muscle Length)

Joint ROM was measured with Jill lying supine on an examination table. Measurements were taken at the end of available passive motion using a 360-degree goniometer. Motion was provided at a slow, steady pace to decrease changes in muscle tension during movement.

JOINT MOTION	LEFT (DEGREES)	RIGHT (DEGREES)
Hip flexion	0 to 123	0 to 127
Hip extension	–15	–10
Hip external rotation	0 to 20	0 to 30
Hip internal rotation	0 to 60	0 to 50
Hip abduction	0 to 30	0 to 40
Hip adduction	0 to 40	0 to 30
Knee flexion	18 to 153	15 to 156
Knee extension	–18	–15
Ankle dorsiflexion	0 to 25	0 to 27
Ankle plantarflexion	0 to 31	0 to 35
Hamstring length— popliteal angle	37 short of full extension	25 short of full extension

Clinician Comment *When measuring hip motions, it is important to note the position of the pelvis.[21] Individuals with CP often have an anterior tilt of the pelvis even when supine. This anterior tilt can result in an inaccurate measurement of the hamstrings. They will measure shorter than they actually are as they are already in a partially lengthened position due to the tilt of the pelvis.*

Hamstring length is traditionally measured using a straight leg raise. This may be difficult to measure in individuals with CP because of increased stiffness, difficulty isolating leg motions, and increased anterior tilt of the pelvis. An alternate measure, the popliteal angle, is often used.[22] This is performed by holding one leg in extension on the mat, then placing the other hip in 90 degrees of flexion with the knee in 90 degrees of flexion. The lower leg is then raised while keeping the hip at 90 degrees. The measurement is taken when the lower leg can no longer be raised. The closer

the lower leg is to full knee extension, or 0 degrees, the longer the hamstrings.

Jill had limitations in hip extension and external rotation with excessive motion in internal rotation. Her knee extension lacked full ROM while her hamstring length was decreased (more on the left than right). Passive range of motion (PROM) is greater than active range of motion (AROM) due in part to decreased strength to actively move the joint. This was especially seen in ankle motions.

Muscle Performance (Including Strength, Power, and Endurance)

Hip flexion, knee extension, knee flexion, and hip abduction strength were measured using a handheld dynamometer (HHD) in a "make" test. Hip flexion, knee extension, and knee flexion were measured sitting on a leg extension machine with a seat belt around the pelvis with the hip and knee at 90 degrees. The dynamometer was placed 2 inches from the top of the patella for hip flexion, 2 inches above the bend in the ankle for knee extension, and 2 inches from the base of the heel on the heel cord for knee flexion. Hip abduction was measured with Jill lying on her side on a mat with her pelvis and trunk stabilized by one examiner. The dynamometer was placed on the lateral aspect of the femur 2 inches above the knee joint. Each muscle group was measured 3 times, with each trial lasting 4 seconds. The highest force produced was recorded.

MUSCLE GROUP	LEFT (POUNDS)	RIGHT (POUNDS)
Hip flexion	29	39
Knee extension	30	48
Knee flexion	4.0	6.3
Hip abduction	8.9	12.1

Ankle plantarflexion was measured standing using the number of toe raises performed with the knee straight and then bent. Single leg (20 considered Normal; 19 to 10, Good; 9 to 1, Fair) Right (R): 2 able to lift heel 1 inch (not full range); Left (L): 1 able to lift heel 0.5 inch (not full range). Ankle dorsiflexion: unable to lift toes in standing; when supine, note minimal movement of ankle and toe extensors R greater than L.

Abdominal strength was measured with Jill supine on a mat performing a sit-up. With her arms crossed over her chest, she had difficulty lifting her head and shoulders off the mat. She was unable to isolate and use her transverse abdominals (maximal inhalation then forced exhalation causing stomach to flatten toward spine), or obliques or rectus.

Functional strength: When going up the stairs and wearing her AFOs, Jill had difficulty flexing either hip enough to place her foot on the next step. Without her AFOs, she had adequate hip flexion but had difficulty dorsiflexing her foot to clear her toe. With and without her AFOs, she had poor eccentric control for going down the stairs and lowering herself from standing to sitting, and slow controlled movements. Jill had poor contraction around her hip and pelvis for single-leg stance. In regular standing, Jill stood with her hips and knees flexed and internally rotated and had difficulty externally rotating her hips and straightening her knees. Jill had difficulty keeping her pelvis and legs forward while sidestepping. She was unable to sustain trunk and leg strength for activities such as transfers into vans and trucks. She was unable to produce enough force to lift moderate-to-heavy objects in sitting or standing. She was also unable to sustain strength to maintain a stable posture to lift her wheelchair.

Clinician Comment *In adolescents, manual muscle testing (MMT) may be used to assess strength. However, in individuals with CP, it may be difficult for the student to isolate movement because of difficulties with motor control and spasticity. MMT may be beneficial to determine strength that is below normal, but having a normal grade of strength may not translate to having enough strength or force generation to perform functional tasks. Hislop and Montgomery[23] provide a description of muscle activity pattern for typical functional activities for infants and children that may also be used when examining functional strength in older children and adolescents. In adolescents, it is important to be aware of the relationship between the strength of the examiner to that of the student. It is also important to standardize tester, position, and any other conditions to improve reliability between measures. MMT, functional skills, or dynamometry, depending on the purpose of examination, may be used to measure muscle strength.*

An HHD is an objective method for measurement force production in the school or clinic setting. It is a valid and reliable way of measuring isometric strength of a muscle group at a specific joint angle that is used to measure the impact of the strengthening program. When using an HHD, it is important to standardize the position of the individual, placement of the HHD, type of test (make or break), length of each trial (2 to 6 seconds), and examiner administering the test.[24] A make test requires the individual to push as hard as he or she can against the HHD while it is held in one place. The break test requires the examiner to exert tension against the individual while he or she attempts to hold the position. Either test has been shown to be appropriate with children, with the break test resulting in higher force production values and the make test being easier for children to understand and perform.[24]

Jill demonstrated deficits in muscle strength, power, and endurance. It was important to consider not only the patient's ability to produce force for a few seconds (testing situation), but also the ability to produce and sustain force over a period of time. Functionally, she was limited in activities that required sustained as well as controlled contraction. She was able to complete short bursts of strength but did not have the reserves to sustain anaerobic or aerobic activities. The majority of activities that Jill needed to perform required power moves versus endurance: sit to stand, transfers, stair ascending/descending, and single-leg stance. It was critical that her intervention program included training specifically for anaerobic muscle use.

Jill's difficulty with core strength (abdominals) may be related to placement of the ITBP catheter at T8-10. Baclofen may also affect the strength of hip muscles, especially smaller muscles around the hip used for stabilization and external rotation.

Posture

Jill stood in a crouched (hip and knee flexion with hip internal rotation) pattern. She had increased lordosis in her low back and kyphosis in her mid-back. Her head was forward and her shoulders rounded. When wearing her AFOs, she stood forward on the ball of her foot, heels off the ground. This threw her trunk forward, so to counterbalance, she had to pull her upper trunk posterior, which increased her lumbar lordosis.

When sitting, Jill had more weight on the right hip with her legs windswept to the right and her trunk leaning to the left to counterbalance. Her trunk was also collapsed into flexion. Jill stated her preferred posture felt "normal" or in centered alignment. She was not aware of her posture or how to correct her posture so that she was in midline and symmetrical.

Clinician Comment *With CP, there are differences within a limb or the trunk as well as between limbs. Muscle stiffness, joint contractures, and difficulty with timing and sequencing may all contribute to poor alignment. Changes in visual spatial perception, righting reactions, and somatosensory may also impact alignment. Movement and the ability to use functional strength to initiate movement and sustain postures also influence posture.*

Jill's posture was consistent with her limitations in joint ROM and decreased muscle strength. She demonstrated a lack of awareness of where her body was in relation to upright midline positions. This made it difficult for her to correct or fix her alignment on her own.

Gait, Locomotion, and Balance

Gait

Jill had 2 forms of mobility: she could walk for short distances in her classroom or at home, and she wheeled herself in her manual wheelchair for moderate and long distances.

She was independent in propelling herself in her manual wheelchair throughout her school and home environments. She reported she had difficulty wheeling or walking on grass, rough terrains, snow, and ice. When going up or down stairs, Jill would go one step at a time, leading with her right leg. She was able to go up and down a standard curb but would stop before stepping off it.

When walking in the hall, Jill trailed the wall (walked with one hand sliding along the wall) to keep her balance and decrease the amount of energy she used. She could walk 3 to 10 feet without touching a support surface or object. She had used a reverse walker in the past but preferred to now walk without an assistive device. Her gait was different when wearing her AFOs compared with not wearing them. When wearing her AFOs, her hips were internally rotated and flexed with her knees turned in. She would lurch from side to side, shifting her weight through her shoulders instead of her pelvis.

Locomotion

Jill reported she crawled or walked using a support surface to get around her house. She was able to get down to the floor from sitting or standing and vice versa using a support surface or physical assistance. She was able to move from sitting on the floor to lying and then back to sitting by rolling to her side and pushing up with her arms.

Balance

Standing balance: Standing balance was tested without AFOs, on 2 feet with feet together and in single-leg stance. Both tests were conducted under 2 conditions: eyes open and eyes closed. During testing, Jill was allowed to crouch or move her arms to assist her balance. For the single-leg stance, the timing was started when her nonsupporting foot lifted off the ground. For double-leg and single-leg stance, timing was stopped when her supporting foot lifted off the ground.

CONDITION	BOTH FEET (MIN/SEC)	LEFT (MIN/SEC)	RIGHT (MIN/SEC)
Eyes open	05.00.00	00.01.62	00.03.50
Eyes closed	05.00.00	00.02.00	00.02.46

Jill was very crouched during the 5-minute balance trial with her eyes open or closed. Her balance on a single leg was not more than the time needed to take a step. She had difficulty shifting her weight through her hips onto the stance leg and, as a result, was off balance before lifting her opposite leg. Jill tended to lower herself into a crouch rather than use ankle strategies to maintain her balance on 2 feet when balancing without her AFOs. When wearing her AFOs, Jill was forced to use either a hip or stepping strategy, as her ankles were not able to bend in the AFOs.

Clinician Comment *The Gross Motor Function Classification System-Expanded and Revised (GMFCS-E&R) was developed to categorize children with CP based on their self-initiated movement in daily life.[25] The 5 levels emphasize what abilities can currently be performed in typical environments such as home, school, and community. It is different from other tests in that it is interested in what individuals do versus the quality of how they do it. The GMFCS includes youths aged 12 to 18 years as well as the concepts of the World Health Organization's International Classification of Functioning, Disability and Health (ICF). It is a common classification for individuals with CP and reports at what level the individual is functioning.[26] For example, Level I is Walks Without Limitations, while Level V is Transported in a Manual Wheelchair. Jill was classified as Level III as she was capable of walking with a handheld device even though she chose to not use one. In addition, she used a manual wheelchair for mobility at school and in community and required a support surface or physical assistance to get up from the floor.*

Jill had difficulty with balance, which appeared to be related to decreased strength in her legs and trunk. This was determined as she was able to balance on 2 feet with eyes open or closed for 5 minutes but had difficulty with single-leg balance. In addition, when wearing her AFOs, she was unable to use ankle strategies for balance and was forced to use either hip or stepping strategies.

Motor Function

Jill was able to initiate, vary speed, and stop movement of her arms without difficulty. She was also able to initiate movement of her trunk and legs but had difficulty varying speed and stopping movement. She tended to move quickly and had difficulty with timing and sequencing of muscles for slow, controlled movements, especially for eccentric control. Her ability to start, stop, and change directions improved when she was not wearing her AFOs.

Jill was able to anticipate and set her body for movement when sitting but had difficulty when she was standing. For example, when sitting, she was able to catch and throw a large ball with 2 hands, but when standing, she was unable to set her body to allow movement of her arms away from her body, especially over her head to throw. She demonstrated difficulty stabilizing her pelvis and weight shifting through pelvis when standing and walking without support, with or without her AFOs.

Clinician Comment *Individuals with CP frequently have difficulties with planning, initiating, modulating, and stopping movement. Depending on the area of the brain affected, movement may be minimally or significantly affected.*

Jill's difficulties with movement were not severe, but they contributed to a lack of variability in movement and the development of muscle strength and endurance. Her difficulty with movement appeared to be related to muscle weakness or fatigue rather than spasticity or motor planning.

Assistive and Adaptive Devices

Jill used a manual, ultra-light folding wheelchair with swing-away leg rests and a 2-inch foam cushion. Her wheelchair was in good condition and the fit was appropriate. Jill used a backpack that she hung on the push handles of her wheelchair. She also used a small pouch placed next to her right thigh for items she needed quick and easy access to, such as her cell phone, pens, pencils, and student identification.

Clinician Comment *Assessment of the type, condition, and use of a wheelchair was completed by looking at the wheelchair and observing Jill's use of it in various activities and environments. In addition, how Jill used the wheelchair needed to be considered so she had one that would allow her to participate in her preferred activities.*

The lighter the wheelchair, the easier it is to self-propel. Swing-away leg rests allow closer access to furniture or vehicles for transfers. Seating provides a base for posture as well as pressure relief for skin. The ease of wheeling and the ability to transfer or manage the wheelchair independently—including loading the wheelchair into and out of a car—are important considerations in wheelchair selection. A folding wheelchair provides more flexibility over a solid frame manual wheelchair or power wheelchair as it can be easily folded and put in most vehicles for transportation. In the educational setting, these devices would be included under the category of assistive technology.

Orthotic, Protective, and Supportive Devices

Jill wore bilateral, solid-ankle AFOs to support her ankle and foot in standing, to prevent crouched standing, and to assist her in walking. The fit was appropriate and the AFOs were in good condition.

Clinician Comment *Individuals with CP frequently use orthotics to improve alignment, support and protect joints, and improve gait and functional abilities. With CP spastic diplegia, AFOs are frequently prescribed to prevent a crouched posture in standing and walking with hopes of enabling the individual to continue to walk as she ages. There are, however, implications to wearing orthotics that limit ankle motion. These include the following:*

- *Balance strategies: When the ankle is free, Jill is able to use ankle, hip, and stepping strategies. These allow her to maintain static balance without swaying and to stand in one place.*
- *Development of muscles of the lower leg: When the ankle is allowed to move, the muscles are able to work and can be strengthened. An AFO not only restricts ankle motion, it restricts the ability of the leg muscles to expand because of the tight fit of the cuff.*
- *Neuromotor learning: Ankle motion allows for learning appropriate motor programs and timing and sequencing for mobility. It also allows for brain mapping of the ankle and foot.*
- *Functional use: Ankle motion allows for forced use instead of forced disuse of ankle and foot in functional activities. It allows for the use of new patterns of movement and strength that allow external rotation of hips, increased hip and knee extension, ankle plantar and dorsiflexion, movement of the leg over the foot that decreases crouch, circumduction, and excessive internal rotation of hip due to compensation to clear the foot when wearing braces.*

Jill was able to perform toe raises bilaterally and clear her foot when walking. She had baseline strength for movement and was an excellent candidate for a trial without wearing AFOs. These devices are also considered assistive technology in the educational setting.

Self-Care and Home Management

Additional information was obtained through observation and interview with Jill, her mother, and the school staff. Jill was independent in most activities of self-care and home management. She had to allow for the increased time it took her to complete these activities. She got up 2.5 hours before she needed to meet her bus in order to get ready for school and eat breakfast. She bathed and washed her hair in the evening instead of the morning to save time.

Jill reported she was more independent in dressing at home because she would lie down on the floor or her bed to dress. This, however, was not an option at school or in community settings. She was independent in toileting with the exception of needing assistance with pulling some of her pants up all the way.

Clinician Comment *Jill was independent in most self-care activities; however, it would take her at least twice as long to complete tasks compared with her peers. Jill's difficulty with ADL appeared to be related to a lack of flexibility and strength. Strategies that worked at home were not effective in other settings. This made it more difficult for her to participate in desired settings, such as at a friend's home or at school, and being independent at the community health club.*

Work, Community, and Leisure Integration

Jill completed simple chores at home. She did not yet have an after-school job. She reported she attended church and was a member of the youth group. She enjoyed shopping with friends. She reported that she was not able to go as often as she would like because she needed help getting the wheelchair into and out of a car. She reported she was able to wheel herself at the mall but friends would also push her. Jill wanted to get her driver's license so she could drive herself to activities and work.

Jill was looking for a job that could be performed sitting. Jill was able to transport light materials on her lap but would have difficulty with heavy materials. She was able to tolerate a full day of school. She was also able to stand and take breaks to relieve pressure and stiffness from sitting for extended periods of time. She would be able to stock shelves that were within her reach with light- to moderate-weight stock.

Clinician Comment *Jill was a typical teenager who wanted to hang out with her friends, get a job, and drive a car. Having CP affected her physical capacity and mobility as well as speed and efficiency for performing movement activities. Increased physical capacity would allow her to perform tasks at a competitive rate for employment as well as make it easier for her to do social activities.*

Environmental, Home, and Work Barriers

Additional information was obtained through observation and interview with Jill, her mother, and the school staff. Her kitchen was not accessible from a wheelchair, but she could stand at the counter and reach with one hand. She was able to get in and out of a car independently but needed assistance getting in and out of a van or truck. She was unable to place her wheelchair in any vehicle without help.

Jill was able to use the elevator at school independently. She was unable to safely or efficiently use the stairs at school. She was able to evacuate the building with her class when on the ground floor and used an evacuation chair or sling for evacuation from other levels. Jill was unable to ascend or descend bus steps because of difficulty lifting her legs high enough to accommodate the increased height of the bus steps. Jill needed a wheelchair-accessible bathroom and lift bus for transportation.

Jill was interested in a job when she got older. She would need a work environment that was accessible and allowed work from a sitting position.

Clinician Comment *Jill would benefit from education on how to evaluate community settings for access and strategies for evacuation.*

EVALUATION

Diagnosis

Jill was a 15-year-old girl attending ninth grade in her local high school. She had a medical diagnosis of CP, spastic diplegia with a history of multiple orthopedic surgeries, and an ITBP to manage spasticity. She participated in general education with support from special education and related services. She was referred as part of her 3-year special education reevaluation. Jill and her family expressed concerns about being more independent in transfers and mobility. Jill was also interested in getting stronger.

Jill had limitations in strength, endurance, coordination, balance, and flexibility that interfered with her ability to move. She had some difficulty with timing and sequencing of muscles for movement but was able to effectively plan movement. She had decreased physical capacity that affected her walking and participating in activities with her friends. Her primary problem appeared to be a lack of sufficient strength to perform movements and activities. Jill was diagnosed with impaired muscle performance.

Practice Pattern

Based on the history, systems review, and tests and measures, this patient was classified into the Preferred Practice Pattern: Musculoskeletal Practice Pattern 4C: Impaired Muscle Performance.

Clinician Comment *While the framework for Jill's evaluation was the practice pattern of Neuromuscular Impaired Motor Function and Sensory Integrity Associated with Nonprogressive Disorders of the Central Nervous System-Congenital Origin or Acquired in Infancy or Childhood 5C, it was not the pattern that described her assessed impairments best. Jill's function was limited most by impaired muscle performance, not motor function. It is important to put the client in the Preferred Practice Pattern that is appropriate for the primary problem identified for that client, not the client's identified medical diagnosis.*

International Classification of Functioning, Disability and Health Model of Disability

See ICF Model on page 69.

Prognosis

Jill's goals were to attain her highest level of fitness and function through participation in an individualized, high-intensity strength-training class. While Jill demonstrated limitations in joint ROM and decreased strength, she also demonstrated good motor planning skills, motivation, and an excellent work ethic. Her spasticity did not interfere with movement. Her primary problem was decreased strength or

ICF Model of Disablement for Jill

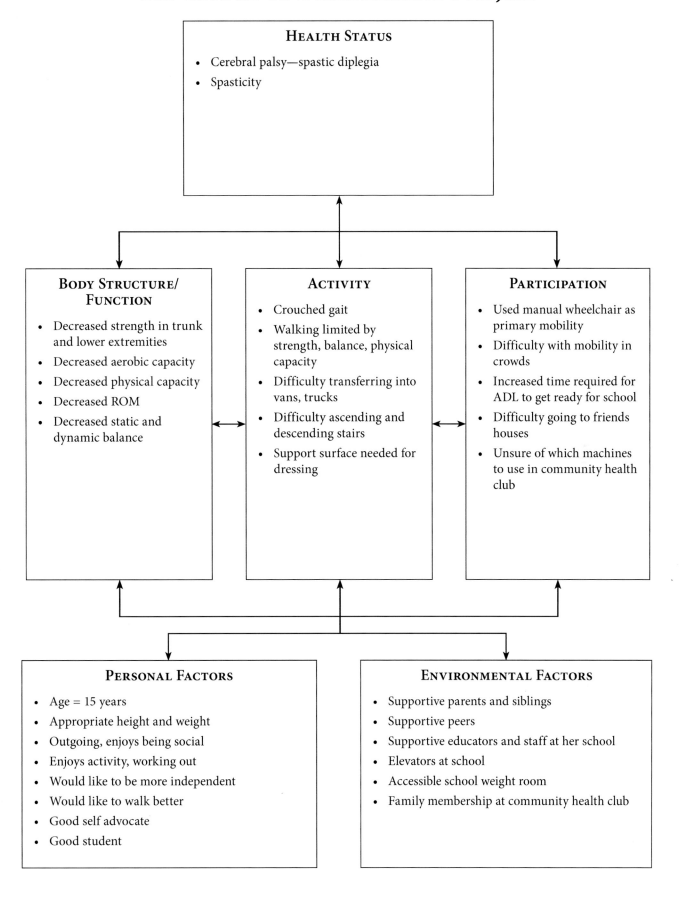

Health Status

- Cerebral palsy—spastic diplegia
- Spasticity

Body Structure/ Function

- Decreased strength in trunk and lower extremities
- Decreased aerobic capacity
- Decreased physical capacity
- Decreased ROM
- Decreased static and dynamic balance

Activity

- Crouched gait
- Walking limited by strength, balance, physical capacity
- Difficulty transferring into vans, trucks
- Difficulty ascending and descending stairs
- Support surface needed for dressing

Participation

- Used manual wheelchair as primary mobility
- Difficulty with mobility in crowds
- Increased time required for ADL to get ready for school
- Difficulty going to friends houses
- Unsure of which machines to use in community health club

Personal Factors

- Age = 15 years
- Appropriate height and weight
- Outgoing, enjoys being social
- Enjoys activity, working out
- Would like to be more independent
- Would like to walk better
- Good self advocate
- Good student

Environmental Factors

- Supportive parents and siblings
- Supportive peers
- Supportive educators and staff at her school
- Elevators at school
- Accessible school weight room
- Family membership at community health club

force production. Jill was an excellent candidate for high-intensity strength and agility training, from which she significantly improved her strength, balance, alignment, and movement patterns. Jill had excellent rehabilitation potential.

PLAN OF CARE

Intervention

Proposed Frequency and Duration of Physical Therapy Visits

Jill participated in the strength-training class offered through the physical education department at her high school. The class met daily for one class period, 65 minutes, with strength training on Monday, Wednesday, and Friday, and cardio, agility, and gait training on Tuesday and Thursday. Her school-based PT developed her program and provided direct, face-to-face service at least 3 days per week. A high school special education paraprofessional with knowledge and background in strength training provided daily direct service. Jill was able to take this class each semester for an entire school year.

Clinician Comment *Fitness programs are safe and beneficial for children and adolescents with CP.[19,27-30] Concerns about strengthening activities making spasticity worse are unsubstantiated.[30,31] Physical education classes offered at the student's school allow for intervention in the natural setting and are often preferred to exercising at a physical therapy clinic.[32-34]*

Many high schools offer strength training classes as part of their physical education curriculum. Working with general and special education staff, the PT is able to develop and provide an individualized program for Jill. In addition to addressing Jill's physical needs, participation in a general physical education class with her peers provided Jill with social interaction that is frequently difficult for adolescents with CP.[35]

Anticipated Goals

1. Jill would improve the flexibility of her hips and knees by 10% over baseline measurements taken at the beginning of the next 2 semesters (14 weeks).

2. Jill would increase the amount of weight she lifted in the weight room by 20% over baseline measurements taken at the beginning of the next 2 semesters (14 weeks).

3. Jill would improve her endurance when walking by 20% as measured by the EEI baseline taken at the beginning of the next 2 semesters (14 weeks).

4. Jill would explore walking with a variety of assistive devices, including walking sticks, forearm crutches, and canes, to determine the feasibility of use in an educational setting (12 weeks).

5. Jill would improve her ability to walk up and down a flight of stairs using one handrail and walking forward alternating steps up and down with standby supervision (12 weeks).

6. Jill would improve her ability to transfer in and out of a variety of vehicles from needing physical assistance to needing standby assistance (20 weeks).

7. Jill would demonstrate a clear understanding of her current and changing evacuation plan and be able to direct staff in all emergencies of drills during the school year (2 weeks).

Clinician Comment *In the educational setting, goals and outcomes are based on the needs identified in the evaluation. Jill had the following identified special education needs:*

- *Jill needs to use assistive technology and modifications in her environment to move safely and independently in the home, school, and community.*

- *Jill needs to improve her overall level of fitness in the areas of flexibility, strength, muscular and cardiovascular endurance, and agility and balance.*

- *Jill needs to improve her mobility in her current and future environments.*

- *Jill needs to improve her ability to transfer in and out of a variety of vehicles and manage her wheelchair with less assistance.*

- *Jill needs an evacuation plan.*

From these needs, specific outcomes and goals were developed, after which her IEP team determined that the expertise of a PT was needed for Jill to attain her fitness and mobility outcomes and goals.

Expected Outcomes (39 Weeks or One School Year)

1. Jill would complete a high-intensity strength training protocol 3 days per week, increasing her weights weekly.

2. Jill would increase the flexibility in her hips to allow her to put her foot on the opposite leg while sitting in her wheelchair in order to put her shoe on her foot.

3. Jill would dress independently for physical education class.

4. Jill would pull her pants up independently after toileting.

5. Jill would walk up or down stairs using a railing to evacuate the building.

6. Jill would walk in her classroom without using any support surface or assistance from students or staff.

7. Jill would walk between close classes.

8. Jill would get in and out of a variety of vans or trucks with standby assistance.

9. Jill would no longer wear AFOs.

10. Jill would participate in her fitness program at her community health club 2 times per week.

11. Jill would maintain or increase her level of fitness through her home fitness program.

Discharge Plan

It was anticipated that Jill would participate in an individualized strength training program for the current school year. These classes met her high school's graduation credit requirement for physical education. Her IEP was in effect for 1 calendar year. Her needs and goals would be updated in 1 year. If Jill decided to continue her participation in strength training, PT services would be available to establish and implement her program during each semester she took the class. Physical therapy services would be discontinued through the educational due process when the educational team determined there was no longer an educational need.

INTERVENTION

Coordination, Communication, and Documentation

Communication occurred with Jill's family regarding her mobility and fitness needs. They discussed a plan to communicate with her physician regarding a trial of Jill not wearing her AFOs. They also discussed a plan for Jill to participate in a fitness program outside of school at their community health club.

Communication occurred with Jill's case manager and teachers regarding accommodations needed for accessing their classrooms, participation in class, and early release. Communication occurred with the school nurse regarding transfers and management of clothing for toileting. Documentation would include all aspects of care, including initial evaluation, progress reports, reexaminations, and discharge summary. Educational requirements were met as described in Jill's IEP.

Coordination and communication with Jill's doctor regarding a 2-month trial without wearing her AFOs occurred with the doctor approving the trial. The trial allowed time for Jill to strengthen her calf and foot muscles and use new movement patterns throughout her day to determine if strengthening would make a difference for her.

With the family's permission, coordination and communication of Jill's fitness program occurred with their community health club.

Clinician Comment *It is important to communicate and coordinate care with Jill's medical team. Before beginning a high-intensity, strength-training program, it is important to make sure there are no contraindications to training. Consulting with her physician regarding programming and interventions at school informed the physician of interventions provided outside the traditional medical model. Requesting a trial is an effective way to evaluate the effectiveness of a proposed intervention, especially when it may be different from the typical course of care.*

When working with a community health club, it is important to obtain permission not only from the family, but also the health club. Since the health club was not a part of the school district or the PT's practice, licensure, liability, and other legal aspects need to be considered before going on site.

Patient-/Client-Related Instruction

Jill received information on general fitness and fitness as related to her CP in education sessions with the evaluating PT. She learned how to manage her energy throughout her day so she could fully participate in her desired activities. She was able to understand how her diagnosis may affect her various body systems and activities as she aged. Following the education sessions, she developed a list of job-demand considerations related to her physical abilities and her mobility. She was instructed in how to evaluate different environments for access, barriers, and evacuation routes.

Procedural Interventions

Therapeutic Exercise
Aerobic Capacity/Endurance Conditioning or Reconditioning

Mode

Walking on treadmill; stationary bike; aerobic activities

Intensity

High-intensity interval training

Duration

10 to 20 minutes depending on activity

Frequency

1 to 2 times per week

Description of the Intervention

With high-intensity interval-training (HIIT), the focus would be on alternating bursts of intense activity with lighter activities. Jill would walk or wheel for 30 seconds at a quick pace and then walk/wheel at a regular pace for 30 seconds. She would continue to alternate between the exercise intensities for 5 and 10 minutes. She would work up to a total workout time of 20 minutes.

Flexibility Exercises

Mode

Stander (standing frame); proprioceptive neuromuscular facilitation (PNF) patterns; yoga patterns

Clinician Comment *It is important to start at a level and intensity that the student can manage before increasing the length of the total activity or the length of the interval. Monitor the student's HR while participating. Walk on a treadmill with hand support, and begin with a slight incline and a slower walking speed for warm-up. Increase intensity by increasing the incline and/or speed. Walk at an intense rate for 30 seconds, slow speed down and walk for 30 seconds, increase speed for 30 seconds, then decrease for 30 seconds and continue for 5 minutes. Monitor HR to determine need for increasing or decreasing intensity. Can also do HIIT with throwing activities, circuits, and agility activities.*

Intensity

Low to moderate

Duration

Stander 15 to 20 minutes; other activities 2 to 5 minutes

Frequency

Stander 2 to 3 times per month; other activities daily

Description of the Intervention

The standing frame would support Jill at her hips and knees while also providing a prolonged stretch to hips, knees, and ankles in a weightbearing position. Movements using PNF patterns or yoga patterns provide inhibition and movement of joints that is slow and gentle.

Strength, Power, and Endurance Training for Head, Neck, Limb, and Trunk Muscles

Mode

Stander (standing frame)

Intensity

Progressive resistance exercise

Duration

10 to 12 repetitions

Frequency

2 to 3 times per month

Description of the Intervention

While standing, the upper body is free to perform strengthening or aerobic activities, such as forward bends with light weights progressing to heavier kettle bells, rotation activities for core strengthening, or medicine ball tossing from overhead.

Strength, Power, and Endurance Training for Head, Neck, Limb, and Trunk Muscles

Mode

Variable resistant machines, manual resistance

Intensity

High intensity to failure for each lift

Duration

10 to 12 repetitions times one set to failure

Frequency

3 times per week—Monday, Wednesday, Friday

Description of the Intervention

Completion of a one-set sequence to failure lifting strategy was used for each lift performed. Focus was on high-intensity work while performing quality repetitions to momentary muscular failure. Weight or amount of resistance was high, 80%, one repetition maximum.

Clinician Comment *Strengthening has been demonstrated to be effective for children and adolescents with CP.[32,33] However, controversy was recently raised as a result of a systematic review that determined the evidence demonstrated that muscle strengthening was not effective.[36] While others debated the findings of the review,[36-40] Verschuren et al proposed that the reason for the lack of evidence was a result of the training protocols used in the studies.[40] They suggest that children and adolescents with CP could use the same guidelines developed by the National Strength and Conditioning Association for those developing typically. Use of higher intensity is needed to obtain gains in strength.[40,41] The National Center on Physical Activity and Disability Exercise/Fitness agrees and has developed a fact sheet for High-Intensity Weight Training for People with Disabilities to guide intervention.[28]*

There are a number of methods for performing strength training.[42-44] High-intensity strength training is recommended as the method to build strength.[40,41,45] When using variable resistant machines or manual resistance for high-intensity strength training, movement is through the full available ROM with tension throughout the range. Movement is slow and controlled in the best alignment possible. Work large muscle groups first, then small muscle groups, then grips followed by abdominals. Begin with either the legs or arms, completing one set before starting the other. Alignment for each lift is critical; physically hold or assist the student to maintain alignment through the entire lift. Technique and form used while lifting are also critical. Whenever possible, DO NOT wear orthotics that limit joint movement or muscle contraction.

A 7-second repetition was used for each repetition that included the following:

- *2 seconds to lift concentrically—positive phase*
- *1-second pause at end of positive phase*
- *4 seconds to lower weight eccentrically—negative phase*

A 1-set sequence was used to reach failure on each lift[28,43-45]:

- *Completed one set of 8 to 12 seven-second repetitions*
- *Worked to muscle failure in positive phase of lift (concentric)*

- *Once reached failure, begin forced repetitions*
  - *Assist with positive phase*
  - *Resist negative phase*
- *Amount of weight lifted is what student can lift without assistance for 8 to 12 repetitions*
- *Weight is increased for the next session when reach 12 repetitions*
- *Weight is decreased for the next session when lift 7 or less repetitions*
- *Limit rest between lifts*
- *Need 48 hours' rest between workouts for same muscle groups*

Strength, Power, and Endurance Training for Core and Ventilatory Muscles

Mode

Active isometric and isotonic progressive exercises

Intensity

Slow, controlled movements through concentric and eccentric phase

Duration

10 to 12 repetitions times one set to failure

Frequency

3 times per week—Monday, Wednesday, Friday

Description of the Intervention

A series of core strengthening exercises were developed with progressive intensity. Training included learning how to activate core muscles to set the pelvis when performing other activities. Breathing exercises were also included as a component of core strengthening as well as to aid appropriate breathing when lifting.

Gait and Locomotion Training

Mode

Walking using a variety of devices including a treadmill and hands-free walker; ascending and descending stairs.

Intensity

Walking at a speed that allows for smooth coordinated control of LE

Duration

20 minutes

Frequency

1 to 2 times per week

Description of the Intervention

Walking on a treadmill without AFOs to facilitate central pattern generators and allow ankle and foot motion. Allow 2 hands on lateral rails, then progress to holding on to horizontal poles with the PT facilitating arm swing. Walking using a hands-free walker without AFOs, focusing on equal stride, and landing on heel while weight shifting through pelvis. May use horizontal poles to facilitate arm swing.

Face forward on stairs using one handrail. Practice lifting and placing foot on step, keeping knee straight ahead while placing other foot on step. Progress from doing one step at a time to alternating steps. When descending stairs, focus on slow, controlled movement to lower self to next step, keeping alignment with feet and knees straight ahead.

Balance, Coordination, and Agility Training

Mode

Balance activities

Intensity

Activities should be performed slowly and controlled with correct alignment of trunk and LE, then increase speed as control improves.

Duration

10 to 20 minutes

Frequency

Once per week

Description of the Intervention

Balance activities initially using walking sticks, then progressing to no-hand support while standing with both feet or one foot on a variety of surfaces, including foam, balance boards, and inflated disc. Start with 2 feet on a stable surface, focusing on alignment and weight shifting through pelvis. Jill would have a mirror available to allow her to see and correct her alignment. Coordination and agility activities using walking sticks or the PT's hands for balance while performing basic stepping drills, speed ladder, and dot drills. Begin with simple activities working on accurate placement, changing direction, and varying speed. Speed ladder and dot drills are performed slowly at first to learn patterns and increase accuracy.

Clinician Comment *The examination showed that Jill's perception of her alignment was not accurate. Using the mirror would provide Jill the opportunity to use visual feedback to self-evaluate her alignment and then correct.*

Functional Training in Work (Job/School/Play), Community, and Leisure Integration or Reintegration, Including Instrumental Activities of Daily Living, Work Hardening, and Work Conditioning

Description of the Intervention

Jill would practice getting in and out of a vehicle. She would start with a variety of cars but then progress in difficulty to vans, SUVs, and trucks. Jill would develop strategies for managing her wheelchair. She would then practice folding and putting her wheelchair into the back seat and trunk of a variety of vehicles.

Jill would develop and implement a fitness program at her community health club. She would communicate with her school PT about her progress and any questions regarding updating her program.

Jill would develop and practice an evacuation plan for school and home.

Prescription, Application, and Fabrication of Devices and Equipment (Assistive, Adaptive, Orthotic, Protective, Supportive, or Prosthetic)

Description of the Intervention

Jill would explore alternative walking devices, including walking sticks, forearm crutches, and canes for walking, as well as how to use them in conjunction with her wheelchair.

REEXAMINATION

Subjective

After 4 weeks of strength training, Jill stated she enjoyed the class and ate lunch with a few of the students from the class. She stated she felt it was easier to walk in the classroom: "I don't need to hold onto my friends or use the desks when I am walking in the room." She also reported she was walking down the stairs at home but would still scoot if she were in a hurry as it was still faster. She felt it was easier to get in and out of her family car, but she still had trouble with her friend's truck.

At the end of the first semester of strength training, Jill stated she was excited about being able to continue the class next semester. She said she was walking a lot more at school, and, "I even walked down the hall to my next class when the halls weren't very crowded and made it without falling!" She said it takes her less time to get dressed after strength training class and, "I can even sit on the bench and put my jeans on."

Objective

Jill participated in class every day during the first semester, missing 1 day in December for a medical appointment. She initially complained of being tired and having sore legs, but this stopped after the second week. Jill participated in all activities and demonstrated a good work ethic in the weight room. She appeared to enjoy the aerobic and agility activities and pushed herself to complete an activity even when it was difficult and she was tired.

Aerobic Capacity/Endurance

EEI in Heartbeats/Meter

Walking independently at regular pace	1.04
Walking independently at fast pace	1.17

Anthropometric Characteristics

Body Fat Percentage

Body fat handheld analyzer	25.2%
Skinfold measurement	24.5%
Height/weight formula (kg/m^2)	20.88%

Body Measurements/Circumference

AREA MEASURED	MEASUREMENT (INCHES) *All measurements are circumference except height and weight*		
		LEFT	RIGHT
Height	61		
Weight	112 pounds		
Shoulders	34$^{3/4}$		
Chest (under arms)	33		
Bicep (flexed)		10$^{3/8}$	10$^{3/4}$
Forearm (wrist flexed)		9$^{1/2}$	10$^{1/8}$
Waist	27		
Hips	35$^{1/8}$		
Thigh (midpoint)		18$^{1/2}$	18$^{3/4}$
Thigh (widest point)		20	20$^{1/4}$
Calf (widest when flexed)		11$^{7/8}$	12$^{1/2}$

Note increased length in gastrocnemius muscle on both legs as muscle belly no longer restricted by AFO.

Range of Motion

JOINT MOTION	LEFT (DEGREES)	RIGHT (DEGREES)
Hip flexion	0 to 130	0 to 139
Hip extension	−11	−7
Hip external rotation	0 to 30	0 to 37
Hip internal rotation	0 to 60	0 to 50
Hip abduction	0 to 30	0 to 40
Hip adduction	0 to 40	0 to 30
Knee flexion	10 to 155	7 to 152
Knee extension	−10	−7
Ankle dorsiflexion	0 to 28	0 to 29
Ankle plantarflexion	0 to 30	0 to 37
Hamstring length—popliteal angle	25 short of full extension	18 short of full extension

Muscle Performance

MUSCLE GROUP	LEFT (POUNDS)	RIGHT (POUNDS)
Hip flexion	36	47
Knee extension	44	46
Knee flexion	8.0	6.7
Hip abduction	24.1	17.9

- **Ankle plantarflexion**: Single leg toe raises with knee straight; L: 5; R: 8.
- **Ankle dorsiflexion**: Lifted toes in standing but could not hold feet up to walk on heels. Active dorsiflexion against gravity, but unable to take any resistance.
- **Abdominal strength**: Completed 5 sit-ups with arms crossed over chest. Completed 4 forced exhalations (transverse abdominals). Completed 2 rotational sit-ups (elbow to opposite knee) with arms behind head.
- **Functional strength**: Walked up stairs with pelvis, legs, and feet forward using one handrail. Walked down stairs in slow, controlled manner. Kept pelvis, legs, and feet forward. Lowered self into chair in slow, controlled manner.

Posture

Jill was able to correct posture when sitting in wheelchair. Stood with heels on floor and knees and hips in a slight crouch.

Gait, Locomotion, and Balance

- **Gait**: Walked in classroom with limited use of friends or support surfaces to balance. Began to walk in hallways without students in them between classes that were close, less than 100 yards away.
- **Locomotion**: Jill reported she was walking most of the time at home.
- **Balance**: Standing balance

CONDITION	BOTH FEET (MIN/SEC)	LEFT (MIN/SEC)	RIGHT (MIN/SEC)
Eyes open	05.00.00	00.04.68	00.05.53
Eyes closed	05.00.00	00.02.45	00.03.36

Motor Function

Increased control to stop, start, and change directions while walking. Movement improves with practice.

Assistive and Adaptive Devices

Tried various canes, crutches, and walkers and determined that forearm crutches were the most adaptable for use with a manual wheelchair.

Orthotic, Protective, and Supportive Devices

Jill no longer needs to wear her AFOs. Her physician discontinued use at Jill's December medical appointment.

Self-Care and Home Management

Jill reported taking less time in the morning to get ready for school. Completed her dressing while sitting on a bench or standing for physical education. Independent in pulling pants up after toileting.

Work, Community, and Leisure Integration

Transferred into cars and some vans independently. Needed assistance with transfers for trucks.

Environmental, Home, and Work Barriers

Evacuated from second floor using stairs to go down following other students.

Assessment

Jill made progress on her all of her goals. She met or exceeded the 20% increase for strengthening and aerobic endurance while walking at a fast pace. Body circumference increased by 0.25 to 1 inch, with the largest increases in her legs. Jill demonstrated an increase in muscle strength, endurance, flexibility, and agility. Functional skills also improved, especially her ability to walk up and down stairs in a controlled manner. Jill's strength training program appeared to be effective in increasing her fitness and functional abilities.

Plan

Jill would benefit from another semester of strength-training class. Jill needs to practice walking in more variable environments to gain confidence to walk in community settings.

REEXAMINATION

Subjective

At the end of 8 weeks of strength training in the second semester of school, Jill reported she was going to her community health club and "working out on the machines" on the weekends. She was excited that she knew which machines to use and how to use them; she "even taught my mom how to use them!"

At the end of the semester, Jill reported she went with her friends to the mall and "we shopped all day and I was able to keep up with them and walk through the stores without worrying that I would fall if I got bumped." She did report she took frequent breaks and a friend would sit and talk with her while others shopped.

Objective

Aerobic Capacity

EEI in Heartbeats/Meter

Walking independently at regular pace	0.71
Walking independently at fast pace	0.94

Anthropometric

Body Fat Percentage

Body fat handheld analyzer	23.4%
Skinfold measurement	22.8%
Height/weight formula (kg/m^2)	21.74%

Body Measurements/Circumference

AREA MEASURED	MEASUREMENT (INCHES) *All measurements are circumference except height and weight*		
		LEFT	RIGHT
Height	61		
Weight	115 pounds		
Shoulders	35$^{1/2}$		
Chest (under arms)	33$^{1/2}$		
Bicep (flexed)		11$^{3/4}$	12$^{1/4}$
Forearm (wrist flexed)		10$^{1/2}$	10$^{7/8}$
Waist	27		
Hips	36		
Thigh (midpoint)		18$^{1/8}$	18$^{3/4}$
Thigh (widest point)		19$^{1/2}$	19$^{7/8}$
Calf (widest when flexed)		12$^{1/2}$	12$^{7/8}$

Range of Motion

JOINT MOTION	LEFT (DEGREES)	RIGHT (DEGREES)
Hip flexion	0 to 137	0 to 143
Hip extension	–8	–5
Hip external rotation	0 to 35	0 to 43
Hip internal rotation	0 to 60	0 to 50
Hip abduction	0 to 35	0 to 40

JOINT MOTION	LEFT (DEGREES)	RIGHT (DEGREES)
Hip adduction	0 to 40	0 to 30
Knee flexion	5 to 154	5 to 155
Knee extension	–5	–5
Ankle dorsiflexion	0 to 24	0 to 25
Ankle plantarflexion	0 to 34	0 to 37
Hamstring length—popliteal angle	30 short of full extension	22 short of full extension

Muscle Performance

MUSCLE GROUP	LEFT (POUNDS)	RIGHT (POUNDS)
Hip flexion	70	79
Knee extension	58	62
Knee flexion	25	28
Hip abduction	28	29

- **Ankle plantarflexion**: Single leg toe raises with knee straight; L: 15; R: 18.
- **Ankle dorsiflexion**: Walked on heels with feet in dorsiflexion for 10 feet.
- **Abdominal strength**: Completed 15 sit-ups with arms crossed over chest. Completed 10 forced exhalations (transverse abdominals). Completed 10 rotational sit-ups (elbow to opposite knee) with arms behind head.
- **Functional strength**: Walked up and down stairs using a reciprocal pattern without a handrail if alone and with a handrail if others on stairs.

Posture

Appropriate alignment when sitting in wheelchair. Stands with hips and knees in slight flexion, slight lumbar lordosis.

Gait, Locomotion, and Balance

- **Gait**: Walked between classes if on the same side of the building. Decreased lateral trunk motions when walking. Used wheelchair for safety in crowded hallways.
- **Locomotion**: Jill reported she walked all the time at home but was cautious when outside on the grass.
- **Balance**: Standing balance

CONDITION	BOTH FEET (MIN/SEC)	LEFT (MIN/SEC)	RIGHT (MIN/SEC)
Eyes open	05.00.00	00.10.15	00.15.07
Eyes closed	05.00.00	00.05.27	00.09.13

Used ankle strategies when standing instead of hip; stood still for periods of time instead of swaying.

Motor Function

Jill walked in the halls with some students present but could not manage large crowds.

Able to anticipate and set her body for throwing activities in standing but had difficulty keeping body set for catching the ball.

Assistive and Adaptive Devices

Jill discontinued use of forearm crutches, stating she did not need them anymore.

Self-Care and Home Management

Jill reported she worked with her mother on simple cooking using the stove and oven.

Work, Community, and Leisure Integration

Jill transferred into most trucks with standby assistance. Jill reported she was taking the driver's education permit class in the fall.

Environmental, Home, and Work Barriers

Jill used the stairs for evacuation, waiting for the crowds to go first and staff to walk beside her to prevent her from being bumped.

Assessment

Jill met and exceeded most of her goals. Jill increased body circumference measurements by an additional 0.25 to 1 inch the second semester. Significant changes in walking and balance as well as functional activities occurred during the semester. Jill demonstrated knowledge in her evacuation plan. Jill developed a fitness program that she used at her community health club.

Plan

Jill needed to maintain or increase her level of fitness over the summer. She planned to go to her community health club 3 times per week over the summer. Jill needed to continue to practice walking in a variety of community settings.

OUTCOMES

Discharge

Jill met the goals and outcomes related to improving her strength and functional abilities. She needed to be able to maintain her newly attained level of fitness through her home program and participation at her community health club. She continued to demonstrate the ability to improve her level of fitness and functional abilities and would be appropriate to continue with strength-training classes at school next year if she chose to continue them. Jill would be discharged from her school-based physical therapy service when she no longer demonstrated educational needs that required the expertise of the PT. This would be determined by her IEP team at her yearly meeting each school year.

REFERENCES

1. Hoch DB, Kaneshiro NK, Zieve D. Cerebral palsy. *PubMed Health*. http://www.ncbi.nlm.nih.gov/pubmedhealth/PMH0001734. Accessed November 29, 2011.

2. Quality Standards Subcommittee of the American Academy of Neurology and the Practice Committee of the Child Neurology Society; Delgado MR, Hirtz D, et al. Practice parameter: pharmacologic treatment of spasticity in children and adolescents with cerebral palsy (an evidence-based review): report of the Quality Standards Subcommittee of the American Academy of Neurology and the Practice Committee of the Child Neurology Society. *Neurology*. 2010;74:336-343.

3. U.S. Department of Education. Building the legacy: IDEA 2004. http://idea.ed.gov. Accessed January 11, 2012.

4. U.S. Department of Education. Questions and answers on secondary transition. *Building the Legacy: IDEA 2004*. http://idea.ed.gov/explore/view/p/%2Croot%2Cdynamic%2CQaCorner%2C10%2C. Accessed January 11, 2012.

5. Sanger TD, Delgado MR, Gaebler-Spira D, et al. Classification and definition of disorders causing hypertonia in childhood. *Pediatrics*. 2003;111:e89-e97.

6. Sheean G. The pathophysiology of spasticity. *Eur J Neurol*. 2002;9(Suppl:1):3-9.

7. Yap R, Majnemer A, Benaroch T, Cantin MA. Determinants of responsiveness to botulinum toxin, casting, and bracing in the treatment of spastic equinus in children with cerebral palsy. *Dev Med Child Neurol*. 2010;52:186-193.

8. Pin TW, McCartney L, Lewis J, Waugh MC. Use of intrathecal baclofen therapy in ambulant children and adolescents with spasticity and dystonia of cerebral origin: a systematic review. *Dev Med Child Neurol*. 2011;53:885-895.

9. Ward AB. Spasticity treatment with botulinum toxins. *J Neural Transm*. 2008;115:607-617.

10. Gough M, Fairhurst C, Shortland AP. Botulinum toxin and cerebral palsy: time for reflection? *Dev Med Child Neurol*. 2005;47:709-712.

11. Gracies JM, Lugassy M, Weisz DJ, Vecchio M, Flanagan S, Simpson DM. Botulinum toxin dilution and endplate targeting in spasticity: a double-blind controlled study. *Arch Phys Med Rehabil*. 2009;90:9-16.

12. Moberg-Wolff E. Potential clinical impact of compounded versus noncompounded intrathecal baclofen, *Arch Phys Med Rehabil*. 2009;90:1815-1820.

13. Gillette Children's Specialty Healthcare. Single event multilevel surgery (SEMLS). http://www.gillettechildrens.org/conditions-and-care/single-event-multilevel-surgery-semls. Accessed June 28, 2014.

14. Novacheck TF, Stout JL, Gage JR, Schwartz MH. Distal femoral extension osteotomy and patellar tendon advancement to treat persistent crouch gait in cerebral palsy. *J Bone Joint Surg Am*. 2009;91(Suppl:2):271-286.

15. Takahasi S, Shrestha A. The vulpis procedure for correction of equinus deformity in patients with hemiplegia. *J Bone Joint Surg Am*. 2002;84(7):978-980.

16. Francisco GE, Saulino MF, Yablon SA, Turner M. Intrathecal baclofen therapy: an update. *PM R*. 2009;1:852-858.

17. Vles JS. Itrathecal baclofen therapy in non-ambulant and ambulant children and adolescents with spasticity of cerebral origin. *Dev Med Child Neurol*. 2001;53:1061; author reply 1062-1063.

18. Rose J, Gamble JG, Lee J, Lee R, Haskell WL. The energy expenditure index: a method to quantitate and compare walking energy expenditure for children and adolescents. *J Pediatr Orthop.* 1991;11:571-578.

19. Fragala-Pinkham MA, Haley SM, Rabin J, Kharasch VS. A fitness program for children with disabilities. *Phys Ther.* 2005;85:1182-1200.

20. Wiart L, Darrah J. Test-retest reliability of the energy expenditure index in adolescents with cerebral palsy. *Dev Med Child Neurol.* 1999;41:716-718.

21. Kendall FP, McCreary DK, Provance PG. *Muscles Testing and Function With Posture and Pain.* 4th ed. Baltimore, MD: Williams & Wilkins; 1993.

22. Katz K, Rosenthal A, Yosipovitch Z. Normal ranges of popliteal angle in children. *J Pediatr Orthop.* 1992;12(2):229-231.

23. Hislop HJ, Montgomery J. *Daniels and Worthingham's Muscle Testing.* 7th ed. Philadelphia, PA: WB Saunders Company; 2002.

24. Jones MA, Stratton G. Muscle function assessment in children. *Acta Paediatr.* 2000;89:753-761.

25. Palisano R, Rosenbaum P, Bartlett D, Livingston MH. Content validity of the expanded and revised Gross Motor Function Classification System. *Dev Med Child Neurol.* 2008;50(10):744-750.

26. Palisano R, Rosenbaum P, Bartlett D, Livingston MH. Gross Motor Function Classification System Expanded and Revised. Hamilton, Ontario: CanChild Centre for Childhood Disability Research, McMaster University; 2007. http://motorgrowth.canchild.ca/en/GMFCS/resources/GMFCS-ER.pdf. Accessed June 1, 2011.

27. American Academy of Pediatrics. Strength training by children and adolescents. *Pediatrics.* 2001;107(6):1470-1472.

28. National Center on Health, Physical Activity, and Disability. High-intensity weight training for people with disabilities. *NCHPAD.* http://www.ncpad.org/24/162/High-Intensity~Weight~Training~for~People~with~Disabilities. Accessed June 1, 2011.

29. Damiano DL. Activity, activity, activity: rethinking our physical therapy approach to cerebral palsy. *Phys Ther.* 2006;86:1534-1540.

30. Fowler EG, Kolobe TH, Damiano DL, et al. Promotion of physical fitness and prevention of secondary conditions for children with cerebral palsy: section on Pediatrics Research Summit Proceedings. *Phys Ther.* 2007;87:1495-1510.

31. Damiano DL. Should we be testing and training muscle strength in cerebral palsy? *Dev Med Child Neurol.* 2002;44:68-72.

32. Eagleton M, Iams A, McDowell J, Morrison R, Evans CL. The effects of strength training on gait in adolescents with cerebral palsy. *Pediatr Phys Ther.* 2004;16:22-30.

33. O'Connell DG, Barnhart R. Improvement in wheelchair propulsion in pediatric wheelchair users through resistance training: a pilot study. *Arch Phys Med Rehabil.* 1995;76:368-372.

34. Unger M, Faure M, Frieg A. Strength training in adolescent learners with cerebral palsy: a randomized controlled trial. *Clin Rehabil.* 2006;20:469-477.

35. Kang LJ, Palisano RJ, Orlin MN, Chiarello LA, King GA, Polansky M. Determinants of social participation—with friends and others who are not family members—for youths with cerebral palsy. *Phys Ther.* 2010;90:1743-1757.

36. Scianni A, Butler JM, Ada L, Teixeira-Salmela LF. Muscle strengthening is not effective in children and adolescents with cerebral palsy: a systematic review. *Aust J Physiother.* 2009;55:81-87.

37. Taylor NF. Is progressive resistance exercise ineffective in increasing muscle strength in young people with cerebral palsy? *Aust J Physiother.* 2009;55:222; author reply 223.

38. Graham HK, Thomason P. Is there sufficient evidence? *Aust J Physiother.* 2009;55:223; author reply 223.

39. Lancaster A, Mudge A, Wu J, Lewis J, Bau K. Should we change practice? *Aust J Physiother.* 2009;55:291; author reply 292.

40. Verschuren O, Ada L, Maltais DB, Gorter JW, Scianni A, Ketelaar M. Muscle strengthening in children and adolescents with spastic cerebral palsy: considerations for future resistance training protocols. *Phys Ther.* 2011;91:1130-1139.

41. van Brussel M, van der Net J, Hulzebos E, Helders PJ, Takken T. The Utrecht approach to exercise in chronic childhood conditions: the decade in review. *Pediatr Phys Ther.* 2011;23:2-14.

42. Taylor NF, Dodd KJ, Damiano DL. Progressive resistance exercise in physical therapy: a summary of systematic reviews. *Phys Ther.* 2005;85:1208-1223.

43. Rhea MR, Alderman BL. A meta-analysis of periodized versus nonperiodized strength and power training programs. *Res Q Exerc Sport.* 2004;75(4):413-422.

44. Willardson JM. The application of training to failure in periodized multiple-set resistance exercise programs. *J Strength Cond Res.* 2007;21(2):628-631.

45. Philbin J. *High-Intensity Training.* Champaign, IL: Human Kinetics; 2004.

CASE 2-2

Kathleen Coultes, PT, PCS

EXAMINATION

History

Current Condition/Chief Complaint

Jack was an obese 11-year-old White male who was referred to outpatient physical therapy. Three weeks prior, he had undergone a left tibia and fibula osteotomy with external fixation. Jack returned to school 1 week prior.

History of Current Complaint

Jack received a diagnosis of Blount disease 3 months prior to his surgery. The monitoring of his status during the 3-month interval documented worsening of the varus deformity (bowing) in his left tibia. It was also noted that he developed a leg length discrepancy of approximately 1.5 cm as a result of the bowing, the left LE shorter than the right. He had increasing complaints of pain and stiffness. Pain would begin after walking more than 5 minutes, sitting still for more than 20 minutes, or any attempt with running.

Jack underwent a left tibia/fibula osteotomy with external fixation and was released from the hospital after a 2-week stay. He was to ambulate with bilateral bariatric axillary crutches with the precaution of toe-touch weightbearing of less than 10 pounds. In addition to the referral to physical therapy at the time of his hospital discharge, a referral was made for a pulmonary consult to follow up on his snoring noted while he was in the hospital. Also, at the time of discharge, a bariatric wheelchair and commode were requested.

Clinician Comment *Blount disease is a skeletal disorder affecting the medial side of the proximal tibial epiphysis.[1] Blount initially reported the acquired varus deformity of the proximal tibia in adolescents. Further classification by Thompson et al led to the description of 2 types of the deformity: juvenile onset of varus deformity* *occurring in children between ages 4 through 10 years, and the true adolescent onset, late onset tibia vara, occurring in children 11+ years of age.[2]*

Generally, there is a history of normal knee alignment prior to the development of the genu varum deformity.[2] The presence of obesity in a growing adolescent can lead to an unequal loading of the tibial plateau, placing undue stress on the medial aspect.[1] This increased pressure on the medial physis leads to a posteromedial growth suppression—the Hueter-Volkmann principle.[1] The growth suppression first produces a varus deformity but then causes a progressive procurvatum of the proximal part of the tibia. Marked tibial varum and tibial torsion can result.

In-toeing during gait worsens as the deformity progresses. This occurs first as a functional accommodation to allow the foot to be placed as close to the line of progression as possible. However, the in-toeing subsequently worsens with progressive tibial torsion.[2]

Social History/Environment

Jack lived at home with his family, including his mother, father, and 2 siblings. His father was disabled and did not work. Jack's mother was employed as a teacher's aide at the school he attended.

Jack was in the sixth grade at an accessible school. His mother reported that Jack's teachers had arranged for Jack to select a classmate to leave class with Jack a few minutes before each classroom period. The classmate would then accompany and assist Jack as he changed classrooms during his school day.

Social/Health Habits

Jack admitted he was not physically active, even prior to the onset of his leg pain. He reported enjoying video games, television, and movies. As his leg pain increased, he reported he avoided walking any more than his daily activities required.

Jack appeared to be tall for an 11-year-old male. His mother reported that Jack's entire family was tall. Jack appeared to be overweight, even for his large frame.

Clinician Comment *Even before his leg began to hurt and limit his weightbearing activities, Jack pursued sedentary leisure activities. Given his sedentary activities and limited weightbearing in the months prior to surgery, as well as the surgery and 2-week hospital stay, Jack was probably deconditioned. Further, obesity has been identified as a precursor to the development of Blount disease. Jack appeared to be overweight. His height and weight needed to be measured to determine his BMI and category for weight.*

The probable obesity and deconditioning were not the only health risks he might face. Youth obesity is a public health

epidemic.[3] Eighteen percent of children and adolescents are reported to be at or above the 95th percentile in weight. There is a prevalence of impaired fasting blood glucose levels recorded in youth at a 7% or higher level. From that statistic, it is not surprising, therefore, that there is an increasing incidence of Type 2 diabetes reported in 12 to 19 year olds.[3] Hyperlipidemia, hypertension, metabolic syndrome, obstructive sleep apnea, asthma. and orthopedic complications, such as a slipped capital femoral epiphysis and Blount disease, are all rising in the pediatric patient populations.[3]

Jack was fortunate to return to an accessible school, and his teachers had developed a plan to help Jack with classroom changes. His mother was also available to help him at school if needed. She reported that one aspect of the teachers' plan had a positive social benefit for Jack: his classmates begged him to be chosen to accompany him so that they, too, could leave class early.

Medical/Surgical History

Past medical history was reported to be insignificant upon initial evaluation. It was reported that Jack has a drug allergy to penicillin. The only surgery reported was the left tibia/fibula osteotomy and placement of the external fixator.

Clinician Comment *The osteotomy consisted of removing a wedge-shaped piece of bone from the medial side of his femur and inserting it into the tibia to replace the posteromedial growth suppression. Pins and screws were utilized to hold the bone wedge in place, with the external fixator further securing the bone from the outside with pins. Use of the external fixator offered the opportunity for further gradual correction of the varus deformity over 3 weeks by distraction osteogenesis. Typically, the frame would be removed about 12 weeks postoperatively when the bone had consolidated.[4] For Jack, the projection for the external fixator's removal would coincide with approximately 2 months into physical therapy.*

Reported Functional Status

Jack reported, and his mother concurred, that he needed a little assistance from family members with all of his self-care activities, including dressing, grooming, and toileting tasks. A family member would assist with management of his left LE during position changes to ensure safety. When asked about household mobility, his mother reported that Jack's dad and siblings were doing a lot for him, rather than making him maneuver around the house independently using either the crutches or wheelchair.

Jack's family members were trained in pin site care prior to his discharge from the hospital. Both Jack and his mom expressed concern that the pin sites could become infected.

Jack reported that he tended to use the wheelchair at school rather than walk with the crutches. He reported that walking with the crutches and trying to limit weightbearing on his left LE to 10 pounds was difficult. He said he was afraid he might fall at school if he used the crutches.

Jack stated that his goal for physical therapy was to be able to walk without the crutches.

Clinician Comment *Jack had a supportive family who was concerned about his safety, comfort, and pin site status during his convalescence. He had supportive teachers who created a plan to help with his mobility that also offered him a bit of social cache. Some of this help, however, may have been interfering with his transition to improved independence with ADL. It was certainly having an impact on his already-reduced activity level.*

Jack was not physically active prior to his surgery. He was in the hospital for 2 weeks. He was probably deconditioned. He tended to use the wheelchair at school. The assistance by a classmate gave him an alternative to self-propelling the wheelchair that would have provided him with some physical activity. Even though using his crutches might have been more difficult than using the wheelchair, the challenge of crutch walking would have, at least, improved his activity tolerance over time.

Walking with the crutches was perceived as challenging—not only physically, but also emotionally—as he did have a fear of falling. As an 11 year old, peer interactions are a strong motivating factor for Jack. He did not want to suffer the embarrassment of falling. He was, therefore, not motivated to use the crutches in school, which was where he was spending the majority of his day. Gaining experience and confidence with crutch walking at home was thwarted by understandable concern for his comfort by his family. Further, the secondary gain of increased attention needed to be considered in attempting to motivate Jack to progress with his independence.

Medications

Jack took Tylenol as needed for pain.

Other Clinical Tests

Radiograph taken preoperatively showed abnormal bone growth patterns in the posteromedial aspect of the left tibia. Prior to his hospital discharge, Jack had experienced swelling in his left calf and associated redness. A Doppler ultrasound of his left LE ruled out a deep vein thrombosis (DVT) prior to discharge.

Clinician Comment *No data were available from the radiology report on the left leg pre- and postoperative mechanical medial proximal tibial angles (mMPTA) in the records brought to the initial physical therapy appointment. An mMPTA angle is used as a basis for degree of deformity calculations in describing the rotational component of tibia varum.[5]*

Doppler ultrasound was used to rule out a DVT because of the presence of swelling in the left calf, with associated redness. Because Jack's level of activity had been significantly decreased postoperatively, DVT needed to be ruled out given his presenting symptoms. An increase in the occurrence of DVT has been reported in adolescents who are obese. Medical intervention to prevent DVT and pulmonary embolism has been recommended in obese adolescents undergoing orthopedic surgeries.[6]

Next, in the examination portion of the evaluation, was the systems review. The limited examination of the systems review aided in the identification of indicated tests and measures as the examination moved forward, as well as establishing that there were no contraindications for Jack to be seen in physical therapy.

Systems Review

Cardiovascular/Pulmonary

HR: 90 bpm

BP: 145/85

Respiratory rate: 15

The recommended outpatient pulmonary evaluation that was recommended at his hospital discharge had not yet occurred.

Clinician Comment *Jack's slightly elevated vital signs could be attributed to being apprehensive about his first outpatient physical therapy session. He had no history of hypertension but did admit to being a little fearful of what was going to happen in the evaluation. Monitoring of Jack's BP in future visits was indicated to rule out any clinically relevant findings.*

One of the comorbidities associated with obesity is sleep apnea. A high prevalence of sleep apnea in morbidly obese patients with late-onset Blount disease has also been reported.[6] Therefore, a high index of suspicion for sleep apnea in snoring adolescents needs to be considered and ruled out. If the sleep apnea is confirmed, then it can be addressed pre- and postoperatively to avoid complications after surgery.[6]

In Jack's case, the snoring was not observed until after his surgery and while he was still in the hospital. The presence of sleep disturbance could have had an impact on Jack's success with rehabilitation. Sleep apnea is known to lead to behavioral and mental problems for children, as well as cardiovascular issues. Excessive sleepiness through the day, decreased academic performance and learning ability, growth disturbances, high BP, and abnormal heart function can all be symptoms related to sleep apnea.[7] Again, monitoring Jack's BP would be indicated. With any endurance complaints in treatment or with physical activity, Jack could be asked if he was feeling sleepy or if his muscles were tired to distinguish between the effects of sleep apnea and deconditioning.

Integumentary

The 2 medial and 2 lateral tibial pin sites from the external fixator were observed to be clean and without sign of infection. The sites were moist and clean. The pins were in good condition where they attached to the external fixator. His mother reported that she was following the pin site cleaning protocol she had been taught. The patient denied specific pain at the pin sites except during knee flexion.

He exhibited intact sensation to light touch throughout his left LE.

Clinician Comment *In a retrospective review of complications associated with tibial osteotomy and external fixation in adolescents with Blount disease, Wilson et al found that wound complications were the most common complication for 53% of surgeries reviewed.[5] Of the 28 complications reported, 20 were at pin sites and 8 were deep infections. This rate of wound complication was increased over previous reports. One difference, however, was that 98% of the patients included in this study were morbidly obese. This suggests pin site infections are yet another possible postoperative complication in obese teens.[5] Consistent monitoring of Jack's pin sites would need to be a component of his physical therapy treatment.*

Musculoskeletal

Gross Symmetry/Posture

Jack held his left LE in extreme external rotation at the hip in the supine, sitting, and standing positions. An increased thoracic kyphosis was evident with associated rounded shoulders and forward head position when he was standing and when sitting. Jack was able to correct his posture easily, however, when given verbal cues. He could maintain the corrected posture with verbal cuing but would return to the "relaxed" poor posture position when not reminded.

Gross Range of Motion/Strength

Both UEs and right LE were without impairments in gross mobility and strength as measured using goniometric measurements and MMT. Trunk strength was within normal limits for age using a sit-up test, with decreased overall tone secondary to excessive soft tissue mass.

The left LE ROM and strength were difficult to assess secondary to Jack's apprehension to actively move the leg and the presence of the external fixator. There was a significant reluctance to actively contract the muscles of the lower leg

for fear of moving or effecting the position of the external fixator. The weight in combination with the bulk of the fixator also contributed to Jack's apprehension to move the left leg. Jack preferred to reposition his left leg passively by using his arms.

Height: 5 feet, 8 inches
Weight: 190 pounds

Neuromuscular

Balance

Impaired balance was noted both in static standing and dynamic weight-shifting movements in standing. His balance was poor +, as tested in supported standing both using crutches and then holding the edge of the plinth. Because of weightbearing restrictions and a reluctance to attempt active LE movements, his fear of falling limited his balance significantly.

Locomotion

As noted in the interview, Jack reported that he struggled to maintain the weightbearing restriction and still manage his crutches for ambulation. He had a strong preference to use the wheelchair and, in addition, to have his friends push him.

Clinician Comment *It was already clear that Jack's gait with the crutches was impaired and needed to be assessed more fully as a test and measure than the limited systems review. The anxiety-producing gait task would be tabled until the tests and measures portion of the examination and placed toward the end.*

Transfers/Transitions

Jack required minimal assistance to position his left LE during position changes and bed mobility tasks during the systems review. His ability to move from sitting to standing in transfers, however, required close supervision to ensure maintenance of his balance as well as limit his weightbearing on the left LE. His mother reported Jack still needed assistance when showering because of his decreased balance. She reported he was independent with dressing and grooming once he was assisted for set-up only.

Communication, Affect, Cognition, Language, and Learning Style

Jack was a pleasant young man. He was alert and oriented but seemed anxious about progressing with his rehabilitation. He was quiet throughout most of the evaluation and tended to defer to his mother. She asked appropriate questions and helped answer questions when the patient was unable to remember. He did not seem to have any barriers to learning. He thought he might learn best from verbal and written instructions as well as pictures when available.

Clinician Comment *In working with adolescents, it is important to determine the style of learning that suits them best. It is even more important to validate and empower them as the primary person responsible for the rehabilitation process. In directing all questions and concerns directly to the patient (provided he or she is at an age to answer), it suggests to him or her that the parent is there for support, but it is the patient him- or herself who will be in control of the session. Empowering the young patient in this manner can make future requirements easier for him or her to take, such as performance of self-stretching or completion of home exercise program. It will also validate to him or her that he or she is being heard, which will build trust between the PT and the child in the rehabilitative process.*

Nothing occurred in the systems review that indicated Jack would not be a candidate for physical therapy. Selection of the tests and measures for the examination was indicated next and would be based on the findings thus far. Because Jack's obesity appeared to be a factor in many aspects of his care and future fitness considerations, his height and weight measures needed to be assessed, as well as the other anthropometric measures of leg length and limb circumference.

His pain needed to be documented as well as any additional environmental, home, school, and play barriers he faced. Measures of ROM and strength were indicated from the deficits noted in the systems review. The overall concern for his deconditioning suggested tests and measures of his aerobic capacity needed to be included, especially regarding the effort required for him to walk with crutches and gait.

Clinician Comment *Jack's obesity was now confirmed, and the impact of his obesity on his physical therapy prognosis needed to be considered. Further, it was important to educate Jack and his parents on the negative impact obesity may have on his future health and wellness. This educational component of physical therapy practice was consistent with the Vision 2020 statement by the American Physical Therapy Association. In it, PTs are identified as practitioners with the knowledge and skills to promote direct, frank, and honest conversations with patients on issues of weight to maximize health and wellness.*

Jack and his mom reported that they had been told by Jack's doctor that Jack may have future weight issues if he continued to gain weight at a rapid pace. It appeared from Jack's BMI that he had weight issues already. The stigma of conversing with youth regarding weight issues can lead to the issue not being addressed. The Vision 2020 statement is clear that the PT needs to consider obesity as an opportunity for education of the patient. The Centers for Disease Control website has resources both for the health care professional and the family/patient.

The most accurate measures of leg length occur with the use of radiographs. Radiograph measures were not available at the time of the PT's evaluation. Because a leg length discrepancy is a hallmark of Blount disease, the attempt to track this measure—even with tape measure estimates—was appropriate to address at the initiation of treatment.

While girth measurements of the left LE were difficult because of the external fixator, subjective documentation was recorded. Subjective observations of the skin color and temperature were noted also.

Tests and Measures

Anthropometric Measures

Based on Jack's height and weight at the time of evaluation, his BMI was 28.9, placing his BMI-for-age at the 98th percentile for boys aged 11 years.[8] In addition, Jack was within the "obese" category for his age.[8]

Leg length measurements, using a tape measure, were taken from the anterior superior iliac spine to the medial malleolus on each leg. The process was more challenging on the left because of the presence of the external fixator. The left LE measured approximately 1.25 cm shorter than the right.

Only slight swelling was noted in the left LE compared to the right. Girth measurements were not taken to confirm this on the first visit because of time and the difficulty posed by the presence of the external fixator on the left. Skin color and temperature throughout the left leg were equal to those on the right.

Pain

A pain assessment using a numeric rating scale revealed Jack reported his lowest pain at a 0/10 intensity and 3/10 for the worst pain intensity. The pain was described as "an ache" with occasional "shooting pains" around the pin sites. Jack reported the pain was random but did seem to intensify with walking and weightbearing.

Clinician Comment *Pain assessment used included a numeric rating scale using whole numbers from 0 to 10 to rate the intensity of the discomfort at a given time. Zero would indicate no pain and 10 would be "take me to the hospital" pain. It is worth noting here that there has been documentation of health care providers' observational ratings being lower than self-ratings by the children.[9]*

In this case, it may have been beneficial to have utilized a pediatric pain rating scale such as the Faces Pain Scale-Revised[10] or the Coloured Analogue Scale.[11] The self-rating by Jack varied greatly throughout the examination, calling into question the validity of using the numeric rating scale with him. He often gave a number that exceeded his previous report of his worst pain. Further, it also appeared as if Jack's fear of the pain that might occur with active movements was the bigger issue.

Whether it was a lack of understanding of the number rating scale or an inability to accurately assess pain, the reliability of Jack's use of the numeric rating scale became irrelevant. The scale was used to help Jack feel as though he was in control of any movement or activity that might cause pain. Throughout the examination, 6/10 became the pain intensity threshold for Jack, above which he had difficulty tolerating. Not exceeding this pain intensity level would become one of the guidelines to be used to define exercise intensity limits in his program.

Environmental, Home, and Work (School/Play) Barrier

Follow-up questions were employed to amplify the information already gained from Jack and his mother in the interview about barriers to his mobility. No additional information was gained except to learn that he climbed stairs at home by sitting on the stairs. He would raise himself up to sit on the adjacent superior stair to move up the stairs. He repeated the process in reverse to descend the stairs. He reported, and his mother concurred, that he did this independently and without pain.

Range of Motion (Including Muscle Length)

For the AROM, Jack moved his left leg independently and was not allowed to assist with his hands. Because of Jack's apprehension of having his left leg moved as well as the larger girth of the leg, the primary PT needed assistance from a colleague to ensure accurate passive measures (PROM).

Measurements for the joint ROM in the left leg were obtained with the patient lying supine on the plinth.

JOINT MOTION	RIGHT	LEFT	
	AROM	AROM	PROM
Knee flexion	0 to 135 degrees	-12 to 109 degrees*	-10 to 111 degrees*
Knee extension	0 degrees	-12 degrees*	-10 degrees*
Ankle dorsiflexion	0 to 20 degrees	-10 degrees	-5 degrees
Plantarflexion	0 to 40 degrees	-10 to 30 degrees	-5 to 35 degrees
*Limited by pain.			

MUSCLE FLEXIBILITY	RIGHT	LEFT
Quadriceps	0 to 135 degrees	Nor tested secondary to pain
Hamstrings (90 to 90)	-20 degrees	-40 degrees
Heel cord	0 to 10 degrees	-10 degrees
Hip flexors (Thomas test position)	-5 degrees	-10 degrees

Clinician Comment *ROM measurements confirmed impairment within the hip and ankle as well as the knee that will need to be addressed. Knee extension and ankle motion would be focal points in the treatment strategies. Identifying and then using a consistent procedure for the ROM measurements now and in reassessments later would allow for comparable measures.*

Muscle Performance (Including Strength, Power, and Endurance)

The only adjustment to standard MMT positions was that all left leg testing was performed with the patient supine on the table.

MUSCLE GROUP	RIGHT	LEFT
UEs	5/5	5/5
Hip flexion	5/5	3+/5
Hip extension	4+/5	3-/5
Hip abduction	4+/5	3-/5
Hip adduction	4/5	3-/5
Knee flexion	5/5	2/5
Knee extension	5/5	2+/5
Ankle dorsiflexion	5/5	3-/5
Ankle plantarflexion	5/5	3-/5
Ankle inversion	4+/5	3-/5
Ankle eversion	4+/5	3-/5

Clinician Comment *MMT was utilized for measuring muscle strength and performance. There are limitations of MMT in the pediatric population because accurate measures require consistent maximal efforts by the subject as well as the subject's understanding of how to reproduce the exact motion being tested. With Jack, he seemed to understand what was being asked but was unwilling to offer maximal effort in testing the left LE.*

While he denied pain with testing, he admitted to being afraid of tearing the skin around the pin sites. In reassessments, the continued presence (or eventual absence) of the external fixator needs to be noted with MMT measures as the fixator may be a significant variable in comparable muscle performance.

In working with an adolescent population, it is important to remember the youth's desire to appear strong and independent to a new adult, particularly when the patient is male and the therapist female. A submaximal effort may be the youth's attempt to avoid a painful level of contraction. Adolescent patients may need extra encouragement to give 100% effort and may be reassured that any pain will diminish as therapy progresses.

Gait, Locomotion, and Balance

Gait

Jack demonstrated his ability to walk using bilateral axillary crutches while attempting to maintain the weightbearing restriction on the left. He required close supervision for safety. He tended to hold his left leg in approximately 25 degrees of external hip rotation. He used a left hip hike and circumduction to advance his left LE during the swing phase of gait. Further, he showed decreased dorsiflexion of the left ankle during swing. During the stance phase of gait, Jack showed decreased hip extension bilaterally. He used a step-to, 3-point gait pattern but required maximal verbal cueing to maintain weight restriction on the left LE. He required close supervision and occasional contact guard to maintain safety in walking.

A scale was utilized to help him see how much actual weight he was putting through his left leg. Initially, he placed 15 and 25 pounds of weight on his left LE. Jack required significant practice while standing in the parallel bars and using the scale before he could consistently avoid exceeding the 10-pound restriction. To help with the carryover of awareness gained in the practice session, he was instructed to just place his toe on the ground when ambulating to limit his weightbearing to an acceptable level.

His bariatric crutches were heavier than standard crutches. With manipulating the heavier crutches as well as the effort of ambulating, he began to exhibit shortness of breath after completing a distance of 50 feet.

Balance

Jack's balance score improved from that noted in the system review to a Fair minus. His overall balance continued to be limited because of his difficulty with manipulating the crutches within the weightbearing restriction. When standing still, Jack held the left LE in flexion and external rotation at the hip, knee slightly flexed, and ankle plantarflexed.

Clinician Comment *The gait of children who are obese is typically altered even without the presence of Blount disease.[12] Children of normal weight tend to place the advancing foot close to the midline of foot progression. This foot placement minimizes weight transfer and decreases energy expenditure in gait.*

For children who are obese, body mass at the thigh limits the ability to adduct the hip. This interferes with the ability to place the foot close to the midline of foot progression, thereby increasing energy expenditure necessary for gait. This wider-than-usual foot placement also results in a varus moment at the knee that increases the pressure on the medial aspect of the proximal tibial physis. This increase in medial pressure inhibits growth in accordance with the Hueter-Volkmann law. As described earlier in this report, this bone growth inhibition leads to the development of Blount disease.[2,13] With the probability that Jack had an altered gait pattern even prior to surgery, it was difficult to assess how his postoperative gait pattern differed. Consideration of preexisting range and strength deficits in the involved extremity associated with an altered gait pattern, because of his obesity, needed to be considered in the development of his treatment program.

For the testing of gait, visual observation was utilized only since it was not safe at the time of the examination to consider standardized tests with Jack, such as the Timed Up and Go test[14] or Berg Balance test[15] given his difficulty with ambulation.

The tests and measures confirmed that Jack had altered anthropometric measures, pain intensity, and environmental barriers to movement. ROM, muscle length, and strength testing further documented his existing impairments. Though not tested directly, his shortness of breath with ambulation suggested decreased aerobic capacity. This along with the comorbidity of obesity and generalized decreased fitness level would affect his gait and balance. He was using bariatric crutches that were larger and heavier than those typically used by patients his same age. The effort of attempting to maintain the weightbearing restriction on his left leg led to a faster increase in his perceived level of exertion for walking.

EVALUATION

Diagnosis

Jack was 3 weeks postoperative from a left tibia/fibula osteotomy to correct altered tibial plateau alignment associated with Blount disease. He had significant limitations in mobility and function because of weightbearing restrictions and the presence of an external fixator. He showed decreased ROM, muscle lengths, and strengths. His mobility was further affected by his obesity and deconditioning.

Practice Pattern

Based on the history, systems review, and tests and measures, this patient was classified into 2 Preferred Practice Patterns:

1. Musculoskeletal Practice Pattern 4I: Impaired Joint Mobility, Motor Function, Muscle Performance, and Range of Motion Associated With Bony or Soft Tissue Surgery

2. Cardiovascular/Pulmonary Practice Pattern 6B: Impaired Aerobic Capacity/Endurance Associated With Deconditioning

International Classification of Functioning, Disability and Health Model of Disability

See ICF Model on page 86.

Prognosis

Jack had a good physical therapy prognosis. He could be expected to make a complete recovery of ROM and strength in his left LE over the course of his treatment. His gait and endurance should return to his prior level. He should be able to return to all previous functional activities consistent with an 11-year-old male with comorbidity of obesity.

Clinician Comment *It is important to note in the prognosis for Jack that he will be somewhat limited in his outcomes by his comorbidity of obesity. As Wilson et al illustrate in the review of complications from tibial osteotomies, there exists a higher prevalence of complications postsurgery in those patients with the presence of obesity.[5] In order to maximize Jack's functional prognosis, it would be indicated to address his obesity and decreased activity levels as well as how both may affect his course of treatment.*

Plan of Care

Intervention

Jack and his family would benefit from continued education regarding Blount disease and his status, plan of care, and discharge plan. A periodic review of pin care techniques was indicated to prevent infection.

Active assisted and AROM exercises for his left LE, including hip flexors, extensors, abductors, and adductors; knee flexors and extensors; and ankle dorsiflexors, plantar flexors, invertors, and evertors, were indicated. His program would be progressed to closed-chain strengthening exercises when weightbearing restrictions were reduced. Progressive resistance exercises would be added as tolerated with the external fixator.

Gait training with bilateral axillary crutches would begin on level surfaces and stairs while also maintaining his weightbearing restriction. When allowed, Jack would be progressed through weightbearing as tolerated and finally to ambulating independently without an assistive device.

An endurance reconditioning program would be addressed with a daily ambulation schedule.

The patient would be instructed in a home exercise program. A paper copy of the exercises with written instructions and drawings would be provided. Frequency for Jack's home exercise program would be recommended as twice daily.

Proposed Frequency and Duration of Physical Therapy Visits

Over the course of 12 weeks, Jack will be seen 2 times per week at school for a total of 24 visits.

Anticipated Goals

1. Jack will move from sitting in his wheelchair to standing in his crutches independently (1 week).

2. Jack will actively flex his left knee to greater than 110 degrees (2 weeks).

3. He will be able to tolerate active assistive ROM left knee extension to at least -10 degrees (2 weeks).

4. Family and patient will demonstrate continued independence with pin care and skin check to avoid infection (2 weeks).

5. He will show active knee extension to at least –10 degrees (3 weeks).

6. Jack will have 3+/5 strength throughout left LE (4 weeks).

7. He will show active knee flexion in his left knee greater than 120 degrees (4 weeks).

8. He will ambulate community distances with bilaterally axillary crutches and following appropriate weightbearing restrictions independently (4 weeks).

9. Jack will show independent performance of a home exercise program with 100% accuracy for all stretching and strengthening procedures (4 weeks).

10. Jack will rate his pain no more than 2 out of 10 with all ADL and perform independently (6 weeks).

11. He will show active knee ROM to 5 to 130 degrees with no report of pain-limiting motion (8 weeks).

12. Family and patient will demonstrate knowledge of risk factors of complications due to obesity with Blount disease (8 weeks).

13. Jack will participate in 30 minutes of cardiovascular endurance activities including biking or elliptical training with 0/10 pain rating (10 weeks).

14. Jack will demonstrate 4+/5 LE strength throughout left LE with MMT (11 weeks).

Expected Outcomes (12 Weeks)

1. Jack will be independent in all ADL as well as school and community ambulation with or without an ambulation device.

2. Jack will be independent with an appropriate fitness activity to ensure continued lifelong weight control.

ICF MODEL OF DISABLEMENT FOR JACK

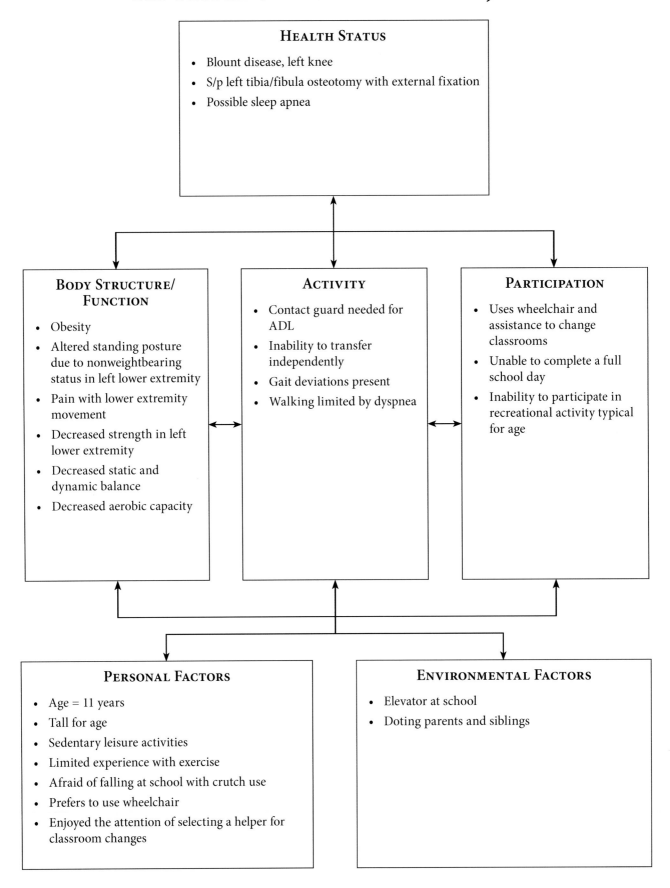

HEALTH STATUS

- Blount disease, left knee
- S/p left tibia/fibula osteotomy with external fixation
- Possible sleep apnea

BODY STRUCTURE/FUNCTION

- Obesity
- Altered standing posture due to nonweightbearing status in left lower extremity
- Pain with lower extremity movement
- Decreased strength in left lower extremity
- Decreased static and dynamic balance
- Decreased aerobic capacity

ACTIVITY

- Contact guard needed for ADL
- Inability to transfer independently
- Gait deviations present
- Walking limited by dyspnea

PARTICIPATION

- Uses wheelchair and assistance to change classrooms
- Unable to complete a full school day
- Inability to participate in recreational activity typical for age

PERSONAL FACTORS

- Age = 11 years
- Tall for age
- Sedentary leisure activities
- Limited experience with exercise
- Afraid of falling at school with crutch use
- Prefers to use wheelchair
- Enjoyed the attention of selecting a helper for classroom changes

ENVIRONMENTAL FACTORS

- Elevator at school
- Doting parents and siblings

Discharge Plan

It was anticipated that Jack would achieve the anticipated goals and expected outcomes at the end of the plan of care. It was expected that he would be discharged to a home program of exercises as well as an identified fitness activity. Jack and his mother understood, and agreed with, the plan of care.

INTERVENTION

Coordination, Communication, and Documentation

Coordinated dialogue with the medical team, educational team, and family regarding progression of care and treatment plan was essential to motivate Jack to maximize his functional independence and remove any secondary gains of remaining dependent for mobility. Ongoing communication with the patient, family, and school staff regarding progression toward goals and any changes in his weightbearing status would be integral. Documentation would include all aspects of care, including initial evaluation, progress reports, reexaminations, and discharge summary.

Patient-/Client-Related Instruction

The patient and his family were given extensive education regarding the plan of care, frequency of visits, and discharge plan as mentioned previously. They also received a review of pin and skin care around the external fixator, following the original instructions given at the hospital prior to Jack's discharge. A written home exercise program was created, along with information on how to begin an endurance reconditioning program using his UEs as well as LEs until weightbearing precautions were lifted. Comorbidities of sleep disturbances and obesity were also discussed. The family was encouraged to pursue the pulmonology consult recommended by the hospital discharge team. Jack received an explanation of what progress he could expect to gain from physical therapy sessions in terms of movement, strength, pain reduction, and progressive weightbearing. Jack reported he understood why physical therapy was necessary and why his follow-through with his home exercise program was critical to his successful return to his previous functional level.

Procedural Interventions

Therapeutic Exercise Prescription

Aerobic Capacity/Endurance Conditioning or Reconditioning

Mode

Walking program and use of an upper body ergometer (UBE)

Intensity

Rate of perceived exertion (RPE) < 8/20, pain intensity < 6/10

UBE: 60 rpm

Duration

Walking: 5 minute walks around the house; UBE: 3 minutes forward, 3 minutes backward

Frequency

Walking: 3 times per day during school days, 6 on weekends; UBE: at physical therapy 2 times per week

Description of the Intervention

Jack was instructed first in a walking program to help increase his endurance for physical activity. Since he had difficulty with ambulation, this activity was supplemented at the school-based physical therapy clinic with the use of a UBE. The UBE was used in the clinic to increase Jack's HR and cardiovascular conditioning because he began with limited ability for repetitive fitness movements with his LEs.

Clinician Comment *RPE was used to define a low level of exertion for Jack rather than a target for him to reach in each session. This patient was not active prior to surgery and admitted to not liking physical activity, preferring more sedentary activities such as watching TV and computer games. While the speed or distance of the walk was not specified, the repetition of the ambulation in 5-minute blocks would serve to increase his overall activity level. For Jack, it was important that he feel the beneficial effect in his exercise tolerance that could occur with even a modest increase in his activity level. Further, his confidence with walking at home would increase and then could be carried over to ambulating in school at a later time.*

Flexibility Exercises

Mode

Assisted and active self-stretching flexibility exercises

Intensity

Slow movements through the entire ROM as able with a hold at end range with no pain sensation, only a stretch

Duration

5 to 10 minutes of flexibility activities daily

Frequency

3 repetitions 2 times per day

Description of the Intervention

A program of flexibility exercises was developed based on the ROM deficits identified in the initial evaluation. The exercises for his school-based physical therapy sessions as well as part of his home exercise program consisted of the following specific stretching and ROM activities for the left LE:

- *Dorsiflexion stretch with use of a towel*: In long sitting, wrap towel around bottom of left foot and pull back into dorsiflexion for a 30-second hold.

- *Knee flexion stretch*: Lying in prone, use a jump rope looped around the left foot and use arms to assist in flexing the knee to tolerance for a 30-second hold.

- *Hamstring stretch*: Sitting on edge of bed, drop right leg off edge and leave left leg on bed, toes pointed to ceiling while reaching with both hands out to the toes. Emphasize keeping left knee completely straight and bending forward at the hip.

Strength and Endurance Training

Training for trunk and leg muscles and home exercise program

Mode

Active and against gravity isometric and progressive isotonic exercises

Intensity

Slow movements through the entire ROM

Duration

20 minutes for entire routine

Frequency

2 sets of 10 repetitions each exercise at least 1 time per day

Description of the intervention

A comprehensive strength and conditioning program was developed that initially consisted of active exercises performed in sitting, prone, and supine positions. When lifting restrictions are lifted, then the exercises would be progressed to standing activities as well as closed kinetic chain activities. The exercises included the following:

- Gluteal sets in supine with 10-second hold

- Quad sets in supine with 5-second hold of the contraction. Because of his difficulty in recruiting the quadriceps for this exercise in the clinic, an inflated BP cuff was positioned under Jack's left leg. To increase the proprioceptive input of a correct quad contraction, he held the dial and monitored the effectiveness of his contraction by watching to see if the needle position changed. Pushing his posterior distal thigh into a towel roll was recommended for his home program.

- Ankle pumps were performed through the entire ROM to assist in dissipating the minimal swelling present in the left knee.

- Assisted heel slides were performed using a rope around the ankle to allow Jack to bring his knee to full available range without assistance from an adult.

- Seated march performed over edge of bed

- Closed kinetic-chain activities would be added when cleared by doctor.

Clinician Comment *As previously stated, Jack's activity level prior to his surgery was decreased as compared to same-aged peers. It was therefore recommended that he perform these exercises at home on both LEs. Care was taken to avoid exercises that would require*

another adult's assistance to reinforce the focus on Jack's gain of functional independence. The less Jack needed to rely on adults, the more responsibility Jack would take to ensure his own progress. This approach eliminated the oft heard excuse with a pediatric client when confronted with poor home program compliance that a parent was not available to help.

Early in the exercise program, it was explained to Jack that the discomfort associated with exercise should never be above a 6/10 rating on a 0 to 10 numeric rating scale. If his pain reached a 6/10 during his school-based program, he was to inform the primary PT, who would modify the activity to decrease the pain intensity felt. This again reinforced to the Jack that, while the PT might direct the course of the session, Jack had active control. It was also explained to Jack that if all of the exercises seem easy or no stretch was felt, the intensity of the exercise needed to be increased for the exercises to be beneficial.

Gait and Locomotion Training

Mode

Walking with appropriate assistive device and obeying weightbearing precautions

Intensity

Walking at a pace that is age appropriate

Duration

10 minutes progressing, up to 30 minutes

Frequency

Daily practice at least 10 minutes

Description of the Intervention

With Jack standing in the parallel bars and his left LE on a scale, he will practice loading his left LE to the weightbearing restricted amount. Jack will progress to walking with the bilateral axillary crutches with appropriate weightbearing through the left leg. As the weightbearing restriction changes, Jack will be progressed to weightbearing as tolerated, and eventually to full weightbearing as indicated by the physician. Emphasis will be placed on increasing step length and improving safety awareness of obstacles in his path. Stair training will be performed when appropriate.

Clinician Comment *Experience suggests that the more learning techniques that can be employed to teach a motor pattern, the more successful a pediatric client might be in achieving the goal. Jack understood that he was not to exceed 10 pounds of weightbearing through his left leg, but he had difficulty identifying what that felt like. By spending time using a visual cue of the scale, he was able to perceive what the 10 pounds of pressure felt like and became better able to adjust his weightbearing when given a verbal reminder. Another motor learning strategy was used when teaching Jack how to recruit his quadriceps in performance of the "quad set" exercise. By handing him the dial of the* *sphygmomanometer and placing the inflated cuff behind his knee, he was given the visual aid of the needle moving, indicating the correct muscular contraction. With a pediatric client, using a visual cue will often lead to decreased frustration and improved outcomes.*

Balance, Coordination, and Agility Training

Mode

Age-appropriate tests of balance, coordination, and agility, such as timed shuttle runs, jump tests, and obstacle courses

Intensity

Moderate to high intensity when cleared by physician

Duration

Up to 5 minutes in duration

Frequency

2 to 3 times per week when cleared to participate

Description of the Intervention

When cleared by the physician for the increased weight-bearing that would be required, balance, coordination, and agility training will be initiated with use of timed shuttle runs, completion of obstacle courses, and upper-level balance training as appropriate for an 11-year-old male.

Functional Training

Training in home and work (job/school/play), community, and leisure integration or reintegration, including ADL, instrumental ADL, work hardening, and work conditioning

Description of the Intervention

- ADL, instrumental ADL, and functional training. Training to include the following:
  - Bed mobility and transfer training
  - Developmental activities appropriate for an 11 year old
  - Simulated school environment, including crowded hallways and school cafeteria
  - Household chores
  - Recreational activities, including simulated physical education tasks
- Injury prevention or reduction
  - Injury prevention education during self-care and home management
  - Injury prevention or reduction with use of devices and equipment including strict adherence to weight-bearing restrictions
  - Safety awareness training during self-care, home, and school management
- Functional training
  - Energy conservation techniques

REEXAMINATION

Jack's progress was monitored at each treatment; however, formal reexaminations occurred at 6 weeks, 4 months, and 6 months from the initiation of physical therapy sessions. These reports were generated prior to Jack's return visits to the referring physician.

Reexamination at 6 weeks

Subjective

"I'm more comfortable walking."

Objective

Pain

As noted previously, Jack reported he was able to walk with his crutches with less pain. The pin site symptoms were reported a 4/10 on the numeric rating scale, especially when bending the left knee during swing phase of gait.

Environmental, Home, and School/Play Barriers

Jack returned to full days of school. He no longer required assistance with transfers, gait, or trips to the bathroom while at school. He ambulated independently with crutches between classrooms but was still given additional time.

He continued to be mostly sedentary when at home. His family still offered him assistance with his needs rather than having him perform them independently.

Range of Motion (Including Muscle Lengths)

Symptoms limited his left knee flexion to 110 degrees. Left knee extension was −6 degrees. Left ankle dorsiflexion (knee bent) was −2 degrees and plantarflexion 35 degrees. His left hip ROM was within functional limits.

Specific muscle length testing showed improved but still limited lengths. His left hamstring length, measured from a vertical 90-degree standard, was −38 degrees. Ankle dorsiflexion measured with the knee straight to assess gastrocnemius length showed −10 degrees. Hip flexor length measured in the Thomas test position showed −8 degrees.

Muscle Performance (Including Strength, Power, and Endurance)

MUSCLE GROUP	MUSCLE GRADE
Hip flexion	3+/5
Hip extension	3−/5
Hip abduction	4/5
Hip adduction	4/5
Knee flexion	4−/5
Knee extension	2+/5
Ankle dorsiflexion	4/5
Ankle plantarflexion	3/5

Gait, Locomotion, and Balance

Jack walked independently with his crutches at school. He was allowed to increase the weightbearing on his left LE to 20 pounds. Though the pin sites remained healthy and without signs of infection, he continued to report decreased ability to comfortably bend his left knee when advancing his left LE forward in gait.

Assessment

Jack was able to show an increase in his overall ambulation ability in the first 6 weeks of physical therapy. He progressed to 20 pounds of weightbearing on his left LE. Jack did not show significant changes in muscle lengths because of continued related symptoms at the pin sites. He did show increased strength in left knee flexors and overall hip strength.

Of the goals anticipated to be met by 6 weeks, he met numbers 1, 3, 4, 5, and 8. Though he made gains with each visit, he did not gain knee flexion greater than 110 degrees (#2) or 120 degrees (#7), or the strength goals for hip and knee extension (#6). He knew his home program, but he had decreased compliance (#9). Goals for pain intensity (#10) and left knee AROM (#11) were thwarted by continued pin site reactivity.

Clinician Comment *Jack made gains, but not as anticipated. The rate of allowed weightbearing was not increased as anticipated because follow-up radiographs did not show the expected bone healing at the rate projected. Increased in weightbearing might have assisted in a more normal gait pattern for his left LE and, thus, left hip and knee strength. The pin site reactivity continued to limit his movement. He was scheduled to attend physical therapy 3 times per week, but with transportation complications, he attended only 1 to 2 times per week.*

Plan

The described physical therapy intervention plan would be continued. The following time changes would be made for his yet-to-be met goals and outcomes.

Anticipated Goals

- #2: Jack will actively flex his left knee to greater than 110 degrees (8 weeks).

- #6: Jack will have 3+/5 strength throughout left LE 6 weeks after the removal of the fixator or weightbearing as tolerated was allowed.

- #9: Jack will show independent performance of a home exercise program with 100% accuracy for all stretching and strengthening procedures (8 weeks).

- #10: Jack will rate his pain no more than 2/10 3 weeks after the fixator is removed.

- #11: He will show active knee ROM to 5 to 130 degrees with no report of pain-limiting motion (12 weeks).

Reexamination at 16 Weeks (4 Months)

Subjective

"It is so much easier to do this [physical therapy] without the fixator."

Objective

Weightbearing Status

Jack remained at 20 pounds weightbearing until the fixator was removed 12 weeks after therapy started. He was then required to go back to a 10-pound weightbearing restriction on his left LE for 5 weeks—a restriction still in place at the time of this reexamination.

Pain

Jack reported his pain level was 0/10. He was also more motivated during rehab sessions.

Environmental, Home, and Work (School/Play) Barrier

Jack was not in school because of the summer break. He spent most of his time at home. His endurance for walking appeared to decrease slightly since he was no longer walking between classes at school. He was able to perform all ADL at home without supervision.

Range of Motion (Including Muscle Length)

LEFT LE	4 MONTHS AROM
Knee flexion	122 degrees
Knee extension	–3 degrees
Ankle dorsiflexion	5 degrees
Ankle plantarflexion	40 degrees
FLEXIBILITY	
Hamstrings (90 to 90)	–34 degrees
Gastrocnemius	–10 degrees
Hip flexors	–5 degrees

Muscle Performance (Including Strength, Power, and Endurance)

MUSCLE GROUP	4 MONTHS (16 WEEKS)
Hip flexion	4/5
Hip extension	3+/5
Hip abduction	4/5
Hip adduction	4/5
Knee flexion	4/5
Knee extension	3+/5
Ankle dorsiflexion	4+/5
Ankle plantarflexion	3/5

Gait, Locomotion, and Balance

Jack was able to demonstrate gait with his crutches and maintenance of the 10-pound weightbearing restriction without difficulty.

> **Clinician Comment** *Pain was no longer an issue for Jack. He was completing his ADL independently at home but walking less overall with summer break. He was meeting the goals for his knee motion. His muscle lengths were not as improved as anticipated with the removal of the fixator, but he was still limited in his gait pattern because of the weightbearing restriction. His overall improvement in ROM, muscle lengths, and strength gave him a good base from which to make further gains.*

Assessment

Jack met the original anticipated goals numbers 1 through 8 as well as numbers 10 and 12. He met expected outcome number 1 using an ambulation device. He was more motivated to be consistent with his home program.

Plan

The projected time interval for achievement of the remaining anticipated goals and expected outcomes were amended. The first expected outcome was changed to "without an ambulation device."

Anticipated Goals

- #1: Jack will show independent performance of a home exercise program with 100% accuracy for all stretching and strengthening procedures (24 weeks).

- #11: He will show active knee ROM to 5 to 130 degrees with no report of pain-limiting motion (20 weeks).

- #13: Jack will participate in 30 minutes of cardiovascular endurance activities, including biking or elliptical training, with 1/10 pain rating (24 weeks).

- #14: Jack will demonstrate 4+/5 LE strength throughout left LE with MMT (24 weeks).

Expected Outcomes (24 Weeks)

1. Jack will be independent in all ADL as well as school and community ambulation without an ambulation device.

2. Jack will be independent with an appropriate fitness activity to ensure continued life-long weight control.

Reexamination at 24 Weeks

Subjective

"I can do everything I used to do [before surgery] and better now, but I get tired more easily." "I think I'm walking funny."

Objective

Weightbearing Status

Weightbearing status was increased to 50% 8 weeks prior, with increase to full weightbearing over 4 weeks.

Pain

Jack continued to report 0/10 pain.

Environmental, Home, and Work (School/Play) Barrier

Jack returned to school in the fall and ambulated throughout the full school day with no restrictions except for physical education. He returned to performing chores at home and was performing his home exercise program and his fitness regime at least 3 times per week.

Range of Motion (Including Muscle Length)

LEFT LE AROM	24 WEEKS
Knee flexion	135 degrees
Knee extension	0 degrees
Ankle dorsiflexion	15 degrees
Ankle plantarflexion	40 degrees
FLEXIBILITY AROM	**24 WEEKS**
Hamstrings (90 to 90)	−25 degrees
Heel cord	5 degrees
Hip flexors	0 degrees

Muscle Performance (Including Strength, Power, and Endurance)

MUSCLE GROUP	24 WEEKS
Hip flexion	4+/5
Hip extension	4/5
Hip abduction	4+/5
Hip adduction	4+/5
Knee flexion	5/5
Knee extension	4+/5
Ankle dorsiflexion	5/5
Ankle plantarflexion	4-/5

Gait, Locomotion, and Balance

Jack had a slightly asymmetrical gait with a slight drop in his center of gravity during stance phase on the left LE when walking without an ambulation aid. He walked better with it.

Assessment

Jack performed his home exercise program and fitness program at home 3 times per week (#9 and #13). Jack had achieved the ROM and muscle length goals (#11). All left LE muscle strength grades were greater than or equal to 4+/5, with the exception of left hip extension and ankle plantar flexion (#14). Pain was absent. His increased ROM and strength allowed him to move with less perceived exertion at home and at school.

At the time of this reexamination, Jack had just been cleared to run. He would benefit from a few additional physical therapy sessions to practice pre-running and running tasks, as well as higher level balance and coordination drills.

Plan

The frequency of treatment sessions would be reduced to once per week. Pre-running and running tasks would be introduced. High-level balance and agility drills would be practiced. Continued education on the importance of fitness and a wellness lifestyle would be included.

Clinician Comment *This case report ties together multiple factors that need to be considered beyond a patient's initial medical diagnosis. Jack was a young man referred to physical therapy for an orthopedic issue but benefitted from a comprehensive treatment approach that included cardiovascular, integumentary, and wellness goals. Pediatric patients have many special circumstances to consider, but adolescent patients in particular can be a challenge to motivate and empower to be an active participant in the process. Through the course of Jack's care, communication between Jack, his family, and his school had to be clear and thorough to ensure follow-through and compliance. Issues that may not be typically addressed by a PT—obesity, explanation of BMI for age, risk factors related to obesity in youth, sleep apnea, and promoting functional independence—needed to be addressed for this patient. Although all goals were not met completely, he was able to resume his previous activities and became educated on how following an active lifestyle would be important for maintenance of good health, now and in the future.*

OUTCOMES

Discharge

While it was recommended Jack continue with physical therapy for 1 additional month, Jack's family chose not to continue the sessions when their insurance coverage would not authorize additional visits. This patient did undergo an extensive course of therapy that lasted over 6 months with sessions occurring 1 or 2 times per week and an extensive home exercise program. Patient and family education were critical components in this case to help control the risk of recurrence or complication.

At the time of discharge, Jack had achieved all anticipated outcomes except a return to running. He had a mildly asymmetrical gait: his left LE strength did not yet equal the right. He was not yet fully participating in physical education.

Near his 12th birthday, Jack was measured at 5 feet, 9 inches tall and 188 pounds. His BMI was calculated to be 27.8, which was in the 97th percentile in BMI for age for a 12-year-old boy. The reduction in his BMI and his BMI-for-age was an outstanding accomplishment for Jack as developing life-long weight control habits was a secondary goal of his program.

At the time of discharge, there had been no follow-up with pulmonary regarding possible sleep apnea despite multiple attempts to encourage Jack's mother to schedule an appointment.

REFERENCES

1. Wills M. Orthopedic complications of childhood obesity. *Pediatr Phys Ther.* 2004;16:230-235.
2. Thompson GH, Carter, JR. Late-onset tibial vara (Blount's disease): current concepts. *Clin Orthop Relat Res.* 1990;(255):24-35.
3. Shulman ST. A sweet solution? And a major philatelic error. *Pediatr Ann.* 2010;39(3):115-116.
4. A patient's guide to Blount's disease in children and adolescents. *eOrthopod* www.eorthopod.com/content/blounts-disease-in-children-and-adolescents. Accessed February 28, 2010.
5. Wilson NA, Scherl SA, Cramer KE. Complications of high tibial osteotomy with external fixation in adolescent Blount's disease. *Orthopedics.* 2007;30(10):848-852.
6. Sabharwal S. Blount disease. *J Bone Joint Surg Am.* 2009;91:1758-1776.
7. Section on Pediatric Pulmonology, Subcommittee on Obstructive Sleep Apnea Syndrome. American Academy of Pediatrics. Clinical Practice guideline: diagnosis and management of childhood obstructive sleep apnea syndrome. *Pediatrics.* 2002;109:704-712.
8. Centers for Disease Control and Prevention. Growth charts. http://www.cdc.gov/growthcharts. Updated September 9, 2010. Accessed February 28, 2010.
9. deTovar C, von Baeyer CL, Wood C, Alibeu JP, Houfani M, Arvieux C. Post-operative self-report of pain in children: interscale agreement, response to analgesic, and preference for a faces scale and a visual analogue scale. *Pain Res Manag.* 2010;15:163-168. Accessed via Pub Med July 21, 2010.
10. Hick CL, von Baeyer CL, Spafford PA, van Korlaar I, Goodenough B. The Faces Pain Scale-Revised: toward a common metric in pediatric pain measurement. *Pain.* 2001;93(2):173-183.
11. McGrath PA, Seifert CE, Speechley KN, Booth JC, Stitt L, Gibson MC. A new analogue scale for assessing children's pain: an initial validation study. *Pain.* 1996;64(3):435-443.

12. McMillan AG, Auman NL, Collier DN, Blaise Williams DS. Frontal plane lower extremity biomechanics during walking in boys who are overweight versus healthy weight. *Pediatr Phys Ther.* 2009;21:187-193.

13. Goshue DL, Houck J, Lerner AL. Effects of childhood obesity on three-dimensional knee joint biomechanics during walking. *J Pediatr Orthop.* 2005;25(6):763-768.

14. Podsiadlo D, Richardson S. The timed "Up & Go": a test of basic functional mobility for frail elderly persons. *J Am Geriatr Soc.* 1991;39(2):142-148.

15. Berg KD, Wood-Dauphinee SL, Williams JI, Maki B. Measuring balance in the elderly: validation of an instrument. *Can J of Public Health.* 1992;83 Suppl 2:s7-s11.

3

System Changes in the Aging Adult

Alison L. Squadrito, PT, DPT, GCS, CEEAA

CHAPTER OBJECTIVES

- Identify the physiologic changes with aging that occur in ventilation, gas exchange, oxygen (O_2) delivery, and cellular O_2 uptake that impact the aerobic capacity of older adults.

- Name the exercise prescription parameters for aerobic capacity training with older adults that have led to effective gains in maximum O_2 consumption (VO_{2max}).

- List the cardioprotective effects seen as a result of exercise for aging adults.

- Describe the age-related changes in the cardiovascular system and the impact they have on an older adult's hemodynamic response to exercise.

- Describe the relationship between O_2 consumption for activities of daily living (ADL), peak VO_2, and functional capacity.

- Name the changes in the aging musculoskeletal system that affect muscle strength and power.

- Discuss what research study results suggest about muscle endurance in aging adults.

- Describe the relationship between muscle performance (strength, power, and endurance) and functional performance of the older adult.

- Using the concept of physical reserve, summarize the impact of function in aging adults with regard to aerobic capacity and muscle performance.

- Summarize what research studies have shown about muscle performance training in aging adults and the impact on physical function.

- Contrast the postural stability control strategies used by aging adults compared to younger adults.

- Discuss how the age-related changes to the 3 components of motor control affect the function (including fall risk) and the quality of life in aging adults.

CHAPTER OUTLINE

- Age-Related Changes in Aerobic Capacity
  - Ventilation
    - Changes in Ventilatory Muscles
    - Changes in the Lung
    - Changes in the Chest Wall
    - Physiologic Measures of Lung Function
  - Gas Exchange
    - Ventilation-Perfusion Matching
    - Diffusion
  - Oxygen Delivery
    - Changes in the Heart
    - Changes in the Blood Vessels
    - Physiologic Measures at Rest
    - Physiologic Measures With Exercise
    - Cellular Oxygen Uptake
  - Benefits of Aerobic Training
  - Summary
- Age-Related Changes in Muscle Performance
  - Age-Related Changes in Skeletal Muscle
    - Muscle Mass
    - Muscle Fiber Type and Size
    - Motor Units

Coglianese D, ed. *Clinical Exercise Pathophysiology for Physical Therapy: Examination, Testing, and Exercise Prescription for Movement-Related Disorders (pp 95-133).*
© 2015 Taylor & Francis Group.

Physical therapists (PTs) interpret examination data and identify abnormal test results to formulate accurate diagnoses and effective treatment plans for their patients and clients. The ability to recognize abnormal findings requires a clear understanding of the expected or normal results of tests and measures. "Normal" often changes as a result of the aging process. Data that might be considered abnormal in a young adult are often considered usual and acceptable in an older individual because of age-associated changes in anatomy and physiology. An appreciation of the expected age-related changes in the body's systems is therefore critical to accurate interpretation of test results and determination of a realistic prognosis and plan of care. As the demographics of the United States population continue to change and the proportion of seniors steadily increases, PTs will be more and more likely to interact with an aging clientele. Thus, knowledge of the physiology of aging will become increasingly pertinent.

Many challenges exist in studying the effects of aging on the body. Primarily, it is difficult to establish age as the sole independent variable in any sample. Rigorous screening is required to exclude subjects with occult disease, significant lifestyle differences, or influential environmental exposures. In addition, research about age-related changes is frequently flawed by lack of the oldest adults (ie, >80 years old) in the sample.

Masoro[1] describes many of the major confounders in study designs that need to be considered when interpreting the results of research on aging. The use of cross-sectional designs to test subjects of different ages at a given point in time is relatively common because it is less expensive and requires less subject commitment over a long period compared to longitudinal studies. Such studies, however, are subject to a cohort or generational effect. That is, individuals born at any particular time are exposed to a specific set of factors (eg, nutritional deficiencies, infections, environmental exposures) that may influence the physiological variables under investigation. If these confounding variables are unknown, the differences between age groups may be erroneously attributed to the effect of aging rather than the effect of the confounding variable.

In addition, cross-sectional study designs increase the risk of selective mortality. When older age groups are studied, the only subjects left to participate are those from the birth cohort who did not have significant risk factors for disease that caused morbidity or mortality at a younger age. Selective mortality may therefore underestimate the rate of change of aging.[2]

The cross-sectional study design is not the only type of research with issues when it comes to accurately documenting the changes of aging. While longitudinal studies may avoid some of the previously described problems, this experimental design has limitations as well. For example, repeated exposure to a measurement can cause subjects to change their performance because they have learned about the measure, not because of a true change in their abilities or perceptions. There also may be significant changes in the lifestyle or environment of the subjects over the course of the study that must be accounted for. Finally, attrition of participants and changes in technology and instrumentation over time can have a significant impact.[1,2]

Despite the difficulties involved in the investigation of the aging process, significant evidence exists that documents age-related changes in anatomy and physiology. This chapter presents the changes in aerobic capacity, muscle performance, and motor control that inevitably occur with advancing age.

AGE-RELATED CHANGES IN AEROBIC CAPACITY

Aerobic capacity is the ability to perform work or participate in activities over time using the body's O_2 uptake, delivery, and energy-release mechanisms.[3] This requires the integrated work of the cardiovascular and pulmonary systems to ensure adequate O_2 delivery to the tissues.

Ventilation is the movement of gas into and out of the lungs. On inspiration, the diaphragm and external intercostals contract to expand the thorax, decreasing intrathoracic pressure and causing atmospheric gas to flow into the lungs. The difference in the partial pressure of O_2 between the alveoli and the blood in the pulmonary capillaries allows O_2 to passively diffuse into capillary blood and be

TABLE 3-1. AGE-RELATED CHANGES IN THE PULMONARY SYSTEM

ANATOMICAL	PHYSIOLOGICAL
Increased	*Increased*
• Collagen cross-linking[4]	• O_2 cost of ventilatory muscles[7]
• Diameter of alveoli and enlarged airspaces[4]	• Ventilation/perfusion (V/Q) mismatch
• Alveolar surface area[5]	*Decreased:*
• Functional residual capacity[4]	• Elastic recoil of the lung[4]
• Residual volume[4]	• Chest wall compliance[2]
Stiffening of the chest wall[4]	• Ventilatory muscle strength[7,8]
Possible changes in alveolar-capillary membrane[6]	• Forced expiratory volume in 1 second (FEV_1) and forced vital capacity (FVC)[2]
	• Diffusion[9]
	Ventilatory fatigue at a lower workload[8]

TABLE 3-2. REFERENCE VALUES WITH LOWER LIMITS OF NORMAL FOR MAXIMAL INSPIRATORY PRESSURE AND MAXIMAL EXPIRATORY PRESSURE

AGE (YEAR)	MIP (CM H_2O) (LLN)	MEP (CM H_2O) (LLN)
20 to 54	Male: 124 (80) Female: 87 (55)	Male: 233 (149) Female: 152 (98)
55 to 59	Male: 103 (71) Female: 77 (51)	Male: 218 (144) Female: 145 (105)
60 to 64	Male: 103 (71) Female: 73 (47)	Male: 209 (135) Female: 140 (100)
65 to 85	Male: 83 (65) Female: 57 (45)	Male: 174 (140) Female: 116 (90)

LLN: lower limits of normal.

Reprinted with permission from Mason RJ, Broaddus VC, Martin T, et al, *Murray and Nadel's Textbook of Respiratory Medicine*, 5th ed, Hegewald MJ, Crapo RO. Pulmonary function testing, Copyright Elsevier 2010.

transported through the pulmonary vasculature to the left side of the heart. The left ventricle pumps the oxygenated blood through the arterial system to the body's tissues where peripheral gas exchange occurs. Metabolically active tissues extract O_2 from the blood for use in aerobic metabolism, a process that creates carbon dioxide (CO_2) as a byproduct. CO_2 is diffused out of the cell into the venous blood for transport to the right side of the heart. The right ventricle is then responsible for pumping venous blood into the lungs for CO_2 to be diffused back into the alveoli and exhaled. The movement of gas out of the lung occurs passively, relying on the recoil of the chest wall and lungs. Efficient functioning of each of these component processes is integral to achieving a functional exercise capacity.

Anatomical and physiological changes occur with aging that affect the ventilation, gas exchange, O_2 delivery, cellular O_2 uptake and, therefore, aerobic capacity of older adults.

Ventilation

Significant anatomic and physiologic age-related changes occur in the pulmonary system that affect the ventilation of older adults. The most important changes are decreased ventilatory muscle strength, decreased elastic recoil of the lung, and decreased chest wall compliance (Table 3-1).

Changes in Ventilatory Muscles

Clinical measurement of maximal inspiratory pressure (MIP) and maximal expiratory pressure (MEP) can quantify the strength of the ventilatory muscles. Tolep and Kelson's[8]

review of the literature provides evidence of an age-related decline in MIP, averaging 15% to 20% between 20 and 70 years. Hautmann et al[7] studied 504 healthy subjects aged 18 to 82 years and found age to be an independent predictor of MIP. Enright and colleagues[10] also found age to be a negative predictor of maximal respiratory pressures in their study of a large sample of ambulatory older adults (n = 4443 for MIP and n = 790 for MEP). Using the data from a healthy subgroup of their sample, the authors derived reference equations to identify normal ranges of MIP and MEP values that are based on age and weight. The investigators note that there is large between-subject variability; therefore, the normal range of MIP and MEP values is wide (Table 3-2).

Tolep and Kelson[8] identified multiple limitations associated with MIP and MEP measurements, including the influence of subject motivation and the inability to isolate individual ventilatory muscles. In addition, the value may reflect elastic recoil properties of the lung and chest wall instead of ventilatory muscle strength when measurements are taken at lung volumes other than functional residual capacity (FRC).[8] For these reasons, they examined the strength of the diaphragm in older subjects compared to young adults by measuring maximum static transdiaphragmatic pressure. They concluded that diaphragmatic strength is reduced by approximately 20% to 25% in older subjects compared to young adults (Figure 3-1). From examination of animal models, the authors suggest that preferential atrophy of type II (fast twitch, oxidative) muscle fibers, changes in myosin heavy-chain content, and decreased capillary density may be responsible for the age-related decline in ventilatory muscle strength. Janssens et al[4] additionally cite impairment

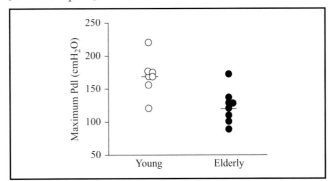

Figure 3-1. Maximum transdiaphragmatic pressures in young and elderly subjects. (Reprinted with permission from *Clin Chest Med*, 14(3), Tolep K, Kelsen SG, Effect of aging on respiratory skeletal muscles, p 372. Copyright Elsevier 1993.)

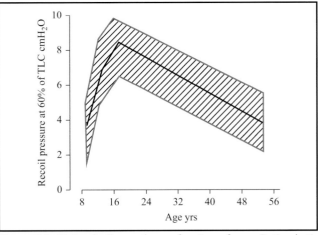

Figure 3-2. Static elastic recoil as a function of age. Static elastic recoil was measured at 60% of total lung capacity. Shaded area shows ± 1 standard deviation of plotted means. (Reprinted with permission from Turner J, Mead J, Wohl M. Elasticity of human lungs in relation to age. *J Appl Physiol.* 1968;25:664-671.)

of the sarcoplasmic reticulum Ca^{2+} pump and a decline in mitochondrial respiratory chain function as possible explanations for impaired ventilatory muscle performance in older adults.

Tolep and Kelsen suggest that, although there are few rigorous studies, preliminary evidence supports preserved ventilatory muscle endurance in healthy older people.[8] They suggest that older adults are more prone to ventilatory fatigue (this occurs when the average pressure during each breath divided by the maximum pressure exceeds 50% to 60%) than young adults because of the close relationship of muscle strength and endurance. At any given workload, older people are functioning at a higher percentage of their maximum capacity due to the age-related decline in maximum strength. Thus, they are less likely to be able to continue contracting for a prolonged period of time.

Clinical evidence has shown an age-related decline in ventilatory muscle strength, which consequently increases the risk of earlier onset ventilatory muscle fatigue at any given workload. In addition, the ventilatory muscles of older adults consume more O_2 at any given workload. These changes decrease ventilatory reserve and the ability to meet the increased O_2 demands of higher levels of activity or the physiologic stress associated with disease.[11]

Changes in the Lung

There is an age-related decline in the elastic recoil of the lung (Figure 3-2) that results in increased lung compliance (ie, change in volume for a given change in pressure).[4] The total amount of collagen and elastin in the lung parenchyma does not change with aging, but the collagen becomes more stable because of the increased number of cross-links. Changes in the orientation and cross-linking of the elastic fibers may explain the decrease in elastic recoil.

Elastic fibers around the respiratory bronchioles and alveoli degenerate, contributing to an increase in the diameter of alveolar ducts and enlargement of the airspaces.[4] Gillooly and Lamb[5] examined the lung tissue of nonsmokers ages 21 to 93 years and found a decrease in the surface area of airspace wall per unit volume of lung tissue beginning in the third decade and continuing throughout life. By the 10th

decade, there was a decrease of approximately 30%. This airspace enlargement is similar to the morphologic changes that occur in emphysema. Unlike emphysema, however, age-related changes in the airways and alveoli occur rather homogeneously throughout the lung, and they are not accompanied by alveolar wall destruction.

Because of the loss of elastic support around the airways, there is also a tendency of the small airways to collapse. Premature collapse may occur during tidal breathing in advanced age.[4,12] The combination of lost elastic recoil and early airway collapse results in air trapping and contributes to the age-related increase in residual volume (the amount of air in the lungs at the end of maximum expiration).[13]

Changes in the Chest Wall

With age, there is stiffening of the chest wall, which is thought to arise from the narrowing of intervertebral disc spaces and calcifications in the rib cage and its articulations, including the costal cartilage and rib-vertebral articulations.[4] This decreases the compliance of the thorax. The change in the compliance of the thorax (which determines the elastic work of breathing during inspiration) is greater than the change in the compliance of the lung (which determines force and rate of expiration). Thus, the net result is a decrease in the total compliance of the ventilatory system with advancing age.[2]

Physiologic Measures of Lung Function

Age-related changes in the ventilatory pump produce alterations in certain lung volumes (Figure 3-3). Total lung capacity remains essentially constant throughout adulthood, but the changes in lung and thorax compliance contribute to an increased FRC (the amount of air in the lungs at the end of a quiet expiration). This causes elderly individuals to breathe at higher lung volumes than their younger counterparts. Both cross-sectional and longitudinal studies have demonstrated that there is also an increase in residual volume (the

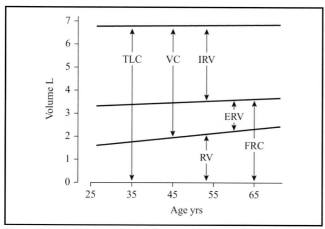

Figure 3-3. Evolution of lung volumes with aging. (Reproduced with permission of the European Respiratory Society. *Eur Respir J. January 1, 1999* 13:197-205.)

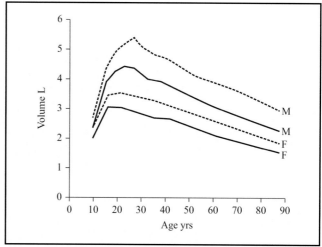

Figure 3-4. Evolution of FEV_1 (solid line) and FVC (dotted line) as a function of age. Average of data from 746 subjects free of cardiorespiratory symptoms and who had never smoked. M: males; F: females. (Reproduced with permission of the European Respiratory Society. *Eur Respir J. January 1, 1999* 13:197-205.)

amount of air left in the lungs after maximum expiration) due to air trapping associated with the lung's decreased elastic recoil and increased compliance. An increase in residual lung volume prevents the diaphragm from reaching its longest resting length at end expiration, which flattens and shortens the diaphragm, decreasing its biomechanical advantage and force-generating capability.

Flow rates are also affected by age (Figure 3-4). Forced expiratory volume in 1 second (FEV_1) and forced vital capacity (FVC) decrease beginning in the mid-30s and demonstrate an accelerated rate of decline with age.[2] Studies that have been conducted to develop regression equations that predict spirometric values based on age have not included sufficient numbers of older subjects to validly identify true age-related ranges. It appears that the extrapolations from younger adults' values have overestimated predicted values for FEV_1, FVC, and FEV_1/FVC in older individuals. Consequently, the usual practice of classifying those who achieve below 80% predicted as abnormal likely results in overdiagnosis of obstructive disease in older adults. Zeleznik[2] reports that the data from the Cardiovascular Health Study suggest a value of 56% to 64% of predicted FEV_1/FVC as the lower limit of normal for those aged 65 to 85 years old instead.

Gas Exchange

The age-related decrease in the lung surface area that is available for diffusion of gases causes an increase in the difference between the partial pressure of O_2 in the alveolar spaces and the arterial blood (the alveolar-arterial pressure difference for O_2, or $AaDO_2$). The result is a decline in the partial pressure of arterial O_2 (PaO_2) of older adults.

Ventilation-Perfusion Matching

Change in the quality of elastin in older adults results in decreased support of the distal airways, which causes collapse and closure of the alveoli at higher lung volumes or earlier in expiration when compared to younger individuals. Because these portions of collapsed lung continue to receive

near optimal perfusion, an increasing mismatch in the ventilation/perfusion (V/Q) ratio develops. V/Q mismatch causes a decline in PaO_2 and the progressive increase in $AaDO_2$ with advancing age.[4,13] Several age-based equations are widely used to predict PaO_2 and $AaDO_2$ values. In her review of the original data that generated these equations, Zeleznik highlights several shortcomings and cautions against using these equations as precise estimates of age-adjusted values.[2] Nonetheless, the majority of evidence supports the presence of an age-related decline in gas exchange that is primarily attributable to a decrement in optimal V/Q matching and results in a lower normal PaO_2.

Diffusion

The rate of diffusion of gases between the alveoli and the capillaries is proportional to the membrane surface area and the difference in gas partial pressure between the 2 sides. It is inversely proportional to the thickness of the membrane.[14] Decreases in V/Q matching, alveolar surface area, density of lung capillaries, and capillary blood volume may all contribute to a decline in diffusion in older age.[12] Stam et al[9] found that the diffusion of carbon monoxide (which is commonly used to study the diffusion properties of the human alveolar-capillary membrane) was decreased in older subjects. The results were normalized for alveolar ventilation to isolate the effect of alterations in the alveolar-capillary membrane on diffusion. The decline observed appears specifically due to age-related changes in the structure of the membrane rather than changes in membrane surface area or ventilation patterns. The results need to be interpreted with caution, however, because of the small number of older subjects ($n = 6$) represented in the sample. It is important to note that an age-related decline in diffusion does not occur with CO_2 and, therefore, an abnormal partial pressure of CO_2 level is always abnormal, regardless of age.[2]

TABLE 3-3. AGE-RELATED CHANGES IN THE CARDIOVASCULAR SYSTEM

ANATOMICAL	PHYSIOLOGICAL
Increased	*Increased*
• Left ventricular wall thickness[15-17]	• Risk of isolated systolic hypertension[32,33]
• Cardiac mass[15-17]	• Reliance on Frank-Starling[21,35,37]
• Myocyte size[18]	*Decreased*
• Amount and cross-linking of myocardial colagen[19]	• Compliance of arteries[20,24]
• Myocardial lipofuscin and amyloid[20]	• Cardiovagal baroreflex sensitivity[26]
• Circumference of heart valves[17,19,21]	• Possible change in resting heart rate[27,28]
• Arterial diameter and wall thickness[20,22,23]	• Heart rate variability[27-31]
Decreased	• Rate of ventricular filling during diastole[21]
• Number of sinoatrial pacemaker cells[24,25]	• VO_{2max}[34]
• Elastin and ↑ collagen in arteries[20,21]	• Maximum heart rate (HR_{max})[35-41]
	• Maximum stroke volume (SV_{max})[36,38,39]

Oxygen Delivery

Once O_2 enters the bloodstream, it is delivered to the body's tissues for utilization in aerobic metabolism. The transport process relies both on the pumping mechanism of the heart and the O_2-carrying capacity of the blood, while the delivery system relies on the dense network of blood vessels. Morphologic and physiologic changes in the cardiovascular and autonomic nervous systems affect the ability of the older adult to meet the body's O_2 delivery demands. The most significant changes affecting O_2 transport and delivery include decreased compliance of the arterial system, a loss of myocytes and atrial pacemaker cells in the myocardium, decreased responsiveness to β-adrenergic stimuli, an increase in the contribution of atrial contraction to end-diastolic volume, and an increased reliance on the Frank-Starling mechanism to maintain cardiac output (CO) at rest and with exercise (Table 3-3).

Changes in the Heart

Several studies have utilized echocardiography to demonstrate a small increase in left ventricular wall thickness and cardiac mass with age.[15-17] Lewis and Maron[21] note that the increase in wall thickness is mild and usually within generally accepted normal limits in absolute terms (ie, < 11 mm). They concluded that even with some age-related increase in left ventricular wall thickness, it would be unusual for a healthy older adult to have a wall thickness > 13 mm, which consequently allows for distinction between the aging heart and one affected by pathological change.

One factor that may contribute to left ventricular wall hypertrophy is the age-related decline in distensibility of the aorta, as that may increase systolic blood pressure (SBP) and, therefore, increase the workload on the heart. The increased work that the heart must perform to overcome the resistance

of a higher afterload may be what stimulates left ventricular hypertrophy.[20,21,23]

When an increase in heart mass does occur, it appears that it may be due to an increase in myocyte size.[18] Additionally, as is seen in the lung parenchyma, there is an alteration in the collagen of the myocardium with age. An increase in the amount of collagen and greater cross-linking may contribute to increased left ventricular wall thickness and greater mass of the heart.[19] There are also greater amounts of myocardial lipofuscin and amyloid in the older heart, though the functional significance of these changes is unknown.[20] As with ventricular wall thickness, this age-related alteration in cardiac structure is distinct from pathological change. For example, the pathological amyloid accumulation associated with primary cardiac amyloidosis has different characteristics than the changes that occur in healthy older adults.[20]

Fibrosis and calcification of the fibrous skeleton of the heart (annular rings and fibrous trigones) also occur.[22] Combined with the age-related alterations in myocardial collagen, this may decrease left ventricular compliance in older adults.[22,23] However, this parameter, which requires simultaneous measurement of pressure and volume, has not been specifically measured in healthy older individuals.

The valves and electrical conduction system of the heart undergo changes with aging as well. All of the heart valves (aortic, pulmonic, bicuspid, and mitral valves) show a progressive increase in circumference throughout life.[17,19,21] The aortic valve demonstrates the greatest enlargement with age, such that it almost equals the mitral valve in size by the tenth decade of life. The aortic and mitral valves also exhibit thickening and calcification of the leaflets, but none of these changes appear to cause any significant valvular dysfunction in the healthy older adult.[21]

Changes in the conduction system of the heart may predispose older adults to arrhythmias.[32] A large decline in the number of sinoatrial pacemaker cells occurs with age so that by age 50, there is a loss of 50% to 75%, of cells and by age 75, fewer than 10% of the cells remain.[14,17] Additionally, there is fibrosis and fatty infiltration in the sinoatrial node.[32] Moderate age-associated cellular loss and fibrosis also occur in the bundle of His. In contrast, the number of atrioventricular nodal cells is relatively well preserved in the older adult.

Changes in the Blood Vessels

Age-related changes in the blood vessels of older adults also affect the ability of the cardiovascular system to transport O_2-rich blood to the tissues. With increasing age, the compliance of the large-sized arteries in the cardiothoracic region declines.[24,33] While this decline in central arterial compliance appears to be an unavoidable effect of aging, the magnitude of the decline can be attenuated by participation in regular, vigorous endurance exercise.[24] The internal radius of the aorta during systole has also been shown to increase on average 9% per decade in subjects aged 19 to 62 years.[26] Finally, there is also an age-related increase in the wall thickness of the large arteries.[24,33]

Alterations in the size and distensibility of blood vessels occurs in the peripheral arteries as well.[20] These changes in the vasculature of the older adult are thought to be due to a diffuse process in the vessel walls that occurs independently from the process of atherosclerosis. Alterations in elastin and collagen are implicated in the age-related changes in blood vessels. Evidence suggests there is elastin degradation, calcification, and disappearance, as well as an increase in the amount of collagen in the arteries of older individuals.[20,21]

According to Lakatta,[20] one implication of the enlargement and decreased distensibility of the aorta is a decline in its volume elasticity and its ability to manage the fluctuations in blood volume that occur during the cardiac cycle. The thoracic aorta stores approximately one-half of the left ventricular stroke volume (SV) during systole, and then, because of the elastic forces of the aortic wall, propels it to the periphery during diastole. Up to the age of 60 years, the age-related increases in the diameter and volume of the aorta allow it to accommodate larger volumes of blood during systole, despite an increase in wall stiffness (and consequent decreased ability to change its radius in response to fluctuations in blood volume). However, beyond the age of 60, volume elasticity decreases significantly. With increasing stiffness, there is a decrease in diastolic aortic elastic recoil and a declining ability to propel blood forward in the arterial system. This change affects not only peripheral blood flow, but it has been shown to also affect coronary blood flow, blood pressure (BP), and left ventricular afterload.

Another ramification of decreased central arterial compliance is that it has been identified as an independent risk factor for future cardiovascular disease.[24] In addition, Seals et al[26] hypothesize that decreased central arterial compliance contributes to the decline in cardiovagal baroreflex sensitivity that occurs with aging. Cardiovagal baroreflex sensitivity is the ability of the arterial baroreceptors located in the large elastic arteries (carotid sinus and aortic arch) to sense alterations in arterial BP and transmit afferent input about these changes to the central nervous system. Such information triggers rapid compensatory adjustments in heart rate (HR) and CO to modify an undesirable BP.

This protective mechanism is known to decline with age. However, Seals et al[26] have demonstrated that the decline can both be delayed to older ages and decreased to about half with moderate to strenuous exercise, perhaps because of the maintenance of improved arterial compliance that occurs with regular exercise. Results from their laboratory indicate that the differences in arterial compliance associated with exercise are positively correlated to the differences in cardiovagal baroreflex sensitivity. The authors suggest that maintenance of cardiovagal baroreflex sensitivity could have significant clinical implications, including improved electrical stability in the aging heart, increased ability to withdraw vagal tone to generate tachycardia in response to acute stress, and decreased arterial BP variability with age.

Physiologic Measures at Rest

Studies investigating age-associated changes in resting HR are not entirely in agreement. Some studies have demonstrated that the resting HR of older adults is comparable to the resting HR of younger individuals.[29,42] These studies, however, did not examine substantial numbers of older patients. This affects the generalizability of the conclusions to individuals in their eighth decade and beyond, the fastest growing subset of our population.

Umetani et al[27] used 24-hour ambulatory Holter echocardiography monitoring to study age and gender effects on HR in 260 healthy subjects, including 62 subjects 60 to 99 years old. They concluded that HR declines gradually in females but not in male subjects (Figure 3-5). Women < 50 years old had significantly higher HR than their male counterparts, but HR was equal in older men and women because of the decline in the female subjects' resting HR with increasing age.

Tasaki et al[28] conducted the first longitudinal study to investigate the change in HR with aging. In contrast to the previously mentioned studies, they found resting HR to increase with advanced age. They obtained two 24-hour Holter monitor recordings for 15 subjects with an interval of 15 years between the 2 recordings. The subjects were 64 to 80 years old at the initial recording, free of any abnormalities on medical testing, and not taking any medications during either testing session. These researchers suggest that age-related changes in HR may be unique to the very old.

Less conflicting information is present in the investigation of HR variability in older adults. There is general agreement that this physiologic function, proposed as a marker of pathology and increased risk of mortality, declines with age.[27-31] This is noted to occur during monitoring of spontaneous variations in HR over a 24-hour period, as well as in response to positional change. The decrease in HR response to position change may be attributable to the age-related decline in baroreceptor reflex function and may predispose older individuals to orthostatic hypotension.[32]

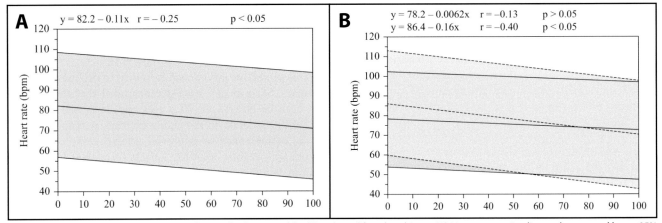

Figure 3-5. Relations between age and HR for (A) all subjects and for (B) male and female subjects. (A) Linear regression line and upper and lower 95% confidence limits are depicted by solid lines. (B) Linear regression line and upper and lower 95% confidence limits are depicted by solid lines for male subjects and dashed lines for female subjects. HR for the cohort as a whole declines gradually with aging (A), but this principally reflects a decline in female HR. Male HR does not decline significantly with age (B). (Reprinted from *J Am Coll Cardiol*, 31, Umetani K, Singer DH, McCraty R, Atkinson M, Twenty-four hour time domain heart rate variability and heart rate: relations to age and gender over nine decades, p 599, Copyright 1998, with permission from Elsevier.)

Systolic function is largely unaffected by aging.[21,22,32] Both SV, the amount of blood ejected from the ventricle with each contraction, and CO (CO = HR × SV) are preserved at rest. In contrast, there are age-related changes in diastolic function. The older person demonstrates a prolonged ventricular relaxation phase and a decreased rate of ventricular filling during diastole. Consequently, a greater proportion of blood enters the ventricle late in diastole.[21] There is also a greater reliance on the contribution of atrial contraction to late diastolic filling and left ventricular end-diastolic volume. Thus, there is no detrimental change in CO with aging, but there are age-related alterations in the patterns of blood flow.

Unlike resting SV and CO, SBP is affected by age-related changes. SBP is equal to the product of CO and the total peripheral resistance (TPR; SBP = CO × TPR). Because of the decline in arterial compliance with age, there is an increase in TPR and, therefore, a tendency for isolated systolic hypertension in older individuals.[32,33]

In summary, the cardiac function of the older adult is relatively well preserved at rest. HR, SV, and CO are maintained, though there are alterations in diastolic filling patterns and a tendency for increased SBP.

Physiologic Measures With Exercise

Though cardiac function at rest is generally unaltered in the older adult, changes in the cardiovascular system do cause limitations in maximal exercise capacity. One of the best measures of cardiovascular fitness and the ability to meet increased O_2 demands is VO_{2max}. VO_{2max} is a measure of the O_2 consumed at maximal levels of exercise and is equal to the product of maximal CO and maximal arteriovenous O_2 content difference (a-vO_{2diff}), a comparison between the O_2 in the arterial and the venous blood, which quantifies the muscle's ability to extract O_2 from the blood. Thus, VO_{2max} can be represented by the equation $VO_{2max} = (HR_{max} \times SV_{max}) \times (\text{a-v}O_{2diff})_{max}$.

VO_{2max} declines with age and has been reported to decline an average of 9% per decade.[34] This information is largely based on the data from cross-sectional studies. Fleg et al[43] conducted a longitudinal study of VO_{2max} and found that longitudinal rates of decline in VO_{2max} in older age decades ($n = 810$, including 24 subjects ≥ 80 years old) were significantly greater than the rates derived from cross-sectional analyses in the same subjects. This suggests that previously reported rates of decline underestimate the decrease in VO_{2max} in older age. Fleg et al[43] also demonstrated that the age-related decline in VO_{2max} is not linear. The rate of decline significantly accelerated with successive age decades. For example, men ≥ 70 years of age showed a 17.6% decline in VO_{2max} (when indexed for fat-free mass) over the 10-year follow-up period, while 40-year-old men lost only an average of 5.1%.

Multiple age-related changes contribute to the reduction in the maximal work capacity of the older adult. One of the most significant age-related changes in the cardiovascular system is the progressive decline in HR_{max}.[35-39] It has been suggested that the HR_{max} can be estimated by the equation $HR_{max} = 220 - \text{age}$, but several studies have shown that this prediction may underestimate the HR_{max} that an older individual can actually achieve.[40] For this reason, Tanaka et al have proposed a new equation to predict HR_{max}.[41] They conducted a meta-analysis of 351 studies and then cross-validated their newly developed equation in a sample of 514 healthy subjects that included sedentary as well as trained individuals. Data from both of these methods support the use of a new equation to predict HR_{max} in healthy adults: $HR_{max} = 208 - (0.7 \times \text{age})$.

The reason for the decline in HR_{max} with age is not entirely clear. It may be related to decreased levels of circulating catecholamines during exercise at any given workload, or to diminished sensitivity and responsiveness to the catecholamines' effect. Catecholamines normally stimulate a chronotropic cardiac response, so either of these mechanisms would result in a lessening of the expected rise in HR.[40]

Though there is not uniform agreement, most investigators suggest that ejection fraction (EF), the percentage of end-diastolic blood volume pumped from the left ventricle during systole, and SV during maximal levels of exercise also decrease with age.[36,38,39] In combination, these decreases cause an age-related decline in CO_{max} and therefore contribute to the progressive decrease in VO_{2max}.

In addition, there are age-related changes in the mechanisms used to increase VO_2 with increases in activity level. Older adults rely more heavily on an increase in SV and less on an increase in HR to enhance CO (recall $CO = HR \times SV$) in the setting of increased O_2 demand.[35,37] To improve SV with higher workloads, older adults increasingly use the Frank-Starling mechanism. That is, they rely more on an increase in end-diastolic volume in the left ventricle in order to increase SV than on an increase in EF. This is supported by the fact that older adults have been shown to have increased end-systolic volumes in addition to end-diastolic volumes. In contrast, young adults generally maintain end-diastolic volumes during exercise that are similar to resting values but demonstrate reduced end-systolic volumes as they improve their EF in response to increasing workloads.[38]

Fleg et al[37] demonstrated gender differences in the cardiovascular response to exercise. As the workload increased, older men demonstrated greater augmentation of EF and higher cardiac volumes (indicating greater use of the Frank-Starling mechanism) than the women did. That is, they relied more on increasing SV to improve CO in the setting of increased O_2 demand when compared to women. In contrast, the female subjects showed a more rapid increase in HR with exercise (though this HR increase was still significantly less than the younger subjects).

Despite limitations in maximum work capacity due to aging, older adults demonstrate relatively well-preserved cardiovascular function when exercising at submaximal workloads. The data of Stratton et al[38] showed a greater increase in BP and a lesser increase in HR in the older subjects at any given workload. There were, however, no age-related differences in EF or end-diastolic volume, end-systolic volume, or SV indices during submaximal exercise. Proctor et al[44] have also shown the ability of older, endurance-trained adults to demonstrate responses to exercise that are comparable to younger subjects. Their data support the ability of older people to utilize increases in CO and SV in response to submaximal exercise that are equal to the responses of younger individuals.

Cellular Oxygen Uptake

In addition to central cardiac changes affecting O_2 transport to the tissues, there are peripheral changes that may contribute to the decline in VO_{2max} of older adults. Older, sedentary adults are less able to extract O_2 from the blood than their younger counterparts, likely because of a lower mitochondrial content and capillary density in their muscles.[35] These characteristics of muscle, however, are significantly affected by fitness level, and the difference identified between old and young subjects may, in actuality, be due largely to effects of declining levels of activity associated with advancing age rather than the aging process itself.

To better study this hypothesis, Proctor and Joyner[45] examined the relationship between appendicular muscle mass, estimated by dual energy X-ray absorptiometry, and treadmill VO_{2max} in chronically endurance-trained subjects. This design eliminated the possibility that differences in cellular O_2 uptake could reflect decreased activity levels or the body composition changes that frequently accompany older age. Their data support a decline in aerobic capacity per unit of active muscle in highly trained older men and women. This can be attributed to either reduced O_2 extraction by the muscles or reduced O_2 transport to the muscles. The authors suggest that, because muscle enzyme activity and capillarization is known to be similar in young and old endurance-trained subjects, this difference between their groups should be ascribed to an age-related reduction in O_2 delivery. Wiebe et al[39] concur. Based on their examination of older endurance-trained women, they suggest that reductions in VO_{2max} are due to changes in maximal HR, SV, and CO, but not maximal a-vO_{2diff}. There are small numbers of subjects in these studies, however, so they should be replicated with a larger sample before drawing firm conclusions about the relative contribution of peripheral changes to the age-related decline in VO_{2max}.

It appears that central changes (ie, HR, SV, and CO) significantly affect an older adult's level of cardiovascular fitness, while the contributions of age-related changes in the skeletal muscle remain inconclusive. It is important to note that decreasing levels of activity, as is often encountered in the older population, contribute to changes in the muscle (eg, decreased capillary density and mitochondrial content) that negatively affect O_2 extraction and work capacity, further reducing the VO_{2max} of sedentary older adults.

Benefits of Aerobic Training

Fortunately, research demonstrates that much of the age-related decline in cardiovascular and pulmonary physiologic function can be attenuated or reversed with regular physical exercise. This finding supports the inclusion of aerobic capacity training in a comprehensive physical therapy plan of care directed toward improving the health and wellness of older clients.

Yerg et al[46] have demonstrated that older athletes sustain better ventilatory efficiency than age-matched sedentary controls. Sedentary older subjects had a significantly higher ventilatory response to submaximal exercise (Ve/VO_2) than elite endurance-trained athletes of similar age. Prolonged endurance training was able to improve the ventilatory efficiency of sedentary subjects to the level of the athletes, suggesting that the decline in older adults may be more related to decreased activity than age. It is beneficial for the older adult to preserve the ability to function with maximum ventilatory efficiency so they can perform ADL without pulmonary limitation and have a large ventilatory reserve for exercise and the stress of illness.

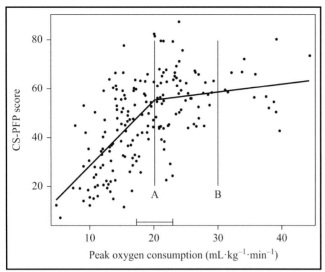

Figure 3-6. Linear regression of peak O_2 consumption (VO_{2peak}) measurements and Continuous-Scale Physical Functional Performance test (CS-PFP) scores. Points A and B represent different physical reserves. If point B loses 8 mL.kg^{-1}.min^{-1} of aerobic capacity, the loss in physical function is a CS-PFP score of approximately 3 units (8×0.32). If point A loses 8 mL.kg^{-1}.min^{-1} of aerobic capacity, the expected drop in function would be a CS-PFP score of approximately 21 units (8×2.67). The solid line designates the 95% confidence interval for the VO_{2peak} measurements. (Reprinted from *Phys Ther.* 2003;83(1):37-48, with permission of the American Physical Therapy Association. Copyright © 2003 American Physical Therapy Association. APTA is not responsible for the accuracy of the translation from English.)

Exercise also has many beneficial effects on the aging cardiovascular system. These are well outlined in a recent position stand published by the American College of Sports Medicine (ACSM).[34] The authors performed an extensive review of the literature and concluded that there is strong evidence from high-quality studies that "aerobic capacity training of sufficient intensity ($\geq 60\%$ of pretraining VO_{2max}), frequency, and length (≥ 3 days/week for ≥ 16 weeks) can significantly increase VO_{2max} in healthy middle-aged and older adults"[34(p 1517)] that is on average 16.3%. They note that larger improvements are observed with longer training periods and that adults ≥ 75 years old may demonstrate smaller improvements in VO_{2max} than younger seniors. The increase in VO_{2max} is attributed to central and peripheral adaptations in men, but only to improved a-vO_{2diff} in women. In addition to gains in VO_{2max}, there has been shown to be a reduction in resting HR and HR at any submaximal workload. Exercise also provides numerous cardioprotective effects including improved lipid profile, arterial compliance, HR variability, body composition, BP, and plasma insulin levels.[34]

Experts from the ACSM and the American Heart Association developed and published recommendations for the type and amount of physical activity required for older adults to maintain or improve health. They suggest moderate intensity aerobic activity for at least 30 minutes 5 days of the week or vigorous exercise for at least 20 minutes 3 days of the week. They define moderate-intensity aerobic activity as a 5 or 6 on a 0 to 10 scale, where sitting is 0 and all-out effort is 10. Vigorous-intensity activity is defined as a 7 or 8.

Summary

The older adult demonstrates decreased ventilatory muscle strength, lung elastic recoil, and chest wall compliance that combine to create less efficient ventilation and increased O_2 cost of breathing. Gas-exchange capacity also declines with age, primarily because of increased V/Q mismatching associated with lessening of the elastic support of alveolar structures. Fortunately, these changes do not significantly affect the physiologic functional ability of the older adult at rest or during daily activities. However, reductions in ventilatory efficiency and gas exchange decrease the reserve capacity of older adults and increase the risk that they will be unable to effectively meet the demands of more intense physical activity or the stresses of pathology when they are superimposed on the changes of advancing age.

The cardiovascular system of the older adult is also affected by age-related changes. Arteries become larger, less compliant, and less able to sense and respond to fluctuations in BP, which predisposes older adults to arrhythmias, orthostatic hypotension, and systolic hypertension. There is less HR variability and delayed diastolic filling in advanced age. Adaptations such as increased reliance on atrial contraction and the Frank-Starling mechanism work together to preserve CO at rest, but CO_{max} declines because of decreases in HR_{max} and SV_{max}. This results in a decline in the maximal exercise capacity of the older adult and causes performance of all ADL to utilize a greater percentage of their VO_{2max}.

If an older adult decreases his or her activity level during a period of illness, deconditioning may cause a reduction in VO_{2max}. Because older adults already have a declining level of cardiovascular fitness, this additional reduction may, in fact, cause the individual to have a VO_{2max} that results in disability. Some ADL may require a level of O_2 consumption that is a high enough percentage of the patient's maximal level to cause significant discomfort, dyspnea, or fatigue. As a result, older adults may need to slow the speed of movements or take frequent rests to decrease the VO_{2max} required for the activity level to still accomplish the task. Some tasks may simply be beyond their capacity to perform.

Cress and Meyer[47] investigated the concept of physical reserve (maximal aerobic capacity in excess of that needed to perform daily functions). Their data on the peak VO_2 of 192 older subjects (69 to 97 years, mean age = 76 years) demonstrated an ability to define a peak VO_2 threshold or "breakpoint" below which individuals experienced functional limitations as measured with the Continuous-Scale Physical Functional Performance test (Figure 3-6). The threshold identified by their work is a VO_{2peak} of 20.1 mL·kg^{-1}·min^{-1}. VO_{2peak} levels below this critical level were associated with a significant decline in physical function.

As shown in Figure 3-6, individuals with a VO_{2peak} well above the aerobic capacity threshold have good physical reserve. That is, a modest decline in their aerobic capacity would not result in a decline in function. In contrast, an older adult with a lower initial VO_{2peak} and less physical reserve would experience the onset of functional limitations with a similar reduction aerobic capacity. Cress and Meyer suggest that this aerobic capacity threshold can therefore be used to help predict the level of support that is needed by older adults given their personal fitness level or to determine the level of fitness that should be achieved and maintained to ensure an adequate physical reserve.

The evidence supports that exercise can attenuate declines in cardiovascular fitness and also that older adults can make substantial gains with training. Even in the absence of significant improvements in cardiovascular fitness, older adults can enhance their health status with increased levels of activity, which warrants the inclusion of aerobic training in the plan of care for the older client.

AGE-RELATED CHANGES IN MUSCLE PERFORMANCE

Muscle performance is the capacity of a muscle or group of muscles to generate forces to perform ADL.[3] Age-related changes in skeletal muscle, including declines in muscle mass, protein metabolism, and number of motor units, result in a loss of muscle strength and power, negatively affecting the ability of the older adult to function (Table 3-4). As with aerobic capacity, the decline in the maximal capability of the musculoskeletal system often causes older adults to perform ADL at a high level of exertion and decreases the functional reserve they have to respond to the stress of exercise or illness.

Age-Related Changes in Skeletal Muscle

Muscle Mass

Loss of muscle mass with advancing age is well documented.[34,48-52] By age 65 years, muscle mass is approximately 25% to 30% less than the peak values measured at 25 to 30 years of age.[48,49] Computed tomography of thigh muscles shows an age-related decrease both in cross-sectional area of the thigh and muscle density beginning at age 30 years.[55] The decline in muscle mass is accompanied by increased amounts of intramuscular fat and connective tissue.[50,51] Lower extremity muscles appear to be more affected by this process than upper extremity muscles.[34,50]

Regular muscle protein turnover maintains the size and quality of skeletal muscles by replacing damaged proteins with newly synthesized proteins.[59] There is an age-related decline in this regenerative process that contributes to decreased muscle mass and strength in older adults.[59] In contrast, the rate of muscle degradation has not been shown to change with age.[66] Altered muscle-building hormone levels and chronic low-level inflammation are also considered causes of the age-related decrease in muscle mass.[67,68]

Muscle Fiber Type and Size

The age-related decrease in muscle mass is thought to be due to a decrease both in the total number of type I (slow-twitch) and type II (fast-twitch) fibers and in the size of type

TABLE 3-4. AGE-RELATED CHANGES IN SKELETAL MUSCLE

ANATOMICAL	PHYSIOLOGICAL
Increased	*Decreased*
• Intramuscular fat and connective tissue[50,51]	• Muscle strength, concentric > eccentric, leg > arm[34,55-58]
• Expression of hybrid fibers[54]	• Muscle quality[56,59,60]
• Size of each motor unit[50]	• Muscle power[61]
Decreased	• Protein metabolism[59]
• Muscle mass[48-52]	• Motor unit firing rate[65]
• Number of type I and II muscle fibers[48,50,53]	Preserved muscle endurance[62-64]
• Size of type II fibers[48,50,53]	
• Number of motor units[50]	

II fibers.[48,50,53] The size of type I fibers appears preserved until very old age.[48]

In addition to the changes in the number and size of muscle fibers, there is an age-related alteration in the expression of myosin heavy-chain isoforms, which are the various structures of the contractile proteins (myosin) found in the sarcomeres of muscle fibers. The isoform affects the function and properties of a muscle fiber. Older adults increasingly express more than one myosin heavy-chain isoform in the same muscle fiber. Recent investigations of single muscle fibers using gel electrophoresis technique indicate the presence of "hybrid" fiber types that contain 2 or more myosin heavy-chain isoforms (eg, I/IIa and IIa/IIx, which compose 50% of older adults' muscle fibers) in addition to "pure" fiber types.[54] Aging muscle contains a significantly larger proportion of hybrid muscle fibers and fewer pure myosin heavy-chain isoforms compared to young adults.[54] Pure type IIx fibers (originally identified as the myosin heavy-chain IIb isoform) become rare in seniors. The age-related decrease in the expression of pure fiber types and the substantial increase in the proportion of hybrid fibers has shown to be reversible with strength training.[69]

Motor Units

The motor unit consists of a single motor neuron and the collection of muscle cells that it innervates. The process of motor unit remodeling is ongoing; denervation at the neuromuscular junction, followed by axonal sprouting and reinnervation, results in continual turnover of synapses. During young adulthood, this process does not cause any change in motor unit size, total number of motor units, or fiber distribution. However, motor unit estimation has demonstrated a

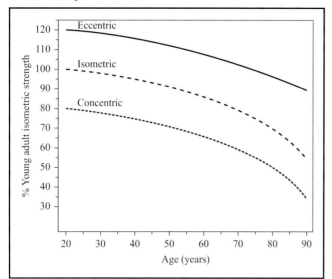

Figure 3-7. Effect of age on maximal strength throughout the human lifespan. (Reprinted from Vandervoort AA. Aging of the human neuromuscular system. *Muscle Nerve.* 2002;5:17-25, with permission of John Wiley and Sons.)

decline in the number of excitable motor units beginning in the seventh decade of life.[50] Research has also demonstrated an increase in the size of the motor unit and a decline in the motor unit firing rate.[65]

Researchers hypothesize that the reduction in the total number of motor units with age is due to healthy motor neurons capturing muscle fibers of failing motor neurons nearby. That is, during the process of motor unit remodeling, strong axonal sprouting and reinnervation result in expansion of some motor neurons' territories; there is the simultaneous degeneration and elimination of motor neurons that have presumably reached the end of their lifespan. Thus, older adults have fewer and larger motor units than their younger counterparts. It has been suggested that innervation of a muscle fiber by a new motor neuron may alter its physiological and biochemical properties, supported by the presence of increased numbers of hybrid muscle fibers in older adults.[48,50]

Effect on Muscle Performance

Muscle Strength

Muscle strength, the force exerted by a single muscle or a group of muscles to overcome resistance under a specific set of circumstances,[3] decreases with age. Muscle strength peaks at about age 30 years and begins to decline by approximately 12% to 15% per decade after age 50 years.[55,56] The rate of decline becomes even greater later in life and is estimated to be up to 30% per decade in those age 70 years and older.[55]

Investigators have demonstrated a greater age-associated loss of concentric strength than eccentric strength, with some research finding no difference at all between the eccentric strength of young and old adults (Figure 3-7).[50,57] Data from the Baltimore Longitudinal Study on Aging did show a

significant age-related decline both in concentric and eccentric peak torque in a large sample of older individuals, but the impact of age on eccentric strength was less than its effect on concentric strength.[56,58] Lindle et al[58] found that the loss of eccentric strength began at least a decade later than the loss of concentric strength. Lynch et al[56] comment that, although their results do not fully support previous reports of preserved eccentric strength in older age, the variance in eccentric strength in their subjects that was explained by age was less than for concentric strength. Thus, the evidence demonstrates that eccentric strength is less affected by age than concentric strength.

The age-related loss of strength has been shown generally to be greater and to occur earlier in the leg than in the arm.[56,70] Because no physiological mechanisms have been identified to explain this, it has been hypothesized that it is due to greater disuse in the leg muscles in older age. The decline in strength has been found both in proximal and distal appendicular muscles.[50]

Decreased muscle mass can explain the majority of the age-related decline in strength. It has been shown, however, that the loss of strength in later decades often exceeds the loss of muscle size. This indicates that the specific force of muscle or muscle quality (ie, strength per unit of muscle mass) also lessens with age. Lynch et al examined age-related changes in muscle quality in 502 older subjects using dual-energy X-ray absorptiometry to estimate muscle mass and an isokinetic dynamometer to measure concentric and eccentric peak torque of the elbow and knee flexors and extensors.[56] Their results demonstrate the presence of an age-related decline in muscle quality both in men and women. Only the muscle quality of the arm in women during eccentric contractions was preserved across the lifespan.

Results of studies investigating muscle quality as determined by normalization of muscle strength for muscle size are not conclusive. Lynch et al attribute the inconsistency in results to differences in the techniques used to measure muscle mass and strength for the determination of muscle quality.[56] Rather than use whole muscle mass, some investigators have studied isolated single muscle fibers to determine specific force, eliminating the question concerning the validity of muscle mass estimations. These studies support a decline in muscle quality with aging.[59,60] As noted previously, reduction in gene transcription or protein synthesis may affect the basic properties of the myosin molecule, thereby lessening the force-generating capacity of muscle fibers in older age.[48,60]

Muscle Power

Muscle power is a measure of the work done (force × distance) per unit of time. While it is dependent on muscle strength and the ability to generate forces, it is also affected by nervous system control and the timing and speed of responses. Research has demonstrated that muscle power begins to decline both in men and women by about age 40 years, and that this age-related loss in power is greater than the strength loss that occurs with advancing age.[61]

Muscle Endurance

Unlike muscle strength and power, muscle endurance, the ability to sustain forces repeatedly or to generate forces over a period of time, is not clearly impaired in older adulthood.[3] In fact, many studies indicate that muscle endurance is unaffected by advancing age. For example, Lindström et al[62] examined the effects of increasing age on knee extensor fatigue and endurance. Twenty-two young subjects and 16 healthy older adults performed 100 repeated maximum dynamic knee extensions on an isokinetic dynamometer (Cybex II, Lumex, Inc). Maximal voluntary contraction was significantly lower in the older adults compared to the young subjects, but the relative muscle force reduction and fatigue rate between the groups was not significantly different.

Bäckman et al[63] also conclude that muscle endurance is preserved in old age. These authors examined the time to exhaustion in the shoulder abductors and hip flexors of 57 women and 62 men aged 17 to 70 years by having the subjects hold their limbs in a static position (90 degrees of shoulder abduction in sitting and 30 degrees of hip flexion in supine) as long as possible. Muscular endurance was extremely variable between individuals but did not decline significantly with age. It is important to note that the sample size was small; there were only 10 subjects over the age of 60 years enrolled in the study.

The results of Schwendner et al[64] agree with the studies described previously. The time to fatigue (performing maximal concentric knee extensions until the force output fell below 50% of maximal voluntary contraction) was no different between young and old women. Older persons with a history of falls did demonstrate significantly decreased muscular endurance when compared to older non-fallers and to young women, though they did not have significantly decreased maximum voluntary contraction when compared to older non-fallers (Figure 3-8).

The evidence suggests that there is no significant difference in the fatigability or endurance of older adults when compared to young adults. It is important to note once again that sample sizes are small and generally include few adults over 75 years of age. Thus, generalization of the results to the very old population should be made with caution. The limitations of cross-sectional studies should be remembered as well when considering the results of these studies.

Though muscle endurance may be preserved with age, older adults are not fully protected from fatigue with daily activities. Because of the age-related loss of strength, movements required during certain functional or mobility activities may require near maximal levels of strength for an older adult. Repetition of these challenging movements to complete the activity will be difficult. Thus, older adults may experience significant fatigue with tasks such as unloading heavy items from grocery bags or climbing stairs. Greater strength capacity allows a person to complete ADL at a lower percentage of maximum and, therefore, to perform the movement repeatedly without undo fatigue.

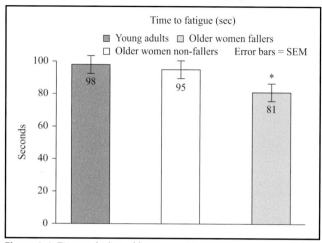

Figure 3-8. Time to decline of force output to < 50% maximum voluntary contraction for 2 consecutive contractions during muscle endurance testing. Time to fatigue was significantly less in older women fallers than in both young women and older women non-fallers. (Reprinted from Schwendner KI, Mikesky AE, Holt WS Jr, Peacock M, Burr DB. Differences in muscle endurance and recovery between fallers and nonfallers, and between young and older women. *J Gerontol A Biol Sci Med Sci.* 1997;52(3):M157, by permission of Oxford University Press.)

Effect on Function

Research has demonstrated that strength affects many different functional activities. Lower extremity strength has been shown to correlate significantly with the time to complete a sit-to-stand transfer in older adults.[71-74] Hernandez et al[75] found that trunk and knee extensor and ankle dorsiflexor and plantar flexor strength contribute to older adults' ability to stoop, crouch, and kneel. The results of studies examining the connection between strength and balance in older adults are less conclusive. For example, Ringsberg et al[76] did not find a significant relationship between maximum isometric leg strength (knee and ankle flexors and extensors) and tests of balance (single-leg stance and stance on a static and moving platform, each performed with both eyes open and eyes closed). In contrast to these results, Wolfson et al[77] concluded that a strong relationship between strength and balance exists. In their study, strength had an independent effect on the odds ratio for frequency of loss of balance during a sensory organization test on a balance platform in healthy, community-dwelling older adults (average age of 80 years). The investigators measured isokinetic peak torque for flexion and extension of the hip, knee, and ankle and for hip abduction and adduction. They calculated the sum of the lower extremity strength measurements and divided by body mass. For each Nm/kg increase in strength, there was a 20% decrease in the odds ratio for a loss of balance on a sensory organization test.

It is likely that the choice of variables (eg, which muscles are tested and which balance tests are chosen) affects the strength of the relationships identified, an idea that is supported by the work of Daubney and Culham.[78] These investigators measured the force generated by 12 lower extremity muscle groups with a handheld dynamometer and balance

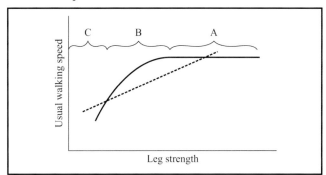

Figure 3-9. Hypothesized relationship between leg strength and usual gait speed. Area A corresponds to the range where strength is sufficient for normal walking and where changes in strength affect physiological reserve but not gait speed. Area B corresponds to the range of marginal or inadequate strength. In Area B, changes in strength cause changes in gait speed, and there exists a curve that quantifies the relationship. In Area C, strength is below the minimum needed to walk at all. (Reprinted from Buchner DM, Larson EB, Wagner EH, Koepsell TD, de Lateur BJ. Evidence for a non-linear relationship between leg strength and gait speed. *Age Ageing.* 1996;25:386-391, by permission of Oxford University Press.)

using a variety of tests, including the Berg Balance scale (BBS), the Timed Up and Go test, and the Functional Reach in adults between the ages of 65 and 91 years. Only ankle muscle force was predictive of the results of the balance tests. Dorsiflexor and evertor force accounted for 58% of the score on the BBS, plantar flexor and invertor force accounted for 48.4% of the Timed Up and Go score, and plantar flexor force accounted for 13% of the Functional Reach score. Because each balance scale incorporates different motions, the contribution of each muscle varies depending on the test performed. Thus, strength appears to contribute to balance scores. However, the relative contribution of each lower extremity muscle group to balance differs depending on the balance measurement that is chosen and the task that is performed.

As just described, Ringsberg et al did not find a significant relationship between muscle strength and balance, but the authors did demonstrate a link between muscle strength and gait performance, a finding that is more consistently supported in the literature.[76,77,79-83] Lower extremity strength has been shown to correlate with gait speed, but the exact relationship between the variables is not clear. Some have suggested a linear relationship.[81,82] If the relationship is linear, then every increase in strength is associated with a faster gait speed. Other investigators have shown a plateau in the correlation, or a curvilinear relationship.[80,83] That is, there comes a point when higher levels of strength are not associated with further increases in gait speed (Figure 3-9). For example, Kwon et al[80] found that levels of knee extensor strength above 130 Nm as measured with a dynamometer at 30 degrees/second were not associated with ongoing increases in comfortable gait speed. If the relationship is curvilinear as Kwon et al suggest, an improvement in strength in a frail, weak patient would be associated with a significant increase in gait speed. In contrast, a healthy senior would show little to no gain in gait speed with increases in strength because

they are beyond the linear portion of the relationship where these variables improve in concert.

As is the case with balance, the contribution of strength to gait speed may be activity dependent. Lamoureux et al[84] found that knee extensor strength (measured one repetition maximum [1-RM]) explained 14.2% to 30.8% of the variance in gait speed when older adults walked along a timed obstacle course designed to represent commonly encountered environmental challenges (stepping over an obstacle, negotiating a raised surface, stepping across an obstacle, and foot targeting). When the investigators progressively increased the challenge of each task, the amount of variance explained by strength also got larger, particularly for stepping over an obstacle and for rising onto a raised surface. The authors suggest that strength is a critical factor in older adults' ability to negotiate community environments, and that it becomes increasingly important as the ambulatory challenges become greater.

More recently, the contribution of muscle power to functional performance has been appreciated.[82,85-87] Puthoff and Nielsen[82] demonstrated that while both strength and power were related to functional limitations and indirectly to disability (the Short Physical Performance Battery, the 6-Minute Walk Test [6MWT], and the Late Life Function and Disability Instrument), power consistently explained more of the variance in the outcomes than strength did. The investigators also examined the effect of the relative intensity level of power and suggest that different tasks require power at different relative intensities. For example, while peak power (defined as the highest power output regardless of the external load at which it was achieved) explained more of the variance in most outcome measures, power at a high relative intensity (90% of 1-RM) explained more of the variance in sit-to-stand transfers than either peak power or power at a low relative intensity (40% of 1-RM). Puthoff and Nielsen[82] therefore recommend clinicians consider training older adults' power at different intensities to maximize performance of all functional skills and to decrease disability.

Puthoff and Nielsen[82] noted that there is a good deal of the variance in the performance of these skills that remains unexplained. Other factors must be considered as possible contributors to the ability to successfully complete functional movements. Lord et al[73] examined the effect of multiple sensorimotor and psychological factors on sit-to-stand performance. They found that visual contrast sensitivity, lower limb proprioception, peripheral tactile sensitivity, reaction time, sway with eyes open on a foam rubber mat, and body weight were independent and significant predictors of sit-to-stand performance. Quadriceps strength was the most important variable in explaining sit-to-stand time, but other measures accounted for half of the explained variance, highlighting the need for a comprehensive examination to identify all factors contributing to an older adult's function.

Puthoff et al[87] recognized that walking ability may be different in a research lab from what it is in the community. Because actual ambulation in daily life is critical to older adults' function, quality of life, and wellness, they sought to understand the contributions of lower extremity strength and power to everyday walking behaviors. Using a pneumatic leg press, they measured the lower extremity strength and power of 30 older adults with mild to moderate functional limitations based on the Medical Outcome Survey (SF-36) physical function subscale. The subjects wore accelerometers that measured total steps, walking distance, and walking speed over a 6-day period. Strength and power (peak, at 40% 1-RM and at 90% 1-RM) were significantly related to walking distance and speed; peak power was related to total number of steps. Again, power demonstrated a stronger relationship to function than strength did. The results of this study provide important evidence about the contribution of muscle performance to actual daily walking and suggest that exercise designed to improve lower extremity strength and power may translate into gains in everyday walking behaviors.

The concept of physical reserve that was described earlier in relation to aerobic capacity also applies to muscle performance. Because of age-related declines in maximum strength and power, older adults have less reserve to draw on during situations of high physiologic stress, such as illness or exercise. As they did with aerobic capacity, Cress and Meyer[47] defined a strength threshold below which individuals demonstrated significant decline in physical function as measured with the Continuous-Scale Physical Functional Performance Test. The authors measured maximal voluntary torque of the knee extensors using an isokinetic dynamometer in 192 elderly subjects. Those with less than 2.5 N·m/(kg·m⁻¹) of knee extensor strength demonstrated significant declines in physical function. Cress and Meyer suggest that this strength threshold can estimate an older adult's physical reserve and predict functional limitation and level of assistance required.

Because most of the studies described are cross-sectional, we cannot conclude that decreased muscle performance causes a decline in function. In reality, the causal relationship is often bidirectional for older adults. An age-related decline in muscle performance, along with other factors, contributes to decreased mobility; consequently, the decline in physical activity further weakens the individual through deconditioning. While it may be hard to tease out the exact nature of this relationship, it is clear that muscle performance is related to functional performance in older adults and, therefore, exercise prescribed to maximize muscle strength, power, and endurance should prove beneficial to maintain optimal physical performance with advancing age.

Benefits of Strength Training

Early studies of strength training in the elderly examined the efficacy of exercise programs that were fairly conservative in terms of the prescription intensity.[88] In the mid-1980s, Frontera et al[89] demonstrated the ability of older healthy men to benefit from high-intensity lower extremity strength training without adverse effects. Twelve men aged 60 to 72 years completed 3 sets of 8 repetitions of knee flexion and extension exercises at 80% of their 1-RM 3 days per week for

a total of 12 weeks. This strength-training regimen resulted in a significant increase both in thigh total muscle cross-sectional area (11.4% as estimated from computed tomography) and strength (107.4% for knee extensor and 226.7% for knee flexors as measured by 1-RM). In addition, vastus lateralis muscle biopsies showed significant increases in the size of both type I and type II fibers of ~30%. Subsequently, Fiatarone et al[90] studied strength training in frail, institutionalized individuals in their 80s and 90s. Their results provided additional evidence that even the oldest individuals can safely participate in high-intensity resistance exercise training and enjoy significant strength gain as a result.

These early studies highlighted that the plasticity of the muscular system is retained in old age. Since then, the results of numerous studies have confirmed the ability of older adults to improve strength with regular exercise, with gains ranging from less than 25% to more than 100%.[34] In their analysis of data pooled from 41 studies of strength training ($n = 1955$ subjects), Latham et al[91] noted a moderate to large beneficial effect of progressive resistance strength training on quadriceps strength. They do note, however, significant variability in the size of the strength gains seen in these studies. This is likely related to differences in factors such as intensity of training, amount of supervision provided, and duration of training, all of which may affect outcome.

Studies that have examined muscle cross-sectional area have shown moderate increases in muscle size resulting from strength training, but these changes are not nearly as substantial as the gains in muscle strength.[50] This finding has led many investigators to believe that the improvements in muscle strength that occur with training are due both to muscle fiber hypertrophy as well as neuromuscular adaptations in motor control pathways (eg, increased motor unit firing frequency and motor unit recruitment rates, and decreased coactivation of agonist and antagonist muscles). For example, Tracy et al[92] studied the effects of 9 weeks of strength training in 23 healthy older men and women. The subjects showed an increase in muscle strength of approximately 30% during 1-RM quadriceps contraction measurements and a 12% increase in muscle volume measured by magnetic resonance imaging. Thus, muscle quality (ie, strength/muscle volume) improved in these subjects, supporting the assertion both that hypertrophy and neuromuscular adaptations contribute to older adults' strength gains after training. Muscle quality increases in older adults are similar to those demonstrated by young adults.[34]

There is some evidence that older adults can also improve their muscle endurance with resisted exercise training, but there is far less research in this area.[34] In contrast, there are multiple investigations that demonstrate that older adults also have the ability to improve their muscle power with resistance exercise training. Ferri et al[93] studied 16 older men (aged 65 to 81 years) who participated in a 16-week low-volume, high-intensity (1 set of 10 repetitions at 80% 1-RM) strength-training program for the plantar flexors and knee extensors. At the conclusion of training, significant increases were found in 1-RM, maximum isometric torque, maximum muscle power, and muscle cross-sectional area. Gains in power resulted from high-intensity strength training at a relatively slow speed. Even greater gains in power can be seen when exercises are performed at high-velocity. Bottaro et al[94] compared 2 groups of older men (aged 60 to 76 years) who exercised twice each week for 10 weeks. Both groups performed 3 sets of 8 to 10 repetitions of exercises at 60% 1-RM. The power training group (PTG) performed the movements as quickly as possible, while the traditional strength training (TST) group performed contractions over 2 to 3 seconds. The groups demonstrated equal gains in strength, but improvements in muscular power were significantly greater in the PTG compared to the TST group (increase in bench press 37% vs 13% and leg press 31% vs 8%, respectively), which is not surprising given the principle of specificity of training.

Older adults clearly have the ability to increase muscle performance, but a more meaningful question is whether those gains translate into improved function. In their systematic review of the literature, Latham et al examined the effects of progressive resistance training on impairment and functional limitation measures in older adults.[91] No clear strength-training effect was identified for measures of standing balance, including timed position holding and balance during more complex activities, such as those on the BBS. Progressive resistance training did have a significant effect on the 6MWT (weighted mean difference 53.7 meters), a moderate to large effect on sit-to-stand time (standardized mean difference –0.67), and a modest beneficial effect on gait speed (weighted mean difference 0.07 meters per second). Though the results are statistically significant, they need to be interpreted considering how much improvement is needed to affect meaningful change in functional mobility for an individual. For example, it must be determined if a gait speed improvement of this size will affect an older client's daily mobility and ability to negotiate the environment.

Unfortunately, when analyzing the results of 14 studies that reported on disability outcomes, Latham et al found no evidence that progressive resistance training had a positive effect on either health-related quality of life or ADL measures.[91] Successful performance of higher-level functional tasks relies on multiple contributing factors, including physical, psychosocial, and cognitive aspects of function. It is possible that strength training alone is not enough to affect physical disability, but that it is a critical element of a comprehensive approach to maximizing older adults' well-being.

Cress et al[95] present another explanation for the lack of significant results when examining the effectiveness of strength training on physical function in healthy older adults. They suggest that commonly used measurement tools may not be able to detect changes in the higher ranges of functional ability that occur as a result of exercise. They sought to determine if the Continuous Scale-Physical Functional Performance (CS-PFP) test, a measure that includes a broad range of activities, would be able to capture changes that occur after a period of exercise intervention. They randomly assigned 49 healthy older adults to a control group or to an exercise group. The subjects in the experimental group

participated in a combined aerobic capacity and strength-training program 3 times per week for 6 months. Compared to the control group, the exercise group showed significant increases in VO_{2max}, muscle strength, and the CS-PFP test. The authors suggest that perhaps the CS-PFP test is better able to capture changes in function than the other familiar measures used (eg, Sickness Impact Profile, SF-36, and 6MWT). They do note that the change in dynamic strength accounted for < 15% of the variance in the change in function as measured by the CS-PFP test. Thus, their results also support the assertion that, while gains in strength may contribute to improved function, there are many additional variables that affect the physical abilities of older adults.

Similar to strength training, power training has not demonstrated the ability to improve standing static balance, but it has resulted in gains in dynamic balance, walking capacity, and functional performance.[96-98] Holviala et al[96] showed that a program of strength and power training did not change timed measures of static balance (standard stance, feet together, and semi-tandem, each with both eyes opened and eyes closed). Subjects did demonstrate significant gains in dynamic balance, however, and these were correlated with increases in power. Significant gains in dynamic balance were observed before there were changes in muscle power. Consequently, the authors note that increased power was only part of the reason for the large improvement in dynamic balance; other factors must also contribute to the changes in this outcome.

Miszko et al[98] found that power training improved function when measured by the CS-PFP test. In fact, their results proved power training to be superior to strength training for improving physical function. The study by Bottaro et al that was described earlier confirmed these results.[94] The subjects in their PTG demonstrated greater improvements on the Senior Fitness Test compared to those in the TST group. This measure, developed by Rikli and Jones,[99] is a battery of tests that examines upper and lower extremity strength and flexibility, balance, and aerobic capacity.

The evidence clearly demonstrates the benefits of strength and power training for older adults. The optimal exercise program is less clear than the need to exercise, however. The exact parameters of intensity, frequency, sets, and repetitions are not yet conclusively established in the literature. Nonetheless, there is evidence that can guide exercise prescription to improve the muscle performance of older adults.

The ACSM has published specific recommendations that outline exercise parameters based on the evidence to date.[28] To improve strength and hypertrophy muscle, they suggest slow to moderate lifting velocity for 1 to 3 sets per exercise with 60% to 80% of 1-RM for 8 to 12 repetitions with 1- to 3-minute rests in between sets for 2 to 3 days per week. The authors of the ACSM position stand note the benefits of power training and advocate inclusion of this in older adults' exercise programs, using 30% to 60% of 1-RM for 6 to 10 repetitions with high-repetition velocity. Muscle endurance training has not been studied as thoroughly, but it appears that exercising with lower loads and higher

TABLE 3-5. AGE-RELATED CHANGES IN SYSTEMS CONTRIBUTING TO MOTOR CONTROL

SENSORY INTEGRITY	CENTRAL PROCESSING	EFFECTOR SYSTEM
Increased	*Increased*	*Decreased*
• Glare sensitivity[102]	• Reaction time[117,120-122]	• Muscle strength[34,56,130]
Decreased	• Execution time[120,122,123]	• Muscle power[61]
• Visual acuity[102]	• Muscle co-contraction[124]	• Range of motion[127,128]
• Contrast sensitivity[102]	• Use of hip strategy[117]	• Postural alignment[129]
• Peripheral vision[102]	• Reliance on stepping[125,126]	Preserved muscle endurance[62-64]
• Dark adaptation[102]	*Decreased*	
• Proprioception[103-109]	• Sensory organization[117,118]	
• Tactile sensitivity[110-112]	• Sensory reweighting[119]	
• Vibratory sense[6]	• Dual-task ability[120]	
• Vestibulo-ocular reflex function[113,114]		
• Otolith function[114-116]		

repetitions can lead to gains in this area of muscle performance and should be considered for inclusion in an exercise program as well.

Not all older adults are willing or able to participate in high-intensity strength training. Even if individuals are not candidates for such an exercise regimen, they should be counseled about the benefits of physical activity. Brach et al[100] found that older adults who lived physically active lives were less likely to have functional limitations compared with individuals who were sedentary. Exercise, however, provided the added benefit of greater physical capacity and functional reserve. The authors suggest that any type of physical activity is better than no activity to protect against functional limitation, but emphasize the ability of exercise (ie, "planned, structured, and repetitive bodily movement for the purpose of improving or maintaining one or more components of physical fitness"(p 502)) to enhance functional reserve in older adults.

Summary

The older adult experiences an age-related decline in muscle strength and muscle power due to decreases in muscle mass and muscle quality, preferential atrophy of type II muscle fibers, and decreased number and function of motor units. In contrast, muscle endurance appears relatively well-preserved into the later decades, though there is still susceptibility to fatigue with ADL due to age-related decline in maximum strength. Losses in muscle performance contribute to worsening balance, slower performance of sit-to-stand transfers, decreased gait speed, and a decline in function. However, a significant proportion of the variance in the performance of these activities remains to be explained by additional physical, psychological, and cognitive variables. Older adults maintain the ability to improve muscle performance with a progressive resistance exercise program and can safely perform high-intensity strength and

power training. This type of intervention can result in gains in function and physical capacity that may improve an older adult's quality of life.

AGE-RELATED CHANGES IN MOTOR CONTROL

Motor control is the ability to initiate, execute, and terminate movements to complete purposeful tasks. Performance of smooth and coordinated movements during dynamic tasks requires adequate sensory input to determine the body's position and path in space, processing of information to plan effective postural adjustments and limb trajectories, and execution of movements through the body's effector system (eg, strength, endurance, range of motion [ROM]).[101] Aging affects each of these areas, and these age-related declines may combine to cause deterioration in coordination, balance, and gait in older adulthood (Table 3-5).

Sensory Integrity

Vision

Vision contributes to motor control by providing environmental cues to use as references for an individual to determine his or her position in space. Body parts' relationships to each other and to the external world can be ascertained through observation. These data are used to understand alignment and location of the body, as well as to identify environmental challenges that may be encountered.

Jackson and Owsley[102] provide a comprehensive review of visual system changes that are part of the normal course of aging. By far, the most common age-related deficit in the visual system is presbyopia, the inability of the lens to accommodate to allow a viewer to focus on objects at near distances. This impairment is typically first noticed in the 40s and is easily managed with corrective lenses. Visual acuity (ie, the smallest spatial detail that can be resolved), declines with increasing age as well, even with corrective lenses. Investigators disagree on the rate of decline and timing of onset of this impairment. Spatial contrast sensitivity (ie, how much contrast a person requires to detect a pattern of a given size) also decreases with age, particularly at higher spatial frequencies and lower levels of light. Excessive and intensive illumination, on the other hand, can also be problematic for older adults. Because of age-related increases in the opacity of the lens and degenerative changes in the cornea, seniors have more problems with glare sensitivity than their young adult counterparts. Visual sensitivity in peripheral visual fields and sensitivity for moving targets both decline. Dark adaptation diminishes after the age of 60 years, as does the "useful field of view." Jackson and Owsley[102] define this term as the *spatial area of the visual field*, over which rapid visual discrimination and identification can take place.

The causes of these problems vary. Some have been attributed to optical changes in the aged eye (eg, increased opacity of the lens, decreased size and responsiveness of the pupil), while others are thought to be due to degeneration of the neural visual pathway.[85] Regardless of their origin, these problems result in an older adult having less accurate available sensory input to optimize motor control, which contributes to impaired balance and increases the risk of falls.[131]

Somatosensation

Proprioception, which includes the awareness of joint position and the awareness of movement at a joint, also declines with advanced age. Multiple investigators have examined age-related changes in proprioception in the lower extremity in a nonweightbearing position. Skinner et al[103] examined the joint position sense of 29 volunteers, aged 20 to 82 years, and found a significant correlation between age and both the ability to reproduce the position of the knee and the ability to detect motion at the knee in nonweightbearing position. Pai et al[104] confirmed a moderate correlation between age and the threshold for detection of joint displacement at the knee. Age-related declines in proprioception have also been identified at the ankle when in a nonweightbearing position.[105,106] In contrast, it appears that proprioception at the hip joint may be preserved.[107]

Research suggests that weightbearing may affect the size of the age-related loss of proprioception at the knee and ankle.[105,108] Thelen et al[105] demonstrated that older women have more difficulty than younger women detecting both the presence and direction of movement of the ankle while standing. They report that the decrease in proprioception that they found in the weightbearing ankle was less than that previously measured with subjects in a nonweightbearing position. The authors suggest that smaller declines in proprioception with weightbearing may be due to the use of sensory input from plantar pressor receptors. Because the calf is in an elongated position, there may also be increased sensory input from calf intrafusal receptors that contributes to better preserved proprioception with weightbearing compared to nonweightbearing.

An additional finding of Thelen et al's[105] work is that the older women were more successful sensing ankle displacements that occurred at faster angular speeds (highest speed was 2.5 degrees/second) compared to slower angular speeds (slowest speed was 0.5 degrees/second). Older women had the most difficulty sensing speeds that were representative of ankle rotational velocities observed during postural sway. In fact, the negative effect of proprioceptive decline on postural sway has been documented. McChesney and Woollacott[109] found that older adults with very poor knee or ankle proprioception (as measured by the amount of movement required to detect passive motion when the joint was moved at a slow speed of 0.4 degrees/second) had significantly greater center of pressure variance, a measure of static postural control, compared to older adults with good proprioception. Impaired proprioception did not, however, affect the subjects' ability to respond to abrupt, unexpected perturbations (movement of the platform 3.80 cm at a speed of 20 cm/second).

Thus, it appears that lower extremity proprioception declines with advancing age, particularly in nonweightbearing positions, and that this reduction may affect postural control. Recent research suggests a relationship with quiet standing, but not with successful response to unexpected perturbations. Further investigation is warranted to fully examine the relationship between impaired proprioception and motor control.

In addition to a decline in proprioception with advancing age, the sensitivity to tactile and vibratory stimuli also declines.[6,110-112] It is not clear whether these age-related declines in sensory integrity are due to alterations in aging skin, a decrease in density and change in receptor morphology, an alteration in number and structure of afferent nerve fibers, or a combination of these factors. The clinical significance of these changes is not firmly established either. Studies consistently demonstrate a loss of these sensory modalities; the difference between young and old is not always large and has, in absence of other impairments, not consistently been linked to functional limitations. It has also been observed that there is great variability in the sensation of older adults, with many older subjects demonstrating levels of tactile and vibratory sensitivity that equal or exceed their younger counterparts.

Vestibular Function

The vestibular system gathers and synthesizes data about head position and motion (velocity and acceleration) to ensure appropriate eye movements for gaze stability and postural responses for balance. In addition, the vestibular system acts as a mediator, resolving conflicting information from the visual and somatosensory systems to facilitate appropriate postural responses.

The vestibular system includes a peripheral sensory apparatus, a central processor, and ocular and spinal motor output mechanisms. The peripheral system consists of otoliths

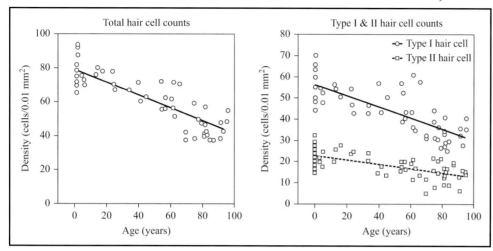

Figure 3-10. Normative hair cell data for crista of the lateral semicircular canal. (Adapted from Velázquez-Villaseñor L, Merchant SN, Tsuji K, Glynn RJ, Wall C 3rd, Rauch SD. Temporal bone studies of the human peripheral vestibular system. Normative Scarpa's ganglion cell data. *Ann Otol Rhinol Laryngol Suppl.* 2000;181:14-19.)

(saccule and utricle) and semicircular canals (anterior, posterior, and horizontal) that provide sensory input to the vestibular nuclei located in the pons and medulla and to the cerebellum, where it is integrated to produce motor outputs through the vestibulo-ocular, vestibulocervical, and vestibulospinal reflexes.

There is a significant, progressive age-related decline in the hair cells (the motion sensors of the periphery) in the peripheral vestibular apparatus (Figure 3-10). In a study by Lopez et al,[132] there was a decrease of 11.6% of hair cell number in the horizontal semicircular canal of adults in their 80s and 25% of adults in their 90s compared to a group of younger adults (42 to 67 years of age). There may also be a loss of hair cells in the otoliths, but this research is not as conclusive. In addition to hair cell loss, there is a decrease in the number of neurons in the vestibular ganglion (Scarpa's ganglion). Park et al[133] found that the average number of nerve cells declined gradually between 30 and 60 years of age and then leveled off.

The exact effect of these anatomical changes on measures of vestibular function is still being determined. The vestibulo-ocular reflex (VOR) stabilizes images on the retina during head movement by generating an eye movement in the direction opposite to the head movement. Multiple studies have documented an age-related decline in the VOR.[113,134] Peterka et al[113] examined the VOR by testing the responses to caloric and sinusoidal rotational stimuli in 216 subjects aged 7 to 81 years. Caloric test parameters did not change with age, but there was a slight progressive change throughout the lifespan in rotation test gain (the magnitude of the eye movement response) and phase (the timing of the eye movement response) with age. The investigators note that only 10% to 15% of the variance in gain data could be explained by age, so factors other than age are contributing significantly to measures of VOR gain. They also report that the magnitude of the changes with age were not large compared to the variability within the population.

In a longitudinal study of the effects of aging on vestibular function, Enrietto et al[114] tested the vestibulo-ocular function of 57 normal older adults (mean age of 82 years)

annually for 5 years. The integrity of the horizontal semicircular canal and the superior vestibular nerve was tested by measuring the VOR during rotational testing. The investigators also tested visual-vestibular interaction by providing additional visual input during the rotary chair testing. The ability to appropriately combine vestibular and visual input requires an intact brainstem and cerebellum. Thus, visual-vestibular interaction testing is useful in identifying central nervous system involvement. A significant decrease in gain and increase in phase lead of the VOR was found. There was also a decline in gain of visual-vestibular responses at low-frequency sinusoidal stimulation over the 5 examinations. The researchers therefore suggest that the age-related declines in vestibular function are likely due to a combination of both peripheral and central vestibular structures.[114]

Research has demonstrated an age-related decline in tests of the function of the otoliths. Both cross-sectional and longitudinal studies have documented a decline in the amplitude of vestibular-evoked myogenic potentials, a measure of saccular function, and/or the corresponding inferior vestibular nerve.[114] Serrador et al[115] report a decline in utricular function as evidenced by a reduction of ocular counter roll (ie, a reflexive ocular torsion in response to head tilt in the roll plane). An additional important finding in their study is a correlation between ocular counter roll and medial-lateral sway as examined during posturography. Since medial-lateral sway has been associated with falls, this raises the possibility that otolith function is also related to fall risk. Decreases in vestibular function as demonstrated in all of the studies described is important to appreciate as vestibular problems can affect an individual's balance and risk of falls.[116]

Central Processing

Sensory input from the visual, somatosensory, and vestibular systems is redundant and, at times, in conflict, requiring the brain to compare the information from these systems to determine the relation of body parts to one another and to the external environment. Afferent input to the brain is integrated, and then an appropriate motor response is planned and executed with consideration of task demands, the environment, the limitations of the effector system, and previous experiences. Research indicates that there are changes that occur with aging that affect the ability of the central nervous system to manage either reduced or conflicting sensory input and to select and execute effective and efficient motor responses.

Sensory Organization

The ability to effectively process and utilize sensory input in advanced age can be challenging to study. The Sensory Organization test has been used frequently to identify older adults' difficulty maintaining quiet stance during conditions of changing sensory input.[117] During this test, postural control is examined under 6 conditions:

1. Normal vision and stable, static platform surface

2. Eyes closed and stable surface (decreased visual input and normal proprioceptive input)

3. Visual surround sway-referenced and stable surface (inaccurate visual input and normal proprioceptive input)

4. Eyes open and platform sway-referenced (normal visual input and inaccurate proprioceptive input)

5. Eyes closed and platform sway-referenced (decreased visual input and inaccurate proprioceptive input)

6. Both visual surround and platform sway-referenced (inaccurate visual and proprioceptive inputs)

Results from this research indicate that older adults have a slight increase in postural sway under normal conditions (ie, eyes open and a firm, static surface) when compared to young adults, though the magnitude of the change is not large enough to threaten postural stability.[117,118]

Older people do, however, demonstrate increased sway and a decreased ability to maintain their balance when sensory input is reduced. This is particularly true in conditions 5 and 6 of the Sensory Organization test when accurate sensory input is reduced from more than one system and seniors are challenged to rely primarily on vestibular input.[117,118] When challenged to stand with abnormal proprioceptive input and either absent or abnormal visual input, 30% to 50% of older adults subjects took a step to regain their balance on the first test trial compared to none of the young adults, suggesting seniors require more sensory input than their younger counterparts to maintain balance.[117,118]

The work of Camicioli et al[124] suggests that balance problems in situations of decreased sensory input are progressive and become even more pronounced in very advanced age. The investigators compared the Sensory Organization test results of "old old" individuals (88 ± 5 years) with those of "young old" subjects (72 ± 3 years). Both groups had difficulty in conditions 5 and 6, when sensory information from 2 systems was reduced. The old old adults also demonstrated difficulty in a situation with inaccurate sensory input from only one of the systems. Specifically, they had significantly greater sway and more frequent falls than younger counterparts in condition 4 (normal vision but inaccurate proprioceptive information). Because the old old adults were unable to use vision to compensate for the loss of accurate proprioceptive information, the researchers suggest there is an age-related increase in reliance on proprioceptive input for balance.

Benjuya et al's[135] research demonstrated decreased reliance on visual information for balance with advancing age. They measured body sway of young and old subjects under 4 conditions: wide base of support with eyes open and eyes closed, and narrow base of support with eyes open and eyes closed. Their data revealed that the reduction in visual input had a greater effect on the postural sway of the younger subjects when compared to the older subjects. The investigators suggest that this is because the older individuals are not relying on the visual system's input for balance as much as the younger adults, so the loss of this information affects their balance to a lesser degree.

Thus, the evidence supports that, in old age, individuals are less able to maintain quiet stance without postural sway in conditions of reduced sensory input on posturography testing. It has been suggested that this can be attributed to a decrease in central processing of sensory information.[124] The possibility exists that, though these subjects were free of known disease and impairment, there were mild age-related declines in the integrity of the peripheral sensory modalities that were not captured on physical exam, and these deficits contributed to age-related changes in Sensory Organization test responses. There is heterogeneity in the aging process, including the aging of the sensory systems. The strength of the visual, somatosensory, and vestibular inputs available for postural control varies from adult to adult. An older adult's stability in different situations is dependent on the strength of the sensory systems of that particular older adult.

The sensory input available to an individual is also dependent on environmental conditions and the information available in different situations. In daily life, the sensory input available to a person changes frequently (eg, walking outside into the bright light from a dark movie theater or walking from a boardwalk onto a sandy beach). Individuals change the relative contribution of each of the senses to postural control as conditions change, a process termed *sensory reweighting*.[119] This process is important to maintain balance. Research suggests that older adults are less able to adapt their use of sensory inputs in response to changes in situation compared with young adults.[119]

The integrity of the sensory systems, patterns of sensory reliance, and sensory reweighting abilities need to be determined during a physical therapy examination. Does an older adult have accurate visual, somatosensory, and vestibular input available? Does he or she effectively use all of the available sensory input, or is there excessive reliance on one system? Is the individual able to change the input relied on in response to changing environmental conditions? Answers to these questions help a PT design the most effective balance training program for an older adult.

Motor Organization

After integrating incoming sensory input, the central nervous system must organize and execute a motor response that is both coordinated and timely. Research indicates that, with age, both the pattern and timing of movements change.

Postural muscles contract to stabilize the body in preparation for a voluntary movement. Early research demonstrated that older adults had difficulty quickly generating these anticipatory postural adjustments when performing voluntary movements.[136] In contrast, Rogers et al[137] found that older adults triggered anticipatory postural events as quickly as younger subjects when asked to generate a voluntary step in response to a visual cue. The time to unload the limb and step was significantly longer in older adults compared with young adults, but there was no difference in the onset of preparatory postural muscle activation.

St. George et al[120] also examined the timing of older adults' voluntary stepping movements in response to a visual stimulus. In their study, subjects were required to step on 1 of 4 foot plates as quickly as possible once it became illuminated. Older adults took longer to initiate a movement, which the authors suggest indicates an age-related decline in central processing of information. In addition, the older adults took longer to reach the foot plate once leg movement had begun. This suggests there is also a decline in the speed of motor execution with age.

An additional and important component of this study was an investigation of the impact of cognitive and motor secondary tasks on stepping ability. The results demonstrated a decline in performance that was dependent on the type of secondary task added. Specifically, subjects performed a visuospatial working memory task immediately prior to illumination of the foot plate. Subjects were also required to step over a low obstacle to reach the foot plate. Initiation and execution times were measured with each of these tasks performed alone as well as when the tasks were performed together. The addition of the memory task increased response times by more than 40% in the older adult group, but by only 7% in the young adult group. Increases in movement execution time were smaller and equal in size in young and old adults. The additional challenge of the obstacle increased movement time by ~40% in all subjects, but it only minimally affected response time. Older adults consistently had more errors in stepping, poorer performance on the memory task, and more contact with the obstacle compared with young adults. The investigators concluded there is an age-related decline in the ability to initiate and execute quick, accurate voluntary steps. The decline is most notable when attention is divided between 2 tasks.

There are additional age-related delays in the onset of muscle activation in reactive balance situations, such as when a force platform is unexpectedly moved.[117] Changes in the patterns of muscle activation have also been noted in response to this challenge. Older adults have been shown to have greater cocontraction of lower extremity musculature compared with young adults when they respond to an unexpected translation of a force platform, a situation that is similar to the experience of a slip while walking.[117,138] They also more frequently contract muscles in a proximal to distal fashion rather than the usual distal to proximal order when compared to young adults.

Individuals rely on ankle, hip, or stepping movements (or a combination) to respond to unexpected challenges to their postural control. Older adults use hip movements more often than young adults, who tend to maintain postural stability in response to small perturbations using ankle muscle activation.[117] Older adults also use a stepping strategy more often and in response to smaller perturbations than the young.[125,126] For example, Hall et al[125] examined younger and older adults' responses to forward and backward translations of a force platform at varying amplitudes and velocities. Older adults generated ankle muscle torques that were similar to the younger subjects' torque in amplitude, rate of development, and scaling to the size and velocity of the perturbation. Despite having the same ankle motor function, older subjects used a stepping strategy to maintain upright more often than the younger adults. It is possible that older adults stepped more frequently because of proximal leg or trunk motor function deficits and an associated inability to rely on a hip strategy, but this remains unknown as those forces were not measured in this study.

Mille et al[126] also studied the effect of external perturbations of various velocities and displacements on the threshold for inducing a stepping response in young (25.3 ± 4.2 years) and old (71.0 ± 7.0 years) subjects. Their work supports the conclusion that seniors step more frequently than young adults in response to both low- and high-velocity displacements. The authors also examined the relationship between multiple sensorimotor factors (vibration sense, touch-pressure sensation, proprioception, visual acuity, ankle plantarflexion strength, and foot voluntary reaction time) and the stepping response. Decreased sensorimotor performance was significantly associated with more frequent stepping. Once age was removed as a factor, however, these associations were no longer present, which suggests that the sensorimotor variables were not directly responsible for the change in stepping behavior seen with advancing age.

The effect of age on upper extremity motor control has also been examined. Fozard et al[121] analyzed both cross-sectional and longitudinal data from 1265 volunteers aged 17 to 96 years and identified an increase in upper extremity reaction time with advancing age. That is, older adults took significantly longer to press a handheld button in response to an auditory stimulus compared with younger adults. The difference in reaction time was more pronounced when the complexity of the task was increased. Beginning at age 20 years, simple reaction time increased at a rate of approximately 0.5 ms/year, and the more difficult disjunctive reaction time (ie, subjects had to decide if they were going to press the button depending on the pitch of the auditory cue) increased at a rate of 1.6 ms/year. Additionally, the variability of responses and number of errors was greater in old age.

Houx and Jolles[122] found age-related slowing mainly in the execution of reaction time tasks, though a slowing in the initiation of a motor response was identified when the task was more complex. In addition to increases in the time to execute upper extremity tasks, research has demonstrated age-related changes in the patterns of movement.[123] Older individuals rapidly reaching for a target spend more time in the deceleration phase, the period of sensory processing that ensures accuracy of movement, than their younger counterparts. There is less evidence to suggest that older adults spend proportionally more time accelerating toward a target. Pohl et al[123] examined the ability of old and young subjects to perform reciprocal tapping with the hand under conditions of differing complexity: tapping a stylus on an 8-cm–wide target, alternating between 8-cm–wide targets placed 37 cm apart, and alternating between 2-cm–wide targets placed 37 cm apart. Older adults demonstrated longer movement times and more than 5 times the number of adjustments in trajectory compared with those in the young group. The older subjects also spent more time reversing direction between targets than the young subjects. Thus, older adults may take longer to reach because of slowing to ensure adequate determination of position in space and added time spent adjusting the path of movement to reach their target. The investigators found that age-related differences became more pronounced in the more difficult conditions.

Wishart et al[139] also found that the performance of older adults on upper extremity coordination tasks was dependent on the speed and complexity of the task. Subjects were asked to complete an upper extremity task in which the mirror image actions of the upper extremities were performed (ie, shoulders both internally or externally rotated at neutral flexion to slide pegs back and forth on steel rods) at 5 different movement speeds. This task was believed to represent an automatic process. The subjects also performed this task with the upper extremities out of phase (ie, moving like windshield wipers), which was believed to be automatic at slow speeds, but a conscious and effortful process at fast speeds. Compared with younger subjects, the older adults demonstrated decreased accuracy and stability of movement at high speeds when performing the more complex task. The researchers suggested that older individuals often perform as well as younger subjects with automatic tasks, but that age-related differences in motor performance become more pronounced when conscious, effortful processing is required.

Effector System

Automatic and voluntary adjustments of the body for stability or mobility occur within the constraints of the effector system. That is, factors such as muscle performance, aerobic capacity, ROM, and posture all affect how motions may be carried out. The age-related changes in aerobic capacity and muscle performance discussed earlier may affect an older adult's ability to perform desired movements once motor plans are created by the central processing system. In addition, age-related changes in ROM and posture may also affect the way an older adult is able to move. ROM decreases with age.[127,128] There is significant variability in how individuals' posture develops with advancing age, but older adults tend to have a greater kyphosis, more posterior hip position, and forward lean at the hips (Figure 3-11). All of these factors must be considered when examining an older adult's performance of functional tasks.

Effect on Function

Cross-sectional and longitudinal data have indicated that changes in upper extremity performance may affect the older adult's ability to perform ADL. Potvin et al[140] and Desrosiers et al[141] examined multiple tests of sensorimotor performance, including gross and fine motor control, strength, coordination, sensory integrity, and reaction time. Age-related declines were documented on almost all tests. In addition, measures of ADL performance were found to decline in older age. It is important to note that the measures chosen by these investigators were timed tests. As older adults took more time to complete a task similar to an ADL, the score they received declined. Thus, it is not known how well the subjects were able to complete the functional tests, only that they required more time to do so.

There are significant age-related changes in gait performance that affect the safety and functional abilities of older adults. Seniors demonstrate slower gait speed, shorter steps, decreased single limb support time, slight hip flexion, anterior pelvic tilt, toeing out of the feet, and decreased ankle plantarflexion power at push-off when compared to younger adults.[142] Himann et al[143] found that the decline in gait speed accelerated after age 62 years. Prior to age 62 years, the normal walking speed decline was demonstrated to be 1% to 2% per decade. After age 62 years, the more rapid decline of 12.4% per decade for females and 16.1% per decade for males was seen. It also has been shown that older adults are less able than younger adults to increase their gait speed from a preferred gait speed to a fast pace of walking.[144] These declines in gait speed may limit an older adult's ability to be functional in the community because certain mobility tasks, such as crossing a street, require an older adult to walk quickly. In fact, Hoxie and Rubenstein[145] found that 27% of 592 pedestrians observed crossing the street were unable to make it to the opposite curb before the light changed, all of them being older adults.

A significant safety concern for older individuals is the increased risk of falling that comes with advanced age.[146] Older adults have delayed, slower, and smaller muscle activation after slips and trips, which may contribute to the inability to recover from these events.[138,147] They also have a decreased ability to terminate gait rapidly compared to younger adults.[148] Priest et al[149] note that variability in stride velocity is a characteristic of unstable gait and predicts falls in older adults. In their study, community-dwelling older women (mean age of 80 years) had significantly more variability in stride velocity compared to young adults. In addition, they found that this variability increased and gait speed

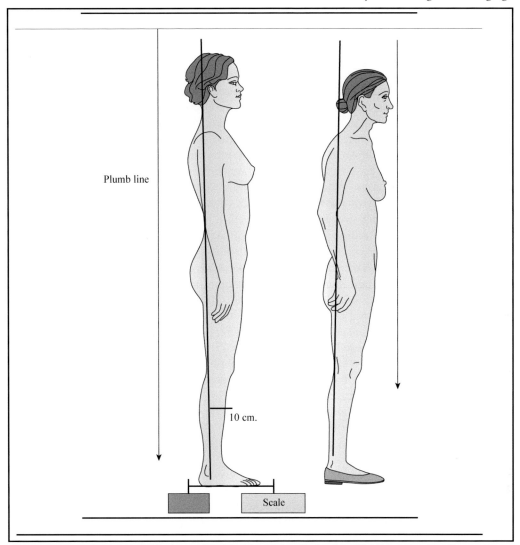

Plumb line

10 cm.

Scale

Figure 3-11. Typical young and old subjects. (Modified from *Aging Clin Exp Res*, 4(3), 1992, pp 219-225, Changes in posture and balance with age, Woodhull-McNeal AP, with kind permission from Springer Science+Business Media B.V.)

decreased in dual-task walking (ie, walking while counting backwards in increments of 3, 4, or 6). Because the addition of a cognitive task has a destabilizing effect on gait, the authors emphasize the need to incorporate such dual-task situations into a rehabilitation intervention. This may be through education about the need to avoid cognitive tasks while walking or through training under dual-task conditions.

Several impairments described previously have been positively associated with falls in community-dwelling older adults, including visual acuity, depth perception, contrast sensitivity, proprioception, vibratory sense, lower extremity strength, reaction time, and postural sway during static stance with eyes open.[131,146,150] Perhaps even more threatening to fall risk than the presence of a single impairment is the effect of multiple impairments. Several authors have noted that a single impairment may explain only a small portion of the fall risk of an older adult or may not significantly increase a senior's risk of being a recurrent faller. Instead, the accumulation of several impairments appears to escalate fall risk more dramatically.[146,151] Thus, an essential component

of the PT's evaluation and plan of care for the older adult at risk for falls is to identify and remediate all correctable impairments and to help the individual compensate for those that cannot be changed.

Benefits of Training

Older adults retain the ability to improve many aspects of motor control with physical activity, exercise, and training. Buatois et al[152] found that older adults who were physically active had improved postural control and better ability to manage situations with sensory conflict on the Sensory Organization test compared to sedentary peers. Current physical activity was the major determinant for measures of postural stability compared to age, gender, body mass index, and past physical activity. Thus, physical activity can minimize age-related declines in sensory organization. It is important to note that it was not just older adults who had been physically active for their entire lives who performed well. Older adults who became active later in life (ie, after retirement) performed significantly better than those who were not currently active. This highlights that a simple change in lifestyle, even made later in life, is valuable for older adults.

Physically active older adults have also demonstrated better reaction times compared with those who described a sedentary lifestyle. Spirduso et al[153] found this difference both with a simple lower extremity response test (pressing a foot switch in response to a visual cue) and a discrimination reaction time test (pressing a foot switch only when the proper color visual cue was presented). An encouraging research finding is that older adults can improve their reaction time with training. Falduto and Baron[154] had 8 older and 8 younger women practice sorting cards for 5 training sessions. At the end of the training, older women demonstrated significantly better sorting ability both in simple and complex conditions.

Lord and Castell[155] implemented a comprehensive 10-week group exercise program for 44 older men and women (mean age = 62.4 years), consisting of walking, lower extremity strength training (using gravity as resistance and targeting ankle dorsiflexors, knee extensors, hip abductors, and the quadratus lumborum), bicycle riding, flexibility, balance exercises, and education regarding safe exercise techniques and proper posture. At the end of this period, the group that exercised demonstrated significant improvements in quadriceps strength, simple lower extremity reaction time, and postural sway (on a firm surface with eyes open and on foam with both eyes open and eyes closed) compared to a control group, demonstrating the reversibility of many impairments found in old age. There were no measures of function or disability in this study, so it is not known how these affected the subjects' functional performance. In a subsequent randomized controlled trial, however, Lord and his colleagues[156] were able to demonstrate that a 22-week exercise program, similar to the one described previously, had a positive impact on the gait pattern of seniors. Older adults had significantly increased gait speed, cadence, stride length, and shorter stride times at the end of the training period, while none of the gait parameters of the control subjects changed.

Of paramount concern to older adults and PTs is the ability to reduce the risk of falling associated with advancing age. Evidence suggests that community-dwelling older adults are able to reduce their risk of falling with training, though the optimal frequency, intensity, duration, and combination of interventions is not completely clear.[146,157,158] In their meta-analysis of 44 randomized controlled trials involving 9603 subjects, Sherrington et al[130] found that exercise reduced fall rates in older adults by 17%. Additionally, they identified 3 characteristics of programs that were associated with better outcomes: inclusion of challenging balance exercises, higher doses of exercise (a minimum of twice per week for 25 weeks), and absence of a walking program. The authors suggest that these findings should be considered when designing an exercise program to reduce the fall risk of an older client. Though the inclusion of moderate- or high-intensity strength training or a walking program did not provide added benefit to the reduction of fall risk, the authors note that these interventions do result in other gains that are important to older adults' health, such as improved fitness and lower BP. Impaired balance may be a greater risk factor for falls, but declines in strength and aerobic capacity do have important implications for function as discussed earlier in the chapter and need to be considered for inclusion in a comprehensive exercise program for an older adult.

In addition to remediating impairments and improving function through training, PTs can help older adults adapt to irreversible problems to improve safety. For example, a clinician can make recommendations for environmental modifications to decrease or minimize the extrinsic risk factors for falls or provide equipment to facilitate performance of ADL (eg, a reacher to obtain objects from high shelves, eliminating the need to climb a step stool). Finally, recognition of risk factors for falls that can effectively be managed by other health care providers should trigger referrals to these clinicians, such as an ophthalmologist for optimal eyewear prescription or a primary care physician for medication modification.

The age-related decline in motor control cannot be avoided, but with training and exercise, older people can lessen the magnitude of the changes that they experience in reaction time, postural sway, gait speed and pattern, and fall risk.

Summary

The ability to initiate, execute, and terminate coordinated and timely movements depends on sensory input from the visual, vestibular, and somatosensory systems; central processing to integrate this afferent information and plan an appropriate motor response; and an expression of that response within the constraints of the body's effector system. Age-related changes occur in each of these components of motor control. Older adults often develop impairments in visual acuity, contrast sensitivity, glare sensitivity, peripheral field vision, and dark adaptation. Proprioception, tactile sensitivity, and vibratory sense also frequently decline in older adulthood. Age-related decreases in vestibular function have been found and are thought to be due to changes both in the peripheral and central vestibular structures.

Older people sway more than young adults during quiet stance and demonstrate decreased ability to maintain their balance in the setting of reduced sensory input during posturography testing. Reaction times are greater, especially as conditions become more complex. The patterns of movement of older adults also change, including increased cocontraction of lower extremity musculature and more frequent reliance on hip or stepping strategies in response to a perturbation.

These changes in the sensory and central processing systems combine with the muscle performance impairments described earlier to slow the performance of older adults during gait and ADL and put them at risk for falls. Though training cannot alleviate these problems, the current evidence demonstrates that multifactorial interventions can improve the coordination, gait, and fall risk profile of older adults.

SUMMARY

An understanding of the inevitable changes that occur at the end of the lifespan is essential for the PT to discriminate between pathology and the normal aging process. An appreciation of the limitations of an older body allows proper interpretation of tests and measures, prognostication, and treatment planning. In the absence of disease, age-related changes in aerobic capacity, muscle performance, and motor control do not generally affect an older person's ability to lead an independent and active life until very advanced age. One of the common threads in this chapter's discussion of age-related changes has been the effect of aging on physical reserve. Declines in maximal fitness, muscle performance, and postural control leave the older adult at risk for functional limitations in the setting of illness, chronic disease, sedentary lifestyle, or particularly challenging task demands. An impairment superimposed on age-related decreases in the maximal capacity of these systems may render an older adult functionally limited.

Another common theme in the data on the physiology of healthy aging is heterogeneity. Human beings do not all age at similar rates nor in the same way. Many researchers note the increased variability of results for older subjects. Reference ranges for normal test result values are broader for older adults than for the young because there is increased variability in performance with advancing age. It cannot be assumed that an older client will or will not demonstrate particular impairments or functional limitations. PTs, therefore, must rely on careful examination to identify what resources an older adult has to rely on to perform their life roles.

Fortunately, older adults retain the ability to improve many of the potential impairments and functional limitations noted in this chapter. With appropriate training, older clients have demonstrated gains in each of the systems reviewed. Thus, a comprehensive physical therapy examination and individualized intervention prescription can facilitate healthy aging and delay or prevent the onset of disability.

REFERENCES

1. Masoro E. Physiology of aging. *Int J Sport Nutr Exerc Metab.* 2001;11:S218-S222.

2. Zeleznik J. Normative aging of the respiratory system. *Clin Geriatr Med.* 2003;19(1):1-18.

3. American Physical Therapy Association. Guide to physical therapist practice. Second edition. American Physical Therapy Association. *Phys Ther.* 2001;81(1):9-746.

4. Janssens JP, Pache JC, Nicod LP. Physiological changes in respiratory function associated with ageing. *Eur Respir J.* 1999;13:197-205.

5. Gillooly M, Lamb D. Airspace size in lungs of lifelong non-smokers: effect of age and sex. *Thorax.* 1993;48:39-43.

6. Martina IS, van Koningsveld R, Schmitz PI, van der Meché FG, van Doorn PA. Measuring vibration threshold with a graduated tuning fork in normal aging and in patients with polyneuropathy. European Inflammatory Neuropathy Cause and Treatment (INCAT) group. *J Neurol Neurosurg Psychiatry.* 1998;65:743-747.

7. Hautmann H, Hefele S, Schotten K, Huber RM. Maximal inspiratory mouth pressures (PI$_{MAX}$) in healthy subjects—what is the lower limit of normal? *Respir Med.* 2000;94:689-693.

8. Tolep K, Kelsen SG. Effect of aging on respiratory skeletal muscles. *Clin Chest Med.* 1993;14(3):363-378.

9. Stam H, Hrachovina V, Stijnen T, Versprille A. Diffusing capacity dependent on lung volume and age in normal subjects. *J Appl Physiol.* 1994;76:2356-2363.

10. Enright PL, Kronmal RA, Manolio TA, Schenker MB, Hyatt RE. Respiratory muscle strength in the elderly. Correlates and reference values. Cardiovascular Health Study Research Group. *Am J Respir Crit Care Med.* 1994;149:430-438.

11. Takishima T, Shindoh C, Kikuchi Y, Hida W, Inoue H. Aging effect on oxygen consumption of respiratory muscles in humans. *J Appl Physiol (1985).* 1990;69:14-20.

12. Janssens JP. Aging of the respiratory system: impact on pulmonary function tests and adaptation to exertion. *Clin Chest Med.* 2005;26:469-484.

13. Sparrow D, Weiss ST. Respiratory system. In: Masoro EJ, ed. *Handbook of Physiology: Aging.* New York, NY: Oxford University Press; 1995.

14. West JB. *Respiratory Physiology: The Essentials.* 6th ed. Baltimore, MD: Lippincott Williams & Wilkins; 2000.

15. Sjögren AL. Left ventricular wall thickness determined by ultrasound in 100 subjects without heart disease. *Chest.* 1971;60:341-346.

16. Gerstenblith G, Frederiksen J, Yin FC, Fortuin NJ, Lakatta EG, Weisfeldt ML. Echocardiographic assessments of a normal adult aging population. *Circulation.* 1977;56:273-278.

17. Kitzman DW, Scholz DG, Hagen PT, Ilstrup DM, Edwards WD. Age-related changes in normal human hearts during the first 10 decades of life. Part II (Maturity): a quantitative anatomic study of 765 specimens from subjects 20 to 99 years old. *Mayo Clin Proc.* 1988;63:137-146.

18. Unverferth DV, Fetters BJ, Unverferth CV, et al. Human myocardial histologic characteristics in congestive heart failure. *Circulation.* 1983;68:1194-1200.

19. Roffe C. Ageing of the heart. *Br J Biomed Sci.* 1998;55:136-148.

20. Lakatta EG. Cardiovascular system. In: Masoro EJ, ed. *Handbook of Physiology: Aging.* New York, NY: Oxford University Press; 1995:413-474.

21. Lewis JF, Maron BJ. Cardiovascular consequences of the aging process. *Cardiovasc Clin.* 1992:22(2):25-34.

22. Cheitlin MD. Cardiovascular physiology—changes with aging. *Am J Geriatr Cardiol.* 2003;12(1):9-13.

23. Thompson LV. Physiological changes associated with aging. In: Guccione AA, ed. *Geriatric Physical Therapy.* 2nd ed. Philadelphia, PA: Mosby Inc; 2000.

24. Tanaka H, Dinenno FA, Monahan KD, Clevenger CM, DeSouza CA, Seals DR. Aging, habitual exercise, and dynamic arterial compliance. *Circulation.* 2000;102:1270-1275.

25. Nichols WW, O'Rourke MF, Avolio AP, et al. Effects of age on ventricular-vascular coupling. *Am J Cardiol.* 1985;55:1179-1184.

26. Seals DR, Monahan KD, Bell C, Tanaka H, Jones PP. The aging cardiovascular system: changes in autonomic function at rest and in response to exercise. *Int J Sport Nutr Exerc Metab.* 2001;11(Suppl):S189-S195.

27. Umetani K, Singer DH, McCraty R, Atkinson M. Twenty-four hour time domain heart rate variability and heart rate: relations to age and gender over nine decades. *J Am Coll Cardiol.* 1998;31:593-601.

28. Tasaki H, Serita T, Irita A, et al. A 15-year longitudinal follow-up study of heart rate and heart rate variability in healthy elderly persons. *J Gerontol A Biol Sci Med Sci.* 2000;12:M744-M749.

29. Craft N, Schwartz JB. Effects of age on intrinsic heart rate, heart rate variability, and AV conduction in healthy humans. *Am J Physiol.* 1995;265:H1441-H1452.

30. Jensen-Urstad K, Storck N, Bouvier F, Ericson M, Lindblad LE, Jensen-Urstad M. Heart rate variability in healthy subjects is related to age and gender. *Acta Physiol Scand.* 1997;160(3):235-241.

31. Schwartz JB, Gibb WJ, Tran T. Aging effects on heart rate variation. *J Gerontol.* 1991;46(3): M99-M106.

32. Pugh KG, Wei JY. Clinical implications of physiological changes in the aging heart. *Drugs Aging.* 2001;18(4):263-276.

33. Jani B, Rajkumar C. Ageing and vascular ageing. *Postgrad Med J.* 2006;82:357-362.

34. Chodzko-Zajko WJ, Proctor DN, Fiatarone MA, et al. ACSM position stand: exercise and physical activity for older adults. *Med Sci Sports Exerc.* 2009;41(7):1510-1530.

35. Rodeheffer RJ, Gerstenblith G, Becker LC, Fleg JL, Weisfeldt ML, Lakatta EG. Exercise cardiac output is maintained with advancing age in healthy human subjects: cardiac dilatation and increased stroke volume compensate for a diminished heart rate. *Circulation.* 1984;69(2):203-213.

36. Ogawa T, Spina RJ, Martin WH, et al. Effects of aging, sex, and physical training on cardiovascular responses to exercise. *Circulation.* 1992;86(2):494-503.

37. Fleg JL, O'Connor F, Gerstenblith G, et al. Impact of age on the cardiovascular response to dynamic upright exercise in healthy men and women. *J Appl Physiol (1985).* 1995;78(3):890-900.

38. Stratton JR, Levy WC, Cerqueira MD, Schwartz RS, Abrass IB. Cardiovascular responses to exercise. Effects of aging and exercise training in healthy men. *Circulation.* 1994;89(4):1648-1655.

39. Wiebe CG, Gledhill N, Jamnik VK, Ferguson S. Exercise cardiac function in young through elderly endurance trained women. *Med Sci Sports Exerc.* 1999;31(5):684-691.

40. Kohrt WM, Brown M. Endurance training of the older adult. In: Guccione AA, ed. *Geriatric Physical Therapy.* 2nd ed. Philadelphia, PA: Mosby Inc; 2000.

41. Tanaka H, Monahan KD, Seals DR. Age-predicted maximal heart rate revisited. *J Am Coll Cardiol.* 2001;37:153-156.

42. Kostis JB, Moreyra AE, Amendo MT, Di Pietro J, Cosgrove N, Kuo PT. The effect of age on heart rate in subjects free of heart disease: studies by ambulatory electrocardiography and maximal exercise stress test. *Circulation.* 1982;65:141-145.

43. Fleg JL, Morrell CH, Bos AG, et al. Accelerated longitudinal decline of aerobic capacity in healthy older adults. *Circulation.* 2005;112:674-682.

44. Proctor DN, Beck KC, Shen PH, Eickhoff TJ, Halliwill JR, Joyner MJ. Influence of age and gender on cardiac output-VO2 relationships during submaximal cycle ergometry. *J Appl Physiol (1985).* 1998;84(2):599-605.

45. Proctor DN, Joyner MJ. Skeletal muscle mass and the reduction of VO_{2max} in trained older subjects. *J Appl Physiol (1985).* 1997;82(5):1411-1415.

46. Yerg JE, Seals DR, Hagberg JM, Hollozy JO. Effect of endurance exercise training on ventilatory function in older individuals. *J Appl Physiol (1985).* 1985;58(3):791-794.

47. Cress ME, Meyer M. Maximal voluntary and functional performance levels needed for independence in adults aged 65 to 97 years. *Phys Ther.* 2003;83(1):37-48.

48. Thompson L. Skeletal muscle adaptations with age, inactivity, and therapeutic exercise. *J Ortho Sports Phys Ther.* 2002;32:44-57.

49. Proctor DN, O'Brien PC, Atkinson EJ, Nair KS. Comparison of techniques to estimate total body skeletal muscle mass in people of different age groups. *Am J Physiol.* 1999;277:E489-E495.

50. Vandervoort AA. Aging of the human neuromuscular system. *Muscle Nerve.* 2002;25:17-25.

51. Delmonico MJ, Harris TB, Visser M, et al. Longitudinal study of muscle strength, quality, and adipose tissue infiltration. *Am J Clin Nutr.* 2009;90:1579-1585.

52. Frontera WR, Hughes VA, Fielding RA, Fiatarone MA, Evans WJ, Roubenoff R. Aging of skeletal muscle: a 12-yr longitudinal study. *J Appl Physiol (1985).* 2000;88:1321-1326.

53. Lexell J, Taylor CC, Sjöstrom M. What is the cause of the ageing atrophy? Total number, size and proportion of different fibre types studied in whole vastus lateralis muscle from 15- to 83-year-old men. *J Neurolog Sci.* 1988;84:275-294.

54. Trappe S. Master athletes. *Int J Sport Nutr Exerc Metab.* 2001;11:S196-S207.

55. American College of Sports Medicine position stand. Exercise and physical activity for older adults. *Med Sci Sports Exerc.* 1998;30(6):992-1008.

56. Lynch NA, Metter EJ, Lindle RS, et al. Muscle quality. I. Age-associated differences between arm and leg muscle groups. *J Appl Physiol (1985).* 1999;86:188-194.

57. Hortobágyi T, Zheng D, Weidner M, Lambert NJ, Westbrook S, Houmard JA. The influence of aging on muscle strength and muscle fiber characteristics with special reference to eccentric strength. *J Gerontol A Biol Sci Med Sci.* 1995;50:B399-B406.

58. Lindle RS, Metter EJ, Lynch NA, et al. Age and gender comparisons of muscle strength in 654 women and men aged 20-93 yr. *J Appl Physiol (1985).* 1997;83:1581-1587.

59. Short KR, Nair KS. Muscle protein metabolism and the sarcopenia of aging. *Int J Sport Nutr Exerc Metab.* 2001;11(Suppl):S119-S127.

60. Frontera WR, Hughes VA, Krivickas LS, Roubenoff R. Contractile properties of aging skeletal muscle. *Int J Sport Nutr Exerc Metab.* 2001;11(Suppl):S16-S20.

61. Metter EJ, Conwit R, Tobin J, Fozard JL. Age-associated loss of power and strength in the upper extremities in women and men. *J Gerontol Biol Sci Med Sci.* 1997;52: B267-B276.

62. Lindström B, Lexell J, Gerdle B, Downham D. Skeletal muscle fatigue and endurance in young and old men and women. *J Gerontol Biol Sci Med Sci.* 1997; 52: B59-B66.

63. Bäckman E, Johansson V, Häger B, Sjöblom P, Henriksson KG. Isometric muscle strength and muscular endurance in normal persons aged between 17 and 70 years. *Scan J Rehabil Med.* 1995;27:109-117.

64. Schwendner KI, Mikesky AE, Holt WS Jr, Peacock M, Burr DB, Differences in muscle endurance and recovery between fallers and nonfallers, and between young and older women. *J Gerontol A Biol Sci Med Sci.* 1997;52:M155-M160.

65. Ling SM, Conwit RA, Ferrucci L, Metter EF. Age-associated changes in motor unit physiology: observations from the Baltimore Longitudinal Study of Aging. *Arch Phys Med Rehabil.* 2009;90:1237-1240.

66. Nair KS. Muscle protein turnover: methodological issues and the effect of aging. *J Gerontol A Biol Sci Med Sci.* 1995;50(Spec No):107-112.

67. Deschenes MR. Effect of aging on muscle fibre type and size. *Sports Med.* 2004;34(12):809-824.

68. Jones TE, Stephenson KW, King JG, Knight KR, Marshall RL, Scott WB. Sarcopenia—mechanisms and treatments. *J Geriatr Phys Ther.* 2009;32(2):39-45.

69. Trappe S, Williamson D, Godard M, Porter D, Rowden G, Costill D. Effect of resistance training on single muscle fiber contractile function in older men. *J Appl Physiol (1985).* 2000;89:143-152.

70. Bemben MG, Massey BH, Bemben DA, Misner JE, Boileau RA. Isometric muscle force production as a function of age in healthy 20- to 74-yr-old men. *Med Sci Sports Exerc.* 1991;11:1302-1310.

71. Brown M, Sinacore DR, Host HH. The relationship of strength to function in the older adult. *J Gerontol A Biol Sci Med Sci.* 1995;50(Spec No):55-59.

72. Corrigan D, Bohannon RW. Relationship between knee extension force and stand-up performance in community-dwelling elderly women. *Arch Phys Med Rehab.* 2001;82:1666-1672.

73. Lord SR, Murray SM, Chapman K, Munro B, Tiedemann A. Sit-to-stand performance depends on sensation, speed, balance, and psychological status in addition to strength in older people. *J Gerontol A Biol Sci Med Sci.* 2002; 57(8):M539-M543.

74. Bohannon RW. Body weight-normalized knee extension strength explains sit-to-stand independence: a validation study. *J Strength Cond Res.* 2009;23(1):309-311.

75. Hernandez ME, Goldberg A, Alexander NB. Decreased muscle strength relates to self-reported stooping, crouching, or kneeling difficulty in older adults. *Phys Ther.* 2010;90:67-74.

76. Ringsberg K, Gerdhem P, Johansson J, Obrant KJ. Is there a relationship between balance, gait performance and muscular strength in 75-year-old women? *Age Ageing.* 1999;28:289-293.

77. Wolfson L, Judge J, Whipple R, King M. Strength is a major factor in balance, gait, and the occurrence of falls. *J Gerontol A Biol Sci Med Sci.* 1995;50(Spec No):64-67.

78. Daubney ME, Culham EG. Lower-extremity muscle force and balance performance in adults aged 65 years and older. *Phys Ther.* 1999:79:1177-1185.

79. Bassey EJ, Bendall MJ, Pearson M. Muscle strength in the triceps surae and objectively measured customary walking activity in men and women over 65 years of age. *Clin Sci (Lond).* 1988;74:85-89.

80. Kwon IS, Oldaker S, Schrager M, Talbot LA, Fozard JL, Metter EJ. Relationship between muscle strength and the time taken to complete a standardized walk-turn-walk test. *J Gerontol A Biol Sci Med Sci.* 2001;56(9):B398-B404.

81. Purser JL, Pieper CF, Poole C, Morey M. Trajectories of leg strength and gait speed among sedentary older adults: longitudinal pattern of dose response. *J Gerontol A Biol Sci Med Sci.* 2001;58(12):M1125-M1134.

82. Puthoff ML, Nielsen DH. Relationships among impairments in lower-extremity strength and power, functional limitations, and disability in older adults. *Phys Ther.* 2007;87:1334-1347.

83. Buchner DM, Larson EB, Wagner EH, Koepsell TD, de Lateur BJ. Evidence for a non-linear relationship between leg strength and gait speed. *Age Ageing.* 1996;25:386-391.

84. Lamoureux EL, Sparrow WA, Murphy A, Newton RU. The relationship between lower body strength and obstructed gait in community-dwelling older adults. *J Am Geriatr Soc.* 2002;50:468-473.

85. Suzuki TS, Bean JF, Fielding RA. Muscle power of the ankle flexors predicts functional performance in community-dwelling older women. *J Am Geriatr Soc.* 2001;49:1161-1167.

86. Bean JF, Kiely DK, LaRose S, Leveille SG. Which impairments are most associated with high mobility performance in older adults? Implications for rehabilitation prescription. *Arch Phys Med Rehabil.* 2008;89:2278-2284.

87. Puthoff ML, Janz KF, Nielson DH. The relationship between lower extremity strength and power to everyday walking behaviors in older adults with functional limitations. *J Geriatr Phys Ther.* 2008;31:24-31.

88. Seguin R, Nelson ME. The benefits of strength training for older adults. *Am J Prev Med.* 2003;25(3Sii):141-149.

89. Frontera WR, Meredith CN, O'Reilly KP, Knuttgen HG, Evans WJ. Strength conditioning in older men: skeletal muscle hypertrophy and improved function. *J Appl Physiol (1985).* 1988;63:1038-1044.

90. Fiatarone MA, O'Neill EF, Ryan ND, et al. Exercise training and nutritional supplementation for physical frailty in very elderly people. *N Engl J Med.* 1994;330:1769-1775.

91. Latham NK, Bennett DA, Stretton CM, Anderson CS. Systematic review of progressive resistance strength training in older adults. *J Gerontol A Biol Sci Med Sci.* 2004;59(1):48-61.

92. Tracy BL, Ivey FM, Hurlbut D, et al. Muscle quality. II. Effects of strength training in 65- to 75-yr-old men and women. *J Appl Physiol (1985).* 1999;86:195-201.

93. Ferri A, Scaglioni G, Pousson M, Capodaglio P, Van Hoecke J, Narici MV. Strength and power changes of the human plantar flexors and knee extensors in response to resistance training in old age. *Acta Physiol Scand.* 2003;177:69-78.

94. Bottaro M, Machado SN, Nogueira W, Scales R, Veloso J. Effect of high versus low-velocity resistance training on muscular fitness and functional performance in older men. *Eur J Appl Physiol.* 2007;99:257-264.

95. Cress ME, Buchner DM, Questad KA, Esselman PC, deLateur BJ, Schwartz RS. Exercise: effects on physical functional performance in independent older adults. *J Gerontol A Biol Sci Med Sci.* 1999;54(5):M242-M248.

96. Holviala JH, Sallinen JM, Kraemer WJ, Alen MJ, Häkkinen KK. Effects of strength training on muscle strength characteristics, functional capabilities, and balance in middle-aged and older women. *J Strength Cond Res.* 2006:20:336-344.

97. Earles DR, Judge JO, Gunnarsson OT. Velocity training induces power-specific adaptations in highly functioning older adults. *Arch Phys Med Rehabil.* 2001;82:872-878.

98. Miszko TA, Cress ME, Slade JM, Covey CJ, Agrawal SK, Doerr CE. Effect of strength and power training on physical function in community-dwelling older adults. *J Gerontol A Biol Sci Med Sci.* 2003;58(2):171-175.

99. Rikli RE, Jones CJ. *Senior Fitness Test Manual.* Champaign, IL: Human Kinetics; 2001.

100. Brach JS, Simonsick EM, Kritchevsky S, Yaffe K, Newman AB; Health, Aging and Body Composition Study Research Group. The association between physical function and lifestyle activity and exercise in the health, aging and body composition study. *J Am Geriatr Soc.* 2004;52:502-509.

101. Chandler JM. Balance and falls in the elderly: issues in evaluation and treatment. In: Guccione AA, ed. *Geriatric Physical Therapy.* 2nd ed. Philadelphia, PA: Mosby Inc; 2000.

102. Jackson GR, Owsley C. Visual dysfunction, neurodegenerative diseases, and aging. *Neurol Clin N Am.* 2003;21:708-728.

103. Skinner HB, Barrack RL, Cook SD. Age-related decline in proprioception. *Clin Orth Rel Res.* 1984;184:208-211.

104. Pai Y, Rymer WZ, Chang RW, Sharma L. Effect of age and osteoarthritis on knee proprioception. *Arthritis Rheum.* 1997;40:2260-2265.

105. Thelen DG, Brockmiller C, Ashton-Miller JA, Schultz AB, Alexander NB. Thresholds for sensing foot dorsi- and plantarflexion during upright stance: effects of age and velocity. *J Gerontol A Biol Sci Med Sci.* 1998;53(1):M33-M38.

106. Vershueren SM, Brumagne S, Swinnen SP, Cordo PJ. The effect of aging on dynamic position sense at the ankle. *Behav Brain Res.* 2002;136:593-603.

107. Pickard CM, Sullivan PE, Allison GE, Singer KP. Is there a difference in hip joint position sense between young and older groups? *J Gerontol A Biol Sci Med Sci.* 2003;58:631-635.

108. Bullock-Saxton JE, Wong WJ, Hogan N. The influence of age on weight-bearing joint reposition sense of the knee. *Exp Brain Res.* 2001;136:400-406.

109. McChesney JW, Woollacott MH. The effect of age-related declines in proprioception and total knee replacement on postural control. *J Gerontol A Biol Sci Med Sci.* 2000;55(11):M658-M666.

110. Thornbury JM, Mistretta CM. Tactile sensitivity as a function of age. *J Gerontol.* 1981;36:34-39.

111. Kenshalo DR Sr. Somesthetic sensitivity in young and elderly humans. *J Gerontol.* 1986;41:732-742.

112. Bruce MF. The relation of tactile thresholds to histology in the fingers of elderly people. *J Neurol Neurosurg Psychiatry.* 1980;43:730-734.

113. Peterka RJ, Black FO, Schoenhoff MB. Age-related changes in human vestibulo-ocular reflexes: sinusoidal rotation and caloric tests. *J Vestib Res.* 1990;1:49-59.

114. Enrietto JA, Jacobson KM, Baloh RW. Aging effects on auditory and vestibular responses: a longitudinal study. *Am J Otolaryngol.* 1999;20:371-378.

115. Serrador JM, Lipsitz LA, Gopalakrishnan GS, Black FO, Wood SJ. Loss of otolith function with age is associated with increased postural sway measures. *Neurosci Lett.* 2009;465:10-15.

116. Marchetti GF, Whitney SL. Older adults and balance dysfunction. *Neurol Clin.* 2005;23:785-805.

117. Woollacott MH. Systems contributing to balance disorders in older adults. *J Gerontol A Biol Sci Med Sci.* 2000;55(8):M424-M428.

118. Wolfson L. Gait and balance dysfunction: a model of the interaction of age and disease. *Neuroscientist.* 2001;7:178-183.

119. O'Connor KW, Loughlin PJ, Redfern MS, Sparto PJ. Postural adaptations to repeated optic flow stimulation in older adults. *Gait Posture.* 2008;28(3):385-391.

120. St. George RJ, Fitzpatrick RC, Rogers MW, Lord SW. Choice stepping response and transfer times: effects of age, fall risk, and secondary tasks. *J Gerontol A Biol Sci Med Sci.* 2007;62(5):537-542.

121. Fozard JL, Vercryssen M, Reynolds SL, Hancock PA, Quilter RE. Age differences and changes in reaction time: the Baltimore Longitudinal Study of Aging. *J Gerontol.* 1994;49:P179-P189.

122. Houx PJ, Jolles J. Age-related decline of psychomotor speed: effects of age, brain health, sex, and education. *Percept Mot Skills.* 1993;76:195-211.

123. Pohl PS, Winstein CJ, Fisher BE. The locus of age-related movement slowing: sensory processing in continuous goal-directed aiming. *J Gerontol B Psychol Sci Soc Sci.* 1996;51(2):P94-P102.

124. Camicioli R, Panzer VP, Kaye J. Balance in the healthy elderly: posturography and clinical assessment. *Arch Neurol.* 1997;54:976-981.

125. Hall CD, Woollacott MH, Jensen JL. Age-related changes in rate and magnitude of ankle torque development: implications for balance control. *J Gerontol A Biol Sci Med Sci.* 1999;54(10):M507-M513.

126. Mille ML, Rogers MW, Martinez, K, et al. Thresholds for inducing protective stepping responses to external perturbations of human standing. *J Neurophysiol.* 2003;90:666-674.

127. James B, Parker AW. Active and passive mobility of lower limb joints in elderly men and women. *Am J Phys Med Rehab.* 1987;68:735-740.

128. Araújo CG. Flexibility assessment: normative values for Flexitest from 5 to 91 years of age. [Article in English, Portuguese] *Arq Bras Cardiol.* 2008;90(4):257-263.

129. Woodhull-McNeal AP. Changes in posture and balance with age. *Aging Clin Exp Res.* 1992;4:219-225.

130. Sherrington C, Whitney JC, Lord SR, Herbert RD, Cumming RG, Close JC. Effective exercise for the prevention of falls: a systematic review and meta-analysis. *J Am Geriatr Soc.* 2008;56:2234-2243.

131. Lord SR. Visual risk factors for falls in older people. *Age Ageing.* 2006;35(Suppl 2): ii42-ii45.

132. Lopez I, Ishiyama G, Tang Y, Tokita J, Baloh RW, Ishiyama A. Regional estimates of hair cells and supporting cells in the human crista ampullaris. *J Neurosci Res.* 2005;82:421-431.

133. Park JJ, Tang Y, Lopez I, Ishiyama A. Age-related change in the number of neurons in the human vestibular ganglion. *J Comp Neurol.* 2001;431:437-443.

134. Ishiyama G. Imbalance and vertigo: the aging human vestibular periphery. *Semin Neurol.* 2009;29:491-499.

135. Benjuya N, Melzer I, Kaplanski J. Aging-induced shifts from a reliance on sensory input to muscle cocontraction during balanced standing. *J Gerontol A Biol Sci Med Sci.* 2004;59(2):166-171.

136. Shumway-Cook A, Woollacott MH. Motor Control: *Translating Research Into Clinical Practice.* 3rd ed. Philadelphia, PA: Lippincott Williams & Wilkins; 2006.

137. Rogers MW, Hedman LD, Johnson ME, Martinez KM, Mille ML. Triggering of protective stepping for the control of human balance: age and contextual dependence. *Brain Res Cogn Brain Res.* 2003;16:192-198.

138. Tang PF, Woollacott MH. Inefficient postural responses to unexpected slips during walking in older adults. *J Gerontol A Biol Sci Med Sci.* 1998;53(6):M471-M480.

139. Wishart LR, Lee TD, Murdoch JE, Hodges NJ. Effects of aging on automatic and effortful processes in bimanual coordination. *J Gerontol B Psychol Sci Soc Sci.* 2000;55(2):P85-P94.

140. Potvin AR, Syndulko K, Tourtellotte WW, Lemmon JA, Potvin JH. Human neurologic function and the aging process. *J Am Geriatr Soc.* 1980;28:1-9.

141. Desrosiers J, Hébert R, Bravo G, Rochette A. Age-related changes in upper extremity performance of elderly people: a longitudinal study. *Exp Gerontol.* 1999;34:393-405.

142. Judge JO, Ounpuu S, Davis RB. Effects of age on the biomechanics and physiology of gait. Clin Geriatr Med. 1996;12:659-678.

143. Himann JE, Cunningham DA, Rechnitzer PA, Paterson DH. Age-related changes in speed of walking. *Med Sci Sports Exerc.* 1988;20:161-166.

144. Shkuratova N, Morris ME, Huxham F. Effects of age on balance control during walking. *Arch Phys Med Rehabil.* 2004;85:582-588.

145. Hoxie RE, Rubenstein LZ. Are older pedestrians allowed enough time to cross intersections safely? *J Am Geriatr Soc.* 1994;42:241-244.

146. Guideline for the prevention of falls in older persons. American Geriatrics Society, British Geriatrics Society, and American Academy of Orthopaedic Surgeons Panel on Falls Prevention. *J Am Geriatr Soc.* 2001;49:664-672.

147. Pijnappels M, Bobbert MF, van Dieën JH. Push-off reactions in recovery after tripping discriminate young subjects, older non-fallers and older fallers. *Gait Posture.* 2005;21(4):388-394.

148. Menant JC, Steele JR, Menz HB, Munro BJ, Lord SR. Rapid gait termination: effects of age, walking surfaces and footwear characteristics. *Gait Posture.* 2009;30:65-70.

149. Priest AW, Salamon KB, Hollman JH. Age-related differences in dual task walking: a cross sectional study. *J Neuroeng Rehabil.* 2008;5:29.

150. Lord SR, Ward JA, Williams P, Anstey KJ. Physiological factors associated with falls in older community-dwelling women. *J Am Geriatr Soc.* 1994;42(10):1110-1117.

151. Duncan PW, Chandler J, Studenski S, Hughes M, Prescott B. How do physiological components of balance affect mobility in elderly men? *Arch Phys Med Rehabil.* 1993;74:1343-1349.

152. Buatois S, Gauchard GC, Aubry C, Benetos A, Perrin P. Current physical activity improves balance control during sensory conflicting conditions in older adults. *Int J Sports Med.* 2007;28:53-58.

153. Spirduso WW, MacRae HH, MacRae PG, Prewitt J, Osborne L. Exercise effects on aged motor function. *Ann N Y Acad Sci.* 1988;515:363-375.

154. Falduto LL, Baron A. Age-related effects of practice and task complexity on card sorting. *J Gerontol.* 1986;41:659-661.

155. Lord SR, Castell S. Physical activity program for older persons: effect on balance, strength, neuromuscular control, and reaction time. *Arch Phys Med Rehabil.* 1994;75:648-652.

156. Lord SR, Lloyd DG, Nirui M, Raymond J, Williams P, Stewart RA. The effect of exercise on gait patterns in older women: a randomized controlled trial. *J Gerontol A Biol Sci Med Sci.* 1996;51(2):M64-M70.

157. Gillespie LD, Gillespie WJ, Robertson MC, Lam SE, Cumming RG, Rowe BH. Interventions for preventing falls in elderly people. *Cochrane Database Syst Rev.* 2003;(4):CD000340.

158. Shumway-Cook A, Gruber W, Baldwin M, Liao S. The effect of multidimensional exercises on balance, mobility, and fall risk in community-dwelling older adults. *Phys Ther.* 1997;77:46-57.

CASE STUDY 3-1

Alison L. Squadrito, PT, DPT, GCS, CEEAA

EXAMINATION

History

Current Condition/Chief Complaint

Ms. Arbor was an 82-year-old White female referred to physical therapy by her primary care physician (PCP) because of increasing difficulty completing her instrumental activities of daily living (IADL).

Ms. Arbor stated she had been going out less frequently over the past 6 months because she was afraid she was going to fall (though she had not fallen yet) and because she became "winded" with community-level activities. Her main goal was to be confident and independent walking in the community and completing all of her IADL.

Social History/Environment

Ms. Arbor lived alone in senior housing and was a widow without children. She had a college education and worked as a secretary until age 65. Ms. Arbor moved into senior housing after her husband died because she did not want to manage a home by herself. She spent her time during the day watching TV, reading, and doing puzzles. She also enjoyed the building's activities, including weekly bingo and bridge games. Ms. Arbor had friends in the building, but their ability to help her was limited because of their own health problems.

Ms. Arbor lived in an apartment in an urban location. Her home was on the 6th floor with elevator access. There were no stairs to enter the building, but the building was on a slight hill. There was a curb to negotiate for vehicle access and a flight of stairs to get to the train stop outside her home.

Social/Health Habits

Ms. Arbor had a glass of wine with dinner several times per week. She had never smoked. Though she had never exercised regularly, she was very willing to begin an exercise program.

Medical/Surgical History

She reports mild osteoarthritis in both knees. Ms. Arbor uses glasses for reading.

Reported Functional Status

Ms. Arbor ambulated without an assistive device in her building and was independent with basic ADL without undue effort or fatigue. She was having more difficulty with community-level ambulation and IADL, however. She reported uncertainty when ambulating outdoors or in a crowded environment and found it increasingly difficult to carry grocery bags. She had begun buying frozen dinners and canned goods so that she would need to go to the store less frequently. Ms. Arbor stated that she was able to walk about one block and then felt too winded to continue without a rest. She had started taking a cab because she was afraid she would not get a seat on the train and would lose her balance when it moved.

Medications

Ms. Arbor reported taking acetaminophen approximately twice per week for knee pain. She takes no other prescription or over-the-counter medications.

Clinician Comment *During the interview, a great deal of information can be gathered that will help the clinician determine an accurate diagnosis, realistic prognosis, and optimal plan of care for a patient. The interview is a time to establish a rapport with the patient, which can influence the patient's experience and engagement in his or her treatment. Through careful questioning and active listening, the PT can gain insight into the patient's values, culture, perception of the problem, and goals, all of which need to be considered when developing a plan of care. If family is present, the dynamics of the relationship can be observed, which can be another influential factor in a patient's care. Knowledge of a patient's life roles, functional requirements, and environment will facilitate development of goals and a plan of care that will best meet the patient's needs. It is also important to understand the impact of a patient's social support system on his or her lifestyle. Lack of social support has been identified as a factor contributing to nursing home placement[1] and a major risk factor for increased morbidity.[2] In the absence of an adequate social network, Ms. Arbor may have been forced to make independent risky trips into the community, raising the likelihood of her falling. Alternatively, she may have chosen to stay home, limiting her ability to access supplies such as groceries and medication.*

The patient's report can help a provider accurately direct the physical examination and choose the most appropriate tests and measures. A directed examination can be less invasive and more efficient for the patient, saving both time and cost.[3] When questioned, Ms. Arbor identifies 2 problems that need to be investigated: fear of falling and shortness of breath.

Falling is a significant problem for older adults. It can have a tremendous effect on function and quality of life and, unfortunately, is an increasingly common problem in advancing age. One-third of individuals over the age of 65 years fall each year, a statistic that worsens with age to the point where 50% of those 85 years and older fall each year. More than 30% of those who fall sustain moderate or severe injuries.[4] After a fall, many older adults restrict their activity because of fear.[5] The resultant deconditioning can further increase a person's risk of falling. The ability to identify an older adult at risk of falling and intervene early presents a wonderful opportunity to preserve function and decrease disability in the individual's later years. Thus, it was very fortunate that Ms. Arbor's PCP referred her to physical therapy before she had fallen.

Many factors can increase fall risk, including impaired vision; decreased lower extremity strength, power, and endurance; poor balance and gait; and cognitive deficits.[6,7] Given Ms. Arbor's reported fear of falling, further testing in these areas was warranted. Ms. Arbor provided important information about balance and gait in her chief complaint. She reported difficulty when outdoors, in crowds, and while carrying bags. Because of these comments, I chose, among other testing, to examine her balance and gait in situations that provide reduced or inaccurate sensory input and/or require her to dual-task.

Ms. Arbor's complaint of shortness of breath with higher level functional activities also needed further evaluation. An examination of her pulmonary system (ie, respiratory rate [RR], breathing pattern, breath sounds, O_2 saturation) was indicated. In addition, her aerobic capacity needed to be measured to identify a possible impairment that may have limited her function.

Systems Review

Cardiovascular/Pulmonary

HR: 78 beats per minute (bpm)

RR: 12 seated at rest

BP: 136/86

Edema: no edema present

Integumentary

No skin disruption, normal skin color and pliability

Musculoskeletal

Gross Symmetry

Thoracic kyphosis in sitting and standing

Gross Range of Motion

Decreased shoulder elevation and ankle dorsiflexion

Gross Strength

Deferred gross testing since more thorough and careful testing of strength was indicated as well as for postural stability

Height/Weight

Height: 62 inches (5 feet, 2 inches)

Weight: 124 pounds (body mass index = 22.7)

Neuromuscular

Gait

Ms. Arbor was cautious with trunk/hip flexion. When asked questions as she walked from the waiting room to the examination room, she significantly slowed her gait speed or stopped to respond.

Locomotion

Independently transferred supine ↔ sit ↔ stand

Balance

No loss of balance during basic mobility skills observed as she walked in the clinic and transferred into and out of chairs and onto and off of the examination table

Motor Function

Decreased ability to control descent into a chair

Communication, Affect, Cognition, Learning Style

Ms. Arbor was oriented to person, place, and time. She engaged easily in conversation and followed all directions well. She was interested in the examination process and asked appropriate questions about the rationale and meaning of the tests performed. She reported some difficulty with memory that she attributed to "old age." She stated that it had never affected her function or safety (eg, forgetting to turn off the stove, missing appointments, not paying bills on time). She believed, however, that she would need written instructions to remember her exercise prescription and educational information.

Clinician Comment *The systems review is a brief, standard examination of all body systems to screen for movement system abnormalities and identify areas that need more specific testing. This information, combined with data collected during the interview, directs the clinician's choice of tests and measures.[8]*

Ms. Arbor's systems review revealed several areas of abnormality. Her BP was in the "prehypertension" range according to the American Heart Association (SBP = 120 to 139 or diastolic BP = 80 to 89), which significantly increases her risk of cardiovascular disease.[9] It was important that her BP was discussed, including the risks associated with the elevated value, the benefits of exercise to help lower it, and the need to work with her PCP to address it. In addition, close monitoring of her BP with exercise was needed.

Because osteoporosis becomes more common in older age, Ms. Arbor's thoracic kyphosis was concerning. It was reasonable to wonder if her loss of vertebral height might be due to compression fractures. Because of this and the impact of impaired posture on balance, further examination of her alignment was indicated. The other finding on her musculoskeletal screen that indicated the need for more testing was her limited shoulder and ankle ROM.

Ms. Arbor stopped walking when she engaged in conversation, which indicated a decreased ability to dual-task and suggested she was at an increased risk of falling.[10] This finding provided further evidence of the need to test her balance in dual-task conditions.

Ms. Arbor noted that she had some memory deficits. Because she did not have any family or friends with her, the reliability of the information she provided could not be determined as well as whether she accurately assessed that it did not affect her safety. Therefore, testing her cognition was indicated. A cognitive impairment would affect her ability to remember instructions and recommendations for her physical training, but, more important, it could prevent her from living safely and independently in the community.

Tests and Measures

Arousal, Attention, and Cognition

Saint Louis University Mental Status Examination (SLUMS) = 27/30[11]

Clinician Comment *The Mini-Mental State Examination (MMSE) is probably the most widely used instrument to screen for dementia. While it is able to identify individuals with dementia, it has been shown to have limited ability to detect mild levels of cognitive impairment, which was necessary in this case.[12] Tariq et al[11] developed the SLUMS to address this limitation. It is a 30-point scale that tests orientation, memory, attention, and executive function. In a comparison of the 2 scales, the MMSE and* the SLUMS were found to have similar ability to detect dementia. Tariq et al[11] conclude that the SLUMS is possibly better at detecting mild neurocognitive disorder, however. The investigators propose that Ms. Arbor's score indicates she had normal cognitive function, which was a reassuring finding.

Aerobic Capacity and Endurance

The 6MWT[13] = 285 meters or 935 feet without rest. Ms. Arbor complained of mild knee aching with ambulation. When asked what kept her from walking farther during the 6 minutes, Ms. Arbor said that she was afraid she would fall if she walked any faster. Her vital signs during the test were as follows:

ACTIVITY	BP	HR	RR	BORG DYSPNEA SCALE[14]
Baseline	136/86	78	12	0
End of test	164/90	106	18	3 (Moderate)
Recovery: 2 minutes	132/84	94	Not taken	0
Recovery: 5 minutes	120/84	80	12	0

Clinician Comment *The 6MWT was chosen to help identify the limitations to Ms. Arbor's community ambulation and to obtain a baseline measure of functional exercise capacity. Ms. Arbor's 6MWT performance was below normal for her age. In his meta-analysis, Bohannon[15] determined the normal 6MWT distance for an apparently healthy woman between the ages of 80 and 89 years to be 382 meters (95% confidence interval 316 to 449). Ms. Arbor's subjective and objective responses to the test helped to identify those factors that might explain her abnormal 6MWT result.*

Analysis of Ms. Arbor's hemodynamic response to activity suggested she was deconditioned. She demonstrated excessive HR and BP increases to the workload she performed. She walked at a speed of 1.8 miles per hour, which approximates a 2.4 metabolic equivalent (MET) activity and an increase in workload of around 1.4 METs compared to her resting state (if we estimate that to be 1 MET, recognizing there is variability in individuals' resting metabolic rates).[16,17] A normal response to exercise is a 10 ± 2 bpm rise in HR and a 10 ± 2 mm Hg rise in SBP per MET.[18] Thus, we can estimate a normal response to this 6MWT to be achievement of an HR of ~92 and an SBP of ~150. Ms. Arbor exceeded these values, suggesting she was in a deconditioned state, which is not surprising given she reported a sedentary lifestyle.

Ms. Arbor reported that, though she was working at approximately 70% of her HR_{max},[19] she was not limited by fatigue or dyspnea. Instead, she felt that her balance problems prevented her from walking faster. Thus, based on her subjective report, it appears that Ms. Arbor's fear of falling was the limiting factor in this test.

Gait, Locomotion, and Balance

- Activities-Specific Balance Confidence (ABC) scale[20-22] = 68% (out of 100%)
- Modified Clinical Test of Sensory Interaction and Balance (modified CTSIB)[23]
  - Condition 1 (firm surface, eyes open) = 30 seconds
  - Condition 2 (firm surface, eyes closed) = 18 seconds
  - Condition 3 (standing on foam, eyes open) = 16 seconds
  - Condition 4 (standing on foam, eyes closed) = immediate loss of balance; required assist to stay upright
- BBS[24,25] = 46/56, difficulty in situations that required a decreased base of support
  - 6-meter comfortable gait speed = 0.84 m/s
  - 6-meter fast gait speed = 1.0 m/s
  - 6-meter gait speed with cognitive task = 0.72 m/s

Ms. Arbor demonstrated decreased step length bilaterally and increasingly flexed posture as she continued walking. She was able to walk and carry a glass of water or a stack of sheets without increased gait deviation, but at a slowed speed. She had repeated lateral deviations in her gait path when walking with horizontal head turns. With light perturbations at her sternum or waist, she utilized a hip strategy to maintain her balance.

Clinician Comment *Ms. Arbor had a significant fear of falling, so the ABC Scale was chosen to quantify her perception of her postural control and functional ability. Her score demonstrated a substantial fear of falling and predicted only a moderate level of functioning.[22] Fear of falling and the perceived negative consequences of falling (ie, loss of functional independence and damage to identity) are correlated with the avoidance of activity.[26] If Ms. Arbor further decreased her activity level, she would have experienced declines in aerobic capacity, muscle performance, and motor control and would have been at an even greater risk of falling. It was hoped that, with a comprehensive physical therapy program, Ms. Arbor would feel more confident with her function and that would be reflected by an increase in this measure, which has been shown to change with rehabilitation intervention.[22]*

The modified CTSIB helped identify what sensory information Ms. Arbor used to maintain her balance while standing still. Ms. Arbor had difficulty in all of the situations that had reduced sensory input. These test results helped identify what activities might be challenging for her and also allowed more specific tailoring of her balance training. For example, Ms. Arbor was unable to safely stand still with her eyes closed, so she was questioned about her ability to stand and wash her hair in the shower. Because this ADL was risky for her, a shower chair was recommended so she could bathe in a more stable position. Ms. Arbor also demonstrated difficulty with dynamic balance in situations that had reduced sensory input, such as walking with head turns. Walking outside her home required Ms. Arbor to negotiate uneven pavement and crowds, situations that decrease the amount of accurate sensory information available. Therefore, training in situations of reduced sensory input was incorporated to address her deficits in these situations.

A cutoff of 45/56 on the BBS has frequently been used to identify if a person is at high risk of falling, but the use of this scale in a dichotomous manner is not appropriate. Muir et al[27] performed the first prospective study to determine the predictive validity of the BBS and found that this cut-off to identify individuals who were going to fall had poor sensitivity. There was some risk associated with all scores on the BBS. Shumway-Cook et al[28] also identified a gradient of risk in their study of the BBS. Based on the model these investigators developed, Ms. Arbor's score of 46, together with the fact that she had never fallen, suggested that she had a 26% chance of falling.

Though Ms. Arbor's gait speed was normal for her age,[29] it did impair her ability to cross the street easily. The stop light was not red long enough for her to reach the other side of the road before it changed back to green. Her speed slowed with the addition of a cognitive or manual task, indicating difficulty walking with confidence and stability in dual-task conditions. These examination results identified additional areas that needed to be addressed during physical therapy.

Ms. Arbor's posture became more flexed with ongoing ambulation, suggesting a muscle endurance impairment in her trunk and lower extremity extensors. This was an important impairment to identify because decreased muscle endurance is not an age-related change,[30,31] and is associated with falls in the elderly.[6,32,33]

Muscle Performance (Strength With Manual Muscle Test)[34]

- Right shoulder flexion and abduction 4/5, elbow flexion and extension 4/5
- Left shoulder flexion and abduction 4/5, elbow flexion and extension 4/5
- Right hip flexion 4/5, hip extension 4/5, hip abduction 3+/5, knee extension 4/5, knee flexion 4/5, dorsiflexion 4/5, plantarflexion 3/5
- Left hip flexion 4/5, hip extension 3+/5, hip abduction 3+/5, knee extension 4/5, knee flexion 4/5, dorsiflexion 4/5, plantarflexion 3/5

Clinician Comment *Ms. Arbor demonstrated impairments in muscle performance that certainly may have affected her functional abilities. Her lower extremity strength may have contributed to her decreased balance and gait speed. While she did not complain of any problems with activities that required upper extremity strength, it was important to include her arms in her resisted exercise program to improve the strength and physical reserve she had for ADL.*

Posture

Ms. Arbor had a fixed thoracic kyphosis. Her protracted scapulae and forward head were partially reversible.

Clinician Comment *Ms. Arbor was able to achieve a more upright posture with cues, indicating a habitual change in posture that could be improved with physical therapy. However, she also had structural changes in her thoracic spine, and there was concern that her abnormal posture might indicate thoracic compression fractures associated with osteoporosis. According to the National Osteoporosis Foundation, 55% of the people 50 years of age and older have osteoporosis.[35] It was suggested she follow up with her PCP about the possibility of having a bone density test and taking medication if appropriate. Back extensor strengthening exercises would improve her posture and decrease her risk of compression fractures.[36] A review of proper body mechanics and suggestions about how to perform ADL without forward bending would be useful for Ms. Arbor since spinal flexion has been shown to increase the risk of compression fractures.[37]*

Range of Motion

Normal ROM,[38-40] except right shoulder flexion = 112 degrees, left shoulder flexion = 118 degrees, bilateral dorsiflexion = 0 degrees, hip extension = 0 degrees, all with firm end feels. Ms. Arbor demonstrated decreased cervical and thoracic rotation bilaterally.

Clinician Comment *Mecagni et al[41] found correlations between total active-assisted ROM of the ankle and the Tinetti gait subscore. Beissner and colleagues[42] found lower extremity ROM was able to predict function as measured by the Physical Performance Test in older adults living in assisted living or skilled nursing facilities. Thus, there is support that Ms. Arbor's loss of lower extremity ROM might have contributed to her functional decline.*

Ms. Arbor's decreased spinal and upper extremity ROM was also affecting her function and postural control. Because of her loss of shoulder flexion and thoracic ROM, Ms. Arbor changed the way she reached for objects overhead. She demonstrated increased reliance on lumbar extension, which increased her risk of losing her balance posteriorly. In addition, because she did not have the shoulder flexion to reach high shelves, she sometimes climbed on a chair to retrieve objects. This was a risky activity that might have caused her to fall.

Sensory Integrity

Ms. Arbor shows intact sensation to light touch throughout and impaired joint position sense at the 4th toe, but intact at the ankle.

Clinician Comment *Ms. Arbor's proprioception was assessed by her ability to sense displacements of her 4th toe.[43] Grasping the digit on its sides, it was moved up and down and randomly stopped in one of these directions (ie, toe flexion or extension), then Ms. Arbor was asked which position her toe was in. Though it is widely used in clinical practice, no studies were located that have examined the reliability or validity of this test.*

This test was performed to identify an impairment that might be contributing to Ms. Arbor's postural instability. Knowing that she had decreased proprioceptive input led to consideration of situations that might be challenging for her. It was hypothesized that Ms. Arbor would be more reliant on her visual and vestibular senses for postural stability because of this loss. Consequently, she might be more likely to lose her balance in situations where information from these systems was reduced, such as walking in the dark. Because this impairment would not improve with physical therapy intervention, Ms. Arbor would have to compensate for it. Consideration was given to having her use a cane to provide sensory input through her upper extremity and stability in the most challenging situations, such as walking on uneven sidewalks with many pedestrians. Ms. Arbor understood the recommendation, but she feared it would make her look old and decided not to use a cane at that point.

Ventilation and Respiration/Gas Exchange

Ms. Arbor's breathing pattern showed no accessory muscle use at rest or with activity.

Her breath sounds included few inspiratory crackles (basal segments of bilateral lower lobes) that did not change with ambulation.

Blood O_2 saturation (SpO_2) = 92% to 93% at rest and with ambulation

Clinician's Comments *Given the age-related changes in the pulmonary system, these results are normal. There was no evidence of pulmonary pathology contributing to Ms. Arbor's dyspnea on exertion. Rather, it seemed that the speed at which Ms. Arbor walked on the 6MWT and in the community required energy expenditure at a*

level that resulted in slight shortness of breath. Ms. Arbor had a decline in her VO_{2max} due to her age as well as her sedentary lifestyle. As a result, the intensity of her walking may have caused her to work at a high enough percentage of her VO_{2max} that it caused her to experience dyspnea.

EVALUATION

Diagnosis

Practice Pattern

Ms. Arbor's subjective complaints and objective findings suggested 2 practice patterns:

1. **Primary Prevention/Risk Reduction for Loss of Balance and Falling**: Ms. Arbor's major complaint was a fear of falling. Her examination confirmed that she was at risk of falling and identified multiple impairments that contributed to her postural instability, including balance, muscle performance, posture, ROM, and sensation. Of primary importance was establishing a comprehensive program to minimize her risk of falling.

2. **Impaired Aerobic Capacity/Endurance Associated With Deconditioning**: As identified on her 6MWT, Ms. Arbor also had an aerobic capacity impairment that needed to be addressed. While this was not as urgent a safety issue as her fall risk, it was affecting Ms. Arbor's function and was important to address with an independent aerobic conditioning program.

International Classification of Functioning, Disability and Health Model of Disability

See ICF Model on page 128.

Prognosis

Research has shown exercise, balance, and gait training to be effective interventions to reduce the risk of falling.[44-46] This evidence, combined with the fact that Ms. Arbor had few comorbidities and excellent motivation, led me to believe that she would reduce her risk of falls and improve her confidence with community activities with a comprehensive physical therapy program. Though Ms. Arbor had several impairments that could not be changed (eg, fixed kyphosis, proprioceptive loss), she also had the potential to improve others with exercise (eg, strength, ROM). In addition to exercise and balance training to address her physical performance, I chose to explore community resources with Ms. Arbor. Because of the environmental challenges in her community, such as hills and busy urban streets, I felt Ms. Arbor might need to modify her methods for completing IADL. For this reason, I believed it was important to provide her information on programs and services in her area that could help her remain independent.

ICF MODEL OF DISABLEMENT FOR MS. ARBOR

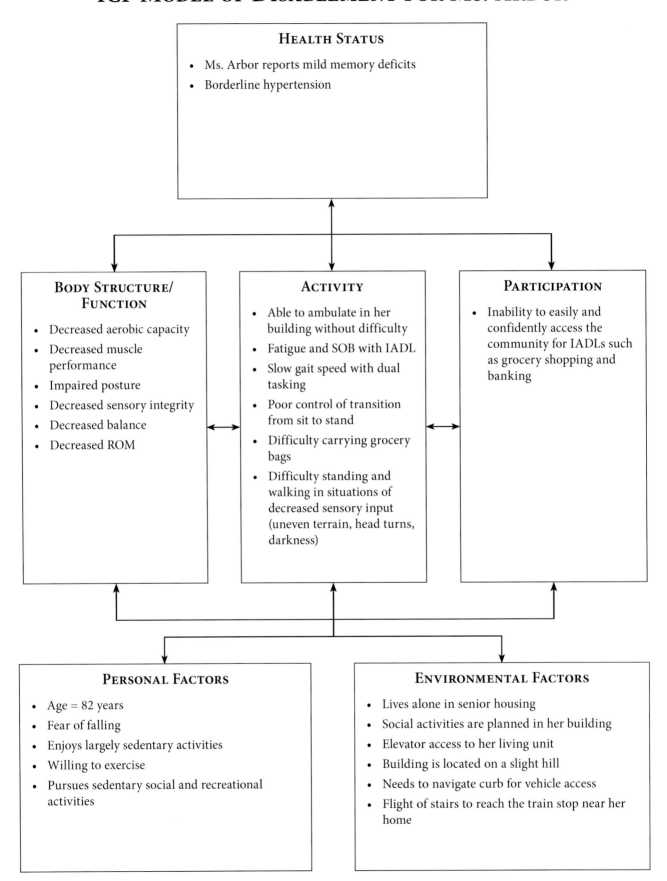

HEALTH STATUS

- Ms. Arbor reports mild memory deficits
- Borderline hypertension

BODY STRUCTURE/ FUNCTION

- Decreased aerobic capacity
- Decreased muscle performance
- Impaired posture
- Decreased sensory integrity
- Decreased balance
- Decreased ROM

ACTIVITY

- Able to ambulate in her building without difficulty
- Fatigue and SOB with IADL
- Slow gait speed with dual tasking
- Poor control of transition from sit to stand
- Difficulty carrying grocery bags
- Difficulty standing and walking in situations of decreased sensory input (uneven terrain, head turns, darkness)

PARTICIPATION

- Inability to easily and confidently access the community for IADLs such as grocery shopping and banking

PERSONAL FACTORS

- Age = 82 years
- Fear of falling
- Enjoys largely sedentary activities
- Willing to exercise
- Pursues sedentary social and recreational activities

ENVIRONMENTAL FACTORS

- Lives alone in senior housing
- Social activities are planned in her building
- Elevator access to her living unit
- Building is located on a slight hill
- Needs to navigate curb for vehicle access
- Flight of stairs to reach the train stop near her home

Plan of Care

Intervention

Therapeutic exercise to address muscle performance, aerobic capacity, flexibility, balance and gait training, and patient education, all as detailed below.

Proposed Frequency and Duration of Physical Therapy Visits

Twelve visits over the course of 6 weeks: 3 times per week for 2 weeks, 2 times per week for 2 weeks, and then 1 time per week for 2 weeks with a final check-in over the phone 1 month after that.

Anticipated Goals

- Patient will be independent with a comprehensive home exercise program with written instructions designed to improve her aerobic capacity, balance, muscle performance, and flexibility so that she may perform her IADL with greater ease and safety (1 week to learn her initial program and ongoing as her exercise prescription was progressed.)
- Patient will demonstrate understanding of community resources available to her to allow her to remain living independently in the community (eg, community transportation options for older adults, grocery delivery, Elder Services) (2 weeks).
- Patient will demonstrate improved functional mobility and aerobic capacity on her 6MWT to allow her to perform IADL with greater ease and less shortness of breath.
- Patient will have improved balance to increase safety with ADL as evidenced by a BBS score ≥ 51/56 (6 weeks).
- Patient will have a fast gait speed of 1.3 m/s to allow her to cross the street safely before the light changes (4 weeks).
- Patient will ambulate at ≥ 0.85 m/s while performing a cognitive task to demonstrate improved ability to function in dual-task situations (4 weeks).
- Patient will have decreased fear of falling as evidenced by an ABC Scale score of 80% (4 weeks).

Expected Outcomes (10 Weeks)

- Patient will be able to complete 2 trips per outing into the community (eg, bank and post office) to complete IADL without complaints of fear of falling or shortness of breath.
- Patient will be able to use the public car service for older adults to go to the grocery store and will walk in the crowded environment while carrying groceries without fear of falling.

Discharge Plan

Ms. Arbor will be discharged from physical therapy with a home exercise program to continue on her own indefinitely.

INTERVENTION

Coordination, Communication, and Documentation

The initial examination findings and plan of care were sent to Ms. Arbor's PCP. In particular, her prehypertensive BP and thoracic kyphosis were noted so that the doctor was aware of the abnormal findings that might require further medical testing and pharmacological treatment.

Patient-/Client-Related Instruction

- Benefits of seeing an eye doctor yearly to ensure an up-to-date eyewear prescription
- Available community resources to assist with IADL: community car service for older adults, grocery delivery, Elder Services, homemaker agencies
- Home modification to improve safety: increase lighting, pick up throw rugs, minimize clutter, obtain night lights, install grab bars in the bathroom
- Strategies to consider to improve safety: allow time for visual accommodation when transitioning from areas with different brightness/lighting, wear sturdy, wide-soled shoes with good tread,[47] do not get up if the train is still moving, have cordless phone with her in the house to avoid rushing to answer the phone
- Body mechanics focused on decreasing spinal flexion
- Benefits of exercise and instruction in an exercise program to continue indefinitely

Procedural Interventions

Therapeutic Exercise

Strength and Power Training

Mode

Strength and power training with body weight, elastic bands, and hand weights for resistance

Intensity

One set of each of the exercises at the following intensities:

- Week 1: ~40% to 60% 1-RM to ensure Ms. Arbor learned proper technique before increasing to the intensity needed for maximum strength gains. Ms. Arbor did not perform 1-RM testing to prescribe the intensity of her exercise program. Instead, her intensity was estimated by having her perform higher numbers of repetitions to fatigue. For example, Ms. Arbor performed wall slides to a depth that caused her to have muscle fatigue and an inability to continue after ~15 to 20 reps, which equates to < 60% 1-RM.[18]

- Week 2: continue at 40% to 60% 1-RM.

- Week 3: increase to 60% to 80% 1-RM. Her intensity was progressed by having her bend her knees further and hold the contraction longer. She performed the exercise in a manner that allowed her to complete ~8 to 12 reps before fatigue, which equates to 60% to 80% 1-RM, the intensity of the exercise desired to maximize her strength gains safely.[18,48]

- Week 4: maintain 60% to 80 % 1-RM for strength training. Add power training at 30% to 60% 1-RM.

- Weeks 5 and 6: as described previously, adjusting the difficulty of the exercises as needed to maintain the desired training intensity.

Duration

Three seconds both for concentric and eccentric contractions for strength training. One second for concentric contraction and 3-second eccentric contraction for power training.

Frequency

Twice per week

Description of the Intervention

- Wall slides: This exercise worked on Ms. Arbor's lower extremity extensor muscle strength, which was important for functional activities such as sit-to-stand transfers and negotiation of curbs. Wall slides allowed her to work on closed-chain, eccentric contractions as used during stand-to-sit transfers, a skill that was difficult for Ms. Arbor to perform with control.

- Standing toe/heel raises: I chose this exercise because ankle muscle strength contributes to balance and gait. Ms. Arbor was instructed to hold very lightly onto a counter or the back of a chair for support as she performed the exercise. By minimizing the amount of upper extremity support she used, this exercise also provided some challenge to her balance. Initially, she was not able to lift her foot off of the floor during the toe raise portion of this exercise because of her decreased dorsiflexion ROM. The exercise was therefore performed with an isometric contraction of her dorsiflexors.

- Bridging: To improve hip extensor and trunk strength, Ms. Arbor performed bridging. When she was able to perform 12 repetitions with good form and controlled, smooth contractions, she progressed to doing single-leg bridges.

- Side lunges: In the clinic, Ms. Arbor performed side stepping with an elastic band around her ankles. As she had difficulty getting a band around her ankles independently, she modified this exercise when doing it at home. She performed hip abduction in sitting with an elastic band around her thighs.

- Seated rowing with resistance from an elastic band: This exercise focused on the recruitment and strength of Ms. Arbor's thoracic extensors. While seated, Ms. Arbor pulled back on an elastic band and held a position of scapular retraction. She progressed by increasing the resistance of the band and the duration that she held the position, and then by performing the exercise in a standing position. This change provided greater challenge to her balance and recruited more back and lower extremity muscles to stabilize her in standing. She was instructed to ensure full retraction so that she also stretched her anterior chest wall with the exercise.

- Elbow flexion and shoulder flexion exercises with hand-held weights

Flexibility Exercises

Mode

Body position and light weight

Intensity

Slow progressive stretch to tolerance using either body or lightweight resistance

Duration

3 repetitions with 60-second hold

Frequency

Twice per week

Description of the Intervention

- Gastroc-soleus and hip flexor stretch while leaning forward against the wall with her spine in neutral. Because a 60-second stretch has been shown to be more effective than a 30-second stretch to gain muscle length in older adults,[49] Ms. Arbor was instructed to hold the stretch initially for as long as tolerated, with the goal of increasing this time to 1 minute.

- Supine shoulder flexion stretch: In supine, Ms. Arbor raised her arms above her head and slowly stretched them back toward the bed. After she was comfortable with holding this position, she held a can of soup to provide a slightly stronger stretch.

Aerobic Capacity Training

Mode

Interval walking

Intensity

5 to 6 on a 0-to-10 scale, where 0 is equivalent to sitting and 10 is all-out effort[50]

Duration

A total of 30 minutes per day, in bouts of at least 10 minutes each

Frequency

At least 5 times per week

Description of the Intervention

She initially walked for 10 minutes, 3 times per day. She progressed to walking for 15 minutes at a time twice per day and eventually to one continuous 30-minute walk.

Clinician Comment *While Ms. Arbor's 6MWT distance ultimately may have been limited by her fear of falling with fast-paced walking, she did achieve a HR that was 70% of her age-predicted HR_{max}, which was an adequate intensity for aerobic capacity training.*

Since she had never exercised before, it was safest for her to begin at a moderate intensity. We had determined that she could safely manage this workload during her exercise test. The ACSM has defined moderate intensity as 5 to 6 on a 0-to-10 scale that they recommend for use with older adults.[50] Ms. Arbor used this as a guideline.

Balance and Gait Training

Mode

Static and dynamic balance activities and gait training with progressively harder challenges

Intensity

Complexity and difficulty of activities progressed based on performance to continue to provide significant challenge to her balance

Duration

Twenty minutes performed during her first 10 physical therapy sessions

Frequency

3 times per week for 2 weeks, then 2 times per week for 2 weeks

Description of the Intervention

The balance and gait program initially included the following:

- Static stance with a narrow base of support, performed with eyes open and eyes closed
- Static stance on foam with eyes open and eyes closed
- Semi-tandem stance with head still and with horizontal and vertical head turns
- Walking with a narrow base of support
- Stance while withstanding external nudges provided at the sternum and hips from all directions

Program progression included activities such as the following:

- Standing and reaching for objects at all heights (including from the floor) and in all directions
- Standing while throwing and catching a ball
- Walking and counting backwards by 3s
- Walking while carrying a glass of water
- Walking with changing speed
- Walking in dim light and from bright to dark and dark to bright spaces
- Walking with horizontal and vertical head turns

Final progression of activities included the following:

- Walking around and over obstacles without a secondary task, while carrying an object, and while performing basic arithmetic
- Carrying objects while walking on uneven surfaces and while carrying weights
- Walking quickly with head turns
- Walking while carrying an object and naming categories of objects (eg, words that begin with the letter "z")
- All activities performed in a complex environment (eg, with people walking by)
- Stair climbing with and without the railing

Clinician Comment *Ms. Arbor's balance program was designed to challenge her with tasks and situations that were difficult for her during her examination, such as balancing on a narrow base of support, walking in dual-task situations, managing situations of reduced sensory input, and walking at a fast speed. Consideration was also given to reported difficulties like negotiation of uneven outdoor surfaces and management of crowded environments. The program initially incorporated more static activities performed without a secondary task and in simple environments. It was progressed by including more dynamic activities, adding cognitive and motor tasks to perform during the balance activities, and eventually increasing the complexity of the environment. Activities were included that required Ms. Arbor to perform more than one task at once, as it has been shown that dual-task ability does not improve with single-task training.[51]*

REEXAMINATION

Subjective

Ms. Arbor reported that she was able to walk with less fear in the grocery store when she was carrying food and managing crowded aisles. She had applied for the senior transportation service and was waiting for approval. She was very excited with her progress.

Objective

Aerobic Capacity

6MWT = 307 meters with a hemodynamic response and dyspnea level similar to that seen on her initial examination. She felt that she could not cover more ground during the 6 minutes because of dyspnea on exertion.

Gait, Locomotion, and Balance

- ABC = 80%
- BBS = 52/56 m, which suggests a fall risk of 7.3%
- Comfortable gait speed = 1.02 m/s
- Fast gait speed = 1.15 m/s
- Gait speed with cognitive task = 0.90 m/s

Range of Motion

- Right shoulder flexion = 138 degrees; left shoulder flexion = 136 degrees

- Right ankle dorsiflexion = 10 degrees; left dorsiflexion = 12 degrees
- Hip extension = 10 degrees bilaterally

Clinician Comment *Ms. Arbor made good progress with physical therapy intervention, demonstrating gains in all areas. Her gains exceeded the minimal detectable change (the minimum amount of change that is not due to measurement error) for those tests with established values (ie, 6MWT, BBS, and gait speed).*[51,52] *This allowed confidence that the improvement in her scores was a true change from her physical therapy intervention and not due to error.*

Assessment

Ms. Arbor's balance, gait, and fear of falling had improved significantly and she was accessing the community more frequently than at the time of initial evaluation. She felt her ability to perform IADL easily was now limited by her fatigue and shortness of breath, despite improvement in her aerobic capacity (as evidenced by her increased 6MWT distance).

Clinician Comment *Her ability to complete her aerobic capacity training at the suggested frequency was dependent on the weather and had been limited because of a great deal of rain. Options were discussed that would help her perform consistent endurance training despite inclement weather. Once she had been approved for the senior transportation service, she would have the ability to get a ride to the mall to complete her walking program there.*

This solution had problems, however, in that she felt she would not go out in the winter weather at all, even if she had to walk only to the car at the sidewalk, because she was afraid she might slip on the ice. In our area, the driver of the transportation service will assist the older adult to the car, so Ms. Arbor said she would consider a trip out once she saw how the service operated. A program on a bike or seated peddler was offered. She declined this offer, as she believed the machine would take up too much room in her small apartment and that she wouldn't enjoy it. Ms. Arbor recognized the benefits of her exercise program and she was very willing to continue it long term. It was understood that the weather, however, might be a limiting factor to completion of aerobic training at the optimal frequency.

Plan

Two sessions were planned to progress her home exercise prescription and ensure she had a good program to follow after discharge from physical therapy.

OUTCOMES

Discharge

At the end of 10 weeks, Ms. Arbor had made clinically significant gains and had met all of the established program goals. She increased her community mobility and overall level of activity. In addition, she had identified community resources she could rely on to help her with her IADL, allowing her to avoid difficult and potentially risky trips into the community that might cause her to fall. Another important outcome was that Ms. Arbor had become a regular exerciser and planned to continue her home exercise program for the rest of her life with the goal of maximizing her function and quality of life as she aged.

REFERENCES

1. Guccione AA. Implications of an aging population for rehabilitation: demography, mortality, and morbidity in the elderly. In: Guccione AA, ed. *Geriatric Physical Therapy.* 2nd ed. St. Louis, MO: Mosby Inc; 2000:5.
2. House JS, Landis, KR, Umberson D. Social relationships and health. *Science.* 1988;241:540-544.
3. Flegel KM. Does the physical examination have a future? *CMAJ.* 1999;161(9):1117-1118.
4. Centers for Disease Control and Prevention. Falls among older adults: an overview. *Home & Recreational Safety.* http://www.cdc.gov/homeandrecreationalsafety/falls/adultfalls.html. Accessed April 30, 2014.
5. Vellas BJ, Wayne SJ, Romero LJ, Baumgartner RN, Garry PJ. Fear of falling and restriction of mobility in elderly fallers. *Age Ageing.* 1997;26(3):189-193.
6. Schwendner KI, Mikesky AE, Holt WS Jr, Peacock M, Burr DB, Differences in muscle endurance and recovery between fallers and nonfallers, and between young and older women. *J Gerontol A Biol Sci Med Sci.* 1997;52: M155-M160.
7. Guideline for the prevention of falls in older persons. American Geriatrics Society, British Geriatrics Society, and American Academy of Orthopaedic Surgeons Panel on Falls Prevention. *J Am Geriatr Soc.* 2001;49:664-672.
8. American Physical Therapy Association. Guide to physical therapist practice. Second edition. American Physical Therapy Association. *Phys Ther.* 2001;81(1):9-746.
9. Chobanian AV, Bakris GL, Black HR, et al. The Seventh Report of the Joint National Committee on Prevention, Detection, Evaluation, and Treatment of High Blood Pressure: the JNC 7 report. *JAMA.* 2003;289(19):2560-2572.
10. Lundin-Olsson L, Nyberg L, Gustafson Y. "Stops walking when talking" as a predictor of falls in elderly people. *Lancet.* 1997;349(9052):617.
11. Tariq SH, Tumosa N, Chibnall JT, Perry MH 3rd, Morley JE. Comparison of the Saint Louis University Mental Status Examination and the Mini Mental State Examination for detecting dementia and mild neurocognitive disorder—a pilot study. *Am J Geriatr Psychiatry.* 2006;14:900-910.
12. Malloy, PF, Cummings JL, Coffey CE, et al. Cognitive screening instruments in neuropsychiatry: a report of the committee on research of the American Neuropsychiatric Association. *J Neuropsychiatry Clin Neurosci.* 1997;9(2):189-197.
13. ATS Committee on Proficiency Standards for Clinical Pulmonary Function Laboratories. ATS Statement: guidelines for the Six-Minute Walk test. *Am J Respir Crit Care Med.* 2002;166:111-117.

14. Wilson RC, Jones PW. Long-term reproducibility of Borg scale estimates of breathlessness during exercise. *Clin Sci.* 1991;80:309-312.

15. Bohannon RW. Six-Minute Walk test: a meta-analysis of data from apparently healthy elders. *Topics Geriatr Rehabil.* 2007;23:155-160.

16. Ainsworth BE, Haskell WL, Whitt MC. Compendium of physical activities: an update of activity codes and MET intensities. *Med Sci Sports Exer.* 2000;32(9 Suppl):S498-S504.

17. ExRx.net. Walk/Run Metabolic Calculator. http://www.exrx.net/Calculators/WalkRunMETs.html. Accessed April 30, 2014.

18. American College of Sports Medicine. *ACSM's Guidelines for Exercise Testing and Prescription.* 8th ed. Baltimore, MD: Lippincott, Williams &Wilkins; 2009.

19. Tanaka H, Monahan KD, Seals DR. Age-predicted maximal heart rate revisited. *J Am Coll Cardiol.* 2001;37:153-156.

20. Powell LE, Myers AM. The Activities-Specific Balance Confidence (ABC) Scale. *J Gerontol A Biol Sci Med Sci.* 1995;50:M28-M34.

21. Myers AM, Powell LE, Maki BE, Holliday PJ, Brawley LR, Sherk W. Psychological indicators of balance confidence: relationship to actual and perceived abilities. *J Gerontol A Biol Sci Med Sci.* 1996;51:M37-M43.

22. Myers AM, Fletcher PC, Myers AH, Sherk W. Discriminative and evaluative properties of the Activities-Specific Balance Confidence (ABC) Scale. *J Gerontol A Biol Sci Med Sci.* 1998;53:M287-M294.

23. Cohen H, Blatchly CA, Gombash LL. A study of the Clinical Test of Sensory Interaction and Balance. *Phys Ther.* 1993;73:346-354.

24. Berg KO, Wood-Dauphinee SL, Williams JI, Maki B. Measuring balance in the elderly: validation of an instrument. *Can J Public Health.* 1992;83(Suppl 2):S7-S11.

25. Berg KO, Wood-Dauphinee SL, Williams JI, Gayton D. Measuring balance in the elderly: preliminary development of an instrument. *Physiother Can.* 1989;41:304-311.

26. Yardley L, Smith H. A prospective study of the relationship between feared consequences of falling and avoidance of activity in community-living older people. *Gerontologist.* 2002;42(1):17-23.

27. Muir SW, Berg K, Chesworth B, Speechley M. Use of the Berg Balance Scale for predicting multiple falls in community-dwelling elderly people: a prospective study. *Phys Ther.* 2008;88(4):449-459.

28. Shumway-Cook A, Baldwin M, Polissar NL, Guber W. Predicting the probability of falls in community-dwelling older adults. *Phys Ther.* 1997;77:576-585.

29. Bohannon RW. Population representative gait speed and its determinants. *J Geriatr Phys Ther.* 2008;31(2):49-52.

30. Lynch NA, Metter EJ, Lindle RS, et al. Muscle quality. I. Age-associated differences between arm and leg muscle groups. *J Appl Physiol* (1985). 1999;86:188-194.

31. Trappe S, Williamson D, Godard M, Porter D, Rowden G, Costill D. Effect of resistance training on single muscle fiber contractile function in older men. *J Appl Physiol* (1985). 2000;89:143-152.

32. Lindström B, Lexell J, Gerdle B, Downham D. Skeletal muscle fatigue and endurance in young and old men and women. *J Gerontol Biol Sci Med Sci.* 1997;52:B59-B66.

33. Bäckman E, Johansson V, Häger B, Sjöblom P, Henriksson KG. Isometric muscle strength and muscular endurance in normal persons aged between 17 and 70 years. *Scan J Rehabil Med.* 1995;27:109-117.

34. Hislop HJ, Montgomery J. *Daniels and Worthingham's Muscle Testing.* 7th ed. Philadelphia, PA: W.B. Saunders Company; 2002.

35. National Osteoporosis Foundation. http://www.nof.org/osteoporosis/diseasefacts.htm#riskfactors. Accessed July 2010.

36. Sinaki M, Itoi E, Wahner HW, et al. Stronger back muscles reduce the incidence of vertebral fractures: a prospective 10 year follow-up of postmenopausal women. *Bone.* 2002;30(6):836-841.

37. Sinaki M, Mikkelsen BA. Postmenopausal spinal osteoporosis: flexion versus extension exercises. *Arch Phys Med Rehabil.* 1984;65(10):593-596.

38. James B, Parker AW. Active and passive mobility of lower limb joints in elderly men and women. *Am J Phys Med Rehabil.* 1989;68:162-167.

39. Chakravarty K, Webley M. Shoulder joint movement and its relationship to disability in the elderly. *J Rheumatol.* 1993;20:1359-1361.

40. Roach KE, Miles TP. Normal hip and knee active range of motion: the relationship to age. *Phys Ther.* 1991;71:656-665.

41. Mecagni C, Smith JP, Roberts KE, O'Sullivan SB. Balance and ankle range of motion in community-dwelling women aged 64-87 years: a correlational study. *Phys Ther.* 2000;80:1004-1011.

42. Beissner KL, Collins JE, Holmes H. Muscle force and range of motion as predictors of function in older adults. *Phys Ther.* 2000;80:556-563.

43. DeMeyer WE. *Technique of the Neurologic Examination: A Programmed Text.* 5th ed. McGraw-Hill Companies Inc; 2004.

44. Gillespie LD, Gillespie WJ, Robertson MC, Lam SE, Cumming RG, Rowe BH. Interventions for preventing falls in elderly people. *Cochrane Database Syst Rev.* 2003;(4):CD000340.

45. Shumway-Cook A, Gruber W, Baldwin M, Liao S. The effect of multidimensional exercises on balance, mobility, and fall risk in community-dwelling older adults. *Phys Ther.* 1997;77:46-57.

46. Sherrington C, Whitney JC, Lord SR, Herbert RD, Cumming RG, Close JC. Effective exercise for the prevention of falls: a systematic review and meta-analysis. *J Am Geriatr Soc.* 2008;56:2234-2243.

47. Menant JC, Steele JR, Menz HB, Munro BJ, Lord SR. Rapid gait termination: effects of age, walking surfaces and footwear characteristics. *Gait Posture.* 2009;30:65-70.

48. Avers D, Brown M. White paper: strength training for the older adult. *J Geriatr Phys Ther.* 2009;32:148-152.

49. Feland JB, Myrer JW, Schulthies SS, Fellingham GW, Measom GW. The effect of duration of stretching of the hamstring muscle group for increasing range of motion in people aged 65 years or older. *Phys Ther.* 2001;81:1100-1117.

50. Chodzko-Zajko WJ, Proctor DN, Fiatarone MA, et al. ACSM position stand: exercise and physical activity for older adults. *Med Sci Sports Exerc.* 2009;41(7):1510-1530.

51. Silsupadol P, Shumway-Cook A, Lugade V, et al. Effects of single-task versus dual-task training on balance performance in older adults: a double-blind, randomized controlled trial. *Arch Phys Med Rehabil.* 2009;90(3):381-387.

52. Perera S, Mody SH, Woodman RC, Studenski SA. Meaningful change and responsiveness in common physical performance measures in older adults. *J Am Geriatr* Soc. 2006;54:743-749.

SECTION II

PATHOPHYSIOLOGY OF DECONDITIONING AND PHYSIOLOGY OF TRAINING

4

Fatigue and Deconditioning

LeeAnne Carrothers, PT, PhD

CHAPTER OBJECTIVES

- Compare and contrast the contribution(s) of anxiety and depression to fatigue.

- Discuss the effects of lifestyle and habits on sleep and fatigue.

- List changes in the cardiovascular, respiratory, and musculoskeletal systems associated with bed rest and how those changes affect response to upright positioning and exercise after cessation of bed rest.

- Describe the effects of systemic illness on the perception of fatigue and tolerance to activity.

- Discuss the energy costs associated with living with a disability and how living long term with a disability increases risk for fatigue.

- Identify objective indicators of deconditioning during examination of patients at rest and in response to activity.

- Distinguish between a normal response to exercise and one that indicates that the patient is deconditioned, and make appropriate modifications to the exercise prescription.

CHAPTER OUTLINES

- Fatigue
  - Psychological Causes
    - Depressive Disorders
      - System Changes With Depression That Lead to Fatigue
        - Cortisol
        - Thyroid Function

- Growth Hormone Levels
- Sleep Cycles
  - Assessing Depression
    - History and Interview
    - Screening Tools
    - Common Presenting Signs
  - Anxiety Disorders
    - Biological Events With Anxiety Disorders
    - Common Presenting Symptoms
  - Substance Abuse
  - Lifestyle Issues Associated with Fatigue
    - Sleep Habits/Hygiene
  - Summary of Fatigue
  - Fatigue Associated With Deconditioning
    - Bed Rest, Zero Gravity, and Head-Down Bed Rest Research
      - Cardiovascular Changes
        - Fluid Balance
        - Loss of Red Blood Cell Mass
        - Cardiovascular Pump Changes
        - Alterations in Oxygen Uptake
      - Musculoskeletal Changes
  - Other Physiological Causes of Fatigue
    - Endocrine System
      - Hypoglycemia
      - Infection and Inflammation
      - Stress
      - Thyroid Disorders
    - Anemia

Coglianese D, ed. *Clinical Exercise Pathophysiology for Physical Therapy: Examination, Testing, and Exercise Prescription for Movement-Related Disorders (pp 137-163).*

- Malnutrition
- Cancer
- Respiratory Distress
- Renal Failure
- Chronic Obstructive Pulmonary Disease
- Aging With a Disability

FATIGUE

Fatigue is a commonly presenting subjective complaint in primary care and community settings, with early studies reporting an adult prevalence of fatigue ranging from 6.7% to 33%, depending on whether the survey was conducted in primary care or community settings.[1-5] It may account for as many as 7 million visits to primary care providers per year in the United States.[6] A 2007 telephone study of nearly 29,000 US adults reported a fatigue prevalence of 37.9% in the 2 weeks preceding the study, accounting for a $136.4 billion loss of productive time.[7] Further, the researchers reported higher rates of fatigue for workers who were female, younger than 50 years old, White (vs Black) and in well-paid jobs with decision-making responsibilities.[7]

Defining fatigue can be difficult because of the variety of nonspecific symptoms experienced by those who struggle with it. Components of fatigue may include difficulty initiating or maintaining previously tolerated activities, feelings of exhaustion associated with usual activities, and/or mental fatigue that manifests itself as difficulty with concentration and memory.[8,9] Evans and Lambert, in their 2007 review of the physiological basis of fatigue, used the definition: "physical and/or mental weariness resulting from exertion, that is, an inability to continue exercise at the same intensity with a resultant deterioration in performance."[10] Other components of fatigue may include weakness, dyspnea, lethargy, and somnolence, though these may simply be symptoms associated with fatigue.

Discerning the causes of fatigue can be daunting, as many conditions share fatigue as a principal symptom. To better understand the patient's complaints of fatigue, the clinician needs to consider the potential psychologic, lifestyle, and physical contributors. What follows is a description of these causes and the mechanisms by which each contributes to fatigue.

Psychological Causes

Depressive Disorders

A 2008 study reported on the prevalence of depression in the United States during the year 2006 based on answers given by nearly 200,000 respondents to the Behavioral Risk Factor Surveillance Survey.[11] The weighted prevalence of lifetime experience of depressive disorder was nearly 16% among respondents aged 18 years or older. Female prevalence was 20.6%, which was approximately twice as high as the prevalence found among males (11%). Based on the results of this study, the authors hypothesized that from the year 2005 to 2050, the total number of US adults with depressive disorder will increase from 33.9 million to 45.8 million, representing a 35% increase. The increase is projected to be greater in the elderly population aged 65 years than in the young population aged <65 years.[12]

Approximately 80% of individuals with depression suffer from sleep abnormalities, ranging from insomnia (most common, with late insomnia or early-morning awakenings being most prevalent) to the less common hypersomnia.[13] Fatigue may be both a symptom of depression and a prognostic indicator. Addington and colleagues, in a 13-year study of community-dwelling adults, found that individuals who reported unexplained fatigue at baseline and follow-up were at significantly increased risk for the development of major depression when compared with those who had no such complaints of fatigue.[14]

Although the exact etiology of depression is still largely unknown, abnormalities in effective use of the neurotransmitters norepinephrine, dopamine, and serotonin in depression are well documented. Decreased levels of these stimulatory neurotransmitters or inability to effectively use available adrenergic neurotransmitters are likely, or at least partially, responsible for the fatigue symptoms associated with depression. Theories about the role of biogenic amines in depression have been generated, in part, from the observation that patients who took monoamine-oxidase inhibitors and tricyclic antidepressants demonstrated increased norepinephrine and serotonin at central adrenergic receptor sites in the limbic system and hypothalamus. Further, since depression-provoking drugs (such as Reserpine) deplete biogenic amines at these sites, it was proposed that naturally occurring depressions might be associated with a deficiency of these substances.[15] According to Nutt,[16] dopamine in particular may be important in the formation of learned pleasurable outcomes. When presented with "normal social interactions," individuals with depression do not experience the typical sense of reward from social interactions, as evidenced by dopamine deficiency in the nucleus accumbens.[17] Further, the relative deficiency of dopamine may be due to chronic stress, which "burns out" dopamine terminals in the prefrontal cortex.[16]

System Changes With Depression That Lead to Fatigue

Cortisol

Cortisol, commonly referred to as the *stress hormone*, may play an important role in the clinical manifestations of depression. Transient exposure to increased levels of cortisol/glucocorticoids plays an important role in the "fight or flight" response and is responsible for such cognitive and emotional functions as regulating energy levels, attention, and cognition. Chronic overexposure to cortisol (whether due to endogenous or exogenous exposure), however, causes many undesired responses, including detrimental effects on arousal, attention, and memory.[18]

According to Thompson and Craighead, altered cortisol secretion can be found in up to 80% of individuals with depression.[19] Individuals with elevated cortisol levels experience depressive symptomatology and dysphoria (a state of feeling "bad or unhappy"), and a tendency to form sad interpretations of events when compared to their nondepressed peers.[18] Individuals with depression further experience alterations in the hypothalamic-pituitary-adrenal (HPA) axis, which leads to stimulation of adrenocorticotropic hormone and thus abnormally increased cortisol release. Cortisol has profound effects on many systems and has been demonstrated to alter mood, learning, and memory in the central nervous system (CNS).[18] Other cortisol-related findings in depression include pituitary and adrenal gland hypertrophy and elevated cerebrospinal fluid corticotropin-releasing factor concentrations,[20] possibly indicating abnormal function of cortisol receptors in the hippocampus.[15]

Thyroid Function

Impairments in the hypothalamic-pituitary thyroid system have been documented in association with depression. Findings include elevated cerebrospinal fluid levels of thyroid-stimulating hormone (TSH), alterations in the thyroid-stimulating response to thyrotropin-releasing hormone, and abnormally high rates of anti-thyroid antibodies.[20] Although abnormalities in thyroid function are well documented in individuals with depression, many of the symptoms of hypothyroidism itself (eg, fatigue, weight gain, difficulty concentrating, and memory disturbances)[21] may mimic those of depression, so screening for levels of thyroid hormones is an important step in the differential diagnosis of depression.

Growth Hormone Levels

People with depression have been demonstrated to have a blunted release of growth hormone during sleep.[15] Additionally, Birmaher et al demonstrated that children and adolescents at risk for major depressive disorder secrete significantly less ($p = 0.007$) growth hormone in response to growth hormone-releasing hormone than their age-matched low-risk peers. These abnormal levels of growth hormone may account for some of the fatigue experienced by individuals with depression and has been identified as a trait marker for depression.[22] Interestingly, increased growth hormone levels were associated with higher fatigue in individuals at least 1 year after traumatic brain injury, although brain-injured

subjects had lower serum cortisol levels.[23] These findings both support (cortisol) and contradict (growth hormone) previous studies on the neuroendocrine systems involved in depression.

Sleep Cycles

The Diagnostic and Statistical Manual of Mental Conditions, Fourth Edition (Text Revision) (DSM-IV-TR) defines circadian rhythm disorder as "a persistent or recurrent pattern of sleep disruption leading to excessive sleepiness or insomnia that is due to a mismatch between the sleep-wake schedule required by a person's environment and his or her circadian sleep-wake pattern."[24(p 629)] Behavioral and lifestyle causes are the most likely causes for these mismatches, including jet lag, work shift disturbances, and phase-delay disturbances (going to bed late and arising late). Other causes for circadian rhythm disturbances may occur because of changes in exposure to ambient light.

Assessing Depression

History and Interview

No medical or laboratory tests are currently in use that definitively diagnose depression. However, laboratory tests are available that validate the neuroendocrine changes associated with depression (eg, Dexamethasone Suppression Test, Corticotropin-Releasing Hormone Test, Serum Thyroxine Concentrations, Thyrotropin-Releasing Hormone Test).[13] Diagnosis is made on the basis of history and interview.

Screening Tools

Several well-validated screening instruments are available, including the Beck Depression Inventory (a 21-item self-report assessment of current depression)[25,26] and the Geriatric Depression Scale (GDS).[27] The GDS excludes somatic complaints from the items for which it screens and is able to distinguish symptoms caused by physical symptoms from depressive symptoms in older adults.[15] The GDS has also been demonstrated to effectively screen for depression in individuals with Parkinson's disease.[28] Interestingly, individuals with fatigue that is psychogenic in nature demonstrate no weakness. Tests of muscle strength and power are normal, as is muscle bulk and tendon reflex activity.[29]

Common Presenting Signs

The *DSM-IV-TR*[24] defines major depression as the presence of 5 or more of the following symptoms during the same 2-week period that represents a significant change in functioning. In addition, the symptoms are severe enough to cause the patient distress and interfere with social, occupation, or other important functioning. Symptoms are as follows:

- Depressed mood most of the day
- Diminished interest or pleasure in activities (anhedonia)
- Significant weight loss or weight gain (+5% total body weight)
- Change in sleep patterns (insomnia or hypersomnia)
- Psychomotor retardation/agitation
- Fatigue or loss of energy nearly every day

- Feelings of worthless or excessive/inappropriate guilt
- Diminished ability to think or concentrate, or indecisiveness
- Recurrent thoughts of death or suicidal ideation

These symptoms in conjunction with the endocrine abnormalities combine to produce a chronic feeling of exhaustion and lack of initiative to participate in physical activity. Individuals suffering from depression describe a sometimes-paralyzing inertia, with even simple activities requiring monumental energy. This sense of inertia, along with the changes in sleep observed in depression, combine to contribute to the fatigue associated with this disorder. An additional factor, which may paradoxically contribute to fatigue associated with depression, is the use of antidepressant drugs.[30]

Anxiety Disorders

There are a number of anxiety disorders that share common symptoms with the depressive disorders, as well as the pathophysiology related to excessive/abnormal sympathetic activation. Theories regarding the development of anxiety come from 2 opposite schools of thought. Strict biological theorists believe that behavioral changes are a result of measurable biological events, while strict behaviorists argue that the measurable biological changes are the results of psychological events. While this presents a set-up for a "chicken or egg" discussion, a discussion of the biological events may provide the best explanation for the fatigue associated with anxiety disorders.

Biological Events With Anxiety Disorders

Increased sympathetic tone has been implicated as a cause for symptoms in individuals with anxiety. According to Retford, CNS anxiety precedes the peripheral manifestations of anxiety, including tachycardia, tachypnea, headache, and diarrhea.[15] These manifestations of anxiety have been tied to an overall increase in sympathetic tone. Neurotransmitters associated with anxiety include norepinephrine, serotonin, and gamma-aminobutyric acid. At a cellular level, individuals with chronic anxiety have increased levels of lactic acid both at rest and with exercise. The increased levels associated with anxiety make the exercise that is necessary to maintain/improve fitness levels and ameliorate fatigue impossible.[31]

Common Presenting Symptoms

Fatigue is a central feature of most anxiety disorders, presumably due to the extreme amounts of energy spent in apprehension and worry. The *DSM-IV-TR*[24] describes the symptoms of generalized anxiety disorder as follows:

- Excessive anxiety and worry
- Difficulty controlling the worry

The anxiety/worry are associated with 3 or more of the following 6 symptoms (with at least some symptoms present for more days than not for at least 6 months):

1. Restlessness/feeling "keyed up" or on edge
2. Being easily fatigued
3. Difficulty concentrating
4. Irritability
5. Muscle tension
6. Sleep disturbance (difficulty falling or staying asleep, or restless unsatisfying sleep)

Regardless of the cause, the sleep disturbances associated with anxiety in combination with the inability to exercise at levels that would both improve fitness and reduce anxiety symptoms makes fatigue a difficult symptom to overcome.

Substance Abuse

Alcohol is often used as a form of self-medication to treat a variety of disorders, including insomnia, anxiety, or stress.[32] Abuse of alcohol may cause or result from sleep disturbances.[33] It contributes to difficulties associated with sleep, including decreased sleep duration and daytime sleepiness.[34] Alcohol is sometimes used as a means of getting to sleep without realizing that it disrupts the normal sleep cycle.[35] Loss of sleep during a single night or multiple nights has been associated with fatigue. Alcohol dependence is frequently associated with chronic insomnia, despite alcohol consumption at bedtime.[32] Sleep induced by alcohol is typically shorter and more fragmented than usual, especially toward the end of the night.[32,35] Despite shortened overall duration, rapid-eye movement (REM) sleep is increased in the second half of the night.[32,35] Frequent awakenings and vivid dreams are common.[32,35]

Sleep disruptive symptoms may persist for many months, even after the individual has stopped drinking.[32] Acute withdrawal of alcohol or other sedatives can cause delayed onset of sleep and REM rebound with intermittent awakening during the night.[32] Interestingly, drinking-related behaviors, heavy smoking (>1 pack per day), and excess caffeine intake are also related to sleep disorders, specifically difficulty falling asleep.[32] Use of other stimulant (ie, sympathomimetic) drugs is also associated with decreased total sleep time and a reduction of non-REM sleep.[32] The fact that disordered sleep is associated both with depressant and stimulant substances is a demonstration of the fragility of the sleep cycle, and that use of such substances should be considered in moderation, especially for the individual who is experiencing difficulty falling or staying asleep.

Lifestyle Issues Associated With Fatigue

Sleep Habits/Hygiene

Fatigue may be due to causes as simple to deal with as behavioral habits related to sleep. Sleep changes are normal with aging (decreased stages 3 and 4 sleep with increased periods of wakefulness),[36] but in younger adults, fatigue due to sleeplessness can often be mitigated with relatively simple behavioral changes. Suggestions for increasing the likelihood of restful sleep adapted from the National Sleep Foundation[37] include the following:

- Avoid stimulating substances (caffeine, nicotine, or other stimulants) in the evenings, or altogether if possible.

- Save the use of one's bed for sleep or sex; avoid watching TV, reading, or listening to the radio.

- Avoid large meals right before bedtime; if spicy foods are irritating, avoid those altogether.

- Avoid napping during the day.

- Attempt to maintain regular exposure to natural daylight—it helps to maintain normal sleep-wake cycles.

- Regular exercise is important, although vigorous exercise in the evenings (especially before bedtime) should be avoided.

- A relaxing pre-bedtime routine should be established (by performing activities such as deep breathing or yoga), but stressful conversations should be avoided around bedtime.

Summary of Fatigue

Given the prevalence and costs associated with the conditions listed previously, significant numbers of Americans are affected by these disorders at a huge cost to productivity and health. The impairments associated with these disorders either prevent individuals from being able to participate in exercise or render them incapable of overcoming the inertia that limits their ability to participate in many life activities, including exercise. As a result, they are additionally at significant risk for the deconditioning related to a sedentary lifestyle and its related comorbidities.

Fatigue Associated With Deconditioning

Individuals who are deconditioned have greater fuel needs for all activities when compared with those who are better trained. In other words, people who are deconditioned will burn more oxygen (O_2) per metabolic equivalent of activity than their more highly trained/conditioned counterparts. One consequence of the increased fuel requirements for daily activities is the perception of activity being more difficult than usual. Additionally, individuals who are deconditioned will report a higher rate of fatigue after completing relatively low-level activities because of the higher energy requirements for completing these tasks. This section will explore the various physiologic mechanisms responsible for the increase in fuel expenditure, and thus fatigue, associated with deconditioning.

Bed Rest, Zero Gravity, and Head-Down Bed Rest Research

Bed rest has evolved from being perceived as a healing intervention to the cause and risk for myriad pathologies, ranging from systemic to cellular. With bed rest, deconditioning happens. These detrimental effects of bed rest are well documented, although the most prolific research into the topic has occurred in the last 50 years. Even Hippocrates commented on the subject: "Should a long period of inactivity be followed by a sudden return to exercise, there will be

an obvious deterioration."[38] Some of the first research studies into the harmful effects of bed rest were conducted in the first half of the 20th century, as researchers noted bone loss in individuals confined to bed rest as a treatment for acute poliomyelitis. Dietrick et al confined 30 healthy medical students to bed rest and documented that simple bed rest, in the absence of pathology, was linked to loss of bone density and increased calcium excretion.[39] World War II physicians noted that soldiers who returned to activity sooner after surgery or injury recovered faster than those who remained in bed to recover,[40] thus hastening a return to community activity and life roles.

Eventually, with the initiation of manned spaceflight in 1961 and previously undocumented effects of microgravity on astronauts, another application evolved for bed rest research. While the use of bed rest as a therapeutic intervention waned in the late 20th century, bed rest studies were continued as a means of documenting the effects of zero-gravity conditions experienced in spaceflight on human anatomy and physiology. Further, these studies had clinical application to the effects of prolonged bed rest as a result of illness or injury. Cosmonauts returning from prolonged space missions in the early 1970s complained of difficulty sleeping in a horizontal position because of the perception of sliding off of the foot of the bed. They attempted to correct this sensation by raising the foot of the bed a little at a time until staying in the horizontal position for sleep felt "normal" again. The Russian researchers observed the behaviors of the cosmonauts and hypothesized that lying with their heads down more accurately replicated what it "felt like to be in space."[40] This led to the question of whether head-down bed rest (HDBR) more accurately replicated the zero-gravity environment experienced in space. Several studies were conducted to answer this question, and HDBR with the head of the bed down 6 degrees was subsequently validated as the best simulation of microgravity.[40,41] Because of the similarity of these 2 scenarios (HDBR and the microgravity experienced in spaceflight), evidence from both types of studies will be included in this review. A summary of the changes experienced after bed rest and spaceflight can be seen in Figure 4-1.

One criticism of the research conducted on the effects of bed rest and/or spaceflight on human physiology is that the studies have small numbers of subjects, and that there are only a few studies that demonstrate the effects of long-term bed rest or spaceflight. Nicogossian et al, in a summary of overall physiologic changes observed after spaceflight, stated that by 1993, only 283 individuals had traveled into space (see Figure 4-1).[42] Ethical considerations limited both the numbers of subjects and the duration of studies because from the early days of the studies, it was known that bed rest and spaceflight caused deleterious changes in the subjects. These studies were difficult logistically as well because of the constraints of spaceflight and mandatory bed rest. In support of this body of research, however, the results reported have been eminently repeatable, as proven by more than 40 years of studies reporting similar results. Studies that have

Figure 4-1. Physiologic changes associated with weightlessness. (Reprinted with permission from Nicogossian A, Sawn C, Huntoon C. Overall physiologic response to spaceflight. In: Nicogossian A, Huntoon C, Pool S, eds. *Space Physiology and Medicine*. 3rd ed. Philadelphia, PA: Lea & Febiger; 1994.)

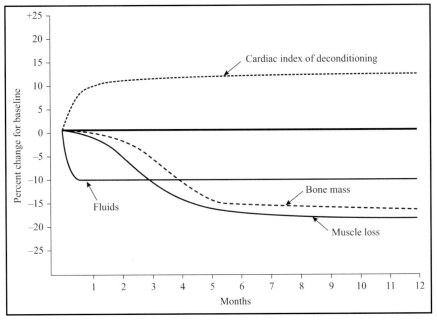

investigated the impact of HDBR have provided significant insight not only into the effects of space travel on human physiology, but also extended and refined essential studies into the harmful effects of immobility and thus bed rest on the cardiovascular, pulmonary, and musculoskeletal systems.

Cardiovascular Changes

The main physiologic effect of bed rest on the cardiovascular system is orthostatic intolerance,[43,44] or the inability to maintain adequate blood pressure (BP)/perfusion during the shift to or maintenance of the upright position after being horizontal. Orthostatic intolerance after bed rest occurs from changes in fluid balance, loss of red blood cell (RBC) mass, and changes in the cardiac structure itself.

Fluid Balance

Immediate changes resulting from assumption of the bed rest position or subsequent to spaceflight include a fluid shift from the lower extremities (LEs) to the thorax, with a change in thoracic fluid volume of ~1 liter, with acute increases in right and left ventricular filling pressures.[45,46] This occurs as the shift of fluid into the central vasculature from the LEs outpaces the ability of the upper extremity capillaries to filter the fluid, redistributing the blood into the central circulation.[47-49] The initial fluid shift results in a transient increase in preload from increased plasma volume.[48] As a result of the increase in preload, there is a transient increase in stroke volume (SV) with an accompanying decrease in heart rate (HR) and total peripheral resistance due to Starling mechanisms and stimulation of carotid and aortic baroreceptors, respectively.[50,51] SV increases in this immediate period have been measured as high as 9.2% after only 6.5 hours.[52]

After this initial response, the increase in preload results in increased cardiac filling and a transient rise in central venous pressure, which stimulates neural and hormonal responses supporting a significant diuresis, with increased urine output and sodium and potassium excretion (Table 4-1).[40]

Early bedrest results in rapid diuresis with marked loss of sodium and potassium.[53] With prolonged bed rest (up to 80 days), overall plasma volume has been demonstrated to decrease as much as 21%.[49] Women have been demonstrated to experience greater losses in plasma volume after short-term spaceflights (5- to 16-day missions) than their male counterparts (19.5 vs 7% [$p = 0.001$]),[54] a factor that likely contributes to the increased orthostatic intolerance observed in women vs men. When diuresis occurs, a new hemodynamic steady state occurs, with a "resetting of aortic and carotid baroreceptors"[55,56] that causes further decreases in SV and cardiac output (CO) in response to diuresis-induced hypovolemia. Perhonen et al demonstrated decreases in SV and CO after as little as 2 weeks of bed rest from 110 ± 20 to 83 ± 11 mL/min ($p = 0.02$) and 7.1 ± 0.7 to 5.9 ± 0.2 L/min ($p = 0.0009$), respectively.[44] Further significant changes were not measured with up to an additional 10 weeks (for a total of 12 weeks) of bed rest.

Loss of Red Blood Cell Mass

In a 1981 summary of changes experienced as a result of 96-day and 140-day spaceflights, Cogoli documented losses of RBC up to 21% and hemoglobin (Hgb) decreases of up to 33%.[57] Losses of RBC mass have been shown within 2 weeks of bed rest,[47,50,58] and continue on a linear basis (% change RBC mass = $0.89 + 0.24 \times$ bed rest days)[59] for up to 60 days and beyond.[50] Losses of 10% to 15% are seen consistently after spaceflight and/or bed rest; recovery to preflight levels of RBC takes up to 4 to 6 weeks.[60]

The etiology of RBC loss is not completely understood, though loss of RBC mass via inhibition of RBC formation seems to be the most likely explanation.[50,60] Several studies have proposed possible explanations for the decrease in RBC, including a drop in erythropoietin (EPO) levels,[61] changes in bone marrow response to EPO,[60] inadequate nutritional intake and decreases in lean body mass,[62] and deconditioning and decreased O_2 demand.[63]

TABLE 4-1. PHYSIOLOGIC CHANGES ASSOCIATED WITH SPACEFLIGHT AND HEAD-DOWN BED REST

	SPACE	HEAD-DOWN BED REST
Height	↑ ± 1.0 cm	↑ ± 1.0 cm
Body mass/weight	↓ 3% to 4%	↓ 3% to 4%
Maximum O_2 consumption (VO_{2max})	Not measured	↓ 25%
Plasma volume	↓ 10% to 15%	↓ 10% to 15%
Urinary calcium	Increases	Increases
Bone density	↓ 1.6%/month	↓ 0.5% to 1.0%/month
Absorption of calcium from the gut	Decreases	Decreases
Risk for renal stones	Increases	Increases
Muscle mass	Decreases	Decreases
Muscle strength	Decreases	Decreases
Insulin resistance	Increases	Increases

Adapted from Fortney S, Schneider V, Greenleaf J. The physiology of bedrest. In: *Handbook of Physiology.* New York: Oxford University Press; 1996:899-939.

Drops in EPO levels are linked to the hemoconcentration (increased hematocrit) that occurs with diuresis/plasma volume losses associated with bed rest,[50] while other studies posit that RBC loss is the result of changes in the bone marrow response to EPO that is caused by bone demineralization and negative calcium balance.[60] Others suggest that inadequate caloric or protein intake during bed rest/spaceflight may be the primary cause for suppression of erythropoesis.[62] Finally, decreases in O_2 demand that occur with deconditioning are thought to be responsible for loss of RBC with bed rest—this was confirmed by Greenleaf et al in 1992, who established that, with the addition of aerobic (vs isokinetic) exercise, RBC mass was maintained despite 30 days of 6-degree HDBR.[63] Regardless of cause, EPO levels return to normal levels within 2 weeks after cessation of spaceflight/bed rest.[61]

Cardiovascular Pump Changes

Changes in cardiac function associated with bed rest occur in 3 distinct phases.[64] In the first 24 hours after assumption of the supine/HDBR position or initiation of spaceflight, the change in pressure that results from the shift to a horizontal position causes transient increases in cardiac filling pressures (venous return) and SV due to Starling mechanisms.[51,65] Over the next 24 to 48 hours, increased pressures on carotid and aortic baroreceptors and an increase in plasma rennin activity[52] stimulates diuresis[40]; the resultant hypovolemia effects a decrease in SV and CO.[50] As bed rest persists, a third stage emerges in which there is a continued drop in CO and SV that results from overall decreased O_2 demand and decrements in active lean muscle mass; decreases in circulating blood volume and shifts in circulation as an accommodation to the headward shift in blood volume contribute to the decreases in CO and SV as well.[50]

Changes in cardiac size have also been observed in bed rest and spaceflight studies. During the first 24 hours of bed rest, the shift to the head down position increases the left-ventricular end-diastolic volume (LVEDV; ie, the volume of the LV at its fullest).[66,67] The increase in LVEDV is an indication of increased overall chamber volumes and reflects the increased preload experienced with the shift to horizontal position. Interestingly, increases in preload reach their highest levels with the assumption of a horizontal position—no further increases in preload are observed after a shift to 6 degrees of HDBR.[64]

After prolonged bed rest and short-term spaceflight, cardiac size decreases have been demonstrated in animal and human models. Studies of rodents have demonstrated a decrease in cardiac myocyte size, which is indicative of cardiac atrophy after as little as 14 days of bed rest.[43,44] Total myocardial protein losses of 9% and 18% have been documented after rat immobilization durations of 30 and 100 days.[68] Decreases in size and number of rat cardiac mitochondria have also been observed during prolonged bed rest,[69] while losses of 23% of total cardiac mass have been observed in as little as 20 days of immobilization.[64,68]

Human studies have revealed similar changes. In a study comparing the effects of spaceflight and bed rest, Perhonen et al[70] noted that LV mass decreased by $8.0 \pm 2.2\%$ ($p = 0.005$) after 6 weeks of bed rest. No significant differences in LV mass existed in controls over the same time period. Control subjects were "freely ambulatory" and performed their usual occupational and recreational activities. After 10 days of spaceflight, LV mass decreased by $12.0 \pm 6.9\%$ ($p = 0.07$).[44] Cardiac atrophy and impaired compliance lead to a reduction in SV and orthostatic intolerance.[43,70] These changes occur as a result of ventricular remodeling and not as a result of hypovolemia alone.[70] Further, no significant differences exist between men and women with regard to cardiac atrophy experienced after bed rest,[71] but women tend to suffer from more severe orthostatic intolerance after bed rest. Possible explanations for this gender difference include a desensitization of beta-adrenergic receptors with bed rest,[72,73] decreased cardiac filling,[74] decreases in SV,[74] low vascular resistance,[54] and gender-specific differences in ventricular size and distensibility.[74]

Perhonen et al[70] set out to determine if observed reductions in SV were due to changes stimulated by bed rest or due to the influence of hypovolemia alone. To that end, LV volume and Starling curves were analyzed after 2 weeks of HDBR and administration of intravenous furosemide. Both interventions led to similar reductions in plasma volume, but SV was reduced more and Starling curves were steeper during orthostatic stress after HDBR. Further, a 20% decrease in LVEDV was observed in the HDBR group, as compared with a 7% decrease with hypovolemia alone, leading the authors to conclude that HDBR leads to ventricular remodeling that is not seen after hypovolemia alone.[70]

Alterations in Oxygen Uptake

Decreases in exercise tolerance after bed rest/spaceflight have been observed in a number of studies[75-79] that identify there is a greater sensation of fatigue, or subjects having to work harder to get less work done. The degree of reduction in maximum O_2 consumption (VO_{2max}) is directly related to the duration of bed rest and pre-bed rest level of aerobic conditioning, but it seems to be independent of age or gender.[75,76,80] Convertino initially proposed that there is a linear decrease in VO_{2max} with bed rest[75] and projected that loss to be ~1%/day. Such a loss would result in a VO_{2max} of 0 after 100 days of bed rest, which does not occur. Capelli and colleagues demonstrated that in a 90-day period of bed rest, most of the decline in VO_{2max} occurs in the first 14 days of bed rest and then decreases at a progressive but slower rate toward the 90th day.[81] Feretti et al demonstrated that bed rest-associated decreases in VO_{2max} result from concurrent actions of 2 factors: a decrease in cardiovascular O_2 transport and a decrease in muscle oxidative capacity that accompanies bed rest-related decreases in muscle mass.[77] Decreases in VO_{2max} cause the individual to experience fatigue and/or breathlessness when performing skills that were well tolerated before the decline in conditioning. The symptoms experienced are a reflection of the increased fuel cost of activities.

Further analysis of bed rest studies of up to 128 days led Capelli and colleagues to hypothesize that the time required for bed rest-related VO_{2max} changes consists of at least 2 components: fast changes related to losses in cardiovascular transport and slower changes related to the decreases in peripheral muscle oxidative potential.[81] Changes in CO were reported in as early as 1968 by Saltin et al.[82] Subsequent studies have demonstrated that HDBR impairs carotid baroreflexes,[55] decreases resting blood catecholamine concentrations,[83] and reduces blood Hgb concentration despite reduced plasma volume.[47] These collective changes may in fact explain the reduced CO at any given exercise intensity after as little as 15 days of bed rest.

Musculoskeletal Changes

Several bed rest studies conducted by Americans and Russians demonstrate a dose-response relationship between the duration of bed rest and the resulting loss of muscle strength.[84,85] Zhang et al described the process of atrophy that occurs because of bed rest, denervation, hindlimb unloading, immobilization, or microgravity as a "highly ordered and regulated process, which is characterized by decreased fiber cross-sectional area (CSA) and protein content, reduced force, increased fatigability, and insulin resistance."[86(p 310)] Further, unlike in illness states, disuse atrophy begins with a "decrease in muscle contractile activity and muscle tension rather than by inflammatory cytokines" and results in a conversion from slow- to fast-twitch muscle fiber types, which predominantly affect anti-gravity muscles when studied in animal models.[86] Dietrick et al, in a study of bed rest with added LE immobilization in waist-to-toe casts, documented an increase in urinary nitrogen excretion (reflecting protein degradation/muscle loss) that peaked at 2 weeks of bed rest at 20% to 43% above baseline.[39] Other studies have replicated the observation of losses in lean body mass in as few as 14 days.[87-89] Tissue losses in these studies were associated with decreases in overall protein synthesis[88,89] and decreases of peak torque of up to 18% to 20%.[90]

Tests of disuse include unilateral limb suspension. Hather el al reported losses of 7% and 14% of muscle CSA at midthigh vs no change reported in the contralateral (control) limb after 4 and 6 weeks, respectively.[91] Losses of muscle mass were greater in the anti-gravity muscles (ie, gastrocnemius and soleus and vastus medialis, oblique, and lateralis) than in their corresponding antagonists (tibialis anterior and hamstrings, respectively).[91] This preferential atrophy of extensor muscles has been extensively documented elsewhere.[92-94] Hides et al demonstrated a significant loss of CSA in the multifidus muscle after 8 weeks of bed rest, with significant losses noted as early as 2 weeks into the period of bed rest. At the same time, anterior abdominal muscles increased in CSA, demonstrating a possible overuse of the trunk flexors during bed rest.[87] In studies of individuals with low-back pain, the evidence points to a selective atrophy of the multifidus muscle when compared to the psoas and erector spinae muscles.[95] The similar pattern of atrophy produced by bed rest may produce conditions in which bed rest makes the individual confined to bed rest more susceptible to the development of low-back pain.

Other studies demonstrate that the predominant and most significant losses of skeletal muscle associated with bed rest/immobilization occur in the LE vs upper extremities.[96] A study of Mir crew members on 4- to 6-month missions showed decreases of ~15% in LE and back muscles. Greatest losses of muscle mass were observed in the lower leg muscles.[93]

Older individuals are particularly susceptible to the changes caused by bed rest/immobilization, a reflection of the lowered physiologic reserve associated with aging. In a 2007 study of 10 days' bed rest in 12 healthy older adults (>65 years old), Kortebein et al demonstrated significant decreases in protein synthesis, lean body mass both overall and in the LEs, and loss of isokinetic LE strength.[90] The older adults showed a 6.3% loss in LE lean body mass ($p=0.001$) after only 10 days of bed rest,[90] which was a greater loss than that experienced by younger adults in a 2004 study after 28 days of bed rest.[97] The sometimes deadly results associated with bed rest and deconditioning for this at-risk age group is reflected in the 2006 report of mortality associated with hip fracture in 606 elderly Brazilian women. The risk for mortality was 21% in the first year.[98]

Vernikos-Danelli et al documented increases in plasma glucose levels for the first 30 days of a 56-day bed rest study of 5 healthy young men, while glucose levels remained unchanged.[99] Stuart et al demonstrated that only 6 to 7 days of bed rest were enough to impair muscle ability to use glucose and that this insulin resistance occurs primarily in skeletal muscle.[100] This finding was further corroborated by Blanc et al, who reported increased insulin-to-glucose levels after only 6 days of HDBR.[101]

Decreases in bone density associated with bed rest/immobility occur because of several factors, including loss of usual weightbearing forces, decreases in longitudinal compression, and loss/decrease of muscle contractions, particularly contractions of postural muscles used in normal gravity. Losses of bone density are dose-dependent (ie, longer periods of spaceflight/bed rest result in greater losses of bone density).[42] Bone density is spared in the upper extremities during bed rest or immobilization,[102,103] with 97% of bone loss originating in the LEs and pelvis.[93] Specific losses of bone density are most significant in long bones, lumbar vertebrae, and the calcaneus with bed rest.

Objective indicators of bone loss, such as urinary calcium and other bone resorption markers, are increased in as little as 4 to 7 days after the initiation of bed rest.[104-106] Further, a 2007 review of skeletal responses to spaceflight indicates that the evidence thus far suggests that complete recovery of bone mineral density may require between 1 to 3 years after bed rest or spaceflight.[96] Bone density changes with bed rest are not fully reversed after 6 months of a return to normal weightbearing activity.[94] In a study investigating potential mitigating factors, LeBlanc et al demonstrated that daily doses of alendronate during 17 weeks of bed rest minimized most of the bone loss changes typically produced by bed rest.[102]

The musculoskeletal alterations described previously produce an individual with decreased muscle strength, fuel utilization, and endurance following even a short period of bed rest.

Other Physiological Causes of Fatigue

Endocrine System

Endocrine system pathologies result in a wide variety of symptoms, as the impact of dysfunction in hormone balance and function can be detrimental to a number of systems.

Hypoglycemia

Hypoglycemia most frequently results from taking hypoglycemic medications or other drugs, including alcohol. It is also associated with a number of other disorders, including sepsis, end-stage organ failure, endocrine disorders, and inherited metabolic disorders. Sometimes hypoglycemia is defined as plasma glucose level <2.5 to 2.8 mmol/L (<45 to 50 mg/dL), but laboratory thresholds for hypoglycemia vary considerably depending on the setting. The presence of Whipple's triad, therefore, provides an important reference point for diagnosis. Whipple's triad includes the following characteristics: "symptoms compatible with hypoglycemia, a low plasma or blood glucose concentration, and resolution of those symptoms after the glucose concentration is raised to normal."[107(p 1904)] Symptoms can be split into 2 categories: those that result from CNS neuronal glucose deprivation and those that are autonomic responses. CNS deprivation of glucose results in symptoms of confusion, fatigue, behavioral changes, seizures, loss of consciousness, and, ultimately, death. Autonomic symptoms include palpitations, tremor, and anxiety (which are triggered by adrenergic activation) as well as cholinergic symptoms (eg, hunger, perspiration, and paresthesia). HR and systolic BP (SBP) are typically elevated in hypoglycemia, but these findings may not be prominent.[107]

Infection and Inflammation

Inflammatory and infectious disorders have potent effects on metabolism and create potential for fatigue. A wide spectrum of microorganisms, when present in the bloodstream, induces the synthesis and release of pyrogenic (fever-causing) cytokines. Cytokines regulate immune, inflammatory, and hematopoietic processes. The increase in white blood cell count seen in infections with an associated increase in the proportion of neutrophils, for example, is the result of the cytokines interleukin (IL) 1 and IL-6. The pyrogenic cytokines include IL-1, IL-6, tumor necrosis factor, ciliary neurotrophic factor, and interferon. Each cytokine is encoded by a separate gene, and each pyrogenic cytokine has been shown to cause fever in laboratory animals and in humans.[108] Levels of proinflammatory cytokines have been associated with several disorders with fatigue as an important symptom, including depression, chronic fatigue syndrome, and fibromyalgia.[109-111] This may also account, in part, for the presence of fatigue as a symptom in a variety of autoimmune disorders, including rheumatoid arthritis, multiple sclerosis, and systemic lupus erythematosus.[112]

Fever, however, can be a manifestation of disease in the absence of microbial infection. Inflammatory processes, trauma, tissue necrosis, or antigen-antibody complexes can induce the production of cytokines, which—individually or in combination—trigger the hypothalamus to raise body temperature to febrile levels.[108] Regardless of whether fever is caused by systemic inflammation or infection caused by a pyrogenic organism, each 1°C rise in body temperature increases basal metabolic rate by 14%,[108,113] increasing the energy demand for any given task.

Figure 4-2. Physiologic changes associated with chronic stress.

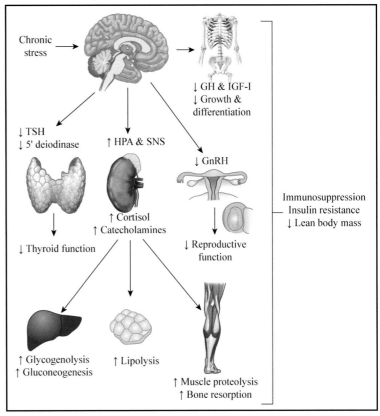

Stress

In 1976, Hans Selye attempted to introduce the concept of stress into physiology, when he defined stress simply as "the rate of wear and tear in the body" and more rigorously as "the state manifested by a specific syndrome which consists of all the nonspecifically induced changes within a biological system."[114] A more recent definition by Christiansen that reflects today's understanding of the complex interplay between an individual and his or her environment states,

> Stress is a process of interchange between an organism and its environment that involves self-generated or environmentally induced changes that, once they are perceived by the organism as exceeding available resources (internal or external), disrupt homeostatic processes in the organism-environment system.[115]

This disruption in processes has physiologic consequences; 2 main physiologic processes occur in the face of stress: autonomic hyperreactivity and immunosuppression.

The neuroendocrine (autonomic and HPA axis) systems, when activated in response to short-term stress, ensure that energy substrates are available to meet the increased metabolic demands of the individual. When an individual is faced with chronic stress, however, chronic activation of the "stress response" can have a deleterious effect on a number of systems. Prolonged duration and amplified magnitude of these activities, however, may lead to erosion of lean body mass and tissue injury (Figure 4-2) as well as dysregulation of immune regulatory responses via the HPA axis.[112] This dysregulation, characterized by a decrease in cortisol secretion, has been associated with increased immune and inflammatory responses, also demonstrated to be contributors to fatigue.[116,117] Autonomic dysregulation in the presence of chronic stress, characterized by increases in resting and exercise HRs and/or reduced HR variability, may also account for immune system hyperactivity and resultant fatigue.[112] Finally, excess stress or the inability to handle the challenges of a stressful life has been linked to depression, anxiety, and coronary artery disease (CAD), each of which has the ability to contribute to the development of fatigue.

Thyroid Disorders

Hypothyroidism is a common endocrine dysfunction—it affects more than 1% of the general population and about 5% of individuals aged 60 years and older. Primary symptoms include weakness, cold intolerance, fatigue, constipation, weight gain, depression, menorrhagia, and hoarseness. Laboratory findings associated with hypothyroidism include low levels of thyroid hormone (T_4) and radioactive iodine uptake, anemia, and elevated TSH. Other objective findings include the presence of a goiter (enlarged thyroid), dry skin, bradycardia, and decreased deep tendon reflexes.[118]

An excess of thyroid hormones causes hyperthyroidism. Common causes include a toxic diffuse goiter (Graves' disease), thyroiditis, iodine-induced hyperthyroidism, oversecretion of pituitary TSH, and excess exogenous thyroid hormone. Presenting symptoms include tremor, palpitations, weight loss, dyspnea on exertion, difficulty concentrating, bowel irritation/diarrhea, and fatigue. Objective physical exam findings include tachycardia and elevated BP (increase in SBP > diastolic BP [DBP]), muscle weakness, resting tremor, and cardiac arrhythmias (eg, atrial fibrillation) on electrocardiogram (EKG). Laboratory tests for hyperthyroid include screening for free T_4 levels, thyroid antibodies, or thyroid-stimulating immunoglobulins.[119]

Both hypo- and hyperthyroid conditions have a negative impact on skeletal muscle, known as *thyroid myopathies.* The exact etiology of the effect on muscle is as of yet unknown. Research to date demonstrates that thyroxine interferes with contraction but does not affect transmission of impulses in the peripheral nerve along the sarcolemma or across the myoneural junction. In hyperthyroidism, the changes in muscle augment the speed of the contractile process and slow its duration, with resultant fatigability, weakness, and diminished endurance. Conversely, in hypothyroidism, muscle contraction and relaxation are slowed.[120]

Anemia

Defined as a reduction in circulating RBCs, anemia is clinically measured as reduction in RBC count, Hgb concentration, or hematocrit. Hgb concentration is measured as the concentration of O_2-carrying pigment in whole blood, and is expressed as grams/liter of blood or grams of Hgb per mL of whole blood. Hematocrit is measured as the percentage of RBCs that occupy a sample of whole blood, while RBC count is the measure of the number of RBCs in a specified volume of whole blood (millions of RBC/μL).[121] The most common cause of anemia is iron deficiency.[122] primary etiologic factors for iron deficiency anemia include dietary insufficiencies/poor absorption and hemorrhage (including blood loss from the gastrointestinal system, trauma, tumor, and menstrual loss).

In chronic conditions like cancer, renal failure, or infection with HIV, low Hgb levels may result from inadequate production of RBCs by the bone marrow and reduced production of EPO by the kidneys.[123] Anemia associated with these conditions is reported to negatively affect work and sleep, as well as physical and emotional well-being.[124,125] It has also been shown to be a potent predictor of survival in individuals with heart failure, AIDS, renal failure, and various cancers, despite controlling for known prognostic factors like age, gender, and other comorbidities.[126-128] The anemia associated with these conditions has been demonstrated to respond favorably (improved Hgb and health-related quality of life) to treatment with EPO alfa.[129] For individuals with anemia, the overwhelming symptoms of fatigue that are associated with even low levels of activity can be daunting when facing simple activities associated with activities of daily living (ADL).

Malnutrition

Malnutrition is a frequent component of acute and chronic illness and is found in ~50% of all hospitalized adults. Increases in in-hospital morbidity and mortality among medical and surgical patients are associated with malnutrition, as is an increased frequency of hospital admissions among the elderly.[130] Weight loss and/or undernutrition occur when energy expenditures exceed caloric intake, and they can occur as a result of inadequate intake or increased metabolic demand. Criteria for diagnosis of malnutrition includes the presence of one or more of the following criteria:

- Unintentional loss of ~10% of usual body weight in the preceding 3 months
- Body weight < 90% of ideal for height
- Body mass index (BMI; weight [kg] divided by height [m^2]) < 18.5

Severity is classified according to body weight: body weight < 90% of ideal for height represents risk for malnutrition, < 85% of ideal constitutes *malnutrition,* < 70% of ideal represents *severe malnutrition,* and < 60% of ideal is typically incompatible with survival. Although fatigue is not specifically named as a complication of malnutrition, the term *failure to thrive* is used to describe a constellation of symptoms including weakness, progressive functional decline, and weight loss. There is typically a triggering event, such as a loss of social support, a bout of an acute illness, or the addition of a new medication.[131] This event may serves as a precursor to a major loss of function for the elderly individual, putting the capability for independent living at risk.[131,132]

Cancer

Improved treatments for cancer and resultant increases in survivability have changed the perception of cancer from being a death sentence to a chronic illness with associated health management needs designed to improve/maintain quality of life. The National Comprehensive Cancer Network describes the fatigue associated with cancer as "a distressing persistent, subjective sense of tiredness or exhaustion related to cancer or cancer treatment that is not proportional to recent activity and interferes with usual functioning."[133] Recent studies of individuals with cancer reveal fatigue rates as high as 70% to 80%.[134-137] Physical activity is often difficult to sustain and, in some cases, even minimal exertion causes symptoms like dyspnea.[138] Oncologists report a belief that pain interferes with patient function more severely than fatigue (61% vs 37%), but patients reported that fatigue had a more devastating affect on their daily lives than pain (61% vs 19%).[139] Fatigue and cancer pain often coexist, and the greater fatigue reported by individuals who complain of pain may in part be a side effect of pain medications,[140] although one study reported that more than 50% of cancer patients report significant difficulties with sleep.[141] Analgesics used to treat cancer pain often cause sleep disturbance, leading to greater daytime fatigue.[140] Although use of analgesics for pain control contributes to fatigue, studies show that pain alone is a significant predictor of fatigue in cancer patients, regardless of analgesic use.[142]

Other causes of fatigue in cancer result both from processes associated with the cancer itself and treatments for the cancer.[136] Frequent causes include anemia, cachexia, and deconditioning.[10] When cancer-related fatigue is caused by deconditioning, physicians often prescribe more rest and relaxation, leading to further deconditioning and exacerbation of fatigue-related symptoms.[10] Rest, sleep, or relaxation, however, do not return perceived sense of vigor or strength back to normal. Symptoms of fatigue may abate to a degree with rest, but perceived stamina and strength do not return to normal.[138] Studies of function revealed that performance in function-related tasks (6-Minute Walk tests [6MWT], a 50-foot walk, or forward reach) was lower in individuals with lymphoma than age- and gender-matched controls, and performance was linked with self-reports of fatigue in these subjects.[143]

Despite the inclination to rest when fatigued or even following physician instructions to do so, exercise is an effective intervention for preventing and/or minimizing cancer-related fatigue. Stricker and colleagues, in a 2004 review of the evidence on exercise as an intervention for cancer-related fatigue, found exercise to be an effective intervention.[144] Two separate studies[145,146] demonstrated that exercise in cancer survivors was inversely related to fatigue and anxiety. In addition, Courneya further demonstrated that exercise during treatment reduced symptoms of depression and number of days hospitalized.[145] Schwartz, in a study of women undergoing treatment for breast cancer, found that women who exercised during treatment reported less fatigue than their nonexercising counterparts and greater decrements in fatigue reported with each treatment cycle.[147] Benefits of exercise on mitigating fatigue occur when exercise is performed during and after treatment for cancer,[148] emphasizing the point that exercise can help decrease fatigue regardless of when that exercise is initiated in the course of treatment. In addition, a study of 85 women[149] who exercised while undergoing chemotherapy treatments demonstrated decreased depression scores in addition to increased physical activity scores. Improvements in depression can help to mitigate the subjective experience of fatigue in these individuals and can positively contribute to quality of life.

Respiratory Distress

Individuals in respiratory distress may suffer from hypercapnia (increased carbon dioxide [CO_2]), which is defined as a $PaCO_2 > 45$ mm Hg, and results from alveolar hypoventilation.[150] It may or may not be accompanied by hypoxemia (decreased O_2), depending on the cause. Distress can result from a number of causes, including ventilatory muscle fatigue, acute pulmonary infections or chronic airway obstruction that impairs gas exchange, splinting from pain caused by thoracic or abdominal trauma or incision, reduced ventilatory drive from drugs (recreational and therapeutic, analgesics being the most common), and diseases/disorders of the neuromuscular system impairing the mechanics of breathing and the ventilatory pump.[151] The patient with hypercapnia resulting from hypoventilation or impaired gas exchange may complain of symptoms of lethargy, headache, or confusion. Degree of symptoms is directly related to the severity of hypercapnia, and at higher levels of hypercapnia, seizures or coma can result.[150] In less severe cases of hypercapnia associated with hypoventilation, the individual may complain of simple fatigue or report a decreased energy level or exercise tolerance.

Objective signs of respiratory distress include nasal flaring, increased ventilatory rate (VR; >22 to 26 breaths/minute), increased use of accessory muscles of ventilation (particularly at rest), active contraction of abdominal muscles on expiration, intercostal or sternal retraction, and a paradoxical breathing pattern.[152] The most common laboratory test for documenting the status of gas exchange is the arterial blood gas, from which information can be gleaned about O_2, CO_2, pH, and bicarbonate levels in arterial blood.[153]

Renal Failure

Fatigue is the most frequently reported symptom experienced by individuals on hemodialysis.[125,154-157] Chronic renal failure (CRF) results in a decrease in Hgb concentration due to an overall decrease in RBC lifespan.[158] Other factors implicated in CRF-related anemia include a decline in erythropoiesis due to uremic substrates and a deficiency of EPO.[159] Administration of exogenous synthetic EPO does not result in significantly improved VO_{2max}, as the difficulty with O_2 extraction reflects a decreased ability to move O_2 from muscle capillaries to the mitochondria.[160-162] A decrease in overall muscle mass occurs with CRF,[163] characterized by increased insulin resistance[164] and a decline in muscle quality, known as *uremic myopathy*.[160] The myopathy associated with CRF causes a decrease in strength that occurs because of a decline in contractile tissue as opposed to an inability to effectively use the available muscle.[163]

Aerobic exercise performed both on non-dialysis and dialysis days results in improvements in VO_{2max} and increased exercise times until exhaustion,[165] although better improvements in exercise capacity are observed when exercise is performed on non-dialysis days. Further, aerobic exercise in patients undergoing hemodialysis has been reported to increase Hgb, augment insulin sensitivity, decrease risk factors for cardiovascular disease (BP and lipid profile), and improve quality of life.[166]

Chronic Obstructive Pulmonary Disease

Reduction of exercise capacity was demonstrated by Oga et al to be the best predictor of mortality in chronic obstructive pulmonary disease (COPD), regardless of age or airflow limitation.[167] Skeletal muscle changes that occur in COPD include decrements in strength, muscle mass, and mitochondrial enzyme activities, and they are coupled with excessive lactate accumulation during exercise.[168] Significant accumulation of skeletal muscle lactate often occurs early in submaximal exercise and is independent of LE circulation at rest and during exercise.[169] Pepin and colleagues reported that the difficulties with physical functional performance reported by individuals with COPD can be attributed to the discomfort (predominantly dyspnea and LE fatigue) provoked by activity.[170] In a 22-month study that documented the symptoms in 74 patients with COPD, fatigue showed the greatest increase over time of the symptoms tracked during the test period. At baseline, 19% and 50% reported mild and severe fatigue, respectively. At follow-up, 30% reported mild fatigue and 62% reported moderate or severe fatigue

($p = 0.001$).[171] Interestingly, in this same study, participants with COPD reported significant ($p = 0.03$) increases in feelings of depression over the same time period, which could compound sensations of fatigue in this population.[171]

While hypotheses exist that these changes are due to a COPD-related systemic disease or specific myopathy, the evidence of such a systemic myopathic process is equivocal to date. Wagner, in his 2006 review of the evidence related to skeletal muscle function in COPD, reports that decrements in muscle activity and mass are due to the inactivity-induced peripheral muscle deconditioning experienced by this population.[169,172] In the population of individuals with COPD (as well as other chronic conditions), a vicious cycle develops—performance of an activity leads to an undesired or unpleasant experience (in this case shortness of breath or dyspnea). The person associates the activity with the unpleasant experience and thus avoids it. Avoidance of the activity results in deconditioning, and an increased energy cost for the activity. It then takes less provocation for the symptoms to result; continued avoidance results in a significant deterioration of functional status and physiological reserve (Figure 4-3).

Aging With a Disability

Individuals living long term with a physical disability are at particular risk for the development of fatigue. First observed in individuals who had poliomyelitis in the 1940s and 1950s, new functional losses were observed in individuals who had lived successfully with polio for many (20+) years, some of whom had years of stable function.[173,174] Average onset of symptoms occurs at reported averages of 20 to 35 years after initial infection.[173,174] These losses were characterized by losses of previously regained function with new onsets of pain, fatigue, weakness, and depression.[174] In the mid-1980s, the phrase *post-polio syndrome* (PPS) was coined at the Warm-Springs Georgia Rehabilitation Center to describe the constellation of functional losses experienced by this population.[175] Fatigue and weakness were the 2 most common symptoms experienced by those aging with polio.[173,174,176,177] Studies have reported that 91% of individuals with PPS experience new or heightened fatigue, while 41% report symptoms severe enough to interfere with work, and 25% reporting that fatigue interferes with performance of ADL.[174,178,179] Up to 42% of individuals with PPS report new breathing problems, and many require additional ventilatory support. The largest percentage of those with PPS who require ventilatory support had ventilatory compromise as part of their initial experience with polio, but some individuals with PPS require ventilatory support despite no such previous history.[174]

Initial studies were based on the assumption that the functional losses were as a result of a pathophysiologic process unique to having had the poliovirus. Indeed, muscle changes were observed in those with PPS, including motor unit enlargement and overuse failure of the nerve axon sprouts.[173,180] First treatments considered for the weakness associated with PPS revolved around vigorous exercise in hopes of restoring strength and thus restoring function. It

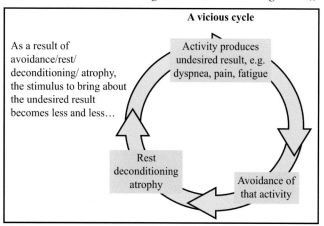

Figure 4-3. Stimulus and avoidance.

was soon discovered, however, that overexertion made the weakness and symptoms worse rather than better.[173,177] Mild to moderate exercise, on the other hand, has been reliably demonstrated to improve strength and function in those with PPS.[176,181,182] Best results for treating fatigue in this population have been achieved with energy conservation strategies, including pacing, use of bracing, frequent rest periods, and use of assistive technology.[173,176]

Further research indicated that the functional losses experienced by those with PPS were not, in fact, unique to polio. As life expectancy has increased for individuals without disabilities because of improvements in medical care, so has the life expectancy for individuals with disabilities (the most frequently studied group is composed of individuals with spinal cord injury).[183] Like the phenomena that occurred in people with PPS, people with physical disabilities (spinal cord injury, cerebral palsy, spina bifida, etc) experience age-related losses of function with new onsets of pain, fatigue, and weakness.[184,185] The onset of these new issues can result in progressive losses of functional independence as the person with a disability ages.[184] As in PPS, the key to management of symptoms experienced by individuals aging with a disability lies in energy conservation. If possible, mild to moderate exercise can play a role in maintenance of function, but the preservation of function is key. Appropriate evaluation and management of new symptoms (eg, pain, depression) and seeking strategies to conserve and thus preserve function can accomplish this.

EXAMINATION OF PATIENTS WITH SYMPTOMATIC FATIGUE AND SIGNS OF DECONDITIONING

In each of the physiologic and psychological conditions described, the complicated interactions of symptomatic fatigue and its interrelationship with physiologic deconditioning have been presented. Often, it is difficult

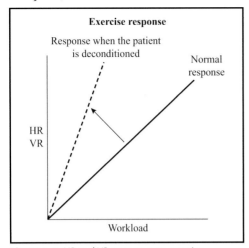

Figure 4-4. HR and VR responses to exercise.

to separate the precipitating factors from the consequential results. It is essential, however, to separate out the fixed pathology from the malleable impairments and functional limitations to accurately manage the impairments and reduce the limitations.

History

Examination of these patients proceeds by taking an accurate history that consists of a comprehensive inventory of past and present conditions requiring medical interventions, past surgeries, family history, current/past medications, social/occupational history, and history of past or current substance use/abuse (to include smoking history). This can occur via a structured interview in combination with analysis of data collected via the health history form.

Systems Review

The systems review is a brief physical examination conducted to glean information about areas that may require further examination or testing. This hands-on examination consists of a brief check of the integumentary, cardiovascular, pulmonary, neurologic, and musculoskeletal systems for indications that more in-depth examination is warranted. In the case of individuals with complaints of fatigue or signs of deconditioning, the systems review may reveal the following: a faster resting HR/VR, difficulty breathing (evidenced by increased work of breathing), a lower BP than usual, evidence of muscle disuse/atrophy, limited range of motion, peripheral edema, and skeletal muscle weakness (manifested by a decreased ability to perform functional tasks/maintain balance).

Initiation of exercise for patients who are deconditioned requires careful scrutiny on the part of the clinician, especially with regard to the cardiac and/or pulmonary system. When determining whether to initiate exercise for patients who are deconditioned, the clinician must evaluate the patient's condition at rest and then determine whether the patient has the capacity to respond to increased demands.

The clinician must have a working knowledge both of the normal response to exercise and what is expected in a patient who is deconditioned. For the patient who is deconditioned, the clinician will likely observe a higher than normal HR and VR at rest and with response to activity. Typically, both HR and VR increase proportionally to workload, but the degree of response to activity can be greatly exaggerated when a person who is deconditioned exercises (Figure 4-4). This is true particularly in the early stages of the initiating exercise after prolonged bed rest. The intensity of exercise required to produce an abnormal exercise response will vary from patient to patient, with the general proviso that the longer the patient has been immobile, the less exercise will be required to produce an abnormal response. In addition, the older the patient is at the initiation of exercise, the more pronounced the abnormal response will be, reflecting greater sensitivity to deconditioning and with losses of physiologic reserve associated with aging.

When monitoring HR response, the clinician should be mindful of the patient's age-predicted HR_{max}, as the patient's HR may be significantly elevated both at rest and with exercise. It is not uncommon for a patient who is severely deconditioned to have resting HRs in the low 100s, for example. Even minor increases in activity may therefore cause the patient's HR to elevate to unsafe levels (depending on the patient's age). As HR increases and thus O_2 demand, the clinician should also be alert for indications of myocardial ischemia, especially onset of angina or arrhythmias (or worsening of a previously stable cardiac rhythm).

Evaluation of the patient's ventilatory status is critical as well. A careful examination of the patient's ventilatory and respiratory status will assist the clinician in his or her decision of whether to initiate or continue activity. Signs of ventilatory muscle fatigue/distress include VR > 20, use of accessory muscles of ventilation, sternal/intercostal retractions, forced use of abdominals on expiration, and/or a paradoxical breathing pattern (in which ventilatory muscle fatigue produces a breathing pattern in which the patient's abdominal contents fall with inspiration and rise with expiration). Presence of any of these signs at rest can be considered relative contraindications to the initiation of exercise. As a general guideline for evaluation of respiratory status, pulse oximetry can provide valuable information about the patient's ability to deliver O_2 to his or her RBCs (and consequently to peripheral tissues), with normal being ≥ 96%. Resting or exercise levels of O_2 saturation (as measured by pulse oximetry) below 92% reflect arterial partial pressures of O_2 that approach levels of O_2 found in venous blood; initiation or continuation of exercise under these circumstances should therefore occur only given careful consideration of the patient's history and current clinical presentation.

In the presence of any of these objective vital sign indicators of unstable cardiac or pulmonary systems, incremental initiation of carefully monitored activity may be necessary. If exercise produces one or more of the previously mentioned signs, especially in the context of poor subjective tolerance to activity, exercise should be discontinued until the patient recovers back to resting levels. The amount of time from the onset of illness/injury to the initiation of therapy can help the clinician decide whether (or when) it is safe to resume activity. Data gathered from exercise sessions (as they occur) can also provide valuable information of when and how vigorously to progress activity based on patient response.

Tests and Measures

This portion of the examination uses specific and objective tests and measures focused on low-level aerobic capacity (eg, 6MWT,[186] Stair Climb Power test,[187,188]) and functional performance (eg, Timed Up and Go[189]). Performance on these tests not only can provide useful objective information about current preintervention functioning, but also can document functional improvements made due to intervention(s).

Diagnosis

Deconditioning

Pattern 6B: Impaired Aerobic Capacity/Endurance Associated With Deconditioning.[190]

Prognosis

The patient's prognosis is highly dependent on a number of factors, including age, time of immobility, and other comorbidities. The patient's physiologic response to activity and the ability to tolerate incrementally greater workloads (or lack thereof) can also provide valuable insight into how well and how far the patient might progress.

REFERENCES

1. Cathebras P, Robbins JM, Kirmayer LJ, Hayton BG. Fatigue in primary care. *J Gen Intern Med.* 1992;7:276-286.

2. Sugarman J, Berg A. Evaluation of fatigue in a family practice. *J Fam Practice.* 1984;5:643-647.

3. Fukuda K, Dobbins JG, Wilson LJ, Dunn RA, Wilcox K, Smallwood D. An epidemiologic study of fatigue with relevance for the chronic fatigue syndrome. *J Psychiat Res.* 1997;31(1):19-29.

4. Wijeratne C, Hickie I, Brodaty H. The characteristics of fatigue in an older primary care sample. *J Psychiat Res.* 2007;62(2):153-158.

5. Bates D, Schmitt W, Buchwald D, et al. Prevalence of fatigue and chronic fatigue syndrome in a primary care practice. *Arch Intern Med.* 1993;153:2759-2765.

6. Schappert S. *National Ambulatory Medical Care Survey: 1989 Summary.* Bethesda, MD: National Center for Health Statistics; 1989.

7. Ricci JA, Chee E, Lorandeau AL, Berger J. Fatigue in the U.S. workforce: prevalence and implications for lost productive work time. *J Occup Environ Med.* 2007;49(1):1-10.

8. Chen MK. The epidemiology of self-perceived fatigue among adults. *Prev Med.* 1986;15:74-81.

9. Gonzalez R. Fatigue and chronic fatigue syndrome. In: McPhee S, Papadakis M, Tierney L, eds. *Current Medical Diagnosis & Treatment 2007.* 46th ed. New York, NY: McGraw-Hill; 2007.

10. Evans W, Lambert C. Physiological basis of fatigue. *Am J Phys Med Rehabil.* 2007;86 (Suppl):S29-S46.

11. Centers for Disease Control and Prevention. *Behavioral Risk Factor Surveillance System Survey Data.* Atlanta, GA: U.S. Department of Health and Human Services; 2006.

12. Heo M, Murphy CF, Fontaine KR, Bruce ML, Alexopoulos GS. Population projection of US adults with lifetime experience of depressive disorder by age and sex from year 2005 to 2050. *Int J Geriatr Psychiatry.* 2008;23:1266-1270.

13. Loosen P, Beyer J, Sells S, et al. Mood disorders. In: Ebert M, Loosen P, Nurcombe B, eds. *Current Diagnosis and Treatment in Psychiatry.* New York, NY: McGraw Hill; 2000.

14. Addington A, Gallo J, Ford D, Eaton W. Epidemiology of unexplained fatigue and major depression in the community: the Baltimore ECA follow-up, 1981-1994. *Psychol Med.* 2001;31(6):1037-1044.

15. Retford DC, ed. *Kaplan and Saddock's Synopsis of Psychiatry: Behavioral Sciences, Clinical Psychiatry.* 7th ed. Baltimore, MD: Williams & Wilkins; 1994.

16. Nutt D. Consensus statement and research needs: the role of dopamine and norepinephrine in depression and antidepressant treatment. *J Clin Psychiat.* 2006;67(Suppl 6):46-49.

17. Stamford JA, Muscat R, O'Connor JJ, et al. Voltammetric evidence that subsensitivity to reward following chronic mild stress is associated with increased release of mesolimbic dopamine. *Psychopharmacology (Berl).* 1991;105(2):275-282.

18. Erickson K, Drevets W, Schulkin J. Glucocorticoid regulation of diverse cognitive functions in normal and pathological emotional states. *Neurosci Biobehav Rev.* 2003;27(3):233-246.

19. Thompson F, Craighead M. Innovative approaches for the treatment of depression: targeting the HPA axis. *Neurochem Res.* 2008;33:691-707.

20. Musselman DL, Betan E, Larsen H, Phillips LS. Relationship of depression to diabetes types 1 and 2: epidemiology, biology, and treatment. *Biol Psychiatry.* 2003;54(3):317-329.

21. Jameson L, Weetman A. Disorders of the thyroid gland. In: Kasper D, Braunwald E, Fauci A, et al, eds. *Harrison's Principles of Internal Medicine.* 16th ed. New York, NY: McGraw-Hill; 2005.

22. Birmaher B, Dahl RE, Williamson DE, et al. Growth hormone secretion in children and adolescents at high risk for major depressive disorder. *Arch Gen Psychiatry.* 2000;57(9):867-872.

23. Bushnik T, Englander J, Katznelson L. Fatigue after TBI: association with neuroendocrine abnormalities. *Brain Inj.* 2007;21(6):559-566.

24. American Psychiatric Association. *Diagnostic and Statistical Manual of Mental Disorders: DSM-IV, Fourth Edition, Text Revision.* 4th ed. Washington, DC: American Psychiatric Association; 2000.

25. Beck AT, Beck RW Screening depressed patients in family practice: a rapid technic. *Postgrad Med.* 1972;52:81-85.

26. Beck AT, Steer RA, Carbin MG. Psychometric properties of the Beck Depression Inventory: twenty-five years of evaluation. *Clinical Psychology Review.* 1988;8(1):77-100.

27. Yesavage JA, Brink TL, Rose TL, et al. Development and validation of a geriatric depression screening scale: A preliminary report. *J Psychiatr Res.* 1982-1983;17(1):37-49.

28. Weintraub D, Oehlberg K, Katz I, Stern M. Test characteristics of the 15-item Geriatric Depression Scale and Hamilton Depression Rating Scale in Parkinson disease. *Am J Geriatr Psychiatry.* 2006;14(2):169-175.

29. Lloyd A, Gandevia S, Hales J. Muscle performance, voluntary activation, twitch properties and perceived effort in normal subjects and patients with the chronic fatigue syndrome. *Brain.* 1991;114(Pt 1A):85-98.

30. Ropper A, Samuels M. Fatigue, asthenia, anxiety, and depressive reactions. In: Ropper A, Samuels M, eds. *Adams and Victor's Principles of Neurology.* 9th ed. New York, NY: McGraw-Hill; 2010.

31. Ropper A, Brown R. Fatigue, asthenia, anxiety, and depressive reactions. In: Adams R, Victor M, Ropper A, eds. *Adams and Victor's Principles of Neurology.* 8th ed. Baltimore, MD: McGraw-Hill; 2005.

32. Clark C, Moore P, Bhatti T, Seifritz E, Gillin J. Sleep disorders. In: Ebert M, Loosen P, Nurcombe B, eds. *Current Diagnosis and Treatment in Psychiatry.* New York, NY: McGraw-Hill; 2000.

33. Neumann T, Neuner B, Weiss-Gerlach E, Spies C. Complaints about sleep in trauma patients in an emergency department in respect to alcohol use. *Alcohol.* 2008;43(3):305-313.

34. Roehrs T, Roth T. Sleep, sleepiness, sleep disorders and alcohol use and abuse. *Sleep Med Rev.* 2001;5(4):287-297.

35. Eisendrath S, Lichtmacher J. Psychiatry. In: Gonzales R, Zeiger R, eds. *Current Medical Diagnosis and Treatment.* New York, NY: McGraw-Hill; 2008.

36. Eisendrath S, Lichtmacher J. Psychiatry. In: McPhee S, Papadakis M, Tierney L, eds. *Current Medical Diagnosis and Treatment 2008.* Baltimore, MD: McGraw Hill; 2007.

37. Thorpy M. Sleep hygiene. 2007. http://sleepfoundation.org/ask-the-expert/sleep-hygiene. Accessed November 2, 2007.

38. Chadwick J, Mann W. *The Medical Works of Hippocrates.* Oxford, England: Blackwell; 1950.

39. Dietrick J, Whedon G, Shorr E, Toscani V, Davis B. Effect of immobilization on metabolic and physiologic functions in normal men. *Am J Med.* 1948;4:33-35.

40. Pavy-Le Traon A, Heer M, Narici M, Rittweger J, Vernikos J. From space to Earth: advances in human physiology from 20 years of bed rest studies (1986-2006). *Eur J Appl Physiol.* 2007;101(2):143-194.

41. White P, Nyberg J, White W. A comparitive study of the physiologic effects of immersion and recumbence. Paper presented at: 2nd Annual Biomedical Research Conference; February 17-18, 1966; Houston, TX.

42. Nicogossian A, Sawn C, Huntoon C. Overall physiologic response to space flight. In: Nicogossian A, Huntoon C, Pool S, eds. *Space Physiology and Medicine.* 3rd ed. Philadelphia, PA: Lea & Febiger; 1994.

43. Levine BD, Zuckerman JH, Pawelczyk JA. Cardiac atrophy after bed-rest deconditioning: a nonneural mechanism for orthostatic intolerance. *Circulation.* 1997;96(2):517-525.

44. Perhonen MA, Franco F, Lane LD, et al. Cardiac atrophy after bed rest and spaceflight. *J Appl Physiol (1985).* 2001;91(2):645-653.

45. Buckey JC Jr, Gaffney FA, Lane LD, et al. Central venous pressure in space. *J Appl Physiol (1985).* 1996;81(1):19-25.

46. White RJ, Blomqvist CG. Central venous pressure and cardiac function during spaceflight. *J Appl Physiol (1985).* 1998;85(2):738-746.

47. Fortney S, Hyatt K, Davis J, Vogel J. Changes in body fluid compartments during a 28-day bed rest. *Aviat Space Environ Med.* 1991;62(2):97-104.

48. Greenleaf JE. Physiological responses to prolonged bed rest and fluid immersion in humans. *J Appl Physiol Respir Environ Exerc Physiol.* 1984;57(3):619-633.

49. Gharib C, Güell A, Pourcelot L, Bost R. Circulatory and hormonal changes induced by microgravity [article in French]. *J Physiol (Paris).* 1985;80(3):182-188.

50. Fortney S, Schneider V, Greenleaf J. The physiology of bedrest. In: *Handbook of Physiology.* New York, NY: Oxford University Press; 1996:899-939.

51. Sagawa K, Maughan L, Suga H, Sunagawa K. Physiologic determinants of the ventricular pressure volume relationship. In: Sagawa K, Maughan L, Suga H, et al, eds. *Cardiac Contraction and the Pressure-Volume Relationship.* New York, NY: Oxford University Press; 1988:110-170.

52. Maillet A, Pavy-Le Traon A, Allevard AM, et al. Hormone changes induced by 37.5-h head-down tilt (-6 degrees) in humans. *Eur J Appl Physiol Occup Physiol.* 1994;68(6):497-503.

53. Vernikos J. Metabolic and endocrine changes. In: Sandler H, Vernikos J, eds. *Inactivity: Physiologic Effects.* New York, NY: Academic; 1986:99-121.

54. Waters WW, Ziegler MG, Meck JV. Postspaceflight orthostatic hypotension occurs mostly in women and is predicted by low vascular resistance. *J Appl Physiol (1985).* 2002;92(2):586-594.

55. Convertino VA, Doerr DF, Eckberg DL, Fritsch JM, Vernikos-Danellis J. Head-down bed rest impairs vagal baroreflex responses and provokes orthostatic hypotension. *J Appl Physiol (1985).* 1990;68(4):1458-1464.

56. Eckberg D, Fritsch J. Carotid baroreceptor cardiac-vagal reflex responses during 10 days of head-down tilt. *Physiologist.* 1990;33(1 Suppl):S177.

57. Cogoli A. Hematological and immunological changes during space flight. *Acta Astronaut.* 1981;8(9-10):995-1002.

58. Scianowski J, Kedziora J, Zolynski K. Red blood cell metabolism in men during long term bed rest. *Int J Occup Med Environ Health.* 1995;8(4):315-319.

59. Kimzey S, Leonard J, Johnson P. A mathematical and experimental simulation of the hematological response to weightlessness. *Acta Astronaut.* 1979;6(10):1289-1303.

60. Talbot J, Fisher J. Influence of space flight on red blood cells. *Fed Proc.* 1986;45(9):2285-2290.

61. Gunga HC, Kirsch K, Baartz F, et al. Erythropoietin under real and simulated microgravity conditions in humans. *J Appl Physiol (1985).* 1996;81(2):761-773.

62. Dunn C, Lange R, Kimzey S, Johnson P, Leach C. Serum erythropoietin titers during prolonged bedrest; relevance to the "anaemia" of space flight. *Eur J Appl Physiol Occup Physiol.* 1984;52(2):178-182.

63. Greenleaf JE, Vernikos J, Wade CE, Barnes PR. Effect of leg exercise training on vascular volumes during 30 days of 6 degrees head-down bed rest. *J Appl Physiol (1985).* 1992;72(5):1887-1894.

64. Sandler H. Cardiovascular effects of weightlessness and ground-based simulation. *NASA Technical Memorandum 88314,* Washington, DC: National Aeronautics and Space Administration; 1988.

65. Gaffney FA, Nixon JV, Karlsson ES, Campbell W, Dowdey ABC, Blomqvist CG. Cardiovascular deconditioning produced by 20 hours of bedrest with head-down tilt (-5 degrees) in middle-aged healthy men. *Am J Cardiol.* 1985;56(10):634-638.

66. Blomqvist C, Nixon J, Johnson RJ, Mitchell J. Early cardiovascular adaptation to zero gravity simulated by head-down tilt. *Acta Astronaut.* 1980;7(4-5):543-553.

67. Nixon JV, Murray RG, Bryant C, et al. Early cardiovascular adaptation to simulated zero gravity. *J Appl Physiol Respir Environ Exerc Physiol.* 1979;46(3):541-548.

68. Kovalenko Y, Gurovskiy N. Circulatory system change during hypokinesia. *Hypokinesia.* Moscow, Russia: Meditsina; 1980:107-208.

69. Romanov V. Quantitative evaluation of ultrastructural changes in the rat myocardium during prolonged hypokinesia [article in Russian]. *Kosm Biol Aviakosm Med.* 1976;10(7):50-54.

70. Perhonen MA, Zuckerman JH, Levine BD. Deterioration of left ventricular chamber performance after bed rest: "Cardiovascular deconditioning" or hypovolemia? *Circulation.* 2001;103(14):1851-1857.

71. Dorfman TA, Levine BD, Tillery T, et al. Cardiac atrophy in women following bed rest. *J Appl Physiol (1985).* 2007;103(1):8-16.

72. Edgell H, Zuj KA, Greaves DK, et al. WISE-2005: adrenergic responses of women following 56-days, 6 degrees head-down bed rest with or without exercise countermeasures. *Am J Physiol Regul Integr Comp Physiol.* 2007;293(6):R2343-R2352.

73. Shoemaker JK, Hogeman CS, Khan M, Kimmerly DS, Sinoway LI. Gender affects sympathetic and hemodynamic response to postural stress. *Am J Physiol Heart Circ Physiol.* 2001;281(5):H2028-H2035.

74. Fu Q, Arbab-Zadeh A, Perhonen MA, Zhang R, Zuckerman JH, Levine BD. Hemodynamics of orthostatic intolerance: implications for gender differences. *Am J Physiol Heart Circ Physiol.* 2004;286(1):H449-H457.

75. Convertino V. Cardiovascular consequences of bed rest: effect on maximal oxygen uptake. *Med Sci Sports Exerc.* 1997;29(2):191-196.

76. Convertino V, Goldwater D, Sandler H. Bedrest-induced peak VO_2 reduction associated with age, gender, and aerobic capacity. *Aviat Space Environ Med.* 1986;57(1):17-22.

77. Ferretti G, Antonutto G, Denis C, et al. The interplay of central and peripheral factors in limiting maximal O_2 consumption in man after prolonged bed rest. *J Physiol.* 1997;501(Pt 3):677-686.

78. Greenleaf J. Intensive exercise training during bed rest attenuates deconditioning. *Med Sci Sports Exerc.* 1997;29(2):207-215.

79. Greenleaf JE, Bernauer EM, Ertl AC, Trowbridge TS, Wade CE. Work capacity during 30 days of bed rest with isotonic and isokinetic exercise training. *J Appl Physiol (1985)*. 1989;67(5):1820-1826.

80. Convertino V, Bloomfield S, Greenleaf J. An overview of the issues: physiological effects of bed rest and restricted physical activity. *Med Sci Sports Exerc*. 1997;29(2):187-190.

81. Capelli C, Antonutto G, Kenfack M, et al. Factors determining the time course of VO₂(max) decay during bedrest: implications for VO₂(max) limitation. *Eur J Appl Physiol*. 2006;98(2):152-160.

82. Saltin B, Blomqvist C, Mitchell J, Johnson R, Wildenthal K, Chapman C. Response to exercise after bed rest and after training. *Circulation*. 1968;38(5 Suppl):1-78.

83. Gharib C, Maillet A, Gauquelin G, et al. Results of a 4-week head-down tilt with and without LBNP countermeasure: I. Volume regulating hormones. *Aviat Space Environ Med*. 1992;63(1):3-8.

84. Fuglsang-Frederiksen A, Scheel U. Transient decrease in number of motor units after immobilisation in man. *J Neurol Neurosurg Psychiatry*. 1978;41(10):924-929.

85. MacDougall J, Elder GS, DG, Moroz J, Sutton JR. Effects of strength training and immobilization on human muscle fibres. *Eur J Appl Physiol Occup Physiol*. 1980;43(1):25-34.

86. Zhang P, Chen X, Fan M. Signaling mechanisms involved in disuse muscle atrophy. *Med Hypotheses*. 2007;69(2):310-321.

87. Hides J, Belavy D, Stanton W, et al. Magnetic resonance imaging assessment of trunk muscles during prolonged bed rest. *Spine*. 2007;32(15):1687-1692.

88. Ferrando AA, Lane HW, Stuart CA, Davis-Street J, Wolfe RR. Prolonged bed rest decreases skeletal muscle and whole body protein synthesis. *Am J Physiol Endocrinol Metab*. 1996;270(4):E627-E633.

89. Biolo G, Ciocchi B, Lebenstedt M, et al. Short-term bed rest impairs amino acid-induced protein anabolism in humans. *J Physiol*. 2004;558(2):381-388.

90. Kortebein P, Ferrando A, Lombeida J, Wolfe R, Evans WJ. Effect of 10 days of bed rest on skeletal muscle in healthy older adults. *JAMA*. 2007;297(16):1772-1774.

91. Hather BM, Adams GR, Tesch PA, Dudley GA. Skeletal muscle responses to lower limb suspension in humans. *J Appl Physiol (1985)*. 1992;72(4):1493-1498.

92. LeBlanc AD, Schneider VS, Evans HJ, Pientok C, Rowe R, Spector E. Regional changes in muscle mass following 17 weeks of bed rest. *J Appl Physiol (1985)*. 1992;73(5):2172-2178.

93. LeBlanc A, Lin C, Shackelford L, et al. Muscle volume, MRI relaxation times (T2), and body composition after spaceflight. *J Appl Physiol (1985)*. 2000;89(6):2158-2164.

94. Bloomfield S. Changes in musculoskeletal structure and function with prolonged bed rest. *Med Sci Sports Exerc*. 1997;29(2):197-206.

95. Hides J, Richardson C, Jull G. Multifidus muscle recovery is not automatic after resolution of acute, first-episode low back pain. *Spine*. 1996;21(23):2763-2769.

96. LeBlanc AD, Spector E, Evans HJ, Sibonga J. Skeletal responses to spaceflight and the bed rest analog: a review. *J Musculoskele Neuronal Interact*. 2007;7(1):33-47.

97. Paddon-Jones D, Sheffield-Moore M, Urban RJ, et al. Essential amino acid and carbohydrate supplementation ameliorates muscle protein loss in humans during 28 days bedrest. *J Clin Endocrinol Metab*. 2004;89(9):4351-4358.

98. Vidal E, Coeli C, Pinheiro R, Camargo K. Mortality within 1 year after hip fracture surgical repair in the elderly according to postoperative period: a probabilistic record linkage study in Brazil. *Osteoporos Int*. 2006;17(10):1569-1576.

99. Vernikos-Danellis J, Leach C, Winget C, Goodwin A, Rambaut P. Changes in glucose, insulin, and growth hormone levels associated with bedrest. *Aviat Space Environ Med*. 1976;47(6):583-587.

100. Stuart CA, Shangraw RE, Prince MJ, Peters EJ, Wolfe RR. Bed-rest-induced insulin resistance occurs primarily in muscle. *Metabolism*. 1988;37(8):802-806.

101. Blanc S, Normand S, Pachiaudi C, Fortrat J-O, Laville M, Gharib C. Fuel homeostasis during physical inactivity induced by bed rest. *J Clin Endocrinol Metab*. 2000;85(6):2223-2233.

102. LeBlanc A, Driscol T, Shackelford L, et al. Alendronate as an effective countermeasure to disuse induced bone loss. *J Musculoskelet Neuronal Interact*. 2002;2(4):335-343.

103. LeBlanc A, Schneider V, Evans HE, D, Krebs J. Bone mineral loss and recovery after 17 weeks of bed rest. *J Bone Miner Res*. 1990;5:843-850.

104. Inouye M, Tanaka H, Moriwake T, Oka M, Sekiguchi C, Seino Y. Altered biochemical markers of bone turnover in humans during 120 days of bed rest. *Bone*. 2000;26(3):281-286.

105. Arnaud S, Sherrard D, Maloney N, Whalen R, Fung P. Effect of 1-week head-down tilt bed rest on bone formation and the calcium endocrine system. *Aviat Space Environ Med*. 1992;63:14-20.

106. Lueken S, Arnaud S, Taylor A, Baylink D. Changes in markers of bone formation and resorption in a bed rest model of weightlessness. *J Bone Miner Res*. 1993;8:1433-1438.

107. Cryer PR, Davis SN, Shamoon H. Hypoglycemia in diabetes. *Diabetes Care*. 2003;6:1902-1912.

108. Dinarello C, Reuven P. Fever and hyperthermia. In: Fauci A, Braunwald E, Kasper D, et al, eds. *Harrison's Principles of Internal Medicine*. 17th ed. New York, NY: McGraw-Hill; 2010.

109. Dantzer R, O'Connor JC, Freund G, Johnson R, Kelley K. From inflammation to sickness and depression: when the iimmune system subjugates the brain. *Nat Rev Neurosci*. 2008;9(1):46-56.

110. Raison C, Capuron L, Miller AH. Cytokines sing the blues: inflammation and the pathogenesis of depression. *Trends Immunol*. 2006;27(1):24-31.

111. Maes M, Yirmyia R, Norsberg J, et al. The inflammatory & neurodegenerative (I&ND) hypothesis of depression: leads for future research and new drug developments in depression. *Metab Brain Dis*. 2009;24:27-53.

112. Silverman M, Heim C, Nater U, Marques A, Sternberg E. Neuroendocrine and immune contributors to fatigue. *PM R*. 2010;2(338):338-346.

113. Barrett K, Barman S, Boitano S, Brooks H. Digestion, absorption, & nutritional principles. In: Barrett K, Barman S, Boitano S, Brooks H, eds. *Ganong's Review of Medical Physiology*. 23rd ed. New York, NY: McGraw-Hill; 2010.

114. Seyle H. *Stress in Health and Disease*. Boston, MA: Butterworth; 1976.

115. Christensen J. Stress & disease. In: Feldman M, Christensen J, eds. *Behavioral Medicine: A Guide for Clinical Practice*. 3rd ed. New York, NY: McGraw-Hill; 2010. http://accessmedicine.mhmedical.com.proxy.westernu.edu/content.aspx?bookid=373&Sectionid=39732031. Accessed May 10, 2014.

116. Chorousos G. Stress and disorders of the stress response. *Nat Rev Endocrinol*. 2009;5:374-381.

117. Raison C, Miller A. When not enough is too much: the role of insufficient glucocorticoid signaling in the pathophysiology of stress-related disorders. *Am J Psychiatry*. 2003(160):1554-1565.

118. Fitzgerald P. Endocrine disorders. In: McPhee S, Papadakis M, Tierney L, Gonzales R, Zeiger R, eds. *Current Medical Diagnosis and Treatment 2008*. New York, NY: McGraw-Hill; 2008.

119. Hueston W, Carek P, Allweiss P. Endocrine disorders. In: South-Paul J, Matheny S, Lewis E, eds. *Current Diagnosis and Treatment in Family Medicine*. 2nd ed. New York, NY: McGraw-Hill; 2008.

120. Ropper A, Brown R. The metabolic and toxic myopathies. *Adam's and Victor's Principles of Neurology*. 8th ed. New York, NY: McGraw-Hill; 2005.

121. Schrier SL. Approach to the adult patient with uremia. In: Mentzer WC, ed. UpToDate. Waltham, MA: UpToDate. Accessed May 10, 2014.

122. Linker C. Hematology. In: McPhee S, Papadakis M, Tierney L, eds. *Current Medical Diagnosis and Treatment 2008*. New York, NY: McGraw-Hill; 2008.

123. Adamson J, Longo D. Anemia and polycythemia. In: Kasper D, Braunwald E, Fauci A, et al, eds. *Harrison's Principles of Internal Medicine*. 16th ed. New York, NY: McGraw-Hill; 2005.

124. Groopman JE. Fatigue in cancer and HIV/AIDS. *Oncology (Williston Park)*. 1998;12(3):335-344; discussion 345-346, 351.

125. McCann K, Boore JR. Fatigue in persons with renal failure who require maintenance haemodialysis. *J Adv Nurs.* 2000;32:1132-1142.

126. Caro J, Salas M, Ward A, Goss G. Anemia as an independent predictor for survival in patients with cancer: a systematic, quantitative review. *Cancer.* 2001;91:2214-2221.

127. Ezekowitz J, McAlister F, Armstrong P. Anemia is common in heart failure and is associated with poor outcomes: insitghts from a cohort of 12, 065 patients with new-onset heart failure. *Circulation.* 2003;107:223-225.

128. Al-Ahmad A, Rand W, Manjunath G. Reduced kidney function and anemia as risk factors for mortality in patients with left ventricular dysfunction. *J Am Cardiol.* 2001;38:955-962.

129. Kimel M, Leidy NK, Mannix S, Dixon J. Does epoetin alfa improve health-related quality of life in chronically ill patients with anemia? Summary of trials of cancer, HIV/AIDS, and chronic kidney disease. *Value Health.* 2008;11(1):57-75.

130. Halstead C. Malnutrition and nutrition. In: Kasper D, Braunwald E, Fauci A, et al, eds. *Harrison's Principles of Internal Medicine.* 16th ed. New York, NY: McGraw-Hill; 2007.

131. Johnston C, Harper G, Landefield C. Geriatric disorders. In: McPhee S, Papadakis M, Tierney L, eds. *Current Medical Diagnosis and Treatment.* New York, NY: McGraw-Hill; 2008.

132. Gladwell M. *The Tipping Point: How Little Things Can Make a Big Difference.* Boston, MA: Back Bay Books; 2002.

133. Mock V. Cancer-related fatigue 2007. National Comprehensive Cancer Network. Clinical Practice Guidelines in Oncology. http://www.nccn.org/professionals/physician_gls/pdf/fatigue.pdf. Accessed February, 7, 2008.

134. Henry DH, Viswanathan HN, Elkin EP, Traina S, Wade S, Cella D. Symptoms and treatment burden associated with cancer treatment: results from a cross-sectional national survey in the U.S. *Support Care Cancer.* 2008;16(7):791-801.

135. Teunissen SC, Wesker W, Kruitwagen C, de Haes HC, Voest EE, de Graeff A. Symptom prevalence in patients with incurable cancer: a systematic review. *J Pain Symptom Manage.* 2007;34(1):94-104.

136. Cella D, Peterman A, Passik S, Jacobsen P, Breitbart W. Progress toward guidelines for the management of fatigue. *Oncology (Williston Park).* 1998;12(11A):369-377.

137. Jacobsen P, Hann D, Azzarello L, et al. Fatigue in women receiving adjuvant chemotherapy for breast cancer: characteristics, course, and correlates. *J Pain Symptom Manage.* 1999;18:233-242.

138. Reddy S, Elsayem A, Talukdar R. Pain management and symptom control. In: Hagop MK, R, Wolff C, eds. *The MD Anderson Manual of Medical Oncology.* New York, NY: McGraw-Hill; 2006.

139. Vogelzang NJ, Breitbart W, Cella D, et al. Patient, caregiver, and oncologist perceptions of cancer-related fatigue: results of a tri-part assessment survey. The Fatigue Coalition. *Semin Hematol.* 1997;34(3 Suppl 2):4-12.

140. Moore P, Dimsdale J. Opiods, sleep and cancer-related fatigue. *Med Hypotheses.* 2002;58:77.

141. Anderson K, Mendoza T, Valero V. Minority cancer patients and their providers: pain management attitudes and practice. *Cancer.* 2000;88:1929.

142. Hwang S, Chang V, Rue M, Kasimis B. Multidimensional independent predictors of cancer-related fatigue. *J Pain Symptom Manage.* 2003;26:604.

143. Lee JQ, Simmonds MJ, Wang XS, Novy DM. Differences in physical performance between men and women with and without lymphoma. *Arch Phys Med Rehabil.* 2003;84(12):1747-1752.

144. Stricker C, Drake D, Hoyer K, Mock V. Evidence-based practice for fatigue management in adults with cancer: exercise as an intervention. *Oncol Nurs Forum.* 2004;31(5):963-976.

145. Courneya K. Exercise in cancer survivors: an overview of research. *Med Sci Sports Exerc.* 2003;35(11):1846-1852.

146. Burnham T, Wilcox A. Effects of exercise on physiological and psychological variables in cancer survivors. *Med Sci Sports Med.* 2002;34:1863-1867.

147. Schwartz AL. Daily fatigue patterns and effect of exercise in women with breast cancer. *Cancer Pract.* 2000;8(1):16-24.

148. Schneider C, Hsieh C, Sprod L, Carter S, Hayward R. Effects of supervised exercise training on cardiopulmonary function and fatigue in breast cancer survivors during and after treatment. *Cancer.* 2007;110(4):918-925.

149. Midtgaard J, Tveterås A, Rorth M, Stelter R, Adamsen L. The impact of supervised exercise intervention on short-term postprogram leisure time physical activity level in cancer patients undergoing chemotherapy: 1- and 3- month follow-up on the body & cancer project. *Palliat Support Care.* 2006;4(1):25-35.

150. Strapczynski J. Respiratory distress. In: Tintinalli J, Kelen G, Stapczynski J, Ma O, Cline D, eds. *Tintalli's Emergency Medicine: A Comprehensive Study Guide.* 6th ed. New York, NY: McGraw-Hill; 2004.

151. Malone D, Adler J. The patient with respiratory failure—Preferred Practice Pattern 6F. In: Irwin S, Tecklin J, eds. *Cardiopulmonary Physical Therapy: A Guide to Practice.* 4th ed. St. Louis, MO: Mosby; 2004.

152. Tecklin J. The patient with ventilatory pump dysfunction/failure—Preferred Practice Pattern E. In: Irwin S, Tecklin J, eds. *Cardiopulmonary Physical Therapy: A Guide to Practice.* 4th ed. St. Louis, MO: Mosby; 2004.

153. Levitzky M. The regulation of acid-base status. In: Levitzky M, ed. *Pulmonary Physiology.* 7th ed. New York, NY: McGraw-Hill; 2007.

154. Barrett B, Vavasour H, Major A, Parfrey P. Clinical and psychological correlates of somatic symptoms in patients on dialysis. *Nephron.* 1990;55(1):10-15.

155. Curtin RB, Bultman DC, Thomas-Hawkins C, Walters BAJ, Schatell D. Hemodialysis patients' symptom experiences: effects on physical and mental functioning. *Nephrol Nurs J.* 2002;29(6):562.

156. Merkus MP, Jager KJ, Dekker FW, de Haan RJ, Boeschoten EW, Krediet RT. Physical symptoms and quality of life in patients on chronic dialysis: results of The Netherlands cooperative study on adequacy of dialysis (NECOSAD). *Nephrol Dial Transplant.* 1999;14(5):1163-1170.

157. Jablonski A. The multidimensional characteristics of symptoms reported by patients on hemodialysis. *Nephrol Nurs J.* 2007;34(1):29-37.

158. Ly J, Marticorena R, Donnelly S. Red blood cell survival in chronic renal failure. *Am J Kidney Dis.* 2004;44(4):715-719.

159. Eschbach JW, Varma A, Stivelman JC. Is it time for a paradigm shift? Is erythropoietin deficiency still the main cause of renal anaemia? *Nephrol Dial Transplant.* 2002;17(Suppl 5):2-7.

160. Moore G, Parsons D, Stray-Gundersen J, Painter P, Brinker K, Mitchell J. Uremic myopathy limits aerobic capacity in hemodialysis patients. *Am J Kidney Dis.* 1993;22(2):277-287.

161. Marrades R, Alonso J, Roca J, et al. Cellular bioenergetics after erythropoietin therapy in chronic renal failure. *J Clin Invest.* 1996;97(9):2101-2110.

162. Sala E, Noyszewski EA, Campistol JM, et al. Impaired muscle oxygen transfer in patients with chronic renal failure. *Am J Physiol Regul Integr Comp Physiol.* 2001;280(4):R1240-R1248.

163. Johansen KL, Shubert T, Doyle J, Soher B, Sakkas GK, Kent-Braun JA. Muscle atrophy in patients receiving hemodialysis: effects on muscle strength, muscle quality, and physical function. *Kidney Int.* 2003;63(1):291-297.

164. Lee SW, Park GH, Lee SW, Song JH, Hong KC, Kim MJ. Insulin resistance and muscle wasting in non-diabetic end-stage renal disease patients. *Nephrol Dial Transplant.* 2007;22(9):2554-2562.

165. Konstantinidou E, Koukouvou G, Kouidi E, Deligiannis A, Tourkantonis A. Exercise training in patients with end-stage renal disease on hemodialysis: comparison of three rehabilitation programs. *J Rehabil Med.* 2002;34(1):40-45.

166. Moinuddin I, Leehey D. A comparison of aerobic exercise and resistance training in patients with and without chronic kidney disease. *Adv Chronic Kidney Dis.* 2008;15(2):83-96.

167. Oga T, Nishimura K, Tsukino M, Sato S, Hajiro T. Analysis of the factors related to mortality in chronic obstructive pulmonary disease: role of exercise capacity and health status. *Am J Respir Crit Care Med.* 2003;167(4):544-549.

168. Casaburi R. Deconditioning. In: Fishman A, ed. *Pulmonary Rehabilitation.* Vol 91. New York, NY: Decker; 1996:213-230.

169. Maltais F, Jobin J, Sullivan MJ, et al. Metabolic and hemodynamic responses of lower limb during exercise in patients with COPD. *J Appl Physiol (1985).* May 1 1998;84(5):1573-1580.

170. Pepin V, Saey D, Laviolette L, Maltais F. Exercise capacity in chronic obstructive pulmonary disease: mechanisms of limitation. *COPD.* 2007;4(3):195-204.

171. Walke LM, Byers AL, Tinetti ME, Dubin JA, McCorkle R, Fried TR. Range and severity of symptoms over time among older adults with chronic obstructive pulmonary disease and heart failure. *Arch Intern Med.* 2007;167(22):2503-2508.

172. Wagner PD. Skeletal muscles in chronic obstructive pulmonary disease: deconditioning, or myopathy? *Respirology.* 2006;11(6):681-686.

173. Perry J. Aging with poliomyelitis. In: Kemp BJ, Mosqueda L, eds. *Aging with a Disability: What the Clinician Needs to Know.* Baltimore, MD: Johns Hopkins University Press; 2004:175-196.

174. Bartels M, Omura A. Aging in polio. *Phys Med Rehabil Clin N Am.* 2005;16(1):197-218.

175. Halstead L. Diagnosing post-polio syndrome: inclusion and exclusion criteria. In: Silver J, Gawne A, eds. *Postpolio Syndrome.* Philadelphia, PA: Hanley and Belfus; 2004:1-20.

176. Jubelt B, Agre JC. Characteristics and management of postpolio syndrome. *JAMA.* 2000;284(4):412-414.

177. Schanke A, Stanghelle J. Fatigue in polio survivors. *Spinal Cord.* 2001;39:243-251.

178. Parsons P. *Data on Polio Survivors from the National Health Review Survey.* Washington, DC: US Printing Office; 1989.

179. Bruno R, Frick N. Stress and type A behavior as precipitants of post polio sequelae. In: Halstead L, Weichers D, eds. *Research and Clinical Aspects of the Late Effects of Poliomyelitits.* White Plains, NY: March of Dimes; 1987:145-156.

180. Grimby G, Stålberg E, Sandberg A, Sunnerhagen K. An 8-year longitudinal study of muscle strength, muscle fiber size, and dynamic electromyogram in individuals with late polio. *Muscle Nerve.* 1998;21(11):1428-1437.

181. Ermstoff B, Wetterqvist H, Kvist H, Grimby G. The effects of endurance training on individuals with post-poliomyelitis. *Arch Phys Med Rehab.* 1996;78(8):107-118.

182. Arge J, Rodríguez A, Franke T. Strength, endurance and work capacity after muscle strengthening exercise in postpolio subjects. *Arch Phys Med Rehab.* 1997;78:681-686.

183. DeVivo MJ, Krause JS, Lammertse DP. Recent trends in mortality and causes of death among persons with spinal cord injury. *Arch Phys Med Rehabil.* 1999;80(11):1411-1419.

184. Kemp B, Mosqueda L. Introduction. In: Kemp B, Mosqueda L, eds. *Aging with a Disability: What the Clinician Ought to Know.* Baltimore, MD: Johns Hopkins University Press; 2004:1-5.

185. Kingbeil H, Baer H, Wilson P. Aging with a disability. *Arch Phys Med Rehabil.* 2004;85(3):S68-S73.

186. Rasekaba T, Lee AL, Naughton MT, Williams TJ, Holland AE. The Six-Minute Walk test: a useful metric for the cardiopulmonary patient. *Intern Med J.* 2009;39:495-501.

187. Bean J, Kiely D, LaRose S, Alian J, Frontera W. Is stair climb power a clinically relevant measure of leg power impairments in at-risk older adults? *Arch Phys Med Rehab.* 2007;80(5):604-609.

188. Roig M, Eng J, MacIntyre DL, Road JD, Reid WD. Associations of the Stair Climb Power Test with muscle strength and functional performance in people with chronic obstructive pulmonary disease: a cross-sectional study. *Phys Ther.* 2010;90(12):1774-1782.

189. Shumway-Cook A, Brauer S, Woolacott M. Predicting the probability for falls in community-dwelling older adults using the Timed Up & Go test. *Phys Ther.* 2000;80(9):896-903.

190. American Physical Therapy Association. *Guide to Physical Therapist Practice.* 2nd ed. Alexandria, VA: American Physical Therapy Association; 2001.

CASE STUDY 4-1

Kerri Lang, PT, DPT

EXAMINATION

History

Current Condition/Chief Complaint

Mr. Biscotti, a 68-year-old male, was referred for outpatient physical therapy by his primary care physician to address the patient's complaints of decreased endurance and weakness. Mr. Biscotti stated that he wanted to be able to walk longer distances without getting tired and "put the cane away for good." The physician script also indicated that Mr. Biscotti had previously had a myocardial infarction (MI).

Clinician Comment *Mr. Biscotti presented as a patient suffering the effects of deconditioning with the possible complication of a previous cardiac event. Actually, the physician script read, "PT for s/p MI with decreased endurance and weakness." So, was Mr. Biscotti primarily a deconditioned patient or a cardiac patient whose cardiac status limited his physical activity? That could not yet be determined but pointed the way for additional information that needed to be gathered.*

Next, it might have been tempting to pursue the medical aspects of his history to determine when the MI occurred, what was the extent of myocardium damage, and what interventions were used. Medical history, though important, is only one aspect of the information needed from the patient interview.

Social History/Environment

Mr. Biscotti had earned a high school degree and owned a produce shop. Until 5 months ago, he worked 50 to 60 hours per week. Work tasks included beginning his day at 4:00 AM to select the fruits and vegetables, then lifting the crates onto the truck and hauling the produce to the store. Occasionally, he helped with setting up the store and assisting customers. More often, however, he supervised these 2 latter tasks in order to have time to complete the office tasks necessary for the business.

Mr. Biscotti lived with his wife of 45 years. He reported she was in good health, though she had to occasionally modify her activities because of mild bilateral knee pain. His wife prepared all of the meals and completed all housecleaning tasks. Mr. Biscotti reported he had a supportive family. In addition to his wife, he noted that he had 3 grown daughters who all lived within a 15-mile radius of his home and were available to assist with his care when needed.

Mr. Biscotti lived on the second and third floors of a 2-family home. He reported he needed to ascend 30 "outside" stairs, with a hand rail on the right, to enter his home. He had only 13 stairs to ascend to get to his bedroom on the third floor of the building, but there were rails on both sides.

Clinician Comment *There are interesting regional differences to consider in patient interviews. Whereas one area in the country may be known for the great number of revolving doors to navigate, in Mr. Biscotti's region, it is the 2- or 3-family residential dwellings that need to be considered.*

True 2- and 3-family residences were built in the late 1800s and early 1900s to accommodate the large families of mill workers in mill towns. Typically, there are 4 to 5 steps, often without rails, to reach a front porch area and the front door. The front door will lead to an entry with additional doors. One door will be the entrance door to the home on the first floor. Behind a second door will be a flight of stairs to the front door of the second-floor home. Sometimes an additional door on the second-floor landing will lead to another flight of stairs to a third-home unit on a third floor. More often, however, if a third floor exists, it becomes the additional living space for the second-floor home. The latter is the situation for Mr. Biscotti's home and are the stairs that lead to the floor with his bedroom. The 30 stairs to which he referred as "outside stairs" are outside of his living area but inside the building.

This contrasts with another residential situation found in the same region. Patients may have a living area in a large house that has been divided into smaller units. Secondary exits to units on upper floors may be metal fire escape-type staircases placed on the outside of the building.

Social/Health Habits

Mr. Biscotti reported that he did not smoke and had never smoked. He reported he would occasionally have an alcoholic beverage when he would eat out for dinner.

Mr. Biscotti did not have a regular exercise program nor had he ever followed a regular program. He reported that he was active enough with his work tasks and with watching his grandchildren when they would visit.

Clinician Comment *From the interview thus far, it was learned that Mr. Biscotti needed to be able to climb stairs easily to get into his home as well as navigate within his home. He did not have experience with a regular exercise program, which has been shown to affect follow-through with a recommended regular exercise program in other patient groups.[1] Something happened 5 months prior that changed Mr. Biscotti's activity level.*

Medical/Surgical History

Mr. Biscotti reported that he had yearly physicals with his primary care physician with no significant medical history except an episode of gout. His mother died of pneumonia, and Mr. Biscotti's father died of a heart attack in his mid-70s.

Five months prior, while working around his home, Mr. Biscotti reported he began to perspire profusely and felt lightheaded. When the symptoms did not decrease after sitting down to rest for 10 minutes, he was taken by ambulance to the emergency room of a small local hospital.

From medical reports Mr. Biscotti brought with him to the initial physical therapy appointment, it could be determined that when an EKG showed changes associated with an acute MI, though the changes were not specified, heparin and Integrilin (eptifibatide) were administered to him in the emergency room.

Following a transfer to a larger regional hospital, he underwent a left heart catheterization, left ventriculography, and coronary angiography. He was diagnosed with CAD and an acute inferior wall MI, then treated with angioplasty including stinting of the mid and distal circumflex artery and second circumflex marginal artery.

A post-procedure echocardiogram confirmed the stunt placement and documented an ejection fraction (EF) of 40% to 45%. In addition, he showed mild mitral and tricuspid valve regurgitation and borderline left ventricular hypertrophy.

His troponin level on admission (128 ng/mL) had decreased to 72.9 ng/mL at discharge 2 days later. During the hospitalization, he was diagnosed with diabetes mellitus (DM) and hypertension. He was discharged with the following medications: Lipitor (atorvastatin), Toprol (metoprolol succinate), Zestril (lisinopril), Plavix (clopidogrel bisulfate), aspirin, Glucophage (metformin Hcl), and nitroglycerine; the latter as needed.

After his hospital discharge, Mr. Biscotti met with a dietician for instruction in diabetes management strategies, including monitoring blood sugar levels, making appropriate food choices, and beginning regular exercise.

Clinician Comment *Mr. Biscotti seemed unaware that he had a number of risk factors for CAD or heart attack as identified by the American Heart Association.[2] As a male over 65 years of age, with a family history of heart disease, he had all the risk factors that could not have been changed. Based on his perception (prior to his MI) that his medical status was unremarkable and that he was active enough, he might have judged that he had none of the risk factors that could have been modified; namely, use of tobacco, high cholesterol, high BP, physical inactivity, obesity, and DM. After his MI, the need to assess the modifiable risk factors was indicated.*

Chest pain is a well-known symptom indicator of a possible MI.[3] The World Health Organization cites chest pain as a diagnostic criteria for an acute MI.[4] In a cohort of patients diagnosed with an acute MI, however, 33% of the patients did not present with chest pain before admission to the hospital. When compared to the cohort, these patients were older, more likely to be female, or had a higher prevalence for DM.[5]

Mr. Biscotti arrived at the emergency room in distress but without chest pain. He was not elderly or female and did not have a diagnosis of DM at that time, so he did not even fit the characteristics noted in the study above. Fortunately, an EKG was administered and the diagnosis of an acute MI was made quickly. This allowed the timely administration of a prophylactic regimen of medications to diminish additional ischemia[6] while he was being transported to another medical center.

The normal rate for an EF, the percentage of blood that is pumped out of the ventricle with each heartbeat, is 55% to 70%.[7] At 40% to 45%, Mr. Biscotti's EF is lower than normal, but not so low as to increase his 30-day mortality rate or readmission into the hospital for failure.[8]

Mr. Biscotti's experience with altered glucose metabolism associated with an acute MI is not unusual. In a prospective study with more than 10,000 patients, 57% of patients admitted to the hospital for an acute MI with no prior history of DM had abnormal glucose metabolism at discharge.[9] In a similar cohort, 45% of patients discharged after an acute MI had impaired glucose metabolism. Less than 35% of these patients returned to normal glucose levels 3 months after discharge.[10]

Reported Functional Status

Mr. Biscotti reported that he needed to sit to dress but dressed independently. Bathing required the use of a bench in the tub for showering. He reported he was reluctant to try standing to shower. Prior to his hospitalization, he took baths but doubted that he'd be able to rise from the bathtub.

The only transfer for which he reported any difficulties in ADL was rising from, or sitting down onto, his home toilet. He was unable to do either without grabbing onto or leaning into an adjacent vanity for support.

Mr. Biscotti reported he could walk without the use of his straight cane but found he needed it when climbing or ascending stairs, or when he got fatigued. He was unable to climb the 30 stairs to his second-floor home without resting several times. He reported he became short of breath (SOB) and hunched over by the time he reached the second-floor landing and the entrance to his home.

He had reduced his work hours to 20 to 30 hours a week, leaving more of the customer service aspects of the business to his daughter and son-in-law, who worked for him. He still rose at 4:00 AM every morning to select the fruits and vegetables for the store but was no longer involved with transferring the produce to the store.

Mostly, he supervised the store's workers and operation and completed the business office tasks for the store. He found he needed to rest during his work day. He lived close enough to be able to go home to rest. However, to avoid the exertion required to climb the stairs to get into his home, he tended to rest in a recliner in the office at work.

He did not want to stop working but recognized that he might need to accept working reduced hours.

Other Relevant Information

Mr. Biscotti reported that he attended a cardiac rehabilitation program for 3 months. He noted he was inconsistent with keeping the 3 times per week schedule. He stopped when his insurance coverage ended for the program.

Clinician Comment *Patients who understand the role of exercise after an MI were more likely to participate in a cardiac rehabilitation program.[11] Mr. Biscotti was inconsistent in attendance at his cardiac rehabilitation program. He believed he was active enough with ADL, instrumental ADL (IADL), and work tasks. It did not appear, however, that he met the recommended standard of moderate activity for 30 minutes per day for 5 or more days per week to bring health benefits to his cardiovascular system, or 60 minutes 5 days per week for weight management.[12] Further, he did not appear to understand the beneficial effects of exercise not just for his cardiovascular system and, thus, his survival,[13] but for improved management of his diabetes as well.[14]*

As central as exercise appeared to be to manage Mr. Biscotti's health and improve his function, a systems review needed to be completed to determine whether he was a candidate for physical therapy and then to guide the selection of tests and measures if the examination was to move forward.

Systems Review

Cardiovascular/Pulmonary

Seated resting values: HR, 57 beats per minute (bpm); BP, 122/68 mm Hg; resting rate, 15 breaths per minute.

No edema was observed in bilateral LE. He had shown mild difficulty in carrying on a conversation when walking from the waiting area to the treatment room. By counting the number of syllables the patient uttered between breaths while walking, a dyspnea index of 2 to 3 was estimated. No dyspnea was noted in the patient's conversation during the interview.

Integumentary

No discoloration or breaks in the integument were seen. Continuity of skin color appeared normal and general pliability was normal.

Musculoskeletal

Height: 5 feet, 9 inches; Weight: 197 pounds (BMI 29.1)

His extremity and trunk range of motion were symmetrical and appeared unimpaired to gross active movements. He did show increased effort needed at end ranges of lifting each arm overhead as well as full extension of each knee, so strength appeared impaired. Mr. Biscotti's sitting and standing posture showed an increased forward lean of his trunk.

Neuromuscular

Locomotion

Impaired—Mr. Biscotti remained stooped forward after rising from the chair in the waiting area and walked to the treatment room using a slow cadence, shuffling gait. He carried his cane.

Transfers/Transitions

Impaired—Mr. Biscotti already reported that he had difficulty moving between sitting and standing with his toilet at home. Mr. Biscotti was observed requiring the assist of the arms of the chair in the waiting area to rise to standing and did not lower himself smoothly into the chair in the treatment room.

Balance

Impaired—Mr. Biscotti did not lose his balance or misstep when walking to the treatment room from the waiting area. His shuffling gait and wide-based stance in standing suggested his balance was impaired.

Motor Function

No impairment noted.

Communication, Affect, Cognition, Language, and Learning Style

Mr. Biscotti is oriented to person, place, and time. No communication problems were detected. His emotional and behavioral responses were appropriate. No learning barriers were identified. He preferred to have pictures and demonstration of exercises.

He would benefit from education regarding use of his assistive device, the role physical therapy can play with regard to his goals as well as cardiac and blood sugar health, and an exercise program. In addition, he would benefit from instruction in monitoring his response with exercise.

Clinician Comment *As shown previously, gathering information about a patient can begin with the introduction in the waiting area. Observations of the patient's movements, along with information gained in the interview, is combined with the brief examination of the systems review to guide the clinician's choice of tests and measures once the clinician has confirmed that the patient is an appropriate candidate for physical therapy.*

The system review did not uncover any findings that would exclude Mr. Biscotti as a candidate for physical therapy. In fact, the findings from the systems review combined with information from the interview assisted the selection of tests and measures to consider.

Mr. Biscotti's BMI places him in the overweight category[15] as well as at moderate risk for heart disease[2] or, in his case, continued heart disease. An exercise program at the level required to begin to assist with weight control as well as blood sugar levels required that his aerobic capacity and endurance be determined.[13]

He reported, and was observed, having difficulty moving between sitting and standing. Given that he also used increased effort with end-range extremity movements and reported difficulty on stairs, his muscle performance needed to be tested more thoroughly.

It was not clear whether he continued to sit to shower because of impaired balance or because sitting to bathe matched closer with his previous habit of tub bathing. Because of this question about his balance, as well as the observed wide-based stance, his balance needed to be assessed further.

It was also not clear whether he was able to use his cane effectively, nor was it known whether his forward posture could be corrected with verbal prompting or was due to a muscle performance impairment in postural muscle or a balance strategy.

Mr. Biscotti needed tests and measures to determine his aerobic capacity and endurance, muscle performance, balance, posture, and gait. The 6MWT was selected along with extremity manual muscle testing (MMT), Berg Balance Scale, posture screen, and gait observation. It was decided to start with the posture screen followed by the MMT to serve as an activity warm-up to the more vigorous 6MWT. Though he might be fatigued after the 6MWT, waiting to test his balance under fatigued circumstances may show a more realistic picture of his balance with functional tasks.

Mr. Biscotti was instructed in the Borg Rate of Perceived Exertion (RPE) scale before any testing was initiated. Using the RPE during the tests and measures would provide another method, in addition to vital signs, to monitor his response to the activities, and it also allowed him to gain experience using the scale before the 6MWT. The Borg scale was designed to have the RPE number chosen by the patient to reflect the actual working HR (RPE × 100 = HR).[16] Mr. Biscotti's Toprol medication could be expected to diminish his adaptive HR rise with exercise, but the RPE has still been a useful tool with cardiac patients.[17] The 6MWT has been found to be an effective tool to evaluate functional capacity even in patients with an EF < 40%.[18]

Tests and Measures

Posture

Tests were performed to determine whether Mr. Biscotti's trunk forward lean in sitting and standing was due to structural changes and could not be corrected, or due to habit. In sitting and standing, Mr. Biscotti was shown and asked to practice a "slump and then sit tall" movement. The same was repeated in standing. In both instances, he was able to correct his posture, with minimal verbal cues, to one with balanced spinal curves and aligned shoulder girdle and head/neck position. He reported an RPE of 10/20.

Muscle Performance (Including Strength, Power, and Endurance)

To ensure Mr. Biscotti did not hold his breath during MMT, he was instructed to count to 3 with the therapist during the resisted portion of each test. With Mr. Biscotti positioned in supine, side-lying, prone, and then standing, the following muscle strength grades were identified with MMT:

	RIGHT	LEFT
Iliopsoas	4–/5	4–/5
Gluteus maximus	3+/5	3/5
Gluteus medius	4–/5	4–/5
Hip adductors	4–/5	4–/5
Quadriceps	4–/5	4–/5
Hamstrings	4–/5	4–/5
Gastrocnemius	3+/5	3+/5

In hook lying, he was unable to perform a short-range sit-up or bridge. He reported an RPE of 12.

Clinician Comment *Mr. Biscotti was able to correct his posture with minimal verbal cuing in sitting and standing. Therefore, his altered posture was not structural.*

Having Mr. Biscotti avoid breath-holding with MMT minimized any CO and BP changes with isometric exercise.[19] MMT showed strength deficits throughout bilateral LEs, with the greatest deficit in left gluteus maximus (3/5), followed by the left gluteus maximus and bilateral gastrocnemius (3+/5). The decrease in hip and ankle strength needed to be considered when testing his balance performance.

Mr. Biscotti was able to use the Borg scale effectively. As anticipated, his RPE of 12 did not match the formula to predict HR. His predicted rate would have been 120 bpm based on an RPE of 12, but it was actually measured at 62 bpm. Again, the RPE has been found to be an effective measure of exertion in cardiac patients.[17]

Aerobic Capacity and Endurance

6MWT: After instruction, Mr. Biscotti walked 350 feet in 6 minutes with an RPE of 14. Immediately after stopping, he showed a HR of 99 bpm and BP of 132/64 mm Hg.

Clinician Comment *Mr. Biscotti showed an adaptation in HR and BP with increased activity from his resting values, but walked only a distance of 350 feet. Even considering the evidence that patients with an EF ≤ 40% cover less distance and, of those patients, the patients who also had DM covered even less distance, 350 feet is low.[20] He began the test walking at a slow speed and took frequent standing rests as if he wasn't certain that he could complete the test. When told he had 1 minute remaining, he increased his speed and did not take any breaks. Had he been more familiar with his ability to walk continuously for 6 minutes, he may have performed differently on the test. Nonetheless, 350 feet on the 6MWT became the baseline measure.*

Gait, Locomotion, and Balance

Gait

During the 6MWT, Mr. Biscotti walked with a slow cadence and short step length. There was little evidence of initial contact, loading response or propulsion during the stance phase of gait, bilaterally. This resulted in a shuffling gait. As he continued to walk, his corrected and erect posture began to show more and more of a forward lean.

Locomotion

Mr. Biscotti had been observed earlier having difficulty rising and moving between standing and sitting.

Balance

In a single-leg stance (SLS) test, Mr. Biscotti was able to maintain SLS on the right for 12 seconds, and on the left for less than 5 seconds. He scored 44/56 on the Berg Balance Scale (BBS). He was reluctant to perform the tasks of placing alternate feet on a step, maintaining a tandem stance position, or standing on one foot. He needed supervision to attempt standing with eyes closed and with feet together.

Clinician Comment *Muscle weakness at the hips and LEs was a risk factor for falls.[21] A score on the BBS below 45/56 suggested an increased risk for Mr. Biscotti for multiple falls, but it is not as significant as a score below 40/56.[22] Mr. Biscotti did have weakness in hip extensors and in his LEs, but he did not report a history of imbalance or falls. The latter, along with an improved performance on the BBS, would place him at a lower risk for falls.[23]*

EVALUATION

Diagnosis

Practice Pattern

Based on the information from the patient interview and findings from the systems review, tests, and measures,

Mr. Biscotti was classified into Cardiovascular/Pulmonary Pattern 6B: Impaired Aerobic Capacity/Endurance Associated with Deconditioning.

International Classification of Functioning, Disability, and Health Model of Disability

See ICF Model on page 161.

Prognosis

Mr. Biscotti had a good prognosis to improve his functional walking status, including stairs, as well as increase his ease with position changes. He could expect improved confidence with weightbearing tasks that challenged his balance.

Plan of Care

Intervention

Mr. Biscotti would benefit from instruction in the importance of regular exercise to address his deconditioning, cardiovascular risk management of weight control, and blood sugar management. Instruction would continue on self-monitoring techniques to assess his response to exercise. Exercise sessions would include aerobic reconditioning, therapeutic exercises for core and extremity musculature strengthening, and gait and balance activities.

Proposed Frequency and Duration of Physical Therapy Visits

Mr. Biscotti was to be seen 2 times per week for 6 weeks. Treatment session would begin with a 30-minute length until he was gradually able to tolerate a 60-minute session.

Anticipated Goals

1. Mr. Biscotti would be able to self-correct his posture during treatment sessions (1 week).
2. Mr. Biscotti would tolerate an initial strengthening, balance, and endurance program (2 weeks).
3. He would tolerate continuous aerobic activity for 20 minutes without rest (2 weeks).
4. He could maintain a standing position with simulated upper extremity movements as for showering (3 weeks).
5. He would show an increased ease with transfers on/off a chair the same height as his toilet at home (3 weeks).
6. Mr. Biscotti would ambulate at least 600 feet on a level surface, without an ambulation device, in 6 minutes.
7. He would be able to climb a full set of stairs without rest or SOB, using rails (5 weeks).

Expected Outcomes (6 Weeks)

1. Patient would report full independence with ADL and IADL.
2. Mr. Biscotti would report the ability to climb the 30 stairs to his home without rest with an RPE ≤ 12/20.

Discharge Plan

It was anticipated that Mr. Biscotti would achieve the anticipated goals and expected outcomes at the end of the plan of care and would be discharged to a home program of exercises and regular walking.

INTERVENTION

Coordination, Communication, and Documentation

The initial evaluation including plan of care was sent to Mr. Biscotti's referring primary care physician with plans for regular updates on Mr. Biscotti's progress toward the stated goals. All aspects of his physical therapy care were documented in Mr. Biscotti's outpatient physical therapy record.

Patient-/Client-Related Instruction

Mr. Biscotti received instruction in, and practiced, self-monitoring techniques to be used during exercise sessions. He was instructed in energy conservation strategies, including slower pace on stairs, marking time, and the correct use of his cane. Review of the printed materials and reinforcement of self-management techniques from his session with the dietician were integrated into his physical therapy sessions.

Procedural Interventions

Therapeutic Exercise

Aerobic Capacity/Endurance Conditioning or Reconditioning

Mode
Recumbent bike, upper body ergometer (UBE)
Intensity
RPE for warm-up = 7 to 8/20; for interval work = 9 to 12/20
Duration
2- to 3-minute warm-up, 5 to 10 minutes for interval work
Frequency
2 times per week
Description of the Intervention
Easy pedaling for LEs or upper extremities during warm-up. Increased speed in pedaling for LEs in timed intervals, alternating with slower speed pedaling later in treatment session.

Strength, Power, and Endurance Training

Training for head, neck, limb, pelvic floor, trunk, and ventilatory muscles
Mode
Active movements

ICF Model of Disablement for Mr. Biscotti

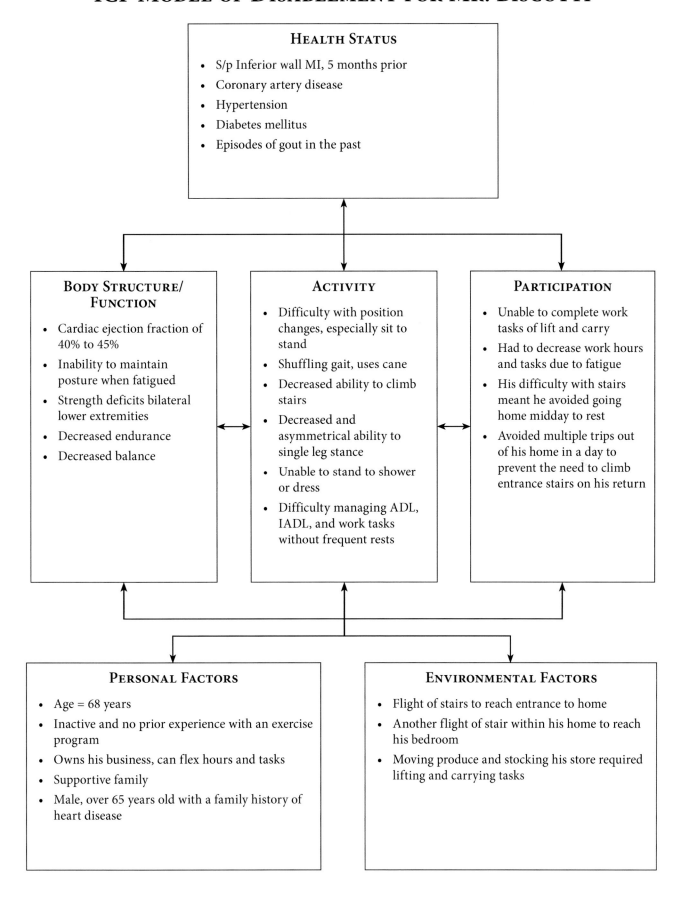

Health Status

- S/p Inferior wall MI, 5 months prior
- Coronary artery disease
- Hypertension
- Diabetes mellitus
- Episodes of gout in the past

Body Structure/Function

- Cardiac ejection fraction of 40% to 45%
- Inability to maintain posture when fatigued
- Strength deficits bilateral lower extremities
- Decreased endurance
- Decreased balance

Activity

- Difficulty with position changes, especially sit to stand
- Shuffling gait, uses cane
- Decreased ability to climb stairs
- Decreased and asymmetrical ability to single leg stance
- Unable to stand to shower or dress
- Difficulty managing ADL, IADL, and work tasks without frequent rests

Participation

- Unable to complete work tasks of lift and carry
- Had to decrease work hours and tasks due to fatigue
- His difficulty with stairs meant he avoided going home midday to rest
- Avoided multiple trips out of his home in a day to prevent the need to climb entrance stairs on his return

Personal Factors

- Age = 68 years
- Inactive and no prior experience with an exercise program
- Owns his business, can flex hours and tasks
- Supportive family
- Male, over 65 years old with a family history of heart disease

Environmental Factors

- Flight of stairs to reach entrance to home
- Another flight of stair within his home to reach his bedroom
- Moving produce and stocking his store required lifting and carrying tasks

Intensity

Low repetitions (3 sets of 5 repetitions) initially, then increasing repetitions (2 sets of 10 repetitions)

Duration

10 to 12 minutes

Frequency

2 times per week

Description of the Intervention

Standing exercises using a bar for support to complete active hip movements, short range squats, step-ups, and step-overs. Theraband exercises for upper extremities. Leg curls using a multigym. Mat exercises for core strengthening, including bridging and abdominal muscle setting with LE exercise is supine and side-lying.

Gait and Locomotion Training

Mode

Forward and backward walking, and sideways stepping

Intensity

Lengths of a 50-foot hallway, RPE < 12/20

Duration

10 to 15 minutes combined with balance activities

Frequency

2 times per week

Description of the Intervention

Forward and backward walking, and sideways stepping with bilateral handheld support, decreasing to single-hand then no-hand support in a 50-foot hallway, with seated rests after each length.

Balance, Coordination, and Agility Training

Mode

Walking on an obstacle-strewn path, static weightbearing positions

Intensity

Just enough difficulty to gently challenge his balance but not cause frequent balance losses

Duration

10 to 15 minutes combined with walking activities

Frequency

2 times per week

Description of the Intervention

Walking a 50-foot obstacle course with walking around or stepping over obstacles with bilateral hand support initially, then decreasing to single-hand then no-hand support. Also practiced SLS on balance cushions.

REEXAMINATION

Mr. Biscotti was reassessed 2 weeks after his initial evaluation.

Subjective

He reported, "I don't think I need to come to physical therapy anymore."

Objective

He reported that he was able to transfer on and off the toilet without using the bathroom vanity for leverage. He no longer used the shower chair and stood for showers without difficulty. He had not attempted a bath but noted that he was able to step over obstacles that were as high as the tub sides without difficulty. Though it was not an initial goal, he noted that he was able to get up from the exercise mat without help. He reported that the squats and step-downs in his physical therapy sessions still were his most demanding tasks and judged his effort during these tasks as RPE = 14/20.

He thought he was able to walk as much as he did before his MI. He no longer used the cane on level surfaces or stairs. Mr. Biscotti reported that if he took 2 short standing rests on the stair landings when ascending stairs at home, he could control his breathing. If he rushed or avoided the rests, he noted SOB. He had started regular walking at the local mall for 20 to 30 minutes and had already done so 5 times since beginning physical therapy. He reported sitting down or standing to rest, which might also occur when stopping to talk with someone he knew. He continued to work modified hours at 20 hours per week.

Aerobic Capacity and Endurance

His resting vital signs were HR = 56 bpm; BP = 132/66; RPE = 10/20

He completed the 6MWT without SOB and covered 800 feet. He reported his RPE while walking as 12/20. His post test vitals were HR = 79 bpm; BP = 140/62.

Strength

MMT was delayed because of time until the 1 month reevaluation.

Gait, Locomotion, and Balance

Gait

He no longer shuffled his feet when walking and had a near normal gait cadence. He still showed a decreased loading response and propulsion with a more whole foot-loaded gait pattern, but he modestly improved from the initial observations. He was able to maintain erect posture throughout the 6MWT.

Locomotion

As Mr. Biscotti noted himself, he was no longer observed having difficulty moving from sitting to standing or during more extensive position changes during treatment.

Balance

Mr. Biscotti's SLS on the right was 22 seconds, and left 16 seconds. A repeat BBS had him earning a 54/56 score.

Assessment

Mr. Biscotti reports marked improvement in his functional status. He accomplished all of the anticipated goals for the 2-week time period except tolerating continuous aerobic activity for 20 minutes without rest (#3). In fact, he had met all of the remaining anticipated goals except climbing a full set of stairs without rest or SOB (#7), projected to be met by 5 weeks.

The expected outcome goal for full independence with ADL and IADL was met, but not the stair-climbing goal for home.

Plan

To begin the transition to independent exercise, Mr. Biscotti's plan of care was amended to decrease physical therapy sessions to once per week for 3 weeks, with the stated expectation that he would continue his mall-walking program 3 times per week.

OUTCOMES

Mr. Biscotti returned for one visit and did not schedule additional visits. Calls to his home were not returned. Therefore, no final reevaluation was performed.

When Mr. Biscotti did not return for the remainder of his plan of care, the referring physician was sent a report based on the reevaluation status at 2 weeks, and Mr. Biscotti was discontinued from physical therapy.

REFERENCES

1. Iverson MD, Fossel AH, Ayers K, Palmsten A, Wang HW, Daltroy LH. Predictors of exercise behavior in patients with rheumatoid arthritis 6 months following a visit with their rheumatologist. *Phys Ther.* 2004;84:706-716.

2. American Heart Association. Understand your risk of heart attack. http://www.heart.org/HEARTORG/Conditions/HeartAttack/UnderstandYourRiskofHeartAttack/Understand-Your-Risk-of-Heart-Attack_UCM_002040_Article.jsp. Updated June 19, 2014. Accessed June 29, 2014.

3. American Heart Association. Warning signs of heart attack, stroke, and cardiac arrest. http://www.heart.org/HEARTORG/Conditions/911-Warnings-Signs-of-a-Heart-Attack_UCM_305346_SubHomePage.jsp. Accessed June 29, 2014.

4. Gillum RF, Fortmann SP, Prineas RJ, Kottke TE. International diagnostic criteria for acute myocardial infarction and acute stroke. *Am Heart J.* 1984;108:150-158.

5. Canto JG, Shlipak MG, Rogers WJ, Malmgren JA. Prevalence, clinical characteristics, and mortality among patients with myocardial infarction presenting without chest pain. *JAMA.* 2000;283:3223-3229.

6. Zafari AM. Myocardial infarction. *Medscape.* http://emedicine.medscape.com/article/155919-overview. Updated May 27, 2014. Accessed June 29, 2014.

7. Grogan M. Ejection fraction: what does it measure? Mayo Clinic. Sept. 19, 2008. http://www.mayoclinic.org/ejection-fraction/expert-answers/faq-20058286. Updated February 20, 2013. Accessed February 13, 2010.

8. Bhatia SR, Tu JV, Lee DS, Austin, PC. Outcome of heart failure with preserved ejection fraction in a population-based study. *N Engl J Med.* 2006;355:260-269.

9. Conaway DG, O'Keefe JH, Reid KJ, Spertus J. Frequency of undiagnosed diabetes mellitus in patients with acute coronary syndrome. *Am J Cardiol.* 2005;96:363-365.

10. Norhammar A, Enerz A, Nilsson G, Hamsten A. Glucose metabolism in patients with acute myocardial infarction and no previous diagnosis of diabetes mellitus: a prospective study. *Lancet.* 2002;359:2140-2144.

11. Cooper AF, Weinman J, Hankins M, Jackson G, Horne R. Assessing patients' beliefs about cardiac rehabilitation as a basis for prediction attendance after acute myocardial infarction. *Heart.* 2007;93:53-58.

12. Haskell WL, Lee IM, Pate RR, et al. Physical activity and public health: update recommendation for adults from the American College of Sports Medicine and the American Heart Association. *Circulation.* 2007;116:1081-1093.

13. Balady GJ, Williams MA, Ades PA, et al. Core components of cardiac rehabilitation/secondary prevention programs: 2007 update a scientific statement from the American Heart Association Exercise, Cardiac Rehabilitation, and Prevention Committee, the Council on Clinical Cardiology; the Councils on Cardiovascular Nursing, Epidemiology and Prevention, and Nutrition, Physical Activity, and Metabolism; and the American Association of Cardiovascular and Pulmonary Rehabilitation. *Circulation.* 2007;115:2675-2682.

14. American Diabetes Association. Physical activity/exercise and diabetes. *Diabetes Care.* 2004; 27(Suppl 1): S58-S62.

15. National Heart, Lung, and Blood Institute. Calculate your body mass index. http://www.nhlbi.nih.gov/guidelines/obesity/BMI/bmicalc.htm. Accessed April 17, 2010.

16. Borg GA. Perceived exertion: a note on "history" and methods. *Med Sci Sports.* 1973;5:90-93.

17. Scherer S, Cassady S. Rating of perceived exertion: development and clinical applications for physical therapy exercise testing and prescription. *Cardiopulm Phys Ther J.* 1999;10(4):143-147.

18. Demers C, McKelvie RS, Negassa A, Yusuf S. Reliability, validity and responsiveness of the six minute walk test in patients with heart failure. *Am Heart J.* 2001;142:698-703.

19. O'Connor P, Sforzo CA, Frye P. Effect of breathing instruction on blood pressure responses during isometric exercise. *Phys Ther.* 1989;69:757-761.

20. Tibb AS, Ennezat PV, Chen JH, et al. Diabetes lowers aerobic capacity in heart failure. *J Am Coll Cardiol.* 2005;46:930-931.

21. Kenny RA, Rubenstein LZ, Martin FC, Tinetti ME. *Guideline for the Prevention of Falls in Older Persons.* New York, NY: American Geriatrics Society Panel on Falls in Older Persons; April 15, 2001.

22. Muir SW, Berg K, Chesworth B, Speechley M. Use of the Berg Balance Scale for predicting multiple falls in the community-dwelling elderly: a prospective study. *Phys Ther.* 2008;88:449-459.

23. Shumway-Cook A, Baldwin M, Polissar NL, Gruber W. Predicting the probability for falls in community-dwelling older adults. *Phys Ther.* 1997;77:812-819.

5

Principles of Training and Exercise Prescription

Skye Donovan, PT, PhD, OCS and LeeAnne Carrothers, PT, PhD

CHAPTER OBJECTIVES

- List the general exercise benefits that are possible for an adult who follows the exercise recommendation from the joint Centers for Disease Control and Prevention (CDC) and American College of Sports Medicine (ACSM) expert panel.

- Compare and contrast the oxidative and nonoxidative pathways for adenosine triphosphate (ATP) production.

- Identify the event duration benefits of the 3 major substrates for fuel.

- Name and describe the 3 principles of training.

- Summarize the physiologic changes that occur in the cardiovascular/pulmonary system to acute versus chronic exercise interventions.

- List the chronic adaptations in response to exercise that occur in the musculoskeletal system.

- Discuss what is known about the relationship between exercise and the immune system and exercise and depression.

- Identify and define the components of exercise prescription.

- Give 2 examples of exercise prescription modification for a varied pathology.

CHAPTER OUTLINE

- Metabolic Fuel
  - Chronic Adaptations to Exercise
    - Oxidative Training
      - Nonoxidative Training
  - Clinical Relevance
- Principles of Training
  - Overload
  - Specificity
  - Reversibility
- System Changes With Exercise
  - Cardiovascular and Pulmonary Systems
    - Specific Adaptations to Exercise
      - Blood Volume
      - Cardiac Muscle
      - Blood Pressure
    - Pulmonary System
    - Considerations for Patient Care
  - Musculoskeletal System
    - Specific Adaptations to Exercise
      - Motor Recruitment
      - Muscle Hypertrophy
      - Muscle Fatigability
      - Bone Growth
    - Considerations for Patient Care
  - Immune System
    - Changes With Exercise
    - Considerations for Patient Care
  - Psychological Factors, Specifically Depression
    - Changes With Exercise
    - Considerations for Patient Care

Coglianese D, ed. *Clinical Exercise Pathophysiology for Physical Therapy: Examination, Testing, and Exercise Prescription for Movement-Related Disorders (pp 165-207).*
© 2015 Taylor & Francis Group.

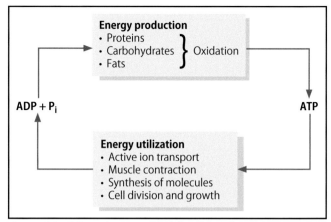

Figure 5-1. ATP as the central link between energy-producing and energy-utilizing systems of the body. ADP, adenosine diphosphate; P_i, inorganic phosphate. (Adapted from Hall JE, Guyton AC. *Guyton and Hall Textbook of Medical Physiology.* 12th ed. St. Louis, MO: Saunders Company; 2011.)

In recent years, there has been a growing interest in health and wellness, specifically the impact exercise and physical activity have on the prevention of chronic diseases. After a review of the evidence related to clinical, physiological, and epidemiologic factors associated with exercise, an expert panel from the CDC and ACSM made the following recommendation: "Every US adult should accumulate 30 minutes or more of moderate-intensity physical activity on most, preferably all, days of the week."[1(p 407)] Moderate-intensity activity (defined as requiring 3 to 6 metabolic equivalents [METs]) was chosen for its ability to produce lasting health benefits, even if there are not observable changes in maximum oxygen consumption (VO_{2max}).[2] Exercise serves as an important source both of primary and secondary prevention[3] for diseases such as cancer, coronary artery disease (CAD), obesity, diabetes, and hypertension (HTN), in addition to affecting multiple other diseases.[4,5] This prevention occurs through risk factor reduction in the form of reduced blood pressure (BP), decreased insulin needs/increased glucose tolerance, maintenance of normal blood lipids, and reduced total body fat.[2,6]

Exercise should be considered as medicine with benefits including (but not limited to) longevity, quality of life, socialization, weight control, disease prevention, and disease management. A major benefit of regular exercise is reduced morbidity and mortality associated with cardiovascular disease (CVD) and cancers. Lee and Skerrett[7] demonstrated that 1000 kcal per week of exercise decreased mortality rates by 30%, with a further 20% decrease with more than 2000 kcal/week. There is also strong evidence to support that exercise leads to improved cardiorespiratory and muscular fitness, prevention of falls, reduced depression, and better cognitive function.[8] Finally, several studies report an improved sense of well-being, better work and sport performance, and reductions in anxiety and depression.

This chapter provides an overview of the relevance of physiologic principles of training as they relate to exercise prescription. While the previous chapter presented system changes with deconditioning, this chapter will explore the "reversibility" of deconditioning through the use of exercise. Using a systems basis, the impact of exercise on the cardiorespiratory, musculoskeletal, and metabolic function is explored in this chapter. A section of the chapter will present aspects of endurance and strength training, and how the body responds according to the type of training employed. It is important to note that there are significant effects on the various systems by other training types (known as *exercise modes*), such as flexibility and balance, that will not be discussed in this chapter.

Finally, this chapter highlights the importance of thoughtful and accurate exercise prescription. Physical therapists (PTs) are experts in formulating exercise programs to meet the needs of their clients and patients. This chapter will discuss guidelines for screening for exercise readiness and recommendations for creating a thorough exercise prescription for various patient/client populations. Benefits of an appropriate exercise prescription include improving function and encouraging optimal health both in healthy individuals and those individuals with disease and dysfunctions. Although understanding principles of exercise physiology is straightforward, the application of those principles to patient populations is less so. This chapter explores exercise from the clinician's point of view, paying particular attention to the integration of physiologic principles into exercise prescription and treatment plans.

METABOLIC FUEL

The body uses 3 major substrates for fuel: fats, carbohydrates, and proteins. These substrates are broken down through various metabolic pathways into ATP to power the body for different levels of activity (Figure 5-1). Conventionally, the term *calorie* is used to denote units of energy. One calorie is the amount of energy required to use 1 g of water 1°C. Fat provides 9.4 kcal while carbohydrates and proteins provide only 4.1 kcals. At any level of activity, a combination of the 3 substrates is being used to provide energy; however, various conditions dictate their relative contributions.

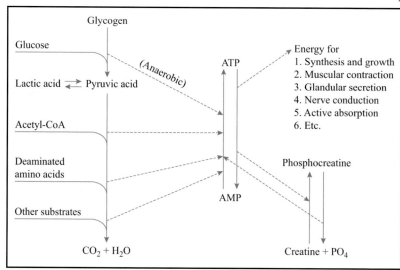

Figure 5-2. Overall schema of energy transfer from foods to the adenylic acid system and then to the functional elements of the cells. (Adapted from Hall JE, Guyton AC. *Guyton and Hall Textbook of Medical Physiology.* 12th ed. St. Louis, MO: Saunders Company; 2011.)

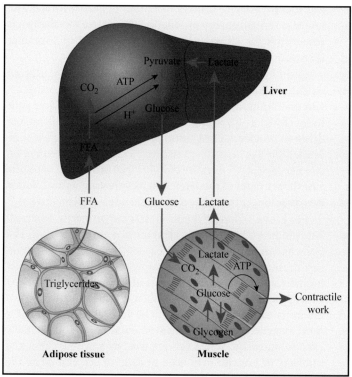

Figure 5-3. Interorgan energy transfers. (Adapted from Levy MN, Stanton BA, Koeppen BM. *Berne & Levy Principles of Physiology.* 4th ed. St. Louis, MO: Mosby; 2006.)

At rest, the majority of energy needs are derived from a combination of carbohydrates and fats. Each type and level of exercise requires different substrates and is dictated by substrate availability and metabolic efficiency. The metabolic systems that generate ATP can be divided into oxidative and nonoxidative pathways (Figure 5-2). Glycogenolysis, glycolysis, and conversion of creatine phosphate (PCr) to ATP make up the nonoxidative pathways. These pathways are rapid and are able to generate only small amounts of ATP, but can do so in the absence of or under low concentrations of oxygen (O_2). Conversely, the oxidative pathway is slower to turn on but is capable of a much greater energy yield. After initial oxidation, carbohydrates, fats, and proteins enter into the Krebs cycle and electron transport chain (located in

the mitochondria) to generate high amounts of ATP. These critical differences in timing and energy yield account for the contributions each pathway plays in exercise. It is important to note that the 2 systems do not work in isolation; rather, all of the metabolic pathways are working together during any activity.

Whole-body proportion of fat and fat-free mass also contributes to metabolic drive (Figure 5-3). Skeletal muscle has much higher metabolic activity than adipose tissue. Skeletal muscle is a key player in insulin-regulated glucose uptake, accounting for as much as 80% of whole-body glucose uptake.[9] Preservation of skeletal muscle mass has been associated with increased insulin sensitivity.[10] Likewise, it has been shown that many metabolic diseases are linked to

TABLE 5-1. SKELETAL MUSCLE FIBER TYPE AND METABOLIC PREFERENCE PROFILE

FIBER TYPE	TYPE I	TYPE IIA	TYPE IIB
Metabolic nomenclature	Slow oxidative	Fast oxidative glycolytic	Fast glycolytic
Diameter	Small	Intermediate	Large
Glycolytic enzyme activity	Low	Intermediate	High
Oxidative enzyme activity	High	Intermediate	Low
Intensity/timing of exercise	Low; unlimited	35% VO_{2max}; intermediate	65% VO_{2max}; short term
Resistance to fatigue	High	Intermediate	Low

Adapted from Thompson WR, Gordon NF, Pescatello LS, eds. *ACSM's Guidelines for Exercise Testing and Prescription.* 8th ed. Philadelphia, PA: Wolters Kluwer, Lippincott Williams & Wilkins; 2010.

abnormally functioning mitochondria. Kelley et al[11] describe that mitochondria-deficient skeletal muscle is present in type 2 diabetics and obese insulin-resistant individuals as compared with controls.

Sedentary lifestyle and aging both contribute to decreased insulin sensitivity. Studies examining obesity demonstrate impaired glucose oxidation, decreased insulin sensitivity, and mitochondrial dysfunction concurrent with excess adipose tissue.[12] It has been shown that weight loss through diet in the absence of physical activity improves insulin sensitivity and whole body metabolism.[13] The addition of exercise, however, has a unique and important impact on whole-body metabolism. This section explores the role aerobic (endurance) and anaerobic (strength/interval training) training has on altering metabolism.

Skeletal muscle largely dictates whole-body metabolism. The individual fibers that make up larger muscles are classified by their metabolic profile. Type I fibers are oxidative (slow), and Type II fibers are glycolytic (fast). There are also the intermediate Type IIa fibers, which are glycolytic-oxidative. The Type I fibers utilize aerobic metabolism and therefore can remain activated for slower, sustained exercise. They are also resistant to fatigue. Type II fibers generate energy from the nonoxidative, glycolytic pathway. These fibers fatigue quickly and are used mainly for rapid bursts of activity. There are no muscles in the body that are made of one type of fiber; all muscles are mixed-fiber type. The percentage of fiber type determines whether the muscle is used for high-force, short-term activity or low-load, long-term activity (Table 5-1).

Given equal access to substrates and activity of metabolic enzymes, the intensity and duration of exercise determines which metabolic pathway is activated. During intense, short-duration muscular effort, the body relies mostly on carbohydrates to generate ATP through nonoxidative metabolism. The nonoxidative ATP-PCr system is used during short, intense bursts of exercise less than 30 seconds in duration, and glycolysis kicks in for bouts lasting 30 seconds to 2 minutes.[14] They are usually stored as glycogen in muscle and liver and are the primary energy source for muscle. Carbohydrates are necessary to complete high-intensity exercise. Longer, less intense exercise utilizes oxidation of carbohydrates and fat for sustained energy production. Oxidative metabolism is responsible for activities lasting greater than 2 to 5 minutes (Figure 5-4).

Carbohydrates are a useful fuel to provide ATP via glucose oxidation; however, they have limits to their storage capacity. Circulating glucose is taken up into muscle and liver cells to be stored as glycogen, which can then rapidly be broken down to provide ATP. A limiting factor of glycogen use is its limited storage capacity, measuring less than one-tenth of fat storage capacity.[14] Maximized glycogen stores can typically sustain activities of moderate intensity lasting up to 2 hours; activities longer than that require glucose supplementation.[15]

For events of longer duration, fats are primarily oxidized. Fats produce a high-energy yield but at a greater O_2 cost. The body has an unlimited storage capacity for fat, but the breakdown process requires many steps and more O_2 than carbohydrate oxidation. Fat is less readily available. It is stored as triglycerides and must be broken down to free fatty acids before it can be metabolized. The increased time and O_2 need associated with fat oxidation comes at a price, namely exercise intensity. When fats are used as a primary fuel, the intensity of exercise may need to drop to accommodate the increased O_2 needed to metabolize the fats; however, the length of exercise is virtually unlimited.

The role of proteins is not to provide substantial energy for cellular activity but to act as the building blocks for the body's tissues. Although protein is not a major fuel, its metabolic contribution is affected by training. With exercise, more proteins participate in gluconeogenesis to provide glucose to the cells.[16] In general, the most important changes in protein metabolism are the rates of muscle protein synthesis and protein breakdown. Evidence has shown that exercise can improve whole-body protein levels. This anabolic result is due to the effect exercise has on insulin levels and protein synthesis rates. Insulin has been shown to inhibit muscle protein breakdown.[17] Also important in stimulating protein anabolism is the availability of appropriate substrates such as amino acids and carbohydrates.[17]

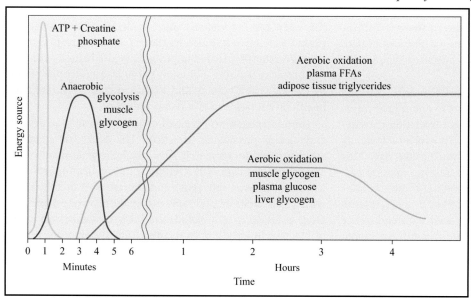

Figure 5-4. Energy sources during exercise. (Reprinted with permission from *Berne & Levy Principles of Physiology*, 4th ed, Levy MN, Stanton BA, Koeppen BM. Copyright Mosby 2006.)

Chronic Adaptations to Exercise

Oxidative Training

Endurance (aerobic) training is usually defined as low-intensity, long-duration training. This type of training primarily affects the cardiovascular/pulmonary system. From a strict metabolic standpoint, endurance-type exercise increases mitochondrial function, thereby increasing oxidative capacity.[18] It is well documented that exercise increases mitochondrial protein synthesis.[19-21] With aerobic training, mitochondria exhibit increases in their size, number, and enzyme activity. These mitochondrial changes enhance the Krebs cycle, oxidative phosphorylation, and the electron transport chain, which ultimately supplies ATP. This increase in mitochondrial function is supported by a concurrent increase in genes that encode mitochondrial proteins.[22] Hawley and Holloszy[12] provide evidence that a single bout of exercise generates a signal to elevate mitochondrial biogenesis.

All substrate utilization is improved with training, but it has its greatest effect on the capacity to oxidize fats. Exercise increases mobilization of free fatty acids, resulting in elevated circulating free fatty acids, which in turn increases the use for metabolic fuel.[23] Exercise has been shown to increase fatty acid transport in the mitochondria, sarcolemma, and at the plasma membrane in human skeletal muscle.[24] These results suggest that exercise-induced increases in skeletal muscle fatty acid oxidation are supported in part by fatty acid transport.[25] Enhanced fatty acid oxidation allows glucose substrates to be relatively preserved. This so-called *glycogen-sparing effect* enables the body to maintain its glucose/glycogen stores, which plays a role in delaying muscle fatigue.[26]

Endurance exercise also improves carbohydrate metabolism. Insulin sensitivity is improved with exercise, as evidenced by increased expression of the insulin-sensitive glucose transporter, GLUT4. Both the number and concentration of GLUT4 transporters increases in skeletal muscle in response to exercise.[27-29] This increase in GLUT4 promotes cellular glucose uptake, the first step in carbohydrate metabolism and glycogen synthesis. Overall, endurance training increases liver and muscle glycogen reserves, and decreases glycogen depletion—both of which help stave off fatigue.[16]

Nonoxidative Training

Nonoxidative training can be defined as short, high-intensity interval training. It is important to note that strength training falls into this category. In general, exercise most enhances oxidative metabolism as opposed to glycolytic metabolism. In order to improve glycolytic capacity, training needs to specifically match the event. Activities relying on anaerobic metabolism would benefit by engaging in high-intensity, brief-duration training. The anaerobic system relies on ATP-PCr and lactic acid to provide energy. A training program that stresses these systems will produce the desired results, namely enhanced speed and performance.

Sprint training has been shown to target glycolytic enzyme activity. With increased glycolytic enzymes (lactate dehydrogenase, phosphofructokinase, and glycogen phosphorylase), utilization of glucose and glycogen is more efficient.[30] Glycogenolysis rates are increased with interval training, allowing substrate to be released faster in trained than in untrained muscle.[30] Interval training has also been shown to increase ATP-PCr turnover.[31] Short bouts of sprint training have been shown to increase both myokinase and creatine phosphokinase, resulting in more rapid breakdown of PCr.[32] In addition, trained muscle maintains higher storage of ATP and PCr as compared with untrained muscle.[12,33] A study investigating strength training demonstrated trained muscle exhibited increased PCr and glycogen storage and subsequent increased ability to generate ATP.[34] An unavoidable consequence with anaerobic training is the build-up of lactic acid. Despite the improvements in ATP generation, there also need to be lactate-handling changes that occur in muscle for enhanced performance in anaerobic activities. Both the muscle's capacity for lactate and speed of lactate clearance are improved with exercise. It has been shown that with training, less lactate accumulates in muscle for a given workload; whether it is decreased production or increased clearance is yet to be elucidated.[35]

Recent studies demonstrate that sprint interval training promotes similar metabolic adaptations to endurance training. Both types of training increase lipid oxidation through increased mitochondrial enzyme activity, which secondarily promotes glycogen and PCr sparing during exercise. This evidence suggests that high-intensity training may be sufficient and a more time-efficient method to promote similar changes than endurance training.[36] The key to short, intense bouts of training mimicking changes seen with endurance training is the subject's need to endure a significant metabolic stress.[37]

Clinical Relevance

Not to overshadow training specificity, it is important realize that all metabolic pathways are used to some extent during different activities, albeit their percentage of contribution may be minimal. There is merit in stressing each of the metabolic pathways by incorporating various types of training for meeting goals. For example, it is important for the sprinter to engage in aerobic training to establish an appropriate aerobic base. This will allow the athlete to withstand the more intense anaerobic training needed for his or her event.[23] Likewise, the older adult whose goal is to ambulate community distances would benefit from some anaerobic training to assist with more taxing tasks such as climbing stairs.

PRINCIPLES OF TRAINING

Exercise is a perceived stress to the body that triggers an adaptive response resulting in physiologic benefits. With repeated exposure to exercise, the body is able to adjust to the challenge (eg, by improved strength, O_2 capacity, and flexibility). The manner in which the body responds to exercise is dependent on how and to what degree exercise is performed. Three principles—overload, specificity, and reversibility—govern response to exercise and are the foundation for effective exercise prescriptions. A recent publication reviewed the use of exercise prescription for breast cancer survivors and found that, of the 29 papers reviewed, none of them applied all of the principles of training (specificity was applied by 64%, progression by 41%, overload by 31%).[38] PTs must have a thorough understanding of these principles in addition to the role they play across the wellness spectrum for their patients and clients.

Overload

The overload principle states that, in order for the body to change in response to exercise, it must receive a load higher than what it is normally exposed to. In other words, the body and its systems must undergo relative stress to promote changes. It is also important to stress the difference between intensity needed to promote health benefits vs high-performance training. For many patients, exercise prescribed by the PT is at a volume and workload commensurate with health promotion and risk factor reduction.

Initial exposure to overload commonly results in fatigue and altered physiologic function. The body has immediate reactions to increased load, including localized skeletal muscle damage with strength training, disproportionate increases in heart rate (HR) and shortness of breath (SOB) with aerobic activity, and rapid metabolic substrate depletion. Once exercise is terminated, the body undergoes an array of changes in an effort to recover from the imposed stress. These changes include (but are not limited to) increasing the number of red blood cells (RBCs) and mitochondria, repair of skeletal muscles, and activation of antioxidant enzymes. This recovery is more of an adaptation that will allow the body to sustain greater levels of similar type of stress. In effect, the body is attempting to acclimate to the imposed demands and to better prepare the body for the next bout of exercise.

This beneficial remodeling is dependent on appropriate selection of exercise specific to the patient/client. Exercise below the adequate intensity threshold will not elicit the adaptation response and will not promote beneficial changes. Overload is commonly described as high-force contractions or metabolic stress demands placed on the body. Metabolic stress, namely substrate availability and rate of depletion, is greatest in endurance activities, where high force contractions are usually used in short bursts of activity or in strength training.[39] The overload principle also states that intensity must increase over time to continue to promote and sustain change. It is important to note that intensity does not have to be on a steady unending climb; rather, incorporating periods of relative rest and changing mode of exercise may be a better way to get desired results.

The ACSM recommends training intensities of 60% to 70%[1] repetition maximum (RM) for strengthening and 60% to 80% of VO_{2max} for cardiovascular fitness in healthy adults.[2] PTs should view these recommendations as guidelines and modify as needed for varying patient populations. Appropriate monitoring before, during, and after exercise is necessary to determine the appropriate training load for patients. Conventional methods of monitoring include HR, BP, resting rate (RR), and rate of perceived exertion (RPE).

This illustrates the importance both of establishing baseline and incorporating progression into PT exercise prescriptions. Clinicians must adequately stress the system to produce change, but also do so in a safe manner in order to protect the patients. Initially, the demand placed on the body systems should be greater than at rest but not so difficult that the patient will decompensate and not be able to complete the exercise bout. PTs must prudently alter rehabilitation programs to either increase resistance, sets, repetitions, or total time of exercise. As the patient improves, the intensity of the exercise should increase to meet the anticipated goals leading to the expected outcomes established by the PT and the patient.

Specificity

Different types of exercise exert different physiologic benefits, which is the underlying principle of specificity. It stands to reason that adaptations occur in only systems that are actively stressed. The type and robustness of the adaptations are also specific to the training stimulus. The explicit gains from exercise are restricted to the location and/or system receiving the imposed demand. For instance, resistive upper extremity (UE) exercises do not improve lower extremity (LE) strength, nor does strength training improve aerobic capacity.

Specificity is addressed within the framework of exercise prescription by the mode of exercise selected by the PT. In choosing the right mode of exercise, the PT can alter systems of the body that will ultimately produce the best functional improvements. For example, individuals who require improvements in range of motion (ROM) will benefit most from flexibility training as opposed to endurance or strength training. It is extremely important to select activities that will match desired outcomes. From a broader perspective, it is important to realize that functional tasks incorporate many individual skills. For example, gaining community ambulation function may require exercise modes to improve strength, aerobic endurance, balance, and flexibility.

There is little transfer of skill from one training program to another, which encourages the use of task-specific training. From a rehabilitation perspective, it is imperative to prescribe exercises that will promote carryover to functional activities. For example, for a person with chronic obstructive pulmonary disease (COPD), light resistance training will help strengthen accessory breathing muscles, while endurance training will help with ambulating community distances. As noted in a study by Ries et al,[40] balance training significantly improved balance performance and decreased risk of falls in patients with Alzheimer's disease.[40] This is especially interesting because it implies that cognition regarding the exercises does not need to play a role in promoting adaptations. Other studies demonstrate the restricted transfer of skill to other systems outside of those specifically trained. Young describes that, although strength training improves body mass and muscle hypertrophy, it has little impact on sports performance.[41] This review article also states that sports-specific exercise prescription is necessary to achieve maximal performance. Another example is noted in a paper by Potdevin et al[38] describing plyometric training that was employed in swimmers. It was shown that only the dive and turns (plyometric activities during swimming) improved with this type of training, and there was no effect on kick propulsion or stroke refinement.[38]

Prescribing the type of exercise includes many variables such as deciding what metabolic system to stress, type of contraction utilized, and patient position for exercise. It is also important to consider what types of exercise the patient enjoys and to incorporate those into the prescription. The PT is well trained to creatively design exercises that will best benefit the patient while recognizing the implications of the training on overall function.

Reversibility

Reversibility refers to the temporary nature of the benefits of exercise; the benefits of exercise are not maintained if exercise is discontinued. The loss of physiologic adaptations with the termination of or a gross reduction in training is defined as *detraining*. A decrease in either the intensity or the frequency in training may result in physiologic decline. In order to sustain the beneficial changes associated with exercise, a maintenance plan of persistent and regular exercise must be carried out.

Termination of endurance training induces negative changes in the cardiovascular system, including decreased blood plasma volume, cardiac contractility, left ventricular (LV) mass, and VO_{2max}. A rapid decline in aerobic capacity is seen with detraining, including a 10% to 17% decrease in stroke volume (SV) seen in just 12 to 21 days,[42-44] and a 3.6% to 14% reduction in VO_{2max} in 2 to 4 weeks.[42,43,45-53] There are also accompanying metabolic changes such as a decrease in mitochondrial number and enzyme activity resulting in a diminished oxidative capacity.[54] Insulin sensitivity and glycogen storage capacity is also reduced, negatively affecting carbohydrate metabolism.[48,55-60] Cessation of strength training results in loss of power, force, and speed. Fiber cross-sectional area also declines, primarily in Type II fibers with disuse over several weeks.[48,61] Importantly, all of these changes can be avoided by engagement in proper maintenance programs.

In order to prevent detraining, an exercise program must either sustain the intensity or frequency of the prior level of exercise. Despite a one-third to two-thirds decrease in training duration, healthy adults are able to maintain aerobic capacity while keeping the intensity of their work elevated.[54] The same is true for strength training; exercising only 1 to 2 times per week but using an intense workload will maintain strength for up to 20 weeks.[54] Maintenance programs can be designed to prevent atrophy and loss of strength or to preserve aerobic capacity, flexibility, and function. The PT must consider this fact not only while treating the patient, but, more important, on discharge. It is crucial to educate the patient on the reversibility of exercise benefits. PTs should encourage patients to engage in exercise of an appropriate intensity that will sustain health and to find an enjoyable exercise routine that will help with long-term compliance.

SYSTEM CHANGES WITH EXERCISE

Cardiovascular and Pulmonary Systems

The cardiorespiratory system has many roles in the body. It serves as an O_2 and nutrient delivery system, aids

TABLE 5-2. CHRONIC ADAPTATIONS IN THE CARDIOVASCULAR SYSTEM IN RESPONSE TO EXERCISE

- Increased venous return
- Increased contractility
- Decreased resting HR
- Increased SV and cardiac output
- Increased coronary perfusion
- Increased blood volume
- Increased blood flow
- Decreased resting SBP
- Increased O_2 extraction

in thermoregulation and immune function, and helps rid the body of unwanted materials. During exercise, incredible demands are placed on the body, many of which are met by the cardiorespiratory system. Fortunately, this system responds readily to exercise and is able to adapt according to the needs of the body.

PTs recommend exercise to a wide variety of patient populations because of the beneficial effects on the cardiorespiratory system (Table 5-2). Engaging in cardiovascular (aerobic) training promotes an increase both in health and fitness. In addition, exercise may be used as an intervention for a variety of cardiovascular disorders and also as a preventive measure against chronic disease.

Regular exercise improves venous return and heart contractility, while beneficially lowering systolic BP (SBP).[62] Both the intensity and the duration of exercise are important factors in dictating changes in the cardiorespiratory system. Moderate to vigorous activity is beneficial in the prevention of CVD.[63,64] Currently, the ACSM recommends healthy adults engage in cardiovascular exercise at a "moderate to vigorous activity for a minimum of 30 minutes at least 5 days per week."[2(p 8)] Vigorous exercise has the greatest impact on the cardiorespiratory system but moderate exercise can benefit those who are not medically stable enough to undergo vigorous intensity exercise.[65] A study by Zheng et al substantiates that walking at an intensity of 8 METs 30 minutes per day/5 times per week reduces the risk of congestive heart disease by 19%.[66] Most adaptations occur in this system in response to aerobic exercise. While there are some changes noted with anaerobic and resistance training, those effects are negligible compared to aerobic activity. There are important acute and long-term changes resulting from exercise therapy. This section will primarily focus on the chronic adaptations (see Figure 5-1).

Specific Adaptations to Exercise

Blood Volume

Blood is made of up several elements that aid in O_2 delivery (RBCs and hemoglobin), immunity (white blood cells), coagulation (platelets), temperature regulation, and pH balance. Regular exercise improves the O_2 transport system by increasing total blood volume, the number of RBCs, and hemoglobin.[67] While plasma volume increases immediately in response to exercise, RBC and hemoglobin volume take days to weeks to increase.[67] This increase in O_2 delivery capacity allows the body to respond to the increased demand of exercise.

Cardiac Muscle

Chronic exercise also allows the heart to maintain a lower HR for a given workload than that of an untrained individual. With training, the heart undergoes long-term changes in contractility and decreased overall myocardial VO_2, reducing demand, accounting for lower HR. After 10 to 20 weeks of habitual training, resting HR has been shown to decrease by 5 beats per minute (bpm) with the potential to decrease 1 to 2 bpm every 1 to 2 weeks in sedentary individuals.[14] This change is beneficial because a lower resting HR increases physiologic reserve, which will be available to the body in times of stress. This decreased resting HR does not, however, compromise the overall blood supply to the body. A slower HR allows for increased filling of the LV. Increased filling beneficially places the wall of the LV on a slight stretch, allowing the LV to more effectively eject, through the Frank-Starling effect.[68] This improved contractility results in an increased SV, defined as the amount of blood ejected from the left ventricle with each contraction. Improved SV is often noted as a hallmark of cardiovascular endurance. With chronic exercise, elevated SV is present even at rest; a sedentary individual has an average SV of 65 mL, whereas a trained individual can average 110 mL.[23] Regular training allows for increased cardiac output (CO) at rest, largely due to increased SV and not HR, as training decreases resting HR. Increased SV also depends on the volume of blood that returns to the heart, the capacity of the LV, and the resistance (afterload) the heart needs to work against.

The size of the myocardium, especially the LV, has the capacity to enlarge with regular aerobic training. Usually only noted in endurance-trained athletes, both the wall thickness and the internal chamber diameter increase in response to stresses endured by the LV. The thickened wall has more muscular mass and therefore is more powerful and augments LV contractility. The increased chamber diameter is caused by the increase in ventricular filling secondary to increased plasma volume and diastolic filling. These adaptations are particularly beneficial to deliver O_2 to exercising tissue.

Myocardial contractility improves with interval training even with severe CVD.[69] Cardiac rehabilitation programs have been shown to significantly decrease cardiac mortality

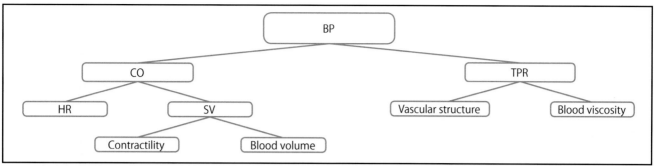

Figure 5-5. BP regulation.

up to 25% as compared with usual care.[70,71] Evidence indicates that with adherence to a cardiac rehabilitation program, changes in fitness, risk, and quality of life can continue to be seen for up to 5 years after the initial event.[72]

Blood Pressure

Habitual exercise benefits the hemodynamic system in many ways, of which the most profound is overall BP-lowering capability (Figure 5-5). A meta-analysis conducted in 2002 demonstrated that all frequencies, intensities, and types of aerobic exercise lowered BP both in normotensive and hypertensive subjects of varying ethnic groups and body weight.[73] Exercise influences various factors that play a role in determining BP, including decreasing amounts of circulating norepinephrine, increasing vasodilatory substances, reducing insulin resistance, and directly affecting the kidney.[74-78] The exact mechanism of how regular exercise lowers BP is unknown. The first of 2 hypotheses states that exercise training reduces HR and CO at rest and that contributes to lower BP. An alternative theory supports the concept that immediate hypotension that follows individual exercise sessions can have an additive response by repeating bouts on successive days, resulting in ultimately lower BP.[79-81]

It is well established that exercise is a highly successful strategy to prevent and treat HTN.[81,82] Sedentary individuals have a 35% to 70% greater risk of developing HTN as compared with age-matched subjects who were physically active.[83-85] Chronic HTN is the primary risk factor for the development of coronary vascular disease.[83-85] Sedentary lifestyle has been shown to be an independent risk factor relating to cardiovascular mortality.[86-90] Increased activity is the best way to decrease risk of CAD.[90-92]

Aerobic exercise in hypertensive subjects lowers BP in all ages and genders.[80,82,93] Multiple studies report that regular physical activity lowers both SBP and DBP by 8 to 10 mm Hg in patients with HTN.[86,94-96] Over a period of 16 weeks, patients with severe HTN who engaged in regular exercise exhibited a decrease in SBP and diastolic BP (DBP), LV mass, and the need for HTN-lowering drugs.[78] The clearest benefits are achieved by exercise set at an intensity of 40% to 60% VO_{2max}.[1,90,91]

Pulmonary System

Exercise training over time does not favor notable benefits to the respiratory system in healthy subjects as opposed to what is seen in the heart and circulatory system. The pulmonary system has been described as being "overbuilt," in that a large respiratory reserve already exists to allow the body to withstand and meet the demands of heavy exercise.[23] Despite this reserve, there are modest improvements seen with long-term training. Improved respiratory strength and endurance have been reported to take 6 to 10 weeks to occur and are seen across all age groups with land- and water-based exercise.[23] In those with diminished lung capacities, long-term exercise is especially beneficial, promoting changes in an accelerated time frame.

Clinicians use exercise in patients with respiratory disorders with the goal of improving aerobic capacity and submaximal exercise tolerance. Resistance training of ventilatory pump muscles using intensity of 30% maximum inspiratory pressure has been shown to improve respiratory muscle strength.[97] This intensity has been cited to be the minimal resistance needed to promote functional improvements. Additionally, UE resistance exercises, which stress accessory breathing muscles, have been noted to positively affect quality of life while decreasing fatigue in those suffering from COPD.[98] A recent study by Kortianou et al[98] suggests that interval training is also a good method to train the pulmonary system. Integrating periods of rest allowed patients to exercise at a higher intensity than they were able to when completing a continuous exercise session, which then equated to the same total work. In patients with COPD, exercise has been shown to improve surfactant levels, which helps to reduce surface tension in the alveoli, making it easier to breathe.[99] Additionally, it has been shown that exercise may help with desensitization toward dyspnea and increasing overall exercise capacity.[97]

Considerations for Patient Care

Ultimately, the goal of training the cardiorespiratory system is to enable patients to return to activities of daily living within the limits imposed by their disease. In order to maximize cardiorespiratory endurance, the exercise program must sustain a considerable increase in O_2 consumption and should use a large amount of muscle mass. Examples of exercise modes that accomplish this are cycling, brisk walking, jogging, and swimming. The ideal frequency of this endurance-promoting exercise is 20 to 60 minutes per day, 3 to 5 times per week. Intensity should be above the

TABLE 5-3. ATHEROSCLEROTIC CARDIOVASCULAR DISEASE RISK FACTOR THRESHOLDS

POSITIVE RISK FACTORS DEFINING CRITERIA

Age	Men ≥45 years; women ≥55 years
Family history	Myocardial infarction, coronary revascularization, or sudden death before 55 years of age in father or other male first-degree relative, or before 65 years of age in mother or other female first-degree relative
Cigarette smoking	Current cigarette smoker or those who quit within the previous 6 months or exposure to environmental tobacco smoke
Sedentary lifestyle	Not participating in at least 30 minutes of moderate intensity (40% to 60% O_2 uptake reserve) physical activity on at least 3 days of the week for at least 3 months
Obesity[a]	Body mass index ≥30 kg/m^2 or waist girth > 102 cm (40 inches) for men and > 88 cm (35 inches) for women
HTN	SBP ≥140 mm Hg and/or DBP ≥90 mm Hg, confirmed by measurements on at least 2 separate occasions, or on antihypertensive medication
Dyslipidemia	Low-density lipoprotein cholesterol (LDL-C) 130 mg/dL^{-1} (3.37 mmol/L^{-1}) or high-density lipoprotein cholesterol (HDL-C) 40 mg/dL^{-1} (1.04 mmol/L^{-1}) or on lipid-lowering medication. If total serum cholesterol is all that is available, use 200 mg/dL^{-1} (5.18 mmol/L^{-1})
Prediabetes	Impaired fasting glucose fasting plasma glucose 100 mg/dL^{-1} (5.50 mmol/L^{-1}) but 126 mg/dL^{-1} (6.93 mmol/L^{-1}) or impaired glucose tolerance 2-hour values in oral glucose tolerance test 140 mg/dL^{-1} (7.70 mmol/L^{-1}) but 200 mg/dL^{-1} (11.00 mmol/L^{-1}) confirmed by measurements on at least 2 separate occasions

NEGATIVE RISK FACTOR-DEFINING CRITERIA

High-serum HDL-C	≥ 60 mg/dL^{-1} (1.55 mmol/L^{-1})

It is common to sum risk factors in making clinical judgments. If HDL is high, subtract 1 risk factor from the sum of positive risk factors, because high HDL decreases CVD risk.

[a]Professional opinions vary regarding the most appropriate markers and thresholds for obesity; therefore, allied health professionals should use clinical judgment when evaluating this risk factor.

Reprinted with permission from Thompson WR, Gordon NF, Pescatello LS, eds. *ACSM's Guidelines for Exercise Testing and Prescription.* 8th ed. Philadelphia, PA: Wolters Kluwer, Lippincott Williams & Wilkins; 2010.

training threshold but below that which induces abnormal clinical signs and symptoms. This intensity typically falls between 50% to 80% VO_{2max} for a healthy adult.[2] Note that the PT may need to adjust accordingly to baseline fitness level; someone of low fitness may start (and see gains) at 40% to 50% VO_{2max} and may exercise only for a much shorter time frame (eg, 5 to 7 minutes). To see continued gains, the program should be progressed at the rate of a 10% increase in volume per week.

Baseline exercise testing and monitoring throughout training are of paramount importance. The ACSM recommends that individuals with 2 or more risk factors undergo a graded exercise test before starting an exercise regimen of vigorous intensity, while those who have known CVD require an exercise test both for moderate and vigorous activities (see Tables 5-1, 5-3, and 5-4). Additionally, the ACSM recommends males over the age of 40 years and females over the age of 50 years also receive a graded exercise test before engaging in vigorous activity.[2] All other patients are appropriate for a submaximal field test, given there are no absolute contraindications to exercise (Table 5-5). Field tests are easy to administer, are inexpensive, and require little equipment, making them suitable for use in various clinical settings.

Field tests enable the PT to estimate the patient's workload (VO_2) based on simple measurement techniques including HR and distance traveled. While VO_2 is important to determine, it is technically difficult, expensive, and burdensome to patients, again highlighting the role of field testing in the clinic. Selection of the appropriate cardiorespiratory endurance field test is dependent on the patient presentation and reliability/validity data for those tests in the given population. Some of the most common field tests used to determine cardiorespiratory fitness include the Rockport 1-Mile Walk Test, the 6-Minute Walk Test (6MWT), and the YMCA Step Test. Detailed instructions for these tests, including stratification tables, can be found in ACSM publications.[2] Proper monitoring is an important part of field testing before, during, and after the test. HR, RPE, BP, and workload are often used as methods of monitoring for field tests.

TABLE 5-4. ACSM MAJOR SIGNS OR SYMPTOMS SUGGESTIVE OF CARDIOVASCULAR, PULMONARY, OR METABOLIC DISEASE

SIGN OR SYMPTOM	CLARIFICATION/SIGNIFICANCE
Pain, discomfort (or other anginal equivalent) in the chest, neck, jaw, arms, or other areas that may result from ischemia	One of the cardinal manifestations of cardiac disease, in particular CAD Key features favoring an ischemic origin include the following: • Character: Constricting, squeezing, burning, "heaviness" or "heavy feeling" • Location: Substernal, across mid-thorax, anteriorly; in one or both arms, shoulders; in neck, cheeks, teeth; in forearms, fingers in interscapular region • Provoking factors: Exercise or exertion, excitement, other forms of stress, cold weather, occurrence after meals Key features against an ischemic origin include the following: • Character: Dull ache, "knife-like," sharp, stabbing, "jabs" aggravated by respiration • Location: In left submammary area; in left hemithorax • Provoking factors: After completion of exercise, provoked by a specific body motion
SOB at rest or with mild exertion	Dyspnea (defined as an abnormally uncomfortable awareness of breathing) is one of the principal symptoms of cardiac and pulmonary disease. It commonly occurs during strenuous exertion in healthy, well-trained persons and during moderate exertion in healthy, untrained persons. However, it should be regarded as abnormal when it occurs at a level of exertion that is not expected to evoke this symptom in a given individual. Abnormal exertional dyspnea suggests the presence of cardiopulmonary disorders, in particular LV dysfunction or COPD.
Dizziness or syncope	Syncope (defined as a loss of consciousness) is most commonly caused by a reduced perfusion of the brain. Dizziness and, in particular, syncope during exercise may result from cardiac disorders that prevent the normal rise (or an actual fall) in CO. Such cardiac disorders are potentially life threatening and include severe CAD, hypertrophic cardiomyopathy, aortic stenosis, and malignant ventricular dysrhythmias. Although dizziness or syncope shortly after cessation of exercise should not be ignored, these symptoms may occur even in healthy persons as a result of a reduction in venous return to the heart.
Orthopnea or paroxysmal nocturnal dyspnea	Orthopnea refers to dyspnea occurring at rest in the recumbent position that is relieved promptly by sitting upright or standing. Paroxysmal nocturnal dyspnea refers to dyspnea, beginning usually 2 to 5 hours after the onset of sleep, which may be relieved by sitting on the side of the bed or getting out of bed. Both are symptoms of LV dysfunction. Although nocturnal dyspnea may occur in persons with COPD, it differs in that it is usually relieved after the person relieves him- or herself of secretions rather than specifically by sitting up.
Ankle edema	Bilateral ankle edema that is most evident at night is a characteristic sign of heart failure or bilateral chronic venous insufficiency. Unilateral edema of a limb often results from venous thrombosis or lymphatic blockage in the limb. Generalized edema (known as *anasarca*) occurs in persons with nephrotic syndrome, severe heart failure, or hepatic cirrhosis.
Palpitations or tachycardia	Palpitations (defined as an unpleasant awareness of the forceful or rapid beating of the heart) may be induced by various disorders of cardiac rhythm. These include tachycardia, bradycardia of sudden onset, ectopic beats, compensatory pauses, and accentuated SV resulting from valvular regurgitation. Palpitations also often result from anxiety states and high CO (or hyperkinetic) states, such as anemia, fever, thyrotoxicosis, arteriovenous fistula, and the so-called *idiopathic hyperkinetic heart syndrome*.

(continued)

TABLE 5-4 (CONTINUED). ACSM MAJOR SIGNS OR SYMPTOMS SUGGESTIVE OF CARDIOVASCULAR, PULMONARY, OR METABOLIC DISEASE

SIGN OR SYMPTOM	CLARIFICATION/SIGNIFICANCE
Intermittent claudication	Intermittent claudication refers to the pain that occurs in a muscle with an inadequate blood supply (usually as a result of atherosclerosis) that is stressed by exercise. The pain does not occur with standing or sitting, is reproducible from day to day, is more severe when walking upstairs or up a hill, and is often described as a cramp, which disappears within 1 to 2 minutes after stopping exercise. CAD is more prevalent in persons with intermittent claudication. Patients with diabetes are at increased risk for this condition.
Known heart murmur	Although some may be innocent, heart murmurs may indicate valvular or other CVD. From an exercise safety standpoint, it is especially important to exclude hypertrophic cardiomyopathy and aortic stenosis as underlying causes because these are among the more common causes of exertion-related sudden cardiac death. Although there may be benign origins for these symptoms, unusual fatigue or SOB also may signal the onset of or change in the status of usual activities of cardiovascular, pulmonary, or metabolic disease. These signs or symptoms must be interpreted within the clinical context in which they appear because they are not all specific for cardiovascular, pulmonary, or metabolic disease.

Adapted from Gordon S, Mitchell BS. Health appraisal in the non-medical setting. In: Durstine JL, King AC, Painter PL, eds. *ACSM's Resource Manual for Guidelines for Exercise Testing and Prescription.* 2nd ed. Philadelphia, PA: Lea & Febiger; 1993:219-228.

PTs often use HR to determine appropriate exercise intensity. Calculating a patient's maximum HR (HR_{max}) is clinically relevant as it is a direct correlate to percentage workload. A common equation used to estimate an individual's maximal HR is $HR_{max} = 220 - age$ (in years); however, this equation yields as much as a 10 mm Hg error.[100,101] In addition, this estimate cannot be used for children younger than age 16 years.[102] Many clinicians instead choose to use the Karvonen formula to determine HR reserve (HRR) calculated as $HRR = HR_{max} - HR_{rest}$.[23] Exercise intensity is then prescribed at a range of HR_{max} or HRR. The ACSM recommends exercising at 45% to 75% of HRR or 65% to 90% HR_{max} for optimal cardiorespiratory benefits.

Musculoskeletal System

The musculoskeletal system is one of the areas of the body with the most robust adaptations to exercise. It has been well documented that exercise increases bone density, skeletal muscle size, motor recruitment, and metabolism. In line with the fundamental exercise principles of specificity and overload, in order for the musculoskeletal system to change, the exercise must be specifically targeted to the muscle group and its supporting structures and must impose an appreciable load. Physiologic changes will occur in response both to strengthening and endurance training, and each training type will have its own unique effect. Depending on the mode of exercise, variable changes will occur in skeletal muscle (Table 5-6). Endurance training improves fatigue resistance, while strength training increases force-generating capability. Additional adaptations induced by training include increased recruitment, bone density, and muscle size.

Bone mass is influenced by multiple factors, including genetics, hormonal and nutritional status, and activity status. Bones have the ability to adapt to mechanical stimuli (eg, increased load) and maintain the potential to remodel throughout life, which is described as Wolff's law.[103] The major force that is responsible for bone remodeling is ground reaction force (eg, landing from a jump). High-intensity loading is common in jumping and gymnastics activities exhibiting ground reaction forces up to 7.5 times greater than low-intensity activities such as walking.[104] The intensity, duration, and frequency of loading in the form of ground reaction forces contribute to the magnitude of bone remodeling. Animal studies have demonstrated that only a modest number of high-intensity loading activities (5 repetitions of jumping from a height) per day led to increased bone mass.[105] These studies also note that there are no added benefits when the number of repetitions was increased to 10.[105,106] The animal studies described employed supraphysiologic strain, which might not be able to be replicated in humans; it does, however, highlight important concepts that warrant further research. It has been shown that muscular contraction also contributes positively to bone growth; however, its magnitude is difficult to determine.[107] Resistance training has been shown to increase bone mass but only at an intensity that also promotes muscular hypertrophy.[107]

Specific Adaptations to Exercise

Motor Recruitment

The motor unit, composed of the motor neuron and the fiber(s) it innervates, is the fundamental unit of the musculoskeletal system. Firing of the motor unit requires integration of motor and sensory information from the central and

TABLE 5-5. CONTRAINDICATIONS TO EXERCISE TESTING

ABSOLUTE

- A recent significant change in the resting electrocardiogram suggesting significant ischemia, recent myocardial infarction (within 2 days), or other acute cardiac event
- Unstable angina
- Uncontrolled cardiac dysrhythmias causing symptoms or hemodynamic compromise
- Symptomatic severe aortic stenosis
- Uncontrolled symptomatic heart failure
- Acute myocarditis or pericarditis
- Suspected or known dissecting aneurysm
- Acute systemic infection, accompanied by fever, body aches, or swollen lymph glands.

RELATIVE[a]

- Left main coronary stenosis
- Moderate stenotic valvular heart disease
- Electrolyte abnormalities (eg, hypokalemia, hypomagnesemia)
- Severe arterial HTN (ie, SBP of >200 mm Hg and/or a DBP of >110 mm Hg) at rest
- Tachydysrhythmia or bradydysrhythmia
- Hypertrophic cardiomyopathy and other forms of outflow tract obstruction
- Neuromuscular, musculoskeletal, or rheumatoid disorders that are exacerbated by exercise
- High-degree atrioventricular block
- Ventricular aneurysm
- Uncontrolled metabolic disease (eg, diabetes, thyrotoxicosis, or myxedema)
- Chronic infectious disease (eg, mononucleosis, hepatitis, AIDS)
- Mental or physical impairment leading to inability to exercise adequately

[a]Relative contraindications can be superseded if benefits outweigh risks of exercise. In some instances, these individuals can be exercised with caution and/or using low-level end points, especially if they are asymptomatic at rest.

Reprinted with permission from Thompson WR, Gordon NF, Pescatello LS, eds. *ACSM's Guidelines for Exercise Testing and Prescription.* 8th ed. Philadelphia, PA: Wolters Kluwer, Lippincott Williams & Wilkins; 2010.

---

peripheral nervous system to promote the desired motor response. The motor neuron activates the appropriate number of motor units to provide the necessary force required by the movement. Motor unit activation is of critical importance in performance of activities, with higher levels of activity requiring increased recruitment of motor units. The majority of recruitment occurs according to motor unit size, with small Type I having a lower recruitment threshold than the larger Type IIa and IIb motor units. There is evidence to support high threshold activity may occur in the absence of low threshold activity in limited situations such as in elite athletes requiring enhanced muscle action.[101]

Training can improve motor unit recruitment and is thought to be the initial adaptation seen in muscle in response to exercise. Enhanced muscular performance in the absence of increased strength is proposed to be of neurogenic origin. Improvements occur within the first 2 weeks of training and, although the evidence is not confirmed, these benefits can be from learning, enhanced mapping of the primary motor cortex, increased motor recruitment, morphologic changes

TABLE 5-6. CHRONIC ADAPTATIONS IN THE MUSCULOSKELETAL SYSTEM IN RESPONSE TO EXERCISE

- Increased skeletal muscle strength
- Increased motor control and motor learning
- Enhanced mapping of the primary motor cortex
- Increased motor recruitment
- Increased firing frequency
- Decreased coactivation of agonist and antagonists
- Increased muscle cross-sectional area
- Increased collagen synthesis
- Increased collagen stiffness
- Increased motor recruitment

at the neuromuscular junction, increased firing frequency, and decreased coactivation of agonist and antagonists.[108,109] There are central mechanisms at play for all skilled movements. Practicing these movements or components of these movements increases performance through neural adaptations. Task-specific learning allows for appropriate balance, biomechanics, and postural support to complete exercises that can in turn enhance skill. Practice also improves ability to contract muscles in desired patterns and allows for carryover from one limb to another.[110,111] Further supporting the idea of central control of movement is that mental imagery and mental (imagined) practice enhance muscle contraction and performance of skilled movements.[112]

Muscle Hypertrophy

Skeletal muscle mass continues to increase until early adulthood (ages 18 to 25 years), which is associated with normal growth and maturation processes, but steadily declines with advancing age.[14] This progressive loss of skeletal muscle mass, known as *sarcopenia*, is seen in aging and disease. The relative decrease in muscle mass has deleterious effects on whole-body metabolism, strength, and heat production. In order to prevent sarcopenia, skeletal muscle protein synthesis must outpace skeletal muscle protein breakdown. Increased muscle mass is achieved largely through hypertrophy. Skeletal muscle is not capable of initiating cell division and proliferation to repair and replace damaged muscle fibers. Skeletal muscle, although mitotically silent, remains plastic and able to respond to a wide variety of stimuli. Exercise is one of the most powerful stimuli inducing muscular protein synthesis.

Transient hypertrophy is seen with an acute exercise bout (one session) because interstitial edema and muscles will return to their original size after several hours. Chronic hypertrophy is a longer-standing morphologic change in the muscle that is supported by increased protein synthesis. This growth is induced by longer-term strength training and also from the influence of anabolic hormones, namely testosterone.[113-115] Overall, the mechanism of chronic hypertrophy leads to an increased number of contractile myofibril proteins (actin and myosin) that enable greater cross-bridge formation and force development. The increased growth of muscle fibers occurs at the level of the myofibrils, which exhibit the addition of contractile materials at their periphery.[116] It has been postulated that the addition of these proteins is dependent on the activation of mitotically active satellite cells.[117] Another potential mechanism of increasing muscle area is the process of hyperplasia. Evidence of hyperplasia exists from experimental studies using animals and describes myofibril "splitting" after training, leading to frank division of the myofibril and subsequent increase in myofibril number.[118,119] Despite its description in animals, hyperplasia in humans occurs at a very slow rate and contributes only minimally to increased muscle size and therefore is not matched to strength gains.[120-122]

The extent to which each muscle group is loaded will determine the amount and location of hypertrophy. An increase in cross-sectional area of individual fibers occurs and the cross-sectional area of the whole muscle also increases. The increase in contractile tissue leads to enhanced cross-bridge formation, enabling muscle to develop greater levels of tension. Both Type I and Type II fibers are capable of hypertrophy. It is has been shown, however, that resistance training favors hypertrophy of Type II fibers largely because of their enhanced plasticity.[123] Type II fibers have been shown to hypertrophy in just 6 weeks, whereas Type I fibers take longer than 10 weeks.[118,123] Now larger in size and in number, the fibers need to be packed more tightly within the muscle. In order to accomplish this, fibers may alter their angle of pennation. Several studies show evidence of hypertrophy coincident with increased angle of pennation with resistance training.[124-126] Both the increased fiber diameter and the increased angle contribute to increased production of force, which equates to strength gains.

Noted hypertrophy has been documented with 8 to 12 weeks of resistance training[127] but can vary slightly by gender, age, and muscle group. Both genders demonstrate marked increases in strength with resistance training; however, males exhibit greater absolute strength and muscle cross-sectional area than women. This difference in muscle size is relatively confined to the UE. Many studies document that women have a capacity similar to men for strength and muscle size gains in the LEs with strength training.[128-134] The UE dominance exhibited in males is largely due to the higher circulating levels of testosterone and muscle androgen receptors located in the UEs.[135,136]

Muscle Fatigability

Endurance training is of long duration and lower intensity and is geared toward increasing resistance to fatigue. This type of exercise preferentially targets slow oxidative (Type I) and fast oxidative glycolytic fibers (Type IIa), with no appreciable hypertrophy noted. Benefits of endurance training in the musculoskeletal system include an increase in number of mitochondria, mitochondrial enzymes, and substrate availability—all of which affect muscle metabolism, which is discussed in detail in the Metabolism section found earlier in this chapter.

Bone Growth

The crest of bone accumulation occurs at puberty, illustrating the importance of high-intensity[137] exercise in this age range. It is important to note, however, that in cases of hormonal imbalance such as is seen in athletic female triads or in menopause, high-intensity loading exercise cannot attenuate the bone loss associated with estrogen deficiency. Bone loss starts as early as in a person's mid-30s when considering trabecular bone and in their mid-50s in cortical bone and can occur at a rate as fast as 0.5% per year.[138-140] Participation in activities promoting high ground reaction forces (eg, jumping sports) leads to higher bone density and increased propensity to lay down new bone.[141-143] In the absence of these forces, bone integrity suffers as demonstrated by studies surrounding antigravity flight, complete bed rest, and neurological injuries that compromise weight-bearing status.[144]

Considerations for Patient Care

Strength can be determined both statically (isometrics) or dynamically through functional ROM. PTs have various methods to determine strength both from the perspective of a single maximal contraction and muscular endurance. One RM is defined as the greatest load through full ROM and often relates to the gross strength of a single muscle group. Many tests exist to estimate 1-RM from several contractions. For example, the clinician selects a weight of appropriate intensity for the patient to perform between 4 and 12 contractions. The number of completed contractions and the weight are then entered into an equation, resulting in an approximate 1-RM. One such method is the Brzycki equation (1-RM = weight lifted (pounds)/[1.0278 – (repetitions to fatigue $\times$ 0.0278)]), which allows the patient to perform multiple contractions and still evaluate 1-RM.[145] This and other 1-RM estimations are considerably less reliable and valid if the patient is able to complete more than 8 repetitions.

The clinical relevance of determining 1-RM is limited since functional activities require repeated contractions of multiple muscle groups acting together. PTs usually prescribe resistance exercises of 8 to 12 repetitions, which equates to the ACSM recommendation of an intensity of 50% to 75% 1-RM. Resistance training is beneficial for all age groups when the proper techniques and guidelines are followed. For children, the ACSM recommends 1 to 3 sets of 6 to 16 repetitions for major muscle groups at a moderate intensity 2 to 3 nonconsecutive days of the week.[146] The practitioner should realize that significant muscle hypertrophy will not occur before the onset of puberty, and that the benefits of resistance training are to improve coordination, motor response, increased bone density, and the promotion of health through exposure to various modes of exercise. Adults of all ages have the capacity to improve strength and muscle cross-sectional area. The ACSM recommends adults engage in 8 to 10 various muscle-strengthening exercises 2 to 3 times per week. Each muscle group needs to be targeted with 2 to 3 different exercises at an intensity that brings muscle to fatigue (8 to 12 repetitions).[2] In the older adult, the literature is conflicted. There is evidence that at an advanced age the potential for muscle hypertrophy is decreased.[147-149] Other studies cite that age has no effect on hypertrophy.[131,150] Despite the impact aging has on amount of hypertrophy, the ACSM recommends that the older adult engages in muscle strengthening consisting of 8 to 10 exercises at moderate intensity (10 to 15 repetitions) 2 to 3 times per week.[2]

Resistance training most often benefits activities requiring strength and/or power. Endurance is also increased because of an improved economy of performance.[151] Strength increases have been documented early on in resistance training programs, even before physiologic hypertrophy has occurred. This increased improvement is primarily due to neurological recruitment.

It is important to also focus on technique when performing strength training. Correct and accurate body position is required to target the desired muscles for hypertrophy in strength training. A compensatory body position or altered biomechanics may activate different muscles during performance of the exercises. Strength training also affects the supporting elements of the musculoskeletal system, namely tendons. Training has been shown to increase tendon stiffness and also to promote tendon hypertrophy, which may have implications in tendon response to rapid force.[152-154] Beyond increased muscle mass, resistance training is an excellent method of accruing bone strength. Moderate resistance training $\leq$60% 1-RM at least 2 to 3 times per week is necessary to optimize bone density. Additionally, the ACSM recommends high-impact activities (eg, gymnastics, plyometrics, sports that involve running and jumping) for 30 to 60 minutes at least 3 days per week for increased bone strength. It is important to encourage patients who are at risk for osteoporosis to engage in a strength training program early on in their fitness pursuits to maximize benefits. Resistance training is also an excellent intervention for maintaining or increasing bone density with a diagnosis of osteoporosis; it is often safer than plyometric or dynamic exercises as there is a low risk for fractures.

Immune System

The relationship between exercise and the immune system still remains unclear. The immune system is driven by complex interactions of cells, hormones, and chemical messengers both innately derived from the body and those that invade the body from an outside source. Additionally, the neuroendocrine system greatly influences the immune system, further complicating the organization and communication of these pathways (Figure 5-6). Despite the intricate cross-talk of the 3 systems, the overall function of the immune system is clear: to initiate tissue repair when it is damaged. This damage can be in many forms such as direct tissue injury, infection with a pathogen, or exposure to stress. The immune system responds to injury by removing damaged tissue and promoting movement and proliferation of special cells to the area to support tissue healing. These cells have specific roles in the immune response such as inactivating pathogens, destroying infected cells, and activating inflammation.

Changes With Exercise

Exercise is considered to be a stress to the immunologic system; the body responds over time by increasing the number and activity of lymphocytes. It has been noted that lymphocytes are increased from 6 to 24 hours after an acute bout of exercise.[155] Evidence suggests that regular exercise promotes resistance to illness, inflammation, and tumor progression.[156,157] Regular exercise elevates the number and activity of cytokines and natural killer (NK), B, and T cells.[23] The increase in NK cells is of particular interest because of their protective effects against viral infections and cancer.[158,159] Moderate exercise has been shown to prevent upper respiratory tract infections[23] and is associated with delayed progression of HIV.[160] In a review by Haaland et

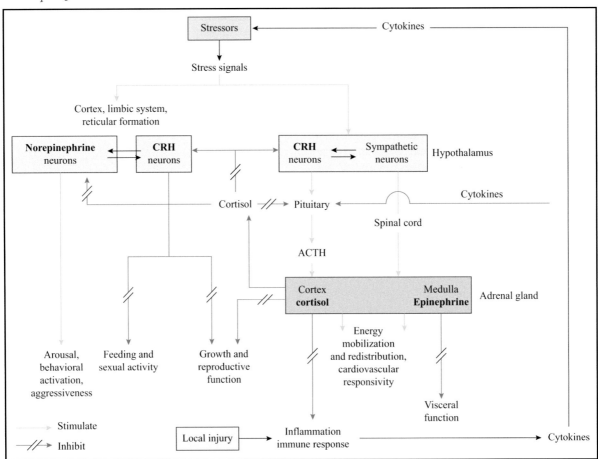

Figure 5-6. Integrated responses to stress mediated by the sympathetic nervous system and the hypothalamic-pituitary-adrenocortical axis. (Adapted from Levy MN, Stanton BA, Koeppen BM. *Berne & Levy Principles of Physiology*. 4th ed. St. Louis, MO: Mosby; 2006.)

al, long-term endurance programs decreased inflammation in patients with heart failure and type 2 diabetes.[156] It has been estimated that regular exercise improves immunity by 15% to 25%. It is debatable, however, how this affects disease susceptibility.[157]

Acute bouts of exercise result in an increase in circulating white blood cells, known as *leukocytosis*.[23] Neutrophils and monocytes (macrophages) have also been noted to increase after exercise proportional to the duration and intensity exercise. A clinically relevant difference is seen in T, B, and NK cells, which are suppressed after exercise, and typically return to normal levels within 24 hours.[157] It is thought that the release of catecholamines during exercise contributes to this drop in B and T cell activity.[160]

A fine line exists between enhancement and suppression of the immune system based on training parameters. Following strenuous exercise the immune system is suppressed for several hours or days, increasing the risk for infection.[23] A study focused on marathon runners and endurance athletes demonstrates a self-reported increase in incidence of upper respiratory tract infections.[161,162] A proposed mechanism for this increased predisposition to infection is the acute decline of NK, B, and T cells following strenuous exercise.[157]

Considerations for Patient Care

The amount of damage the body incurs with exercise is dependent on the intensity, duration, and frequency of the exercise. A fine line exists between enhancement and suppression of immune system based on training parameters. In a position statement published by the *Exercise Immunology Review*, "The general consensus on managing training to maintain immune health is to start with a programme of low to moderate volume and intensity; employ a gradual and periodized increase in training volumes and loads."[163(p 64)] The position statement also warns against excessive training loads that could result in injury or exhaustion while also ensuring adequate rest and recovery. The clinician should also realize that time to exhaustion, internal stress, and immunocompetence are all individual factors that will vary from one patient to the next. Factors that may negatively affect immunocompetence include presence of disease, psychological or physiologic stress, and various medications (eg, chemotherapy). There are no definitive exercise prescriptions for optimizing immune function in patients with chronic diseases. The clinician should be prudent by prescribing appropriate intensity and duration of exercise that would enhance immune function while not exacerbating the patient's confounding medical diagnoses. Lastly, importance should be stressed on adequate recovery time in order to avoid exhaustion and overtraining that could negatively affect the immune system.

Psychological Factors, Specifically Depression

Both aerobic and strength training improve symptoms in those diagnosed with depression.[164,165] It is important to note, however, that regular activity does not prevent the onset of depression. Individuals with depression have been found to have a hyperactive hypothalamic-pituitary-adrenal and with accompanying elevated levels of cortisol (see Figure 5-6). Depression has also been associated with decreased hippocampal expression of various neurotrophic factors (eg, brain-derived neurotrophic factor).[166]

Changes With Exercise

Acute exercise is viewed as a stressor and causes rise in norepinephrine and cortisol through direct activation of the hypothalamic-pituitary-adrenal axis.[23] Those who engage in regular exercise, however, exhibit decreased levels of cortisol in response to acute bouts of exercise or stress.[167-169] It is thought that exercise positively affects hippocampal neurotrophic gene expression and subsequently improves the symptoms of depression. An additional benefit of exercise is the resultant increase in monoamines, tryptophans and B-endorphin levels, which also attenuate symptoms of depression.

Exercise has been used successfully to ameliorate symptoms of depression in health subjects across all age groups.[170-173] Patients who exercised regularly reported symptom reductions similar to those receiving cognitive behavioral therapy.[174,175] Likewise, exercise has been shown to decrease depression accompanying various chronic diseases, including cancer,[176] neuromuscular disorders,[177] cardiac conditions,[178] and COPD.[179]

Considerations for Patient Care

Despite strong evidence for the links between exercise and reduction of clinical depression, its use is still under investigation. More studies on the clinical effects and dosage response to exercise are needed to determine optimal prescription parameters. It is known that overtraining mimics depressive symptoms, so treatment plans should employ appropriate rest, recovery, and variety of activity. Currently, exercise should be used as an adjunct to psychological and pharmacologic interventions, and patient response should be monitored closely.

EXERCISE PRESCRIPTION

General Considerations

The benefits of exercise both for fitness and general health and well-being are well documented.[2,180] Exercise programs are created to improve overall health, reduce risk for the development or progression of disease, and promote physical fitness in a manner that ensures safety for the participant. Each person will have his or her own definition of fitness; it will be specific to his or her personal view of optimal health and well-being whether that involves disease prevention or minimizing disability. A well-designed exercise program can provide a means for increasing independence and overall function.

The program needs to consider the patient's baseline health status, abilities, and desired goals. The PT should also consider the patient's familiarity with the mode of exercise, access to equipment, and time constraints. Each exercise prescription should be unique to the individual for whom it is prescribed, taking into account the specific health needs, interests, and clinical status of that person.[2] Customized exercise programs that are patient- and function-focused will help improve compliance and prevent injury. Despite the vast variability in the factors and resultant exercise prescriptions described earlier, all programs should have one common predominant feature: they are specifically individualized to the needs, desires, and stated goals of the person who plans to follow the program.

The broad categories of exercise include cardiovascular training, strength, flexibility, speed, agility, and balance.[2] Ideally, the exercise prescription is determined from data obtained in an objective assessment of the individual response to exercise, be it by standard exercise testing protocol or by a previously presented functional or field test. Both categories of testing can be used to help diagnose, assign risk stratification, and set appropriate guidelines and goals for patients and clients. Many options exist to stratify patients in various states of fitness and disease or dysfunction. Using tests with high validity and reliability will produce more meaningful interpretation. However, ease of use, cost, time of administration, and appropriateness for the patient are also critical factors to consider.

Fitness tests range from medically monitored clinical exercise tests to field tests conducted in a variety of settings. Commonly used tests include the use of treadmills, cycle ergometers, upper body ergometers, and steps. Certainly the test chosen must be justified by past medical history and screening and/or physical examination. The practitioner should have a general familiarity with many fitness tests in order to select the most appropriate one based on mode of exercise, end point of test, and safety considerations. Additionally, the clinician should be aware of tests for various ages and levels of ability, as those criteria often require modifications of standard fitness tests. The clinician should also monitor the patient throughout the test and have proper equipment and personnel to accomplish this effectively. Various monitoring techniques include HR, BP, electrocardiogram (ECG), VO_2, RR, and RPE. Each fitness test should also allow for a warm-up or practice period before the test and cool down period after the test to maximize results and for the safety of the patient. Testing should be terminated if

TABLE 5-7. WHEN TO STOP AN EXERCISE TEST (ACSM RECOMMENDATIONS)

- SOB/wheezing
- Intermittent claudication
- Angina
- Chronotropic incompetence
- HR fails to increase with increased exercise intensity and subject wants to stop
- SBP > 250 mm Hg or DBP > 115 mm Hg
- Cyanosis, lightheadedness, nausea, pallor
- Severe fatigue
- Subject requests to stop or testing equipment fails

Reprinted with permission from Committee Members; Gibbons RJ, Balady GJ, Bricker JT, et al. ACC/AHA 2002 guideline update for exercise testing: summary article. *Circulation.* 2002;106(14):1883-1892.

any of the identified criteria for cessation of an exercise test are met, as listed in the ACSM resource guide (Table 5-7).

The information gained from the fitness test will allow for a thorough, adequate, and specific exercise prescription. The essential components to exercise prescription are described by the FITT principle: frequency, intensity, type (mode), and time. An important addition to the FITT principle is progression of the prescribed activity, which fosters continued gains and achievement of patient goals. It is important to note the rate of progression is highly variable among individuals and is dependent on functional status.

When designing a specific exercise program, the ACSM recommends that clinicians consider the specific health needs of the individual when creating or modifying a program for that person. Specifically, variability of perceptual and physiologic responses to exercise necessitates careful titration of duration and intensity of exercise as well as the need to ensure patient safety. Additionally, each exercise session should include a warm-up, focused exercise, cool down, and stretching.[2] Time should also be devoted to educating the patient in goal-setting, self-monitoring techniques, and independent progression of exercises. In doing so, the patient will be empowered to continuously exercise for the benefits of improved health and function. Finally, the best exercise program will be the one that is the most successful in bringing about long-term health changes associated with exercise, which requires a balance of behavioral change techniques and solid exercise science to support attainment of the individual goals.[2]

Mode

The greatest benefit (measured as changes in VO_{2max}) attained from exercise occurs when exercise "uses large muscle groups over prolonged periods in activities that are rhythmic and aerobic in nature (walking, running, hiking, cycling, stair climbing, etc)."[2(p 163)] The mode of exercise selected to attain these qualities should reflect the individual's goals and specific functional deficits, as well as skill level and enjoyment of the activity. Careful attention to these factors is likely to improve compliance and thus chances for success.[181,182]

Intensity

The ACSM recommends a broad range of training intensities depending on the activity. For cardiorespiratory training, they range from a level corresponding to 55% to 90% of HR_{max}, 40% to 85% of O_2 uptake reserve ($VO_2R = VO_{2max} - VO_{2rest}$), or 50% to 85% of HRR ($HRR = HR_{max} - HR_{rest}$).[2] Higher intensities of exercise are appropriate and safe to improve cardiorespiratory fitness in healthy/fit individuals, while intensities as low as 40% to 49% HRR have been demonstrated to bring about changes in sedentary or deconditioned individuals.

Duration

Early ACSM recommendations for exercise duration promoted continuous exercise for durations of 30 to 60 minutes, which proved to be somewhat daunting for many individuals, especially those who were sedentary or just beginning an exercise program. The most recent ACSM/CDC guidelines[183] reflected a consensus desire to include the most number of Americans and to reflect a continuum of activity recommendations. Their recommendation stated that adults should "accumulate"[146] minutes of moderate intensity exercise per week vs performing continuous activity. As an individual gains endurance and exercise tolerance, exercise duration can be increased with the goal of increasing exercise time. For individuals who have been sedentary or deconditioned, an important goal is to attain durations of 30 to 40 minutes of continuous ambulation, which provides the individual with the endurance necessary to achieve community ambulation.[184-186]

Frequency

Fitness goals may be attained for those who are deconditioned or sedentary with only twice-weekly exercise, though optimal benefits can be attained with 3 to 5 sessions per week. An analysis of the potential benefits of increasing exercise frequency beyond 5 days per week demonstrates that there is a greater likelihood of injury and only minimal benefits to be attained. When determining appropriate exercise frequency for a patient, intensity of exercise should also be considered. For individuals exercising at higher intensities (60% to 80% HRR), fewer bouts of exercise (twice weekly) are adequate to attain desired changes. Individuals who are sedentary or deconditioned when beginning an exercise program and exercising at lower intensities may not only require more frequent weekly exercise sessions, but they also may need to perform multiple short bouts of exercise each day to meet their training goals. Frequency and duration of exercise can be adjusted to attain a goal of 45 minutes of continuous activity. Once the individual is able to tolerate 45 minutes of continuous activity, only then should intensity be increased.[186]

Exercise Prescription and Movement-Related Disorders

Exercise is vital to the maintenance of health and wellness. It is also a valuable intervention to slow the rate of change brought about by disease as well as to aid the recovery of health, function, and well-being lost by patients because of injury or illness. Initiating and progressing exercise programs for individuals who are ill or recovering, however, requires careful consideration. Exercise prescriptions need to factor in not just individual desires and goals, but the pathophysiological effect system disorders have on exercise tolerance. For individuals with acute or chronic movement-related disorders that limit exercise tolerance, a parameter based on an age-related HR_{max} or percentage of VO_{2max} may not be appropriate. For these individuals, the onset of disorder-specific signs or symptoms determine the intensity, frequency, and duration of exercise, as well as measured individual variations, in exercise tolerance.

The chapters in the next section of the text will provide the variations in normal physiology—the pathophysiology—for movement-related disorders in patients treated by PTs. The monitoring strategies to be used during exercise for these patients are based on the specific pathophysiology for each disorder, but a few generalities can be offered here. A patient with CAD, for example, will not be appropriately treated by an exercise prescription where the intensity is based solely on an age-defined HR_{max}. Instead, a new HR_{max} will have been determined by the HR identified when symptoms or ECG changes occurred in an exercise stress test. SOB and leg fatigue may be a parameter for the intensity or duration of exercise during an exercise session for a patient with a gas-exchange disorder. Even standard exercise monitoring measures of HR and BP will show a greater than expected rise in patients who are deconditioned, and these signs need to be considered in the parameters for the prescription.

Just as the symptoms patients experience with exercise are related to the pathophysiology of their disorders, these are often the same symptoms patients associate with being "sick." A patient with cardiac disease would likely have angina or SOB associated with exercise, just as a patient with pulmonary disease could likely have difficulty breathing even at rest, much less with exercise. It can be a daunting task for the clinician to introduce the idea of exercise, with the possible generation of distressing symptoms, as part of the physical therapy plan for these patients. Although exercising may be anxiety-provoking for patients, a carefully planned and safely implemented program has the potential to improve the patient's confidence that exercise—with all of its benefits to restore health, function, and well-being—is possible without symptom provocation.

SUMMARY

Exercise is an important intervention to promote beneficial morphologic, physiologic, and metabolic change in the body. These changes are highly specific and can be modified depending on intensity, mode, and duration of exercise. Exercise adaptations are readily reversible and are affected by cessation of training, increased age, and presence of disease. Individual differences based on heredity, prior training experience, and health status affect the amount of physiologic change induced by exercise.

As the chapter content in the next section will show, the PT is able to prescribe an appropriate and individualized exercise intervention based on knowledge of disorder pathophysiology, thorough patient examination, and careful consideration of individual patient needs. Well-considered exercise prescriptions for patients can enhance fitness, promote health, and ensure safety as well as encourage long-term compliance.

REFERENCES

1. Pate RR, Pratt M, Blair SN, et al. Physical activity and public health. A recommendation from the Centers for Disease Control and Prevention and the American College of Sports Medicine. *JAMA.* 1995;273(5):402-407.

2. American College of Sports Medicine. *ACSM's Guidelines for Exercise Testing and Prescription.* 8th ed. Philadelphia, PA: Lippincott, Williams & Wilkins; 2010.

3. Lavie CJ, Thomas RJ, Squires RW, Allison TG, Milani RV. Exercise training and cardiac rehabilitation in primary and secondary prevention of coronary heart disease. *Mayo Clin Proc.* 2009;84(4):373-383.

4. Physical activity and cardiovascular health. NIH Consensus Development Panel on Physical Activity and Cardiovascular Health. *JAMA.* 1996;276(3):241-246.

5. Ettinger WH Jr, Burns R, Messier SP, et al. A randomized trial comparing aerobic exercise and resistance exercise with a health education program in older adults with knee osteoarthritis. The Fitness Arthritis and Seniors Trial (FAST). *JAMA.* 1997;277(1):25-31.

6. Whaley M, Kaminsky L. Epidemiology of physical activity, physical fitness and selected chronic disease. In: *ACSM's Resource Manual for Clinical Guidelines for Exercise Testing and Prescription.* Baltimore, MD: Williams & Wilkins; 1998:13-26.

7. Lee IM, Skerrett PJ. Physical activity and all-cause mortality: what is the dose-response relation? *Med Sci Sports Exerc.* 2001;33(6 Suppl):S459-S471; discussion S493-S494.

8. Singh MA. Exercise comes of age: rationale and recommendations for a geriatric exercise prescription. *J Gerontol A Biol Sci Med Sci.* 2002;57(5):M262-M282.

9. DeFronzo RA, Gunnarsson R, Björkman O, Olsson M, Wahren J. Effects of insulin on peripheral and splanchnic glucose metabolism in noninsulin-dependent (type II) diabetes mellitus. *J Clin Invest.* 1985;76(1):149-155.

10. Ivy JL. Muscle insulin resistance amended with exercise training: role of GLUT4 expression. *Med Sci Sports Exerc.* 2004;36(7):1207-1211.

11. Kelley DE, He J, Menshikova EV, Ritov VB. Dysfunction of mitochondria in human skeletal muscle in type 2 diabetes. *Diabetes.* 2002;51(10):2944-2950.

12. Hawley JA, Holloszy JO. Exercise: it's the real thing! *Nutr Rev.* 2009;67(3):172-178.

13. Toledo FG, Menshikova EV, Azuma K, et al. Mitochondrial capacity in skeletal muscle is not stimulated by weight loss despite increases in insulin action and decreases in intramyocellular lipid content. *Diabetes.* 2008;57(4):987-994.

14. Wilmore J. *Physiology of Sport and Exercise.* 4th ed. Champaign, IL: Human Kinetics; 2008.

15. Ivy JL. Muscle glycogen synthesis before and after exercise. *Sports Med.* 1991;11(1):6-19.

16. Abernethy PJ, Thayer R, Taylor AW, et al. Acute and chronic responses of skeletal muscle to endurance and sprint exercise. A review. *Sports Med.* 1990;10(6):365-389.

17. Tipton KD, Wolfe RR. Exercise, protein metabolism, and muscle growth. *Int J Sport Nutr Exerc Metab.* 2001;11(1):109-132.

18. Holloszy JO. Biochemical adaptations in muscle. Effects of exercise on mitochondrial oxygen uptake and respiratory enzyme activity in skeletal muscle. *J Biol Chem.* 1967;242(9):2278-2282.

19. Baar K, Wende AR, Jones TE, et al. Adaptations of skeletal muscle to exercise: rapid increase in the transcriptional coactivator PGC-1. *FASEB J.* 2002;16(14):1879-1886.

20. Irrcher I, Adhihetty PJ, Sheehan T, Joseph AM, Hood DA. PPARgamma coactivator-1alpha expression during thyroid hormone- and contractile activity-induced mitochondrial adaptations. *Am J Physiol Cell Physiol.* 2003;284(6):C1669-C1677.

21. Wright DC, Han DH, Garcia-Roves PM, Geiger PC, Jones TE, Holloszy JO. Exercise-induced mitochondrial biogenesis begins before the increase in muscle PGC-1alpha expression. *J Biol Chem.* 2007;282(1):194-199.

22. Lanza IR, Nair KS. Muscle mitochondrial changes with aging and exercise. *Am J Clin Nutr.* 2009;89(1):467S-471S.

23. Plowman S. *Exercise Physiology for Health, Fitness, and Performance.* 3rd ed. Philadelphia, PA: Wolters Kluwer Health/ Lippincott Williams & Wilkins; 2011.

24. Holloway GP, Bonen A, Spriet LL, et al. Regulation of skeletal muscle mitochondrial fatty acid metabolism in lean and obese individuals. *Am J Clin Nutr.* 2009;89(1):455S-462S.

25. Talanian JL, Holloway GP, Snook LA, Heigenhauser GJ, Bonen A, Spriet LL. Exercise training increases sarcolemmal and mitochondrial fatty acid transport proteins in human skeletal muscle. *Am J Physiol Endocrinol Metab.* 2010;299(2):E180-E188.

26. Rennie MJ, Winder WW, Holloszy JO. A sparing effect of increased plasma fatty acids on muscle and liver glycogen content in the exercising rat. *Biochem J.* 1976;156(3):647-655.

27. Seki Y, Berggren JR, Houmard JA, Charron MJ. Glucose transporter expression in skeletal muscle of endurance-trained individuals. *Med Sci Sports Exerc.* 2006;38(6):1088-1092.

28. Sato Y, Ito T, Udaka N, et al. Immunohistochemical localization of facilitated-diffusion glucose transporters in rat pancreatic islets. *Tissue Cell.* 1996;28(6):637-643.

29. Daugaard JR, Nielsen JN, Kristiansen S, Andersen JL, Hargreaves M, Richter EA. Fiber type-specific expression of GLUT4 in human skeletal muscle: influence of exercise training. *Diabetes.* 2000;49(7):1092-1095.

30. Mougios V. *Exercise Biochemistry.* Champaign, IL: Human Kinetics; 2006.

31. Johansen L, Quistorff B. 31P-MRS characterization of sprint and endurance trained athletes. *Int J Sports Med.* 2003;24(3):183-189.

32. Ross A, Leveritt M. Long-term metabolic and skeletal muscle adaptations to short-sprint training: implications for sprint training and tapering. *Sports Med.* 2001;31(15):1063-1082.

33. Perry CG, Heigenhauser GJ, Bonen A, Spriet LL. High-intensity aerobic interval training increases fat and carbohydrate metabolic capacities in human skeletal muscle. *Appl Physiol Nutr Metab.* 2008;33(6):1112-1123.

34. MacDougall JD, Ward GR, Sale DG, Sutton JR. Biochemical adaptation of human skeletal muscle to heavy resistance training and immobilization. *J Appl Physiol Respir Environ Exerc Physiol.* 1977;43(4):700-703.

35. Harmer AR, McKenna MJ, Sutton JR, et al. Skeletal muscle metabolic and ionic adaptations during intense exercise following sprint training in humans. *J Appl Physiol (1985).* 2000;89(5):1793-1803.

36. Burgomaster KA, Howarth KR, Phillips SM, et al. Similar metabolic adaptations during exercise after low volume sprint interval and traditional endurance training in humans. *J Physiol.* 2008;586(1):151-160.

37. Gibala MJ, Little JP, van Essen M, et al. Short-term sprint interval versus traditional endurance training: similar initial adaptations in human skeletal muscle and exercise performance. *J Physiol.* 2006;575(Pt 3):901-911.

38. Potdevin FJ, Alberty ME, Chevutschi A, Pelayo P, Sidney MC. Effects of a 6-week plyometric training program on performances in pubescent swimmers. *J Strength Cond Res.* 2011;25(1):80-86.

39. Baar K. The signaling underlying FITness. *Appl Physiol Nutr Metab.* 2009;34(3):411-419.

40. Ries JD, Drake JM, Marino C. A small-group functional balance intervention for individuals with Alzheimer disease: a pilot study. *J Neurol Phys Ther.* 2010;34(1):3-10.

41. Young WB. Transfer of strength and power training to sports performance. *Int J Sports Physiol Perform.* 2006;1(2):74-83.

42. Ghosh AK, Paliwal R, Sam MJ, Ahuja A. Effect of 4 weeks detraining on aerobic & anaerobic capacity of basketball players & their restoration. *Indian J Med Res.* 1987;86:522-527.

43. Coyle EF, Hemmert MK, Coggan AR. Effects of detraining on cardiovascular responses to exercise: role of blood volume. *J Appl Physiol (1985).* 1986;60(1):95-99.

44. Martin WH 3rd, Coyle EF, Bloomfield SA, Ehsani AA. Effects of physical deconditioning after intense endurance training on left ventricular dimensions and stroke volume. *J Am Coll Cardiol.* 1986;7(5):982-989.

45. Coyle EF, Martin WH 3rd, Sinacore DR, Joyner MJ, Hagberg JM, Holloszy JO. Time course of loss of adaptations after stopping prolonged intense endurance training. *J Appl Physiol Respir Environ Exerc Physiol.* 1984;57(6):1857-1864.

46. Moore RL, Thacker EM, Kelley GA, et al. Effect of training/detraining on submaximal exercise responses in humans. *J Appl Physiol (1985).* 1987;63(5):1719-1724.

47. Houston ME, Bentzen H, Larsen H, et al. Interrelationships between skeletal muscle adaptations and performance as studied by detraining and retraining. *Acta Physiol Scand.* 1979;105(2):163-170.

48. Houmard JA, Shinebarger MH, Dolan PL, et al. Exercise training increases GLUT-4 protein concentration in previously sedentary middle-aged men. *Am J Physiol.* 1993;264(6 Pt 1):E896-E901.

49. Houmard JA, Hortobágyi T, Neufer PD, et al. Training cessation does not alter GLUT-4 protein levels in human skeletal muscle. *J Appl Physiol (1985).* 1993;74(2):776-781.

50. Ready AE, Eynon RB, Cunningham DA. Effect of interval training and detraining on anaerobic fitness in women. *Can J Appl Sport Sci.* 1981;6(3):114-118

51. Pivarnik JM, Senay LC. Effects of exercise detraining and deacclimation to the heat on plasma volume dynamics. *Eur J Appl Physiol Occup Physiol.* 1986;55(2):222-228.

52. Wibom R, Hultman E, Johansson M, Matherei K, Constantin-Teodosiu D, Schantz PG. Adaptation of mitochondrial ATP production in human skeletal muscle to endurance training and detraining. *J Appl Physiol (1985).* 1992;73(5):2004-2010.

53. Klausen K, Andersen LB, Pelle I. Adaptive changes in work capacity, skeletal muscle capillarization and enzyme levels during training and detraining. *Acta Physiol Scand.* 1981;113(1):9-16.

54. Kraemer W. *Exercise Physiology: Integrating Theory and Application.* Philadelphia, PA: Wolters Kluwer Health/Lippincott Williams & Wilkins; 2012.

55. Mikines KJ, Dela F, Tronier B, Galbo H. Effect of 7 days of bed rest on dose-response relation between plasma glucose and insulin secretion. *Am J Physiol.* 1989;257(1 Pt 1):E43-E48.

56. Mikines KJ, Sonne B, Farrell PA, Tronier B, Galbo H. Effect of training on the dose-response relationship for insulin action in men. *J Appl Physiol (1985).* 1989;66(2):695-703.

57. Mikines KJ, Sonne B, Tronier B, Galbo H. Effects of training and detraining on dose-response relationship between glucose and insulin secretion. *Am J Physiol.* 1989;256(5 Pt 1):E588-E596.

58. Hardman AE, Lawrence JE, Herd SL. Postprandial lipemia in endurance-trained people during a short interruption to training. *J Appl Physiol (1985).* 1998;84(6):1895-1901.

59. McCoy M, Proietto J, Hargreves M. Effect of detraining on GLUT-4 protein in human skeletal muscle. *J Appl Physiol (1985).* 1994;77(3):1532-1536.

60. Vukovich M, Arciero P, Kohrt W, Racette SB, Hansen PA, Holloszy JO. Changes in insulin action and GLUT-4 with 6 days of inactivity in endurance runners. *J Appl Physiol (1985).* 1996;80(1):240-244.

61. Hortobágyi T, Houmard J, Stevenson JR, Fraser DD, Johns RA, Israel RG. The effects of detraining on power athletes. *Med Sci Sports Exerc.* 1993;25(8):929-935.

62. Fagard RH, Cornelissen VA. Effect of exercise on blood pressure control in hypertensive patients. *Eur J Cardiovasc Prev Rehabil.* 2007;14(1):12-17.

63. Gupta S, Rohatgi A, Ayers CR, et al. Cardiorespiratory fitness and classification of risk of cardiovascular disease mortality. *Circulation.* 2011;123(13):1377-1383.

64. Haskell WL, Lee IM, Pate RR, et al. Physical activity and public health: updated recommendation for adults from the American College of Sports Medicine and the American Heart Association. *Med Sci Sports Exerc.* 2007;39(8):1423-1434.

65. Swain DP, Franklin BA. Comparison of cardioprotective benefits of vigorous versus moderate intensity aerobic exercise. *Am J Cardiol.* 2006;97(1):141-147.

66. Zheng H, Orsini N, Amin J, Wolk A, Nguyen VT, Ehrlich F. Quantifying the dose-response of walking in reducing coronary heart disease risk: meta-analysis. *Eur J Epidemiol.* 2009;24(4):181-192.

67. Sawka MN, Convertino VA, Eichner ER, Schnieder SM, Young AJ. Blood volume: importance and adaptations to exercise training, environmental stresses, and trauma/sickness. *Med Sci Sports Exerc.* 2000;32(2):332-348.

68. Levick JR. *Introduction to Cardiovascular Physiology.* 4th ed. London, UK: Edward Arnold Ltd; 2003.

69. Wisløff U, Støylen A, Loennechen JP, et al. Superior cardiovascular effect of aerobic interval training versus moderate continuous training in heart failure patients: a randomized study. *Circulation.* 2007;115(24):3086-3094.

70. Taylor RS, Brown A, Ebrahim S, et al. Exercise-based rehabilitation for patients with coronary heart disease: systematic review and meta-analysis of randomized controlled trials. *Am J Med.* 2004;116(10):682-692.

71. Jolliffe JA, Rees K, Taylor RS, Thompson D, Oldridge N, Ebrahim S. Exercise-based rehabilitation for coronary heart disease. *Cochrane Database Syst Rev.* 2001;(1):CD001800.

72. Sakamoto S, Yokoyama N, Tamori Y, Akutsu K, Hashimoto H, Takeshita S. Patients with peripheral artery disease who complete 12-week supervised exercise training program show reduced cardiovascular mortality and morbidity. *Circ J.* 2009;73(1):167-173.

73. Whelton SP, Chin A, Xin X, He J. Effect of aerobic exercise on blood pressure: a meta-analysis of randomized, controlled trials. *Ann Intern Med.* 2002;136(7):493-503.

74. Reaven GM. Hypothesis: muscle insulin resistance is the ("not-so") thrifty genotype. *Diabetologia.* 1998;41(4):482-484.

75. He J, Klag MJ, Caballero B, Appel LJ, Charleston J, Whelton PK. Plasma insulin levels and incidence of hypertension in African Americans and whites. *Arch Intern Med.* 1999;159(5):498-503.

76. Brown MD, Moore GE, Korytkowski MT, McCole SD, Hagberg JM. Improvement of insulin sensitivity by short-term exercise training in hypertensive African American women. *Hypertension.* 1997;30(6):1549-1553.

77. Kokkinos P, Naravan P, Colleran J, et al. Effects of regular exercise on blood pressure and left ventricular hypertrophy in African-American men with severe hypertension. *N Engl J Med.* 1995;333(22):1462-1467.

78. Brett SE, Ritter JM, Chowienczyk PJ. Diastolic blood pressure changes during exercise positively correlate with serum cholesterol and insulin resistance. *Circulation.* 2000;101(6):611-615.

79. Halliwill JR, Taylor JA, Eckberg DL. Impaired sympathetic vascular regulation in humans after acute dynamic exercise. *J Physiol.* 1996;495 (Pt 1):279-288.

80. Huonker M, Halle M, Keul J. Structural and functional adaptations of the cardiovascular system by training. *Int J Sports Med.* 1996;17(Suppl 3):S164-S172.

81. Pescatello LS, Franklin BA, Fagard R, et al. American College of Sports Medicine position stand. Exercise and hypertension. *Med Sci Sports Exerc.* 2004;36(3):533-553.

82. Kokkinos PF, Narayan P, Papademetriou V. Exercise as hypertension therapy. *Cardiol Clin.* 2001;19(3):507-516.

83. Daviglus ML, Liu K, Pirzada A, et al. Favorable cardiovascular risk profile in middle age and health-related quality of life in older age. *Arch Intern Med.* 2003;163(20):2460-2468.

84. Chobanian AV, Bakris GL, Black HR, et al. The Seventh Report of the Joint National Committee on Prevention, Detection, Evaluation, and Treatment of High Blood Pressure: the JNC 7 report. *JAMA.* 2003;289(19):2560-2572.

85. He J, Muntner P, Chen J, Roccella EJ, Streiffer RH, Whelton PK. Factors associated with hypertension control in the general population of the United States. *Arch Intern Med.* 2002;162(9):1051-1058.

86. Braith RW, Pollock ML, Lowenthal DT, Graves JE, Limacher MC. Moderate- and high-intensity exercise lowers blood pressure in normotensive subjects 60 to 79 years of age. *Am J Cardiol.* 1994;73(15):1124-1128.

87. Powell KE, Thompson PD, Caspersen CJ, Kendrick JS. Physical activity and the incidence of coronary heart disease. *Annu Rev Public Health.* 1987;8:253-287.

88. Morris JN, Clayton DG, Everitt MG, Semmence AM, Burgess EH. Exercise in leisure time: coronary attack and death rates. *Br Heart J.* 1990;63:325-334.

89. Blair SN, Kohl HW 3rd, Paffenbarger RS Jr, Clark DG, Cooper KH, Gibbons KH. Physical fitness and all-cause mortality. A prospective study of healthy men and women. *JAMA.* 1989;262(17):2395-2401.

90. Lee IM, Hsieh CC, Paffenbarger RS Jr. Exercise intensity and longevity in men. The Harvard Alumni Health Study. *JAMA.* 1995;273(15):1179-1184.

91. Blair SN, Kohl HW III, Barlow CE, Paffenbarger RS Jr, Gibbons LW, Macera CA. Changes in physical fitness and all-cause mortality. A prospective study of healthy and unhealthy men. *JAMA.* 1995;273(14):1093-1098.

92. Hein HO, Suadicani P, Gyntelberg F. Physical fitness or physical activity as a predictor of ischaemic heart disease? A 17-year follow-up in the Copenhagen Male Study. *J Intern Med.* 1992;232(6):471-479.

93. Kelley GA, Kelley KA, Tran ZV. Aerobic exercise and resting blood pressure: a meta-analytic review of randomized, controlled trials. *Prev Cardiol.* 2001;4(2): 73-80.

94. Hagberg JM, Montain SJ, Martin WH 3rd, Ehsani AA. Effect of exercise training in 60- to 69-year-old persons with essential hypertension. *Am J Cardiol.* 1989;64(5):348-353.

95. Kokkinos P, Pittaras A, Manolis A, et al. Exercise capacity and 24-h blood pressure in prehypertensive men and women. *Am J Hypertens.* 2006;19(3):251-258.

96. Jennings GL, Deakin G, Dewar E, Laufer E, Nelson L. Exercise, cardiovascular disease and blood pressure. *Clin Exp Hypertens A.* 1989;11(5-6):1035-1052.

97. Ehrman J. *Clinical Exercise Physiology.* 2nd ed. Champaign, IL: Human Kinetics; 2009.

98. Kortianou EA, Nasis IG, Spetsioti ST, Daskalakis AM, Vogiatzis I. Effectiveness of interval exercise training in patients with COPD. *Cardiopulm Phys Ther J.* 2010;21(3):12-19.

99. Doyle IR, Jones ME, Barr HA, et al. Composition of human pulmonary surfactant varies with exercise and level of fitness. *Am J Respir Crit Care Med.* 1994;149(6):1619-1627.

100. Miller WC, Wallace JP, Eggert KE. Predicting max HR and the HR-VO$_2$ relationship for exercise prescription in obesity. *Med Sci Sports Exerc.* 1993;25(9):1077-1081.

101. American College of Sports Medicine. *ACSM's Resource Manual for Guidelines for Exercise Testing and Prescription.* 6th ed. Philadelphia, PA: Wolters Kluwer Health/Lippincott Williams & Wilkins; 2010.

102. Rowland TW, Boyajian A. Aerobic response to endurance exercise training in children. *Pediatrics.* 1995;96(4 Pt 1):654-658.

103. Pearson OM, Lieberman DE. The aging of Wolff's "law": ontogeny and responses to mechanical loading in cortical bone. *Am J Phys Anthropol.* 2004;(Suppl 39):63-99.

104. McNitt-Gray JL. Kinetics of the lower extremities during drop landings from three heights. *J Biomech.* 1993;26(9):1037-1046.

105. Umemura Y, Ishiko T, Yamauchi T, Kurono M, Mashiko S. Five jumps per day increase bone mass and breaking force in rats. *J Bone Miner Res.* 1997;12(9):1480-1485.

106. Rubin CT, Lanyon LE. Regulation of bone formation by applied dynamic loads. *J Bone Joint Surg Am.* 1984;66(3):397-402.

107. Kohrt WM, Bloomfield SA, Little KD, et al. American College of Sports Medicine Position Stand: physical activity and bone health. *Med Sci Sports Exerc.* 2004;36(11):1985-1996.

108. Baratta R, Solomonow M, Zhou BH, Letson D, Chuinard R, D'Ambrosia R. Muscular coactivation. The role of the antagonist musculature in maintaining knee stability. *Am J Sports Med.* 1988;16(2):113-122.

109. Osternig LR, Hamill J, Lander JE, Robertson R. Co-activation of sprinter and distance runner muscles in isokinetic exercise. *Med Sci Sports Exerc.* 1986;18(4):431-435.

110. Shumway-Cook A, Woollacott MH. *Motor Control: Translating Research into Clinical Practice.* 4th ed. Philadelphia, PA: Wolters Kluwer Health/Lippincott Williams & Wilkins; 2011.

111. Schmidt R. *Motor Control and Learning: A Behavioral Emphasis.* 3rd ed. Champaign, IL: Human Kinetics; 1999.

112. Lieber R. *Skeletal Muscle Structure, Function, and Plasticity: The Physiological Basis of Rehabilitation.* 3rd ed. Baltimore, MD: Lippincott Williams & Wilkins; 2010.

113. Wong TS, Booth FW. Protein metabolism in rat gastrocnemius muscle after stimulated chronic concentric exercise. *J Appl Physiol (1985).* 1990;69(5):1709-1717.

114. Wong TS, Booth FW. Protein metabolism in rat tibialis anterior muscle after stimulated chronic eccentric exercise. *J Appl Physiol (1985).* 1990;69(5):1718-1724.

115. Chesley A, MacDougall JD, Tarnopolsky MA, Atkinson SA, Smith K. Changes in human muscle protein synthesis after resistance exercise. *J Appl Physiol (1985).* 1992;73(4):1383-1388.

116. Morkin E. Postnatal muscle fiber assembly: localization of newly synthesized myofibrillar proteins. *Science.* 1970;167(3924):1499-1501.

117. Kadi F, Thornell LE. Concomitant increases in myonuclear and satellite cell content in female trapezius muscle following strength training. *Histochem. Cell Biol.* 2000;113(2):99-103.

118. MacDougall JD, Elder GC, Sale DG, Moroz JR, Sutton JR. Effects of strength training and immobilization on human muscle fibres. *Eur J Appl Physiol Occup Physiol.* 1980;43(1):25-34.

119. Goldspink G, Howells KF. Work-induced hypertrophy in exercised normal muscles of different ages and the reversibility of hypertrophy after cessation of exercise. *J Physiol.* 1974;239(1):179-193.

120. Sjöström M, Lexell J, Eriksson A, Taylor CC. Evidence of fibre hyperplasia in human skeletal muscles from healthy young men? A left-right comparison of the fibre number in whole anterior tibialis muscles. *Eur J Appl Physiol Occup Physiol.* 1991;62(5):301-304.

121. McMall GE, Byrnes WC, Dickinson A, Pattany PM, Fleck SJ. Muscle fiber hypertrophy, hyperplasia, and capillary density in college men after resistance training. *J Appl Physiol (1985).* 1996;81(5):2004-2012.

122. Autopsies and the need for pituitaries. *N Engl J Med.* 1978;298(24):1366-1367.

123. Hakkinen K, Komi P, Tesch P. Effect of combined eccentric and eccentric strength training and detraining on force-time, muscle fiber and metabolic characteristics of leg extensor muscles. *Scand J Sports Science.* 1981;3:50-58.

124. Kanehisa H, Nagareda H, Kawakami Y, et al. Effects of equivolume isometric training programs comprising medium or high resistance on muscle size and strength. *Eur J Appl Physiol.* 2002;87(2):112-119.

125. Kawakami Y, Abe T, Kuno SY, Fukunaga T. Training-induced changes in muscle architecture and specific tension. *Eur J Appl Physiol Occup Physiol.* 1995;72(1-2):37-43.

126. Reeves ND, Narici MV, Maganaris CN. Effect of resistance training on skeletal muscle-specific force in elderly humans. *J Appl Physiol (1985).* 2004;96(3):885-892.

127. Folland JP, Williams AG. The adaptations to strength training: morphological and neurological contributions to increased strength. *Sports Med.* 2007;37(2):145-168.

128. Abe T, DeHoyos DV, Pollock ML, Garzarella L. Time course for strength and muscle thickness changes following upper and lower body resistance training in men and women. *Eur J Appl Physiol.* 2000;81(3):174-180.

129. Cureton KJ, Collins MA, Hill DW, McElhannon FM Jr. Muscle hypertrophy in men and women. *Med Sci Sports Exerc.* 1988;20(4):338-344.

130. Häkkinen K, Kallinen M, Linnamo V, Pastinen UM, Newton RU, Kraemer WJ. Neuromuscular adaptations during bilateral versus unilateral strength training in middle-aged and elderly men and women. *Acta Physiol Scand.* 1996;158(1):77-88.

131. Zachariae F. Preventive health policy [article in Danish]. *Ugeskr Laeger.* 1975;137(43):2542.

132. Colliander EB, Tesch PA. Responses to eccentric and concentric resistance training in females and males. *Acta Physiol Scand.* 1991;141(2):149-156.

133. Lexell J, Downham DY, Larsson Y, Bruhn E, Morsing B. Heavy-resistance training in older Scandinavian men and women: short- and long-term effects on arm and leg muscles. *Scand J Med Sci Sports.* 1995;5(6):329-341.

134. Weiss LW, Clark FC, Howard DG. Effects of heavy-resistance triceps surae muscle training on strength and muscularity of men and women. *Phys Ther.* 1988;68(2):208-213.

135. O'Hagan FT, Sale DG, MacDougall JD, Garner SH. Response to resistance training in young women and men. *Int J Sports Med.* 1995;16(5):314-321.

136. Hubal MJ, Gordish-Dressman H, Thompson PD, et al. Variability in muscle size and strength gain after unilateral resistance training. *Med Sci Sports Exerc.* 2005;37(6):964-972.

137. Bailey DA. The Saskatchewan Pediatric Bone Mineral Accrual Study: bone mineral acquisition during the growing years. *Int J Sports Med.* 1997;18(Suppl 3):S191-S194.

138. Marcus R, Kosek J, Pfefferbaum A, Horning S. Age-related loss of trabecular bone in premenopausal women: a biopsy study. *Calcif Tissue Int.* 1983;35(4-5):406-409.

139. Recker RR, Davies KM, Hinders SM, Heaney RP, Stegman MR, Kimmel DB. Bone gain in young adult women. *JAMA.* 1992;268(17):2403-2408.

140. Riggs BL, Wahner HW, Dunn WL, Mazess RB, Offord KP, Melton LJ 3rd. Differential changes in bone mineral density of the appendicular and axial skeleton with aging: relationship to spinal osteoporosis. *J Clin Invest.* 1981;67(2):328-335.

141. Courteix D, Lespessailles E, Peres SL, Obert P, Germain P, Benhamou CL. Effect of physical training on bone mineral density in prepubertal girls: a comparative study between impact-loading and non-impact-loading sports. *Osteoporos Int.* 1998;8(2):152-158.

142. Khan KM, Bennell KL, Hopper JL, et al. Self-reported ballet classes undertaken at age 10-12 years and hip bone mineral density in later life. *Osteoporos Int.* 1998;8(2):165-173.

143. Morris FL, Naughton GA, Gibbs JL, Carlson JS, Wark JD. Prospective ten-month exercise intervention in premenarcheal girls: positive effects on bone and lean mass. *J Bone Miner Res.* 1997;12(9):1453-1462.

144. Giangregorio L, Blimkie CJR. Skeletal adaptations to alterations in weight-bearing activity: a comparison of models of disuse osteoporosis. *Sports Med.* 2002;32(7):459-476.

145. Brzycki M. Strength testing—predicting a one-rep max from a reps-to-fatigue. *J Phys Ed Rec Dance.* 1993;64(1):88-90.

146. Faigenbaum AD, Kraemer WJ, Blimkie CJ, et al. Youth resistance training: updated position statement paper from the national strength and conditioning association. *J Strength Cond Res.* 2009;23(5 Suppl):S60-S79.

147. Keen DA, Yue GH, Enoka RM. Training-related enhancement in the control of motor output in elderly humans. *J Appl Physiol (1985).* 1994;77(6):2648-2658.

148. Welle S, Totterman S, Thornton C. Effect of age on muscle hypertrophy induced by resistance training. *J Gerontol A Biol Sci Med Sci.* 1996;51(6):M270-M275.

149. Häkkinen K, Newton RU, Gordon SE, et al. Changes in muscle morphology, electromyographic activity, and force production characteristics during progressive strength training in young and older men. *J Gerontol A Biol Sci Med Sci.* 1998;53(6):B415-B423.

150. Ivey FM, Tracy BL, Lemmer JT, et al. Effects of strength training and detraining on muscle quality: age and gender comparisons. *J Gerontol A Biol Sci Med Sci.* 2000;55(3):B152-B157; discussion B158-159.

151. Paavolainen L, Häkkinen K, Hämäläinen I, Nummela A, Rusko H. Explosive-strength training improves 5-km running time by improving running economy and muscle power. *J Appl Physiol (1985).* 1999;86(5):1527-1533.

152. Kongsgaard M, Aagaard P, Kjaer M, Magnusson SP. Structural Achilles tendon properties in athletes subjected to different exercise modes and in Achilles tendon rupture patients. *J Appl Physiol (1985).* 2005;99(5):1965-1971.

153. Sommer HM. The biomechanical and metabolic effects of a running regime on the Achilles tendon in the rat. *Int Orthop.* 1987;11(1):71-75.

154. Birch HL, McLaughlin L, Smith RK, Goodship AE. Treadmill exercise-induced tendon hypertrophy: assessment of tendons with different mechanical functions. *Equine Vet J Suppl.* 1999;30:222-226.

155. Mooren FC, Lechtermann A, Fromme A, Thorwesten L, Völker K. Alterations in intracellular calcium signaling of lymphocytes after exhaustive exercise. *Med Sci Sports Exerc.* 2001;33(2):242-248.

156. Haaland DA, Sabljic TF, Baribeau DA, Mukovozov IM, Hart LE. Is regular exercise a friend or foe of the aging immune system? A systematic review. *Clin J Sport Med.* 2008;18(6):539-548.

157. Walsh NP, Gleeson M, Shephard RJ, et al. Position statement. Part one: immune function and exercise. *Exerc Immunol Rev.* 2011;17:6-63.

158. Brittenden J, Heys SD, Ross J, Eremin O. Natural killer cells and cancer. *Cancer.* 1996;77(7):1226-1243.

159. Biron CA. Expansion, maintenance, and memory in NK and T cells during viral infections: responding to pressures for defense and regulation. *PLoS Pathog.* 2010;6(3):e1000816.

160. Brenner IK, Shek PN, Shephard RJ. Infection in athletes. *Sports Med.* 1994;17(2):86-107.

161. Nieman DC. Exercise, upper respiratory tract infection, and the immune system. *Med Sci Sports Exerc.* 1994;26(2):128-139.

162. Nieman DC. Risk of upper respiratory tract infection in athletes: an epidemiologic and immunologic perspective. *J Athl Train.* 1997;32(4):344-349.

163. Walsh NP, Gleeson M, Pyne DB, et al. Position statement. Part two: maintaining immune health. *Exerc Immunol Rev.* 2011;17:64-103.

164. Paluska SA, Schwenk TL. Physical activity and mental health: current concepts. *Sports Med.* 2000;29(3):167-180.

165. Carek PJ, Laibstain SE, Carek SM, et al. Exercise for the treatment of depression and anxiety. *Int J Psychiatry Med.* 2011;41(1):15-28.

166. Smith MA, Makino S, Kvetnanský R, Post RM. Effects of stress on neurotrophic factor expression in the rat brain. *Ann N Y Acad Sci.* 1995;771:234-239.

167. Dienstbier RA. Behavioral correlates of sympathoadrenal reactivity: the toughness model. *Med Sci Sports Exerc.* 1991;23(7):846-852.

168. Luger A, Deuster PA, Kyle SB, et al. Acute hypothalamic-pituitary-adrenal responses to the stress of treadmill exercise. Physiologic adaptations to physical training. *N Engl J Med.* 1987;316(21):1309-1315.

169. Wittert GA, Livesey JH, Espiner EA, Donald RA. Adaptation of the hypothalamopituitary adrenal axis to chronic exercise stress in humans. *Med Sci Sports Exerc.* 1996;28(8):1015-1019.

170. Martinsen EW. Physical activity in the prevention and treatment of anxiety and depression. *Nord J Psychiatry.* 2008;62(Suppl 47):25-29.

171. Blumenthal JA, Babyak MA, Moore KA, et al. Effects of exercise training on older patients with major depression. *Arch Intern Med.* 1999;159(19):2349-2356.

172. Singh NA, Clements KM, Singh MA. The efficacy of exercise as a long-term antidepressant in elderly subjects: a randomized, controlled trial. *J Gerontol A Biol Sci Med Sci.* 2001;56(8):M497-M504.

173. DiLorenzo TM, Bargman EP, Stucky-Ropp R, Brassington GS, Frensch PA, LaFontaine T. Long-term effects of aerobic exercise on psychological outcomes. *Prev Med.* 1999;28(1):75-85.

174. Lawlor DA, Hopker SW. The effectiveness of exercise as an intervention in the management of depression: systematic review and meta-regression analysis of randomised controlled trials. *BMJ.* 2001;322(7289):763-767.

175. Manber R, Allen JJ, Morris ME. Alternative treatments for depression: empirical support and relevance to women. *J Clin Psychiatry.* 2002;63(7):628-640.

176. Segar ML, Katch VL, Roth RS, et al. The effect of aerobic exercise on self-esteem and depressive and anxiety symptoms among breast cancer survivors. *Oncol Nurs Forum.* 1998;25(1):107-113.

177. Brosse AL, Sheets ES, Lett HS, Blumenthal JA. Exercise and the treatment of clinical depression in adults: recent findings and future directions. *Sports Med.* 2002;32(12):741-760.

178. Beniamini Y, Rubenstein JJ, Zaichkowsky LD, Crim MC. Effects of high-intensity strength training on quality-of-life parameters in cardiac rehabilitation patients. *Am J Cardiol.* 1997;80(7):841-846.

179. Emery CF, Schein RL, Hauck ER, MacIntyre NR. Psychological and cognitive outcomes of a randomized trial of exercise among patients with chronic obstructive pulmonary disease. *Health Psychol.* 1998;17(3):232-240.

180. Whaley M, Kaminsky L. Epidemiology of physical activity physical fitness and selected chronic disease. In: *ACSM's Resource Manual for Clinical Guidelines for Exercise Testing and Prescription.* Baltimore, MD: Williams and Wilkins; 1998:13-26.

181. Hughes AR, Mutrie N, Macintyre PD. Effect of an exercise consultation on maintenance of physical activity after completion of phase III exercise-based cardiac rehabilitation. *Eur J Cardiovasc Prev Rehabil.* 2007;14(1):114-121.

182. Howley ET. Type of activity: resistance, aerobic and leisure versus occupational physical activity. *Med Sci Sports Exerc.* 2001;33(6 Suppl):S364-S369; discussion S419-S420.

183. Centers for Disease Control and Prevention. Physical activity: how much physical activity do adults need? http://www.cdc.gov/physicalactivity/everyone/guidelines/adults.html. Accessed October 29, 2011.

184. Tucker D, Molsberger SC, Clark A. Walking for wellness: a collaborative program to maintain mobility in hospitalized older adults. *Geriatr Nurs.* 2004;25(4):242-245.

185. Roach KE, Ally D, Finnerty B, et al. The relationship between duration of physical therapy services in the acute care setting and change in functional status in patients with lower-extremity orthopedic problems. *Phys Ther.* 1998;78(1):19-24.

186. Irwin S. Primary prevention and risk factor reduction for cardiovascular and pulmonary disorders—Preferred Practice Patterns 6A. In: *Cardiopulmonary Physical Therapy: A Guide to Practice.* 4th ed. St. Louis, MO: Mosby; 2004:254-269.

CASE STUDY 5-1

Lola Sicard Rosenbaum, PT, DPT, MHS

EXAMINATION

History

Current Condition/Chief Complaint

Mr. Cedar, an obese 51-year-old White male, was referred to physical therapy by his primary care physician (PCP) for an aquatic exercise program to improve his activity tolerance without aggravating his arthritic knee pain. He reported that he wanted to be able to take walks with his grandchildren or play with them without getting so tired.

Social History/Environment

He was previously employed as a police officer, but accepted a medical retirement 3 years ago because of deteriorating cardiac health.

Several months prior to the physical therapy appointment, he was awarded custody of his 2 preschool-aged grandchildren. He was designated as the primary caregiver since his wife worked outside their home.

He lived in a private home with 4 outside stairs with no railing, and one flight of inside stairs with railings. His grandchildren's bedrooms were on the second floor and Mr. Cedar complained of difficulty climbing up and down stairs.

Mr. Cedar smoked cigarettes in the past but quit 4 years prior. He reported alcohol use of 2 to 3 beers 2 days per week.

Family History

Mr. Cedar's father was still living and diagnosed with CAD, HTN, diabetes mellitus (DM), and hyperlipidemia. Mr. Cedar reported CAD "runs in my family." His mother and both sets of grandparents died from CAD complications, either stroke or cardiac pathology.

Medical/Surgical History

Mr. Cedar had 2 previous cardiac catheterizations and was diagnosed with severe CAD. He had a myocardial infarction (MI) and coronary artery bypass graft prior to his catheterizations. He was also diagnosed with hyperlipidemia, HTN, morbid obesity, dyspnea, and recurrent angina.

Mr. Cedar wanted to improve his cardiac health but was not able to continue in a standard cardiac rehabilitation program because of bilateral knee pain, left greater than right. He underwent a left knee arthroscopy and was diagnosed with osteoarthritis (OA).

Reported Functional Status

He reported difficulty with self-care and home management. He reported SOB with dressing, getting breakfast, doing housework, or caring for his 2 young grandchildren.

He was able to play board games with his grandchildren, but not able to play ball, go for walks, or play any active games.

Mr. Cedar reported difficulty with locomotion and movement. His knee symptoms and fatigue increased with walking greater than 50 feet on level ground, or uneven terrain, as well as with using stairs or ramps.

He stated he was not able to participate in any exercise beyond daily activities because of SOB and fatigue.

Clinician Comment *A significant cardiac history along with a patient report of fatigue beyond expectations for an activity would be a red flag for careful monitoring when examining a patient for consideration of an exercise program.[1] In addition, Mr. Cedar had significant comorbidities of HTN, arthritis, and obesity. These needed to be considered when determining whether he would be an appropriate aquatics physical therapy candidate. Further, it was possible that Mr. Cedar's dyspnea and fatigue with activity were due to underlying heart failure. Heart failure, along with his HTN, would be an important consideration with aquatic treatment as the presence of either might designate the level of water immersion he would tolerate.*

A 100-cm column of water exerts a pressure of 76 mm Hg on a person's body surface. This pressure compresses superficial veins, resulting in a blood volume shift to the heart and thorax. This blood volume shift is not significant on immersion to the iliac crest but can increase significantly on immersion up to the neck.[2] Immersion past the xiphoid process can produce hemodynamic problems in a patient with moderate MI or heart failure. Unfortunately, the patient is not aware of the hemodynamic deterioration taking place in deeper water, and a patient can maintain a false sense of well-being. Immersion to the xiphoid process does not affect mean pulmonary artery pressure or pulmonary capillary pressure. Immersion to the neck or in a supine position increases both pulmonary artery and capillary pressure, resulting in LV overload and increased SV, both of which are dangerous in moderate MI and heart failure patients.[2]

Aquatic therapeutic exercise for patients with moderate to severe MI or heart failure can be allowed provided the patient remains in an upright position immersed no deeper than the xiphoid process. Water-based therapy with the appropriate modifications, therefore, can be as safe as land-based physical therapy in the treatment of middle-aged males with cardiovascular impairments.[2]

Heart failure is a difficult disease to define. The American Heart Association lists 4 stages of heart failure[3]:

1. *Stage A: At risk to develop heart failure without evidence of heart dysfunction.*

2. *Stage B: Evidence of heart dysfunction without symptoms.*

3. *Stage C: Evidence of heart dysfunction with symptoms.*

4. *Stage D: Symptoms of heart failure despite maximal therapy.*

Though easier to recognize in the moderate to severe stages, heart failure is often missed in the early stages when a patient may complain of dyspnea but not have evidence of LV systolic dysfunction.[4] Dyspnea, fatigue, and ankle edema are physical signs of heart failure that are sensitive but nonspecific and of low predictive value since they occur in many other diseases. Orthopnea and paroxysmal nocturnal dyspnea are specific signs of heart failure but have low sensitivity because heart failure has to be quite advanced before they occur.

Mr. Cedar's body mass index (BMI) of 53.75% indicates extreme obesity and more than doubles his risk of heart failure.[5] Other clinical clues from Mr. Cedar's history were the presence of a previous MI, HTN, dyspnea, and fatigue. The possibility of early heart failure needed to be considered as the interview continued.

Medications

Mr. Cedar's current medications were Synthroid (levothyroxine sodium), Lasix (furosemide), Plavix (clopidogrel bisulfate), Prevacid (lansoprazole), acetylsalicylic acid (ASA), Zetia (ezetimibe), Lopressor (metoprolol tartrate), Xanax (alprazolam), Diovan (valsartan), and Aleve (naproxen).

Clinician Comment *Mr. Cedar was taking many prescription medications, taking a few over-the-counter medications, and occasionally used alcohol. Mr. Cedar has a veritable cocktail of prescription medications to which he occasionally adds an alcoholic drink or over-the-counter medication, such as Advil. Using 2 different online drug interaction checkers,[6,7] more than 10 possible interactions between his medications and social drinking were identified, which, in turn, may affect his status for physical therapy treatment.*

Since Mr. Cedar was at risk for a drug interaction,[8] he needed to be advised to tell his physicians and pharmacists about all of his medications. Filling all of his medications at the same pharmacy that has a conscientious drug-drug interaction monitoring program was advised.[9]

His prescription medications and their indications are as follows:

- *Synthroid: used as replacement or supplemental therapy in congenital or acquired hypothyroidism of any etiology*
- *Lasix: used in the management of edema.*
- *Plavix: used to reduce the risk of MI in patients with atherosclerosis documented by recent ischemic stroke, recent MI, or established peripheral arterial disease*
- *Prevacid: used for short-term treatment and symptomatic relief of gastroesophageal reflux disease*
- *Zetia: used as a cholesterol absorption inhibitor*
- *Lopressor, a beta adrenergic blocking agent: used alone or in combination with other classes of antihypertensive agents in the management of HTN*

- *Xanax, a benzodiazepine: used for the management of anxiety disorders or for the short-term relief of symptoms of anxiety or anxiety associated with depressive symptoms*
- *Diovan, an ace inhibitor: used alone or in combination with other classes of antihypertensive agents (eg, thiazide diuretics) in the management of HTN*

Reviewing Mr. Cedar's medications helped to identify medical conditions he had not mentioned when originally asked, such as hypothyroidism, anxiety, depression, and gastroesophageal reflux disease. It was important to stress that the 2 medications to manage his HTN needed to be taken consistently.

Other Clinical Tests

An addendum to Mr. Cedar's referral to physical therapy indicated that he had undergone a recent treadmill stress test, during which he maintained a normal ECG with no evidence of exercise-induced ischemia. His report of varying treadmill speeds and inclines, as well as the assessment of ischemia (in his case, absent) suggests he underwent a symptom-limited maximal exercise stress test. The normal ECG result along with BP, O_2 saturation (SpO$_2$), and HR monitoring reasonably rules out left- or right-sided heart failure and unmanaged HTN.[10]

Clinician Comment *Mr. Cedar was a medically retired, obese, middle-aged male with a cardiac history and an arthritic left knee. His goal was to improve his ability to care for his dependent grandchildren. Because of his arthritic knees, aquatic physical therapy might be an ideal treatment to improve his activity tolerance. The stress test findings suggested that his dyspnea was not due to heart failure or a gas-exchange disorder. Further confirmation of this could be achieved in a full systems review. It could be anticipated that auscultation would confirm the absence of an S3 heart sound associated with heart failure.[11] Clear lung sounds and normal SpO$_2$ would eliminate restrictive lung disease or a gas-exchange disorder as the cause of his dyspnea.[10] A full systems review would determine whether Mr. Cedar would be an appropriate candidate for physical therapy.*

Systems Review

Cardiovascular/Pulmonary System

Resting: HR: 70; BP: 134/84; RR: 22; SpO$_2$ 96%; S1S2 sounds only: no S3 heard, breath sounds clear

Edema: impaired. Mild edema noted bilateral ankles, which was not pitting edema.

Clinician Comment *Mr. Cedar had presented himself for his physical therapy initial evaluation approximately 20 minutes early so he would have time to recover from his walk from the parking lot to the waiting room. After walking with him the 150 feet from the waiting room to the treatment room, his SOB was noted. His SOB abated after a short rest while sitting in a chair with back support.*

Mr. Cedar sat, rested, and answered patient interview questions for approximately 10 minutes before vital signs were taken. This met the guideline recommendation for taking resting BP measures of at least 5 minutes rest prior.[12] An aneroid device was used and a large-size cuff positioned on his right arm and lined up with the lines drawn on the cuff to indicate proper circumference. He was positioned with his back and arm supported.

Clear breath sounds and the absence of S3 heart sound were confirmed at rest but remained to be assessed with activity.

Integumentary System

Presence of scar formation 24 cm long in midsternal area was noted.

Continuity and pliability of skin was within normal limits (WNL).

Musculoskeletal System

Gross symmetry: WNL
Gross ROM: WNL, slight decrease in left knee flexion
Gross strength: 3/5, no break testing done
Height: 69 inches (1.75 m); weight: 364 pounds (165 kg); BMI: 53.75, very obese

Clinician Comment *Mr. Cedar's multiple-year history of arthritis in his left knee, lack of exercise, and decreased function suggested that he had muscle weaknesses in one or both of his LEs. Manual muscle testing (MMT) is used by PTs to test strength. Sustained and repetitive isometric exercise can cause an increase in CO and a disproportionate rise in SBP, DBP, and mean BP.[13] The sustained hold for 1 to 3 seconds against resistance required by the patient to determine MMT grades above 3/5 is a precaution in certain patient populations, but does not need to be avoided.[14] Clear instructions to avoid breath holding during the resisted effort can minimize the CO and BP changes noted earlier.[15]*

Mr. Cedar's strength was assessed by asking him to move his extremities through a full ROM against gravity, but his strength at end range was not break tested. Without the applied resistance, the optimal MMT grade that could be assigned was 3/5, which corresponded to the ability to contract the tested muscle through a full ROM against gravity.[16]

Mr. Cedar's obesity is an issue. In this instance, his BMI was determined. Other clinical tests conducted by PTs during an examination that would indicate obesity include waist to height, waist circumference, hip circumference, waist:hip ratio, and abdominal height in supine (as measured from the table).[17] Patients may also undergo more elaborate testing to determine the extent of their obesity, including dual-energy X-ray absorptiometry, bioimpedance, skinfold thickness, and plethysmography. Despite the fact that PTs may not actually conduct these tests, they should be aware of how to interpret their findings and use the results to enhance patient treatment.

Neuromuscular System

Gait: He ambulated independently, without an assistive device. An antalgic gait pattern was noted with decreased left stance time. Walking speed appeared slower than normal.

Locomotion: He transferred independently but slowly using bilateral UEs to assist sit to stand and vice versa.

Balance: Normal bilateral stance, impaired single-leg stance, bilaterally

Motor function: No gross deficits noted.

Communication, Affect, Cognition, Learning Style

No deficits were noted in communication, affect, and cognition. He was able to make his needs known, was oriented ×3, and demonstrated a normal emotional response. He reported he learned best by demonstration with written instructions. No learning barriers were noted.

Education Needs

He would benefit from education regarding his disease processes as well as the role exercise would play to manage and control disease progression. Instruction in self-monitoring of HR, RPE, and respiratory rate during exercise was indicated.

Clinician Comment *Mr. Cedar walked independently without the use of an assistive device. During the interview, he reported function limiting left knee pain; however, his observed ability to walk was hampered more by SOB and the need for frequent rests. Mr. Cedar's knee pain was a contributing factor to his functional limitations, but his impaired aerobic capacity and endurance were probably a greater limiter of his function. The results of the systems review indicated that further testing of Mr. Cedar's aerobic capacity and endurance was needed, in addition to exploration of his LE joint mobility, ROM, and performance in gait. Since he showed an impaired ability to perform a single-leg stance on either LE, further testing of his balance was indicated to determine if he was at risk for falls.*

Tests and Measures

Aerobic Capacity and Endurance

Two-minute walk test (2MWT): Distance walked 125 m (410 feet); BP: 144/80; HR: 88; RR: 32; SpO_2: 96%; S1 and S2 heart sounds only; complained of SOB and sweating. Borg Rating of Perceived Exertion was 15/20. Mr. Cedar complained of left anterior knee pain afterwards.

Clinician Comment *A clinical decision needed to be made on whether to use the 2MWT or the 6MWT with Mr. Cedar. The 6MWT has been shown to be the test of choice when using a functional walk test for clinical purposes.[18]*

The 6MWT can be conducted at the patient's rate. If the 6MWT had been the selected tool, Mr. Cedar could have stopped to rest by leaning against the wall. With rests, he may have completed the test. If he had not, then the time and distance could have been noted in his chart. Being able to complete the entire test could have then become one of his goals for therapy.

The 2MWT has not been studied as extensively as the 6MWT. The 2MWT, however, showed moderate correlation with measures of physical function in patients before and after coronary bypass surgery and may prove to be the recommended test for cardiac patients, or for patients whose comorbidities make the completion of the 6MWT difficult.[19]

Mr. Cedar experienced dyspnea with the short walk from the waiting area to the treatment room. This observation, along with his comorbidities of CVD, LE OA, and obesity, led to the selection of the 2MWT.

During the 2MWT, Mr. Cedar's HR and BP were adaptive as expected to the increased activity. He rated the effort as "hard," which corresponds to 15/20 on the Borg RPE scale. He became dyspneic, but his normal range of SpO_2 was maintained. After walking, an S3 heart sound remained absent and breath sounds clear. Therefore, it was reasonable to conclude that, for this level of exercise, he showed no gas-exchange or cardiac pathology. The SOB and effort were probably due to deconditioning of the exercising muscles in the LEs and possibly those of the ventilatory pump.

Joint Integrity and Mobility

Goniometric ROM: right knee 0 to 115 degrees (obesity limited); left knee 0 to 100 degrees

Patellar mobility: Decreased on left as compared to right, crepitus noted left.

Joint mobility: Unable to assess secondary to obesity.

Edema: Bilateral ankle edema. Used a tape measure with figure-of-eight wrap: right 56.5 cm; left 57.5 cm.

Clinician Comment *Use of the figure-of-eight ankle measurements is a tool for determining if physical therapy interventions are having an effect on ankle edema. Figure-of-eight ankle measurements have been shown to be reliable, valid, and an efficient measurement of ankle edema as compared to the gold standard of water displacement volumetry.[20]*

Gait, Locomotion, and Balance

Gait: Mr. Cedar ambulated on level surfaces without an assistive device but with a slow pace, wide base of support, and slight decrease in left stance time. While ambulating, Mr. Cedar reported 3 to 4/10 pain intensity in his left knee. During the 2MWT, Mr. Cedar exhibited SOB after walking 2 minutes with a respiratory rate of 32 respirations per minute. His walking speed of 1.0 m/s (39.3 in/s) is slightly below the normal walking speed for a 50-year-old male of 1.4 m/s (55.1 in/s).[21]

Locomotion: No further testing was conducted.

Balance: Berg Balance Score 45/56, low fall risk

Single-leg stance time: right LE 5 sec; left LE 3 sec; eyes opened

Clinician Comment *The tests and measures confirm that Mr. Cedar is more limited by his aerobic capacity than by his knee pain. He was able to complete the 2MWT with relatively low pain but with notable SOB. After 2 minutes of slower-than-normal walking for his age, Mr. Cedar rated his perceived exertion as 15/20, which is defined as "hard" or "heavy" work. His reported knee pain rating was 2 to 3/10 at rest with increases to 3 to 4/10 when ambulating. His painful left knee ROM was 15 degrees less than his right knee. A Timed Up and Go Test was not performed but would have been an effective measure of locomotion. Mr. Cedar's Berg Balance Scale score and single-leg stance times confirm he is at a low risk for falls. Limitations in balance may be a result of knee pain.*

EVALUATION

Diagnosis

Based on the history, systems review, and tests and measures mentioned previously, Mr. Cedar was classified into 2 practice patterns. His major pattern is Cardiopulmonary Pattern 6B: Impaired Aerobic Capacity/Endurance Associated With Deconditioning. His secondary pattern is Musculoskeletal Pattern 4E: Impaired Joint Mobility, Motor Function, Muscle Performance, and Range of Motion Associated With Localized Inflammation.

International Classification of Functioning, Disability, and Health Model of Disability

See ICF Model on page 192.

ICF MODEL OF DISABLEMENT FOR MR. CEDAR

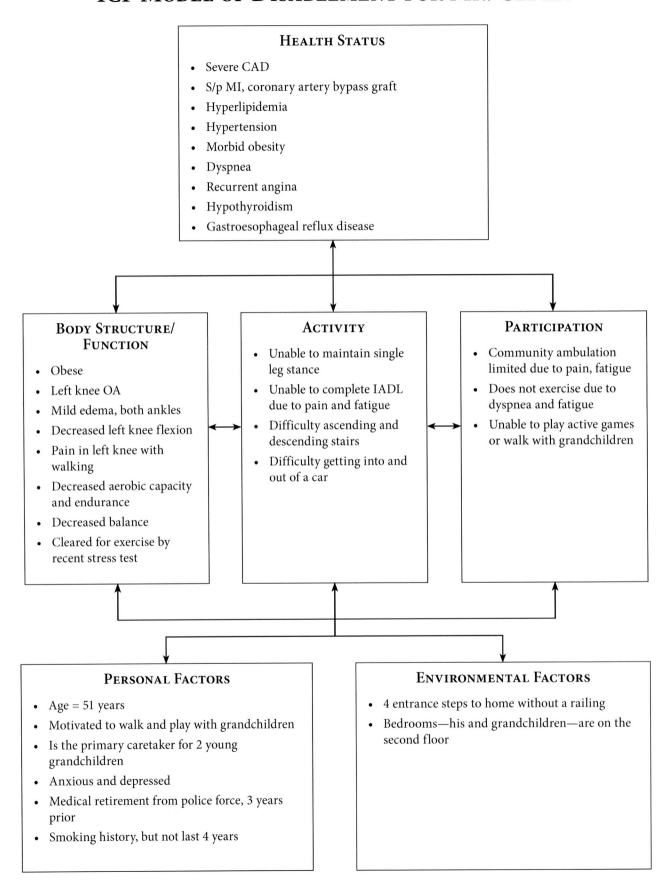

HEALTH STATUS

- Severe CAD
- S/p MI, coronary artery bypass graft
- Hyperlipidemia
- Hypertension
- Morbid obesity
- Dyspnea
- Recurrent angina
- Hypothyroidism
- Gastroesophageal reflux disease

BODY STRUCTURE/ FUNCTION

- Obese
- Left knee OA
- Mild edema, both ankles
- Decreased left knee flexion
- Pain in left knee with walking
- Decreased aerobic capacity and endurance
- Decreased balance
- Cleared for exercise by recent stress test

ACTIVITY

- Unable to maintain single leg stance
- Unable to complete IADL due to pain and fatigue
- Difficulty ascending and descending stairs
- Difficulty getting into and out of a car

PARTICIPATION

- Community ambulation limited due to pain, fatigue
- Does not exercise due to dyspnea and fatigue
- Unable to play active games or walk with grandchildren

PERSONAL FACTORS

- Age = 51 years
- Motivated to walk and play with grandchildren
- Is the primary caretaker for 2 young grandchildren
- Anxious and depressed
- Medical retirement from police force, 3 years prior
- Smoking history, but not last 4 years

ENVIRONMENTAL FACTORS

- 4 entrance steps to home without a railing
- Bedrooms—his and grandchildren—are on the second floor

Clinician Comment *Before moving forward in the evaluative process to establish the prognosis, plan of care, and intervention, a consultation with Mr. Cedar's physician was indicated. Though Mr. Cedar was referred with a musculoskeletal diagnosis, his systems review and tests and measures identified that his major limitation was deconditioning.*

Further, the indoor pool available for Mr. Cedar's program had a water depth of 1.07 m to 1.37 m (3.5 to 4.5 feet). Mr. Cedar was 1.75 m (5.75 feet) tall. With water walking and exercises performed in standing, Mr. Cedar would not be submerged past his xiphoid process. Nonetheless, his primary physician was consulted to ensure she was aware of the caution with regard to an aquatic program.

Mr. Cedar's physician was not surprised with the report of findings that defined Mr. Cedar's deconditioned status. She reaffirmed his clearance for monitored exercise from the recent stress test. Though she stated that she was not aware of the hemodynamic implications of immersion past the xiphoid process for some patients, she concurred with the conclusion that he would not be at risk, even with HTN, given his height and the pool depth.

Prognosis

Mr. Cedar gained 60 pounds in 3 years and was deconditioned from lack of exercise. His left knee pain hindered his ability to walk for exercise. A monitored exercise program was indicated, as well as intervention for his knee pain. His obesity and knee pain impeded his progress in a cardiac rehabilitation program. Mr. Cedar would improve his aerobic capacity and endurance as well as strengthen his supporting knee musculature in a monitored aquatic exercise program. Over the course of 12 weeks, it could be expected that Mr. Cedar would demonstrate improved aerobic capacity/endurance and joint mobility, motor function, and ROM to achieve a higher level of functioning in home, community, and leisure environments.

Clinician Comment *Patients with cardiac disease and symptomatic arthritis of the knee can improve levels of functional capacity that are comparable to changes observed in patients with cardiac disease only.[22] Cardiac rehabilitation results in significant improvement in the cardiovascular risk profile at all levels of BMI, independently of weight loss, and can achieve significant improvements in exercise capacity and metabolic profile, even without weight loss.[23] When comorbidities are recognized and the exercise interventions appropriately modified, the presence of activity limitation may be associated with a greater potential for improved prognosis and outcomes from physical therapy.*

Mr. Cedar had comorbidities of HTN, arthritis, cardiac disease, and obesity. Modifying his exercise interventions

was as simple as prescribing a monitored aquatics exercise program instead of a land-based program. Would water-based physical therapy be as effective as land-based physical therapy for Mr. Cedar?

Both issues of cardiovascular impairments and OA were addressed in a study by Foley et al.[24] A total of 105 subjects over 50 years old with LE arthritis were randomized into 1 of 3 groups: hydrotherapy (n = 35), gym (n = 35), or control (n = 35). Both exercising groups had 3 exercise sessions per week for 6 weeks. At the beginning and end of the exercise program, a single, trained, blinded-to-group PT performed all outcome assessments. Outcomes included the 6MWT, muscle strength dynamometry, the Western Ontario and McMaster Universities Osteoarthritis Index (WOMAC), total drugs, the SF-12 quality of life, the Adelaide Activities Profile, and the Arthritis Self-Efficacy Scale. The participants in the groups had a mean age that was older than Mr. Cedar, but more than one-third of each group had comorbid conditions of cardiac conditions and/or obesity. The water-based group demonstrated a significant gain in muscle strength compared with the control group, but less than the land-based group. The water-based group, however, showed a significant increase in physical function over both the land-based and control groups.

Since progressive overloading of the muscles and loading through the eccentric phase of muscle contraction is not possible in water, the researchers attempted to balance the intensity of exercise. Higher and faster repetitions were used in the water, and the water group was subject to the continuing effects of water movement while moving through their exercise program. The land-based group exercising on gym equipment had pauses and rests that may have accounted for decreased aerobic benefit as compared with the aquatics group. The aerobic effect as a result of aquatic exercise was supported by Meyer and Bucking.[2] Mr. Cedar was deconditioned but was unable to tolerate a land-based program because of his knee pain. It could be anticipated that water-based physical therapy would be as effective as land-based physical therapy to address his OA knee pain, balance,[25] and deconditioning.

Plan of Care

Intervention

Patient-/client-related instruction regarding deconditioning, heart failure, and arthritis. Instruction will also include normal HR, BP, and respiratory response to exercise, as well as self-monitoring techniques, including use of RPE scale.

Aquatics physical therapy program to include cardiac and respiratory conditioning, balance training, ROM, therapeutic exercise, and strength and endurance training for ventilatory muscles.

Instruction in home exercise or fitness center program.

Proposed Frequency and Duration of Physical Therapy Visits

Aquatic exercise program 2 to 3 times per week for 8 to 12 weeks.

Anticipated Goals

1. Patient will be able to use the RPE scale to report his exercise effort (1 week).

2. Patient will demonstrate knowledge of appropriate BP, HR, and respiratory response to exercise (2 weeks).

3. Patient will be able to participate in 30 minutes of aquatics physical therapy at an RPE level from 9/20 to 12/20 (3 weeks).

4. Patient will be able to complete a 2MWT without SOB (4 weeks).

5. Patient will show increased left knee flexion by 10 to 15 degrees (6 weeks).

6. Patient will show reduced LE edema by 1 to 2 cm on figure-eight measure (6 weeks).

7. Patient will increase his single LE stance by 6 to 8 seconds (8 weeks).

8. Patient will report his left knee pain intensity has decreased by 2 levels (8 weeks).

9. Patient will be able to participate in 60 minutes of exercise (land- and water-based) with 20 minutes at the RPE level from 12/20 to 14/20 (12 weeks).

10. Patient will be able to complete a 6MWT without SOB or fatigue (12 weeks).

Expected Outcomes (Upon Discharge)

1. Patient will be independent in a home- or fitness center-based exercise program.

2. Patient will resume cooking and cleaning tasks without significant fatigue.

3. Patient will report he can walk 20 minutes with his 2 dependent grandchildren without significant fatigue.

4. Patient will report no loss of balance or falls with stair climbing or walking on uneven ground.

5. Patient reports he can flex left knee to get in and out of automobile without difficulty and stoop to pick up grandchildren's toys on the floor.

Clinician Comment *Increased survival and optimal quality of life are 2 major objectives of health care. Quality of life can be defined as the patient's ability to enjoy normal life activities. Mr. Cedar's functional status as a result of his cardiac and arthritis problems significantly affected his quality of life. Health-related quality of life instruments measure the patient's perception of the functional effect of an illness and the results of the therapeutic intervention.*

A health-related quality of life instrument would focus on a population with a specific condition or disease, such as a cardiac population with anginal symptoms. The specific instruments allow responsiveness and sensitivity to be maximized and detect small changes that the patient and PT consider important.[26]

Outcome measures to quantify the effects of physical therapy interventions include joint-specific and disease-specific rating instruments. The disease-specific instruments report a more global picture of outcomes from the patient's perspective. An example of a joint-specific instrument would be the Lysholm Knee Rating Scale,[27] and an example of a disease-specific instrument would be the WOMAC.[28]

The WOMAC is a disease-specific, self-administered, widely used instrument that measures symptoms and physical disability. It was originally developed for people with OA of the hip or knee to measure changes in health status after some kind of treatment intervention.

The WOMAC has been shown to be effective instruments for measuring outcomes in populations with arthritis of the knee.[29] The WOMAC would have been an appropriate measure to use with Mr. Cedar. Mr. Cedar did not complete a subjective, impairment-specific outcome instrument for either his dyspnea and fatigue or his OA knee status.

Discharge Plan

It was anticipated that Mr. Cedar would achieve the anticipated goals and expected outcomes at the end of the plan of care and would be discharged to a home exercise program.

INTERVENTION

Coordination, Communication, and Documentation

The findings of Mr. Cedar's examination were discussed with him. All elements of his management were documented. Through his PCP, he was referred to a dietitian for instruction in weight control guidelines and appropriate nutrition and food choices to aid his effort in weight loss and risk factor reduction.

Patient-/Client-Related Instruction

Education regarding his current condition, impairments, and functional limitations were discussed with Mr. Cedar. The importance of following the designed home exercise program, including progressive walking or biking, was stressed with Mr. Cedar, as well as the need to continue exercising after his course of physical therapy ended in order to maintain gained aerobic conditioning. Mr. Cedar was informed of the danger of drinking alcohol while taking prescription medications.

Procedural Interventions

Therapeutic Exercise

Aerobic Capacity/Endurance Conditioning or Reconditioning

Mode

Water walking

Intensity

RPE between 9/20 and 12/20

Duration

10 to 15 minutes

Frequency

2 to 3 times per week

Description of the Intervention

Walk forward, backward, and sideways in the water, varying step length and step height. Increased speed, ankle weights, and/or resistance board or dumbbells held in UEs may be added to increase RPE as conditioning improves. Walking will be performed in a 25-meter pool with submersion no deeper than chest level.

Flexibility Exercises

Mode

Muscle lengthening and stretching

Intensity

To a position of mild discomfort

Duration

30 to 60 seconds for 2 to 3 repetitions

Frequency

2 to 3 times per week

Description of the Intervention

Hamstring, hip flexor, gastrocnemius, and soleus stretching. For all stretches, he will isolate the muscle to be stretched, then stretch the muscle to a position of mild discomfort and hold for 30 to 60 seconds, concentrating on breathing deeply and regularly while stretching. The water level for all stretches should be approximately waist high.

- Hamstring stretch: Standing on the right LE with his back to the wall of the pool, perform a straight leg raise with the left LE until the left LE is on stretch. Place a buoyant noodle around the ankle of the left LE and keep the left knee straight and the left ankle dorsiflexed. Allow the buoyancy of the water acting on the noodle to stretch the left hamstrings. Repeat with the right LE.

- Hip flexor stretch: Standing on the right LE facing the wall of the pool, bend the left knee toward the buttocks. Place a buoyant noodle around the left ankle. Keep the knees together and the hips extended and allow the buoyancy of the water acting on the noodle to stretch the left hip flexors. Repeat with the right LE.

- Gastrocnemius and soleus stretch: Perform this stretch in the water as would be done on land.

Strength, Power, and Endurance Training for Limb, Pelvic-Floor, Trunk, and Ventilatory Muscles

Mode

Active resistive isotonic exercises

Intensity

Using buoyant devices and increasing velocity over time

Duration

10 to 15 repetitions

Frequency

2 to 3 times per week

Description of the Intervention

Using the resistance of the water and buoyant devices such as dumbbells for UE and noodles for LE, move the extremity through the water at increasing speeds for each muscle group, concentrating on breathing deeply and regularly while exercising. Progress to using water weights on LEs and water resistance gloves on UEs. All exercises will be performed with submersion no deeper than chest level.

Gait and Locomotion Training

Mode

Water walking

Intensity

Self-paced

Duration

10 minutes

Frequency

2 to 3 times per week

Description of the Intervention

Walk in water chest deep holding dumbbells or noodle in UE with heel-toe gait pattern, concentrating on taking equal step lengths and swing-through motions. UEs are stationary, initially progressing to no-hand holds with proper arm swing with each step.

Balance, Coordination, and Agility Training

Mode

Posture awareness training and standardized exercise approaches to task-specific performance training

Intensity

Challenge beyond usual positions/length of time

Duration

10 to 15 minutes

Frequency

2 to 3 times per week

Description of the Intervention

Single-leg stance activities, tandem walking, crossover walking. While standing at rail in water at chest level, lift one leg off the floor in a stork stance. Maintain this position without hand hold for 20 to 30 seconds. Move both UEs through various motions and activities (ie, throwing and catching a ball) while maintaining single-leg stance. Repeat for the opposite LE. Walk forward and backward on straight line in pool, placing one foot directly in front of or behind the other. Walk sideways in pool, crossing leading LE in front of the stance extremity, then on the next step, cross-behind stance extremity.

Informed Consent

Mr. Cedar helped formulate, and agreed with, the proposed plan of care.

OUTCOMES

Reexamination

Reexamination took place at monthly intervals until discharge. After 4 weeks of twice weekly aquatics physical therapy, Mr. Cedar was able to use the RPE scale to report his exercise effort and understood what his appropriate BP, HR, and respiratory response should be to exercise. He was able to participate in 30 minutes of aquatics physical therapy at an RPE level from 9/20 to 12/20. He walked 135 meters but was not yet able to complete the 2MWT without SOB.

His 8-week reassessment showed that he was able to complete 160 meters in the 2MWT test without SOB, his left knee pain intensity was decreased by 2 levels, and his left knee flexion was increased by 10 degrees from 100 to 110. His LE edema was reduced by 1.5 cm and he could balance on a single LE for 10 to 15 seconds. Mr. Cedar reported that he was able to walk to his mailbox, an approximately 4- to 5-minute walk, without SOB or fatigue. He was progressing toward his physical therapy discharge goals as planned.

Discharge

Mr. Cedar was discharged from physical therapy at 10 weeks, which was earlier than intended secondary to insurance and monetary issues. At that time, he had not achieved his 12-week goals of being able to participate in 60 minutes of exercise (land- and water-based) with 20 minutes of the exercise performed at the RPE level from 12 to 14/20.

He did not meet the goal of completing a 6MWT without SOB. He was able to walk continuously for 6 minutes, but with mild SOB. He attributed the SOB during the test to his attempt to walk faster than his normal walking pace. He was instructed to continue to work toward achieving these goals by continuing to participate and progress his home exercise program.

Mr. Cedar did achieve the expected outcomes of independence in a home- or fitness center-based exercise program, resumption of cooking and cleaning tasks without significant fatigue, no loss of balance or falls while traversing stairs and uneven ground, and adequate flexion in his left knee to get in and out of automobile without difficulty and stoop to pick up his grandchildren's toys on the floor. His expected outcome of being able to walk 20 minutes with his 2 dependent grandchildren without significant fatigue was not achieved. He was discharged to a water exercise and land walking program at a local fitness center with written instructions.

REFERENCES

1. Goodman CC, Boissonnault WG, Fuller KS. *Pathology: Implications for the Physical Therapist.* 2nd ed. Philadelphia, PA: Saunders; 2003.
2. Meyer K, Buking J. Exercise in heart failure: should aqua therapy and swimming be allowed? *Med Science Sports Exerc.* 2004;36(12):2017-2023.
3. Bonow RO, Bennett S, Casey DE Jr, et al. ACC/AHA Clinical Performance Measures for Adults With Heart Failure: a report of the American College of Cardiology/American Heart Association Task Force on Performance Measures (Writing Committee to Develop Heart Failure Clinical Performance Measures): endorsed by the Heart Failure Society of America. *Circulation.* 2005;112(12):1853-1887.
4. Struthers AD. The diagnosis of heart failure. *Heart.* 2000;84:334-338.
5. Kenchaiah S, Evans JC, Levy D, et al. Obesity and the risk of heart failure. *N Engl J Med.* 2002;347:305-313.
6. Medscape. Drug interaction checker. http://reference.medscape.com/drug-interactionchecker. Accessed March 20, 2010.
7. Drug Digest. Check interactions. http://www.drugdigest.org/wps/portal/ddigest. Accessed March 20, 2010.
8. Juurlink D, Mamdani M, Kopp A, et al. Drug-drug interactions among elderly patients hospitalized for drug toxicity. *JAMA.* 2003;289:1652-1658.
9. Sandson N. Drug-drug interactions: the silent epidemic. *Psych Services.* 2005;56(1):22-24.
10. DeTurk WE, Cahalin LP. Evaluation of patient intolerance to exercise. In: DeTurk WE, Cahalin LP, eds. *Cardiovascular and Pulmonary Physical Therapy: An Evidence-Based Approach.* New York, NY: McGraw-Hill; 2004:361-378.
11. Cahalin LP. Chapter 10. Cardiovascular evaluation. In: DeTurk WE, Cahalin LP, eds. *Cardiovascular and Pulmonary Physical Therapy: An Evidence-Based Approach.* New York, NY: McGraw-Hill; 2004:297.
12. Pickering TG, Hall JE, Appel LJ, et al. Recommendation for blood pressure measurement in humans and experimental animals: Part 1: blood pressure measurement in humans: a statement for professionals from the Subcommittee of Professional and Public Education of the American Heart Association Council on High Blood Pressure Research. *Hypertension.* 2005;45(1):142-161.
13. Vincent KR, Vincent HK. Resistance training for individuals with cardiovascular disease. *J Cardiopulm Rehabil.* 2006;26:207-216.
14. Clarkson HM. *Musculoskeletal Assessment: Joint Range of Motion and Manual Muscle Strength.* 2nd ed. Baltimore, MD: Lippincott Williams & Wilkins; 2000.
15. O'Connor P, Sforzo CA, Frye P. Effect of breathing instruction on blood pressure responses during isometric exercise. *Phys Ther.* 1989;69:757-761.
16. Kendall FP, McCreary EK, Provance PG, et al. *Muscles: Testing and Function with Posture and Pain.* 5th ed. Baltimore, MD: Lippincott Williams & Wilkins; 2005.
17. Heyward VH. *Advanced Fitness Assessment & Exercise Prescription.* 6th ed. Champaign, IL: Human Kinetics; 2010.
18. Solway S, Brooks D, Lacasse Y, Thomas S. A qualitative systematic overview of the measurement properties of functional walk tests used in the cardiorespiratory domain. *Chest.* 2001;119:256-270.
19. Brooks D, Parsons J, Tran D, et al. The two-minute walk test as a measure of functional capacity in cardiac surgery patients. *Arch Phys Med Rehabil.* 2004;85(9):1525-1530.
20. Rohner-Spengler M, Mannion AF, Babst R. Reliability and minimal detectable change for the figure-of-eight-20 method of measurement of ankle edema. *J Orthop Sports Phys Ther.* 2007;37(4):199-205.

21. Fitz S, Lusardi M. White paper: "walking speed: the sixth vital sign". *J Geriatr Phys Ther.* 2009;32(2):46-49.

22. Woodard CM, Berry MJ, Rejeski WJ, Ribisl PM, Miller HS. Exercise training in patients with cardiovascular disease and coexistent knee arthritis. *J Cardiopulm Rehabil.* 1994;14:255-261.

23. Shubair MM, Kodis J, McKelvie RS, Arthur HM, Sharma AM. Metabolic profile and exercise capacity outcomes: their relationship to overweight and obesity in a Canadian cardiac rehabilitation setting. *J Cardiopulm Rehabil.* 2004;24(6):405-413.

24. Foley A, Halbert J, Hewitt T, Crotty M. Does hydrotherapy improve strength and physical function in patients with osteoarthritis—a randomized controlled trial comparing a gym based and a hydrotherapy based strengthening programme. *Ann Rheum Dis.* 2003;62:1162-1167.

25. Douris P, Southard V, Varga C, Schauss W, Gennaro W, Reiss A. The effect of land and aquatic exercise on balance scores in older adults. *J Geriatr Phys Ther.* 2003;26(1):3-6.

26. Oldridge NB. Outcome assessment in cardiac rehabilitation: health-related quality of life and economic evaluation. *J Cardiopulm Rehabil.* 1997;17(3):179-194.

27. Kocher MS, Steadman JR, Briggs KK, Sterett WI, Hawkins RJ. Reliability, validity, and responsiveness of the Lysholm Knee Scale for various chondral disorders of the knee. *J Bone Joint Surg Am.* 2004;86;1139-1145.

28. Tegner Y, Lysholm J. Rating systems in the evaluation of knee ligament injuries. *Clin Orthop.* 1985;190:43-49.

29. Angst F, Aeschlimann A, Michel BA, Stucki G. Minimal clinically important rehabilitation effects in patients with osteoarthritis of the lower extremities. *J Rheumatol.* 2002;29(1):131-138.

CASE STUDY 5-2

Mary Jane Myslinski, PT, EdD

EXAMINATION

History

Current Condition/Chief Complaint

Ms. Caster, a 56-year-old female, was referred to a wellness center by her PCP to begin a fitness program. Ms. Caster stated she worked long hours, felt fatigued when she came home, and then was unable to perform many of her household tasks. She reported she was "out of shape" and was largely sedentary.

The patient had completed an exercise stress test 1 week prior and brought the report with her. She was "cleared for vigorous exercise" according to the script from her PCP.

Clinician Comment *Ms. Caster was referred to a hospital-based fitness and wellness center by her PCP. New fitness clients at this center were evaluated by a PT. With the findings from the initial examination, the PT determined if the client required physical therapy to address impairments prior to beginning a fitness program. If so, then the patient was scheduled for outpatient physical therapy until ready to begin a fitness program. The evaluating PT*

could also assess that any impairments might be addressed within the scope of a monitored fitness program.

Based on Ms. Caster's age (over 55 years) and her single risk factor known thus far (sedentary lifestyle), she would be placed into the moderate risk stratification category according to the ACSM for participation in an exercise program (Figure 5-7). Generally, her age and single risk factor alone would not require a stress test, though she would need a physician's clearance for vigorous exercise according to the ACSM guidelines. To answer the question, "What prompted the stress test?" the interview needed to continue. As well, results from a participation screening questionnaire could have been administered and reviewed. Even though she was cleared by her physician for exercise, it would be useful to identify how Ms. Caster described the nature of her fatigue.

Social History/Environment

Ms. Caster had earned a college degree in finance and had worked in the banking field for more than 30 years. In her current position as a manager of a commercial bank, she worked 40 to 60 hours per week. She reported that the majority of her work tasks were completed while sitting at her desk, using her computer or phone. She engaged in little physical movement during the work day since she rarely left her desk, even to take a lunch break.

Ms. Caster lived with her husband of more than 30 years. They had 2 grown children and 3 grandchildren. Each of her children lived out of state and she lamented that she no longer had her children as a support system. Her husband was an investment banker and worked more than 80 hours per week, including weekends. She was the sole caretaker of the house and performed all household duties such as food shopping, laundry, and cleaning. Ms. Caster had a large home, 3600 square feet, with 2 stories and a finished basement. The bedrooms were on the second floor and the laundry room was on the main level. Her home office was located in the finished basement.

The grounds of her home had a built-in swimming pool with a cabana, a multi-level deck with Jacuzzi and gas grill, and extensive gardens. Ms. Caster reported she gardened as "therapy" but hired a pool company to maintain the pool. She reported that her weekends were very busy with the normal upkeep of the house. She often felt overwhelmed with the impossibility of what she needed to accomplish at home. She also noted she had little time to herself.

Clinician Comment *Based on this information, it appeared that Ms. Caster had a large house to maintain with little help. Her children lived out of state and her husband worked even more hours at his job than she did at her own demanding job. Making time for a fitness program may pose a challenge for her.*

Figure 5-7. Risk stratification for exercise testing. (Adapted from Pescatello LS, Arena R, Riebe D, Thompson PD, eds. *ACSM's Guidelines for Exercise Testing and Prescription.* 9th ed. Philadelphia, PA: Wolters Kluwer, Lippincott Williams & Wilkins; 2014.)

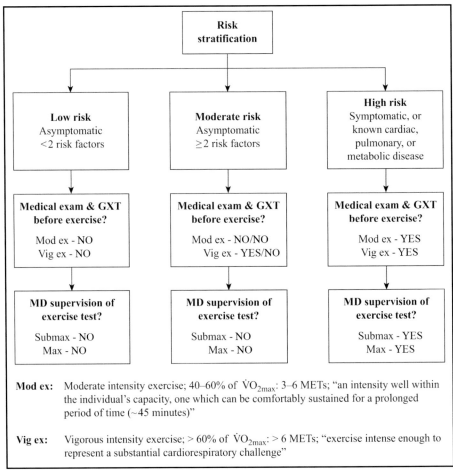

Social/Health Habits

Ms. Caster reported she did not smoke nor had she ever smoked. She reported drinking an occasional alcoholic beverage, generally a glass of red wine, when her husband was home and not working. She reported that she and her husband seldom took vacations because of their work schedules. In fact, her last vacation was 9 years ago. She stated she didn't cook on work nights but would stop for takeout.

Ms. Caster reported she did not have a regular exercise program because of her busy work schedule and home maintenance schedule. She was an avid exerciser prior to the purchase of her current home 8 years ago. Before then, she would exercise 4 to 5 times per week with aerobic and anaerobic program components. Ms. Caster reported she had gained about 30 pounds over the course of 5 years, mostly in her abdomen. She also noticed a decrease in her overall muscle mass. She reported that she had gone up 4 clothing sizes. She had a more recent weight gain of another 15 pounds over the past 2 months.

Clinician Comment *Based on the interview so far, we have learned a lot about Ms. Caster and her lifestyle choices. It appears that prior to the purchase of her*

current home, she was living a much healthier lifestyle. It also sounded as if her children had been her support system to help her cope with her husband's extensive work hours. It also appeared that the lack of exercise and her eating choices in the past years have led to a significant amount of weight gain. The health risks of abdominal weight gain, especially after menopause (if appropriate for Ms. Caster), needed to be kept in mind.[1] Also, her body fat and BMI were not known at this point. Once these are known, more information about the type of fat distribution, thus the health risks, could be identified.

She did not have a smoking history. She drank only red wine, which might have imparted some health benefit. One glass of red wine for females may protect against coronary heart disease and will increase antioxidants.[2,3] Her rapid recent weight gain of 15 pounds was a concern.

Medical/Surgical History

Ms. Caster reported that she had physicals with her PCP nearly every 4 years. She had yearly physicals with her gynecologist. She had a hysterectomy at age 36 and was in menopause.

Four months prior, Ms. Caster noted the onset of chest palpitations and increased fatigue after another significant weight gain of 15 additional pounds. She defined the fatigue as being tired after work, which did not allow her to accomplish all of the home maintenance tasks she needed to do. She reported that she ate quickly with her husband, when he was home, and then she worked to get her "chores" done. She reported feeling exhausted around 10:00 at night and would need to go to sleep. To make up for not getting enough done the evening prior, she would be up at 4:00 AM every day to get more done at home before leaving for work.

She mentioned the onset of chest palpitations and fatigue at her gynecologist's appointment. Her doctor also noted an elevation in Ms. Caster's BP from previous visits. Ms. Caster reported her BP was 150/90 at that visit. Her gynecologist referred her to a cardiologist to evaluate the heart palpitations and to manage the HTN.

Ms. Caster reported she saw the cardiologist and had a cardiac work up of ECG, Holter monitor, nuclear stress test, and blood work. When these reports were forwarded to her PCP with the cardiologist's appraisal, Ms. Caster's PCP subsequently referred her to the fitness and wellness center.

Family Medical History

Ms. Caster's mother was still living but had a history of CAD, triple coronary artery bypass graft surgery, MI, and peripheral arterial disease of both LEs. Her father was deceased but also had an extensive cardiac history of a quadruple coronary artery bypass graft, pacemaker, and defibrillator insertion. He also developed type 2 DM along with many in his family.

Clinician Comment *More was known about the medical factors that led to the stress test. More risk factors for CAD, as identified by the American Heart Association[4] and the ACSM Risk Stratification for CAD, had emerged. Ms. Caster had HTN, a strong family history of heart disease, and episodes of heart palpitations. This put her into the high-risk category according to the ACSM risk stratification. Based on the ACSM preparticipation screening algorithm, medical examination and exercise testing prior to the start of moderate or vigorous exercise was recommended.[5] Moderate exercise is defined as activities of 3 to 6 METs and vigorous above 6 METs.[5]*

Ms. Caster was in menopause. Therefore, some of the weight gain could be explained, but she was at increased risk for heart disease and osteoporosis because of the decrease in estrogen.[6,7] It was not yet known if she was on hormone replacement therapy or if she had a bone mineral density test to determine the presence of osteoporosis or osteopenia.

According to the Eighth Report of the Joint National Committee on Prevention, Detection, Evaluation, and Treatment of High Blood Pressure (JNC8), Ms. Caster had BP that fits under recommendation 2 and 3 in JNC8. She

might benefit from a thiazide-type diuretic, possibly in combination with another medication.[8]

More was also known about Ms. Caster's definition of fatigue. Fatigue is physical and/or mental exhaustion that can be triggered by stress, medication, overwork, or symptom of a disease.[9] Since the latter was ruled out by the physician examination and stress testing, it was anticipated that an exercise program would assist in alleviating some of the fatigue Ms. Caster reported.[5,10]

Reported Functional Status

She complained again about her daily fatigue and her concern that she should be able to accomplish more things in her day. She reported annoying aches and pains in her knees, especially when she took repeated trips up and down the stairs or was on her knees while cleaning.

She stated she had no other issues related to function. She was able to perform all of the individual activities related to daily living without difficulty. She felt restricted only because of the noted fatigue. If needed, she could push past the fatigue and accomplish more if she wished.

Medications

Ms. Caster reported that she took Diovan HCT 160 mg/12.5 mg daily for the last year to manage her HTN. With the recent rise in her BP, one option for improved control was an increase in her medication. She did not wish to increase her medications, however, until she had tried exercise and weight loss to improve control of her BP. She took over-the-counter supplements of calcium and vitamin D3. She did not take hormone replacements.

Clinician Comment *Diovan HCT (valsartan and hydrochlorothiazide) is a combination of valsartan, an orally active, specific angiotensin II receptor blocker acting on the AT_1 receptor subtype, and hydrochlorothiazide, a diuretic.[11]*

The overall frequency of adverse reactions is neither dose-related nor related to age, gender, or race. In clinical trials, the most common reason for discontinuation of Diovan HCT was because of complaints of headache and dizziness.

Diovan HCT was the type of drug that the JNC8 recommended for Stage I HTN. There were no known adverse exercise/drug interactions, making exercise safe with this drug.[5]

Other Clinical Tests

Ms. Caster reported she had undergone a bone mineral density test, as ordered by her gynecologist, with a normal result. Radiographic studies of both knees showed possible early-stage arthritis. The results of the blood chemistry, ECG, Holter monitor, and nuclear stress test results are shown as follows:

Blood chemistry	• Hemoglobin: 15 mL/dL
	• Fasting blood glucose: 90 mg/dL
	• Triglyceride: 200 mg/dL
	• Cholesterol: 260 mg/dL
	• LDL: 150 mg/dL
	• HDL: 47 mg/dL
ECG (obtained from physician)	Short run of supraventricular tachycardia (SVT)
Holter monitor (obtained from physician)	Short run of SVT
Nuclear stress test results (obtained from physician)	1. No ST depression
	2. MET level: 7 METS (VO$_{2max}$ – 20 to 24.7 mL/kg/min)
	3. Completed stage 2 of the Bruce protocol
Nuclear stress test results (obtained from physician)	4. Patient's complaints: fatigue, patient requested to stop
	5. Resting HR: 90 bpm
	6. Resting BP: 150/90 mm Hg
	7. Peak HR: 160 bpm
	8. Peak BP: 180/90 mm Hg
Strength test	• Upper body using 1-RM bench press: 70 pounds
	• Lower body using 1-RM leg press: 150 pounds
	• Muscular Endurance test
	• Push-up test: 3 completed

Clinician Comment *Based on the bone mineral density test, osteoporosis was not a precaution in her exercise prescription. Considerations for the early arthritis in her knees should be factored into the exercise choices for her program.*

When reviewing the Holter monitor and the ECG results, it was noted that Ms. Caster had short runs of SVT. SVT is a type of supraventricular arrhythmia that is fairly common, often repetitive, occasionally persistent, and rarely life-threatening.[12] Patients who experience SVT are often asymptomatic and have symptoms only during the burst of SVT. Symptoms can include palpitations, fatigue, lightheadedness, chest discomfort, dyspnea, presyncope, or more rarely, syncope.[12] This arrhythmia is generally brought on by caffeine, anxiety, alcohol, nicotine, recreational drugs, or hyperthyroidism. It is rarely caused by exercise.[12]

Her stress test was normal with normal exercises responses. The HR and SBP increased as expected, and the DBP remained the same.[10] She achieved 100% of her age-predicted HR$_{max}$ during the stress test. No sign of ischemia, in the form of ST depression, was noted. The stress test was valid since she requested to stop after she had already achieved her age-predicted HR$_{max}$.[5] Her predicted VO$_{2max}$ was between 20 and 24.7 mL/kg/min based on the MET level she achieved on the Bruce Protocol.[5] Based on her VO$_{2max}$, she falls into the 15th percentile for her age and gender. According to research, a VO$_2$ below the 20th percentile for age and gender is indicative of a sedentary lifestyle and is associated with an increased risk of death from all causes.[13]

Based on the norms for the strength tests,[5] she was in the 15th percentile for upper body (poor) and in the 15th percentile for the lower body (well below average). Her muscular endurance test put her into the fair category.

Other Relevant Information

Ms. Caster stated that she'd been thinking about starting an exercise program even before she was referred by her PCP. She said she really wanted to "get back in shape," lose weight, and make her muscles "less flabby." She believed she could fit exercise back into her busy schedule since the wellness center was across the street from where she worked.

Clinician Comment *Based on this interview, the client had more fitness goals than functional goals. Physical fitness is defined as a set of attributes such as cardiorespiratory endurance, skeletal muscular endurance, strength, power, speed, flexibility, agility, balance, reaction time, and body composition.[14] She had expressed a desire to lose weight, change her body composition, and increase her aerobic endurance as well as her muscular endurance and strength. These parameters will need to be measured and then incorporated in the fitness prescription for this client.*

It is also important to determine a client's readiness for change. This can be accomplished by understanding and using the Transtheoretical Model to promote physical activity.[15] Based on the information Ms. Caster gave, she appeared to be in the second stage of the model: contemplation. This meant that she was thinking about increasing her physical activity but had not taken any steps toward this goal. To assist the client with this goal, the clinician can encourage the client to get started in a variety of ways. Encouragement can take the form of suggesting enrollment in an appropriate exercise class or simply to identify the barriers to getting started and discuss how to overcome them. In this case, Ms. Caster walked over to the fitness and wellness center, located near her work site, during her lunch time.

The purpose of the information gathered in the system review is to further ensure that Ms. Caster is a candidate for physical therapy or the fitness program to which she has been referred.

Systems Review

Cardiovascular/Pulmonary/Fitness

Resting vital signs: HR = 90 bpm; BP = 150/90 mm Hg; respiratory rate = 14 breaths per min

Integumentary

No abnormalities of the skin were noted; no abnormal moles, no skin discoloration, no open cuts or wounds. Skin was intact.

Musculoskeletal

Height = 5 feet, 4 inches
Weight = 180 pounds
BMI = 30.9

Gross UE and LE and trunk active ROM was WNL. Strength was generally 4/5 throughout. Posture exam revealed the presence of a forward head posture with rounded shoulders. Muscle length tests found tight hamstrings, bilaterally, as well as tight pectoralis minor muscles. All joints were intact, including the knees.

Neuromuscular

Cleared, no impairments were noted.

Communication, Affect, Cognition, Language, and Learning Style

Ms. Caster was an educated, intelligent, and pleasant woman. No impairments were noted. She was motivated to start her exercise program and requested individualized sessions until she was comfortable with the program.

Clinician Comment *Based on the resting vital signs, Ms. Caster was classified as being in Stage I HTN. Her resting HR was slightly elevated, but still considered to be WNL. Generally, a normal resting HR is between 60 and 100 bpm, with a more conservative number range between 60 and 90 bpm. Her measured normal respiratory rate was normal, as would have been expected for someone without a history of pulmonary disease or cardiac disease.*

Her BMI was greater than would be expected for good health. She showed muscle length and strength deficits. Her posture was not optimum. The neuromuscular and integument reviews were clear.

There were no findings that contraindicated participation in physical therapy. The tests and measures would assist with the evaluation on whether existing impairments could be addressed within the scope of a fitness program rather than formal physical therapy treatment.

In planning the tests and measures portion of the examination, it was determined to confirm the stress test findings with a measure of her aerobic capacity that could be used to compare outcomes, but the stress test was not repeated. Because Ms. Caster had a stress test prior to the fitness program and it was negative, insurance would not pay for another full stress test simply to be used later to determine outcomes. Additional anthropometric measures would be gathered. The extent of muscle length deficits as well as test muscle strengths would be measured. A pain profile for her knees would be useful and would be completed.

Tests and Measures

Aerobic Capacity and Endurance

The YMCA Submaximal Bike test was administered with VO_{2max} extrapolation to be used as an outcome measure. Her HR_{submax} was 139 bpm, Peak BP was 170/90, RPE was 8, and extrapolated VO_{2max} was 22 mL/kg/min. She had no adverse responses.

Clinician Comment *The YMCA Submaximal Bike test is one of the most popular assessment techniques to estimate VO_{2max}.[5] This test was used because it is a more fitness-based test and not a functional measure of how far a client can walk. The ACSM has extensive research and instructions on this test, including its validity and reliability.[5] Ms. Caster's response to the Submaximal test was normal, but it confirmed her low fitness level in the area of cardiopulmonary endurance. She did achieve the 85% of age-predicted HR_{max}, which is the stopping point for a Submaximal test. As has been discussed in the Chapter 4 cases, her RPE did not reflect her actual HR but is still a valid measure of exertion.[16]*

Anthropometric Measurements

Body fat: 38% (caliper method)
Somatotype: endomorphic
Regional fat distribution: android-type obesity
Waist circumference measure: 89 cm

Clinician Comment *The client's BMI placed her into obesity class I, and her waist circumference measurement placed her into the very high disease risk classification.[5] The BMI, or Quetelet index, assesses weight relative to height and is calculated by BMI = body mass (kg)/stature (m²).[10] It is important to note that BMI fails to distinguish between body fat, muscle mass, or bone; therefore, other methods of body composition should be used to calculate body fat. Based on the caliper method for measure of body composition, her body fat was 38%, which put her into the obese category for older women.[10]*

Based on the BMI and body composition measure, this client is obese and faces many risks for disease. A study by Field et al[17] showed that the risk of developing diabetes, gallstones, HTN, heart disease, and stroke increased with severity of overweight among both sexes. They also found that the risk of developing chronic diseases was evident among adults in the upper half of the healthy weight ranges of BMI 22.0 to 24.9. They concluded that a BMI between 18.5 and 21.9 was required to minimize the risk of disease. That BMI range might be very difficult for Ms. Caster to achieve, but a decrease in weight by 10% does confer a health benefit and decreases the risk of disease.

She also has an increased risk of disease, given her regional fat distribution. The android-type obesity or central-type obesity marks an increase in the fat deposits in the internal viscera.[10] Central fat deposition reflects an altered metabolic profile that increases the risk for hyperinsulinemia, glucose intolerance, type 2 DM, endometrial cancer, hypertriglyceridemia, hypercholesterolemia, HTN, and atherosclerosis. Looking at her blood chemistry, she already presented with an increased triglyceride, cholesterol, and LDL and a lower HDL. Given these issues, she was at risk for developing metabolic syndrome.[18]

Metabolic syndrome is defined as "a constellation of interrelated risk factors of metabolic origin—metabolic risk factors—that appear to directly promote the development of atherosclerotic cardiovascular disease."[18(p 2735)] The risk factors for developing this syndrome include abdominal obesity, insulin resistance, physical inactivity, and hormonal imbalance. She presented with normal glucose, but if she did not correct her behavior, she was at risk of developing insulin resistance given her current health status as well as her family history. Therefore, Ms. Caster might benefit from a referral to a registered dietician.

Posture

Ms. Caster presented with marked forward head posture, rounded shoulders, and slightly protracted scapulas.

Clinician Comment *Her posture reflected what clinicians sometimes call "computer posture" because it is a posture that is seen in someone who works on the computer all day and does not take breaks. This posture exam was conducted using a visual assessment, which was more subjective than measures taken from a plumb line.[19]*

Muscle Length Tests

Ms. Caster had shortness in her hamstrings and pectoralis minor muscles. A straight leg raise test documented hamstring length at 60 degrees, bilaterally. The tightness in the pectoralis minor muscles was classified as moderate based on the distance of the shoulder from the table and from the amount of resistance offered by the muscles to downward pressure on the shoulder.

Clinician Comment *Muscle length testing is important to determine what fitness exercises the client may or may not perform until the muscle lengths are WNL. To not consider muscle length with regard to exercises chosen may increase a muscle imbalance. Further, shortened muscles can contribute to other injuries such as low back pain with shortened hamstrings or arm pain with decreased length in pectoralis minor muscles.*

Normal length for the hamstrings is 80 degrees on a straight leg raise test. The pectoralis minor is considered normal when the full shoulder girdle and shoulder rests on the mat when the client is lying in supine.[19] When a length deficit is present, the short muscles need to be stretched. Later, the lengths need to be reexamined and judged to be restored to normal length before exercises that can further shorten the muscles can be started by the client. The muscle length tests for Ms. Caster were conducted in a manner to spot substitutions or other length imbalances.[19]

Muscle Performance (Including Strength, Power, and Endurance)

Ms. Caster presented with weakness in both her UEs and LEs in the systems review. To ensure a full and accurate survey of extremity musculature, MMT was performed while she was positioned supine, side lying, prone, and then standing. The following muscle strength grades were identified:

	RIGHT	LEFT
Shoulder flexion	3+/5	3+/5
Shoulder extension	3+/5	3+/5
Shoulder abduction	3+/5	3+/5
Abdominals	3/5	3/5
Hip flexion	4/5	4/5
Hip extension	4/5	4/5
Knee extension	4/5	4/5
Knee flexion	3+/5	3+/5
Plantarflexion	4/5	4/5

Clinician Comment *MMT showed strength deficits throughout bilateral LEs and UEs as suggested by the strength deficits noted in the systems review. Although these strength deficits are less than those noted in the system review fitness exam, her decreased strength still needed to be addressed in the exercise program both to maintain bone stock and improve function.*

It is worth noting that strength testing can give false measurements if not performed correctly.[10] For example, use of only 1 or 2 1-RM attempts underestimates the "true" 1-RM by as much as 11% because of learning improvement.

Pain

Using the numeric rating scale, Ms. Caster rated her knee pain as 2/10 when she went up and down stairs and 3/10 when she knelt down on her knees.

Clinician Comment *Ms. Caster's low pain intensity could be expected because of the mild arthritis in her knees as noted in the radiology report. Pain will be another vital sign monitored during her exercise session to avoid having exercises exacerbate her knee arthritis. The numeric rating scale uses a 0 to 10 intensity scale, where 0 indicates no pain and 10 is the worst pain ever. The client is asked to rate pain using this scale during exercise as another indicator of exercise intensity.*

EVALUATION

Diagnosis

Practice Pattern

Based on the information from the client interview, systems review, and indicated tests and measures, Ms. Caster was classified into 2 cardiovascular/pulmonary practice patterns: 6A—Primary Prevention/Risk Factor Reduction for Cardiopulmonary Disorders, and 6B—Impaired Aerobic Capacity/Endurance Associated With Deconditioning.

International Classification of Functioning, Disability, and Health Model of Disability

See ICF Model on page 204.

Clinician Comment *It was concluded that Ms. Caster had no findings on the tests and measures that required physical therapy treatment prior to beginning a fitness program. Her impairments should be able to be addressed with a well-designed and monitored fitness program at the fitness and wellness center.*

Further, Ms. Caster's own goals also matched those of a fitness program, namely improved cardiorespiratory endurance, skeletal muscular endurance, strength, power, speed, flexibility, agility, balance, reaction time, and body composition.[14]

Prognosis

Ms. Caster had an excellent prognosis to increase her aerobic capacity, improve her posture, and increase her muscular strength and endurance with a fitness program. She could also anticipate that she would improve her fitness profile, including improve her lipid panel, decrease her weight, improve her BP, improve her posture, and change her body composition, thus decreasing the risk factors for cardiovascular, metabolic, and systemic diseases.

Plan of Care

Intervention

Ms. Caster would benefit from a progressive fitness program to address her poor fitness level. The program would include aerobic and anaerobic exercise (anaerobic exercise in the form of resistive training), a flexibility program, and postural education. She would also benefit from a cardiovascular risk management program of weight control, BP, and lipid management, as well as stress management. Education in prevention of osteoporosis and metabolic syndrome would be included. She may benefit from referrals to a registered dietician and stress management counselor.

Proposed Frequency and Duration of Physical Therapy Visits

Ms. Caster would arrange to work out at the fitness and wellness center 3 to 5 times per week for 30 to 60 minutes to start. She would start with one-on-one training and progress to independent sessions after 1 month.

Clinician Comment *Her insurance covered $300.00 per year for a fitness center. This will be used to offset the cost of the entire program.*

Anticipated Goals

1. Ms. Caster will be able to monitor her HR accurately and independently (1 week).

2. Ms. Caster will show 100% compliance with a 3 times per week fitness program (2 weeks).

3. Ms. Caster would demonstrate correct posture when walking on the treadmill (2 weeks).

4. Ms. Caster would tolerate aerobic activity for 30 minutes (2 weeks).

5. Ms. Caster will tolerate the addition of resistance training, 2 sets of 10 repetitions at 50% of her maximum (3 weeks).

6. Ms. Caster would demonstrate an understanding of risk factor reduction for cardiac and metabolic diseases (4 weeks).

ICF Model of Disablement for Ms. Caster

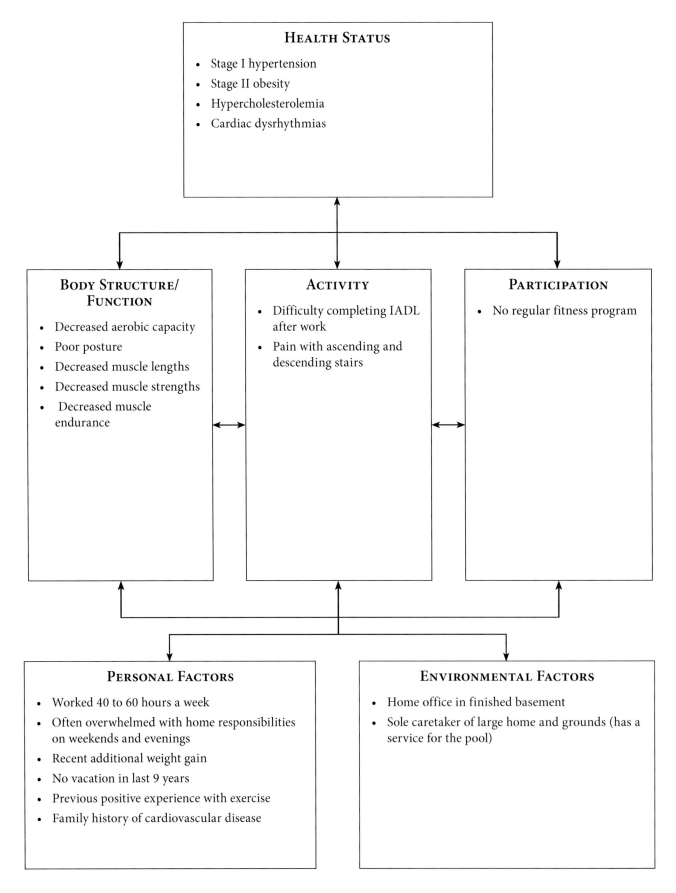

Health Status

- Stage I hypertension
- Stage II obesity
- Hypercholesterolemia
- Cardiac dysrhythmias

Body Structure/ Function

- Decreased aerobic capacity
- Poor posture
- Decreased muscle lengths
- Decreased muscle strengths
- Decreased muscle endurance

Activity

- Difficulty completing IADL after work
- Pain with ascending and descending stairs

Participation

- No regular fitness program

Personal Factors

- Worked 40 to 60 hours a week
- Often overwhelmed with home responsibilities on weekends and evenings
- Recent additional weight gain
- No vacation in last 9 years
- Previous positive experience with exercise
- Family history of cardiovascular disease

Environmental Factors

- Home office in finished basement
- Sole caretaker of large home and grounds (has a service for the pool)

7. Ms. Caster would be independent in her exercise program, demonstrating proper technique and understanding of progression (4 weeks).

8. Ms. Caster would have 0/10 pain with steps and kneeling (6 weeks).

Expected Outcomes: 3-Month Mark

1. Ms. Caster would show a decrease in her resting HR and resting BP to normal values.

2. Ms. Caster would achieve a 20% increase in her aerobic capacity.

3. Ms. Caster would demonstrate an increase in muscle strength and endurance by 40%.

4. Ms. Caster would be able to perform all exercises and daily activities with no complaints of fatigue.

5. Ms. Caster would achieve optimal results on her lipid panel.

6. Ms. Caster would achieve a 24-pound weight loss.

7. Ms. Caster would demonstrate a significant change in body composition with a 7% decrease in her body fat.

8. Ms. Caster would demonstrate continued compliance in her fitness program.

Clinician Comment *The opportunity to improve her impairments with a fitness program at the fitness and wellness center also allowed Ms. Caster a longer time interval to make the needed gains with monitoring than might have been approved by her insurance carrier for physical therapy treatment. Initial fitness goals can be achieved in 3 months.[10] It can take up to 1 year or more to achieve optimal goals based on the person's needs and the initial fitness level. For example, weight loss should only occur at a 2-pound per week loss to maintain lean tissue. Lipid panels can show changes but can take 3 to 6 months to show significant changes.*

Discharge Plan

It was anticipated that Ms. Caster would achieve the anticipated goals and expected outcomes at the end of the fitness program plan of care. She would need to continue regular exercise sessions at the fitness and wellness center to achieve optimal outcomes and then to maintain her new fitness level.

INTERVENTION

Coordination, Communication, and Documentation

The initial examination findings and evaluation, including the fitness program plan of care, was sent to Ms. Caster's referring PCP and to her cardiologist. Accompanying the report to her PCP was a request to have Ms. Caster referred to a registered dietitian and a stress management counselor.

HRs and RPE along with the exercises completed would be documented in the fitness chart by Ms. Caster. At the end of each exercise session, Ms. Caster and the fitness program monitor would review the session and adjust Ms. Caster's program as indicated for the next session.

Clinician Comment *Some insurance companies will pay for fitness benefits. Also, some plans consider obesity a disease and will cover the services of a dietician. If Ms. Caster was referred to, and evaluated by, a dietician, it could be anticipated that the dietician would send a report documenting weight loss, body composition, and blood profile goals to the PCP and cardiologist. Along with progress notes, the dietician would also send requests for repeat blood profiles to the physicians.*

Patient-/Client-Related Instruction

Ms. Caster would receive instruction in HR and RPE monitoring. She would be shown, and would practice, the use of the equipment with correct proper body form. Additional educational sessions were planned for use of a proper warm-up and cool-down and the importance of maintaining the defined target heart range. Exercise responses to monitor for her safety would be identified for her as well as how to minimize the effects of delayed onset muscle soreness. As her program progressed, the educational topics on osteoporosis and metabolic syndrome would be presented.

Procedural Interventions

Therapeutic Exercise Prescription

Aerobic Capacity/Endurance Conditioning or Reconditioning

Mode
Dual-action bike, elliptical, treadmill—any aerobic equipment the client favors except a single-action bike

Intensity
HR = 132 bpm; RPE < 11/20

Duration
20 to 30 minutes of aerobic exercise to start and progress accordingly

Frequency
3 to 5 times per week; start with 3 days per week and progress

Description of the Intervention
Ms. Caster was instructed to exercise on the dual-action bike using the following stages:

- Warm-up for 5 to 10 minutes on the bike at a lower intensity

- Training zone for 20 to 60 minutes at identified HR intensity
- Cool-down for 5 to 10 minutes by slow biking or walking, followed by gentle stretching as outlined in her flexibility program

Clinician Comment *A dual-action bike was selected for Ms. Caster because she had HTN. Single-action bikes can increase the BP response because of increased vascular constriction from nonworking muscles.*

Ms. Caster's HR_{max} (160 bpm) was identified from the stress test. This allowed a more accurate calculation for her target HR range for exercising than using the age-predicted formula for the HR_{max} of 220 – age. Tanka et al[20] did formulate another way to determine HR_{max} that is more exact but unnecessary for Ms. Caster since hers was identified in the stress test.

The Karvonen formula was used to calculate her target HR for exercising at 60% of her HR_{max}: target HR = [(HR_{max} – resting HR) × 60%] + resting HR; target HR = [(160 – 90) × 0.6] + 90 = 132 bpm

RPE was used as a measure of her perceived work and monitored along with her HR.[21]

Flexibility Exercises

Mode
Muscle lengthening and stretching
Intensity
To a position of mild discomfort
Duration
30 seconds for 2 repetitions
Frequency
Twice a day
Description of Intervention

- Hamstring and pectoralis minor stretches: She will isolate the muscle to be stretched and work up to holding the stretch for 30 seconds.

- Hamstring stretch: Patient will sit on one of the benches located against the gym wall, where she is able to sit with her back maintained straight against the wall, then she will slowly extend her knee as much as possible without changing her buttocks and back position.[19]

Strength, Power, and Endurance Training for Head, Neck, Limb, Pelvic-Floor, Trunk, and Ventilatory Muscles

Mode
Weight machines initially then progressing to free weights
Intensity
60% to 70% of 1-RM. Rest intervals will be 2 to 3 minutes for core exercises and 1 to 2 minutes for multi-joint using heavy loads. Velocity was to be slow to moderate.

Duration
1 to 3 sets, 8 to 12 repetitions to start
Frequency
2 to 3 times per week
Description of the Intervention
When able, the exercises will begin with light eccentric work and progress to concentric. Large muscle group exercises will precede those for small muscle groups. Multiple-joint exercises will occur before single joint. There will be a rotation of exercises in a session of upper and lower body exercises. Ms. Caster will be shown and reminded to maintain correct body position.

Clinician Comment *There are many methods in strength training. The description noted previously relies on the recommendations for resistive exercises by Kraemer et al.[22]*

REEXAMINATION

Ms. Caster was assessed 1 month after starting her fitness program.

Subjective

"I am amazed at my progress."

Objective

Client reported a weight loss of 10 pounds and one drop in dress size. She was less fatigued and able to complete tasks when she returned to home. Knee pain was gone with stairs. Ms. Caster was keeping regular appointments with a dietician and a stress management counselor. Ms. Caster thought both practitioners had been helpful. She was very compliant with her fitness program. She was tolerating slow but consistent progression in her program.

Aerobic Capacity and Endurance

Resting vital signs were: HR = 87 bpm; BP = 140/82
Submaximal Bike test would be repeated at 3 months from program initiation.

Muscle Length

Pectoralis minor and hamstring length were normal, bilaterally.

Strength

Strength increased to 5/5 throughout and the 1-RM increased by 30% for UEs and LEs. Muscular endurance also improved by increasing her to the 30th percentile.

Anthropometric Measurements

BMI: 29.2
Weight: 170 lbs
Body fat: 34%
Waist circumference measure: 79 cm

Assessment

Client showed excellent progress the first month. Significant changes were noted in her resting vital signs. An increase in strength and muscular endurance were noted. Significant changes were also noted in the anthropometric measurements. Muscle lengths were normal and the postural dysfunction was corrected. Ms. Caster reported she no longer had knee pain during functional activities. Ms. Caster still had Stage I HTN but she had reduced her BMI to the overweight category. Her risk for disease dropped from the very high risk category to the increased risk category. Her body fat measures kept her in the obese category.

Plan

Ms. Caster was kept on her basic fitness program. Her program would be reviewed with her monthly and progressed accordingly. She would exercise at the fitness and wellness center independently. The education sessions were to continue until completed as planned. The expected outcomes remained as those established in the initial fitness program plan of care.

OUTCOMES

At 3 months, a review of Ms. Caster's fitness record showed that she continued to exercise regularly at the fitness and wellness center with a steady progression of her program. Based on the reports filed in her fitness record, all the expected outcomes established in the initial fitness program plan of care had been achieved.

REFERENCES

1. Mayo Clinic. Belly fat in women: taking—and keeping—it off. http://www.mayoclinic.org/healthy-living/womens-health/in-depth/belly-fat/art-20045809. Accessed July 2, 2010.
2. Klatsky A, Armstrong MA, Friedman GD. Red wine, white wine, liquor, beer and risk for coronary artery disease hospitalization. *Am J Cardiol.* 1997;80:416-420.
3. Pignatelli P, Ghiselli A, Buchetti B, et al. Polyphenols synergistically inhibit oxidative stress in subjects given red and white wine. *Atherosclerosis.* 2006;188:77-83.
4. American Heart Association. Coronary artery disease - coronary heart disease. http://www.heart.org/HEARTORG/Conditions/More/MyHeartandStrokeNews/Coronary-Artery-Disease---Coronary-Heart-Disease_UCM_436416_Article.jsp. Accessed July 2, 2010.
5. Pescatello LS, Arena R, Riebe D, Thompson PD, eds. *ACSM's Guidelines for Exercise Testing and Prescription.* 9th ed. Philadelphia, PA: Wolters Kluwer, Lippincott Williams & Wilkins; 2014.
6. WebMD. Menopause. http://www.webmd.com/menopause/default.htm. Accessed July 3, 2010.
7. National Osteoporosis Foundation. NOF's clinician's guide to the prevention and treatment of osteoporosis. *Bone Source.* http://nof.org/hcp/resources/913. Accessed July 3, 2010.
8. James PA, Aparil S, Carter BL, et al. 2014 evidence-based guideline for the management of high blood pressure in adults report from the panel members appointed to the eighth joint national committee (JNC8). *JAMA.* epub Dec 18, 2013. doi:10.1001/jama.2013.28447.
9. Fatigue. Answers. http://www.answers.com/topic/fatigue. Accessed July 8, 2010.
10. McArdle WD, Katch FI, Katch VL. *Exercise Physiology Energy, Nutrition, and Human Performance.* 7th ed. Philadelphia, PA: Lippincott Williams & Wilkins; 2010.
11. Gladson B. *Pharmacology for Physical Therapists.* Philadelphia, PA: Elsevier; 2008.
12. Blomström-Lundqvist C, Scheinman MM, Aliot EM, et al. ACC/AHA/ESC guidelines for the management of patients with supraventricular arrhythmias—executive summary. A report of the American College of Cardiology/American Heart Association Task Force on Practice Guidelines and the European Society of Cardiology Committee for Practice Guidelines (Writing Committee to Develop Guidelines for the Management of Patients With Supraventricular Arrhythmias) developed in collaboration with NASPE-Heart Rhythm Society. *J Am Coll Cardiol.* 2003;42(8)1493-1531.
13. Blair SN, Kohl HW 3rd, Barlow CE, Paffenbarger RS Jr, Gibbons LW, Macera CA. Changes in physical fitness and all-cause mortality: a prospective study of healthy men and unhealthy men. *JAMA.* 1995;273:1093-1098.
14. Pollock M, Chairperson. ACSM position stand: the recommended quantity and quality of exercise for developing and maintaining cardiorespiratory and muscular fitness and flexibility in healthy adults. *Med Sci Sport Exerc.* 1998;30:6-28.
15. Pekmezi D, Barbera B, Marcus B. Using the transtheoretical model to promote physical activity. *ACSM's Health & Fitness Journal.* 2010;14:8-13.
16. Borg GA. Perceived exertion: a note on history and methods. *Med Sci Sports.* 1973;5:90-93.
17. Field AE, Coakley EH, Must A, et al. Impact of overweight on the risk of developing common chronic diseases during a 10-year period. *Arch Intern Med.* 2001;161:1581-1586.
18. Grundy SM, Cleeman JI, Daniels SR, et al. Diagnosis and management of the metabolic syndrome: an American Heart Association/National Heart, Lung, and Blood Institute scientific statement. *Circulation.* 2005;112:2735-2752.
19. Kendall FP, McCreary EF, Provance PG. *Muscles Testing and Function.* 4th ed. Baltimore, MD: Williams & Wilkins; 1993.
20. Tanka H, Monahan K, Seals R. Age-predicted maximal heart rate revisited. *J Am Coll Cardiol.* 2001;37:2001-2005.
21. Eston RG, Thompson M. Use of rating of perceived exertion for predicting maximal work rate and prescribing exercise intensity in patients taking atenolol. *Br J Sports Med.* 1997;31:114-119.
22. Kraemer WJ, Adams K, Cafarelli E, et al. Progression models in resistance training for healthy adults. *Med Sci Sports.* 2002;34:203-208.

SECTION III

PATHOPHYSIOLOGICAL CONSIDERATIONS AND CLINICAL PRACTICE

6

Individuals With Cardiovascular Pump Dysfunction

Daniel Malone, PT, PhD, CCS and Scot Irwin, PT, DPT, CCS

CHAPTER OBJECTIVES

- Review the statistics and physiologic processes that make it likely that a physical therapist (PT) will encounter a patient with primary or secondary cardiovascular pump dysfunction.

- List the survival prognostic factors identified in the study by Proudfit et at.[1]

- Answer the question, "What is known about the effect risk factors have on vessel tissues that lead to the development of coronary artery disease (CAD)?"

- Outline the sequence of events that can occur in an artery that can lead to an eventual occlusion or thrombosis.

- Describe the mechanical and metabolic factors, as well as the neural influences, that determine coronary artery blood flow.

- Outline the sequence of events during exercise that may lead to cardiac ischemia in a patient with an obstructive lesion.

- Discuss the sequence of events that lead to an acute myocardial infarction (MI) and the findings that confirm that an infarction has occurred.

- Identify the evidence that suggests risk factor reduction may favorably alter arterial lesions.

- Compare and contrast the sequence of events, signs, and symptoms for right vs left congestive heart failure.

CHAPTER OUTLINE

- Epidemiology
- Pathology/Pathophysiology
- Coronary Artery Disease
  ○ Atherosclerosis
  ○ Mechanisms of Atherogenesis: Relationship to Risk Factors
  ○ Hemodynamics of Coronary Artery Flow in Normal and Diseased States
- Cardiac Pump Ischemia
  ○ Pathophysiology of Ischemia
  ○ Acute Myocardial Infarction
  ○ Reversal and Retardation of Progression of Atherosclerosis
- Heart Failure
  ○ Congestive Heart Failure
  ○ Differences Between Left- and Right-Sided Heart Failure
  ○ Distinguishing Between Left- and Right-Sided Failure
  ○ Summary of Cardiac Pump Disorder Pathophysiology
- Patient Examination: History, Systems Review, Tests, and Measures
  ○ History and Interview
  ○ Systems Review
  ○ Test and Measures

Coglianese D, ed. *Clinical Exercise Pathophysiology for Physical Therapy: Examination, Testing, and Exercise Prescription for Movement-Related Disorders (pp 211-246).*
© 2015 Taylor & Francis Group.

This chapter will provide a brief description of the most common pathologies associated with cardiovascular pump dysfunction, CAD, and heart failure. This will include a review of the pathophysiological consequences of these diseases and their impact on patients' aerobic capacity and subsequent functional abilities. An overview of examination considerations and intervention strategies will be presented. The chapter will conclude with the critical thinking required to examine, evaluate, and treat a patient with a cardiac pump disorder.

EPIDEMIOLOGY

Cardiovascular pump dysfunction may result from myriad pathophysiological processes (Box 6-1). Regardless of the medical diagnosis and the etiology of the cardiac pump dysfunction, the practitioner must be able to appropriately identify the limitations and alterations in the oxygen (O_2) transport system to determine the most efficacious intervention(s) for the patient.

The impairments resulting from cardiovascular pump dysfunction have a direct effect on an individual's maximum O_2 consumption, an individual's aerobic capacity, and ultimately, on O_2 transport. Any pathology that reduces or limits cardiac output (CO) will impair aerobic capacity. Cardiac dysfunction can progress to the point that it may limit even the least demanding of daily activities.

BOX 6-1. PHYSIOLOGICAL PROCESSES THAT MAY RESULT IN CARDIOVASCULAR PUMP DYSFUNCTION

• Alcohol abuse	• Contusions
• Autonomic nervous system dysfunction	• Dysrhythmias
	• Heart failure
• Cancer	• Inflammation of myocardial and pericardial structures
• Chronic diabetes (Type I or Type II)	
• Chronic hypertension	• Ischemia
• Conduction disturbances	• MIs
	• Surgery
• Congenital malformations	• Valvular disorders

This list is not exclusive; it is only a selection.

Although mortality has decreased, the incidence of cardiovascular pump dysfunction and failure is growing steadily in the United States.[2] Over the last decade, the number of individuals surviving heart surgeries, transplants, CAD, MI and heart failure has increased, but the burden of these disease processes remains high. The cost of heart failure care alone in the United States exceeds $20 billion per year. Heart failure is the most common discharge diagnosis for hospitalized Medicare patients and the fourth most common discharge diagnosis for all patients hospitalized in the United States.[3-5] Greater than 5 million patients have been diagnosed with heart failure and 670,000 new cases are diagnosed annually. Given these statistics, therapists working in any environment are likely to encounter patients with a primary or secondary diagnosis that may include cardiovascular pump dysfunction.

PATHOLOGY/PATHOPHYSIOLOGY

The most common cardiac diagnoses are a result of CAD and heart failure. CAD may be treated conservatively (medically) or surgically (eg, coronary artery bypass grafting, angioplasty, stenting, or atherectomy).

Heart failure is usually treated through the use of medications, but diagnosis of either heart failure or CAD requires long-term follow up. As heart failure progresses, activities of daily living (ADL) and quality of life will become impaired, life expectancy will be limited, and the patient may become a candidate for heart transplantation or mechanical assistance (eg, left ventricular [LV] assist device). Although CAD and heart failure are primarily diseases of adulthood, the pediatric specialist should also be aware that congenital cardiac anomalies can also have detrimental effects on cardiac pump function.

BOX 6-2. DATA POINTS COMMONLY USED TO FORM A TREATMENT PROGRAM FOR CORONARY ARTERY DISEASE

- Clinical monitoring
- Exercise testing
- Results from special studies
- Echocardiography
- Angiography/ventriculography
- MRI
- Patient history
- Physical examination

BOX 6-3. RISK FACTORS ASSOCIATED WITH THE DEVELOPMENT AND PROGRESSION OF ATHEROSCLEROSIS

- Physiology
- Age
- Male sex
- Lifestyle
- Cigarette smoking
- Sedentary lifestyle
- Medical indicators
- Increased serum levels of low-density lipoprotein cholesterol (LDL-C) and triglycerides
- Decreased serum levels of high-density lipoprotein cholesterol (HDL-C)
- Elevated homocysteine and fibrinogen levels
- Hypertension
- Diabetes

In addition to the direct effect of the numerous cardiovascular pathologies on the heart's contractile function, the clinician must also be concerned with the effects of electrical abnormalities on cardiac pump function. A heart that is free of any apparent pathology can develop an electrical abnormality resulting in blood clot formation, leading to stroke (atrial fibrillation), acute orthostasis/shortness of breath (SOB; ventricular tachycardia or supraventricular tachycardia), or sudden death (ventricular fibrillation or third-degree heart block). The interventions by the PT will vary depending upon their examination findings, the goals of the patient, and the progression of the pathology.

CORONARY ARTERY DISEASE

Atherosclerosis

An understanding of the natural history of CAD is important to the clinician for risk stratification and understanding the patient's prognosis. Ideally, awareness of diagnostic subsets of patients with CAD, along with the data accumulated from various examinations or tests (Box 6-2) will provide the basis for an individualized treatment program.

Atherosclerosis affects the large- and medium-size arteries throughout the body; its nomenclature depends on the location of the plaques:

- In the extremities, aorta, or iliac arteries (a common manifestation of systemic atherosclerosis): peripheral arterial disease or peripheral arterial occlusive disease

- In the vessels of the heart: CAD

The exact etiology of atherosclerosis is not fully understood; however, there are certain factors that have been shown to increase the likelihood of the disease process occurring in a given person (Box 6-3).

CAD is generally considered to be a progressive disease that can develop and manifest as early as the second decade of life,[6,7] but the disease process begins in early childhood.

Though the natural history of the disease is difficult to document because of intervening variables (eg, medical and surgical therapy, risk factor changes, aging, the presence or absence of other coexisting illnesses), mortality and morbidity rates are primarily dependent upon 2 factors:

1. Ventricular function (ejection fraction)

2. Total atherosclerotic load (number of vessels occluded)

Those aside, it is important to have some indication of whether certain factors relative to the severity of the disease at the time of initial evaluation predict the likelihood of future coronary events (eg, progression of symptoms, recurrent MI, or cardiac death). For example, women have been shown to have significantly higher mortality rates than men after their first MI.[8]

As noted in Chapter 1, there are 2 major epicardial, or surface, coronary arteries: the right coronary artery and the left main coronary artery. The left coronary system is the major source of blood supply to the LV, perfusing up to 60% to 70% of the LV muscle mass. The precise perfusion distribution patterns of the coronary arteries vary among patients.

Most of the literature describing the progression of cardiovascular disease postdiagnosis is limited by short follow-up study periods; an exception to this trend is the work of Proudfit et al.[1] The Proudfit study involved a 10-year follow-up period of 601 nonsurgical patients. The number of coronary arteries involved, especially the left anterior descending (LAD) artery, was an important prognostic factor, with 10-year survival rates for patient with single-vessel, double-vessel, and triple-vessel disease being 63%, 45%, and 23%, respectively.[1] The presence of a 50% or greater lesion in the left main coronary artery, also associated with

TABLE 6-1. LAYERS OF AN ARTERY

LAYER	PHYSIOLOGY
Intima (inner layer)	Lined with endothelial cells Supported by connective tissue
Media (middle layer)	Consists mainly of smooth muscle cells
Adventitia (outer layer)	Consists of collagenous elastic fibers and small blood vessels (vasa vasorum)

multi-vessel disease, was another important prognostic factor limiting survival.[9] Ventricular function, quantified as the ejection fraction, is also associated with prognosis. Patients with poor LV function and low ejection fractions (less than 35%) had lower survival rates than those with small areas of damage and normal ventricular function. Patients with a ventricular aneurysm or with ejection fractions less than 40% have 10-year survival rates of 10% to 18%.[10] Other factors, independent of the number of coronary vessels diseased and ventricular function, associated with poor prognosis include the following:

- Severity of functional impairment imposed by angina pectoris
- Electrocardiogram (ECG) evidence of LV hypertrophy or conduction defects
- Persistence of risk factors such as cigarette smoking, diabetes, and hypertension[1]

Functional performance during a 6-minute walk test (6MWT) has also been shown to be an important predictor of survival in patients with heart failure.[11]

Mechanisms of Atherogenesis: Relationship to Risk Factors

Atherosclerosis is a disease process that potentially can affect the majority of the medium and large arteries throughout the body, including the vertebral, basilar, carotid, coronary, femoral, and popliteal arteries, and the thoracic and abdominal aortas. Its effects are varied; atherosclerotic changes in the aorta include thinning of the media with weakening of the vessel wall, and aneurysm formation (with possible rupture), whereas the major change in the coronary artery is a stenotic, occlusive lesion. The following information will focus on the particular atherosclerotic process that leads to the type of occlusive lesions that form in the coronary arteries.

It is clear that there are certain factors that increase the likelihood of developing CAD or vein graft atherosclerosis after bypass surgery. However, a cause-and-effect relationship between the risk factors and atherosclerosis cannot be assumed on the basis of the epidemiological studies alone. Salel et al[12] investigated the relationship between a risk factor

index (score derived from total number of risk factors) and the presence or absence of coronary disease found at the time of angiography. The study highlighted the significant relationship between the risk factors and the presence of CAD. The study also demonstrated that patients with multi-vessel disease had significantly higher risk factor indexes than patients with single-vessel disease. The exact relationship between the risk factors and atherogenesis is still not specifically determined, but current evidence points to a long-term, progressive cycle of inflammation, lipid accumulation, scarring, smooth muscle cell proliferation, and endothelial cell dysfunction as the basis of athersclerosis.[13]

As noted in Chapter 1 (see Figure 1-16), arteries consist of 3 distinct layers (tunicae; Table 6-1). Veins, like arteries, have 3 layers, but the amount of smooth muscle tissue and elastic tissue is considerably less, most likely because veins function in a low-pressure system.

There is evidence that the major component of the atherosclerotic plaque is LDL-C. Despite overwhelming evidence that LDL is an atherogenic lipoprotein, the precise mechanisms of atherosclerosis remain unknown. Current concepts hypothesize that LDL-C filters and accumulates into the intima (insudate) when the permeability of the vascular endothelium increases due to injury (Table 6-2). When LDL begins to accumulate, endothelial cells increase production of adhesion molecules and inflammatory proteins, which in turn augments the adhesion and subsequent egress of macrophages into the subendothelium.[14] The artery responds with smooth muscle cell proliferation, increased collagen formation, and inflammatory reactions that lead to the development of obstructive atherosclerotic lesions.[15]

This damage to the arterial endothelial layer allows insudation and adherence of several macromolecules such as LDL and fibrinogen, both of which are believed to be key factors in the atherogenic process. It is well documented that hypoxia and elevated levels of serum carbon monoxide alter arterial permeability,[16] which suggests one way cigarette smoking plays a direct role in atherogenesis. Hypertension (probably as a result of direct trauma) and angiotensin II also have been shown to damage the endothelial cells and therefore alter permeability of the endothelial layer. Catecholamines (epinephrine, norepinephrine, serotonin, bradykinin), which can be elevated by stress or cigarette smoking, also cause endothelial damage.[17]

Once the endothelium has been damaged, one potential cascade of events follows the course depicted in Figure 6-1.[17] This may eventually predispose the individual to plaque rupture or thrombosis. In short, the endothelium is damaged by various factors as listed in Table 6-1. Once damaged, an injury response occurs with inflammation, cell necrosis, phagocytic activity, and scarring. LDLs are not completely digested by the phagocytes and large pools of lipids become deposited in the smooth muscle. These lipids are activated when oxidized and further facilitate an inflammatory response. The arterial reaction to this accumulation is to surround the pools of LDL with collagen (fibrous caps).[18] These caps are thin-walled and exposed to the shear forces of blood

TABLE 6-2. SUMMARY OF VARIOUS FACTORS THAT HAVE BEEN SHOWN TO ALTER ENDOTHELIAL PERMEABILITY TO LIPOPROTEINS AND MACROPHAGES

SUBSTANCE OR PHYSICAL CONDITION	MECHANISM INVOLVED	CLINICAL CONDITION
Hemodynamic forces; tension, stretching, shearing, eddy currents	Separation or damage to endothelial cells, increased permeability, platelet sticking, stimulation of smooth muscle cell proliferation	Hypertension
Angiotensin II	"Trap-door" effect	Hypertension
Carbon monoxide or decreased O_2 saturation	Destruction of endothelial cells	Cigarette smoking
Catecholamines (epinephrine, norepinephrine, serotonin, bradykinin)	Hypercontraction, swelling, and loss of endothelial cell and platelet agglutination	Stress, cigarette smoking
Metabolic products	Endothelial cell damage	Homocystinemia, uremia
Endotoxins and other similar bacterial products	Endothelial cell destruction, platelet sticking	Acute bacterial infections
Ag-Ab complexes, immunological defects	Platelet agglutination	Serum sickness, transplant rejection, immune complex diseases, lupus erythematosus
Virus diseases	Endothelial cell infection and necrosis	Viremias
Mechanical trauma to endothelium	Platelet sticking, increased local permeability	Catheter injury
Hyperlipidemia with increase in circulating lipoproteins (cholesterol, triglycerides, phospholipids) and free fatty acids	Platelet agglutination in areas of usually hemodynamic damage, over "fatty streaks"	Chronic nutritional imbalance (high-fat and high-cholesterol diets), familial hypercholesterolemia, diabetes, nephrosis, hypothyroidism

Reprinted with permission from Braunwald E, ed. *Heart Disease: A Textbook of Cardiovascular Medicine*. Philadelphia, PA: WB Saunders; 1984.

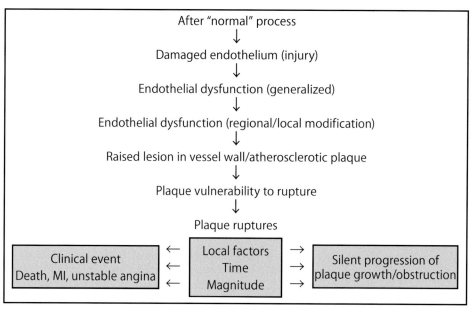

Figure 6-1. Sequence of events leading to adverse outcomes in CAD if cardiovascular risk factors persist. FMD, flow-mediated dilation; IVUS, intravascular ultrasound sonography; QIMT, quantitative intima media thickening. (Adapted with permission from Barth JD. Which tools are in your cardiac workshop? Carotid ultrasound, endothelial function, and magnetic resonance imaging. *Am J Cardiol*. 2001;87(4A):8A-14A.)

Figure 6-2. (A) Diagram of area of endothelial damage or injury; the major initial phase of atherogenesis. (B) Secondary phase of atherogenesis involving platelet aggregation; a phase that probably precedes smooth muscle cell proliferation. (C) Diagram of smooth muscle cell proliferation and migration from the media to the intima. (D) Insudation of LDL-C within the inner layers of the arterial wall. (Adapted from Ross R, Glosmet JA. The pathogenesis of atherosclerosis. *N Engl J Med.* 1976;295(7):369-377.)

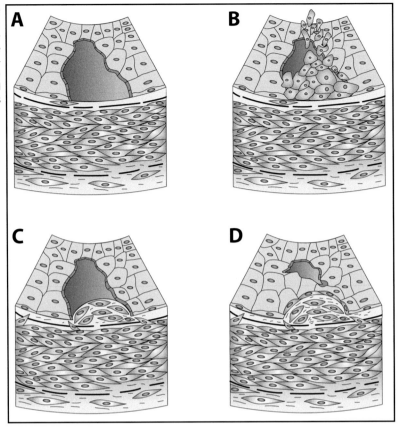

flow. When the caps break, the oxidized lipids are exposed to thrombogenic factors in the blood stream, platelets, and fibrinogen. This can lead to thrombosis or embolic obstruction of the narrowed lumen.

There is also evidence that certain blood components, such as platelets and monocytes, play a role in the pathogenesis of atherosclerosis.[19] Part of the normal activity of platelets is to adhere to damaged, irregular, or injured arterial intimal surfaces, and when they aggregate, the preliminary step in forming a clot has started. In fact, hyperlipidemia, cigarette smoking, and glucose intolerance have been shown to increase the tendency for platelet aggregation.[20] Repeated aggregation is believed to contribute to the progression of the atherosclerotic process. Plaque fissures may be sites where this aggregation takes place. The work of Ross and Glosmet[18,21] has confirmed that platelet aggregation and degeneration occurs at the site of intimal injury and that a platelet-derived growth factor is released at these sites. Platelet-derived growth factor has been shown to stimulate increased cholesterol synthesis and LDL-C binding to the smooth muscle cells, as well as stimulating proliferation of smooth muscle cells contributing to the pathogenesis of atherosclerosis (Figure 6-2).[18]

The actions of HDLs should be considered when one is examining risk factors in the pathogenesis of atherosclerosis. There is evidence that HDL-C protects against the formation of atherosclerotic plaques by removing cholesterol and cholesterol esters from smooth muscle cells in the arterial wall and blocking the atherogenic action of LDL on the smooth muscle cells of the intima. Epidemiological studies have consistently shown low levels of serum HDL to be a strong risk factor for CAD.

There is growing scientific evidence relating the major risk factors directly to the pathogenesis of atherosclerosis. These data underscore the importance of therapeutic modalities aimed at risk factor reduction that are used in both primary and secondary prevention programs.[22]

Hemodynamics of Coronary Artery Flow in Normal and Diseased States

It is important to understand the normal determinants of myocardial O_2 (MO_2) supply and demand to fully appreciate the consequences of hemodynamically significant atherosclerotic occlusions in the coronary arteries. CAD manifests itself in 3 ways: angina, infarction, and sudden death. The risk for developing one or more of these manifestations is correlated with the extent (number of coronary vessels occluded) and severity (percentage narrowing) of the occlusions.

The average resting coronary blood flow in humans is 75 mL of blood/min per 100 g of myocardium; this can increase to as high as 350 mL of blood/min per 100 g at maximal exercise.[23] Coronary blood flow or supply depends on the driving pressure through the coronary artery and the resistance to flow along the coronary vascular bed. During ventricular contraction (the systolic phase of the cardiac cycle), the extravascular pressure from the LV increase, which subsequently increases subendocardium pressures compressing the coronary arteries, increasing vascular resistance (see Chapter 1, Blood Flow section on p 15) and resulting in severely restricted blood flow to the subendocardial zones and minimal flow to the subepicardial regions of the LV. Therefore, the driving pressure for filling the coronary arteries is primarily determined by the pressure during ventricular relaxation or the diastolic phase of the cardiac cycle. The systemic blood pressure (BP) provides a driving force that promotes retrograde blood flow into the coronary arteries, and this coronary blood flow is impeded by ventricular pressure and coronary vascular resistance. The forces that impede coronary blood flow are least during ventricular diastole, resulting in phasic coronary blood flow to the LV. In the normal person, the LV end-diastolic pressure is low (5 to 10 mm Hg) and has little or no adverse effect on the net driving pressure (systemic diastolic BP [DBP] minus LV end-diastolic pressure; Figure 6-3).[23] Because the right ventricle develops less pressure, the changes in coronary vascular resistance are also less and coronary blood flow is more constant throughout the cardiac cycle.

The vascular resistance to flow depends on the tone of the smooth muscle of the arteries, resulting in coronary vasodilation or constriction and the length of the arteries. A third factor in determining coronary flow is duration of diastolic filling time. Since the coronary arteries fill during diastole and diastole comprises two-thirds of the cardiac cycle at rest, filling time does not impede coronary artery filling at rest. However, during exercise, as the heart rate (HR) increases, the time span of systole remains fairly constant, while diastolic filling time can decrease as much as 35% to 40%.[24] The reduced filling time in the normal person even during maximal exercise is not a limit to coronary blood flow.

Normally, the myocardium extracts 75% of the O_2 (an O_{2diff}, or arterial and central venous O_2 difference) from the coronary blood supply both at rest and with exercise. Therefore, any increase in MO_2 demand must be matched by an increase in coronary blood supply.[1] The factors that determine MO_2 demand are HR, systemic systolic BP (SBP), myocardial wall tension, and rate pressure generation in the LV. At rest, the average MO_2 demand is 10 mL of O_2/min/100 g of myocardium, and with exercise the MO_2 can exceed 50 mL of O_2/min/100 g. Coronary blood flow is auto regulated by both neural and metabolic influences. A potent metabolic coronary vasodilator is hypoxia, which leads to the release of vasodilator substances from the smooth muscle cells of the coronary arteries (eg, adenosine, bradykinin, carbon dioxide).[25] It is assumed that the vasodilatory influence of hypoxia overrides the vasoconstricting influence of the alpha adrenergic fibers that innervate the coronary vessels during exercise.[26] The coronary arteries are also innervated by beta1 and beta2 adrenergic fibers, which vasodilate the vessels but play a relatively minor role in the regulation of coronary blood flow. The endothelial cells of the coronary tree secrete a hormone (adenosine) that acts as a potent vasodilator. Endothelial secretory function may become dysfunctional in the presence of inflammation and plaque formation.[14]

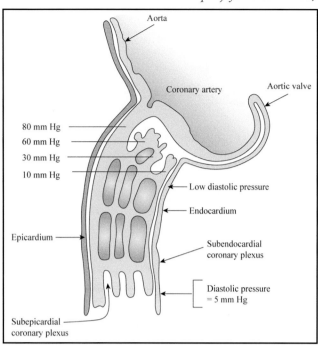

Figure 6-3. Scheme of epicardial, subepicardial, and subendocardial branches. (Adapted from Ellestad MH. Physiology of cardiac ischemia. In: *Stress Testing.* 3rd ed. Philadelphia, PA: FA Davis; 1986.)

The coronary blood flow (O_2 supply to the heart) is determined by mechanical factors such as the driving pressure, extravascular pressure, and diastolic filling time; metabolic factors such as hypoxia; and, to a lesser degree, neural influences resulting from innervation of both alpha and beta adrenergic fibers. The O_2 demand is a function of HR, mean arterial BP (afterload), ventricular wall tension, and contractility. When atherosclerosis is present, coronary artery BP is decreased beyond the site of the atherosclerotic lesion (Figure 6-4).[23]

The greater the number and/or length of lesions, the lower the downstream pressure and blood flow. The resultant problem is that fixed coronary atherosclerotic lesions may decrease coronary flow ability to below cardiac muscle demand levels. What degree of stenosis is hemodynamically significant? Logan[27] demonstrated that, at low flow rates (10 to 30 mL/min), resistance to flow was minimal; however, at flow rates of 30 to 100 mL/min, resistance increased 2- to 3-fold. More importantly, he demonstrated that lesions involving less than 70% to 80% stenosis had fairly constant curves of flow vs percent stenosis, but with lesions greater than a range of 70% to 80% stenosis, minimal increases in luminal narrowing resulted in pronounced increases in resistance to flow and decrease in flow beyond the stenosis. Due to the physiology of laminar blood flow, the longer an atherosclerotic lesion, the greater the resistance and the worse the overall hemodynamic effect. As shown in Figure 6-5, a diffuse, lengthy, 50% lesion could impair coronary flow as much as or more than a discrete 70% lesion. Sequential lesions can also have more of a bearing on flow and coronary driving pressure than a single discrete lesion, depending on the percent stenosis.

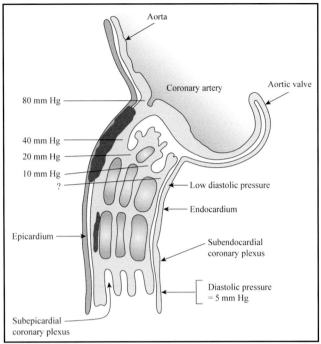

Figure 6-4. Fall in diastolic coronary artery driving pressure beyond the area of obstruction. Note the fall in pressure as the blood flows toward the endocardium. (Adapted from Ellestad MH. Physiology of cardiac ischemia. In: *Stress Testing.* 3rd ed. Philadelphia, PA: FA Davis; 1986.)

The idea that all atherosclerotic lesions are fixed and rigid is somewhat misleading. In fact, there is evidence that coronary lesions are dynamic and variable, depending on the degree of vasomotor tone at the lesion site. Coronary plaque fissures create opportunities for intermittent episodes of platelet aggregation, which may result in ischemia and thrombus formation. Sharp increases in vasomotor tone leading to a localized or diffuse spasm of a coronary artery (with or without a fixed lesion) have been shown to reduce coronary flow significantly, resulting in one of several clinical manifestations including resting angina, MI, or sudden death. Evidence suggests that coronary spasm often occurs in persons with atherosclerotic lesions, and the degree of spasm is more severe at the site of the atherosclerotic lesion than it is at adjacent uninvolved areas of the same artery in the same person.[28] An interrelationship exists between the vasomotor tone of an artery and the integrity of the endothelium, the presence of vasoactive substances, and certain components in the blood, including catecholamines thromboxane A2 (a substance derived from phospholipids of agglutinated platelets), serotonin, and histamine.[29] Persons with periodic coronary spasm that results in myocardial ischemia often exhibit certain characteristic signs or symptoms that include, but are not limited to, a variant angina pattern often involving discomfort at rest and a variable threshold for exertional discomfort, cyclic symptom patterns such as recurrent nocturnal or early morning discomfort, and ST segment elevation with or without symptoms.

ISCHEMIC CASCADE

Resting coronary blood flow adequate

Normal end-diastolic pressure (gradient normal)

Endocardial ischemia begins as oxygen demand exceeds supply

Increased myocardial oxygen demand (HR × SBP)

Fixed coronary flow (obstructive disease)

Increase Ca^{2+} retention in the endocardial myocytes ($\downarrow$ relaxation)

$\uparrow$ Preload due to $\uparrow$ venous return from exercise

$\uparrow$ End-diastolic pressure (worsens pressure gradient)

Worsens ischemia

Figure 6-5. Ischemic cascade created by obstruction of the coronary arteries and increasing MO_2 demand.

CARDIAC PUMP ISCHEMIA

Pathophysiology of Ischemia

Why is the heart so much more susceptible to ischemia and infarction than other areas of the human body? There are over 600,000 MIs in the United States each year. The heart has 3 distinct disadvantages contributing to the increased susceptibility to ischemia and infarction. First, the heart has only a small capability to function anaerobically. It is primarily an aerobic muscle that has constant, high rates of O_2 and nutritional demand. Secondly, the heart receives its blood supply primarily in diastole, not during systole like the rest of the body. This means that the DBP is the driving force for circulatory distribution, not the systolic pressure. Finally, the heart receives blood from the external surface—epicardial arteries—which then must pass through an extensive network of capillaries to the internal or endocardial areas.

The reader is encouraged to study Figure 6-4 carefully. The relationship between coronary artery blood flow and normal blood flow is uniquely depicted by this figure. Note there is a diastolic pressure reading inside the LV of 5 mm Hg. The normal end-diastolic pressure is 4 to 12 mm Hg. This is the pressure being exerted by the volume of blood in the LV just prior to systole. This blood volume does not provide O_2, glucose, or waste removal to the heart muscle.

This requires the circulating DBP to exceed the end-diastolic pressure in the ventricle in order to assure perfusion of the endocardial myocytes. Regardless, the perfusion of the endocardial tissues has to overcome the pressure gradient between the DBP and the LV end-diastolic pressure as it decreases from the epicardium to the endocardium. This pressure gradient relationship is insignificant to a normal nonoccluded coronary vascular tree, but with even small occlusions of the epicardial arteries, the pressure gradient can diminish significantly (see Figure 6-4).

Prior to exercise, a patient may have sufficient coronary artery blood flow to meet MO_2 demand. With the onset of exercise, there is an increase in MO_2 demand, HR, and BP. This increased demand may not be met due to the resistance in coronary artery blood flow and the reduction in net driving pressure beyond the obstructions. This usually results in an endocardial, regional ischemia and contractile dysfunction. This reduction in contractility in turn leads to an increase in end-systolic volumes and ultimately end-diastolic volumes, which may cause increases in end-diastolic pressure. The rise in end-diastolic pressure further reduces the net coronary artery driving pressure and worsens the ischemia. As the myocardium becomes ischemic, it does not relax completely, a condition that leads to a prolonged period of systole and thus shorter diastolic filling time, decreased compliance of the LV, and increased LV end-diastolic pressure that further decreases the net coronary driving pressure, all of which leads to more severe ischemia. Ischemia is often accompanied by dysrhythmias, and dysrhythmias are a common cause of sudden death.[30]

The hemodynamic consequences of a coronary lesion depend on the degree of luminal narrowing, the severity and frequency of plaque fissures ulcerations, the degree of calcification or soft plaque formation, the length of the stenosis, the coronary blood flow rate, and the degree of vasomotor tone of the affected artery. In a person with a hemodynamically significant obstructive lesion, exercise with the associated increases in the HR and SBP (MO_2 demand) results in increased extravascular pressure, insufficient coronary flow, and increased LV filling pressures, resulting in decreased coronary perfusion pressures, myocardial ischemia, and potentially, dysrhythmias. This series of events is depicted in Figure 6-5.[23]

Acute Myocardial Infarction

Myocardial cell death (infarction) may result from prolonged ischemia, which is the result of complete occlusion of a coronary artery vessel, vasospasm, or plaque rupture and embolism. There are numerous possible mechanisms that lead to coronary artery occlusion, including the following:

- Progression of the atherosclerotic lesion to complete occlusion
- Near total obstruction coupled with a thrombosis, resulting in total obstruction of the vessel
- Near total obstruction coupled with coronary spasm
- Near total obstruction coupled with prolonged, relatively high MO_2 demands
- Plaque rupture with thrombosis or embolism

Myocardial cell necrosis is followed by an inflammatory response, cell absorption, and eventually scar formation.

The exact site and extent of necrosis depend on the anatomic distribution of the artery, the adequacy of collateral circulation, presence and extent of previous infarction, and factors that influence the MO_2 demand, such

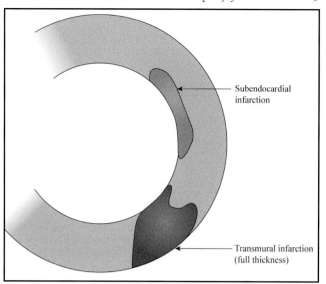

Figure 6-6. Illustration of subendocardial and transmural infarctions in a single-plane view.

as catecholamine release rates, activity of the autonomic nervous system, the SBP, and the LV end-diastolic volume and pressure. There are generally 2 types of MIs: transmural infarction, also called a *Q wave infarction*, which extends through the subendocardial tissue to the epicardial layer of the myocardium, and subendocardial infarction, also called a *non-Q wave infarction*, which involves only the innermost layer of the myocardium and, in some cases, portions of the middle layer of tissue, but does not extend to include the epicardial region of the myocardium (Figure 6-6).

The diagnosis of acute MI is made from the combination of several findings, including clinical history of signs and symptoms, elevation of specific serum markers in the blood, presence of an acute injury pattern on the 12 lead ECG, and positive findings of special radioisotope studies. It is important to recognize that all of the previously mentioned findings are not necessarily evident in every acute MI and that, in most cases, the changes in serum markers and the 12 lead ECG are relied on most heavily.

The classic symptoms of an acute MI involve severe central chest or retrosternal discomfort (unstable, resting angina). The nature of the discomfort varies but most commonly is described as either pain, pressure, or heaviness that the patient states is "like a heavy weight on my chest." The discomfort often will radiate to several areas, including the neck or jaw, one or both upper extremities, and the midscapular region. Infarction symptoms usually persist for prolonged periods of time (hours) but may wax and wane and are not relieved by nitroglycerin. Associated signs and symptoms commonly include dyspnea, diaphoresis, lightheadedness, nausea, apprehension, weakness, vomiting, and hypotension. The clinician must be aware, however, that the so-called classic symptoms described do not always accompany an infarction and that the nature, location, and intensity of discomfort, along with the associated signs and symptoms, can vary widely among patients. Finally, MIs can

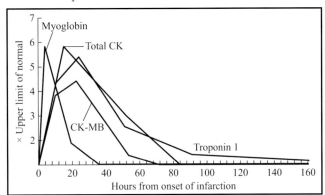

Figure 6-7. Serum markers indicative of MI. The relative rate of rise, peak values, and duration of cardiac marker elevations above the upper limit of normal for multiple serum markers following acute MI. (Reprinted with permission from Porth CM, Hennessey CL. Alterations in cardiac function. In: Porth CM, ed. *Pathophysiology.* 6th ed. Philadelphia, PA: Lippincott Williams & Wilkins; 2002.)

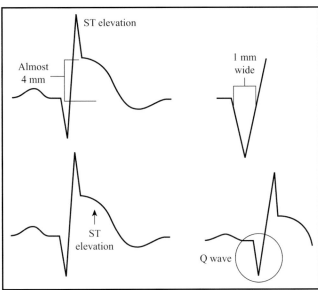

Figure 6-8. Illustration of a classic acute infarction pattern seen in a single-lead ECG tracing.

occur without symptoms; in fact, based on postmortem and epidemiological studies, 20% to 25% of all infarctions are "silent" or asymptomatic.

The use of serum markers to diagnose an acute MI is based on several assumptions that are still somewhat controversial. First, it is assumed that elevation of a specific marker occurs only with cell death and not in instances of prolonged ischemia. Second, the rise in the marker is not attributable to damage in other major organs. Finally, there is a direct relationship between the amount of rise in the marker and the size of the infarction.

The 3 serum markers that are characteristically elevated when an acute MI has occurred are myoglobin; creatine kinase (CK), formerly called *creatinine phosphokinase* (CK-MB), a cardiac specific isoenzyme of CK; and troponin I. The serum levels of all of these markers will increase within the first 36 hours of an infarction (Figure 6-7).[31] The myoglobin levels are the first to rise and they peak during the first 4 to 8 hours after the infarct. CK also rises early after infarction but may remain elevated for several days after the infarct. CK-MB rises more gradually and follows a pattern resembling CK by dissipating within 3 days. Troponin I rises with CK but may remain elevated for several days after the infarct. False positive rises in the CK and CK-MB can occur in patients with myositis, muscular dystrophies, and pericarditis. The clinical significance of these changes for the therapist working in an acute care setting is as follows: Prior to increasing activity levels with a patient, it is prudent to check the latest serum levels. If the serum markers are spiked, the patient may have extended their infarction or had another infarction that has gone undocumented. Although this is a rare phenomenon, it is better to know their current serum marker status than to just assume that the other medical staff will tell you to hold rehabilitation. The other clinically significant information that can be obtained from the markers is that, in general, the higher the level of CK and CK-MB, the larger the area of infarction. The patient's prognosis is directly related to the extent of tissue damage and the degree of additional coronary artery obstruction.

The acute changes in the 12 lead ECG that occur as a result of an MI depend on the type of infarction (transmural vs subendocardial) and the area of infarction. By definition, subendocardial infarctions result in new T wave inversion, ST segment depression, or both that persist for 48 hours with no new Q wave changes or R wave losses. Transmural infarctions usually result in ST segment elevation associated with T wave inversion in leads specific to the area of infarction.[32]

In addition, evolutionary changes in the ECG pattern of a patient with a transmural infarction induce a significant Q-wave (greater than 0.04 seconds in duration and greater than 25% of the amplitude of the R wave) and, in some cases, decreased R wave voltage (Figure 6-8). Reciprocal ST segment depression often occurs in undamaged areas opposite the area of infarction. Studies indicate that ECG changes establish the correct diagnosis 85% of the time in men. Postmortem studies indicate that the sensitivity of acute ECG changes in infarction patients is 60% and the false positive rate is 42%. The most common causes of "false positive" 12 lead ECG changes include cardiomyopathies, cerebrovascular accidents, pulmonary emboli, hyperkalemia, idiopathic hypertrophic subaortic stenosis, and 12 lead conduction abnormalities such as left bundle branch block and Wolff-Parkinson-White syndrome. It is often 24 or more hours before the acute ECG changes described previously appear.

Reversal and Retardation of Progression of Atherosclerosis

The concept that the normal progression of atherosclerosis can be altered and, in some cases, reversed is no longer theoretical. There is evidence that risk factor reduction has a major impact on the disease process both for those with known coronary disease and for those at high risk of developing hemodynamically significant coronary atherosclerosis.

TABLE 6-3A. FUNCTIONAL AND THERAPEUTIC CLASSIFICATIONS OF HEART DISEASE FROM THE NEW YORK HEART ASSOCIATION

FUNCTIONAL CAPACITY CLASSIFICATION	THERAPEUTIC CLASSIFICATION
Class I: No limitation of physical activity. Ordinary physical activity does not cause undue fatigue, palpitation, dyspnea, or anginal pain	Class A: Physical activity need not be restricted
Class II: Slight limitation of physical activity. Comfortable at rest, but ordinary physical activity results in fatigue, palpitation, dyspnea, or anginal pain	Class B: Ordinary physical activity need not be restricted, but unusually severe or competitive efforts should be avoided
Class III: Marked limitation of physical activity. Comfortable at rest, but less than ordinary activity causes fatigue, palpitation, dyspnea, or anginal pain	Class C: Ordinary physical activity should be moderately restricted, and more strenuous efforts should be discontinued
Class IV: Unable to carry on any physical activity without discomfort. Symptoms of cardiac insufficiency or of the anginal syndrome may be present even at rest; any physical activity increases discomfort	Class D: Ordinary physical activity should be markedly restricted
	Class E: Patient should be at complete rest and confined to bed or chair

(continued)

Evidence shows that arterial lesions can be favorably altered by a reduction in hypertension, hypercholesterolemia, and hyperglycemia.[33-35]

Multiple studies have provided impressive clinical evidence, indicating that lipid lowering is an effective prevention intervention.[36-38] Additionally, diet modification has been shown to reduce coronary lesion size accompanied by decreased arterial lipid content in primates.[39,40] There have also been several human studies involving coronary angiography that have demonstrated that lipid lowering through diet or medical therapy results in a decreased incidence of coronary lesion progression and an improved clinical course.[41,42] Additionally, Blankenhorn et al[43,44] have demonstrated that aggressive lipid lowering and elevation of HDL led to a decreased incidence of lesion progression, but a treated group of post-coronary artery bypass grafting patients also demonstrated a significantly higher incidence of lesion regression.

The angiographic evidence of the beneficial effects of aerobic exercise on coronary progression is by no means as extensive. However, Kramsch et al[45] have published evidence that moderate exercise carried out over a period of 3 or more years and associated with improvements in HDL, LDL, and triglyceride levels resulted in decreased degree of atherosclerosis, decreased lesion size and collagen accumulation, and increased heart size and vessel lumen. These authors concluded that regular aerobic exercise may prevent or retard the development of coronary atherosclerosis, especially if it is initiated before an atherogenic diet.

The evidence is now clear that aggressive management of dyslipidemia, hypertension, glucose intolerance, and regular moderate levels of aerobic exercise can significantly moderate the course and outcome of the pathophysiology of atherosclerosis and its subsequent manifestations.

HEART FAILURE

Heart failure may be defined as the inability of the heart to pump sufficient amounts of blood to meet the physiologic demands of the body.[46] Heart failure is a common coexisting condition in patients with strokes, diabetes, chronic obstructive pulmonary disease (COPD) and the multitude of potential combinations of these diseases and other chronic disease states. The advancements in cardiac care have created an ever-growing population of individuals living with heart failure.[47] In fact, heart failure is the final common pathway for virtually all forms of heart disease, including CAD/ischemic heart disease, HTN, cardiomyopathies, valve disorders, arrhythmogenic diseases, and congenital heart disease.[15] This requires that the rehabilitation professional recognize and quickly assess the presence of worsening failure or the onset of acute heart failure. Heart failure may be classified based on the severity of the patient's symptoms and functional limitations by the New York Heart Association. The New York Heart Association classification system is a well accepted scale for heart disease and heart failure and should be familiar to all health care providers who may see patients with heart diseases (Table 6-3).

Heart failure is a medical condition that can be slow in development and progressive in nature, but it may also be characterized by acute exacerbations. Clinically, heart failure may be categorized by several terms, including high output/low output or right-sided/left-sided, but the most frequent description is systolic heart failure (failure of the ventricular pump) or diastolic heart failure (limited ability to fill properly). Regardless of etiology, the common manifestations of the disease result from an inadequate CO. The most common causes of heart failure in the adult population in the United States are ischemic heart disease and chronic hypertension.

TABLE 6-3B. GUIDELINES FOR RISK STRATIFICATION FROM THE AMERICAN HEART ASSOCIATION WHEN CONSIDERING AN EXERCISE PROGRAM

AHA CLASSIFICATION	NYHA CLASS	EXERCISE CAPACITY	ANGINA/ISCHEMIA AND CLINICAL CHARACTERISTICS	ECG MONITORING
A: Apparently healthy			Less than 40 years of age; without symptoms, no major risk factors, and normal GXT	No supervision or monitoring required
B: Known stable CHD, low risk for vigorous exercise	I or II	5 to 6 METs	Free of ischemia or angina at rest or on the GXT; EF=40% to 60%	Monitored and supervised only during prescribed sessions (6 to 12 sessions); light resistance training may be included in comprehensive rehabilitation programs
C: Stable CHD with low risk for vigorous exercise, but unable to self-regulate activity	I or II	5 to 6 METs	Same disease states and clinical characteristics as class B but without the ability to self-monitor exercise	Medical supervision and ECG monitoring during prescribed sessions; nonmedical supervision of other exercise sessions
D: Moderate-to-high risk for cardiac complications during exercise	≥III	<6 METs	Ischemia (≥4.0 mm ST depression) or angina during exercise; 2 or more previous MIs; EF <30%	Continuous ECG monitoring during rehabilitation until safety established; medical supervision during all exercise sessions until safety established
E: Unstable disease with activity restriction	≥III	<6 METs	Unstable angina; uncompensated heart failure; uncontrollable arrhythmias	No activity recommended for conditioning purposes; attention directed to restoring patient to class D or higher

CHD, coronary heart disease; EF, ejection fraction; GXT, graded exercise test; NYHA, New York Heart Association.
Adapted from American College of Sports Medicine. *Guidelines for Exercise Testing and Prescription.* 6th ed. Baltimore, MD: Williams & Wilkins; 2000.

Chronic ischemic disease will result in ischemic cardiomyopathy with ventricular dilatation and volume overload, while patients with chronic hypertension will exhibit hypertrophy due to elevated afterload, termed *pressure overload*, and concentric hypertrophy. As the heart's contractile function deteriorates, multiple compensatory mechanism attempt to increase blood volume and raise cardiac filling pressure to maintain the CO and raise BP (Figure 6-9).

As CO falls, LV pressure rise. This pressure is transmitted from the LV into the left atrium and then to the pulmonary venous vasculature. As noted in Chapter 1, the pulmonary venous system is normally a low-pressure system. As pulmonary venous hydrostatic pressures increase, fluid may be pushed out of the venous capillaries into the interstitial space and eventually into the lung itself, resulting in pulmonary edema. This rise in pressure is eventually reflected in a rise in pulmonary artery pressure. The right heart, which is significantly smaller in cross-sectional area and not designed to pump against elevated pressures, will also begin to fail. The right ventricular end-diastolic pressure begins to rise and the result is elevations in right atrial pressures and increases in peripheral venous pressures and peripheral edema (see

Figure 6-9). In this way, the LV causes the right ventricle to fail.

Congestive Heart Failure

Congestive heart failure, as the name suggests, is failure of the heart causing congestion in the chest, often resulting in the patient complaining of an inability to take a deep breath or dyspnea on exertion. Some of the most common signs and symptoms of left-sided failure or congestive heart failure are shown in Table 6-4.

Pulmonary edema occurs at the base of lungs first in the upright position, and the associated crackles are best heard in the posterior bases early in an acute exacerbation of heart failure. As the failure worsens, the edema will ascend (from bases toward apices) and eventually (end stage), the patient may develop frothy pink-tinged sputum and bubbly respiration known as the *death rattle*. A dry nonproductive cough is common. Cough in the middle of the night if the patient has been lying horizontal for a prolonged period is described as night cough or paroxysmal nocturnal dyspnea. When a patient assumes the horizontal position, venous return is

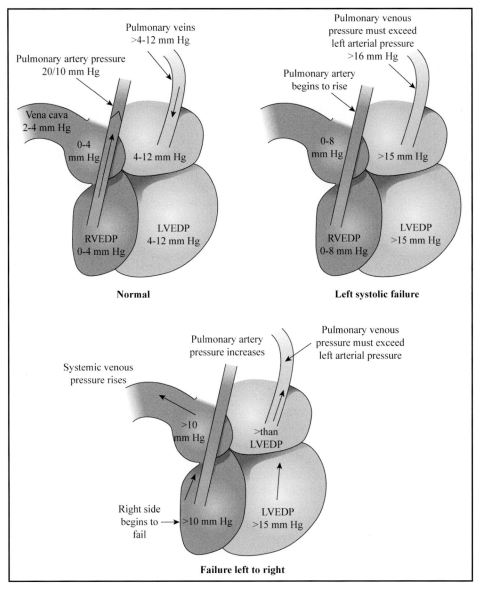

Figure 6-9. Illustration of normal and abnormal pressure changes that occur as a result of left heart failure. (LVEDP, LV end-diastolic pressure; RVEDP, right ventricular end-diastolic pressure.)

enhanced. If the heart is unable to increase CO in the presence of this increasing volume, then decompensation and pulmonary edema develop, leading to cough and the sensation of dyspnea and the patient is awakened.

Another sign of heart failure or decompensation is a third heart sound (S3). This sound is thought to be the result of an increase in ventricular wall stiffness (a decreased ventricular compliance). The rapid inflow of blood during early diastole is met by a noncompliant ventricular wall, creating a soft extra sound. An S3 may be a normal sound in children and athletes but is usually pathological in adults over age 40 years.[46,48]

Orthopnea, SOB when lying flat, is also a common symptom due to heart failure and may be further described by the number of pillows required to alleviate the symptom (eg, 1-, 2-, or 3-pillow orthopnea). Exercise intolerance is due to multiple factors. Exercise requires an increase in CO to augment O_2 delivery to the exercising muscle. A failing heart may have

TABLE 6-4. MOST COMMON SIGNS AND SYMPTOMS OF LEFT-SIDED FAILURE OR CONGESTIVE HEART FAILURE

• Pulmonary edema	• Exertional hypotension
• Dry cough	• Sudden weight gain
• Nocturnal dyspnea	• Cardiac enlargement by chest x-ray and hypertrophy on a 12 lead ECG
• S3	
• Orthopnea	
• Exertional dyspnea at low levels of exercise (2 to 4 METs)	• High resting HRs > 100
	• SOB at rest

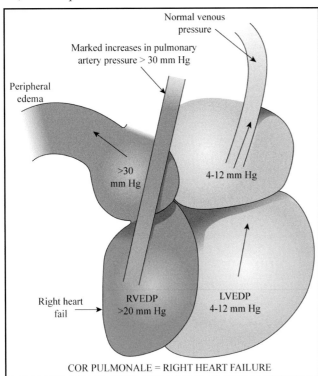

Normal venous
pressure

Marked increases in pulmonary
artery pressure > 30 mm Hg

Peripheral
edema

>30
mm Hg

4-12 mm Hg

Right heart
fail

RVEDP
>20 mm Hg

LVEDP
4-12 mm Hg

COR PULMONALE = RIGHT HEART FAILURE

Figure 6-10. Illustration of pressure changes that occur as a result of advanced COPD that leads to cor pulmonale (right heart failure).

a normal CO at rest but is not capable of increasing CO to any substantial degree with increasing demand. Additionally, the peripheral resistance of the vasculature is increased compared to normal, further limiting O_2 delivery.[49] Heart failure is also associated with altered skeletal muscle. Specifically, there is atrophy, muscle fiber transitions from type I to type II-like muscle fibers, and reduced mitochondria and capillary density.[50,51] Patients with heart failure will also demonstrate altered pulmonary responses to exercise with limited pulmonary reserve.[52-54] The combination of these alterations in exercise responses limit the activity and exercise performance of patients with heart failure.

Sudden weight gain (ie, 6 to 10 pounds or more in 1 to 2 days) results from the body's attempt to increase CO by retaining sodium and subsequent fluid retention and blood volume expansion (see Chapter 1, Frank-Starling Reflex section on p 13). Finally, pathological findings on the ECG (LV hypertrophy), chest x-ray findings (pulmonary engorgement and cardiomegaly), and echocardiography (ejection fraction) are used to confirm the diagnosis of congestive heart failure.

Differences Between Left- and Right-Sided Heart Failure

How does left-sided heart failure differ from right-sided heart failure? As previously noted, right-sided heart failure commonly occurs as a result of left-sided failure. The pressure changes on the left are transmitted via the closed vascular network of the lung to the pulmonary arteries.

An elevation in the pulmonary artery pressure will have a similar effect on the right ventricle that elevations in systemic pressures (hypertension) has on the LV, an increase in ventricular afterload. The greatest difference being, as seen in Figures 6-1 through 6-9, is that the right ventricle has significantly less cross-sectional area (muscle mass) than the left and cannot as easily tolerate even increases in ventricular afterload. The signs and symptoms of right-sided failure are peripheral edema and poor exercise tolerance. The edema usually manifests itself in the lower extremities initially and then can progress up into the abdomen (ascites), and liver. Whenever a patient has bilateral lower-extremity edema, the clinician should always rule out the possibility of right-sided failure before initiating any anti-edema interventions. Attempting to reduce the edema by using pressure garments, pressure pumps, or gravity may increase the right heart pressures, cardiac wall tension, and MO_2 demand. This can worsen the patient's failure and put undo stress on the failing ventricles.

There are many additional causes of right-sided failure besides left-sided failure; these include but are not limited to chronic or acute pulmonary hypertension, cor pulmonale, right ventricular infarct(s) and valvular dysfunctions (tricuspid and pulmonary semi-lunar valves regurgitation and stenosis). Cor pulmonale is right-sided heart failure resulting from pulmonary disease. This may be commonly encountered as a secondary diagnosis in patients with COPD. The primary cause of the right-sided heart failure is chronic elevations in pulmonary artery pressures as a result of chronic hypoxia and pulmonary hypoxic vasoconstriction and resultant vascular remodeling (Figure 6-10).

Distinguishing Between Left- and Right-Sided Failure

The signs and symptoms of selective right-sided failure are similar to left-sided failure, namely peripheral edema and limited exercise tolerance. Right-sided failure is not congestive heart failure because pulmonary edema does not develop. However, similar to left-sided failure, there is failure to sustain CO resulting in inadequate tissue/organ perfusion and exercise intolerance. The signs and symptoms of right-sided failure with exercise include hypotension, due to reduced LV filling, no pulmonary edema (no crackles), and usually no audible S3. Thus, the clinician that monitors the patient's responses to exercise may be able to differentiate a patient suffering exclusively from right-sided failure from one suffering from left-sided failure because of the difference in signs and symptoms. It is also imperative that the clinician who is treating a patient with the diagnosis of COPD and cor pulmonale monitor the patient's BP and pulse oximetry responses to exercise. This will assist in identifying a patient with SOB because of heart failure (cor pulmonale) from a patient who is SOB strictly from pulmonary disease (eg, COPD).

Summary of Cardiac Pump Disorder Pathophysiology

The adequacy of coronary blood flow to the myocardium depends on the balance between supply and demand. Atherosclerotic changes in the coronary arteries can significantly decrease coronary supply because of luminal narrowing. Supply can be further compromised by increased vasomotor tone in the coronary arteries, leading to acute spasm of the artery. The possible consequences of an imbalance between supply and demand include myocardial ischemia with or without symptoms, MI, or sudden death. The diagnosis of an acute MI is based on a combination of findings. Clinical symptoms, serum markers of cardiac damage, and changes in the 12 lead ECG are all used to determine the diagnosis of MI.

CAD is a progressive process. The prognosis of a patient with coronary disease depends primarily on the number of vessels diseased and the degree of LV dysfunction as a result of infarction or ischemia. Angiographic evidence exists, demonstrating that risk factor reduction, including improvement of lipid levels and regular aerobic exercise, does alter the progression of coronary atherosclerosis and, in some cases, leads to regression of the disease process. Further study is needed to uncover the various ways in which risk factor reduction alters the normally progressive course of atherosclerosis.

Due to the significant advances in the treatment of all heart conditions, we are seeing an ever-growing population of individuals living with heart failure. Recognizing the signs and symptoms of heart failure are important to the rehabilitation professional who may be working with patients with secondary morbidities (stroke, hypertension, diabetes). An ability to use the findings from an examination of the patient with cardiac and pulmonary diseases to differentiate left- and right-sided heart failure is useful in determining the most appropriate selection of interventions for each individual.

PATIENT EXAMINATION: HISTORY, SYSTEMS REVIEW, TESTS, AND MEASURES

The history, systems review, and tests and measures are key components to the clinician's evaluation. For those patients with cardiovascular pump dysfunction, these components revolve around any medical diagnoses or comorbidities that may create increases in O_2 consumption demands or interfere with O_2 transport within the body. Common comorbidities are COPD, type II diabetes, chronic hypertension, age, renal disease, and any neuromusculoskeletal impairments that require an increased demand on the cardiovascular system for even normal daily activities.

History and Interview

The patient's history should include but is not limited to age; gender; race; and past medical history with particular emphasis on previous MIs, cardiac surgeries, and hospital admissions for angina, heart failure, or syncope. A careful review of the patient's risk factors should also be completed at this time. Those individuals with the greatest number of risk factors for CAD have an increased risk for progression of the disease. The clinician should probe carefully about family history and smoking history. A simple question like, "Do you have a family history of heart disease?" is often answered with a quick no, whereas a few additional questions like, "Has anyone in your family ever had a heart attack or high BP?" will bring a more elucidating response. Another often missed risk factor is cigarette smoking. Patients will say they are not smokers when they are or when they just quit. Again, a more probing request is to ask, "Have you every smoked?" Establishment of the patient's risk factors will assist in directing the patient's and families' education programming.

A thorough review of the patient's current medications can be very revealing. The most common medications used when someone has CAD are beta blockers, nitrates, ACE inhibitors, and calcium channel blockers. Patients with heart failure will often be prescribed cardiac glycosides (Digitalis), ACE inhibitors, low doses of beta blockers, and diuretics (Lasix). An understanding of the mechanism of action of the medications and their potential side effects can help explain examination findings.

A review of the patient's social and work history may provide information regarding activity/exercise tolerance. During this portion of the examination, the therapist should ask the patient about his or her goals and determine his or her chief complaint. The therapist should understand that patients may often experience denial, especially if they have just recently had an MI or episode of angina.

Identification of the patient's family will help with discharge and educational interventions. Heart disease prevention should include the children of patients with heart disease. The data on the incidence of heart disease in families are clear, and if the risk factors are present in childhood, then they will progress into adulthood.[55,56] The patient's support system and work requirements will often direct the goals of therapy. For example, a patient who works using primarily his or her upper extremities needs to be trained using upper extremity equipment and monitoring. One of the more common effects of CAD is depression, which may lead to a poor prognosis.[57] It is important to recognize other confounding factors that would promote psychological dysfunction, such as being a widow or living alone.

Systems Review

A brief gross inspection of the neuromusculoskeletal systems can be completed on most patients with a primary physical therapy diagnosis of cardiovascular pump dysfunction by doing a gross manual muscle test. The integumentary

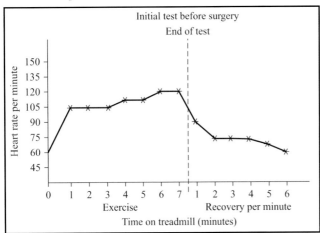

Figure 6-11. HR response to Bruce Protocol Treadmill test in Patient A, a 45-year-old man, before surgery. Patient completed 6 minutes and 6 seconds of the Bruce Protocol. He was limited by angina. Resting HR was 54 bpm, and maximum HR was 118 bpm. Resting BP was 164/98, and maximum BP was 244/126. He demonstrated moderate systolic and severe progressive diastolic hypertension with exercise. No ST-segment changes were found in any of the 6 leads: V1, V5, V6, X, CM4, and Y. No dysrhythmias occurred. His medications were nitroglycerine as needed and Dyazide (triamterene and hydrochlorothiazide). An S4 was auscultated.

system can be examined by inspection and is rarely contributory to the PT diagnosis unless the patient has undergone a surgical procedure. In patients with severe burns, the cardiovascular system demands may be so great that the functional limitations are a result of cardiovascular limits and not integumentary embarrassment. The cardiopulmonary system can also be grossly examined by obtaining resting and activity associated HR, respiratory rate, BP, lung sounds, O_2 saturation, symptoms, perceived exertion, and heart sounds. A more detailed explanation of the importance of these measures is included in the test and measures section to follow.

Test and Measures

The definitive test for the rehabilitation professional in examination and evaluation of the patient with any pathology that affects cardiovascular system is the exercise test—a measure of aerobic capacity/endurance. The format for this test can range from the maximum symptom-limited treadmill exercise test with thallium scanning or echocardiography to a simple self-care evaluation involving minimal demands on cardiovascular reserves.

The primary ingredients in any exercise test though are as follows:

1. A known measurable workload or O_2 consumption requirement (ie, speed, grade, kilogram-meters, METS)

2. Repeated measurement during the test of HR, BP, ECG, and symptoms

3. Heart sounds assessment before and after testing

4. Instant interpretation of the data being obtained from numbers 1 and 2

Prior to the exercise test, the therapist should have reviewed any other tests that may be available on the patient. This includes echocardiography, angiography, chest x-ray, 24-hour ECG monitoring, and laboratory values, (cardiac enzymes, 12 lead ECG, blood gases, glucose, hemoglobin, cholesterol, and any renal function studies). The significance of each of these variables will be clarified as a part of the patient case presented at the end of this chapter. Instant interpretation requires the therapist to understand both the normal and abnormal responses to exercise.

To understand the abnormal responses often observed in clinical environments, one must have a sound understanding of normal human responses. To the purist, the term *abnormal* is a misnomer, because a clear-cut definition of "normal" has not been established. Normal values may range from those less than average to those above average. This makes it difficult to distinguish normal variations from true aberrations.

There are several established normal physiological responses to exercise. For example, HR and SBP rise as the workload is increases. Normally, CO is the primary limitation to maximum O_2 consumption and determines the maximal physical work capacity. Furthermore, numerous articles describe the angina threshold (the point at which a patient first perceives angina) as a fixed phenomenon based on MO_2 demand, which is strongly correlated to the product of HR and SBP, the rate pressure product.[58] Various pathological conditions and treatments (including medications) can create demonstrable changes in normal HR, BP, and anginal responses during exercise.

Heart Rate Response

Normal

At normal and submaximal levels of exercise, CO and HR responses increase linearly as the workload and O_2 consumption demands increase. At near maximum and maximum levels of exertion, however, the HR response becomes less linear and increases disproportionately to the workload imposed (Figure 6-11). If the workload is applied using arm work exclusively, the HR and BP responses are significantly higher for any given workload. The maximum workload achievable with arm work is significantly lower than with leg work. These 2 concepts are important to keep in mind when treating debilitated patients with primary or secondary cardiopulmonary dysfunction. Although arm work appears to be significantly easier, the work on the heart may be higher with relatively arm work versus even moderate levels of leg work (Figure 6-12).

Normal resting HR ranges from 60 to 100 bpm. Below 60 bpm is called *bradycardia*. Above 100 bpm is called *tachycardia*. Although a resting HR of less than 60 bpm is described as bradycardia, significant hemodynamic consequences do not become apparent until the resting HR approaches 40 bpm. As noted in Chapter 1, CO is defined as HR multiplied by stroke volume (SV) (CO= HR x SV). In order to maintain a CO of 4 to 6 L/min (normal range for

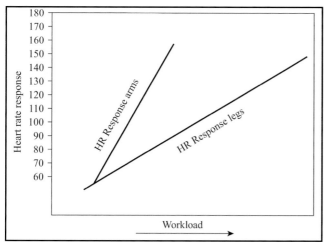

Figure 6-12. Relationship between the HR response to arm work relative to leg work.

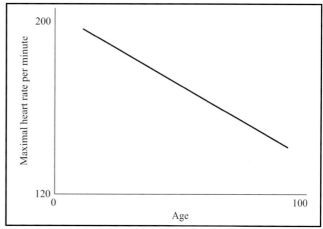

Figure 6-13. Maximum HR decreases with increase in age.

resting CO) at an HR of 40 bpm, the client's SV would have to be 100 to 150 mL per beat. The majority of patients with clinically significant heart disease do not have the contractile strength required to achieve this level of SV. Their CO falls below the levels required to provide adequate O_2 delivery to the tissues (heart failure). Many patients with CAD are prescribed beta-blocking medications, which reduce resting and exercise HRs. Even when these medications are present, a resting HR near or below 40 bpm should be considered a red flag and the appropriate actions immediately implemented to prevent further untoward events.

In addition to the effects that a low resting HR has on CO, it may indicate another problem such as heart block. Second- and third-degree heart blocks are potentially life threatening and are closely associated with low but regular HRs at rest. These blocks indicate that there is a conduction abnormality impacting the signal transmission from the SA node through the AV node to the ventricles. The clinician is encouraged to routinely assess the client's resting HR and rhythm even when the primary diagnosis for referral or clinic visit is not because of a cardiac or pulmonary origin. The adult resting HR is, under normal conditions, a very stable variable and does not vary as a function of age.[59]

Clearly, pathophysiological considerations will cause changes, but that is all the more reason to routinely assess each patient's resting HR. Drastic changes in the resting HR, up or down, may be the result of any number of associated pathological conditions (heart failure, autonomic nervous system dysfunction, anemia, conduction system blocks, supraventricular and ventricular dysrhythmias, hormone imbalances, MIs, systemic infections, and a wide variety of medications). For example, your patient is referred for home health rehabilitation for a total knee replacement. His resting HR on the first visit is a regular 78 bpm. On a subsequent visit 1 week later, the patient's HR is 54 to 60 bpm. This may have been the result of a change in medications (beta-blocker). If so, there is a significant reason for the addition of this drug. On the other hand, what if his resting HR was greater than 100 bpm? The patient may be experiencing a drop in

hemoglobin, anxiety, fever, hormonal imbalance, or myriad other negative possibilities.

Heart Rate Responses to Exercise

An adult's maximum attainable HR decreases with age. A useful but limited formula for predicting a maximum HR is to subtract the patient's age from 220 (Figure 6-13).

The accuracy of this formula is limited because of the effects of medications, abnormal HR responses, and the wide range of individual variations in maximum HR response ($\pm 10\%$ to 15%).[60] This variability is especially prevalent in women. Clinical experience has demonstrated that women, especially those over age 50 years have significantly higher maximum HRs than is predicted by the formula. The 220 – age formula should not be used to assess HR responses of patients on medications (beta-blockers or sympathomimetics) or post-cardiac transplant. Beta-blockers blunt the resting and exercise HR, and sympathomimetics (bronchodilators) have nearly the opposite effect. Many patients post-heart transplant have denervated hearts (no autonomic nervous system input). Thus, their resting and exercise HR responses are markedly abnormal compared to a normally innervated heart. On the other hand (for clinical guidance), for individuals not on cardiac medications, the formula provides a gross indication of the intensity of work being performed. It is preferable to obtain a patient's true maximum HR by performing a maximum symptom-limited exercise test.

Abnormal

In the clinical setting, a small subset of patients with CAD demonstrates a clearly abnormal HR response to exercise. This phenomenon has been described by Ellestad,[61] Miller et al,[62] and others.[46,63] Although each describes slightly different criteria for the response, and thus a slightly different population of patients, they agree that this response is a sign of an advanced pathological condition. Generally, the following criteria are observed:

- Low resting HR (50 to 70 bpm)
- Poor physical condition (untrained)

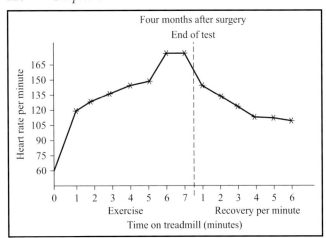

Figure 6-14. HR response to Bruce Protocol Treadmill test in Patient A, 8 weeks after bypass surgery. Patient completed 6 minutes and 7 seconds of the Bruce Protocol. He was limited by leg pain. Resting HR was 62 bpm and maximum HR was 160 bpm. Resting BP was 176/110, and maximum BP was 292/120. He demonstrated severe SBP and DBP response throughout the test. He had no angina or ST-segment changes. One PVC occurred during exercise. He was not using medications. An S4 was auscultated.

- Advanced CAD
- Maximum symptom-limited HR achieved during exercise testing is well below the person's predicted maximal HR, obtained by subtracting the individual's age from 220
- Men between the ages of 40 and 60 years
- Not using chronotropic inhibiting/exciting medications (chronotropic means influencing the rate of the heart beat)
- Poor, slow HR increase in response to incremental increases in exercise workload
- Poor exercise tolerance

An example of this phenomenon in a patient tested before and after bypass surgery (see Figures 6-11 and 6-14). A summary interpretation of each of these tests follows the graph. Each exercise test was performed using a standardized exercise testing protocol.

It is extraordinary that this patient's exercise tolerance was unchanged despite a 42 bpm increase in his maximum HR between the first test before surgery and the second test 8 weeks after surgery. In effect, this patient had a 36% increase in his HR reserve but essentially no change in his physical work capacity.

The following findings were recorded on his catheterization:

- 25% narrowing of the left main coronary artery
- Less than 50% narrowing at the junction of the proximal and middle thirds of the LAD artery, plus a somewhat narrowed appearance throughout its length
- About 75% stenosis at the origin of the second posterolateral branch of the circumflex and mildly irregular throughout

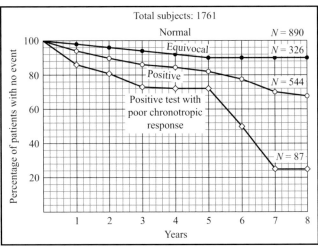

Figure 6-15. Abnormal rate response. Life-table display of incidence of MI. Notice the higher incidence of infarction in those with poor chronotropic response to exercise. (Adapted from Ellestad MH. Physiology of cardiac ischemia. In: *Stress Testing.* 3rd ed. Philadelphia, PA: FA Davis; 1986.)

- Right coronary artery 75% stenotic at the ostium and midpoint
- Hemodynamically, the right ventricle and atrium had greatly elevated end-diastolic and systolic pressures
- LV end-diastolic pressure was greatly elevated
- Ejection faction was normal
- The LV contractile pattern was normal

An abnormal HR response to exercise testing using the criteria listed may be the only abnormality found on the exercise test. This finding often signifies advanced CAD and a poor prognosis. In an otherwise normal individual, a slow gradual increase in HR with large increases in workload would signify someone with extremely good levels of physical fitness. This is clearly not the case with this subset of cardiac patients.

Mechanisms

There appears to be a close relationship between the patient's HR response and ischemia. (Note that there were no ST-segment changes on either test.) The first test, which vividly demonstrates chronotropic incompetence, illustrates the need to watch all factors involved in exercise testing, not just the ST segments.

Ellestad,[61] confirmed by Brener and others,[46,63] found that this decreased response is an ominous sign of advanced CAD associated with accelerated rates of mortality and morbidity (Figures 6-15 and 6-16), especially when compared with patients with normal HR responses.

If ischemia is the cause of this decreased HR response, the body's defense mechanism is appropriate because a reduced HR facilitates improved coronary blood flow and decreases MO_2 demand. A lower HR lengthens the diastolic filling time, enhancing LV perfusion. Alternatively, an increased diastolic filling time may cause large increases in end-diastolic volume, especially during exercise. Volume increases are well tolerated by a normal, well perfused

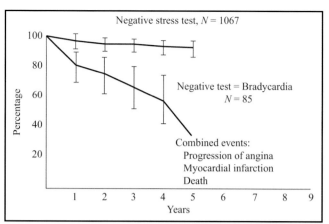

Figure 6-16. Combined events bradycardia. Those with bradycardia (pulse fell below 95% confidence limits for age and sex) and normal ST segments have a high incidence of combined events (similar to those with ST-segment depression). (Adapted from Ellestad MH. Physiology of cardiac ischemia. In: *Stress Testing*. 3rd ed. Philadelphia, PA: FA Davis; 1986.)

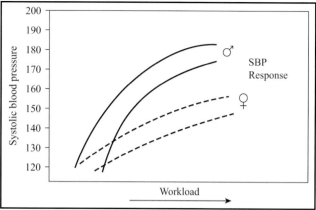

Figure 6-17. Comparison of SBP responses between men and women.

myocardium, but in the ischemic myocardium, volume changes are associated with increased pressures and thus decreased subendocardial perfusion (see Figure 6-4) As the reader may note from the patient example, his end-diastolic pressure was greatly elevated—20 mm Hg—at rest (normal is 0 to 12 mm Hg). One could speculate that the rising end-diastolic pressure that undoubtedly occurred with increased venous return during exercise may have somehow been the impetus to a reflex inhibition in HR.[61] The pathological chronotropic incompetence exhibited during a progressive increase in workload should not be taken lightly by clinicians, but instead interpreted as a highly abnormal, pathological response to exercise.[46]

There are no normal conditions wherein an individual's HR decreases with an increase in workload. Clinical conditions that may alter the normal HR response include second- or third-degree heart block, bigeminal rhythms (premature ventricular contraction [PVC] every other beat) and sick sinus syndrome. A decrease in HR with increasing levels of exercise is always a red flag for the clinician. The client should discontinue his or her exercise program, and the cause of the decreased HR should be determined and the physician notified. No further exercise training should be carried out until the patient is cleared to resume exercise by his or her cardiologist.

Summary of Clinical Significance

1. Failure to perform symptom-limited, maximum exercise tests may mask the patient with abnormal HR responses.

2. A slow HR at rest and a slow HR response to exercise does not always signify a good state of fitness.

3. Abnormal HR response to exercise may be an ominous sign, predictive of severe CAD.

4. Patients who exhibit an abnormal HR response to exercise should be monitored carefully and medically supervised closely if they are enrolled in a cardiac rehabilitation program.

5. A decrease in HR with an increase in O_2 demand (exercise workload) is associated with potentially serious dysrhythmias and conduction defects and is a contraindication to continued exercise.

Blood Pressure Response

Normal

In normal adult men, BP responses to increasing levels of exertion is not nearly so clearly described as their HR response. Systolic pressure rises with increasing levels of workload, and diastolic pressure either rises slightly (less than 10 mm Hg), remains the same, or drops slightly (less than 10 mm Hg). In healthy individuals who can achieve or exceed their predicted maximum HRs, the systolic pressure may rise steadily during the submaximal workloads and then plateau or even fall at peak exercise. This is not an abnormal finding. Generally, the SBP response to exercise in adult women is less pronounced than that found in men (Figure 6-17).

The primary reason that BP responses are difficult to interpret is that the auscultatory method of obtaining BP during exercise can be unreliable. It requires good clinical skill to obtain any BP readings when someone is exercising on a treadmill or free walking, but reliable readings are difficult to obtain because of the excessive extraneous noise and the arm movement that occurs during an exercise session. At low levels of exercise, it is possible to get fairly reliable and reproducible data, but accurate readings are increasingly difficult at high levels of exercise.[64] An arterial indwelling pressure sensor would be the most accurate means of obtaining BPs, but this is highly impractical to the PT.

SBP rises during exercise because the increase in CO is greater than the decrease in peripheral vascular resistance (Figure 6-18). The normal physiological response to exercise is a dramatic redistribution of blood flow away from the nonworking muscles and organs to the working muscles. With lower extremity exercise in normal adults, this will cause a decrease in overall peripheral vascular resistance. As noted in Chapter 1, the mean arterial pressure (MAP) is the average pressure over a cardiac cycle and is considered

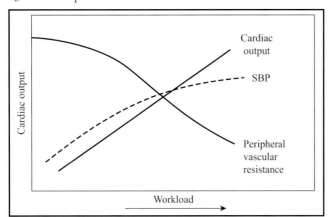

Figure 6-18. Relationship between CO, peripheral vascular resistance, and SBP with increasing levels of exercise.

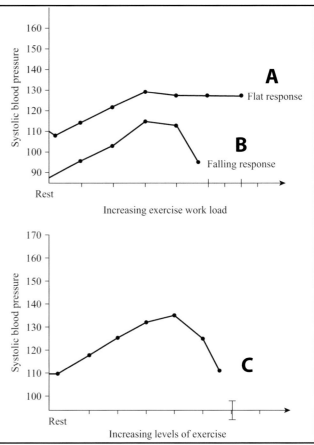

Figure 6-19. (A) Abnormal SBP response to exertion. Flat response. (B) Poor response with an abnormal fall at peak exercise. (C) Abnormal SBP response to exertion. Striking fall in SBP with exercise despite a normal response at submaximal levels of exertion.

to be the perfusion pressure of the organs of the body. MAP is directly proportional to the product of CO and peripheral vascular resistance (MAP = CO × TPR) and, clinically, MAP is estimated by adding the DBP to the pulse pressure (PP = SBP – DBP) in the equations: MAP ∼ DBP + 1/3 (PP). MAP includes the relationship between SBP and DBP, and the clinician should keep this relationship in mind when interpreting BP responses to exercise. In well-conditioned athletes and in younger persons, the DBP may fall precipitously during exercise, creating a wide pulse pressure. This phenomenon is rarely seen with patients or persons over 40 years of age. Additionally, there is no evidence that a drop in DBP with exercise has any relationship to adverse pathological conditions.

Abnormal

Significant abnormalities in BP responses to increasing levels of exertion occur both in SBP and DBP. Both abnormalities often represent the existence of significant pathological conditions and should be recognized, interpreted, and incorporated into each patient's examination and evaluation.

Systolic Abnormality

There are 3 abnormal SBP responses that occur during increasing levels of exertion. The first is the flat response, in which the pressure may rise slightly but fails to continue to rise and remains generally below 140 mm Hg (Figure 6-19A). The second is a response in which the systolic pressure is low to start (less than 110 mm Hg), rises slightly, and then begins to fall despite increases in HR and workload (Figure 6-19B). The third and clinically most common response, especially in patients following an infarction, is a normal submaximal response with a precipitous fall in SBP at higher workloads (Figure 6-19C). This response is often associated with pronounced ST-segment depression, cardiomyopathies, and large infarctions with poor ejection fractions. In order for a fall in SBP with increasing HR to be significant, it must be at least a 20-mm Hg drop. Lesser drops may be clinically significant, but they need to be related to other clinical signs and symptoms (SOB and the development of an S3).

Bruce et al[65] and Ben-Ari et al[66] have found that this response is highly indicative of serious pathological conditions. They found that patients not on medications, with poor SBP responses and peak systolic pressures less than 140 mm Hg, had a much higher incidence of sudden death. In addition, they found that this response was most commonly found in 3 patient groups: those with severe obstructive CAD, which caused pronounced ischemia with exertion but with normal ventricular function; those with cardiomegaly or gross myocardial damage and poor ventricular function; and those with a combination of these 2 conditions.[67]

The abnormal SBP response should not remove a patient for consideration in a cardiac rehabilitation program, but the exercise prescription must be adjusted to accommodate this abnormality. Patients with these responses must be monitored closely.

Mechanisms

When we look at the normal SBP response, it is common to see a person's BP flatten or fall at peak exercise. As noted in Chapter 1, BP = CO × TPR. Theoretically, as HR exceeds 190 bpm, the filling time for the ventricle decreases to a point at which SV actually falls. As SV falls, CO declines (CO = HR × SV), but peripheral vascular resistance continues to fall so that a decrease in systolic pressure results. This normal response provides context to explain the mechanism of abnormal BP responses.

An ischemic ventricle, a ventricle with a large scar, or a failing ventricle will quickly achieve a maximum SV. Normally, during progressive incremental increases in exercise workloads, venous return rises, causing elevation in the end-diastolic volume. In the normal heart, this elevation in volume is met by increased contractility (see Chapter 1, Frank-Starling Reflex section on p 13) with a resultant increase in ejection fraction. On the other hand, patients with severe pathological conditions (ischemia, large infarcts, heart failure) are not able to increase contractility. SV does not increase and in fact may fall. A decreasing SV limits increases in CO. Because systolic pressure is a result of the relationship between CO and peripheral vascular resistance, an abnormal CO response with a normal fall in peripheral vascular resistance during exercise may cause a fall in SBP.[65,67,68]

A fall in systolic pressure is often associated with additional signs and symptoms of inadequate CO, including SOB, deep ST-segment depression or elevation, angina, and pallor. After exercise, patients may exhibit an S3. Care should be taken not to overinterpret a flat or falling systolic response in middle-aged women or a patient on antihypertensive or beta-blocking medications. These patients may exhibit this response, but unless there are additional signs or symptoms, it may not be significant.

The clinician should be sure that the BP fall occurs with an increase in workload. It is normal for SBP to flatten and fall with prolonged (30 to 45 minutes) bouts of exercise at the same workload (Figure 6-20). This should not be considered an abnormal response. The decline in SBP is explained by the decline in peripheral resistance as a result of an increase in body temperature. Blood flow has been redistributed to the skin to assist in maintaining or lowering the core temperature, and this has caused a further decline in peripheral vascular resistance with little or no increase in CO.

Summary of Clinical Significance

1. Abnormal SBP responses are exhibited by patients with severe ischemia, poor ventricular function, or a combination of these pathological conditions.

2. This abnormality is commonly associated with other significant signs and symptoms including angina, SOB, pallor, and S3s.

3. Patients who demonstrate falling SBP have higher annual morbidity and mortality rates than those with normal BP responses.

4. An abnormal SBP response with accompanying signs and symptoms is a clinical indication to discontinue exercise and contact the referring physician.

5. These patients can still undergo exercise conditioning, but must be closely monitored for signs of ventricular dysfunction and the advent of serious dysrhythmias.

Diastolic Abnormalities

The second, less commonly cited, abnormal BP response is a persistent rise in diastolic pressure with increases in

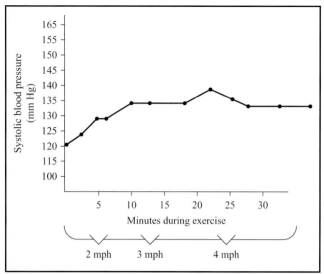

Figure 6-20. Normal flattening of SBP due to prolonged exercise at the same workload.

exercise workloads. The normal DBP response to exercise is to have DBP fall slightly (10 to 20 mm Hg) in younger persons or to rise slightly, fall slightly, or remain the same in older persons.[69,70]

A common sequel to a progressive rise in diastolic pressure with exercise is for the diastolic pressure to remain elevated several minutes after exercise. There is no literature that describes the significance of this finding, but in the author's clinical experience it is an abnormal finding. An abnormal DBP response occurs when the diastolic pressure rises 15 to 20 mm Hg or more above 90 mm Hg with increasing levels of exercise. A patient's actual abnormal response and the generally accepted normal response are depicted in Figure 6-21. Patients who exhibit this response may have CAD even in the absence of ST-segment changes.[71]

Mechanisms

The cause or causes for progressive DBP responses to exercise are open to speculation, and humoral, neurological, or hemodynamic factors could be the cause. It is of interest, though, to speculate that patients exhibiting the progressive diastolic response to exercise may have a reflex mechanism that senses a need for increased coronary blood flow. This as yet unidentified mechanism may exert an influence on the peripheral vascular tree to increase diastolic pressures and thereby cause an increase in coronary artery driving pressure. The cause or causes may also be simple coincidence. Patients with severe coronary disease generally have some additional peripheral vascular disease, which can dramatically affect systolic and diastolic pressures.

Again, a rise in progressive diastolic pressure with exercise is a clinical sign that adds to each patient's data base and should be recognized and incorporated into exercise test interpretations and individualized exercise training programs. If the diastolic pressure rises more than 20 mm Hg above 90 during increasing levels of exercise, the exercise should be terminated and the patient's physician notified.

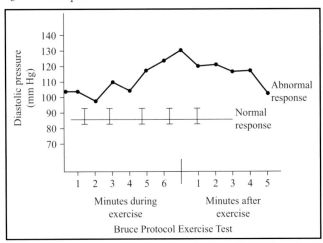

Figure 6-21. Abnormal DBP response to the Bruce Protocol maximum symptom-limited exercise test. Patient E was a 47-year-old man who completed 7 minutes and was limited by leg fatigue and SOB. Resting BP standing was 176/104 mm Hg, and maximum BP was 246/126 mm Hg. He exhibited 2 mm of ST-segment depression in 4 leads and mild angina 4 minutes after exercise. He had frequent multifocal PVCs throughout the test and an S4 after exercise.

Summary of Clinical Significance

1. A progressive rise in DBP with exercise may indicate severe CAD.
2. The rise should be at least 20 mm Hg or more above 90 mm Hg and persist after exercise testing or training.

Angina

Angina is classically described as a chest discomfort caused by an impaired blood supply (ischemia) to cardiac muscle. This impairment results in an imbalance between MO_2 supply and demand. It is a well documented finding that a patient's threshold for angina is roughly equivalent to a fixed, clinically measurable product of his or her HR multiplied by his or her SBP, the rate pressure product, and is linearly correlated with MO_2 demand.[23,58,72] Angina that recurs at a fixed rate-pressure product is referred to as *chronic stable angina*. There are 2 other types of angina: unstable and variant. Variant angina, also called *Prinzmetal's angina*, is caused from vasospasm of a coronary artery. Variant angina can occur any time and may lead to infarction, but it is not common and is usually treated with vasodilating medications. Unstable angina is angina that occurs at rest or wakes a patient during the night. This form of angina is also referred to as *preinfarction angina* and is an ominous symptom of impending myocardial damage. Chronic stable angina that begins to occur at lower and lower rate-pressure products may also be considered unstable angina.

Chronic stable angina may be defined as any discomfort that occurs above the waist that is reproduced by eating, emotional distress, or exercise and relieved by rest or nitroglycerin. Patient descriptions of chronic stable angina is variable. Descriptions include but are not limited to tightness, burning, pressure, aching, hurting, soreness, difficulty taking a deep breath, squeezing, and "I can't really describe it." Most patients do not use the word *pain* when describing their angina. They may use it when describing the discomfort associated with an MI, but they rarely use the word *pain* when describing the discomfort associated with activity. Although this symptom is most often associated with the chest in male patients, in female patients, the anatomical site for the discomfort can vary widely. Typical distribution patterns for the discomfort are depicted in Figure 6-22.

Any clinician working with patients with known heart disease should attempt to determine if they have or have had angina. Once this has been determined, the clinician should only refer to that patient's angina using the word(s) he or she used to describe his or her symptom. The patient will not respond or understand your requests to tell him or her about any anginal symptoms if you use words that do not describe his or her angina. This can be critical when exercise training patients or when initially getting patients up early after their MIs or bypass surgery.

It is also important to help the patient differentiate non-anginal pains from angina of cardiac origin. Chest, jaw, and shoulder discomforts occur for a multitude of reasons. Potential causes of noncardiac chest pain include but are not limited to costochondritis, pleurisy, gall bladder dysfunction, cervical impingements, and dental diseases. These noncardiac causes of chest pain are not reproducible with exercise, eating, or emotional distress and are not relieved by nitroglycerin. Many patients who are early postinfarction, angioplasty, or bypass surgery may not clearly understand their angina, but a clear explanation of differences between angina and other chest wall pains will assist the patient in better defining and living with their symptoms. From this point on, anyone working with the patient should use the term *aching* when asking about the patient having any symptoms, especially with increasing levels of exercise.

Although angina is a common symptom of people with heart disease, it is not always so easy to determine if your patient is having this symptom. Careful review of the patient's prior history with close attention to the description of his or her symptoms is helpful. Remember that angina does not always present itself as a discomfort in the chest and most patients do not describe it as a pain (see Figure 6-22).

Angina Threshold

Many current practitioners have found that patients with chronic stable angina can improve their exercise tolerance and maximum pre-angina working capacity, but patients with angina are unable to exceed their angina threshold or rate-pressure product.

One of the more rewarding clinical improvements is when a patient exceeds his or her angina threshold. Through careful screening and monitored exercise training, some patients can raise their angina threshold and rate-pressure product before experiencing angina. There is even a small percentage of patients who actually eliminate their angina completely. Those who are capable of increasing or eliminating their angina threshold commonly have the following characteristics:

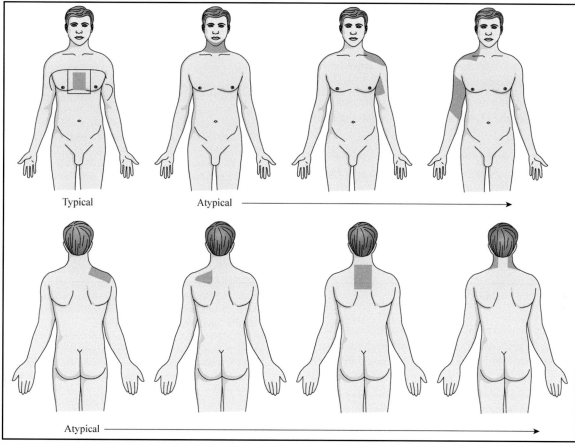

Figure 6-22. Typical and atypical anginal patterns.

- Inoperable CAD or patients who refuse surgery
- Highly motivated and compliant with their exercise program, diet, and risk factor modification
- Chronic, stable angina
- Capable of walking through their angina within the first 3 months of their training program

Walk-through angina is angina that occurs during a training session at a specific workload but gradually diminishes and finally goes away despite the fact that the workload is the same or even slightly higher. This is not recommended unless there is approval by the physicians and the patients have a clear understanding of their angina symptom. It is common for patients with chronic stable angina to experience angina when they begin their exercise training program. With careful instruction and monitoring, they should learn to train at a level that is just below their angina threshold. The time to onset of angina can be lengthened by having the patient prolong their warm-up time. As the training program progresses and the patient's exercise intensity and tolerance improves, they may begin to experience walk-through angina.

Increasing or eliminating angina thresholds in patients with CAD is not a quick process. It often takes 12 to 24 months of training and must be combined with risk factor modification, including but not limited to lowering BP, decreasing cholesterol levels, and eliminating smoking.

Mechanisms

As with the other abnormal findings, it is difficult to explain how a person's angina threshold can be increased or eliminated. These patients still exhibit ST-segment depression at the same rate-pressure product as they did before their exercise training program, and the depth of the depression is unchanged. This indicates that ischemia may still be present, but the discomfort that previously accompanied it is gone.

Although unproven, there are numerous potential explanations for the occurrence of this phenomenon, including the following:

- Increased oxidative enzymes in the heart muscle
- Improved coronary blood flow through the development of collateral arteries[73,74]
- Accommodation of the pain stimulus created by the ischemia via the central nervous system
- Decreased atherosclerotic load and improved stability of coronary artery smooth muscle[73]

Regardless of the cause for increasing or eliminating angina thresholds, the therapist conducting a cardiac rehabilitation program for patients with reproducible angina thresholds should consider this threshold as a symptom that can be successfully treated and, in some cases, eliminated completely with proper exercise conditioning and risk factor modification.

Summary of Clinical Significance

1. Angina symptoms are best described by the patient.

2. The therapist should carefully determine the patients with angina and use their terminology when asking them about their symptoms.

3. Descriptions of angina are as varied as individuals and may not follow the classic descriptions depicted in the media.

4. Angina may be successfully treated by exercise training.

5. Angina threshold measured by multiplication of the HR and SBP is not a fixed value.

6. Further research into the mechanisms of elimination of angina in humans through exercise training is necessary.

SUMMARY

Patients with cardiovascular pump dysfunction or failure encompass the largest cohort of individuals in the American health care system. The application of the basic principles of monitoring (HR, BP, ECG, symptoms, and heart sounds) will provide the rehabilitation professional with the objective measures required to develop safe, effective and individualized exercise interventions. To ensure the ability to achieve the patient and program goals, a thorough understanding of the physiological effects of ischemia, medications, dysrhythmia, and bed rest on cardiovascular function is required.

REFERENCES

1. Proudfit WL, Bruschke AV, Sones FM Jr. Natural history of obstructive coronary artery disease: ten-year study of 601 nonsurgical cases. *Prog Cardiovasc Dis*. 1978;21(1):53-78.

2. Roger VL, Go AS, Lloyd DM, et al. Heart disease and stroke statistics--2011 update: a report from the American Heart Association. *Circulation*. 2011;123(4):e18-e209.

3. American Heart Association. *2002 Heart and Stroke Statistical Update*. Dallas, TX: American Heart Association; 2001.

4. Wenger NK, Froelicher ES, Smith LK, et al. Cardiac rehabilitation as secondary prevention. Agency for Health Care Policy and Research and National Heart, Lung, and Blood Institute. *Clin Pract Guidel Quick Ref Guide Clin*. 1995;(17):1-23.

5. Jessup M, Brozena S. Heart failure. *N Engl J Med*. 2003;348(20):2007-2018.

6. Enos WF, Holmes RH, Beyer J. Coronary artery disease among United States soldiers killed in action in Korea: preliminary report. *JAMA*. 1953;152(12):1090-1093.

7. McNamara JJ, Molot MA, Stremple JF, Cutting RT. Coronary artery disease in combat casualties in Vietnam. *JAMA*. 1971;216(7):1185-1187.

8. National Heart, Lung, and Blood Institute. *Morbidity and Mortality: 1996 Chartbook on Cardiovascular, Lung and Blood Diseases*. Bethesda, MD: US Department of Health & Human Services, National Institutes of Health; 1996.

9. Conley MJ, Ely RL, Kisslo J, Lee KL, McNeer JF, Rosati RA. The prognostic spectrum of left main stenosis. *Circulation*. 1978;57(5):947-952.

10. Haim M, Hod H, Reisin L, et al. Comparison of short- and long-term prognosis in patients with anterior wall versus inferior or lateral wall non-Q-wave acute myocardial infarction. Secondary Prevention Reinfarction Israeli Nifedipine Trial (SPRINT) Study Group. *Am J Cardiol*. 1997;79(6):717-721.

11. Cahalin LP, Mathier MA, Semigran MJ, Dec GW, DiSalvo TG. The six-minute walk test predicts peak oxygen uptake and survival in patients with advanced heart failure. *Chest*. 1996;110(2):325-332.

12. Salel AF, Fong A, Zelis BS, Miller RR, Borhani NO, Mason DT. Accuracy of numerical coronary profile. Correlation of risk factors with arteriographically documented severity of atherosclerosis. *N Engl J Med*. 1977;296(25):1447-1450.

13. Libby P. Coronary artery injury and the biology of atherosclerosis: inflammation, thrombosis, and stabilization. *Am J Cardiol*. 2000;86(8B):3J-8J; discussion 8J-9J.

14. Smith JK. Exercise and atherogenesis. *Exerc Sport Sci Rev*. 2001;29(2):49-53.

15. Braunwald E. *Heart Disease: A Textbook of Cardiovascular Medicine*. 5th ed. Philadelphia, PA: WB Saunders Company; 1997.

16. Astrup P, Kjeldsen K, Wanstrup J. Enhancing influence of carbon monoxide on the development of atheromatosis in cholesterol-fed rabbits. *J Atheroscler Res*. 1967;7(3):343-354.

17. Barth JD. Which tools are in your cardiac workshop? Carotid ultrasound, endothelial function, and magnetic resonance imaging. *Am J Cardiol*. 2001;87(4A):8A-14A.

18. Ross R, Glomset JA. The pathogenesis of atherosclerosis (first of two parts). *N Engl J Med*. 1976;295(7):369-377.

19. Lam JY, Latour JG, Lespérance J, Waters D. Platelet aggregation, coronary artery disease progression and future coronary events. *Am J Cardiol*. 1994;73(5):333-338.

20. Sullivan JM, Heinle RA, Gorlin R. Studies of platelet adhesiveness, glucose tolerance and serum lipoprotein patterns in patients with coronary artery disease. *Am J Med Sci*. 1972;264(6):432-513.

21. Ross R. The pathogenesis of atherosclerosis. In: Santamore WP, Boe A, eds. *Coronary Artery Disease*. Baltimore, MD: Urban & Schwarzenberg; 1982.

22. West of Scotland Coronary Prevention Study Group. The baseline risk factors and their association with outcome in the West of Scotland Coronary Prevention Study. *Am J Cardiol*. 1997;79(6):756-762.

23. Ellestad MH. Physiology of cardiac ischemia. In: *Stress Testing*. 3rd ed. Philadelphia, PA: FA Davis; 1986.

24. Duncker DJ, Bache RJ. Regulation of coronary blood flow during exercise. *Physiol Rev*. 2008;88(3):1009-1086.

25. Guyton AC, Hall JE. *Textbook of Medical Physiology*. Philadelphia, PA: WB Saunders Company; 2000.

26. Shimizu S, Bowman PS, Thorne G 3rd, Paul RJ. Effects of hypoxia on isometric force, intracellular Ca(2+), pH, and energetics in porcine coronary artery. *Circ Res*. 2000;86(8):862-870.

27. Logan SE. On the fluid mechanics of human coronary artery stenosis. *IEEE Trans Biomed Eng*. 1975;22(4):327-334.

28. Freedman B, Richmond DR, Kelly DT. Pathophysiology of coronary artery spasm. *Circulation*. 1982;66:705-709.

29. Maseri A. Coronary artery spasm and atherosclerosis. In: Santamore WP, Boe A, eds. *Coronary Artery Disease*. Baltimore, MD: Urban & Schwarzenberg; 1982.

30. Franklin BA, Bonzheim K, Gordon S, Timmis GC. Snow shoveling: a trigger for acute myocardial infarction and sudden coronary death. *Am J Cardiol*. 1996;77(10):855-858.

31. Porth CM. *Pathophysiology*. 6th ed. Philadelphia, PA: Lippincott Williams & Wilkins; 2002.

32. Saw J, Davies C, Fung A, Spinelli JJ, Jue J. Value of ST elevation in lead III greater than lead II in inferior wall acute myocardial infarction for predicting in-hospital mortality and diagnosing right ventricular infarction. *Am J Cardiol*. 2001;87(4):448-540, A6.

33. Franklin BA, Kohn JK. Delayed progression or regression of coronary atherosclerosis with intensive risk factor modification. Effects of diet, drugs, and exercise. *Sports Med*. 1996;22(5):306-320.

34. Beckett NS, Peters R, Fletcher AE et al. Treatment of hypertension in patients 80 years of age or older. *N Engl J Med*. 2008;358:1887-1898.

35. Rydén L, Standl E, Bartnik M, et al. Guidelines on diabetes, pre-diabetes, and cardiovascular diseases: executive summary. The Task Force on Diabetes and Cardiovascular Diseases of the European Society of Cardiology (ESC) and of the European Association for the Study of Diabetes (EASD). *Eur Heart J*. 2007;28(1):88-136.

36. Frick MH1, Elo O, Haapa K, et al. Helsinki Heart Study: primary-prevention trial with gemfibrozil in middle-aged men with dyslipidemia. Safety of treatment, changes in risk factors, and incidence of coronary heart disease. *N Engl J Med*. 1987;317(20):1237-1245.

37. Nissen ST. Effect of intensive lipid lowering on progression of coronary atherosclerosis: evidence for an early benefit from the Reversal of Atherosclerosis with Aggressive Lipid Lowering (REVERSAL) trial. *Am J Cardiol*. 2005;96(5A):61F-68F.

38. Deedwania P, Stone PH, Bairey Merz CN, et al. Effects of intensive versus moderate lipid-lowering therapy on myocardial ischemia in older patients with coronary heart disease: results of the Study Assessing Goals in the Elderly (SAGE). *Circulation*. 2007;115(6):700-707. Epub 2007 Feb 5.

39. Armstrong ML, Megan MB. Lipid depletion in atheromatous coronary arteries in rhesus monkeys after regression diets. *Circ Res*. 1972;30(6):675-680.

40. Armstrong ML, Warner ED, Connor WE. Regression of coronary atheromatosis in rhesus monkeys. *Circ Res*. 1970;27:59.

41. Arntzenius AC, Kromhout D, Barth JD, et al. Diet, lipoproteins, and the progression of coronary atherosclerosis. The Leiden Intervention Trial. *N Engl J Med*. 1985;312(13):805-811.

42. Nikkilä EA, Viikinkoski P, Valle M, Frick MH. Prevention of progression of coronary atherosclerosis by treatment of hyperlipidaemia: a seven year prospective angiographic study. *Br Med J (Clin Res Ed)*. 1984;289(6439):220-223.

43. Blankenhorn DH, Kramsch DM. Reversal of atherosis and sclerosis. The two components of atherosclerosis. *Circulation*. 1989;79(1):1-7.

44. Blankenhorn DH, Nessim SA, Johnson RL, et al. Beneficial effects of combined colestipol-niacin therapy on coronary atherosclerosis and coronary venous bypass grafts. *JAMA*. 1987;257(23):3233-3240.

45. Kramsch DM, Aspen AJ, Abramowitz BM, Kreimendahl T, Hood WB Jr. Reduction of coronary atherosclerosis by moderate conditioning exercise in monkeys on an atherogenic diet. *N Engl J Med*. 1981;305(25):1483-1489.

46. Brener SJ, Pashkow FJ, Harvey SA, Marwick TH, Thomas JD, Lauer MS. Chronotropic response to exercise predicts angiographic severity in patients with suspected or stable coronary artery disease. *Am J Cardiol*. 1995;76(17):1228-1232.

47. Wilson PW. An epidemiologic perspective of systemic hypertension, ischemic heart disease, and heart failure. *Am J Cardiol*. 1997;80:3J-8J.

48. Perloff JK. *Physical Examination of the Heart and Circulation*. 3rd Edition. Philadelphia, PA: WB Saunders Company; 2000.

49. Sullivan MJ, Knight JD, Higginbotham, Cobb FR. Relation between central and peripheral hemodynamics during exercise in patients with chronic heart failure. Muscle blood flow is reduced with maintenance of arterial perfusion pressure. *Circulation*. 1989;80:769-781.

50. Sullivan MJ, Green HJ, Cobb FR. Skeletal muscle biochemistry and histology in ambulatory patients with long-term heart failure. *Circulation*. 1990;81:518-527.

51. Massie BM, Simonini A, Sahgal P, Wells L, Dudley GA. Relation of systemic and local muscle exercise capacity to skeletal muscle characteristics in men with congestive heart failure. *J Am Coll Cardiol*. 1996;27(1):140-145.

52. Walsh JT, Andrews R, Johnson P, Phillips L, Cowley AJ, Kinnear WJ. Inspiratory muscle endurance in patients with chronic heart failure. *Heart*. 1996;76(4):332-336.

53. Meyer FJ, Borst MM, Zugck C, et al. Respiratory muscle dysfunction in congestive heart failure: clinical correlation and prognostic significance. *Circulation*. 2001;103(17):2153-2158.

54. Buller NP, Poole-Wilson PA. Mechanism of the increased ventilatory response to exercise in patients with chronic heart failure. *Br Heart J*. 1990;63(5):281-283.

55. Davis PH, Dawson JD, Riley WA, Lauer RM. Carotid intimal-medial thickness is related to cardiovascular risk factors measured from childhood through middle age: the Muscatine Study. *Circulation*. 2001;104(23):2815-2819.

56. Berenson GS; Bogalusa Heart Study Investigators. Bogalusa Heart Study: a long-term community study of a rural biracial (Black/White) population. *Am J Med Sci*. 2001;322(5):293-300.

57. Milani RV, Lavie CJ, Cassidy MM. Effects of cardiac rehabilitation and exercise training programs on depression in patients after major coronary events. *Am Heart J*. 1996;132:726-732.

58. Kitamura K, Jorgensen CR, Gobel FL, Taylor HL, Wang Y. Hemodynamic correlates of myocardial oxygen consumption during upright exercise. *J Appl Physiol*. 1972;32(4):516-522.

59. Gillum RF. Epidemiology of resting pulse rate of persons ages 25-74—data from NHANES 1971-74. *Public Health Rep*. 1992;107(2):193-201.

60. Tanaka H, Monahan KD, Seals DR. Age-predicted maximal heart rate revisited. *J Am Coll Cardiol*. 2001;37(1):153-156.

61. Ellestad MH. Chronotropic incompetence. The implications of heart rate response to exercise (compensatory parasympathetic hyperactivity?). *Circulation*. 1996;93(8):1485-1487.

62. Miller TD, Gibbons RJ, Squires RW, Allison TG, Gau GT. Sinus node deceleration during exercise as a marker of significant narrowing of the right coronary artery. *Am J Cardiol*. 1993;71(4):371-373.

63. Lauer MS, Francis GS, Okin PM, Pashkow FJ, Snader CE, Marwick TH. Impaired chronotropic response to exercise stress testing as a predictor of mortality. *JAMA*. 1999;281(6):524-529.

64. Nagle FJ, Naughton J, Balke B. Comparisons of direct and indirect blood pressure with pressure-flow dynamics during exercise. *J Appl Physiol*. 1966;21:317-320.

65. Bruce RA, T DeRouen, Peterson DR. Noninvasive predictors of sudden cardiac death in men with coronary heart disease: predictive value of maximal stress testing. *Am J Cardiol*. 1977;39(6):833-840.

66. Ben-Ari E, Fisman EZ, Pines A, Dlin R, Kessler G, Kellermann JJ. Significance of exertional hypotension in apparently healthy men: an 8.9-year follow-up. *J Cardiopulm Rehab*. 10:92, 1990.

67. Iskandrian AS, Kegel JG, Lemlek J, Heo J, Cave V, Iskandrian B. Mechanism of exercise-induced hypotension in coronary artery disease. *Am J Cardiol*. 1992;69(19):1517-1520.

68. Mazzotta G, Scopinaro G, Falcidieno M, et al. Significance of abnormal blood pressure response during exercise-induced myocardial dysfunction after recent acute myocardial infarction. *Am J Cardiol*. 1987;59(15):1256-1260.

69. Myers JN. The physiology behind exercise testing. *Prim Care*. 1994;21(3):415-437.

70. Berne R, Levy M. *Physiology*. 4th ed. St. Louis, MO: Mosby; 1998.

71. Sheps DS, Ernst JC, Briese FW, Myerburg RJ. Exercise-induced increase in diastolic pressure: Indicator of severe coronary artery disease. *Am J Cardiol*. 1979;43(4):708-712.

72. Go BM, Sheffield D, Krittayaphong R, Maixner W, Sheps DS. Association of systolic blood pressure at time of myocardial ischemia with angina pectoris during exercise testing. *Am J Cardiol*. 1997;79(7):954-956.

73. Niebauer J, Hambrecht R, Marburger C, et al. Impact of intensive physical exercise and low-fat diet on collateral vessel formation in stable angina pectoris and angiographically confirmed coronary artery disease. *Am J Cardiol*. 1995;76(11):771-775.

74. Schwarz F, Schaper J, Becker V, Kübler W, Flameng W. Coronary collateral vessels: their significance for left ventricular histologic structure. *Am J Cardiol*. 1982;49(2):291-295.

CASE STUDY 6-1

Scot Irwin, PT, DPT, CCS

EXAMINATION

History

Current Condition/Chief Complaint

Ms. Damask was a 68-year-old Black female referred to physical therapy for a functional assessment shortly after transferring from the coronary care unit (CCU) to the CCU step-down unit. She had been admitted to the CCU via the emergency room with the diagnosis of an acute anteroseptal MI 5 days prior to the referral to physical therapy. It was anticipated that she would be discharged from the hospital in 2 days.

History of Current Complaint

On the day of her admission, Ms. Damask reported she was performing her normal housework when she felt a dull "pressure-like" discomfort in her jaw and neck. She noted that the discomfort did not abate when she rested. Over the next 10 to 30 minutes, the discomfort worsened and she noticed that she was getting sweaty and nauseated. She called the local hospital and an emergency team was sent to her home. The patient did not remember anything else until she woke up in the CCU at the local general hospital.

The emergency medical technician's notes indicated that the patient was found unconscious but breathing with a very fast irregular pulse of 116 bpm. Her SBP could not be measured by auscultation but was 66 mm Hg by palpation. She was attached to a portable ECG monitor and appropriate emergency procedures were implemented. She was transported to the hospital emergency room.

Upon arrival at the emergency room, she was in atrial fibrillation with a pulse of 108 bpm. She had multifocal premature ventricular dysrhythmias with occasional runs of ventricular tachycardia. She had signs of LV failure, including crackles in her lung bases, and S3 and mild SOB at rest. She had positive troponin levels that indicated a large infarction. Ms. Damask was diagnosed with an acute anteroseptal MI. Thrombolytic therapy was considered but the attending physician thought that she was outside the time frame for optimal results. She was admitted to the CCU.

On her second day postinfarction, the patient underwent cardiac catheterization with the following findings: extensive CAD involving the proximal right coronary artery (70% occluded), LAD (100% occluded just distal to the first septal perforator and some minor plaque formation distally), and the circumflex artery (50% occluded).

Ms. Damask's ejection fraction was 32%. Her LV end-diastolic pressure was 18 mm Hg. Her initial chest x-ray showed mild cardiomegaly with some signs of pulmonary edema.

Clinician Comment *What is known about Ms. Damask and her medical status thus far? Ms. Damask is female and women have lower mortality rates following admission with heart failure than men.[1] Her CAD involved multiple vessels and especially her LAD coronary artery, which provides blood to the anterior and septal portions of the LV. In the CCU, she initially had prolonged episodes of both angina and heart failure, which defined her cardiac condition as "complicated." Because of the area and size of the infarction, she was at a high risk for failure and life-threatening ventricular dysrhythmia.*

A review of the patient's medical record and the therapist's interview provided the following additional historical information.

Social History/Environment

Ms. Damask reported that she lived alone in her 2-story home. Her bedroom was on the second floor. She had been widowed 6 years prior; her husband died from a heart attack when he was in his late 50s. Ms. Damask had been a full-time homemaker for her entire adult life. She had 2 cats and 1 dog. Ms. Damask was active in her church and had several female friends in her neighborhood.

Her 2 adult daughters lived nearby. Both daughters were married, had children, and worked outside the home. Her 4 grandchildren were of various ages. She helped her daughters by providing day care for the 2 youngest grandchildren as well as afternoon care for the older children.

Social/Health Habits

Ms. Damask reported that she had been in great health all of her life and her 2 daughters confirmed this. The patient had never smoked, but her husband smoked 2 packs per day for their entire married life of 38 years. She reported that she had never followed a regular exercise program. Ms. Damask appeared to be overweight.

Medical/Surgical History

Until this admission, her medical history was unremarkable except for 2 normal pregnancies, a hysterectomy in her early 50s, and hypertension. She was diagnosed with hypertension on a routine physical when she was 40 years old and had been treated with a variety of medications over the last 18 years. These medications included diuretics, beta-blockers, and, most recently, an ACE inhibitor. Her BP had been well controlled over the prior year with the ACE inhibitor.

Ms. Damask reported that her mother and father died from heart failure.

Clinician Comment *Though she reported great health, Ms. Damask had several risk factors for CAD. She had a 38-year history of secondhand smoke, an 18-year history of hypertension, and a family history of heart disease. She did not exercise regularly and appeared overweight.*

Reported Functional Status

Ms. Damask reported she was fearful of attempting any activity. She reported she had not been out of bed since she was admitted to the hospital. While in the hospital, she had been using a bedpan for toileting. The nursing staff had been performing most of her daily hygiene.

Prior to her admission, she was independent with all ADL and IADL. Her daughters confirmed that she was managing well on her own. All were hopeful that she could return to her prior level of function. Ms. Damask reported that she enjoyed caring for her grandchildren, though she was concerned that she would not be able to do so anymore.

She would like to be discharged to her home. If discharged to home, she would need to be able to climb the stairs to her bedroom. Each daughter expressed willingness to have her convalesce at one of their homes, but it was not clear if either had a ground floor bedroom to offer her.

Clinician Comment *Ms. Damask expressed fear of activity and concern that she might not be able to continue to care for her grandchildren. Fear is a very typical early postinfarction response, especially when the patient has experienced a near-death experience. A primary benefit of early safe mobilization for Ms. Damask, along with education for her and her family, would be to prevent her from becoming psychologically crippled by her fear of her disease.*

To return to her previous normal daily activities, she would need to acquire an exercise tolerance of about 4 to 5 METs, including at least one trip up and down a flight of stairs in a day.

Medications

In the CCU step-down unit, Ms. Damask's medications were a beta-blocker, digitalis, diuretic, ACE inhibitor, and aspirin. The patient's ventricular dysrhythmia and atrial fibrillation had not returned since cardioversion and the administration of the beta-blocker.

Clinician Comment *Ms. Damask was taking medications that relieved her signs and symptoms of acute congestive failure, namely the digitalis and the diuretic. She was taking a low-dose beta-blocker, which has been found to reduce the risk of life-threatening dysrhythmias for patients in heart failure.[2] Beta-blockers are also prescribed to most patients following an MI because they reduce mortality and morbidity.[3]*

Other Clinical Tests

The review of the medical record revealed that the latest chest radiograph showed the pulmonary edema had resolved but the cardiomegaly remained. Her initially raised troponin levels had returned to a normal level. Her glucose levels were mildly elevated at 136 mg/dL. Her hematocrit and hemoglobin were within normal ranges. Elevated cholesterol and triglycerides were recorded with no apparent treatment for the high cholesterol.

She still had occasional ventricular ectopy at rest with some couplets, but no runs of ventricular tachycardia. She had no overt signs of heart failure, but the cardiologist's examination continued to detect an S3 with a mild systolic murmur (I/VI) in the midclavicular line. No reports of angina had been recorded for the 24 hours prior to the physical therapy referral.

Clinician Comment *Since her hemoglobin and hematocrit were within normal limits, Ms. Damask could be expected to have adequate O$_2$ carrying capacity for activity. What was not yet known was whether she would be able to show adequate SV for activity without a compensatory rapid rise in her HR or develop dysrhythmia.*

Cardiomegaly by chest X-ray is an ominous finding. Cardiomegaly is defined as the patient's cardiac silhouette being greater than half the width of her chest cavity. Usually, the heart's dimension is less than half the width of the chest, and this degree of change in heart size is strongly associated with long-standing hypertension as one potential cause of Ms. Damask's heart failure.

The system review was next and would help determine if Ms. Damask was a candidate for physical therapy. She had multi-vessel CAD. Though she had not had angina for the 24 hours prior to the physical therapy referral, her specific descriptors for her angina symptoms needed to be identified. As well, she needed to be guided to report the reappearance of the symptoms if any occurred during the therapy session.

She had a moderate to poor ejection fraction. The ejection fraction is a strong predictor of mortality and morbidity. It is inversely related with the incidence of systolic heart failure—the lower the ejection fraction, the higher the risk of failure. This meant that the therapist should be closely monitoring Ms. Damask's breath sounds and SBP during any exercise activities. Before activity could be considered, however, Ms. Damask's breath sounds needed to be evaluated and found absent of pulmonary edema signs (crackles).

Systems Review

Cardiovascular/Pulmonary

HR: 60 bpm
She had a loud S3 gallop
Resting BP: 116/76 mm Hg
Her lungs were clear but her breath sounds were distant.
Edema: No evidence of peripheral edema

Integumentary

Her skin was clear and intact.

Musculoskeletal

Gross symmetry/posture: She was able to sit at the side of her bed with symmetrical and nearly erect posture

Gross range of motion: Extremities and trunk showed full and symmetrical movements with no report of pain.

Gross strength: Normal, in bilateral upper and lower extremities and trunk, and without apparent impairment

Height: Her medical record indicated she was 5'4"

Weight: 170 pounds, also from the medical record

Neuromuscular

Balance: No difficulty with sitting balance

Locomotion: Not attempted in systems review

Transfers: Not attempted in systems review

Transitions: No impairment or difficulty with bed mobility

Communication, Affect, Cognition, Language, and Learning Style

Ms. Damask was alert, cooperative, and oriented. She was able to report most of her medical history with modest supplementation by her daughters. She reported no chest pain or the previously noted presenting symptoms of pressure in her neck and jaw.

Ms. Damask was initially fearful about sitting up at the side of the bed. She was pleasant and polite, even when expressing her initial misgivings with the suggested activity. She again expressed that she wanted to go home, to her own home. She was concerned, none-the-less, that she might not be able to return to her previous activities.

Clinician Comment *Her resting HR and BP were in acceptable ranges. The S3 is consistent with her history of heart failure. Auscultation of the chest reveals that the pulmonary edema and subsequent crackles have resolved and the distant breath sounds may be due to her obesity or pulmonary changes associated with her long exposure history to secondhand smoke.*

Even though Ms. Damask was cooperative with the bed mobility and sitting activity, her concerns about her status with activity meant she would require reassurance when the examination required higher-intensity activity.

The examining therapist decided to use a low-level activity assessment with self-care items to measure Ms. Damask's aerobic capacity. Items assessed can include, but are not limited to, dressing, hygiene, grooming, and the transfers or short-distance walking required to complete each. A low-level activity assessment is a patient's first exercise test.

A low-level activity assessment can be appropriately performed on patients with a multitude of medical diagnoses, including angioplasty, bypass surgery, stenting, heart transplant, heart valve surgery, and cardiomyopathy. The primary objective—examination of the patient's cardiac responses to increasing levels of activity—remains, regardless of the medical diagnosis. The clinical measurements do not change, with the exception of adding breath sounds and O_2 saturation measurements with pulmonary patients.

Ms. Damask would remain connected to the ECG monitor during the activities providing immediate data on HR and heart rhythm. The evaluating therapist would take and record BP and heart sounds as well as monitor Ms. Damask's verbal and nonverbal reaction to the activities.

It was anticipated that her HR would rise with the increase in activity. As stated previously, the rate at which her HR increased would reflect her heart's ability to adapt to increased activity with increased SV. Although she was on 2 antihypertensive medications (ACE inhibitor and beta-blocker), her SBP could be expected to rise in relation to any elevation in her HR with exercise. If the systolic pressure fell with an increasing HR, however, and she developed SOB, there was a strong probability that the exertion exceeded her heart's ability to maintain CO. These would be signs that she was going into overt heart failure, as would the development of postexercise crackles, indicating pulmonary edema.

The decision whether to include short-distance ambulation would be based on Ms. Damask's tolerance with the initial activities.

Tests and Measures

Aerobic Capacity

Ms. Damask's vital signs were recorded while she was sitting inclined in bed, sitting at the side of the bed, and standing and during ADL activities of dressing, teeth brushing, and walking. The results were as follows:

	HR	BP	ECG	SX	HS
Rest	66	116/76	NSR	none	S3
Sitting	66	104/70	NSR	none	S3
Standing	72	96/66	NSR	dizzy	S3
ADL activity Dressing Teeth brushing	72 to 78	102/70	rare PVC	none	S3
Ambulation 150 feet in 1 min	78 to 84	102/68	6 to 8 PVCs	SOB	S3
HS, heart sounds; NSR, normal sinus rhythm; Sx, symptoms					

Clinician Comment *Ms. Damask had a fairly flat BP response with increasing levels of activity. Her HR increase was a little high considering she was on a beta-blocker. Many patients on beta-blockers during the early postinfarction period may have little or no HR change with activity. The development of SOB with a very slow walking speed was also a concern. This finding, along with the blunted BP response, suggested marked impairment of her cardiac function. The therapist stopped the ambulation because of the increasing dysrhythmia frequency and SOB combined with the patient's recent cardiac event.*

There were 3 possible causes of her SOB:

1. *The exercise exceeded her LV performance ability. The venous return and end-diastolic volume exceeded the pumping ability of the LV and blood started to back up in her lungs (ie, heart failure).*

2. *The SOB was an angina equivalent, and the ventricle, which was experiencing further ischemia in the presence of depressed contractility, resulting in heart failure.*

3. *Her responses were a result of the combination of both of the explanations above, along with the dampening effects of her medications.*

The antihypertensive may be limiting the rise in BP and her HR is accelerating to augment CO and subsequently the BP.

The clinical finding was that Ms. Damask's cardiac impairment was significant enough to limit her walking velocity. Note that the aerobic capacity chart includes not just the distance walked, but also the time it took to cover that distance. Noting the time and distance allows the walking velocity to be calculated. Walking velocity is a functional measure. If Ms. Damask was able to walk 150 feet but it took her 5 minutes to do so, then her walking would not have been functional. She would have been walking at less than 1 mile per hour. She could not cross a street within the usual duration of a walk signal or make it to a bathroom in an adequate amount of time to avoid an accident. In addition, the walking velocity becomes a defined workload against which to measure a patient's response and note changes.

What was the significance of the dysrhythmias with walking for Ms. Damask? An increased frequency of PVCs at any time is a finding that requires documentation and close monitoring. Any time this occurs, it is worthy of written and verbal communication with the patient's nursing and medical staff. If coupling or tripling of PVCs were to occur, then any activity should be immediately terminated and followed up with immediate verbal, and then written, notification of the medical team.

EVALUATION

Diagnosis

Practice Pattern

Based on the patient history, systems review, and measured aerobic capacity, Ms. Damask was classified into Preferred Practice Pattern: Cardiovascular/Pulmonary Practice Pattern 6D: Impaired Aerobic Capacity/Endurance Associated With Cardiovascular Pump Dysfunction or Failure.

International Classification of Functioning, Disability and Health Model of Disability

Please refer to the ICF Model on p 240.

Prognosis

It was anticipated that Ms. Damask would be able to meet goals to prepare her to continue a progressive activity and walking program at home within safe and defined parameters.

Plan of Care

Intervention

Ms. Damask would benefit from an inpatient physical therapy program of monitored ambulation including warm-up movements, ambulation, and cool down. Ms. Damask would be shown, and would practice, self-monitoring skills. A home program of activity would also be identified for her to follow when she is discharged. Ms. Damask and her family would benefit from participation in a series of educational sessions.

PATIENT AND FAMILY EDUCATION TOPICS
Structure and function of the heart
Heart disease and risk factors
Cardiac medications (individual)
Effects of exercise training
Self-monitoring: HR, angina, SOB (perceived exertion)
Dietary considerations (cholesterol, fats, sugar) (Individualized)
Lifestyle adjustments (psychosocial impact of heart disease)
Emergency procedures (CPR course for family members)

Proposed Frequency and Duration of Physical Therapy Visits

Ms. Damask would be seen twice per day until she is discharged from the hospital, anticipated to be in 2 days.

ICF Model of Disablement for Ms. Damask

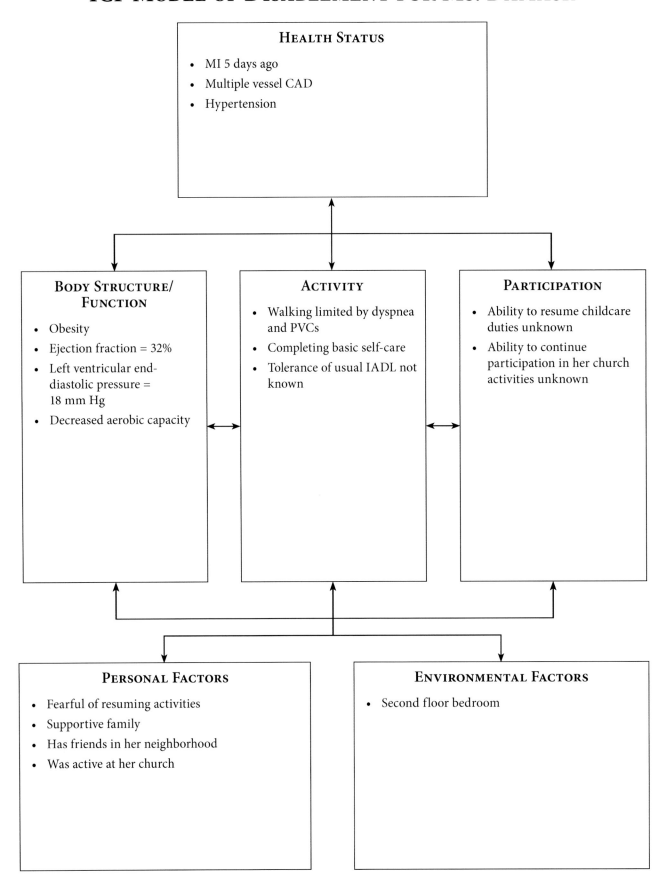

HEALTH STATUS

- MI 5 days ago
- Multiple vessel CAD
- Hypertension

BODY STRUCTURE/ FUNCTION

- Obesity
- Ejection fraction = 32%
- Left ventricular end-diastolic pressure = 18 mm Hg
- Decreased aerobic capacity

ACTIVITY

- Walking limited by dyspnea and PVCs
- Completing basic self-care
- Tolerance of usual IADL not known

PARTICIPATION

- Ability to resume childcare duties unknown
- Ability to continue participation in her church activities unknown

PERSONAL FACTORS

- Fearful of resuming activities
- Supportive family
- Has friends in her neighborhood
- Was active at her church

ENVIRONMENTAL FACTORS

- Second floor bedroom

Anticipated Goals

1. Ms. Damask would be able to identify, and complete, components of a low-intensity exercise program including warm up (easy extremity and trunk movements in sitting), monitored progressive ambulation, and cool down (first follow-up session).

2. She would be able to set an ambulation pace without dyspnea or exceeding 72 to 78 bpm (second session).

3. Ms. Damask would be able to accurately, and independently, count her pulse to identify her HR during a therapy session (third session).

4. Ms. Damask would be able to pace herself to climb up and down a flight of stairs using a standing rest every 2 to 4 steps (fourth session).

5. Ms. Damask would be making progress toward activity tolerance to walk 500 feet in 2 minutes without dyspnea and with an HR up to 72 to 78 bpm.

Expected Outcomes (4 Sessions Over 2 Days)

1. Ms. Damask would be independent in a self-monitoring activity program for home.

Discharge Plan

It was anticipated that Ms. Damask would be able to meet the anticipated goals and expected outcome before her discharge from the hospital in 2 days. Further, it was anticipated that she would be referred to an outpatient cardiac rehabilitation program to begin 2 weeks after discharge.

Clinician Comment *The plan of care is consistent with phase I cardiac rehabilitation. The general goal of phase I rehabilitation is to enable the patient to tolerate ADL, including self-care activities, stair climbing, toileting, and walking functional distances (typically 1 to 5 METs of activity), with minimal to no cardiovascular symptoms and appropriate vital sign responses Since hospital lengths of stay are short, education is of paramount importance, and this is a time to introduce risk factor and behavior modification in addition to a home exercise program. It is well established that risk factor modification and living a more "heart healthy" lifestyle can reduce secondary complications and future coronary events.*

INTERVENTION

Coordination, Communication, and Documentation

The PT evaluating and then treating Ms. Damask would coordinate the planned treatment session with Ms. Damask's hospital schedule and other medical providers. Clear communication with the members of Ms. Damask's medical team and her family regarding the program and progression toward goals will be carried out. Documentation in her medical record would include all aspects of care including initial evaluation, session progress notes, reexaminations, and discharge summary.

Patient-/Client-Related Instruction

Ms. Damask and her family members would be encouraged to attend any of the educational series sessions during Ms. Damask's hospitalization. Continuing cardiac rehabilitation once she is discharged would also be recommended.

Additional individual instruction would be centered on recognizing the signs and symptoms of heart failure. Ankle swelling, nocturnal cough, increased SOB at lower levels of activity, or angina with activity should be noted and reported to Ms. Damask's physician.

One or 2 of her family members would be encouraged to accompany her during at least one ambulation session while she is an inpatient to learn the pacing and self-monitoring techniques Ms. Damask will need to follow on her home program. In addition, Ms. Damask would be instructed to have someone with her during walking sessions once she is home for the first 6 weeks.

Clinician Comment *As noted in the intervention table on p 239, several of the general educational topics require individualization. A group discussion of medications is difficult and not fruitful if a patient is not on the medications discussed. In general, the patient's family will retain far more information than the patient will. It is important to supplement any educational information with booklets, handouts, websites, and video material. All of this information is available from the American Heart Association.*

Procedural Interventions

Therapeutic Exercise

Aerobic Capacity/Endurance Conditioning or Reconditioning

Mode
Monitored progressive walking, inpatient
Intensity
HR should exceed 72 to 78 bpm
Duration
~30-minute physical therapy session
Frequency
2 sessions per day
Description of the Intervention
Ms. Damask's vital signs would be monitored while she completed a routine of warm-up exercises consisting of easy active extremity and trunk movements while seated.

Ambulation in a hallway with marked distances would follow. She would be instructed to walk at a comfortable pace within her tolerance with rests as needed. Vital sign monitoring would continue throughout the session at regular intervals, including 5 minutes and 10 minutes after the activity has ended. Ms. Damask will be shown, and will then practice, self-monitoring of HR, symptoms, and walking pace.

Aerobic Capacity/Endurance Conditioning or Reconditioning

Mode

Self-monitored walking—home program

Intensity

HR only to 72 to 78 bpm, and gradually increase to the pace of 500 feet in 2 minutes

Duration

Short interval of walking, 3 to 5 minutes, after warm-up exercises

Frequency

2 to 3 times per day, 3 to 5 days per week[4-6]

Description of the Intervention

Ms. Damask would be instructed to continue with the identified active movements while seated for a warm-up activity prior to walking. The short interval walking may take place in her home or outside. Once she is able to walk 500 feet in 2 minutes, then she would continue to maintain that velocity for gradually increasing distances.

Clinician Comment *Ms. Damask and her family should understand that more is not necessarily better with her exercise program. Exercising several days in a row may cause secondary joint, back, or leg trauma that will preclude her from exercising on subsequent days. The goals for this part of her rehabilitation would be to learn how to exercise, make exercise a part of her life, and monitor her own signs and symptoms with activity.*

Patient instruction in an unmonitored home exercise program requires that the patient is accurate and reliable in monitoring pulse and symptoms. Preferably, a patient should exercise with someone at all times during the healing phase, defined as discharge to 6 weeks after an infarction. If the patient and family do not appear to be reliable, then a supervised program recommendation is necessary. Transtelephonic monitoring in the home has been shown to be safe with elderly cardiac patients.[7]

Patients should avoid walking up inclines or in poor weather conditions during the healing phase. Either can challenge exercise tolerance. A solution may be to walk indoors at a mall, gym, or home.

HR, on a self-monitored home program, should not exceed the baseline established with the low-level activity assessment for any activities. If the patient notices that he or she is getting short of breath with any activity, that activity should be curtailed or the intensity should be decreased to a level where he or she is not short of breath. The duration of ambulation should be progressively increased from 2 minutes until the patient can ambulate continuously without symptoms, at an HR of 72 to 78 bpm or less for 20 minutes. Work toward increasing duration before any changes in intensity.[6,8,9]

HOSPITAL DISCHARGE

The results from the low-level activity assessment were documented in Ms. Damask's medical record and brought to the attention of the nursing and medical staff. The medical staff decided to alter the dosage of her beta-blocker and ACE inhibitor medications due to the excessive HR increase and flat BP response. Ms. Damask was discharged to the home of one of her daughters that afternoon. A referral was made for outpatient cardiac rehabilitation to be initiated 2 weeks after her hospital discharge.

Clinician Comment *The evaluating therapist had no opportunity to provide further intervention for Ms. Damask. Fortunately, Ms. Damask was referred to an outpatient program. Women, especially elderly women, are less likely to be referred for cardiac rehabilitation than their male counterparts.[4]*

REEXAMINATION AND EVALUATION (OUTPATIENT)

Subjective

"I'm still anxious about how I'm doing; I don't know how much I can do for myself at home."

Objective

Four weeks after Ms. Damask's discharge from the hospital, she was examined for home physical therapy. The inpatient physical therapy evaluation was available for review by the examining PT. The following updates were noted:

- Ms. Damask reported she had had no episodes of angina or acute SOB.

- She had been walking a couple of times per day in her living room for about 5 minutes each session without incident.

- Her HR had remained below 78 bpm every time she walked and whenever she checked it during other activities.

- She was taking the same medications as when she was discharged from the hospital.

- Her physician had referred her to a cardiac surgeon for an evaluation for bypass surgery. She did not want to proceed with a surgical intervention yet due to fear of the surgery and concerns about the expense.

- She was uncertain of how to safely increase her activities for herself and her home.

- She wanted to safely return to her previous activity level, including caring for her grandchildren. She also wanted to resume attending church socials without SOB.

The PT confirmed that Ms. Damask's status for the systems review matched the findings identified when she was an inpatient. A 2-pound weight gain was noted; Ms. Damask weighed 172 pounds. The PT decided that an updated measure of Ms. Damask's exercise tolerance was needed. The therapist determined that the most appropriate testing protocol for Ms. Damask was the 6MWT.

Clinician Comment *It was important to monitor Ms. Damask's weight. Remember she was at high risk for developing heart failure at rest due to the extent of her infarction and coronary involvement. A rapid weight gain of 6 to 10 pounds in less than 48 hours is a sign of heart failure. For accurate weight comparisons, as many of the variables that affect weight need to be controlled (eg, the weight of clothing, time of day, and time interval since the last meal).*

Why a 6MWT? This test has been used extensively to examine patients with cardiac dysfunction and failure.[10-12] In one study, the distance walked during this test was predictive of peak O_2 consumption and survival of patients with congestive heart failure.[10] This test is performed by asking the patient to walk as far as he or she can in 6 minutes. Walking needs to occur on a measured, level surface and with close monitoring of the patient's HR, BP, ECG (if available), symptoms, and heart sounds. If the patient needs to stop and rest, that is allowed, but the 6-minute clock continues to run.

If a patient is unable to walk due to musculoskeletal or neurological involvement, then other forms of aerobic exercise may be used such as biking or swimming. Another mode of exercise may be used if that is the patient's preference. If, however, an alternative mode of exercise is indicated or preferred, then the exercise test should be conducted using that mode of exercise. Conversion of a 6MWT to an exercise prescription for a biking or swimming exercise program is not appropriate. This is especially true for those patients with heart failure because their symptoms may vary greatly depending on the mode of exercise used for testing.[12,13]

Aerobic Capacity

As the following table shows, Ms. Damask completed the test and walked a total of 1150 feet without any assistance or assistive devices. The therapist pushed a wheelchair as Ms. Damask walked. Ms. Damask sat in the wheelchair to rest during the fourth minute. Ms. Damask walked faster during the third minute of the test with the result that her HR was

higher and she experienced the most symptoms during that minute. During the assessment of the patient's pulse, the therapist noted some occasional "skips." These skips were not frequent and did not cause any symptoms.

INITIAL 6-MINUTE WALK TEST RESULTS				
Minute	HR	BP	EKG	Symptoms
1	66	130/88	N/A	None
2	78	146/82	N/A	None
3	90	138/80	N/A	Leg fatigue; SOB; patient requested rest break
4 (rest)	78	136/78	N/A	"Ready to walk again"
5	84	142/84	N/A	None
6	84	136/78	N/A	None

The calculated velocity of the walk was calculated from 1150 feet walked in 6 minutes. At a steady pace, this would convert to 11,500 feet in an hour, or 2.17 mph.

Assessment

Ms. Damask was 4 weeks post-large MI with significant inpatient complications of angina, heart failure, and decreased exercise tolerance. Her ejection fraction and CAD indicated moderate to severe cardiac dysfunction. Her exercise tolerance at discharge was poor.

Her reassessed exercise tolerance was limited by SOB and leg fatigue. Her HR and BP responses were normal. The slight fall in her systolic pressure with the increase in HR during the third minute of her 6MWT might have been significant, especially in light of her SOB. Her pulse findings were only significant to the extent that she continued to have ventricular ectopy with exercise. Even as an averaged velocity, 2.17 mph was barely a functional velocity for someone attempting to cross an urban street at a signaled cross walk.

The practice pattern and ICF Model of Disability remained largely as that defined during her inpatient evaluation. Her prognosis to meet an updated plan of care was good.

Clinician Comment *There are many methods to assess exercise tolerance of patients with heart failure. A diversity of opinion exists about the most accurate and meaningful methods. The controversy revolves around the best method of identifying those patients who should be considered for transplantation by using measures of O_2 consumption. For the PT, the important factor is that a patient's exercise tolerance in heart failure is not merely a matter of the peak O_2 consumption, especially in women.[1] Chronic heart failure patients are often limited by breathlessness, and leg fatigue before they achieve their maximum O_2 consumption. Chronic heart failure causes secondary changes in exercise tolerance because of the long-term effects on arterial* blood flow and the loss of oxidative enzymes in muscle.[14] In addition, there are secondary changes that occur in the lung that cause the patients to experience dyspnea at low levels of exercise when CO is not the limiting factor.

Ms. Damask's prognosis was good to excellent to return to her previous level of function. She might never achieve the intensity, frequency, and duration of exercise required to modify her major CAD risk factors. She may, however, improve her level of exercise tolerance beyond her preinfarction level.

There is some evidence that supports the use of home-based exercise programs[15] in patients post-bypass surgery and with heart failure.[16] There is some controversy about the application of home-based programs for those patients with congestive heart failure,[17] but since the goal is to achieve a lifetime program of exercise, home-based programming will eventually be necessary.

Plan of Care

Intervention

The education program started in the hospital will continue with Ms. Damask and her family. The information covered will be individualized for Ms. Damask during her physical therapy sessions but still includes topics from the hospital education series. See the intervention table on p 231.

Ms. Damask would continue with progressive walking but a new exercise prescription would be identified.

Clinician Comment *The patient and family will only retain a small percentage of the information unless it is repeated several times over the course of her rehabilitation. The educational materials, (booklets, videotapes, CDs, and advanced reading material) are all available from the American Heart Association or their website.[18]*

The mode of aerobic exercise training for Ms. Damask initially was walking. Walking was specifically applicable to her normal activities and was easily accommodated into her routine. Prior to accepting this mode of exercise, she should obtain a comfortable, durable pair of walking shoes.

Proposed Frequency and Duration of Physical Therapy Visits

Her first 2 exercise sessions following the establishment of a new exercise prescription would be supervised and monitored. If the prescription allowed her to exercise without complaint during these supervised sessions, then she would begin self-monitored sessions. The supervised sessions would continue 2 times per week for 6 weeks.

Anticipated Goals

1. Ms. Damask would be able to tolerate a new exercise prescription without complaints (1 week).

2. Ms. Damask would have clear written guidelines for a home walking program with the new exercise prescription (2 weeks).

3. Duration of her walking session would gradually increase until she was able to walk continuously for 30 minutes (4 weeks).

4. Ms. Damask would be able to tolerate increases in her exercise prescription (4, 8, and 12 weeks).

Expected Outcomes (16 weeks)

Ms. Damask would report she had returned to at least her preinfarction level of function.

Clinician Comment *Compliance with her medical and rehabilitation programs will lead to numerous positive outcomes for Ms. Damask. The application of a program of aerobic training for a patient with cardiac dysfunction should result in an increase in aerobic and functional ability,[19] decrease in elevated homocysteine levels,[20] improvement in New York Heart Association Classification with reduction in symptoms,[16,21] improvement in quality of life,[21] reduction in body mass index,[22] increases in HDL levels, reduction in triglycerides, improvement in glucose tolerance and resting glucose levels, reduction in anxiety, and less depression. Perhaps most interesting in this health care market is the dramatic reduction in cost of care.[23] Exercise training for patients with chronic heart failure reduced hospital admissions and increased life expectancy by almost 2 years over a 15-year period.[23]*

Procedural Intervention

Therapeutic Exercise

Aerobic Capacity/Endurance Conditioning or Reconditioning

Mode
Walking
Intensity
HR not to exceed 84 bpm

Clinician Comment *The intensity of the exercise was determined from the results of her 6MWT. Ms. Damask was symptomatic and had a slight fall in her BP when her HR reached 90 bpm.*

Since Ms. Damask's exercise tolerance was so limited, the use of a target HR to determine intensity was somewhat irrelevant. It was more important for the therapist to review the results of Ms. Damask's exercise test and identify the HR at which Ms. Damask became symptomatic. Ms. Damask and her family would be instructed that 84 bpm would be the HR Ms. Damask should not exceed. Ms. Damask and her family would be instructed to note any activity that caused her to become short of breath and identify her HR.

Linking HR to activity intensity can become important feedback to the patient and the therapist about whether the patient's condition is worsening or remaining the same. It is also a wonderful way for the patient to experience positive reinforcement about the effects of his or her exercise program on symptoms and function. The patient can identify those activities that he or she was unable to perform prior to the exercise program that he or she will be able to perform asymptomatically as he or she improves.

Duration

5 minutes

Frequency

3 times per day, 4 days per week

Clinician Comment *The frequency and duration for the new exercise prescription was determined with another walking session. Ms. Damask ambulated on a level surface with standby assistance at a pace of less than 2 mph and an HR of less than 84 bpm. She was not symptomatic nor were there any palpable "skipped beats" until she had been walking for 5 minutes, and then she reported leg fatigue and asked to rest. The therapist had a wheelchair available while Ms. Damask walked so sitting rest breaks were available. She rested for 2 minutes before her HR was back to 66 bpm and she was ready to resume. Ms. Damask repeated walking for 2 more intervals for a total of 3 walks of 5 minutes each. Each time, the reason for stopping was her leg fatigue. The total duration of exercise was 15 minutes and the distance walked was less than 0.5 mile. Therefore, Ms. Damask's new exercise prescription had frequency and duration assigned as 3 times per day for 5 minutes, 4 times per week.*

Reexamination

Objective

Aerobic Capacity

Ms. Damask had been exercising in her home for 5 weeks. She had achieved an exercise tolerance of 30 minutes of continuous walking at a velocity of 2.25 mph. With the report of improved exercise tolerance to her physician, he had her undergo a low-level exercise test.

During the exercise test, she was able to complete 6 minutes of treadmill walking at a velocity of 1.7 mph with a 5% grade. The test was terminated with her complaints of leg fatigue and SOB, which occurred at an HR of 96 bpm. She had some ventricular ectopy but no couplets or ventricular tachycardia. Her BP response was again very flat with a maximum BP of 146/78 mm Hg during the fourth minute of exercise and another peak of BP at 138/78 mm Hg after

the fifth minute of exercise. She had no angina or significant ST-segment changes during the test.

Assessment

The results of the exercise test allowed the exercise prescription for her home walking program to be progressed. The frequency of her supervised home health physical therapy appointments could be reduced. Referral to outpatient cardiac rehabilitation was considered at this time.

Plan

Procedural Interventions

Aerobic Capacity

Mode

Walking

Intensity

Walking pace of 2.8 mph, but HR was not to exceed 96 bpm

Duration

30 minutes of continuous walking

Frequency

4 to 5 days per week; supervised sessions were decreased to once per week for 4 weeks, then to once per month

Clinician Comment *Should Ms. Damask have had a resistance-training program as a component of her interventions? The literature supports supplementation of aerobic exercise with resistance exercise in patients with heart failure.[16,17] However, most of this literature has been completed on men, and longitudinal studies are yet to be completed. If added, resistance training should be limited until the patient has been completely cleared by her physician. A program of resistance training would need to be accepted as a lifetime goal of the patient. If a resistance-training program was initiated and then stopped, the beneficial effects would be lost.*

There is evidence that indicates that combining aerobic and resistance exercise is more beneficial to ventricular function (increased ejection fraction, decreased LV end-diastolic volume) than aerobic training alone.[24] The therapist and patient should be mindful that compliance with a resistance-training program is more difficult because of the need for standardized equipment. If the patient is motivated and has demonstrated good compliance, a resistance-training program can be instituted. As with any exercise prescription, and especially with patients with heart failure, careful monitoring of the responses to initial resistance training should be obtained prior to continuing any program. Arm work, especially above the level of the heart, can cause acute increases in BP and HR that may well exceed those levels obtained during aerobic activities.

For Ms. Damask, resistance training was not an option. She had no means of follow-up other than at the hospital, which was too far from her home.

OUTCOMES

Discharge

After 16 weeks of supervised and self-monitored progressive ambulation, Ms. Damask achieved her goal of returning to her previous level of function. She was able to return to her independent living status and resume babysitting. She maintained her routine aerobic exercise program at a local YWCA.

Her physician had her undergo a hospital-based follow-up 6MWT with telemetry rather than symptom-limited maximum treadmill test. The latter would have been preferred if she had required a diagnostic and prognostic work-up. The 6MWT was sufficient, however, to document her progress.

As the following table shows, she walked 1600 feet in 6 minutes. She attained an average speed of just over 3 mph. Her only complaint was that she was mildly short of breath. She continued to have some ventricular ectopy, but even that was at a lower frequency than on her initial test.

DISCHARGE 6-MINUTE WALK TEST RESULTS				
Minute	*HR*	*BP*	*EKG*	*Symptoms*
Rest	60	118/78	NSR	None
1	66	122/80	NSR	None
2	78	144/86	NSR	None
3	90	146/82	NSR	None
4	96	146/78	Rare unifocal PVC	Mild SOB
5	96	140/80	Rare unifocal PVC	Mild SOB
6	96	140/78	Rare unifocal PVC	Mild SOB

Clinician Comment *Was this marked level of improvement in exercise tolerance realistic? The reality is that the worse the patient's initial level of exercise tolerance, generally, the greater percentage improvement can be expected and achieved. Part of the improvement in the test results was attributable to Ms. Damask becoming familiar with the test. The 6MWT's reliability improves with repeated testing, as does the patient's performance. Patient familiarity with the test needs to be considered when interpreting improvements.*

REFERENCES

1. Philbin EF, DiSalvo TG. Influence of race and gender on care process, resource use, and hospital-based outcomes in congestive heart failure. *Am J Cardiol.* 1998;82(1):76-81.
2. Goldstein S. Clinical studies on beta blockers and heart failure preceding the MERIT-HF Trial. Metoprolol CR/XL Randomized Intervention Trial in Heart Failure. *Am J Cardiol.* 1997;80:50J-53J.
3. Packer M, Bristow MR, Cohn JN, et al. The effect of carvedilol on morbidity and mortality in patients with chronic heart failure. *N Eng J Med.* 1996;334(21):1349-1355.
4. Lavie CJ, Milani RV. Effects of cardiac rehabilitation and exercise training on exercise capacity, coronary risk factors, behavioral characteristics, and quality of life in women. *Am J Cardiol.* 1995;75(5):340-343.
5. Meyer K, Stengele E, Westbrook S, et al. Influence of different exercise protocols on functional capacity and symptoms in patients with chronic heart failure. *Med Sci Sports Exerc.* 1996;28(9):1081-1086.
6. Meyer K. Exercise training in heart failure: recommendations based on current research. *Med Sci Sports Exerc.* 2001;33(4):525-531.
7. Sparks KE, Shaw DK, Jennings HS III, Quinn LM. Cardiovascular complications of outpatient cardiac rehabilitation programs utilizing transtelephonic exercise monitoring. *Cardiopulm Phys Ther.* 1998;18(5):363.
8. Certo C. Guidelines for exercise prescription in congestive heart failure. *Cardiopulm Phys Ther.* 2001;12:39.
9. Smith KL. Exercise training in patients with impaired left ventricular function. *Med Sci Sports Exerc.* 1991;23(6):654-660.
10. Cahalin LP, Mathier MA, Semigran MJ, Dec GW, DiSalvo TG. The six-minute walk test predicts peak oxygen uptake and survival in patients with advanced heart failure. *Chest.* 1996;110(2):325-332.
11. Delahaye N, Cohen-Solal A, Faraggi M. Comparison of left ventricular responses to the six-minute walk test, stair climbing, and maximal upright bicycle exercise in patients with congestive heart failure due to idiopathic dilated cardiomyopathy. *Am J Cardiol.* 1997;80(1):65-70.
12. Gualeni A, D'Aloia A, Gentilini A, et al. Effects of maximally tolerated oral therapy on the six-minute walking test in patients with chronic congestive heart failure secondary to either ischemic or idiopathic dilated cardiomyopathy. *Am J Cardiol.* 1998;81(11):1370-1372.
13. Meyer K, Foster C, Georgakopoulos N, et al. Comparison of left ventricular function during interval versus steady-state exercise training in patients with chronic congestive heart failure. *Am J Cardiol.* 1998;82(11):1382-1387.
14. Okita K, Yonezawa K, Nishijima H, et al. Muscle high-energy metabolites and metabolic capacity in patients with heart failure. *Med Sci Sports Exerc.* 2001;33(3):442-448.
15. Arthur HM, Smith KM, Kodis J, McKelvie R. A controlled trial of hospital versus home-based exercise in cardiac patients. *Med Sci Sports Exerc.* 2002;34(10):1544-1550.
16. Oka RK, De Marco T, Haskell WL, et al. Impact of a home-based walking program and resistance training program on quality of life in patients with heart failure. *Am J Cardiol.* 2000;85(3):365-369.
17. Caldwell MA, Dracup K. Team management of heart failure: the emerging role of exercise, and implications for cardiac rehabilitation centers. *J Cardiolpulm Rehab.* 2001;21(5):273-279.
18. American Heart Association. *2001 Heart and Stroke Statistical Update.* Dallas, TX: American Heart Association; 2002.
19. Delagardelle C, Feiereisen P, Krecké R, et al. Objective effects of 6 months endurance and strength training program in outpatients with congestive heart failure. *Med Sci Sports Exerc.* 1999;31(8):1102-1107.
20. Ali A, Mehra MR, Lavie CJ, et al. Modulatory impact of cardiac rehabilitation hyperhomo-cystinemia patients with coronary artery disease and "normal" lipid levels. *Am J Cardiol.* 1998;82:1543-1545.
21. McConnell TR, Mandak JS, Sykes JS, Fesniak H, Dasgupta H. Exercise training for heart failure patients improves respiratory muscle endurance, exercise tolerance, breathlessness and quality of life. *J Cardiopulm Rehab.* 2003;23(1):10-16.
22. Yu CM, Li LS, Ho HH, Lau CP. Long-term changes in exercise capacity, quality of life, body anthropometry, and lipid profiles after a cardiac rehabilitation program in obese patients with coronary heart disease. *Am J Cardiol.* 2003;91(3):321-325.
23. Georgiou D, Chen Y, Appadoo S, et al. Cost effectiveness analysis of long-term moderate exercise training in chronic heart failure. *Am J Cardiol.* 2001;87(8):984-988; A4.
24. Delagardelle C, Feiereisen P, Autier P, Shita R, Krecke R, Beissel J. Strength/endurance training versus endurance training in congestive heart failure. *Med Sci Sports Exerc.* 2002;34(12):1868-1872.

Scot Irwin, now deceased, was the original author for this chapter and case. Both were adapted from selected chapters in Irwin & Tecklin: *Cardiopulmonary Physical Therapy: A Guide to Practice,* 4th Edition, St. Louis, MO: Mosby; 2005. We are grateful to Elsevier for permission to include Scot's work in this book and especially to Kathy Falk for her assistance.

Individuals With Peripheral Vascular Disorders

Cheryl L. Brunelle, PT, MS, CCS, CLT

CHAPTER OBJECTIVES

- Discuss the distinction between claudication in limbs with peripheral arterial disease (PAD) and limb ischemia conditions.

- Identify correlating factors with the diagnosis of PAD.

- Summarize the physiologic progression of PAD.

- Discuss the relationship between deep venous thrombosis (DVT) and post-thrombotic syndrome.

- Compare and contrast the progression of chronic venous disease (CVD) with that of PAD.

- Discuss the relationship between PVD, depression, revascularization, and quality of life measures.

- Identify the difference in symptom presentation with elevation, dependent limb position, and walking in PAD versus CVD.

- Outline the sequence for measuring ankle brachial index (ABI) and identify what can be learned from this measure.

- Name the tests included in a vascular lab work-up for PAD versus CVD.

- Outline how risk factor management for PAD is similar to that for cardiovascular disease.

- Identify the effective exercise intervention differences in a patient with PAD and a patient with CVD.

CHAPTER OUTLINE

- Peripheral Arterial Disease
  - Clinical Definitions and Classification
  - Epidemiology
  - Pathophysiology
    - Race and Genetics
    - Age
    - Gender
    - Smoking
    - Diabetes
    - Hypertension
    - Dyslipidemia
    - Impaired Renal Function
    - Physical Activity
    - Other Risk Factors
    - Nonatherosclerotic Causes of Peripheral Arterial Disease
  - Prognosis
- Chronic Venous Disease
  - Clinical Definitions and Classification
  - Epidemiology
  - Pathophysiology
  - Prognosis
- Physical Therapy Examination and Diagnosis
  - The Subjective Exam
  - The Objective Exam
    - Systems Review
      - Cardiovascular and Pulmonary
      - Integumentary Integrity
      - Musculoskeletal

Coglianese D, ed. *Clinical Exercise Pathophysiology for Physical Therapy: Examination, Testing, and Exercise Prescription for Movement-Related Disorders (pp 247-281).*
© 2015 Taylor & Francis Group.

In recent years, collaboration of various global vascular societies has provided several clinical practice guidelines and consensus documents[1-5] that have significantly shaped the practice of health care professionals treating those with peripheral vascular disease (PVD), thereby greatly affecting the care of these patients. Literature supporting examination and interventions that are utilized by physical therapists (PTs) in these populations has been evolving, more so in the population with PAD than in that with CVD. There is sufficient evidence to guide the physical therapy examination of patients with PAD and CVD and to support various interventions in these populations. As will be further discussed, the prevalence of these diseases is high, they present significant risks of morbidity and serious cardiovascular events, and many of these patients are asymptomatic. It is imperative, therefore, that the PT is able to appropriately examine for, diagnose, and provide intervention for patients with these diseases.

Although PVD encompasses pathologic conditions of blood vessels supplying the extremities and the vital abdominal organs,[5] this chapter will be limited to discussion of PAD and CVD of the lower extremities (LEs), as both can lead to significant functional disability, morbidity, and impaired quality of life.

The goals of this chapter include increasing the PT's understanding of the pathophysiology of PAD and CVD and helping the PT examine, diagnose, and choose evidence-based interventions for patients with PAD and CVD.

PERIPHERAL ARTERIAL DISEASE

Clinical Definitions and Classification

PAD represents stenotic, occlusive, and aneurysmal diseases of the aorta and its branch arteries.[2] A resting ABI of 0.90 or less is most often used as a hemodynamic definition of LE PAD.[3]

The Trans-Atlantic Inter-Society Consensus (TASC) anatomic classification of aortoiliac (inflow) and femoral-popliteal (outflow) lesions allow vascular surgeons to classify lesions based on location and morphology. Lesions are classified by location, size, and number from Lesion Type A to Type D, and indicate the treatment of choice for best outcome. For example, Type A aortoiliac lesions indicate unilateral or bilateral stenoses of the common iliac artery, or unilateral or bilateral short (< 3 cm) stenoses of the external iliac artery, and are preferentially treated endovascularly, which yields excellent results in these kinds of lesions.[3]

Some patients with PAD experience claudication, which is LE pain produced by exercise and relieved within 10 minutes of rest,[3] defined as *intermittent claudication* (IC) or "claudication." PAD may lead to critical limb ischemia (CLI), which is characterized by LE ischemic rest pain, ulceration, or gangrene. Left untreated, CLI would lead to major limb amputation.[2] Acute limb ischemia (ALI) is a form of CLI that arises when a sudden decrease in limb perfusion threatens tissue viability.[2] Patients with ALI may present with the "5 Ps": pain, pulselessness, pallor, paresthesia, and paralysis. ALI is treated as a medical emergency.[2]

The Fontaine stages and Rutherford categories are used to classify the symptoms of PAD (Table 7-1).

Epidemiology

The prevalence of PAD and its most common disabling symptom, IC, varies in the literature, and there is a paucity of recent data. A study published in 2004[6] found that the estimated prevalence of PAD among 2174 adults 40 years and older was 4.3%, which corresponded to approximately 5 million individuals in the United States. In those older than age 70 years, the prevalence rose to 14.5%. The prevalence of PAD increased dramatically with age and disproportionately affected Black people.[6] This study did not discuss the presence or absence of IC among these individuals; however,

TABLE 7-1. STAGING OF ARTERIAL DISEASE: FONTAINE STAGES VS RUTHERFORD CATEGORIES

FONTAINE STAGES OF PAD		RUTHERFORD CATEGORIES OF PAD		
Stage	*Clinical*	*Grade*	*Category*	*Clinical*
I	Asymptomatic	0	0	Asymptomatic
IIa	Mild claudication	I	1	Mild claudication
IIb	Moderate to severe claudication	I	2	Moderate claudication
III	Ischemic rest pain	I	3	Severe claudication
IV	Ulceration or gangrene	II	4	Ischemic rest pain
		III	5	Minor tissue loss
		III	6	Major tissue loss

Reprinted with permission from *J Vasc Surg*, 45(1 Suppl S), Norgren L, Hiatt W, Dormandy J, Nehler M, Harris K, Fowkes FG, Inter-society consensus for the management of peripheral arterial disease (TASC II), pp S5-S67, Copyright Elsevier 2007.

in previous studies, approximately 25% to 33% of patients with PAD had IC.[7] The clinician should not assume that patients with PAD not experiencing claudication have normal LE function.[2] People with IC may experience significant functional disability; loss of quality of life because of claudication; or severe impairment, morbidity, and/or mortality because of CLI.[8,9] Hiatt et al[8,10] reported that patients with IC had maximal oxygen (O_2) consumption equal to 50% of age-matched controls, indicating a level of impairment similar to patients with New York Heart Association class III heart failure. Patients with PAD are more likely to have advanced systemic atherosclerosis,[11,12] and they are at increased short-term risk for cardiovascular events and death in comparison to age-matched cohorts.[2] Despite significant functional impairment, increased risk, and available effective treatments, between 10% and 50% of patients with IC have never consulted a doctor about their symptoms.[3]

Pathophysiology

PAD is primarily caused by atherosclerosis,[2] in which plaque progressively obstructs the lumen.[13] Narrowing of the arteries reduces blood flow to the limbs, which leads to O_2 deprivation to the working muscles, resulting in IC,[5] and symptoms usually occur distal to the narrowed arteries. In severe cases, the blood flow is inadequate at rest, resulting in leg pain, termed *resting claudication*.[12] Symptoms of PAD may include pain, aching, cramping, weakness, or fatigue.[5] There are patients who do not experience symptoms of claudication despite significant atherosclerotic blockage, although the same long-term progression and complications result as when patients are symptomatic.[5] Over time, occlusion of vessels may lead to skin changes, including ulcers and necrosis.

Risk factors for atherosclerosis, and therefore PAD, are discussed next. Some risk factors in the development of PAD are also traditional risk factors for coronary artery disease (CAD). Risk factors other than atherosclerosis account for some cases of PAD and are discussed.

Race and Genetics

The National Health and Nutrition Examination Survey found that Blacks were 2.8 times as likely as Whites to have PAD.[6] It is possible, therefore, that genetic factors play a role in the development of PAD. The San Diego population study included 2404 multicultural males and females 29 to 91 years of age. Family history of PAD (defined as any first-degree relative with PAD) was associated with a 1.83-fold higher risk of PAD, and a 2.42-fold higher risk of severe PAD (ABI < 0.70), and the authors concluded that family history of PAD is independently associated both with prevalence and severity of PAD.[14] It is possible that a combination of genetic and environmental factors led to the development of PAD; however, the authors did not find any statistically significant interaction of sex, race or ethnicity, body mass index (BMI), pack-years of smoking or ever smoking, or diabetes with family history of PAD. There was limited power in these calculations, so they should be viewed with caution.[14] Another study examining a multi-ethnic Asian population supports the role of genetics and found that subjects with PAD were more likely to be of Malay or Indian ethnicity than those without PAD. In a large population-based study of twins in Sweden, including 1464 twins with PAD, traditional cardiac risk factors (diabetes, hypertension, hyperlipidemia, and previous or current smoking) were significantly more prevalent in twins with PAD than in those without PAD.[15]

Age

Incidence and prevalence of PAD increases dramatically with increasing age.[3,16]

Gender

The effect of gender on the prevalence of PAD is controversial. Some studies have found the prevalence greater in males,[17] whereas other studies have found a more equal distribution between genders or greater prevalence in females.[3,16,18,19]

Smoking

Smoking is highly correlated with PAD,[6,20] and smokers are diagnosed with PAD approximately 10 years earlier than nonsmokers. The risk of PAD is affected by whether a person is a current smoker, a former smoker, or has never smoked. The National Health and Nutrition Examination Survey found that current smoking is highly associated with PAD.[6] The number of cigarettes smoked, or the cumulative pack-years, increases the severity of PAD.[3,16] This modifiable risk factor deserves much attention, as the prevalence of smoking in the United States remains high, with 19% of adults aged 18 years and older reporting that they are current smokers, and 21% reporting that they are former smokers.[21]

Diabetes

Diabetes is highly associated with PAD,[6,19] and patients with diabetes are approximately twice as likely to have IC than those without diabetes.[3] PAD in these patients is more aggressive in terms of large vessel involvement and peripheral sensory neuropathy, and these patients are 5 to 10 times more likely to require amputation than those without diabetes.[3]

Hypertension

As with any CVD, hypertension is positively associated with PAD.[3,6,16,19]

Dyslipidemia

High total cholesterol levels are positively associated with PAD,[3,6] and effective treatment reduces the progression of PAD and incidence of IC.[3] Elevated total cholesterol, low-density lipoprotein cholesterol, triglycerides, and lipoprotein(a) have been identified as independent risk factors for PAD.[3,16,17]

Impaired Renal Function

The results of the National Health and Nutrition Examination Survey found that patients with impaired kidney function are twice as likely to have PAD (odds ratio 2.17, 95% confidence interval 1.10 to 4.30).[6] In a multi-ethnic Asian population, patients with PAD were more likely to have renal impairment than those without PAD.[19]

Physical Activity

In a group of 1381 subjects, those reporting no lifetime history of regular recreational physical activity had a significantly lower ABI than those who reported a history of regular recreational physical activity.[16] In another study, lack of recreational physical activity within the year prior to examination was significantly correlated with lower ABI in patients with IC. It was unclear whether the lack of activity was due to patients' inability to participate, or the sedentary nature of the patients.[22] A sedentary lifestyle was found to be a predictor of PAD in elderly patients in another recent study.[17]

Other Risk Factors

Elevated levels of C-reactive protein, a marker of inflammation, have been found to be associated with PAD.[3,6] Several recent studies have shown that impaired walking ability in patients with PAD is related to higher levels of certain inflammatory markers (C-reactive protein, interleukin-6, and soluble vascular cell adhesion molecule-1).[23,24] Several studies have found hyperhomocysteinemia to be a strong, independent risk factor for PAD and CAD.[3] Hypercoagulable states, specifically increased plasma fibrinogen and high hematocrit levels, have been reported in patients with PAD, and both seem to lead to a poor prognosis.[3]

Nonatherosclerotic Causes of Peripheral Arterial Disease

There are several causes of PAD other than atherosclerosis, and these should be considered as appropriate, allowing for accurate diagnosis and therefore best management. These may include thromboembolic, inflammatory, or aneurysmal disorders; trauma; cysts; entrapment syndromes; or congenital abnormalities.[2]

Prognosis

Physiologic progression of PAD is identical whether a patient is symptomatic or not.[3] In the majority of patients with PAD who initially present with claudication, symptoms stabilize. Approximately 25% will significantly deteriorate clinically and only 1% to 3.3% will need major amputation over a 5-year period.[3] The prognosis for the limb is poor without immediate revascularization in patients who initially present with CLI.[13] In patients who are not surgical candidates, or whose revascularization has failed, approximately 40% will require amputation within 6 months, and 20% will die.[3] In patients who undergo below-knee amputations, approximately 60% heal by primary intention, 15% after secondary procedures, 15% need to be converted to above-knee amputations, and 10% of patients die in the postoperative period.[3] Over a 5-year period, patients with PAD are at increased risk for myocardial infarction, stroke, and vascular death in comparison to age-matched norms.[2] In a literature review, Hooi et al found that IC, an ABI ≤0.90, or other abnormal noninvasive test results were independent prognostic factors for cardiovascular death in patients with noncritical ischemia secondary to PAD.[25] Overall 5-year mortality for patients with PAD is 15% to 30%, with the majority of deaths secondary to cardiovascular causes.[2]

CHRONIC VENOUS DISEASE

Clinical Definitions and Classification

CVD includes medical conditions of long duration involving a range of abnormalities of the venous system manifested by symptoms and/or signs requiring investigation and care.[1] The Clinical-Etiology-Anatomy-Physiology (CEAP) classification system for CVD was developed to facilitate communication between practitioners and to assist in standardizing language for research and treatment purposes (Table 7-2).

TABLE 7-2. CLASSIFICATION OF CHRONIC VENOUS DISEASE		
CLASSIFICATION	**NOTATION**	**DESCRIPTION**
Clinical	C_0	No visible or palpable signs of venous disease
	C_1	Telangiectasias or reticular veins
	C_2	Varicose veins
	C_3	Edema
	C_{4a}	Pigmentation and/or eczema
	C_{4b}	Lipodermatosclerosis and/or atrophie blanche
	C_5	Healed venous ulcer
	C_6	Active venous ulcer
	C_S	Symptoms including ache, pain, tightness, skin irritation, heaviness, muscle cramps, as well as other complaints attributable to venous dysfunction
	C_A	Asymptomatic
Etiological	E_c	Congenital
	E_p	Primary
	E_s	Secondary (post-thrombotic)
	E_n	No venous etiology identified
Anatomical	A_s	Superficial veins
	A_p	Perforator veins
	A_d	Deep veins
	A_n	No venous location identified
Pathophysiological	P_r	Reflux
	P_o	Obstruction
	$P_{r,o}$	Reflux and obstruction
	P_n	No venous pathophysiology identifiable

Reprinted with permission from *J Vasc Surg*, 40(6), Eklöf B, Rutherford RB, Bergan JJ, Revision of the CEAP classification for chronic venous disorders: consensus statement, pp 1248-1252, Copyright Elsevier 2004.

Chronic venous insufficiency (CVI) describes advanced CVD, in which subcutaneous and skin changes lead to chronic changes such as edema, pigmentation, lipodermatosclerosis, or ulcerations.[1]

Epidemiology

CVD is the most common vascular disorder, although estimates of prevalence vary in the literature.[26] In a cross-sectional study of a multi-ethnic sample of 2211 adults in San Diego, California, 81.1% and 27% of the study population was found to have visible or functional venous disease, respectively. It is not clear whether prevalence of CVD is higher in males or females, but it does increase with age.[26] A study completed in Bulgaria found that among 26,785 subjects aged 18 years and older attending their general practitioner's office for routine consultation, 44% were found to have CVD. Prevalence increased with age and BMI.[27] In the Edinburgh Vein Study, 9.2% and 6.6% of male and female subjects, respectively, were classified as having CVI. This value increased with age, and in the 55-to-64 age group, 25.25% and 12.27% of men and women, respectively, were classified as having CVI.[28]

Pathophysiology

The signs and symptoms of CVD occur secondary to prolonged venous hypertension in the LEs. Venous pressure in the leg is determined by the weight of the column of blood from the foot to the right atrium and the pressures generated by the LE skeletal muscle pump. Venous pressures in the leg may reach 80 to 90 mm Hg during static standing when there is no muscle contraction; therefore, the pressure in the leg is determined by the weight of the column of blood from the foot to the right atrium. Skeletal muscle contraction of the leg (eg, during activity) transiently increases the venous pressures of the deep venous system in the leg. When venous valves are functioning normally, venous blood flows toward the heart because of the muscle pump, and the deep and superficial venous systems are emptied, thereby decreasing the pressure in the venous system to less than 30 mm Hg.[29]

When venous valves or the muscle pump are malfunctioning, blood flow is abnormally redirected from the deep to the superficial venous system, resulting in increased superficial venous pressures.[29,30] This increases capillary permeability near the skin and may lead to accumulation of fluid, leukocytes, and extravasated red blood cells in the interstitial space.[31] These elevated pressures, when prolonged, can trigger inflammation and structural changes in the venous valves and walls, leading to valvular incompetence, eventual valvular destruction and weakness, and reduced elasticity of the venous walls.[29] Local tissue inflammation and damage, lipodermatosclerosis (pigmentation, induration, and fibrosis or scarring of the skin at or above the level of the malleoli), edema, and ulcers may occur.[28,29,31,32] Ulceration is therefore the end of a continuum of physiologic changes resulting from prolonged venous hypertension, and the patient with CVD remains at high risk for recurrent wounds, delayed wound healing, cellulitis, and lymphedema.[31]

There are several risk factors for CVD, including age,[27,28,33] family history of venous insufficiency,[27,33,34] obesity,[27,33,35,36] smoking,[34,37] decreased activity (eg, frequent or regular standing for prolonged periods or low reported levels of physical activity),[34] LE trauma, thrombosis, and pregnancy.[27,33]

Excess abdominal mass associated with obesity increases abdominal pressure, which results in reduced blood flow in the pelvic veins.[35] LE trauma may directly damage the venous system and/or cause LE impairments resulting in immobility of the limb and, therefore, an inadequate muscle pump. Sequelae of DVT include recurrence and post-thrombotic syndrome, which presents as peripheral venous disease, secondary to venous hypertension associated with diminished blood flow distal to the clot (Box 7-1) Incidence is high after DVT; a recent study found that 23% to 60% of patients develop post-thrombotic syndrome within 2 years of an acute DVT of the LE.[38] Post-thrombotic syndrome includes a continuum of signs and symptoms of CVD.[39]

Prognosis

Causative factors contributing to time course, severity of disease, and formation of ulceration in CVD remain somewhat elusive. Labropoulos et al[40] tracked 116 limbs in 90 patients with CVD for up to 43 months with duplex ultrasound and clinical examination. Changes in reflux on ultrasound (new or extension of previously documented sites) were found in 31 limbs, whereas changes in symptoms or progression of CEAP staging was noted in only 13 limbs. It was noted that progression of CVD may not be identified by physical examination, and repeat duplex ultrasound should be performed and used for surveillance in order to document progression and to make treatment decisions. Chiesa et al[33]

found that frequency of valve incompetence correlated with worsening of symptoms when signs of disease were present. Therefore, when early signs of venous disease (eg, spider veins) are noticed on examination, patients could be referred to care earlier, allowing for initiation of treatment prior to progression of the disease. CVI leads to venous ulcers in a substantial number of cases, with up to 80% of LE ulcers being venous in origin.[41] Venous ulcers are highly prone to recurrence, with recurrence rates of up to 72% reported in the literature[42] and delayed healing.[43] Cost associated with the treatment of venous stasis ulcers is high. Olin et al[43] found that of 78 patients presenting with venous stasis ulcers, 14 patients accounted for 18 hospitalizations for ulcer care, and mean cost per patient in the study was $9685 over a 1-year period. In another study,[44] the mean annual cost to treat patients with delayed venous ulcer healing was between $20,041 (with Graftskin, a living human skin graft) and $27,493 (with an Unna Boot, a commonly prescribed nonelastic compression system). As these studies were completed in 1999 and 2000, these costs would be much higher in current monetary value. These values did not account for indirect costs, such as loss of work, early retirement, loss of independence, and emotional suffering associated with these ulcers.[43]

PHYSICAL THERAPY EXAMINATION AND DIAGNOSIS

Given the often insidious presentation of PAD and CVD, association with known risk factors, and associated morbidity of both, it is prudent that the PT is able to identify those patients who are at high risk and may need further testing for the purposes of diagnosis and treatment. Through a comprehensive screening examination, indication for further tests and measures may be identified, and patients whom the examiner suspects of having PAD or CVD can be referred for important early intervention and serial monitoring, and/or patients with PAD or CVD can be treated appropriately. Examination of patients for PVD can be daunting for the PT; however, knowledge of the etiology, pathophysiology, and clinical presentations of PAD and CVD should guide the clinician through the examination process. The most appropriate practice pattern in the *Guide to Physical Therapist Practice*[45] for patients with PVD may be impaired aerobic capacity/endurance associated with cardiovascular pump dysfunction or failure. An outline of examination in this population, including patient/client history, systems review, and tests and measures is further discussed in the *Guide*.[45]

The Subjective Exam

Every physical therapy examination should begin with a comprehensive subjective history (provided the patient is able to provide it), which can guide the examiner to appropriate tests and measures based on the patient's presentation.

Box 7-1. Deep Vein Thrombosis: Clinical Summary and Management

DVT of the LE is classified as either distal (confined to the calf veins) or proximal (involving the popliteal, femoral, or iliac veins) thrombosis. This section is limited to the discussion of proximal DVT of the LE, as this presents increased risk to the patient and is well established in the literature. Patients with acute proximal DVT are at significant risk for developing post-thrombotic syndrome, which presents as CVI, as a result of residual venous impairment and damaged venous valves.[1]

Risk factors for DVT may include but are not limited to immobility, recent surgery, LE trauma, prior venous thromboembolism, obesity, malignancy, use of oral contraceptives or hormone replacement therapy, pregnancy or postpartum status, and stroke.[2]

Signs and symptoms of DVT may include swelling, pain, and erythema of the involved extremity, although the location of symptoms may not indicate the site of thrombosis.[2] A recent meta-analysis, however, revealed that individual clinical findings are not predictive of DVT.[3] If DVT is suspected, further diagnostic testing is required to confirm a diagnosis. This usually consists of compression ultrasonography, which has very high sensitivity, reported in the literature at approximately 95%.[4]

Once a diagnosis of acute proximal LE DVT is made, in absence of any contraindications, the patient is anticoagulated. Options include low molecular weight heparin, unfractionated heparin, and warfarin. Low molecular weight heparin is dosed based on body weight alone, and laboratory studies are not routinely required to confirm therapeutic anticoagulation.[5] Therapeutic anticoagulation status of unfractionated heparin is monitored with partial thromboplastin time, and that of warfarin with international normalized ratio. Therapeutic anticoagulation should be confirmed by the PT before treatment.

Management of the patient with symptomatic acute proximal DVT who is therapeutically anticoagulated should include early ambulation and compression (calf or thigh length, 30 to 40 mm Hg at the ankle). Together, these treatments reduce pain and edema significantly faster than bed rest or no compression, limit thrombus progression, and do not increase the risk of pulmonary embolism.[1,6-9] Compression established with early ambulation and continued for 2 years is well established in the literature to significantly reduce the risk of post-thrombotic syndrome. In a recent study, 46% of patients not treated with compression stockings developed post-thrombotic syndrome, compared to 26% of patients treated with compression stockings, indicating a high risk of developing the syndrome after acute proximal DVT, and a 54% relative risk reduction with compression.[10]

REFERENCES

1. Blättler W, Partsch H. Leg compression and ambulation is better than bed rest for the treatment of acute deep venous thrombosis. *Int Angiol.* 2003;22(4):393-400.
2. Landaw SA, Bauer KA. Approach to the diagnosis and therapy of lower extremity deep vein thrombosis. http://www.uptodate.com/contents/approach-to-the-diagnosis-and-therapy-of-lower-extremity-deep-vein-thrombosis. Updated January 9, 2014. Accessed September 21, 2012.
3. Goodacre S, Sutton A, Sampson F. Meta-analysis: the value of clinical assessment in the diagnosis of deep venous thrombosis. *Ann Intern Med.* 2005;143(2):129-139.
4. Hamper UM, DeJong MR, Scoutt LM. Ultrasound evaluation of the lower extremity veins. *Radiol Clin North Am.* 2007;45:525-547.
5. Rydberg EJ, Westfall JM, Nicholas RA. Low molecular weight heparin in preventing and treating DVT. *Am Fam Physician.* 1999;59(6):1607-1612.
6. Partsch H. Immediate ambulation and leg compression in the treatment of deep vein thrombosis. *Dis Mon.* 2005;51:135-140.
7. McCollum C. Avoiding the consequences of deep vein thrombosis. *BMJ.* 1998;317:696-697.
8. Jünger M, Diehm C, Störiko H, et al. Mobilization versus immobilization in the treatment of acute proximal deep venous thrombosis: a prospective, randomized, open, multicentre trial. *Curr Med Res Opin.* 2006;22(3):593-602.
9. Partsch H, Blättler W. Compression and walking versus bed rest in the treatment of proximal deep venous thrombosis with low molecular weight heparin. *J Vasc Surg.* 2000;32(5):861-869.
10. Musani MH, Matta F, Yaekoub AY, Liang J, Hull RD, Stein PD. Venous compression for prevention of postthrombotic syndrome: a meta-analysis. *Am J Med.* 2010;123:735-740.

There has been increasing discussion in recent years regarding the effect of PVD on quality of life. The literature supports significant relationships between depression and impaired quality of life and PAD. Remes et al[46] found that patients with PAD who had undergone percutaneous transluminal angioplasty and/or one or more surgical revascularization had significantly lower scores on the Geriatric Depression Scale and on the Self-Reported Life Satisfaction score than age-matched controls. Cherr et al[47] found that 36.1% of patients undergoing intervention for PAD were diagnosed with depression when screened prior to surgery. Those patients with depression at the time of revascularization were more likely to have failure of the revascularization and were at significantly higher risk of recurrent symptomatic PAD.

TABLE 7-3. GRADING OF PITTING EDEMA

GRADE	DESCRIPTION OF EDEMA	TIME TO RETURN TO BASELINE
0	None	
1+	Trace	< 10 seconds (rapid)
2+	Mild	10 to 15 seconds
3+	Moderate	1 to 2 minutes
4+	Severe	2 to 5 minutes

Reprinted with permission from *Critical Care Nursing: Diagnosis and Management*, 6th ed, Urden LD, Stacy KM, Lough ME, Copyright Mosby Elsevier 2010.

As in PAD, there is substantial evidence that CVD affects health-related quality of life, and investigators are increasingly including quality of life measures as outcomes of treatment for CVD.[48] A multinational study looking at quality of life in varicose veins[49] found that the SF-36 physical and SF-36 mental scores were significantly lower in patients with varicose veins than in the general population, and that quality of life worsens with clinical severity of the disease. This finding was consistent with the finding of another study, in which SF-36 Physical Component Summary Scores and VEINES-QOL and VEINES-Sym scores decreased significantly with increasing CEAP class.[50] Palfreyman[51] found that patients with a current or healed venous ulcer have a significantly reduced self-reported quality of life as compared to the general population, and 65% reported signs and symptoms of depression. Many patients with CVI fear amputation or death due to their vascular disease and are unaware that these are not generally outcomes of isolated venous insufficiency.[52]

During the subjective history, patients should be questioned very specifically about baseline mobility in terms of activities of daily living (ADL) and instrumental activities of daily living (IADL), employment, regular exercise, and distance walked, as well as about their living environment, recreational interests, and activities. Discussion and clarification of symptoms is imperative, and limitations to baseline mobility should be noted (eg, spinal stenosis may limit walking at baseline, although this is unrelated to the limitations caused by the discomfort of dependency in patients with CVD). This baseline should be compared to the patient's report of current abilities and limiting factors. If the patient reports a decline in function, reasons for this decline should be clarified. For example, if the patient states that he or she no longer drives, the examiner should question the patient as to when and why he or she stopped driving. These types of questions can elicit information that can help guide the examination. For example, if a patient stopped driving as he or she is having difficulty feeling the foot pedals, the examiner would be sure to incorporate LE sensation testing into the exam. The patient should specifically be questioned about how current symptoms (eg, leg pain with walking or

at rest, drainage of venous wounds) are affecting ADL and IADL, recreational activities and interests, and quality of life. When asked how the current symptoms are affecting activities and quality of life, the therapist can often perceive what the patient's goals may be. Clarification of the patient's symptoms and course, functional limitations, discussion of how these are affecting the patient's life, and establishment of the patient's own goals should be the aims of the discussion.

On interview, the patient with PAD may complain of pain that interferes with sleep, worsens with LE elevation, and improves with LE dependency. In patients with claudication, pain may increase with walking after certain distances and then is relieved quickly with rest.[53] In contrast, patients with CVD may complain of worsening pain with dependency, which is relieved with elevation of the leg, walking, and compression.[52] Patients should be asked about any symptoms of CVD, including tingling, aching, burning, pain, muscle cramps, swelling, throbbing, heaviness, itching skin, and restless or tired legs.[1,54] These symptoms may worsen throughout the course of the day, especially if patients are required to stand for long periods of time (eg, during work hours),[54] and improve at night with sleeping. Risk factors for PAD and/or CVD should be reviewed, as appropriate, to elicit whether the patient may be at risk.

The decision of whether to conduct a peripheral vascular examination should be made based on identification of risk factors, the patient's subjective history of symptoms and limitations, and/or after screening integumentary integrity during the physical therapy examination.

The Objective Exam

Systems Review

Cardiovascular and Pulmonary

Resting blood pressure (BP), heart rate (HR), and respiratory rate should be measured. Any signs of edema should be noted. Patients with CVD often present with edema that may be pitting in early stages but may become nonpitting as the skin becomes more fibrotic as the disease progresses. If edema is present, the examiner should note its location and move on to tests and measures of anthropometric characteristics, specifically, palpation, grading, and measurement of edema, as indicated. Edema should be palpated for pitting, which is graded as shown in Table 7-3.

If edema is present and objective change over time needs to be monitored and/or intervention for edema is considered, girth measures should be obtained. At minimum, landmarking using a reproducible bony landmark, with measurement at equal intervals proximal or distal to that landmark, should be used to allow for reproducibility. For example, circumferential measurement every 10 cm proximal to the center of the lateral malleolus is reproducible even in most patients with moderate to severe edema. Girth measurements using limb circumference are often used to calculate limb volumes in patients with edema, to make treatment decisions, and to document change over time. Typically, calculating limb

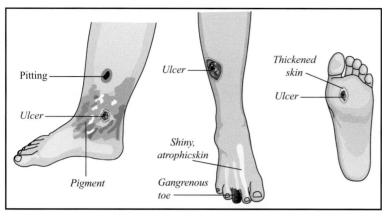

Figure 7-1. Summary of the presentation of venous (left) and arterial (center and right) ulcers. (Reprinted with permission from Bates B. *A Guide to Physical Examination and History Taking.* 4th ed. Philadelphia, PA: J.B. Lippincott Company; 1987.)

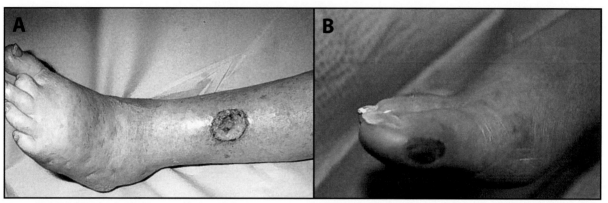

Figure 7-2. (A) Typical arterial ulcer. Location is pretibial (a potential pressure point), without signs of CVD, with a defined edge, pale, and dry. (Reprinted with permission from *Diseases of the Skin*, 2nd ed, White G, Cox N, Copyright Elsevier 2006.) (B) Typical arterial ulcer. Location is over a bony prominence, very distal, with a defined edge, dry, with some periwound edema. (Reprinted with permission from *Acute & Chronic Wounds: Current Management Concepts*, 3rd ed, Bryant R, Nix D, Copyright Elsevier 2007.) *(continued)*

volume from circumferential measures taken in equal intervals from a bony landmark has been studied, comparing with the gold standard of water volumetry. Circumferential limb measures using a segment length of 10 cm from a bony landmark provide volume estimates that are highly correlated with that of water displacement volume and are sufficient for routine limb measurement and for estimates of limb volume changes over time.[55-57]

Integumentary Integrity

Inspection of the integumentary integrity of the LEs should be conducted with shoes and socks off, pant legs rolled up above the knees at the very least, and with the patient in supine and standing.

Venous and arterial ulcers present very differently, and the clinician can usually denote the etiology of the ulcer from a careful clinical exam (Figure 7-1).

Areas of pressure points should be noted, observing for areas of callous, which may indicate areas susceptible to wounds (Figure 7-2A). Areas of bruising should also be noted, which may indicate recent trauma, in which case interventions regarding skin protection should be discussed in light of potential risk of wounds. Temperature of the skin, including left-right symmetry and proximal-distal differences, should be noted. Areas of decreased perfusion may

be cold; areas of infection may feel very warm to touch. Any trophic changes, which are general changes indicative of vascular impairment, should be noted on the LEs. These may include dry, shiny, or hairless skin, or thickened, hypertrophic toenails. Color of the skin should be noted, and if any of these findings are abnormal, further testing may be warranted.

Limbs of patients with arterial insufficiency may be discolored (pale, red, blue, or dusky purple), may lack hair growth, and the distal extremity may be cool to the touch.[53,58] Arterial wounds will appear commonly on or below the ankle, specifically around areas of bony prominences (Figure 7-2B), such as the lateral malleoli, tips of the toes, metatarsal heads, or in areas of bunions.[53,58] These wounds generally have a defined edge (are "punched out" in appearance), are pale, dry (without significant drainage), and painful to touch. Signs of venous insufficiency such as hemosiderin staining, stasis dermatitis, or lipodermatosclerosis are absent.[53,59]

Patients with suspected venous insufficiency should be examined in the standing position to allow for maximal venous distention and for visualization from the front, back, and sides.[31,54] Spider veins or telangiectasia (Figure 7-2C) present as fine-lined networks of red, blue, or purple veins on the LEs and indicate broken capillaries.[5]

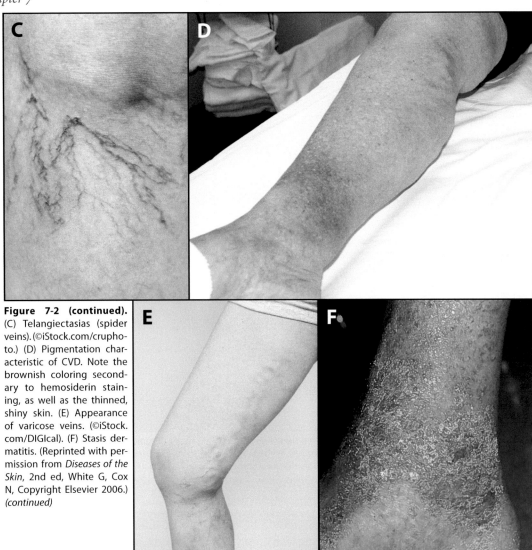

Figure 7-2 (continued).
(C) Telangiectasias (spider veins). (©iStock.com/crupho-to.) (D) Pigmentation characteristic of CVD. Note the brownish coloring secondary to hemosiderin staining, as well as the thinned, shiny skin. (E) Appearance of varicose veins. (©iStock.com/DIGIcal). (F) Stasis dermatitis. (Reprinted with permission from *Diseases of the Skin*, 2nd ed, White G, Cox N, Copyright Elsevier 2006.) *(continued)*

Thinned skin and hemosiderin staining (Figure 7-2D) may be apparent at the ankle, lower leg, and foot. Hemosiderin staining is brown discoloration in a circumferential pattern between the malleoli and calf that results from breakdown of red blood cells into the interstitial space from the capillaries.[53]

Irregularities or bulges on the surface of the skin suggest the presence of varicose veins (Figure 7-2E), which may be tender to palpation[31] and are easily visible in the standing position.[5]

Moderate to severe edema that may feel hardened or woody may be apparent in patients with long-term venous disease, and untreated varicosities will become thickened and hard. These patients are at risk of developing stasis dermatitis (Figure 7-2F), which presents as an erythematous, pruritic plaque[60] that may be very itchy and worsened with scratching.

Lipodermatosclerosis (Figure 7-2G) may eventually develop, which presents starting at the medial ankle, progressing to the entire lower leg in advanced cases as heavily pigmented, fibrotic, and edematous. The pigmented area will be hardened and fibrotic on palpation.

Eventually, venous ulcers may develop.[5] Inspection for any openings in the skin should be meticulous. Venous ulcers are typically located below the knee and above or around the ankles and are irregular in shape and draining, sometimes excessively (Figure 7-2H). This discharge will be expected to improve dramatically with appropriate wound care, elevation, and compression.

In any vascular examination, odor of the wounds or of the skin should be noted, which may indicate fungal or bacterial infection. If there is demarcation of painful erythema and rubor, with or without systemic signs of infection, this may indicate cellulitis (Figure 7-2I). In these cases, referral to a physician for timely diagnosis and treatment of infection should be mobilized.

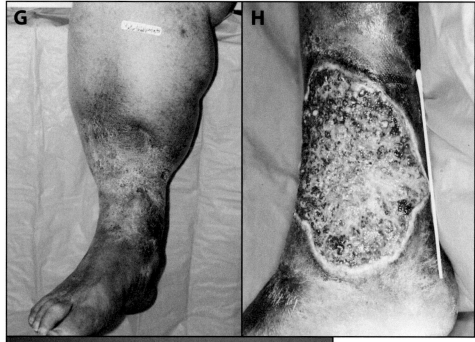

Figure 7-2 (continued). (G) Lipodermatosclerosis. Note the pronounced pigmentation, edema, and fibrosis. (Reprinted with permission from Alguire PC, Mathes BM. Chronic venous insufficiency and venous ulceration. *J Gen Intern Med.* 1997;12(6):374-383.) (H) A typical venous ulcer. Note the medial, circumferential location on the calf, the irregular border, and moist wound bed. (Reprinted with permission from Alguire PC, Mathes BM. Chronic venous insufficiency and venous ulceration. *J Gen Intern Med.* 1997;12(6):374-383.) (I) Cellulitis. Note the demarcation of the erythema, which would be painful to the touch. (Reprinted with permission from *Diseases of the Skin*, 2nd ed, White G, Cox N, Copyright Elsevier 2006.)

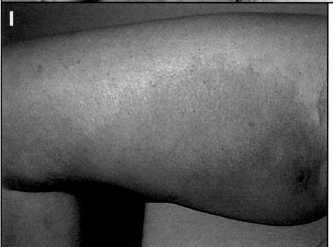

If there are any wounds found on examination in patients at risk of or with known vascular disease, examination by a physician is warranted as soon as possible.

Musculoskeletal

The systems review should include screening of gross range of motion, gross strength, and height and weight. Ankle range of motion and calf muscle strength and endurance are worthy of specific mention as they pertain to patients with CVD, as will be discussed in the Therapeutic Exercise Prescription section of Procedural Interventions in the Case Study at the end of the chapter (see p 279).

Neuromuscular

Balance, gait, and functional mobility (transfers, ambulation), as well as motor function, should be screened. Given potential impairments in several contributing factors to gross motor movements and motor function, including vision, LE sensation, range of motion, and strength, impairments in these areas are common among patients with PVD.

Tests and Measures

Aerobic Capacity and Endurance

Cardiovascular signs and symptoms in response to increased O$_2$ demand with exercise or activity (ADL, IADL, and/or exercise) should be monitored. These may include BP; HR or rhythm; or angina, claudication, and/or exertion scales. Given the associated cardiovascular risk in this population, close monitoring of hemodynamic response to activity is warranted. Activity should mimic the maximum activity the patient needs to accomplish in his or her everyday life to fulfill ADL and IADL, as well as recreational and vocational interests, as appropriate. This part of the examination should rely on the patient's reports of baseline and current function, and further highlights the importance of a comprehensive subjective history.

The PT may decide, based on the patient's report and the results of examination thus far, to examine aerobic capacity, which is often measured during walking, potentially on

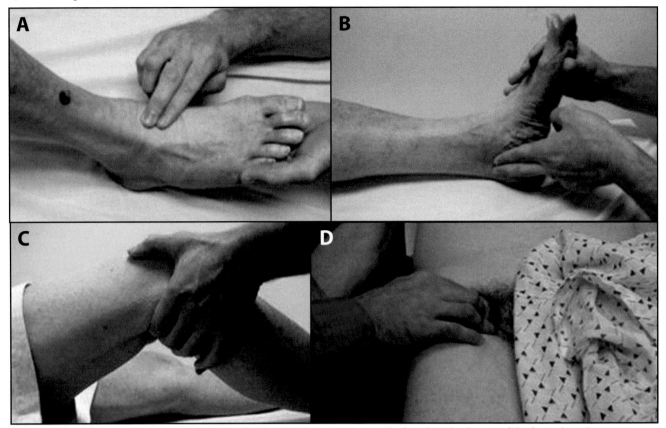

Figure 7-3. Palpation of pulse points. (A) Dorsalis pedis. The dorsalis pedis artery can be found on the dorsum of the foot, where the artery passes over the navicular and cuneiform bones just lateral to the extensor hallucis longus tendon. (B) Posterior tibial posterior. The posterior tibial artery runs posterior to the medial malleolus and the tendons of tibialis posterior and flexor digitorum longus. (C) Popliteal, which can be felt on deep palpation in the popliteal fossa with the knee slightly flexed. (D) Femoral; with the thigh slightly flexed and laterally rotated, the femoral artery runs from the midpoint of the pubic symphysis and the anterior superior iliac spine. (Images A, B, and C reprinted with permission from Paul Gaspar and Robert Snow. Image D reprinted with permission from Moore K, Agur AMR. *Clinically Oriented Anatomy.* 2nd ed. Philadelphia, PA: Wolters Kluwer; 1992.)

TABLE 7-4. GRADING OF PERIPHERAL PULSES

GRADE	DESCRIPTION
0	Absent
1	Diminished
2	Normal
3	Bounding

Reprinted with permission from *J Vasc Surg*, 31(1), Dormandy JA, Rutherford RB, Management of peripheral arterial disease (PAD), S1-S296, Copyright Elsevier 2000.

level ground or on a treadmill. The American College of Cardiology (ACC)/American Heart Association (AHA) recommends that a 6-Minute Walk Test (6MWT) is reasonable to measure functional limitation in patients who are not able to conduct treadmill testing.[2]

Appropriate hemodynamic monitoring should be conducted throughout the aerobic capacity testing. If the patient complains of claudication pain during the test, both pain-free and maximum distances walked and limiting factors to further walking should be noted, including location of pain. Amount of time for resolution of symptoms should be noted.

Circulation

Measurement of physiological responses to position change may be warranted and may be useful in isolating physiologic responses to activity, as discussed previously. For example, if a patient's BP and HR are measured with him or her sitting prior to activity and then again standing at peak activity, if the BP dropped, it should not be construed as an inappropriate hemodynamic response to activity. Clarification that the patient had an appropriate response to position change would be required prior to concluding a failure response to activity. To isolate the hemodynamic response to activity, this would ideally include measures of standing resting BP and HR prior to activity, then standing peak BP and HR.

The PT will commonly examine pulses as part of the vascular examination of the LE. The ACC/AHA recommends that all patients at risk of lower-extremity PAD should undergo a comprehensive pulse examination, including femoral, popliteal, dorsalis pedis, and posterior tibial sites, in addition to inspection of the feet (Figure 7-3).

Pulses should be graded numerically (Table 7-4).

A handheld Doppler device, if available, can be used to assess pulses if palpation proves difficult. A normal arterial pulse assessed with a Doppler is triphasic. In the presence of arterial disease, the arterial signal is impaired and may be biphasic or monophasic, or in the most severe cases, it may be absent.[13]

Capillary refill time (CRT) has been used as part of the clinical assessment of peripheral arterial perfusion for many years. As for pulses, the PT may incorporate this into the vascular examination. To measure CRT, the examiner presses the finger or toe pad until the skin blanches. Pressure is removed, and the time it takes blood to refill the blanched area is observed. Normal CRT is less than 3 seconds, and longer times may indicate arterial insufficiency.[61] Schriger and Baraff[62] found that CRT in healthy adults varies with age and sex (being significantly longer in older adults and women), and the cut-off times for normal capillary refill continue to be debated in the literature. Although abnormal capillary refill may indicate impaired peripheral perfusion, it should not be relied on as the sole indicator of peripheral arterial status, but rather one component of a comprehensive clinical exam.

The ABI is an index that compares systolic BP at the ankle to that at the brachial artery, and it is a measure of arterial perfusion of the LEs. When clinicians feel a patient may be at risk of PAD based on subjective history, identification of risk factor(s), and/or clinical examination, measurement of the ABI may be considered. The ABI has sensitivity ranging from 79% to 95% and specificity consistently >95% in the literature in detecting PAD in patients undergoing diagnostic testing.[2] Current guidelines recommend that the resting ABI be measured in patients with exertional leg symptoms, nonhealing wounds, increasing age (65 to 70 years), 50 years or older with cardiovascular risk factors, or subjects with a Framingham risk score between 10% and 20%.[3,4]

When measured at rest, the patient should, when able, assume the supine position for 5 to 10 minutes prior to measurement.[13,63] At that time, usually with a Doppler probe, BP is measured in both arms at the brachial artery and, if different values are found, the highest brachial value is used for both left and right ABI calculation. The ankle BP is taken on both sides using the dorsalis pedis and posterior tibial artery (Figure 7-4).

The higher of the dorsalis pedis or posterior tibial ankle BP on each side is divided by the higher of the 2 brachial pressures to establish a right and a left LE ABI (Figure 7-5).[3]

Normal ABI values range from 1.00 to 1.40, and an abnormal ABI is defined as ≤0.90. ABI values of 0.91 to 0.99 are considered "borderline" and values >1.40 indicate noncompressible arteries (as would be found with calcification).[4] Resting or exercising ABI values of <0.90 or <0.85, respectively, are universally accepted to indicate a diagnosis of PAD in adults over 55 years of age.[64] An ABI of 0.7 to 0.89 is considered mild, 0.4 to 0.69 moderate, and less than 0.4 severe PAD.[13] Calcification of the arteries, as is common in patients with diabetes or renal insufficiency, will falsely elevate and therefore invalidate ABI measurements, and they should not be used for diagnostic purposes in that case.[3]

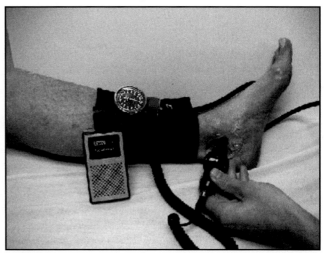

Figure 7-4. Measuring the ankle pressure at the posterior tibial artery using a Doppler probe. (Reprinted with permission from Paul Gaspar and Robert Snow.)

Some patients may undergo an ABI with exercise if resting ABI is within normal limits and PAD is still suspected. Protocols for exercise testing for evaluation of IC and PAD are discussed elsewhere.[65,66] After exercise, BP measurement at the ankle is repeated in supine within 30 seconds of stopping activity. In patients with PAD, ankle systolic pressure falls with exercise, often cannot be recorded, and does not recover to baseline for several minutes.[5] A decrease in ankle pressure with exercise of 15% or 20 mm Hg indicates PAD.[3,63]

Although the ABI is often measured in a vascular lab, the PT may choose to measure it if he or she feels it is indicated to help diagnose or rule out PAD or to help with treatment decisions such as compression management.

Pain

Examination of pain is an important part of the vascular examination. Based on the subjective history and objective examination, pain patterns may lead to further testing or to suspicion of a certain diagnosis. For example, LE pain with walking that is relieved with rest, in absence of other causes, may be attributed to claudication. Lack of pain in an ulcer of a patient who is diabetic, along with other observations of the wound, may indicate venous origin of the ulcer. A Visual Analog scale or the Claudication Pain Rating scale (refer to the Exercise section in Intervention for PAD) may be appropriately used for this population. The PT needs to consider causes of pain other than PVD and examine as appropriate as part of the differential diagnosis of PVD.

Summary: The Clinical Examination and Peripheral Arterial Disease

One should consider that the noninvasive clinical examination (skin inspection, palpation, pulses) is somewhat limited in its ability to accurately identify patients who have PAD. A recent systematic review of studies compared

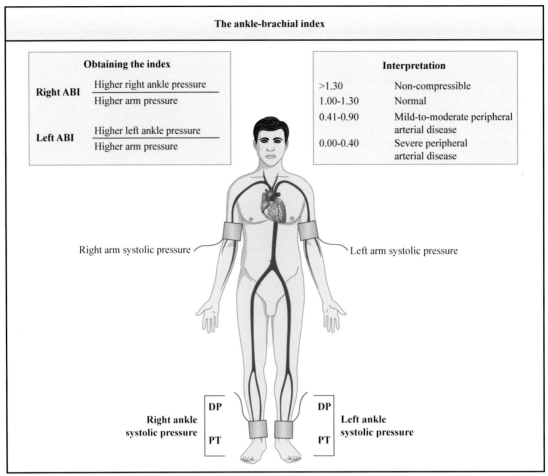

Figure 7-5. Calculation of the ABI. (Adapted from Salameh MJ, Ratchford EV. Update on peripheral arterial disease and claudication rehabilitation. *Phys Med Rehabil Clin N Am.* 2009;20(4):627-656.)

clinical examination components (skin examination, pulse examination, auscultation of bruits) to ABI, duplex, or angiography in order to assess the accuracy and precision of the clinical examination for PAD.[58] The examiners concluded that absence of claudication did not reduce the likelihood of PAD, although the presence of claudication increased the likelihood of PAD. As previously discussed, a relatively small percentage of patients with PAD have claudication; therefore, the absence of complaints of claudication should not be used to rule out a diagnosis of PAD or to make a decision not to continue with a vascular examination. A limb that is cooler to the touch than the opposite limb, discolored skin, and wounds or sores all increase the likelihood of PAD, but the absence of these factors, with the exception of normal skin color, does not lessen the likelihood of PAD. Therefore, presence of cooler temperature, skin discoloration, and wounds or sores may help the clinician hypothesize about the likelihood of PAD given the risk factors and the rest of the examination, but again, absence of these factors should not rule out PAD for the clinician, especially if risk factors are present. Reduced or absent femoral, posterior tibial, or dorsalis pedis pulse increases the likelihood of PAD at least moderately, and the absence of any pulse abnormality decreases the likelihood of PAD at least moderately.[58] Abnormal CRT

is associated with moderate to severe PAD, but not in those with diabetes.[58] When individual clinical examination findings were combined, if all were normal, likelihood of PAD was lower than if one or more individual findings were abnormal. It has been suggested that in the absence of any risk factors for PAD, if clinical examination findings are all normal, no further testing is required.[67]

Medical Diagnosis

Peripheral Arterial Disease

In most cases, patients with PAD can be accurately diagnosed with noninvasive diagnostic techniques. As previously discussed, ABI is helpful in the diagnosis of PAD, and this may be measured in a vascular lab setting as part of a formal diagnostic work-up or for surveillance. Toe pressures and toe-brachial index (TBI) may be useful in patients with diabetes, renal failure, or other disorders resulting in arterial calcification, as they provide an accurate measurement of pressures in vessels that do not typically become calcified.[2,3] The toe pressure is normally ~30 mm Hg less than the ankle pressure, and an abnormal TBI is <0.70.[3] A specialized cuff is required to measure TBI, usually in a noninvasive vascular laboratory.[3]

Segmental limb pressures (SLPs) are measured throughout the LE in the same method as at the ankle. A sphygmomanometer cuff and Doppler probe are used to measure systolic pressures at different levels of the thigh and calf, and location of lesions are isolated by pressure gradients between different levels.[3] Pulse volume recordings (PVRs) use a cuff inflated to ~60 to 65 mm Hg (to detect volume changes without occluding the arteries), connected to a plethysmograph, which detects and records changes in limb volume throughout the arterial pulse cycle.[3] Amplitude of the waveform will decrease with severity of PAD within the same patient. Tracings should not be compared between patients, as individual cardiac and peripheral vascular factors affect the amplitude of PVR tracings. These may be used to establish diagnosis, localize occlusions and severity, and follow change over time after revascularization procedures within the same patient.[2] SLPs and PVRs are often used together, which increases accuracy and ensures that patients with calcified arteries who may have elevated SLP will be appropriately recognized by PVRs.[3]

If further anatomic localization of the lesion is necessary beyond information provided by the previously mentioned noninvasive tests, in order to make definitive decisions regarding intervention, duplex ultrasonography, magnetic resonance angiography (MRA), computed tomography angiography, or contrast angiography may be completed, depending on availability, cost, and skill. Contrast angiography, with visualization from the level of the renal arteries to the pedal arteries, remains the gold-standard imaging technique for PAD. This is an invasive evaluation with contrast, and despite the risks and its invasive nature, remains the evaluation of choice in many cases.[3] Intervention may be completed during angiography in some cases (eg, during acute ischemia).

Chronic Venous Disease

On clinical examination, LE edema and pigmentation or other skin changes support the diagnosis of CVD in absence of systemic causes of venous hypertension. In order to plan an intervention, the anatomic site of reflux needs to be identified, and venous duplex scanning is best for this purpose.[31] The Society for Vascular Surgery and the American Venous Forum (SVS/AVF) recommends duplex scanning of the deep and superficial veins of the LEs in all patients with chronic disease. In this examination, pulsed-wave Doppler transducers are used to evaluate reflux in the deep and superficial veins with the patient standing. All deep veins of the leg are examined from the inguinal region distally in 3 to 5 cm intervals, followed by the superficial veins. Four components are included in a venous duplex study: (1) visibility, (2) compressibility, (3) venous flow, including duration of reflux, and (4) augmentation. Operational definitions of reflux, pathologic veins, and valvular incompetence are discussed in the *Clinical Practice Guidelines*.[1] The SVS/AVF recommends that venous air plethysmography be used in patients with advanced CVD (CEAP classes 3 to 6) if duplex scanning does not elicit definitive pathophysiology. Air plethysmography measures passive venous refill and drainage, and

outflow, which can isolate impairments in the calf muscle pump, reflux, and venous obstruction.[1] In patients with more advanced CVD, computed tomography venography, magnetic resonance venography, ascending and descending contrast venography, and intravascular ultrasonography may be used as appropriate.[1]

TREATMENT

Medical and physical therapy interventions for PAD and CVD are discussed together in this section. Evidence-based physical therapy interventions for PAD may include patient education for cardiovascular risk reduction, skin and wound care, and exercise prescription. In CVD, the PT is paramount in the areas of education regarding skin and wound care, exercise prescription, and compression.

Peripheral Arterial Disease

Cardiovascular Risk Reduction

As previously discussed, PAD shares several risk factors with cardiovascular disease, and therefore a strong emphasis is placed on reduction of cardiovascular risk factors in the treatment of PAD. These may include pharmacotherapy aimed at controlling lipids; hypertension; risk of thrombosis; and interventions aimed at reducing obesity, smoking cessation, and diabetes management.

The ACC/AHA recommends that for patients with PAD who are hypertensive, antihypertensives should be given to maintain systolic BP less than 140 mm Hg for those without diabetes, and less than 130 mm Hg for those with diabetes or chronic renal disease. Patients with PAD may require multiple agents to control hypertension.[2,3]

Antiplatelet therapy, including aspirin, and/or clopidogrel, is recommended for patients with atherosclerotic LE PAD,[2,3] and combination therapy may be used for patients with symptomatic atherosclerotic PAD.[4]

The aim of glucose control in patients with diabetes and PAD is to maintain the hemoglobin A_{1C} below 7%.[2,3]

Patients with PAD who smoke should be asked about tobacco use, counseled to stop smoking, and assisted in developing a plan to quit, which may include pharmacotherapy and/or referral to a formal smoking cessation program.[2-4] A recent study found that long-term smokers with PAD who were randomly assigned to an intensive formal smoking cessation intervention were significantly more likely to be confirmed abstinent at 6 months than those assigned to minimal care (verbal advice and a list of community resources).[68]

The PT's role in cardiovascular risk reduction in this population is paramount. The PT may be the health care professional with whom the patient has the most frequent contact and therefore has access to the patient for monitoring and frequent reassessment. The PT should incorporate patient education regarding the importance of medication compliance, smoking cessation, healthy nutrition, and

TABLE 7-5. CLAUDICATION PAIN RATING SCALE

PAIN RATING	DESCRIPTION
1	Definite discomfort or pain, but only at initial or models levels (established, but minimal)
2	Moderate discomfort or pain from which the patient's attention can be diverted (eg, by conversation)
3	Intense pain (short of grade 4) from which the patient's attention cannot be diverted
4	Excruciating and unbearable pain

Reprinted with permission from Pescatello LS, Arena R, Riebe D, Thompson PD, eds. *ACSM's Guidelines for Exercise Testing and Prescription.* 9th ed. Baltimore, MD: Wolters Kluwer/Lippincott Williams & Wilkins; 2014.

meticulous skin care. Any barriers to cardiovascular risk reduction in these areas should be identified and addressed (eg, impaired vision affecting medication management and skin care). Consults should be mobilized as appropriate and may include that for smoking cessation, to a nutritionist, or for appropriate footwear (eg, referral to a pedorthist for custom footwear).

A recent study of 391 patients with PAD from a Canadian urban academic teaching hospital examined the extent to which risk factors were managed according to the AHA/ACC guidelines for PAD. Only 37.4% of those patients in the study with hypertension had adequate BP control, 49% of patients with diabetes had adequate glucose control, and 38.7% of those prescribed statins did not have adequate cholesterol control. The authors concluded that, although atherosclerotic risk factors are prevalent in patients with PAD, many patients receive suboptimal risk reduction treatments and/or are not meeting risk factor control goals with treatment.[69] The goal of these interventions is to reduce the risk of cardiovascular events in individuals with atherosclerotic LE PAD, and effective strategies to encourage adherence to established guidelines need to be developed.[69]

Exercise

Little is known about the effects of exercise in patients with asymptomatic PAD.[70] However, in patients with IC, there is much evidence to support the benefits of supervised exercise programs in improving maximum and pain-free walking distance.[71] Efficacy of unsupervised exercise programs is less extensively studied; however, in 2 recent studies, one found that a supervised exercise program was superior to a home-based program in terms of walking times,[72] and the other study found no significant difference in terms of walking times between home-based and supervised exercise programs.[73] A Cochrane review from 2008 found a significantly greater benefit of an exercise program in terms of maximum walking time than that seen with angioplasty at 6 months.[74]

The mechanisms by which exercise may improve walking distances and times for patients with claudication are not fully understood at this point, but may include the following:

- Improved endothelial vasodilator responses[75-77]
- Improved peripheral blood flow.[75,78,79] Improvements in blood flow, when identified, have not correlated with improved functional parameters (eg, walking distance) with exercise.[70,76]
- Improved mitochondrial function and muscle characteristics (cross-sectional area and fiber type)[76]
- Suppression of chronic inflammation[76]
- Adaptation in pain threshold with exercise[80]
- An increase in stroke volume and decrease in peripheral resistance during exercise[80]

Central mechanisms have been postulated given improvements in walking performance through an upper extremity aerobic exercise program.[80,81]

Evidence suggests that patients who can safely exercise should partake in programs that include walking for 30 to 50 minutes 3 to 5 times per week. Patients should walk at an intensity that elicits symptoms within 3 to 5 minutes, continue to walk at moderate intensity, and stop if symptoms become severe on the Claudication Pain Rating scale (Table 7-5).[66,71] Duration of a supervised program should be at least 12 weeks in order to ensure increases in maximum and pain-free walking distance.[3]

Although patients with IC often present with comorbidities that may limit exercise tolerance, they often do not preclude participation in a safe and effective exercise program. In this case, many patients would not only be appropriate candidates for an exercise program, but in fact would significantly benefit from one. The PT should prescribe an exercise program individualized to the patient and consider the patient's goals, comorbidities, and response to exercise. In many cases, interval walking would be indicated with the goal of 30 to 50 minutes of work-rest cycles per session, as many patients would not tolerate constant walking for this duration. After completion of a supervised walking program, strategies to enhance long-term adherence with a home walking program should be incorporated.[82]

It should be noted that, in patients with arterial compromise, elevation may further impede flow and symptoms may be worsened with elevation of the LEs. Therefore, elevation of the extremities should be discouraged. In fact, dependency of extremities affected by PAD may help to alleviate symptoms.

In the case of an arterial wound on the weightbearing surface of the foot, discussion with the vascular team is important to determine the best approach to offloading the wound during activity. Offloading the area of a diabetic ulceration,[83] caused by excessive pressure in combination with arterial insufficiency, usually results in healing.[83] For many patients with PAD, impairments associated with significant comorbidities may make it difficult to ambulate safely in a nonweightbearing fashion, even with assistance and an assistive device. For some patients, bed to wheelchair transfers and wheelchair locomotion may be the best option while the wound is healing. Other options for pressure relief may be considered, depending on availability and feasibility. Armstrong et al[84] found that the total contact cast (TCC) heals more wounds more quickly than a half-shoe or a removable cast walker (RCW) and is considered by many the gold standard of offloading devices.[85] However, a technician with specific training or experience should apply any TCC because improper application can lead to further ulceration. Assessment and care of the wound on a daily basis is not possible, and patients may find bathing and sleeping difficult in a TCC. For these reasons, TCCs are not routinely used.[84,85] Other offloading devices have been used for pressure relief; however, they have demonstrated limited success in adequately offloading diabetic wounds. Armstrong et al[86] found that, although patients with diabetic wounds were more active while wearing an RCW, only 28% of daily activity occurred while subjects wore the device. This indicates that compliance with RCW wear for offloading the diabetic ulcer is low. More recently, it has been shown that making the RCW nonremovable (for example wrapping it with a cohesive bandage or plaster) forces adherence to pressure reduction, and both proportion and rate of wound healing were significantly improved.[87,88] If these pressure-relieving devices are not feasible or are unavailable, the best approach is nonweightbearing on the sole of the foot with the ulcer, if possible, to allow for wound healing. The PT needs to consider balancing the risk of limiting mobility in a patient with multiple comorbidities and at significant risk of deconditioning, with the risk of infection, necrosis, and amputation from a nonhealing ulcer on the sole of the foot.

The PT should consider that patients on bed rest because of CLI, those undergoing limb salvage procedures, and/or those who may undergo an amputation may have significant vascular compromise throughout the body and/or several comorbidities that have already led to a progressive decline in aerobic capacity, muscle performance, and baseline function.[89] The PT should intervene during efforts at limb salvage procedures in anticipation that, after a period of decreased mobility, with or without amputation, the patient will need to mobilize. The PT should consider an exercise prescription that will result in maximum aerobic capacity, muscle performance, and range of motion. Close communication with the vascular team may be warranted, and the PT should ensure that O_2 demand in the already ischemic extremity is not increased and that the patient is not being put at risk through exercise intervention.

A return to independent ambulation is a major challenge to the population postamputation. All levels of amputation, from transmetatarsal or transfemoral, place increasing demands on the proximal limb and increase energy demands centrally. These demands increase as the level of amputation becomes more proximal.[89] O_2 consumption during ambulation at 1.24 miles per hour (2 km per hour) for patients post-unilateral transtibial and transfemoral amputations is 123% and 155%, respectively; that of the patient without a LE amputation. Use of assistive devices in this population increases O_2 consumption as compared to ambulation without an assistive device.[90] If the patient undergoes an amputation, mobility will require greater energy expenditure than at baseline, and the patient will have lost sufficient strength and aerobic capacity without intervention in the meantime.

Some patients may not return to independent ambulation after LE amputation but may mobilize in a wheelchair. This may be the case for many patients' status post-bilateral transfemoral amputations given that the O_2 costs of prosthetic ambulation with various assistive devices is significantly greater than that of independent wheelchair propulsion or mobility without amputation.[91,92] Self-paced wheelchair propulsion is significantly faster than self-paced prosthetic ambulation in this population, and for these patients, wheelchair propulsion may simply be more feasible and functional, making it the preference for locomotion.[92]

Skin and Wound Care

As previously discussed, meticulous skin hygiene and monitoring is encouraged in every patient with PAD given the risk of wounds and infection and the potential for impairments in sensation. Any wound, no matter how small, should be addressed urgently.[2] The PT should consistently educate the patient in this area, determine barriers to compliance, and monitor the skin for changes. Discussion regarding appropriate wound care for arterial ulcers is beyond the scope of this chapter and should be deferred to a wound care specialist.

Pharmacotherapy

Pharmacotherapy for Claudication

Treatments aimed at reduction of cardiovascular risk factors to prevent cardiovascular events associated with atherosclerosis will not significantly decrease claudication symptoms. Drugs aimed at decreasing the pain of claudication are separate from those used to decrease cardiovascular risk.[3] The ACC/AHA and TASC II working group recommends cilostazol to improve symptoms and walking distance in patients with IC associated with PAD. Cilostazol is a phosphodiesterase III inhibitor with vasodilatory, metabolic, and antiplatelet effects, and is the most evidence-based drug and the main pharmacologic agent currently used for IC in patients with PAD.[3,13] This medication should not be used for patients with heart failure.[2] Pentoxifylline, a methylxanthine derivative that has antiplatelet effects and lowers fibrinogen levels, may be considered as a second-line alternative to cilostazol. However, its clinical effectiveness is not established.[2,13]

Pharmacotherapy for Critical Limb Ischemia

In patients with CLI, when revascularization has failed or is not an option, pharmacotherapy that may produce improvements in circulation, with the goal of overcoming severely reduced perfusion to the distal microcirculation, may be considered.[3] Treatment with prostanoids, such as prostaglandin E-1 or iloprost, may be considered to reduce ischemic pain and facilitate ulcer healing.[2] These drugs prevent platelet and leukocyte activation and protect the vascular endothelium.[3]

Revascularization

Recall that in most cases, claudication does not progress to limb-threatening ischemia; therefore, surgery is generally reserved for those patients whose symptoms are lifestyle limiting, unresponsive to exercise, and/or pharmacotherapy, with a reasonable symptomatic and medical prognosis.[2]

On the other hand, without timely revascularization, CLI may result in loss of limb or death.[93] For example, in the case of ALI, surgical revascularization may be indicated in a threatened limb or in limbs with dramatic motor and sensory deficits of short duration (hours)[2,3] in order to prevent worsening of limb ischemia. CLI is commonly associated with multilevel disease and secondary to chronic impaired perfusion,[94] and revascularization may be considered if signs of CLI are present or if there is a nonhealing neuroischemic ulcer despite optimum conservative management. The primary goal of revascularization is limb salvage or amputation-free survival[3] through reestablishing pulsatile flow to the distal extremity.[93] A successful revascularization would result in a pain-free, functional extremity.[3]

Several factors will determine the surgical option chosen (ie, endovascular or open surgical procedures), including the premorbid condition of the patient and the extremity, expected durability of the reconstruction, adequate aortoiliac flow (inflow), anatomy of an occlusion, contraindications, and local practice.[2,3] Intervention for proper aortoiliac flow (inflow) may be ensured prior to intervening on the more distal stenosis, and, in some cases, this is sufficient to heal superficial ulcers or resting claudication[94] without further intervention. Endovascular procedures for aortoiliac occlusive disease have been associated with significantly lower complication rates, shorter length of stay, and lower hospital costs[95] than open procedures. The approach for an endovascular procedure is commonly through the common femoral artery, or, if needed, through the brachial artery. In both of these cases, the site can be easily compressed following catheter removal, minimizing postprocedural complications.[94] Open procedures include several types of bypass surgeries, with nomenclature indicating the area of the arterial tree that is blocked and therefore bypassed in the procedure. For example, a femoral popliteal bypass (commonly called *fem-pop*) bypasses the blocked portion of the femoral artery through open visualization of the femoral artery, and a graft using blood vessels or synthetic materials is attached above the blockage at the femoral artery and below the blockage at the popliteal artery. The majority of limb salvage surgery addresses the outflow circulation or that distal to the aortoiliac tree, which is the femoral popliteal circulation.[94] After revascularization, limb salvage procedures may take place that may involve wound débridement or amputation of parts of the foot once demarcation occurs, with the goal of salvaging some or all of the foot.

Catheter-based pharmacologic endovascular thrombolysis is often the treatment for ALI, and balloon embolectomy or angioplasty may also be considered.[2,3] Percutaneous aspiration thrombectomy (uses catheters and suction with a syringe to remove emboli or thrombi) and percutaneous mechanical thrombectomy (devices trap, dissolve, and evacuate thrombi) are other endovascular procedures that may be used in conjunction with pharmacologic thrombolysis to speed up clot lysis, especially when time to revascularization is critical.[2,3] Data from randomized studies in patients with ALI suggest that catheter-directed thrombolysis results in lower mortality and less complex surgical procedures and may reduce risk of reperfusion injury compared with open surgery.

Major amputation (above the ankle) may be required when life-threatening infection sets in, resting pain is uncontrolled, or necrosis has made the foot nonviable.[3] Given the severity of these end-stage issues, incidence of major amputations is limited. For some patients with CLI (eg, those who are very high risk for surgery)[3] or who have necrosis of the weightbearing portions of the foot, irreversible contracture, irreversible loss of function in the limb, uncontrolled ischemic resting pain despite pharmacologic management, sepsis, or very limited life expectancy,[2] primary amputation may be required. Secondary amputation may be required when revascularization is no longer possible or the limb continues to deteriorate despite what appears to be a patent revascularization.[3] Incidence of major LE amputation in ALI is up to 25%, and the site of amputation is often more proximal than that in CLI as the muscles of the calf are often not viable. The primary goal of amputation is to obtain primary LE healing as distally as possible; therefore, the site of amputation is chosen based on the lowest level of transaction at which healing is expected to occur.[3]

Other Treatments

Most notably, stem cell therapy for CLI is emerging in the research, with publication of first results in 2011. This therapy may be a useful adjunct to current therapies and is an option for patients with CLI who are not appropriate for revascularization. Further research is needed with more rigorous methodology to confirm current encouraging literature in terms of safety and clinical outcomes such as improved pain, decreased incidence of major amputation, improvement of ABI, and transcutaneous partial pressure of O_2.[96-100] Intermittent mechanical calf compression has been recently studied as an intervention for claudication as compared with medical therapy alone. Significantly increased claudication distance and postexercise ABI were found at 1 month and maintained or further improved at 3 months. Postexercise ABI remained stable 3 months after discontinuation of therapy.[101] Further research is required in this area, and one should refer to the discussion around cautious use of compression in patients with PAD, found in the compression section for treatment of CVD next. A Cochrane review concluded that, in patients with diabetic arterial ulcers, hyperbaric O_2 significantly decreased the risk of major amputation; however, methodological shortcomings of the included studies were noted and further research is required.[102]

Chronic Venous Disease

Treatment of venous disease is aimed at ameliorating symptoms of the disease and/or improving the cosmetic appearance of the limbs. The initial treatment of CVD is conservative and consists of skin care, elevation, exercise, and compression. The PT can be instrumental in all of these areas. Pharmacologic management, surgery, and wound care are reserved for situations where patients remain symptomatic despite more conservative measures.

Skin and Wound Care

Patients with CVD are at significant risk of wounds and infections. The PT should incorporate education regarding skin and wound care into the plan of care for every patient with CVD, and barriers to learning or compliance should be identified and addressed. An important goal for these patients is to maintain skin integrity, thereby avoiding ulceration and infection. It is important to keep areas affected by venous insufficiency clean and well moisturized daily to maintain skin health and avoid itching, thereby avoiding the chance of trauma to the skin caused by scratching. Any areas of compromise, including redness or open areas, no matter how small, should be addressed by a health care professional as soon as possible. Treatment of infection (only if present), compression, and meticulous wound care are the mainstays of treatment for venous ulceration.[1,32] Discussion of appropriate wound care for venous ulceration is beyond the scope of this chapter and should be deferred to a wound care specialist.

Compression

The use of compression is a mainstay of treatment for CVD, and its mechanism of action, although not fully understood, is direct compensation for ambulatory venous hypertension.[1] Buhs et al[103] found that 20 to 30 mm Hg thigh-high compression garments help preserve venous caliber and prevent dilation in the deep, superficial, and perforating venous system of the LEs during daily activities. Ibegbuna et al[104] found that Class II compression garments significantly improved venous dynamics by reducing residual volume fraction in patients with CVD during walking. There are several kinds of ambulatory compression, including multilayer short stretch wraps, elastic or nonelastic compression garments, impregnated paste gauze wraps (Unna boots), and pneumatic compression devices. There are several options available for patients who have difficulty donning or doffing the garment, including donning devices or custom-fitted stockings with Velcro or zippers, which, unfortunately, are significantly more expensive than off-the-shelf garments. Despite numerous compression options available, compliance with high-grade compression (> 30 mm Hg) is poor, and in some cases, one must consider lower levels of compression in order to achieve compliance[105,106]; it is likely that some compression is better than none. Appropriate tension of elastic compression is disputed in the literature; however, the SVS/AVF recommends graded prescription stockings with an ankle pressure of 20 to 30 mm Hg (Class I) for patients with varicose veins. The SVS/AVF recommends compression as the primary treatment for venous ulcers, and evidence suggests that compression of 30 to 40 mm Hg is more effective than lower levels of compression at enhancing ulcer healing and preventing ulcer recurrence.[1,32,107] It has been proven that venous ulcers heal more quickly with compression than without.[108] Once ulcer healing is achieved, lifelong compression may be recommended to prevent recurrence.[52] In a recent Cochrane Review,[106] noncompliance with compression was associated with ulcer recurrence.

Although there is no convincing evidence that intermittent pneumatic compression improves ulcer healing when compared to continuous compression or when added to compression garment use,[109] these devices may be helpful for patients for whom compression garments are not tolerated or not feasible. These devices consist of an air pump to intermittently inflate/deflate single or multiple bladders in nylon sleeves that envelope the limb, either to knee or hip height.[109] Medicare and Medicaid will cover pneumatic compression for patients with CVD who have refractory venous ulcers after 6 months of conservative treatment, including compression, wound care, exercise, and elevation.[110]

Prescription of compression for venous disease should be performed only by health care professionals with appropriate skills and training because several complications of inappropriately measured or applied garments have been reported.[1,111] Some PTs are trained and skilled in this area and will provide effective compression management, whereas others will mobilize a referral to a local certified lymphedema therapist or wound care clinic. Compression should not be provided in the presence of cellulitis until symptoms of the infection, specifically pain and erythema, have subsided.[112] Every patient for whom compression is considered should be clinically examined for signs of arterial insufficiency, and, if found, consideration of further testing to rule out moderate to severe arterial insufficiency may be prudent. Compression should be used only with caution and meticulous monitoring in patients with arterial disease, as the application of external compression at high pressures will reduce blood supply to the skin and may lead to damage.[53,108] Compression should be combined with leg exercises and walking as activation of the calf muscle pump is more effective with compression during activity.[104] For this reason, adherence to compression and development of a compression plan of care that is comfortable and feasible for each patient is paramount. Any patient undergoing compression management should be closely monitored and educated regarding donning and doffing, situations that would warrant immediate discontinuation of compression and consultation with a health care professional, care of compression garments, and when and how to obtain new garments. Stockings should be replaced every 6 to 12 months with daily wear to avoid loss of pressure.[31,53]

Elevation and Exercise

The literature concerning the appropriate exercise prescription for patients with CVD is much less advanced or definitive than that for exercise in patients with PAD. It is a common theme in the literature, however, that patients should be counseled in weight loss, exercise, and elevation of the legs as much as possible.[1,54] The PT should consider appropriate patient education and exercise prescription for all patients with CVD.

Leg elevation, with ankles at or above the level of the heart, improves venous blood flow compared with dependency of the legs, thereby directly counteracting venous hypertension experienced by patients with CVD in the dependent position. In one study, leg elevation 30 cm above the heart significantly increased the blood flow velocity by 41% in liposclerotic skin of patients with CVI.[113] Another study[114] found that elevation above the level of the heart at least 1 hour per day for 6 or more days per week in Class II (20 to 30 mm Hg) or Class III (30 to 40 mm Hg) compression was significantly associated with a lower risk of venous ulcer recurrence. Although elevation of this level may be difficult for some patients given musculoskeletal comorbidities (eg, back pain or hip osteoarthritis), patients should be strongly advised to avoid dependency whenever possible, elevating the ankles at least to slightly above the level of the hip, which would allow gravity to assist in venous drainage centrally. Working on positioning strategies for patients with discomfort with leg elevation should be routinely incorporated into the plan of care. For patients for whom prolonged or frequent elevation is not practical given the nature of their work, short periods of elevation throughout the day may also be beneficial.

As previously discussed, an impaired calf muscle pump can significantly contribute to development of LE edema and other symptoms of CVD.[115] The goal of exercise in CVD is to improve the calf muscle function and the pressures generated by the LE skeletal muscle pump. Studies have found that patients with CVD have a significant impairment of calf muscle function when compared to healthy controls. There are impairments of peak torque/body weight (strength) and total work (endurance)[116] and in ulcerated limbs secondary to venous insufficiency, significantly poorer ejection fractions, and greater residual volume fractions than in limbs with healed ulcers or no history of ulceration.[117]

Patients with leg ulcers have reported low levels of physical activity. In one study of self-reported physical activity in 150 patients with leg ulcers secondary to venous insufficiency, only 13% of patients reported that they walked for 30 minutes or more at least 5 days of the week. Thirty-five percent of patients reported that they had not walked for 10 minutes at least once the week prior to the interview, and only 35% of patients reported that they performed exercises for the lower legs.[115] It is difficult to know whether a sedentary lifestyle has led to progression of venous disease in these individuals or whether the symptoms of venous disease have led to avoidance of activity. In one study, 83% of subjects with a leg ulcer avoided movements or activities based on fear, and patients with low reported physical activity had significantly stronger fear-avoidance beliefs and more severe pain than those with high reported physical activity.[118] These findings speak to the importance of patient education surrounding the benefits of exercise and compression in CVD, and addressing the individual fear-avoidance beliefs of each patient as appropriate.

In the few studies that have examined the effects of exercise in patients with CVD, calf muscle pump function and muscle strength and endurance have improved significantly with exercise. Kan and Delis[119] conducted a study comparing an exercise program of supervised isotonic calf muscle exercise consisting of plantarflexion against a 4-kg resistance for 3 sets of 6 minutes daily (number of repetitions started with 75% of the maximal number of repetitions reached at baseline during 6 minutes at 1 repetition/second), with a 5-minute rest in between, for 7 consecutive days. Both the exercise and the control group received ulcer dressings and compression bandaging. After 7 days, patients in the exercise group showed significantly improved ejected venous volume and ejection fraction in the calf compared with the control group. Calf muscular endurance in the exercise group increased significantly by 135%. This was a small study (exercise group $n = 10$, control group $n = 11$) lacking power, and the significance of the changes is surprising given the duration of the program; however, statistical significance was reached, and the results of this study are promising and certainly warrant more stringent research in this area.

In another study,[120] 31 patients with CVD were randomized into control and exercise groups, and all subjects were treated with compression garments. The exercise group received 3 months of supervised exercise, followed by 3 months of unsupervised exercise. The exercise program was designed by a PT, individualized for each patient, and included lower limb and trunk stretching and strengthening with resisted exercises 2 days per week, progressing in repetitions, sets, and resistance throughout the 3 months. Inclined treadmill walking was incorporated in each session of the supervised component, and subjects were encouraged to continue uphill walking and were taught the principles of exercise progression to continue during the unsupervised component of the exercise program. It should be noted that comorbid conditions were frequent in this study and included obesity, coronary heart disease, heart failure, angina, hypertension, dyspnea, asthma, diabetes, arthritis, and DVT. Despite these multiple comorbidities, compliance to the exercise regimen was good (mean 18 ± 1.6 days out of 22 sessions for the supervised phase, and 63 ± 7.3 days out of a possible 90 days). It should also be noted that reported compliance with compression (Class II: 30 to 40 mm Hg) was excellent in this study, with 89% of patients wearing their compression garments for 6.24 days per week. This rate of compliance is very high as compared to other studies but was not further discussed by the authors. Both calf muscle function (residual volume fraction and ejection fraction) and strength improved significantly in the exercise group as compared with the control group after exercise intervention; however, there were no changes observed in quality of life or disease severity. Again, this study lacked power given its sample size, but the findings were statistically significant and warrant further research in this area. As would be expected, in both of these studies, the amount of venous reflux, which reflects the state of the venous valves, remained unchanged after the exercise intervention. Physiologic change is not a goal of exercise intervention in the population with CVD.

Back et al[121] found that ankle range of motion was significantly lower in patients with CVD as compared to that in age-matched controls, and ankle range of motion was significantly correlated to calf muscle ejection fraction, residual volume fraction, and clinical severity of CVD. Although there are no studies examining the effects of an intervention to improve ankle range of motion in this population, given these findings, any impairment in ankle range of motion in this population should likely be addressed.

Given the lack of strong literature in this area, limited recommendations regarding exercise prescription in the population with CVD can be made. It seems as though a combination of exercises aimed at strength and endurance of calf musculature would be best, including some resistance training, stretching, and endurance training through walking. Compression in conjunction with activity should be prescribed and encouraged throughout treatment. Recommended intensity, frequency, and duration of programs are not clear in this population; however, consideration of each patient's impairments, and the literature surrounding exercise and comorbidities (eg, heart failure, osteoarthritis) in that population would be warranted. Best care for exercise prescription, development of plans for effective and feasible compression regimens, and determinants for adherence to compression and exercise in the population with CVD are all areas in the literature that require more development.

Pharmacology

There are several venoactive drugs used in CVI; some for symptom relief, some for acceleration of healing of venous ulcers. Although the precise mechanism of action is unknown, the main principle of these drugs is to improve venous tone and capillary permeability.[31] The SVS/AVF[1] recommends the use of venoactive drugs together with compression for symptomatic CVD, and pentoxifylline or micronized purified flavonoid fraction together with compression to accelerate venous ulcer healing. There has been much discussion in the literature concerning use of horse-chestnut seed extract (HCSE). A recent Cochrane review[122] suggests that HCSE is a safe and effective short-term treatment for CVD; however, it recommends that stronger literature is required to confirm its effectiveness. These findings are consistent with those of other studies on the use of HSCE in CVD.[123-126] The consensus exists in the literature that larger and more rigorous clinical trials are needed to improve existing recommendations surrounding the pharmacological treatment of CVD.[127]

Surgery

Surgery for varicose veins is generally reserved for patients who require symptomatic relief.[54] For those requiring surgery, open surgical treatment of varicose veins with venous ligation and stripping of the great or small saphenous veins and excision of large varicose veins has been the mainstay of treatment for more than 100 years. Other less invasive surgery for varicose veins includes phlebectomy, or removal or avulsion of varicosities through small wounds. Results of open surgery have continued to improve, and open surgery continues to be considered safe and effective. In the last 10 years, use of minimally invasive endovenous thermal ablation (EVTA) has dramatically increased, and open surgery has been used less in the United States.[1] EVTA includes endovenous laser ablation and radiofrequency ablation. Ablation, or occlusion, of the varicose vein is accomplished in both cases by causing direct thermal damage to the venous wall by applying heat directly into the vein through a percutaneously applied catheter. This may be performed as an outpatient procedure under ultrasound guidance using percutaneous catheters. Patients have less pain and can return to regular activities faster than with an open surgical procedure.[1] Patient selection for EVTA or open surgery is important, as some patients may not be appropriate for endovenous procedures (eg, those with irreversible coagulopathy, liver dysfunction limiting local anesthetic use, immobility, pregnancy, and breastfeeding).[1] In any surgical procedure for varicose veins, an external compression dressing, usually with an elastic wrap, is applied and will be left in place for 48 to 72 hours, and elevation should be encouraged. Often, graded compression stockings are applied after removal of the primary dressing.[54] Sclerotherapy, or chemical injection into a vein to achieve fibrotic obstruction, may be used to treat superficial varicose veins, residual or recurring varicose veins following surgery, and for thread (spider) veins.[128] There is a chance of recurrence after any treatment for varicosities, and this depends on the severity of the initial varicosities and on the treatment used.[54]

SUMMARY

The prevalence of PVD is high, affecting millions of Americans. Patients with PAD and CVD experience high morbidity and decreased quality of life, and those with PAD are at significantly greater risk of cardiovascular events and death than age-matched norms. The cost associated with treating these diseases is high, including the cost in loss of work hours and emotional suffering incurred by patients. Given the prevalence, impact, and costs associated with PVD, it is imperative that the PT be able to effectively examine for, diagnose, and provide evidence-based interventions for clients presenting with these diseases.

An understanding of the risk factors for, pathophysiology of, and clinical presentation of PAD and CVD can guide the

PT to appropriately examine and diagnose each of these diseases. A comprehensive social history is imperative to reveal risk factors, clarify symptoms, determine the affect on the patient's life, and elicit each patient's goals of treatment.

With consideration of the patient's subjective history and risk factors elicited, as well as any findings in the integumentary examination, the PT can determine whether vascular tests and measures are warranted. A careful clinical examination may result in confirmation of a diagnosis of PAD (eg, by ABI measurement) or may identify those patients at risk and/or requiring further vascular testing to diagnose PAD or CVD. In both cases, the PT can, from the literature, determine best physical therapy intervention for the patient.

The PT's role in educating patients with PAD and CVD is paramount in the areas of risk factor management and skin care. Skin and wound care is extremely important in both populations, and the PT who is trained and experienced in compression management may dramatically affect the care of patients with CVD.

The literature supporting exercise prescription for patients with PAD and CVD continues to evolv, and is more advanced for patients with PAD. Further research is required to determine the best intensity, frequency, type, and duration of exercise for patients with CVD. It is imperative that the PT apply current literature to the exercise prescription for patients with both PAD and CVD in order to develop individualized programs of sufficient intensity and frequency to elicit change.

Although a vast number of patients with PAD and CVD have comorbidities that may limit exercise tolerance, they do not usually preclude the patient from participating in a safe and effective program. Any patient with PVD who can safely exercise should be given an individualized exercise program.

Additional considerations for the PT in this population may include appropriateness of weightbearing on a wound, O_2 demand of an ischemic extremity and exercise prescription, prognostication of energy demands during mobility in patients postamputation, and need for mobilization of referrals to other health care professionals.

PAD and CVD are lifelong diseases, and many of these patients have had symptoms for years while receiving inadequate education or intervention to manage their disease. Evidence shows that with effective intervention, patients can increase exercise tolerance, control signs and symptoms of the disease, and decrease risk of wounds and infection. These outcomes are often in concordance with the verbalized goals of these patients, and many interventions can be taught to the patient to encourage patient autonomy and lifelong compliance. An effective physical therapy outcome would be a patient independent with an appropriate exercise program and with clear knowledge of all physical therapy recommendations. The patient would understand that these diseases are lifelong and progressive and would value the need for prolonged adherence and immediate follow-up at the earliest sign of complications.

References

1. Gloviczki P, Comerota A, Dalsing M, et al. The care of patients with varicose veins and associated chronic venous diseases: Clinical practice guidelines of the Society for Vascular Surgery and the American Venous Forum. *J Vasc Surg.* 2011;53(5 Suppl):2S-48S.

2. Hirsch A, Haskal Z, Hertzer N, et al. ACC/AHA 2005 guidelines for the management of patients with peripheral arterial disease (lower extremity, renal, mesenteric, and abdominal aortic): executive summary a collaborative report from the American Association for Vascular Surgery/Society for Vascular Surgery, Society for Cardiovascular Angiography and Interventions, Society for Vascular Medicine and Biology, Society of Interventional Radiology, and the ACC/AHA Task Force on Practice Guidelines (Writing Committee to Develop Guidelines for the Management of Patients With Peripheral Arterial Disease) endorsed by the American Association of Cardiovascular and Pulmonary Rehabilitation; National Heart, Lung, and Blood Institute; Society for Vascular Nursing; TransAtlantic Inter-Society Consensus; and Vascular Disease Foundation. *J Am Coll Cardiol.* 2006;47(6):1239-1312.

3. Norgren L, Hiatt W, Dormandy J, Nehler M, Harris K, Fowkes FG. Inter-society consensus for the management of peripheral arterial disease (TASC II). *J Vasc Surg.* 2007;45(1 Suppl S):S5-S67.

4. Rooke T, Hirsch A, Misra S, et al. 2011 ACCF/AHA focused update of the guideline for the management of patients with peripheral artery disease (updating the 2005 guideline): a report of the American College of Cardiology Foundation/American Heart Association Task Force On Practice Guidelines: developed in collaboration with the Society for Vascular Medicine, and Society for Vascular Surgery. *J Vasc Surg.* 2011;54(5):e32-e58.

5. Goodman CC, Fuller KS. *Pathology: Implications for the Physical Therapist.* 3rd ed. St. Louis, MO: Saunders Elsevier; 2009.

6. Selvin E, Erlinger T. Prevalence of and risk factors for peripheral arterial disease in the United States: results from the National Health and Nutrition Examination Survey, 1999-2000. *Circulation.* 2004;110(6):738-743.

7. McDermott M, Greenland P, Liu K. Leg symptoms in peripheral arterial disease: associated clinical characteristics and functional impairment. *JAMA.* 2001;286:1599.

8. Hiatt W, Nawaz D, Brass E. Carnitine metabolism during exercise in patients with peripheral vascular disease. *J Appl Physiol (1985).* 1987;62:2384-2387.

9. Mukherjee D, Cho L. Peripheral arterial disease: considerations in risks, diagnosis, and treatment. *J Nat MedAssoc.* 2009;101(10):999-1008.

10. Hiatt W. Medical treatment of peripheral arterial disease and claudication. *N Engl J Med.* 2001;344(21):1608-1621.

11. Shammas NW. Epidemiology, classification, and modifiable risk factors of peripheral arterial disease. *Vasc Health Risk Manag.* 2007;3(2):229-234.

12. Spronk S, White J, Ryjewski C, Rosenblum J, Bosch JL, Hunink MG. Invasive treatment of claudication is indicated for patients unable to adequately ambulate during cardiac rehabilitation. *J Vasc Surg.* 2009;49(5):1217-1225.

13. Salameh MJ, Ratchford EV. Update on peripheral arterial disease and claudication rehabilitation. *Phys Med Rehabil Clin N Am.* 2009;20(4):627-656.

14. Wassell CL, Loomba R, Ix JH, Allison MA, Denenberg JO, Criqui MH. Family history of peripheral artery disease is associated with prevalence and severity of peripheral artery disease: the San Diego population study. *J Am Coll Cardiol.* 2011;58(13):1386-1392.

15. Wahlgren CM, Magnusson PK. Genetic influences on peripheral arterial disease in a twin population. *Arterioscler Thromb Vasc Biol.* 2011;31(3):678-682.

16. Wilson A, Sadrzadeh-Rafie A, Myers J, et al. Low lifetime recreational activity is a risk factor for peripheral arterial disease. *J Vasc Surg.* 2011;54(2):427-432.e1-e4.

17. Escobar C, Blanes I, Ruiz A, et al. Prevalence and clinical profile and management of peripheral arterial disease in elderly patients with diabetes. *Eur J Intern Med.* 2011;22(3):275-281.

18. Aponte J. The prevalence of asymptomatic and symptomatic peripheral arterial disease and peripheral arterial disease risk factors in the U.S. population. *Holist Nurs Pract.* 2011;25(3):147-161.

19. Subramaniam T, Nang E, Lim S, et al. Distribution of ankle-brachial index and the risk factors of peripheral artery disease in a multiethnic Asian population. *Vasc Med.* 2011;16(2):87-95.

20. Conen D, Everett BM, Kurth T, et al. Smoking, smoking cessation, [corrected] and risk for symptomatic peripheral artery disease in women: a cohort study. *Ann Intern Med.* 2011;154:719-726.

21. Schiller JS, Lucas JW, Ward BW, Peregoy JA. Summary health statistics for U.S. adults: National Health Interview Survey, 2010. *Vital Health Stat 10.* 2012;(252):1-207. http://www.cdc.gov/nchs/data/series/sr_10/sr10_252.pdf. Accessed May 15, 2014.

22. Gardner A, Clancy R. The relationship between ankle-brachial index and leisure-time physical activity in patients with intermittent claudication. *Angiology.* 2006;57:539-545.

23. McDermott M, Liu K, Ferrucci L, et al. Circulating blood markers and functional impairment in peripheral arterial disease. *J Am Geriatr Soc.* 2008;56:1504-1510.

24. Nylaende M, Kroese A, Stranden E, et al. Markers of vascular inflammation are associated with the extent of atherosclerosis assessed as angiographic score and treadmill walking distances in patients with peripheral arterial occlusive disease. *Vasc Med.* 2006;11:21-28.

25. Hooi JD, Stoffers HE, Knottnerus JA, van Ree JW. The prognosis of non-critical limb ischaemia: a systematic review of population-based evidence. *Br J Gen Pract.* 1999;49:49-55.

26. Criqui MH, Jamosmos M, Fronek A, et al. Chronic venous disease in an ethnically diverse population: the San Diego population study. *Am J Epidemiol.* 2003;158(5):448-456.

27. Zahariev T, Anastassov V, Girov K, et al. Prevalence of primary chronic venous disease: the Bulgarian experience. *Int Angiol.* 2009;28(4):303-310.

28. Evans CJ, Fowkes FG, Ruckley CV, Lee AJ. Prevalence of varicose veins and chronic venous insufficiency in men and women in the general population: Edinburgh Vein Study. *J Epidemiol Community Health.* 1999;53:149-154.

29. Bergan JJ, Schmid-Schönbein GW, Coleridge-Smith PD, Nicolaides AN, Boisseau MR, Eklöf B. Mechanisms of disease: chronic venous disease. *N Engl J Med.* 2006;355(5):488-498.

30. Alguire PC, Mathes BM. Chronic venous insufficiency and venous ulceration. *J Gen Intern Med.* 1997;12:374-383.

31. Eberhardt RT, Raffetto JD. Chronic venous insufficiency. *Circulation.* 2005;111:2398-2409.

32. Angle N, Bergan JJ. Chronic venous ulcer. *BMJ.* 1997;314(7086):1019-1023.

33. Chiesa R, Marone E, Limoni C, Volonte M, Petrini O. Chronic venous disorders: correlation between visible signs, symptoms, and presence of functional disease. *J Vasc Surg.* 2007;46(2):322-330.

34. Gourgou S, Dedieu F, Sancho-Garnier H. Lower limb venous insufficiency and tobacco smoking: a case-control study. *Am J Epidemiol.* 2002;155(11):1007-1015.

35. Fowkes FG, Lee AJ, Evans CJ, Allan PL, Bradbury AW, Ruckley CV. Lifestyle risk factors for lower limb venous reflux in the general population: Edinburgh Vein Study. *Int J Epidemiol.* 2001;30(4):846-852.

36. Willenberg T, Shumacher A, Amann-Vesti B, et al. Impact of obesity on venous hemodynamics of the lower limbs. *J Vasc Surg.* 2010;52(3):664-668.

37. Criqui M, Denenberg J, Bergan J, Langer R, Fronek A. Risk factors for chronic venous disease: the San Diego population study. *J Vasc Surg.* 2007;46(2):331-337.

38. Ashrani AA, Heit JA. Incidence and cost burden of post-thrombotic syndrome. *J Thromb Thrombolysis.* 2009;28(4):465-476.

39. Cushman M, Callas PW, Denenberg JO, Bovill EG, Criqui MH. Risk factors for peripheral venous disease resemble those for venous thrombosis: the San Diego population study. *J Thromb Haemost.* 2010;8(8):1730-1735.

40. Labropoulos N, Leon L, Kwon S, et al. Study of the venous reflux progression. *J Vasc Surg.* 2005;41(2):291-295.

41. Valencia I, Falabella A, Kirsner RS, Eaglstein WH. Chronic venous insufficiency and venous leg ulceration. *J Am Acad Dermatol.* 2001;44(3):401-421.

42. Nelzén O, Bergqvist D, Lindhagen A. Venous and non-venous leg ulcers: clinical history and appearance in a population study. *Br J Surg.* 1994;81(2):182-187.

43. Olin J, Beusterien K, Childs M, Seavey C, McHugh L, Griffiths R. Medical costs of treating venous stasis ulcers: evidence from a retrospective cohort study. *Vasc Med.* 1999;4(1):1-7.

44. Schonfeld WH, Villa KF, Fastenau JM, Mazonson PD, Falanga V. An economic assessment of Apligraf (Graftskin) for the treatment of hard-to-heal venous leg ulcers. *Wound Repair Regen.* 2000;8(4):251-257.

45. American Physical Therapy Association. *Guide to Physical Therapist Practice.* 2nd ed. Alexandria, VA: American Physical Therapy Association; 2003:738.

46. Remes L, Isoaho R, Vahlberg T, Viitanen M, Rautava P. Quality of life among lower extremity peripheral arterial disease patients who have undergone endovascular or surgical revascularization. *Eur J Vasc Endovasc Surg.* 2010;40(5):618-625.

47. Cherr G, Wang J, Zimmerman P, Dosluoglu H. Depression is associated with worse patency and recurrent leg symptoms after lower extremity revascularization. *J Vasc Surg.* 2007;45:744-750.

48. Hareendran A, Bradbury A, Budd J. Measuring the impact of venous leg ulcers on quality of life. *J Wound Care.* 2005;14(2):53-57.

49. Kurz X, Lamping D, Kahn S, et al. Do varicose veins affect quality of life? Results from an international population-based study. *J Vasc Surg.* 2001;34(4):641-648.

50. Kahn SR, M'lan CE, Lamping DL, Kurz X, Bérard A, Abenhaim LA. Relationship between clinical classification of chronic venous disease and patient-reported quality of life: results from an international cohort study. *J Vasc Surg.* 2004;39(4):823-828.

51. Palfreyman S. Assessing the impact of venous ulceration on quality of life. *Nurs Times.* 2008;104(41):34-37.

52. Raju S, Neglen P. Chronic venous insufficiency and varicose veins. *N Engl J Med.* 2009;360(22):2319-2327.

53. Malone DJ, Bishop Lindsay KL. *Physical Therapy in Acute Care: A Clinician's Guide.* Thorofare, NJ: SLACK Incorporated; 2006:666.

54. Deatrick KB, Wakefield TW, Henke PK. Chronic venous insufficiency: current management of varicose vein disease. *Am Surg.* 2010;76(2):125-132.

55. Latchford S, Casley-Smith J. Estimating limb volumes and alterations in peripheral edema from circumferences measured at different intervals. *Lymphology.* 1997;30(4):161-164.

56. Mayrovitz HN, Macdonald J, Davey S, Olson K, Washington E. Measurement decisions for clinical assessment of limb volume changes in patients with bilateral and unilateral limb edema. *Phys Ther.* 2007;87(10):1362-1368.

57. Sander AP, Hajer NM, Hemenway K, Miller AC. Upper-extremity volume measurements in women with lymphedema: a comparison of measurements obtained via water displacement with geometrically determined volume. *Phys Ther.* 2002;82(12):1201-1212.

58. Khan NA, Rahim SA, Anand SS, Simel DL, Panju A. Does the clinical examination predict lower extremity peripheral arterial disease? *JAMA.* 2006;295(5):536-546.

59. White G, Cox N. *Diseases of the Skin.* 2nd ed. Philadelphia, PA: Mosby Elsevier; 2006.

60. Gosnell AL, Nedorost ST. Stasis dermatitis as a complication of amlodipine therapy. *J Drugs Dermatol.* 2009;8(2):135-137.

61. Bunker Rosdahl C, Kowalski MT. *Textbook of Basic Nursing*. Philadelphia, PA: Wolters Kluwer Health/Lippincott Williams & Wilkins; 2008.

62. Schriger DL, Baraff L. Defining normal capillary refill: variations with age, sex and temperature. *Ann Emerg Med*. 1988;17(9):932-935.

63. American Diabetes Association. Peripheral arterial disease in people with diabetes: consensus statement. *Diabetes Care*. 2003;26(12):3333-3341.

64. Schroll M, Munck O. Estimation of peripheral arteriosclerotic disease by ankle blood pressure measurements in a population study of 60-year old men and women. *J Chronic Dis*. 1981;34:261-269.

65. Gardner AW, Skinner JS, Cantwell BW, Smith LK. Progressive vs. single-stage treadmill tests for evaluaton of claudication. *Med Sci Sports Exerc*. 1991;23(4):402-408.

66. Whaley M, Brubaker P, Otto R, eds. *ACSM's Guidelines for Exercise Testing and Prescription*. 7th ed. Baltimore, MD: Lippincott Williams & Wilkins; 2006.

67. Marcon G, Barbato O, Scevola M, Bettin MG, Zolli M. Unnecessary arterial Doppler examination of the legs. Clinical decision rules may help? *Qual Assur Health Care*. 1991;3:115-122.

68. Hennrikus D, Joseph AM, Lando HA, et al. Effectiveness of a smoking cessation program for peripheral artery disease patients: a randomized controlled trial. *J Am Coll Cardiol*. 2010;56(25):2105-2112.

69. Al-Omran M, Verma S, Lindsay TF. Suboptimal use of risk reduction therapy in peripheral arterial disease patients as a major teaching hospital. *Ann Saudi Med*. 2011;31(4):371-375.

70. Stewart KJ, Hiatt WR, Regensteiner JG, Hirsch AT. Exercise training for claudication. *N Engl J Med*. 2002;347:1941-1951.

71. Bendermacher BL, Willingendael EM, Teijink JA, Prins MH. Supervised exercise therapy versus non-supervised exercise therapy for intermittent claudication. *Cochrane Database Syst Rev*. 2009(1):1-24.

72. van Asselt AD, Nicolaï SP, Joore MA, et al. Cost-effectiveness of exercise therapy in patients with intermittent claudication: supervised exercise therapy versus a 'go home and walk' advice. *Eur J Vasc Endovasc Surg*. 2011;41(1):97-103.

73. Gardner AW, Parker DE, Montgomery PS, Scott KJ, Blevins SM. Efficacy of quantified home-based exercise and supervised exercise in patients with intermittent claudication: a randomized controlled trial. *Circulation*. 2011;123(5):491-498.

74. Watson L, Ellis B, Leng GC. Exercise for intermittent claudication. *Cochrane Database Syst Rev*. 2008;(4):CD000990.

75. Brendle DC, Joseph LJ, Corretti MC, Gardner AW, Katzel LI. Effects of exercise rehabilitation on endothelial reactivity in older patients with peripheral arterial disease. *Am J Cardiol*. 2001;87(3):324-329.

76. Hamburg N, Balady G. Exercise rehabilitation in peripheral artery disease: functional impact and mechanisms of benefits. *Circulation*. 2011;123:87-97.

77. McDermott MM, Ades P, Guralnik JM, et al. Treadmill exercise and resistance training in patients with peripheral arterial disease with and without intermittent claudication: a randomized controlled trial. *JAMA*. 2009;301(2):165-174.

78. Gardner AW, Katzel LI, Sorkin JD, et al. Exercise rehabilitation improves functional outcomes and peripheral circulation in patients with intermittent claudication: a randomized controlled trial. *J Am Geriatr Soc*. 2001;49(6):755-762.

79. Gardner AW, Katzel LI, Sorkin JD, Goldberg AP. Effects of long-term exercise rehabilitation on claudication distances in patients with peripheral arterial disease: a randomized controlled trial. *J Cardiopulm Rehabil*. 2002;22(3):192-198.

80. Zwierska I, Walker RD, Choksy SA, Male JS, Pockley AG, Saxton JM. Upper- vs lower-limb aerobic exercise rehabilitation in patients with symptomatic peripheral arterial disease: a randomized controlled trial. *J Vasc Surg*. 2005;42(6):1122-1130.

81. Bronas U, Treat-Jacobson D, Leon A. Comparison of the effect of upper body-ergometry aerobic training vs treadmill training on central cardiorespiratory improvement and walking distance in patients with claudication. *J Vasc Surg*. 2011;53(6):1557-1564.

82. Brunelle C, Mulgrew J. Exercise for intermittent claudication. *Phys Ther*. 2011;91(7):997-1002.

83. Tamir E, Daniels TR, Finestone A, Nof M. Off-loading of hindfoot and midfoot neuropathic ulcers using a fiberglass cast with a metal stirrup. *Foot Ankle Int*. 2007;28(10):1048-1052.

84. Armstrong DG, Nguyen HC, Lavery LA, van Schie CH, Boulton AJ, Harkless LB. Off-loading the diabetic foot wound: a randomized clinical trial. *Diabetes Care*. 2001;24(6):1019-1022.

85. Wu SC, Armstrong DG. The role of activity, adherence, and off-loading on the healing of diabetic foot wounds. *Plast Reconstr Surg*. 2006;117(7S):248S-253S.

86. Armstrong DG, Lavery LA, Kimbriel HR, Nixon BP, Boulton AJ. Activity patterns of patients with diabetic foot ulceration: patients with active ulceration may not adhere to a standard pressure off-loading regimen. *Diabetes Care*. 2003;26(9):2595-2597.

87. Armstrong DG, Lavery LA, Nixon BP, Boulton AJ. It's not what you put on, but what you take off: techniques for debriding and off-loading the diabetic foot wound. *Clin Infect Dis*. 2004;39(Suppl 2):S92-S99.

88. Armstrong DG, Lavery LA, Wu S, Boulton AJ. Evaluation of removable and irremovable cast walkers in the healing of diabetic foot wounds: a randomized controlled trial. *Diabetes Care*. 2005;28(3):551-554.

89. Satterfield K. Amputation considerations and energy expenditures in the diabetic patient. *Clin Podiatr Med Surg*. 2003;20(4):793-801.

90. Waters RL, Mulroy S. The energy expenditure of normal and pathological gait. *Gait Posture*. 1999;9(3):207-231.

91. Hoffman MD, Sheldahl LM, Buley KJ, Sandford PR. Physiological comparison of walking among bilateral above-knee amputee and able-bodied subjects, and a model to account for the differences in metabolic cost. *Arch Phys Med Rehabil*. 1997;78(4):385-92.

92. Wu YJ, Chen SY, Lin MC, LanC, Lai JS, Lien IN. Energy expenditure of wheeling and walking during prosthetic rehabilitation in a woman with bilateral transfemoral amputations. *Arch Phys Med Rehabil*. 2001;82(2):265-269.

93. Yan BP, Moran D, Hynes BG, Kiernan TJ, Yu CM. Advances in endovascular treatment of critical limb ischemia. *Circ J*. 2011;75(4):756-765.

94. Nawalany M. Endovascular therapy for limb salvage. *Surg Clin North Am*. 2010;90(6):1215-1225.

95. Indes JE, Mandawat A, Tuggle CT, Muhs B, Sosa JA. Endovascular procedures for aorto-iliac occlusive disease are associated with superior short-term clinical and economic outcomes compared with open surgery in the inpatient population. *J Vasc Surg*. 2010;52(5):1173-1179.

96. Gupta R, Losordo DW. Cell therapy for critical limb ischemia: moving forward one step at a time. *Circ Cardiovasc Interv*. 2011;4(1):2-5.

97. Idei N, Soga J, Hata T, et al. Autologous bone-marrow mononuclear cell implantation reduces long-term major amputation risk in patients with critical limb ischemia: a comparison of atherosclerotic peripheral arterial disease and Buerger disease. *Circ Cardiovasc Interv*. 2011;4(1):15-25.

98. Kim A, Kim M, Kim S, et al. Stem-cell therapy for peripheral arterial occlusive disease. *Eur J Vasc Endovasc Surg*. 2011;42(5):667-675.

99. Lawall H, Bramlage P, Amann B. Treatment of peripheral arterial disease using stem and progenitor cell therapy. *J Vasc Surg*. 2011;53(2):445-453.

100. Walter D, Krankenberg H, Balzer JO, et al. Intraarterial administration of bone marrow mononuclear cells in patients with critical limb ischemia: a randomized-start, placebo-controlled pilot trial (PROVASA). *Circ Cardiovasc Interv*. 2011;4(1):26-37.

101. de Haro J, Acin F, Florez A, Bleda S, Fernandez JL. A prospective randomized controlled study with intermittent mechanical compression of the calf in patients with claudication. *J Vasc Surg.* 2010;51(4):857-862.

102. Kranke P, Bennett M, Roeckl-Wiedmann I, Debus S. Hyperbaric oxygen therapy for chronic wounds. *Cochrane Database Syst Rev.* 2004;(2):CD004123.

103. Buhs C, Bendick P, Glover J. The effect of graded compression elastic stockings on the lower leg venous system during daily activity. *J Vasc Surg.* 1999;30(5):830-835.

104. Ibegbuna V, Delis K, Nicolaides A, et al. Effect of elastic compression stockings on venous hemodynamics during walking. *J Vasc Surg.* 2003;37(2):420-425.

105. Marston W. Summary of evidence of effectiveness of primary chronic venous disease treatment. *J Vasc Surg.* 2010;52(14S):54S-58S.

106. Nelson EA, Bell-Syer SE. Compression for preventing recurrence of venous ulcers. *Cochrane Database Syst Rev.* 2012;8:CD002303

107. Partsch H, Flour M, Smith PC. Indications for compression therapy in venous and lymphatic disease consensus based on experimental data and scientific evidence. Under the auspices of the IUP. *Int Angiol.* 2008;27(3):193-219.

108. O'Meara S, Cullum NA, Nelson EA. Compression for venous leg ulcers. *Cochrane Database Syst Rev.* 2009;(1):CD000265.

109. Nelson EA, Mani R, Thomas K, Vowden K. Intermittent pneumatic compression for treating venous leg ulcers. *Cochrane Database Syst Rev.* 2011;(2):CD001899.

110. Centers for Medicare & Medicaid Services. National coverage determination (NCD) for pneumatic compression devices (280.6). http://www.cms.gov/medicare-coverage-database/details/ncd-details.aspx?NCDId=225&ncdver=1&DocID=280.6&bc=gAAAAA gAAAAA&. Accessed May 15, 2014.

111. Bauer NA. The 4 rights of compression therapy for patients with chronic venous insufficiency and venous ulceration. *Home Healthcare Nurse.* 1998;16(7):443-448.

112. Clinical resource efficiency support team (CREST). *CREST Guidelines on the Management of Cellulitis in Adults.* June 2005. http://www.acutemed.co.uk/docs/Cellulitis%20guidelines,%20 CREST,%2005.pdf. Accessed May 14, 2015.

113. Abu-Own A, Scurr J, Coleridge-Smith P. Effect of leg elevation on the skin microcirculation in chronic venous insufficiency. *J Vasc Surg.* 1994;20(5):705-710.

114. Finlayson K, Edwards H, Courtney M. Relationships between preventive activities, psychosocial factors and recurrence of venous leg ulcers: a prospective study. *J Adv Nurs.* 2011;67(10):2180-2190.

115. Heinen MM, van der Vleuten C, de Rooij MJ, Uden CJ, Evers AW, van Achterberg T. Physical activity and adherence to compression therapy in patients with venous leg ulcers. *Arch Dermatol.* 2007;143(10):1283-1288.

116. Yang D, Vandongen YK, Stacey MC. Changes in calf muscle function in chronic venous disease. *Cardiovasc Surg.* 1999;7(4):451-456.

117. Araki C, Back T, Padberg F, et al. The significance of calf muscle pump function in venous ulceration. *J Vasc Surg.* 1994;20(6):872-877; discussion 878-870.

118. Roaldsen KS, Elfving B, Stanghelle JK, Talme T, Mattsson E. Fear-avoidance beliefs and pain as predictors for low physical activity in patients with leg ulcer. *Physiother Res Int.* 2009;14(3):167-180.

119. Kan Y, Delis KT. Hemodynamic effects of a supervised calf muscle exercise in patients with venous leg ulceration. *Arch Surg.* 2001;136(12):1364-1369.

120. Padberg FT Jr, Johnston MV, Sisto SA. Structured exercise improves calf muscle pump function in chronic venous insufficiency: a randomized trial. *J Vasc Surg.* 2004;39(1):79-87.

121. Back TL, Padberg FT Jr, Araki CT, Thompson PN, Hobson RW 2nd. Limited range of motion is a significant factor in venous ulceration. *J Vasc Surg.* 1995;22(5):519-523.

122. Pittler MH, Ernst E. Horse chestnut seed extract for chronic venous insufficiency. *Cochrane Database Syst Rev.* 2012;11:CD003230.

123. Bielanski TE, Piotrowski ZH. Horse-chestnut seed extract for chronic venous insufficiency. *J Fam Pract.* 1999;48(3):171-172.

124. Diehm C, Trampisch HJ, Lange S, Schmidt C. Comparison of leg compression stocking and oral horse-chestnut seed extract therapy in patients with chronic venous insufficiency. *Lancet.* 1996;347(8997):292-294.

125. Ottillinger B, Greeske K. Rational therapy of chronic venous insufficiency—chances and limits of the therapeutic use of horse-chestnut seed extract. *BMC Cardiovasc Disord.* 2001;1(5):5.

126. Pittler MH, Ernst E. Horse-chestnut seed extract for chronic venous insufficiency. A criteria-based systematic review. *Arch Dermatol.* 1998;134(11):1356-1360.

127. Perrin M, Ramelet AA. Pharmacological treatment of primary chronic venous disease: rationale, results and unanswered questions. *Eur J Vasc Endovasc Surg.* 2011;41(1):117-125.

128. Tisi PV, Beverley C, Rees A. Injection sclerotherapy for varicose veins. *Cochrane Database Syst Rev.* 2006;(4):CD001732.

CASE STUDY 7-1

Cheryl L. Brunelle, PT, MS, CCS, CLT; Paul D. Gaspar, PT, DPT, CCS; and Robert M. Snow, PT, DPT, OCS, ATC

EXAMINATION

History

Current Condition/Chief Complaint

Mr. Eagle is a 67-year-old English-speaking, White male. He was referred to physical therapy by his cardiologist for LE IC and limited ability to manage his cardiovascular risk factors.

Mr. Eagle stated that he had episodes of LE claudication for more than 10 years and had never received physical therapy. He reported that claudication was limiting his community level activities and that he was experiencing progressively worsening quality of life.

Clinician Comment *From the consult, Mr. Eagle already carried a long-standing diagnosis of PAD. He reported a lack of intervention for his claudication symptoms, resulting in limitations in activities and participation at the community level. Lack of intervention for claudication is not uncommon and is consistent with the literature.[1] The PT should consider that Mr. Eagle may have a large knowledge gap about his disease and its management; therefore there may be a role for significant education in his plan of care. The PT should, based on the current complaint and reason for consult, plan on including a comprehensive social history to elicit risk factors and baseline and current functional status, and a vascular examination in the initial examination. In this case, clarifying Mr. Eagle's understanding of his disease and its management would be helpful.*

Social History/Environment

Mr. Eagle lived with his wife in a 1-story house with no steps to enter. He had 3 adult children living locally who could help with shopping, but all worked full time and had families of their own to manage. He had 3 siblings who all lived at least 3 hours away. Mr. Eagle had a college education, he had spent more than 40 years in the investment business, and, for the past few years, he and his wife had been working part time from their home (by choice) as financial advisors for small businesses. He enjoyed using the Internet, reading, spending time with his grandchildren on weekends, and going out for dinner with his wife.

Social/Health Habits

Mr. Eagle had been a nonsmoker for 13 years. Previously, he had smoked 2 packs per day for more than 35 years—a 70 pack-year history. He stopped smoking at his physician's request prior to his first carotid endarterectomy. At the time of the appointment, he had not had an alcoholic beverage for 1 year, and prior to that had less than 1 per day. He followed a low-cholesterol diet and drank 2 cups of coffee per day.

Family History

Mr. Eagle's father died of a cerebral vascular accident at 78 years of age. His mother died at 72 years of age during a heart valve replacement surgery. His 2 sisters and 1 brother, ages 56, 60, and 64 years, were in excellent health.

Reported Functional Status

Mr. Eagle reported that he ambulated independently without an assistive device for both household- and community-level distances, and reported no difficulty at the household level. He was able to perform ADL independently. He reported that, at the time of examination, his self-paced walking was limited to less than one block because of bilateral calf claudication. If he stood or sat to rest, the pain would resolve and he could proceed another block. He reported he had no discomfort when standing for prolonged periods.

He reported that, 10 years prior, he had been able to walk 1 mile with mild claudication, and his walking tolerance had declined gradually. At the time of the appointment, he had not been exercising because of claudication pain and in fact would walk outside his home only when necessary. He and his wife went out for dinner only if parking was close to the restaurant and he did not have to walk any distance. He avoided intersections as his walking was too slow to make it across the street before the pedestrian signal ended. His wife and children did their grocery shopping because he could not tolerate the distances needed to walk in the large local grocery store. He continued to go over to his son's house every weekend for Sunday dinner and to play with the children. He could no longer go around the block while his grandson rode his bike, and missed this time with him dearly. He did not walk for exercise or perform any other type of exercise on a regular basis. He reported he would like to be able to exercise and would be willing to participate in a regular exercise program either as an outpatient or independently at home.

Mr. Eagle wanted to improve his walking distance, speed, and comfort. He wanted to get back to going to some of his favorite restaurants with his wife that required parking and walking a distance, partake in a regular exercise program, do the grocery shopping, and be able to walk around the block comfortably next to his grandson.

Clinician Comment *Mr. Eagle was an educated man who was still actively working and whose work had fortunately not been affected by his PAD. His health habits, including low caffeine and alcohol intake, a healthy diet, and his choice to quit smoking at his physician's request years earlier, all spoke of a man who would likely be compliant with recommendations and exercise interventions. He clearly wished to increase his ability to be active and participate in community-level activities, and he was articulating his intention to participate in a structured exercise program. Risk factors for PAD had already appeared in Mr. Eagle's history, including his age, prior smoking history, and a significant family history of cardiovascular disorders. Recall that other risk factors for PAD include diabetes, hypertension, dyslipidemia, or renal issues, and these would need to be discussed as part of the review of Mr. Eagle's medical and surgical history. Clearly, Mr. Eagle was already diagnosed with PAD; however, identification of further risk factors would help to clarify educational needs.*

Mr. Eagle described a progressive decline over the past decade, which has significantly affected his ability to participate in activities that bring him much joy and help him maintain his independence. His quality of life at that point had been significantly affected, which is consistent with the literature in this population. Recall that the literature supports significant relationships between depression and impaired quality of life in patients with PAD and those who have undergone surgical intervention for such.[2,3] The PT may consider use of an outcome measure to measure and monitor the effect of Mr. Eagle's PAD on his quality of life. Mr. Eagle had clear goals in mind that should be incorporated into the physical therapy plan of care.

Medications

- Aspirin
- Lipitor (atorvastatin calcium)
- Norvasc (amlodipine besylate)
- Avapro (irbesartan)
- Cilostazol

Mr. Eagle reported no side effects associated with these medications and no difficulty with medication compliance.

Clinician Comment *Mr. Eagle had been prescribed aspirin as an antiplatelet therapy for cardioprotection, Lipitor to control hyperlipidemia, Norvasc and Avapro* *for control of hypertension, and Cilostazol to control symptoms of IC. Additional risk factors were identified—of note, those shared by PAD and CAD, including hypertension and hyperlipidemia. The PT should assume Mr. Eagle is at high risk of CAD and should plan on close hemodynamic monitoring to establish Mr. Eagle's responses to position change and to activity. Cardiac history would be further elicited in review of his past medical/surgical history.*

Medical/Surgical History

Mr. Eagle has undergone several interventions in an attempt to revascularize his impaired peripheral circulation and improve symptoms. He reported he was diagnosed with PAD and carotid disease 12 years prior to the examination. At that time, he noticed difficulty walking and complained of "flecks" running across his eyes. He underwent a right carotid endarterectomy at that time, and a left carotid endarterectomy 3 years ago. He underwent an angioplasty in the right femoral artery 10 years ago, and the left 9 years ago. He had bilateral common iliac artery and external iliac artery angioplasties with stent placement 1 year ago. He had an angioplasty of the mid-portion of the left anterior descending coronary artery 3 years ago after an adenosine stress test indicated blockage of the left anterior descending coronary artery. He had no symptoms of angina or dyspnea prior to or since the intervention.

Mr. Eagle reported 5 transient ischemic attacks in the past, but none in the 3 years prior to the physical therapy appointment. He had an arterial ulcer on his left heel 18 months prior that healed after 3 to 4 months with restricted weightbearing (crutch walking) and independent wound care at home. He reported no history of orthopedic, pulmonary, rheumatologic, or oncology-related signs, symptoms, or medical care. His only hospitalizations were for the episodes of care related to his cardiac and PVD, mentioned previously, with the exception of a tonsillectomy many years ago.

Clinician Comment *It is clear from his numerous revascularizations that Mr. Eagle not only has advanced PAD, but also CAD. It is unfortunate that Mr. Eagle has not had physical therapy intervention up to this point; however, it is possible that he was independently mobile after each of these revascularizations, and the medical team was not aware of the educational and exercise physical therapy interventions that may have helped Mr. Eagle to manage his disease. Mr. Eagle's significant vascular history and history of an arterial ulcer confirms the need for a comprehensive vascular exam, specifically looking for signs of PAD on integumentary exam, including wounds, circulation of the extremities, and claudication pain within tests and measures. It also confirms the need for examination of aerobic capacity and walking tolerance with close hemodynamic monitoring. The PT should consider, given his established history of CAD and*

cerebrovascular disease, that Mr. Eagle is at high risk of serious cardiovascular events and may have an inappropriate hemodynamic response to mobility. It is possible that if Mr. Eagle had a cardiovascular pump dysfunction during activity, it would likely be asymptomatic given his reports of an absence of cardiac-related symptoms with activity.

Other Clinical Tests

The following measures were reported from noninvasive arterial studies:

ABI	One year prior to physical therapy examination: Right, 0.31; Left, 0.37
MRA	Completed 1 week prior to the physical therapy examination, showed impaired flow in the iliac, femoral, and popliteal arteries
Echocardiogram	Performed 2 years prior to physical therapy examination, showed that Mr. Eagle had a left ventricular ejection fraction of 65% with normal left ventricular systolic function. No wall motion abnormalities were noted; however, mild mitral regurgitation and left atrial dilation were noted. The right heart was within normal limits
Electrocardiogram	One week prior in the cardiologist's office that read normal sinus rhythm, rate 72

Clinician Comment *Mr. Eagle's ABI measurements were taken after his most recent revascularization and indicated bilateral, severe PAD with an ABI of < 0.40 bilaterally. One should consider that these values are 3 years old and could be even lower at this time; however, they would still reflect severe PAD and would not change the clinical decision-making process of the PT. Mr. Eagle's MRA also reflects the severity of his PAD, with multiple continued impairments in flow throughout the LE arterial circulation. His cardiac echocardiogram is helpful in that it is relatively recent. However, given the severity of his vascular issues, one may consider that there could be deterioration within a 3-year time period. There are some early changes on echocardiogram and, again, this test is 2 years old, so it is possible there have been changes since then. This is a resting echocardiogram and in no way insinuates that Mr. Eagle's cardiovascular pump will respond normally to activity or that hemodynamic response to activity will be normal. Together with his lack of any spinal complaints in his history, his markedly abnormal ABIs and MRA indicate that Mr. Eagle's claudication was likely vascular as opposed to neurogenic. The severity of PAD indicated by his*

ABIs identified that compression therapy would not be an appropriate treatment consideration if edema were present because the risk of further impairment of blood flow would be too high. His electrocardiogram was normal at rest; however, this does not imply that rhythm or rate would be normal with activity. In absence of any history of arrhythmias, the PT would monitor hemodynamic response closely given his history, and if any arrhythmias were noted on palpation of HR, immediate referral back to his cardiologist would be warranted.

Systems Review

Cardiovascular/Pulmonary

HR: 72 beats per minute (bpm) and regular

Respiration rate: 16 breaths per minute

BP (brachial, seated rest): 160/86 mm Hg right, 148/84 mm Hg left

Edema: None noted bilaterally in the LEs

Integumentary

Integumentary integrity of the LEs was intact. Trophic changes, including loss of hair and thickening of the toenails, were noted. Mr. Eagle's feet were symmetrically cool, dry, and pale. No signs of venous insufficiency were noted.

Sensation

Intact to light touch and proprioception bilateral LEs.

Musculoskeletal

- Height: 6 feet, 1 inch; Weight: 170 pounds
- Gross range of motion: Within normal limits upper and LEs
- Gross strength: Within normal limits upper and LEs

Neuromuscular

Gait, balance, and motor function were within normal limits. Mr. Eagle was independent without an assistive device for transfers and ambulation.

Communication, Affect, Cognition, Language, and Learning Style

Mr. Eagle was an excellent historian who was alert and oriented times 4. He reported that he did not have a strong learning preference, but enjoyed learning and reading about his condition on the Internet.

Clinician Comment *Mr. Eagle's resting BP is high, which is consistent with his history of hypertension. As previously discussed, ACC/AHA guidelines recommend a systolic BP < 140 mm Hg for patients with PAD without diabetes.[1,4] It is possible that his hypertension is not well controlled, and this should be communicated to his primary care physician (PCP). BP in the right upper extremity was*

greater than that in the left upper extremity, which likely indicates some arterial stenosis in the left arm impeding flow and resulting in a lower BP reading. Any subsequent BPs should be measured in the right upper extremity for accuracy. Not surprisingly given the severity of Mr. Eagle's PAD as indicated by his ABIs, trophic changes were noted in the LEs, indicating vascular insufficiency; coolness, dryness, and pallor indicated arterial insufficiency. Based on Mr. Eagle's chief complaint, social history, reported functional status, and established diagnosis of severe PAD, the PT decided that tests and measures were indicated even before the systems review in this case. In cases in which the patient has not been definitively diagnosed, the PT would complete the systems review and then decide on tests and measures based on a combination of the systems review and the patient's history together. Mr. Eagle gave a good history of his community-level activities, and the PT should examine him based on his reports of the IADL he needs to perform as well as with the knowledge that his walking distance is significantly impaired at baseline. This would allow the examiner to determine whether Mr. Eagle can successfully complete the IADL he needs to complete to be independent, determine his cardiovascular response to these activities to ensure safety, and determine limiting factors that may drive the PT's plan of care. It is unlikely that he will be able to mobilize community distances, and one can anticipate that his main limiting factor will be IC. In this case, walking distance and time should be noted, and claudication pain should be measured during ambulation and throughout recovery.

Tests and Measures

Circulation

Pulses

- Femoral: 1 bilaterally
- Popliteal: Not palpable bilaterally; Dopplerable
- Dorsalis pedis: 1 bilaterally
- Posterior tibial: Left, 1; Right, not palpable; Dopplerable
- CRT: Impaired (> 3 seconds) bilateral great toes

Clinician Comment *If Mr. Eagle did not have a confirmed diagnosis of PAD, recall that reduced or absent pulses throughout the LE would increase the likelihood of PAD.[5] Given that he already has been diagnosed with PAD, palpation of pulses serves as a baseline for the examiner, who will be able to note changes over time (eg, a deterioration in pulses from diminished to absent, or Dopplerable to non-Dopplerable). Given the severity of Mr. Eagle's PAD and his MRA findings of stenosis throughout the LE arterial circulation, it is not surprising that pulses are reduced or absent to palpation. Recall that CRT greater than*

3 seconds is associated with moderate to severe PAD,[5] so it was not surprising to find Mr. Eagle's CRT was impaired. Measurements of ABI were not taken during the physical therapy examination. Mr. Eagle's ABI values from 1 year prior indicated severe PAD, so remeasurement was not likely to add any new information to the examination and therefore would not influence intervention for this patient.

Joint Integrity and Mobility

Clinician Comment *The PT did not feel that tests and measures were indicated to rule out neurogenic claudication as a cause for Mr. Eagle's symptoms. His symptoms were reproducible with a given amount of exercise and relieved with standing still, which is classic in a patient with vascular claudication. A patient with neurogenic claudication may have symptoms at rest or with activity, but symptoms are usually exacerbated with extension of the spine, relieved with flexion of the spine, and thought to be caused by stenosis of the spinal canal.[6] Relief of symptoms with standing still would not be characteristic in a patient with neurogenic claudication; therefore, Mr. Eagle's symptoms are not consistent with neurogenic claudication and no further testing was warranted.*

Aerobic Capacity and Endurance
Six-Minute Walk Test

Average gait speed	0.46 m/sec (1.03 mph)
Average energy expenditure	1.8 metabolic equivalents (METs)
Time to claudication onset	40 seconds
Distance to claudication onset	66 feet (20.1 m)
Maximum walking time	85 seconds
Maximum walking distance	144 feet (43.9 m)
Total walking distance	284 feet (86.6 m), including a 2-minute, 50-second rest break
Resting HR standing	78 bpm
Peak HR	110 bpm
Resting right brachial BP	164/84 mm Hg
Peak right brachial BP	198/96 mm Hg
Postexercise ankle BP	50% lower than resting value, 7 minutes to recover to baseline

Clinician Comment *The 6MWT was chosen because it has established reliability in the population with PAD and its measurements are related to the functional and hemodynamic severity of PAD in patients with IC.[7] Mr. Eagle's 6MWT distance of 284 feet was low compared to the healthy elderly population. One study found that healthy subjects 50 to 85 years of age walked an average distance of 2070 feet during a 6MWT.[8] Mr. Eagle's average gait speed was very low and, in fact, was equivalent to approximately one-third of the average comfortable gait speed of males in their seventh decade.[9] Mr. Eagle's energy expenditure during walking helps to determine whether his hemodynamic response to this activity was appropriate. For every 1 MET of activity above resting (equivalent to 1 MET), systolic BP should be expected to rise 10 mm Hg and HR 10 bpm. Since Mr. Eagle's energy expenditure was equivalent to 1.8 METs, or a 0.8-MET increase beyond resting, one would expect his HR and BP to rise less than 10 bpm or mm Hg, respectively; however, his HR rose 32 bpm, and his systolic BP rose 34 mm Hg, indicating an exaggerated response to activity, which would be consistent with a deconditioned response.*

The absolute value of his HR is not concerning as he is not near his age-predicted maximum HR. The absolute value of his BP at peak activity is high but expected given his deconditioned response superimposed on a resting hypertension. Such a high BP with such low level activity is concerning, and warrants discussion with the physician. If resting BP were better controlled, even with a deconditioned response to activity, absolute peak BPs would be lower. Although Mr. Eagle's hemodynamic response did not indicate a cardiovascular pump dysfunction at this workload, he would need continued monitoring with activity, especially as symptoms are expected to improve and workload may progress. He should not be expected to have the same hemodynamic response at all workloads. Given Mr. Eagle's very low gait speed and deconditioned response to low-level activity, it is clear that, as he reports, his quality of life was significantly affected by his inability to walk at a functional speed or for community distances. Mr. Eagle's ankle BP fell dramatically with exercise and recovered slowly, consistent with the response expected in a patient with PAD as previously discussed.[10]

Work (Job/School/Play/Leisure)
King's College Vascular Quality of Life Questionnaire (VascuQol)

Total score at the evaluation	2.96/7
Physical activity score	2.1/7
Pain score	4/7
Symptom score	4.7/7
Psychological well-being score	2.6/7
Social activity score	2/7

Clinician Comment *The VascuQol is a valid, reliable, and disease-specific outcome measure of quality of life for patients with chronic limb ischemia or PAD.[11] The questionnaire includes 25 items with 7 possible responses listed in the order of decreasing impairment. Each item is scored from 1 (most impaired) to 7 (least impaired). A total score is calculated by dividing the total of the item scores by 25. Each item is classified into 1 of 5 domains: physical activity, pain, psychological well-being, symptoms, and social activity. The domains are scored by totaling the scores of all items in the domain and dividing by the number of questions in the domain. Mr. Eagle's total score of 2.96 indicates significant impact of PAD on his quality of life. His scores are lowest in the domains of physical activity, psychological well-being, and social activity, which are consistent with his subjective history. Because the measure has been shown to be responsive to change[11] and one of Mr. Eagle's main complaints is around his quality of life, he will complete this questionnaire at regular intervals in order to monitor change in quality of life with physical therapy intervention.*

Pain

The Claudication Pain Rating Scale[12] was used to quantify Mr. Eagle's pain during activity. He reported a pain rating of 1 (minimal discomfort) within 40 seconds of slow-paced walking on the 6MWT. His rating increased to a pain rating of 4 (unbearable) at 144 feet before a rest was required.

Clinician Comment *Mr. Eagle independently walked until his pain was unbearable, which often discourages these patients from walking any distance. His pain further supports his significant impairment in walking distance and time and helps the PT to provide an appropriate exercise prescription using the Claudication Pain Rating Scale.*

EVALUATION

Diagnosis

Mr. Eagle was referred to physical therapy with the medical diagnosis of PAD. His subjective complaints and objective findings suggested the following 2 practice patterns.

Impaired Aerobic Capacity/Endurance Associated With Deconditioning

Mr. Eagle's main complaint was claudication limiting his community-level activities, and as a result, he was experiencing progressively worsening quality of life. His examination confirmed that he was deconditioned, as evidenced by his impairment in aerobic capacity on his 6MWT, and his exaggerated hemodynamic response to low-level activity (slow walking on level ground for a short distance). His PAD was directly affecting his quality of life, as evidenced by his scores on the VascuQol. Of primary importance was establishing an individualized, comprehensive exercise program.

Impaired Aerobic Capacity/Endurance Associated With Cardiovascular Pump Dysfunction, Specifically Peripheral Vascular Dysfunction

Mr. Eagle had a long-standing diagnosis of PAD that, by his ABIs and MRA results and significant need for revascularization over the last decade, was severe. His LE skin and circulatory changes, history of arterial ulcer, ankle pressures, and pain ratings during exercise that recovered with rest were evidence of his peripheral vascular system impairment. He also carried diagnoses of CAD and cerebrovascular disease and was therefore at significantly higher risk for cardiovascular events and death as compared to the healthy adult population. He had several cardiovascular risk factors that would be important to address, and he had received no comprehensive education or exercise intervention to address his disease thus far in the course of his disease. It would be important to address these issues with education regarding skin care and risk factor management, as well as a comprehensive exercise program as mentioned previously.

International Classification of Functioning, Disability, and Health Model of Disability

See ICF model on page 277.

Prognosis

Mr. Eagle's prior surgical history, medical history, vascular labs, and physical therapy evaluation all indicated severe PAD. Research has shown that exercise improves walking distance and time in patients with IC,[13-15] and strategies to enhance long-term adherence with a home walking program should be incorporated.[15] Mr. Eagle was motivated to begin a structured exercise program, and it was believed that he would be able to achieve his goals of increased community ambulation and return to social activities through increasing walking time and distance. He had established relationships with his PCP and cardiologist for follow-up care for his PAD and had exhibited excellent compliance with medical recommendations and follow-up since his diagnosis. It was anticipated that he would be compliant with recommendations regarding follow-up for his hypertension and appropriate skin care to decrease his risk of wounds and associated complications.

It was anticipated that he would be able to progress to an independent home walking program and maintenance skin care program once he demonstrated knowledge of risk factor management and independence with his exercise program.

ICF MODEL OF DISABLEMENT FOR MR. EAGLE

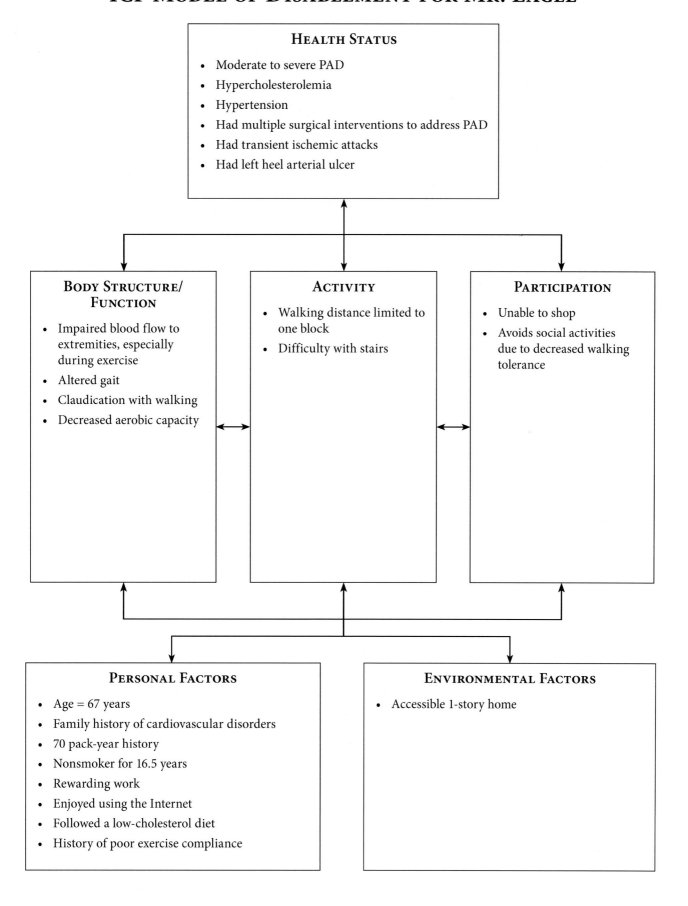

HEALTH STATUS

- Moderate to severe PAD
- Hypercholesterolemia
- Hypertension
- Had multiple surgical interventions to address PAD
- Had transient ischemic attacks
- Had left heel arterial ulcer

BODY STRUCTURE/ FUNCTION

- Impaired blood flow to extremities, especially during exercise
- Altered gait
- Claudication with walking
- Decreased aerobic capacity

ACTIVITY

- Walking distance limited to one block
- Difficulty with stairs

PARTICIPATION

- Unable to shop
- Avoids social activities due to decreased walking tolerance

PERSONAL FACTORS

- Age = 67 years
- Family history of cardiovascular disorders
- 70 pack-year history
- Nonsmoker for 16.5 years
- Rewarding work
- Enjoyed using the Internet
- Followed a low-cholesterol diet
- History of poor exercise compliance

ENVIRONMENTAL FACTORS

- Accessible 1-story home

Plan of Care

Intervention

Therapeutic exercise to address aerobic capacity and patient education, as detailed next.

Proposed Frequency and Duration of Physical Therapy Visits

36 visits, 3 times per week over the course of 12 weeks

Clinician Comment *Evidence shows that patients with IC should partake in walking programs 3 to 5 times per week, and duration of the supervised component of the program should be at least 12 weeks in order to ensure increases in maximum and pain-free walking distance.*[1,13] *If this frequency of care is not feasible, frequency closest to 3 times weekly over 12 weeks would be recommended.*

Anticipated Goals

1. Patient will be independent with a self-paced walking program at least 3 times per week using the Claudication Pain Rating Scale in order to improve aerobic capacity and progress his exercise program into the community (1 week).

2. Patient will demonstrate improved functional mobility and aerobic capacity on his 6MWT to allow him to perform IADL and short-distance community mobility more easily (8 weeks).

3. Patient will improve his maximum walking distance to 500 feet in order to progress toward independent community-level ambulation distances (8 weeks).

4. Maximum walking speed will be equal to or greater than 1.3 m/s (2.90 mph) to allow him to cross the street safely before the light changes in the community (12 weeks).

5. Patient will demonstrate improved quality of life as evidenced by a 20% improvement in his VascuQol total score (total score to at least 4.36) (8 weeks).

6. Patient will verbalize understanding of the benefits of exercise in PAD, the importance of a long-term independent walking program, importance of meticulous skin care to decrease risk of wounds and infection, the importance of continued adherence to cardiovascular risk management interventions and situations necessitating immediate medical care in order to progress his exercise program independently and to control his risk of wounds and cardiovascular events (1 week).

Expected Outcomes (12 weeks)

1. Patient will be able to complete grocery shopping and partake in a weekly outing for dinner with his wife to a restaurant of his choice.

2. Patient will be able to walk around the block comfortably with his grandson, with standing rests as needed.

3. Patient will report improved health-related quality of life.

4. Patient will verbalize understanding of and confidence with independent PAD management.

Clinician Comment *Of paramount importance is that Mr. Eagle understands and independently follows the recommended parameters of his walking program; this will be critical for his long-term independent disease management. The minimal clinically important difference in the 6MWT is 86 meters,*[16] *so Mr. Eagle would need to improve his 6MWT by 100% in order to establish a significant change. This may take at least 8 weeks. Although pain is Mr. Eagle's limiting factor to mobility, this is incorporated into the goals for independent use of the Claudication Pain Rating Scale, maximum walking distance, and improved 6MWT distance, so a specific claudication pain goal is not included. Mr. Eagle verbalized an avoidance of intersections because of his slow gait. Research has shown that the average steady state gait velocity at a pedestrian crosswalk is 1.36 ± 0.24 m/s regardless of intersection width.*[17] *This gait speed was incorporated into the goals so that Mr. Eagle could function more easily in the community and return to going out for dinner with his wife at various downtown restaurants requiring distant parking and negotiation through pedestrian intersections.*

Discharge Plan

It was anticipated that Mr. Eagle would be discharged from physical therapy with an independent exercise program to continue on his own for the long term.

INTERVENTION

Coordination, Communication, and Documentation

The initial examination findings and physical therapy plan of care were sent to Mr. Eagle's cardiologist and PCP. In particular, Mr. Eagle's resting hypertension and hemodynamic response to low-level activity were noted so that the doctor may consider pharmacologic titration of Mr. Eagle's BP medications.

Patient-/Client-Related Instruction

- Encouragement to follow-up with his cardiologist regarding his hypertension as soon as possible, and regarding the importance of medication compliance with antihypertensives

- Information on the pathophysiology, prognosis, and treatment of his disease process through verbal education and the provision of several reputable educational websites for him to review at his convenience, given his interest in using the Internet

- Pain monitoring and exercise pacing using the Claudication Pain Rating Scale

- Strategies for skin care: daily visual inspection, skin hygiene, and moisturizing, immediate medical follow-up in the event of any wound, no matter how small, and appropriate footwear to avoid pressure points and during every exercise session

- Avoidance of LE elevation or compression

- Importance of continuation of nonsmoking status and avoidance of second-hand smoke

Procedural Interventions

Therapeutic Exercise Prescription

Aerobic Capacity Training

Mode
Interval walking

Intensity
Self-paced walking speed to prolong onset of symptoms for as long as possible, with the eventual goal of walking at a speed that elicits symptoms within 3 to 5 minutes. Continue to walk at moderate intensity (2 on the Claudication Pain Rating Scale), and stop if symptoms become intense (3).

Duration
Total walking time initially 15 minutes, progressing to 30 minutes, as tolerated

Frequency
3 to 5 times per week, including supervised sessions

Description of the Intervention
Mr. Eagle will need to perform interval walking initially because his walking ability was severely limited in terms of speed and duration. Given that his maximum walking time on initial exam was 86 seconds, his intervals will be shorter than that as we do not want him to walk to maximum intensity on the Claudication Pain Rating Scale. In the first several weeks of treatment, he may need to walk at least 10 to 15 intervals per day to achieve a walking duration of 15 minutes. As he progresses, length of time of each interval and number of walking intervals will increase to gradually improve his total walking time to 30 minutes daily.

Clinician Comment *Mr. Eagle is new to a structured exercise program, so making it feasible and tolerable for him is very important. Working together with him to establish appropriate interval length based on use of the Claudication Pain Rating Scale, and tolerable number of intervals per day, would hopefully help him to ease into a walking program and maximize adherence. The concern would be if the program were too difficult or too painful, adherence may understandably be an issue. His gait speed beginning the program was very slow, and his time and distance walked was low, making it quite easy to become discouraged by the program. Encouragement that the evidence supports progression of walking time and distance with this type of walking program should help, as well as highlighting small progressions of interval time or number as steps in the right direction. At least 3 sessions per week should be supervised sessions, and encouraging Mr. Eagle to increase independence with another 2 sessions would help to establish independence and confidence with his program. Any barriers to progression to an independent program would likely declare themselves, and they could be addressed appropriately during the episode of care.*

REEXAMINATION

Subjective

Mr. Eagle reported that he was able to walk for longer distances and times without requiring rest. Just the previous week, he had surprised his wife and took her to dinner at their favorite restaurant for the first time in 3 years, which required parking in a lot across the street and negotiating through a pedestrian intersection. He was able to walk around the block with his grandson slowly with minimal to moderate discomfort, and his grandson agreed to walk with him, rather than bike, so that Mr. Eagle could pick a comfortable pace and rest as needed. He had just gone grocery shopping with his wife on the weekend, and was able to pace himself through the store for 1 hour, with minimal discomfort, resting as needed as his wife shopped. He reported that he was managing to walk twice per week on his own in addition to the supervised program at the clinic, and his wife had been walking with him, which was a great motivator for him. His total walking time per independent session was 20 minutes, in intervals of just under 4 minutes. He felt comfortable using the Claudication Pain Rating Scale independently, and carried a copy with him in his pocket as he walked. He reported feeling improvement in his health status and feeling that his quality of life was improving.

Objective

Integumentary	Intact to the LEs, unchanged
Circulation	Pulses and capillary refill unchanged from initial examination
Aerobic capacity and endurance	6MWT
Average gait speed	0.86 m/sec (1.92 mpm)
Average energy expenditure	2.5 METs
Time to claudication onset	1 minute, 15 seconds
Distance to claudication onset	154 feet (46.9 m)
Maximum walking time	3 minutes, 15 seconds
Maximum walking distance	512 feet (148.1 m)
Total walking distance	726 feet (221.3 m), including 2 rest breaks of 56 and 47 seconds
Resting HR standing	76 bpm
Peak HR	98 bpm
Resting right brachial BP	128/84 mm Hg
Peak right brachial BP	148/90 mm Hg
Postexercise ankle BP	50% lower than resting value; 6 minutes, 30 seconds to recover to baseline
Maximal walking speed	1.26 m/sec (2.82 mph)

Work (Job/School/Play/Leisure)

King's College Vascular Quality of Life Questionnaire (VascuQol)

Total score	4.65/7
Physical activity score	4.52/7
Pain score	5/7
Symptom score	5.1/7
Psychological well-being score	4.3/7
Social activity score	4.2/7

Clinician Comment *Mr. Eagle's circulation and integumentary integrity remained unchanged, but it was important to reexamine it to ensure there was no deterioration, and this had been monitored throughout the* episode of care. His aerobic capacity significantly improved with physical therapy intervention, as evidenced by his improvement in 6MWT score and gait speed, which both exceeded the minimal clinically important difference for each measure.[16,18] Mr. Eagle's resting BP was lower at reexamination, which reflected the fact that he had followed up with his cardiologist, who had titrated his antihypertensive regimen. His BP and HR response to this workload was still exaggerated, although less so than at initial examination, and given his resting BP was lower, so was his peak BP. Mr. Eagle's maximal walking speed had not met his goal of 1.3 m/sec, but it was close and he was no longer reporting difficulty negotiating the main pedestrian intersection in his town. His quality of life improved as evidenced not only by his subjective report, but by the VascuQol score at reexamination, which was 157% that at initial examination.

Assessment

Mr. Eagle's aerobic capacity, walking times, and distances had improved and he had returned to community-level activities as compared to initial evaluation. He had met his own personal goals and felt that his quality of life had improved significantly. He had met all of his physical therapy goals with the exception of that for maximum walking speed, although he reported no difficulty negotiating the main pedestrian intersection in his town at the time of reexamination. He was independent with his walking program and could verbalize how to appropriately progress it. He continued to be compliant with all risk factor management recommendations.

Plan

Mr. Eagle was ready for discharge from therapy, with continuation of an independent home exercise program and self-management program.

OUTCOMES

Discharge

Mr. Eagle met all goals established at the time of his initial evaluation, with the exception of maximum walking speed of 1.3 m/sec, and had made clinically significant gains both in walking speed and 6MWT. He was independent with skin care, cardiovascular risk management, and his exercise program. He could verbalize understanding of situations that would require immediate medical follow-up. Mr. Eagle would continue his home exercise program, walking 3 to 5 times per week, with progression to walking at an intensity that elicited onset of claudication symptoms within 3 to 5 minutes, continuing to walk with moderate pain, stopping if the pain becomes intense, for 30 to 50 minutes per session. He was encouraged to continue his program for the long term, if possible, and follow up with physical therapy or with his physician as indicated.

Clinician Comment *Although Mr. Eagle had shown improvements in all areas, he still had impairments in walking speed, aerobic capacity, and quality of life, and was still walking distances less than that required for full community ambulation. Given the severity of Mr. Eagle's PAD, it was anticipated that all of these impairments would continue to improve, although they may not be expected to return to age-matched normative values. Long-term adherence to his self-management plan would be imperative for lifelong disease management. Mr. Eagle had shown compliance with medical recommendations and follow-up since his PAD diagnosis, as well as throughout his physical therapy episode of care; therefore, his motivation and excellent compliance were anticipated to continue.*

REFERENCES

1. Norgren L, Hiatt W, Dormandy J, Nehler M, Harris K, Fowkes FG. Inter-society consensus for the management of peripheral arterial disease (TASC II). *J Vasc Surg.* 2007;45(1 Suppl S):S5-S67.

2. Cherr G, Wang J, Zimmerman P, Dosluoglu H. Depression is associated with worse patency and recurrent leg symptoms after lower extremity revascularization. *J Vasc Surg.* 2007;45:744-750.

3. Hareendran A, Bradbury A, Budd J. Measuring the impact of venous leg ulcers on quality of life. *J Wound Care.* 2005;14(2):53-57.

4. Hirsch A, Haskal Z, Hertzer N, et al. ACC/AHA 2005 guidelines for the management of patients with peripheral arterial disease (lower extremity, renal, mesenteric, and abdominal aortic): executive summary a collaborative report from the American Association for Vascular Surgery/Society for Vascular Surgery, Society for Cardiovascular Angiography and Interventions, Society for Vascular Medicine and Biology, Society of Interventional Radiology, and the ACC/AHA Task Force on Practice Guidelines (Writing Committee to Develop Guidelines for the Management of Patients With Peripheral Arterial Disease) endorsed by the American Association of Cardiovascular and Pulmonary Rehabilitation; National Heart, Lung, and Blood Institute; Society for Vascular Nursing; TransAtlantic Inter-Society Consensus; and Vascular Disease Foundation. *J Am Coll Cardiol.* 2006;47(6):1239-1312.

5. Gosnell AL, Nedorost ST. Stasis dermatitis as a complication of amlodipine therapy. *J Drugs Dermatol.* 2009;8(2):135-137.

6. Comer C, Redmond A, Bird H, Conaghan P. Assessment and management of neurogenic claudication associated with lumbar spinal stenosis in a UK primary care musculoskeletal service: a survey of current practice among physiotherapists. *BMC Musculoskelet Disord.* 2009;10:121.

7. Montgomery P, Gardner A. The clinical utility of a six-minute walk test in peripheral arterial occlusive disease patients. *J Am Geriatr Soc.* 1998;46(6):706-711.

8. Troosters T, Gosselink M, Decramer M. Six minute walking distance in healthy elderly subjects. *Eur Respir J.* 1999;14:270-274.

9. Bohannon RW. Comfortable and maximal walking speed of adults aged 20-79 years: reference values and determinants. *Age Ageing.* 1997;26(1):15-19.

10. Goodman CC, Fuller KS. *Pathology: Implications for the Physical Therapist.* 3rd ed. St. Louis, MO: Saunders Elsevier; 2009.

11. Morgan M, Crayford T, Murrin B, Fraser SC. Developing the vascular quality of life questionnaire: a new disease-specific quality of life measure for use in lower limb ischemia. *J Vasc Surg.* 2001;33(4):679-687.

12. van Asselt AD, Nicolaï SP, Joore MA, et al. Cost-effectiveness of exercise therapy in patients with intermittent claudication: supervised exercise therapy versus a 'go home and walk' advice. *Eur J Vasc Endovasc Surg.* 2011;41(1):97-103.

13. McDermott MM, Ades P, Guralnik JM, et al. Treadmill exercise and resistance training in patients with peripheral arterial disease with and without intermittent claudication: a randomized controlled trial. *JAMA.* 2009;301(2):165-174.

14. Zwierska I, Walker RD, Choksy SA, Male JS, Pockley AG, Saxton JM. Upper- vs lower-limb aerobic exercise rehabilitation in patients with symptomatic peripheral arterial disease: a randomized controlled trial. *J Vasc Surg.* 2005;42(6):1122-1130.

15. Armstrong DG, Lavery LA, Wu S, Boulton AJ. Evaluation of removable and irremovable cast walkers in the healing of diabetic foot wounds: a randomized controlled trial. *Diabetes Care.* 2005;28(3):551-554.

16. Wise R, Brown CD. Minimal clinically important differences in the six-minute walk test and the incremental shuttle walking test. *COPD.* 2005;2(1):125-129.

17. Fugger TJ, Randles B, Stein A, Whiting W, Gallagher B. Analysis of pedestrian gait and perception-reaction at signal-controlled crosswalk intersections. *Transportation Research Record.* 01/2000;1705(1):20-25. DOI:10.3141/1705-04.

18. Puthoff ML. Outcome measures in cardiopulmonary physical therapy: gait speed. *Cardiopulm Phys Ther J.* 2008;19(1):17-22.

8

Individuals With Ventilatory Pump Disorders

Jane L. Wetzel, PT, PhD

CHAPTER OBJECTIVES

- Identify the components of the thoracic cage and the dimensions of movement possible.
- Describe the sequences of muscular contractions and chest wall movements that accompany inspiration and expiration.
- Outline the mechanisms that monitor the levels of arterial carbon dioxide (CO_2) and oxygen (O_2), and the changes in ventilation that are prompted.
- Contrast the effect of altered length-tension of the diaphragmatic muscle fibers in patients with chronic obstructive pulmonary disease (COPD) and patients with neuromuscular weakness.
- List age-related changes that occur in ventilation.
- Discuss anatomical variations or injuries that can contribute to altered chest wall compliance.
- Explain the physiologic basis for interventions to decrease ventilatory load and those to improve ventilatory muscle capacity.
- Discuss the factors that might indicate a life-long management of respiratory impairment needs to occur and identify the possible components of management to be considered.
- Compare and contrast altered ventilatory pump considerations in patients with nonprogressing neuromuscular disorders and those with progressing neuromuscular disorders.

CHAPTER OUTLINE

- Biomechanics of Ventilatory Pump Dysfunction
  - Inspiration
  - Expiration
  - Accessory Muscle Actions
- Neuromuscular Innervation/Central Control of Breathing
- Ventilatory Pump Physiology
- Epidemiology of Ventilatory Biomechanical Pathology
  - Age-Related Changes and Ventilatory Pump Function
  - Incidence and Prevalence of Pathology Affecting Ventilatory Pump Function
    - Chronic Obstructive Pulmonary Disease Pathology Affecting Ventilatory Pump Function
    - Neuromuscular Conditions Affecting Ventilatory Pump Function
    - Musculoskeletal Disorders Affecting Ventilatory Pump Function
- Pathophysiology of Ventilatory Pump Disorders
  - Mechanical and Physiologic Limitations to Ventilation
    - Factors Related to Ventilatory Load
    - Factors Related to Ventilatory Capacity

Coglianese D, ed. *Clinical Exercise Pathophysiology for Physical Therapy: Examination, Testing, and Exercise Prescription for Movement-Related Disorders* (pp 283-335).
© 2015 Taylor & Francis Group.

Ventilation is the movement of air in and out of the lungs. Respiration is the actual exchange of gas at the alveolar capillary interface in the lungs. As gas is exchanged in the lungs, O_2 is transported for use in the creation of energy for muscle contraction. It is the working muscle that determines how much energy is required. The higher the muscular demand, the greater the requirement for ventilation. When a person moves, afferent signals from the muscles send a message for the nervous system to respond in proportion to the amount of motion created and thereby increase the contraction of respiratory muscles.[1] CO_2, a byproduct of metabolism, also increases with activity and stimulates breathing through central and peripheral chemoreceptors.[2] When there is ventilatory pump dysfunction, individuals may have insufficient O_2 to supply energy for movement. They may choose to move more slowly or limit activity to conserve energy. Poor ventilation can also lead to CO_2 retention and respiratory acidosis.[3] In some cases the ability to breathe may be so impaired that there is inadequate ventilation to support resting energy metabolism. These individuals will require mechanical ventilation. Thus, ventilation is essential for life and the ability to enhance ventilatory capacity is critical to support activity and movement.

BIOMECHANICS OF VENTILATORY PUMP DYSFUNCTION

The biomechanics of ventilatory pump function are dependent on the structure and function of the thoracic musculoskeletal and nervous systems. Additionally, lung tissue must be free of disease to ensure proper mechanics of breathing. The thoracic musculoskeletal system has a skeletal portion and a muscular component. The skeletal system, or the thoracic cage, is composed of a rib cage, formed by the 12 pairs of ribs, the sternum (breast bone), costal cartilages, and the 12 thoracic vertebrae. The ribs are articulated to a thoracic spine posteriorly by the costovertebral and costotransverse ligaments.[4,5] The sternum is composed of 3 parts: a manubrium, a body, and the xiphoid process and is loosely supported by its attachment to the clavicles and has flexible costal cartilage articulations with the ribs. The 12 ribs have 3 classifications; true ribs (ribs 1 to 7), false ribs (ribs 8 to 10) and floating ribs (ribs 11 and 12). The true ribs attach directly to the sternum through their own costal cartilages and the false ribs are joined to the rib just above through interchondral cartilaginous attachment. Floating ribs do not attach to the sternum and simply end anteriorly.[4]

The thoracic cage serves to protect the underlying vital organs while remaining flexible and compliant to allow rib cage motion required for inspiration and expiration. The thorax moves in 3 dimensions: anterior-posterior, superior-inferior, and lateral costal expansion.[6,7] Posteriorly, small movements at the costovertebral axis of the first 7 ribs result in larger anterior displacement of the upper chest. The sternum moves anteriorly and superiorly, referred to as pump handle motion. There is also lateral movement in the lower thoracic cage as ribs 8 to 10 move up and out in a bucket handle motion.[5] The inferior division of the thorax has no skeletal floor and depends on diaphragm partitioning of internal organs and respiratory muscle mechanics to support ventilation.[8,9]

The muscle component of the ventilatory pump acts on a flexible thoracic cage to deform the chest wall during quiet inspiration. The muscles attached to the thoracic cage contract in a coordinated way, optimizing muscle fiber length

TABLE 8-1. PRIMARY AND ACCESSORY MUSCLES OF VENTILATION

PRIMARY MUSCLES OF VENTILATION AND SEGMENTAL INNERVATION

Diaphragm (C3 to C5)
- Costal and sternal (C3 to C4)
- Crural (C4 to C5)

Chest wall muscles
- Scalenes (C2 to C7)
- Parasternal intercostal muscles (T1 to T5)
- Interosseous intercostal muscles (T1 to T11)
  - Internal intercostals
  - External intercostals
- Triangularis sterni

Abdominal muscles (T5 to T12)
- Rectus abdominis
- External oblique
- Internal oblique
- Transverse abdominis

ACCESSORY MUSCLES OF VENTILATION

- Scalenes (C2 to C7)
- Sternocleidomastoid (C2 to C3)
- Levator scapulae (C3 to C5)
- Rhomboids (C5)
- Trapezius (C3 to C4)
- Erector spinae (C4 to L5)
- Pectoralis minor (C6 to C8)
- Pectoralis major (C5 to T1)
- Serratus anterior (C5 to C7)
- Latissimus dorsi (C6 to C8)
- Levator costarum (T1 to T12)
- Quadratus lumborum (T12, L1 to L3)

tension and biomechanical efficiency while expanding the chest in multiple dimensions. The muscles acting on the thorax consist of primary muscles of ventilation and accessory muscles (Table 8-1). Three groups of muscles: diaphragm, chest wall muscles (scalene, parasternal, and intercostal muscles), and abdominal muscles work in an interdependent manner as primary muscles of ventilation. Accessory muscles are active during deep inspiration prior to coughing, when metabolic demands are extreme (running or heavy repetitive work) or when severe respiratory disorders increase the work of breathing.[10,11]

Inspiration

The principal muscle of inspiration is the diaphragm, which is responsible for 70% change in tidal volume (TV).[12] The diaphragm rests in a dome shape in the thoracic cavity at the level of the fifth rib at the end of expiration.[13] The diaphragm has 2 halves, a right and left hemidiaphragm each innervated by a separate phrenic nerve.[12] There are 3 parts to each hemidiaphragm: that costal, sternal, and lumbar portion that merge together into a central tendon. The costal portion arises from the lower 4 ribs and lower 6 costal cartilages to form the dome of each of the 2 hemidiaphragms. The sternal portion originates on the posterior surface of the xiphoid process. The lumbar portion arises from the anterolateral aspect of the first 3 lumbar vertebrae, and is composed of the right and left crura. The crural portion of the diaphragm stabilizes the central tendon while the costal fibers shorten during contraction of the diaphragm.[12]

During inspiration the diaphragm contracts and descends in the thoracic cavity, increasing the volume vertically. As the diaphragm continues to descend, it places increased pressure on the internal organs in the abdominal cavity. Intra-abdominal pressure rises as abdominal muscle tone supports the internal organs and opposes further descent of the diaphragm. As intra-abdominal pressure rises significantly, further diaphragm contraction causes the costal fibers to moves the rib cage laterally and anteriorly.[14,15] Thoracic volume increases transversely as well as vertically and finally superiorly in a rhythmic and biomechanically efficient sequence. The thoracic cage expands in a variety of planes (Figure 8-1).[13] As the chest wall expands the intrathoracic pressure is decreased relative to atmospheric pressure and air moves into the lungs.[2]

The chest wall muscles serve to stabilize and oppose negative forces generated by diaphragm descent, while also acting to lift the upper rib cage superiorly.[14,15] The external intercostals attach from the rib above to the costochondral junction of the rib below and continue into the anterior intercostal membrane. The muscle fibers of the external intercostal are angled and can lift the rib below upward toward the rib above and assist in expanding the chest. These actions occur at higher levels of ventilation.[12,15] The scalene muscles insert on the superior surface of the first and second ribs and attach to the transverse processes of the lower 5 cervical vertebrae to lift and expand the rib cage. The parasternal muscles run between the sternum and the costal cartilages and lift the ribs in an anterior direction. Both scalene and parasternal muscles act to prevent retraction of the upper chest due to the negative forces imposed by diaphragm descent.[15] If there is dyssynchronous recruitment of the 3 groups of muscles (diaphragm, chest wall muscles, or abdominal muscles), then ventilation becomes inefficient and abnormal breathing patterns appear.[14] For example, paradoxical breathing, the inward movement of the chest wall during inspiration, results from paralysis of the abdominal and intercostals muscles and dominance of diaphragmatic breathing (Figure 8-2).

Expiration

Quiet expiration is a passive event that does not depend on muscle contraction. Once the respiratory muscles stop contracting, at the end of inspiration, the flexible chest wall relaxes and recoils along with the lung tissue. There is an

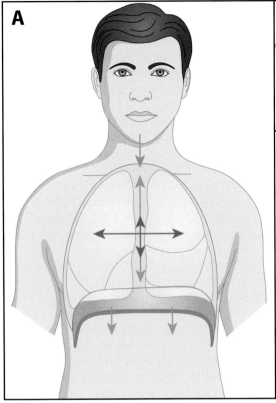

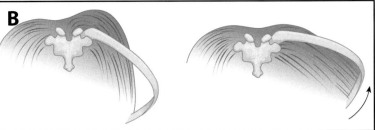

Figure 8-1. Respiratory muscle action on thoracic expansion. (A) Planes of respiration: anterior-posterior, inferior-superior, and lateral. (B) Contraction of the costal fibers of the diaphragm causes rib eversion and elevation. (Adapted from Frownfelter D, Dean E, eds. *Cardiovascular and Pulmonary Physical Therapy: Evidence and Practice.* 4th ed. St. Louis, MO: Mosby; 2006.)

Figure 8-2. Paradoxical breathing patterns. (A) Neck accessory breathing (C2 to C4). (B) Diaphragmatic breathing (C5 to C8). (Adapted from Frownfelter D, Dean E, eds. *Cardiovascular and Pulmonary Physical Therapy: Evidence and Practice.* 4th ed. St. Louis, MO: Mosby; 2006.)

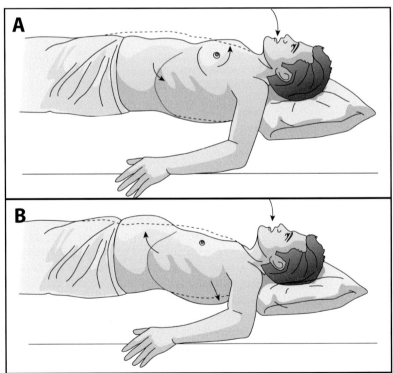

increase in intrathoracic pressure and air leaves the lungs. The elastic tendency of the lungs and chest wall ensure quiet expiration is a passive event. If the chest wall becomes stiff because of poor posture, abnormal muscle tone or pain associated with trauma (rib fractures), arthritis or surgical procedures (sternotomy, thoracic cage incisions), then breathing becomes shallow and the work of breathing is increased.[4,15] Therefore, good inspiratory capacity (IC) and a compliant chest wall and lungs ensure expiratory volume is normal for TV breathing. Aging, immobility, or lung disease may lead to a loss of elasticity in the chest wall and lung tissue with potential decline in passive expiration.[16]

Forced expiration is important in healthy individuals for coughing, shouting loudly, and to produce rapid air flow during exercise. Lungs that lack elastic recoil (aging or disease) may become hyperinflated such that active forced expiration appears at rest or with minimal activity. The abdominal muscles (rectus abdominis, external and internal obliques, and transversus abdominis) and internal intercostals actively contract to increase intra-abdominal and intrathoracic pressure. The action of these muscles forcefully expels air rapidly from the lungs. At the end of forceful expiration, the diaphragm will be extended further into the thoracic cavity.[14] During periods of high ventilatory demand (severe respiratory disorders or exercise) this new position will improve the length-tension of the myofibrils in the diaphragm and optimize breathing.[15] Forced expiration may be further assisted by accessory muscles that compress the chest wall.[10]

Eccentric control of exhalation is important to produce speech.[4] Expiration can be prolonged by gradual release of inspiratory muscle contraction until the chest wall and lungs are near functional residual capacity (FRC). Good eccentric control will allow most adults to vocalize a vowel sound for at least 15 seconds.[17] Volitional eccentric control is also used during pursed-lip breathing and singing and requires intact nervous system over the glottis, the diaphragm, and other inspiratory and expiratory muscles.

Accessory Muscle Actions

Accessory muscle actions are required when the demands of breathing are elevated. Healthy individuals will recruit neck accessory muscles (scalenes and sternocleidomastoid), stabilize the spine, scapula and upper arm (erector spinae, trapezius, rhomboids, and quadratus lumborum) and use the reverse actions of the chest muscles (pectoralis major and minor and serratus anterior) to assist inspiratory effort.[10,12] In addition, the abdominal muscles will increase in intensity and push the diaphragm upward to improve the biomechanical advantage for deep inspiration[14] as well as act to stabilize the trunk for postural control during activity.[18,19] These same muscles assist TV breathing at rest in individuals with respiratory disease or neuromuscular weakness.[4] Expiration may also be assisted by the latissimus dorsi and pectoralis major when other respiratory muscles are compromised.[20,21]

NEUROMUSCULAR INNERVATION/ CENTRAL CONTROL OF BREATHING

Breathing is responsive to activity on an unconscious level. Adjustments are made after a variety of signals communicate with the respiratory center in the medulla. The goal is to maintain homeostasis of the body's pH. Unconscious control can be briefly regulated by volitional control from the cerebral cortex. The volitional control is important for functions that require breath holding (defecation, parturition, and Valsalva maneuver for core stabilization) and eccentric

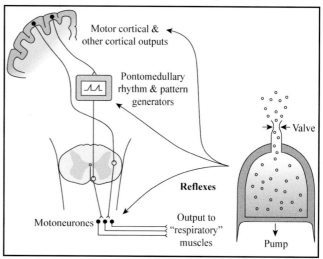

Figure 8-3. Control of respiration. Schematic representation of the control of the muscles of respiration. Direct corticospinal and bulbospinal pathways to respiratory motoneurons and a putative connection between the motor cortex and the pontomedullary respiratory centers are shown. The output from the motoneurons to respiratory muscles includes "pump" muscles that act on the chest wall and "valve" muscles of the upper airway. Feedback from lung, airway, and muscle afferents reaches the 3 levels cortex, medulla, and motoneurons through reflex pathways. (Adapted from Butler JE. Drive to the human respiratory muscles. *Respir Physiol Neurobiol.* 2007;159(2):115-126.)

control of exhalation (for speech, singing) and to build pressure prior to coughing and sneezing. Inspiration for sniffing is also volitional.[22] Each muscle is innervated at a segmental level (see Table 8-1) and may contract at will for volitional breathing or for other functions (eg, arm work). Automatic pathways are distinct from volitional pathways and must be activated rhythmically and repetitively for normal ventilation.[23] Input from reflex pathways from the lungs, airways, and muscle afferents all converge and are integrated to create a precisely timed and appropriate descending respiratory drive (Figure 8-3).

The descending pathways, bulbospinal from the medulla (automatic) or corticospinal (volitional), are coordinated to activate chest wall muscles in a timed sequence that allows the breathing response to vary according to the needs of the individual. Additionally, there is a neuromechanical matching of drive to individual muscles that is organized at the spinal level to allow the most efficient breathing pattern to emerge in the face of pathological conditions or injury to primary muscles of ventilation.[23] Inspiratory drive arises from cyclical firing of neurons in the medulla and is regulated by ascending reflexive nervous system input and chemical stimulation of neurons. Chemoreceptors located on the ventral and lateral surface of the medulla sense the level of CO_2 and hydrogen ion (H+) in the cerebrospinal fluid. As the partial pressure of CO_2 rises, then there will be increased firing of the rate and depth of ventilation.[2,22] Peripheral chemoreceptors in the carotid bodies sense the partial pressure of arterial CO_2 ($PaCO_2$) and also the partial pressure of arterial O_2 (PaO_2). Ventilation increases when there is an elevation of $PaCO_2$ or a decrease in PaO_2 beyond threshold levels. When

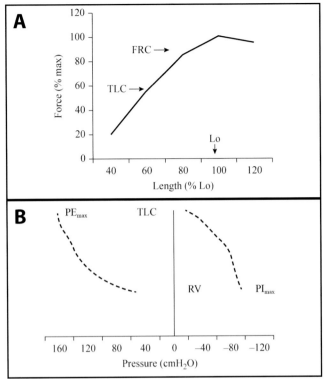

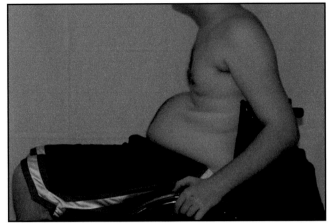

Figure 8-5. Posture and diaphragmatic breathing in a person with abdominal muscle weakness.

Figure 8-4. (A) Diaphragm contractile force and fiber length associated with lung capacities. The relationship between contractile force (percentage of maximum) and resting length (% Lo) for isolated diaphragmatic fibers. Contractile force is greatest close to the resting length (usually higher). As lung volume is increased passively to total lung capacity (TLC), the diaphragm shortens away from its Lo and loses force-generating capacity. (B) Relationship between lung volumes and maximum pressure-generating capacity. At TLC, maximum expiratory pressure (PE$_{max}$) is highest and at residual volume (RV), peak inspiratory pressure (PI$_{max}$) is minimal. (Reprinted from *Clin Chest Med*, 22(4), Flaminiano LE, Celli BR, Respiratory muscle testing, pp 661-677, Copyright 2001, with permission from W.B. Saunders.)

CO_2 is chronically elevated, as occurs with COPD, then the individual becomes more dependent on peripheral chemoreceptor signals from drops in PaO$_2$. This type of breathing control is referred to as hypoxic drive. Together both reflexive and chemical signals work to adjust the descending neural drive rate and depth of breathing. Individuals with COPD have elevated CO_2 and also hyperinflated lungs, which signal an increase in central neural drive. The enhanced central drives recruits more respiratory muscle to assist in managing a high mechanical load during ventilation.

VENTILATORY PUMP PHYSIOLOGY

The muscles of ventilation are influenced by length-tension and force-velocity principles. The force generated by any muscle involved in breathing is a function of its initial resting length as well as the level of neural excitation.[2,10,11] Lung volumes, air pressures, and air flow will affect respiratory muscle mechanics. Measures of lung volume (length) and air pressures (tension) and air flow (velocity) are used to infer respiratory muscle performance.[10] Graphically, the force-length

relationships of respiratory muscles are described using a pressure-volume curve (Figure 8-4).[11] Air pressure generated during maximal inspiration (PI$_{max}$) or expiration (PE$_{max}$) serves as an indication of tension generated by the muscles of inspiration and expiration. Terminology used to describe respiratory physiology and breathing mechanics is provided in Table 8-2 to assist the reader.

The diaphragm position at rest will engage actin and myosin cross bridges such that contraction results in movement through an excursion of 12 to 13 mm as it descends during quiet respiration and 28 to 30 mm during maximal inspiration.[12] At the end of maximal inspiration, the diaphragm is in its shortened position and cannot generate any more force. Once the individual maximally inspires, the lungs are at total lung capacity (TLC) and will hold about 6 L (5 L vital capacity [VC] and 1 L residual volume [RV]) in the young male of average height.[2] Pulmonary function testing is conducted to evaluate ventilation. A variety of lung capacities and volumes may be examined. Maximal forced vital capacity (FVC) is the volume of air that can be maximally inspired and expired. The FVC can be measured and compared to norms for age, height, and gender to evaluate pulmonary status and respiratory muscle function. If the lungs are healthy, the volume of air moved may be used to infer ventilatory muscle performance. However, the diaphragm can lose the ability to generate force if the lungs are hyperinflated, as occurs with lung disease. In this case the diaphragm is flat and muscle fibers in a shortened state so a smaller volume of air is inspired and less air is moved during an FVC maneuver. Likewise if the abdominal muscles are weak or paralyzed (neuromuscular disorders), the abdominal contents fall forward and pull down on the diaphragm and compromise length-tension when the individual is sitting or standing upright (Figure 8-5). The result is a decrease in FVC below what is expected (called "predicted FVC").

Since the diaphragm position is compromised in individuals with either severe COPD or with neuromuscular weakness, there is a loss of optimal length-tension that lowers the volume of air moved (decreased FVC) and pressure generated (decreased PI$_{max}$) during maximal effort.

TABLE 8-2. PULMONARY FUNCTION AND RESPIRATORY PERFORMANCE TERMINOLOGY

TERM AND ABBREVIATION	DEFINITION/RELEVANCE
Vital capacity (VC)	The maximum volume of air that can be expelled after a maximum inspiration (ie, from TLC to RV).
Total lung capacity (TLC)	The total amount of air in the lungs after a maximal inspiration. TLC = RV + ERV + TV + IRV
Inspiratory capacity (IC)	The maximal volume of air that can be inhaled (sum of TV and IRV).
Functional residual capacity (FRC)	The volume of air remaining in the lungs at the end of an ordinary TV expiration. FRC = ERV + RV
Tidal volume (TV)	The volume of air inhaled or exhaled during breathing (at rest or during exercise).
Inspiratory reserve volume (IRV)	The maximum volume of air that can be inhaled to TLC over and above TV inspiration.
Expiratory reserve volume (ERV)	The maximum volume of air that can be exhaled from the end expiratory level or from FRC to RV.
Residual volume (RV)	The volume of air remaining in the lungs after a maximal expiration.
Maximum voluntary ventilation (MVV)	The volume of air breathed when a person breathes as deeply and as quickly as possible for a given time (15 seconds). Usually extrapolated to what could be breathed over 1 minute.
Forced expiratory volume in the first second (FEV_1)	The volume of air released during the first second of a VC maneuver. This indicates the speed of air movement out of the lungs. Used to detect resistance to lung flow or poor expiratory flow.
Peak expiratory flow rate (PEFR)	The fastest speed of airflow in liters per second or liters per minute generated during a maximal VC maneuver. This measure is used to detect any airway restriction or loss of rapid expiratory flow due to decreased speed of expiratory muscle contraction.
Peak cough flow rate (PCFR)	A measure of speed of airflow in liters per second or liters per minute generated during rapid forced expiration such as occurs with coughing. Normal PCFR = 6 to 20 L/sec or 300 to 700 L/min
Partial pressure of carbon dioxide ($PaCO_2$)	The gas pressure of CO_2 found in arterial blood. Normal $PaCO_2$ = 35 to 45 mm Hg
End tidal CO_2 ($ETCO_2$)	Provided the patient has a stable cardiac status, stable body temperature, absence of lung disease, and a normal capnographic trace, $ETCO_2$ approximates the partial pressure of CO_2 in arterial blood ($PaCO_2$.) The measure is taken non-invasively (without needles)
Partial pressure of oxygen (PaO_2)	The gas pressure of O_2 found in arterial blood. Normal PaO_2 = 80 to 100 mm Hg
O_2 saturation of hemoglobin (SaO_2)	The percentage of hemoglobin-carrying sites that are occupied by O_2. Fully saturated = 100%
Diffusion capacity (DLCO)	The ability of the lungs to transfer gas (carbon monoxide) across the alveoli to the pulmonary circulation. Used to detect lung tissue thickening or disease.

(continued)

TABLE 8-2 (CONTINUED). PULMONARY FUNCTION AND RESPIRATORY PERFORMANCE TERMINOLOGY

TERM AND ABBREVIATION	DEFINITION/RELEVANCE
Peak inspiration maximum (PI_{max}) or maximal inspiratory pressure (MIP)	Different terms are used to denote peak or maximal inspiratory pressure generated during a maximal inspiratory maneuver against occluded airflow. The subject inhales maximally from a predetermined lung volume (RV or end tidal volume). A negative pressure is generated and recorded in cubic centimeters or centimeters of H_2O.
Peak expiration maximum (PE_{max}) or maximal expiratory pressure (MEP)	Different terms are used to denote peak or maximal expiratory pressure generated during a maximal expiratory maneuver against occluded airflow. The subject exhales maximally from a predetermined lung volume (TLC or end tidal inspiratory volume). A positive pressure is generated and recorded in cubic centimeters or centimeters of H_2O.
Negative inspiratory pressure/force (NIP/NIF)	A measure of inspiratory muscle strength. The subject inhales against a device that occludes airflow. A negative pressure in generated and recorded in cubic centimeters or centimeters of H_2O. It may or may not be a maximal effort.
Minute ventilation (VE)	The volume of air moved in 1 minute. Typically used to determine the ability of the person to move air in and out of the lungs during exercise. $VE = TV \times RR$
Inspiratory duty cycle; inspiratory time/total time for one breath (Ti/T_{TOT})	Method for detecting the increase in inspiratory muscle activation during the respiratory cycle. Increase in Ti suggests the muscles of inspiration are working harder and have the potential to fatigue. Denotes an increased work of breathing.
Transdiaphragmatic pressure (P_{di})	Difference between pressure generated at the esophageal level (pleural pressure) and pressure generated at the gastric level (abdominal pressure). The difference in pressure suggests the ability of the diaphragm to contract and generate force.
Pressure at the level of the esophagus (sometimes called PPl for pleural pressure [Pes (Ppl)])	A pressure reading taken in the esophagus to detect pressure during various phases of the respiratory cycle and used to infer pleural pressure.
Pressure at the level of the gastric region (sometimes called Pab for intra-abdominal pressure [Pgs (Pab)])	A pressure reading taken in the stomach or gastric region to detect pressure during various phases of the respiratory cycle and used to infer intra-abdominal pressure.
Mouth occlusion pressure ($P_{0.1}$)	Measure used to indicate central respiratory motor drive. Airway pressure developed at the mouth that occurs 0.1 seconds after the onset of inspiration. The airway is occluded at the mouth. The time parameter suggests that this measure occurs before volitional contraction of respiratory muscles and reflects nervous system activation.
Rapid shallow breathing index (RR/TV)	Method used to determine volitional breathing ability. Breaths per minute divided by TV in liters (breaths/min/L). Normal = 50
Ventilatory muscle training (VMT)	Resistive training for the respiratory muscles; includes both inspiratory and expiratory muscle work.
Inspiratory muscle training (IMT)	Resistive training for the muscles responsible for inspiration.
Expiratory muscle training (EMT)	Resistive training for the muscles responsible for expiration.
Threshold loading maximum (TLmax)	The highest resistive load that can be sustained for at least 2 minutes during progressive incremental resistive loading test. Used to define the endurance capacity of the respiratory muscles.

Poor IC leads to poor expiratory capacity since the lung and chest wall recoiling forces are lower. During coughing in individuals with disease or weakness, the abdominal muscles may contract but since there is little air movement into and out of the lungs, the flow generated may not be effective for coughing for some individuals.[24]

Rapid contraction of respiratory muscles is essential for coughing to clearing mucus or other particulate matter. The velocity of respiratory muscle contraction can be examined by measuring air flow, specifically peak expiratory flow rate (PEFR) or peak cough flow rate (PCFR) in liters per second (L/s) or liters per minute (L/min). Normal cough volumes are 2.3 ± 0.5 L with a PCFR of 6 to 12 L/s or 300 to 700 L/min.[24-26] An individual must have a minimum PCFR of 2.7 L/s for effective airway clearance.[4,24] However, if there is lung disease and airway collapse restricts air flow, then the decrease in PEFR is not simply a reflection of respiratory muscle performance. Any drop in flow rate may also indicate a loss of air flow due to restrictions in the outflow of air and may occur with asthma, mucus or dynamic airway collapse from obstructive lung disease or aging.

Another test of flow rate is the forced expiratory volume (FEV). The FEV_1 is the volume of air that may be expelled during the first second of an FVC maneuver. About 80% of the total FVC is usually removed from the lungs during this time. Normally the FEV_1/FVC relationship is between 70% and 85% and values falling below 70% indicate obstructive disease while values above 85% indicate restrictive disease.[27] For individuals with neuromuscular conditions, when the FEV_1/FVC falls below 60%, cough flow rates may be inadequate.[4] All pulmonary functions (FVC, FEV_1, and PEFR) and respiratory pressure measures (PI_{max} and PE_{max}) may also be compared to normative standards for age, height, and gender. These values will be 100% of expected or better if there is no pathology interfering with ventilation. However, values that fall below predicted levels are abnormal. Typically, the lower the percentage predicted, the worse the ventilatory impairment. These values may be reported as FVC% predicted, FEV_1% predicted, PEFR% predicted, PI_{max}% predicted or PE_{max}% predicted and are documented in the pulmonary function test reports.

O_2 requirements for movement are met by increasing ventilation, which is enhanced by increasing TV and respiratory rate (RR). Exercise increases the need for O_2 and the body responds, driving up TV (from .5 to 2 to 3 L per breath) and RR (16 to about 40 breaths per minute) to enhance the minute ventilation (VE).[1] The work of breathing increases according to the rate (RR) and depth of each breath (TV) as well as the level of contractile force and overall inspiratory time (Ti) within the total respiratory cycle (T_{TOT}) or Ti/T_{TOT}. VE increases as activity level is elevated. However, the work of breathing for any given submaximal activity requires a higher VE if the individual is either older or deconditioned or has pathology.[28] Therefore, physiologic monitoring of therapeutic exercise and testing aerobic capacity will also assist in describing any ventilatory limitation and developing a plan of care (POC) to address these.[29]

Ventilatory pump physiology changes and adapts to compensate for alterations in lung compliance (COPD, pulmonary fibrosis, and pulmonary edema), chest wall compliance (kyphoscoliosis, rib fracture, postsurgical pain, developmental or musculoskeletal postural dysfunction) and neuromuscular conditions (Guillain-Barré syndrome [GBS], spinal cord injury [SCI], hemiplegia, cerebral palsy). A variety of disorders may affect ventilatory pump physiology and increase the work of breathing (Table 8-3). An individual with pathology may have the ability to compensate at rest and during routine activity but as O_2 demands are extended during exercise, there is usually increased RR and accessory muscle use once the TV is maximized. The next 2 sections (see Epidemiology of Ventilatory Pump Disorders and Pathophysiology of Ventilatory Pump Disorders sections) will discuss the clinical presentation of common ventilatory pump disorders and potential compensatory breathing actions appearing in individuals presenting with age-related changes, primary lung disease, neuromuscular conditions, and chest wall limitations.

EPIDEMIOLOGY OF VENTILATORY BIOMECHANICAL PATHOLOGY

Age-Related Changes and Ventilatory Pump Function

Age-related changes and pathology (COPD, neuromuscular disease, musculoskeletal disorders) may disrupt the mechanics of normal, efficient breathing. The skeletal, pulmonary, and neuromuscular systems undergo age-related changes that affect the ability to ventilate (Table 8-4).[30] The physiologic changes in the skeletal system include calcification of the costal cartilages, arthritic changes in the joints of the ribs and vertebrae along with decalcification of the ribs. Many older individuals develop a barrel chest and/or thoracic kyphosis.[16,31] In the pulmonary system, there is a reduced lung elastic recoil (alveolar compliance increases) which contributes to early airway closure and decreased FEV_1. Air trapping leads to an elevation of the RV and FRC (Figure 8-6), which results in hyperinflation and flattening of the diaphragm, disrupting the mechanics of breathing. The work of breathing increases as the lungs lose their elasticity and the chest wall stiffens.[32] The inspiratory muscles are less optimally aligned and contract at a higher percentage of maximum during exercise, which drives up the cost of breathing.[33] As a result respiratory muscle strength (PI_{max} and PE_{max}) and endurance (maximum voluntary ventilation [MVV]) are reduced.[30,34-37]

Additionally, there is a loss of pulmonary capillary bed perfusion, increased physiologic dead space and ventilation perfusion mismatch decreasing the gas transfer (diffusion: DLCO) and causing PaO_2 to decline.[38] In the nervous system, both the peripheral and central chemoreceptors lose their

Table 8-3. Clinical Conditions and Ventilatory Pump Dysfunction

Primary Lung Diseases	• Obstructive lung disease
	  ○ Chronic bronchitis
	  ○ Emphysema
	  ○ Cystic fibrosis
	  ○ Bronchiectasis
	  ○ Asthma
	• Restrictive lung disease
	  ○ Adult respiratory distress syndrome
	  ○ Bronchopulmonary dysplasia
	  ○ Pulmonary fibrosis
	  ○ Sarcoidosis
	  ○ Asbestosis
	  ○ Bronchiolitis obliterans
	  ○ Pneumoconiosis
	• Adverse medical conditions
	  ○ Pleural effusions
	  ○ Empyema
	  ○ Pulmonary edema
	  ○ Pulmonary emboli

Neuromuscular Conditions	• SCI • Spinal muscular atrophy • GBS • Multiple sclerosis • Cerebral palsy • Myasthenia gravis • Poliomyelitis/post-polio • Muscular dystrophy • Cerebral vascular accident • Brain injury • Amyotrophic lateral sclerosis • Parkinson's disease
Chest Wall Disorders	• Postural dysfunction • Ankylosing spondylitis • Trauma • Rib fracture • Burns • Postsurgical • Arthritis • Connective tissue disorders

Table 8-4. Age-Related Changes Affecting Ventilation

BODY SYSTEM	SYSTEM CHANGES
Skeletal system	Costal cartilage calcification Narrowing of vertebral discs Barrel chest due to↑ a-p diameter ↑ Kyphosis due to vertebral fx/compression Alter angulation of rib articulations ↑ Chest wall stiffness (↓ compliance)
Pulmonary system	Altered connective tissue structure ↓ Elastic recoil (↑ compliance) ↓ Alveolar-capillary surface area ↓ Small airway diameter (bronchioles) ↓ Force expiratory flow (FEV_1) ↑ RV ↓ FVC ↓ Ventilation-perfusion matching ↓ PaO_2 ↓ DLCO ↑ Pulmonary vascular resistance
Neuromuscular system	↓ PE_{max} (MEP) ↓ PI_{max} (MIP) ↓ MVV ↓ Central drive ($P_{0.1}$) Loss of type II fibers = ↑ work of breathing

fx: fracture.

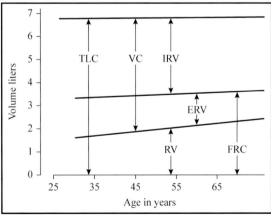

Figure 8-6. Evolution of lung volumes with aging. ERV, expiratory reserve volume; FRC, functional residual capacity; IRV, inspiratory reserve volume; RV, residual volume; TLC, total lung capacity; VC, vital capacity. (Reproduced with permission of the European Respiratory Society. *Eur Respir J, January 1, 1999,* 13(1):197-205.)

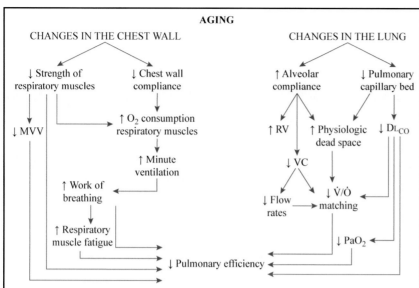

Figure 8-7. Respiratory changes with aging. V/Q: ventilation/perfusion. (Adapted from Hillegass EA, Sadowsky HS, eds. *Essentials of Cardiopulmonary Physical Therapy.* 2nd ed. Philadelphia, PA: W.B. Saunders Company; 2001.)

sensitivity to PaO_2 and PCO_2. The normal PaO_2 declines 5 to 10 mm Hg by age 70 or and averages 75 mm Hg.[34] Because the chemoreceptors lose their sensitivity, the central drive ($P_{0.1}$) at rest is depressed.[39,40] These changes are accelerated after age 65 to 70.[32] Age-related changes affecting ventilation are summarized in Figure 8-7.

Although we begin aging in our 20s, the aging effects on the pulmonary system are not observed to affect function until age 60 or 70.[16,31] Normally, the young, healthy individual can exercise to maximal level without reaching the limits of pulmonary function. VE is elevated during a progressive exercise test by increases in TV and RR. During an exercise test to maximum, TV normally plateaus at about 60% of maximum O_2 consumption (VO_{2max}), after which the increase in VE is achieved by further increases in RR.[1] In the younger individual cardiac output limits further final maximal work rate. This is also true for the older individual although lower HR_{max} and cardiac output result in lower VO_{2max} compared to younger individuals.[41]

After age 70 there is evidence that VE limits may be reached. Even those with superior fitness cannot attenuate age-imposed limitations to pulmonary ventilation at maximal exercise. McClaran et al[32] demonstrated, in a longitudinal study over 6 years, the impact of aging and reduced ventilation on VO_{2max} in 18 fit older individuals (67 to 73 years). During high-intensity exercise, the ventilatory response (VE) was limited because of reduced TV component. As a result of a lower TV during exercise, RR increases to compensate. There is an excessive elevation in CO_2 production (VCO_2) that is due in part to an increased respiratory muscle demand for breathing.[42] Although mild and moderate intensity exercise ($< 60\%$ of VO_{2max}) is not affected by age-related changes in the pulmonary system for the well-trained older individual, there are several reports documenting an increase in the work of breathing during submaximal work for those who are older and sedentary.[16,34]

Compared to younger counterparts, the older individual reaches higher VE than younger counter parts for a specific submaximal activity. The older individual ventilates at a higher lung volume and therefore must work against higher pleural pressures and increased elastic load (due to chest wall stiffness) to sustain a deeper TV in order to achieve the same submaximal work rate.[34] The end-expiratory lung volume will be increased, trapping air and preventing full expiration (hyperinflation). Expiration in the older individual is assisted by higher levels of expiratory muscle contraction. As hyperinflation volumes are increased with progressive work, the diaphragm is flattened and becomes less efficient in generating contractile force. Eventually, as submaximal activity increases in intensity, the frequency of breathing (f or RR) also increases to a greater extent in the older person. The O_2 consumption for the respiratory muscles may require as much as 10% to 12% of the total VO_{2max}.[16,34] Despite the increase in the work of breathing, the elderly may have a diminished sensitivity to increased respiratory load that may or may not translate into higher levels of perceived breathlessness.[43]

The impact of age-related changes to the pulmonary system on acute exercise can be improved with training.[16,44] For those older individuals who are sedentary or not highly trained, aerobic training will lower ventilatory requirement for submaximal exercise and raise the VO_2 max and VE at maximal exercise.[45] These changes are primarily due to improved O_2 uptake in the peripheral muscle, lowering the relative ventilatory requirement.[16] The physiological benefits observed with training in the older individual translate to greater improvements in older individuals with ventilatory pump limitations. Peripheral training effects and enhancement of VE serve as a basis for use of exercise training in many individuals with ventilatory pump dysfunction. Various forms of exercise training play a key role in improving functional status in older individuals who may also have lung tissue disorders.

Table 8-5. GOLD Classification System for Severity of Chronic Obstructive Pulmonary Disease

STAGE	CHARACTERISTICS
0: At risk	Normal spirometry Chronic symptoms (cough, sputum production)
I: Mild COPD	$FEV_1/FVC < 70\%$ FEV_1 greater than or equal to 80% predicted With or without chronic symptoms (cough, sputum production)

II: Moderate COPD	$FEV_1/FVC < 70\%$
	FEV_1 greater than or equal to 30% to <80% predicted
	    IIa: FEV_1 greater than or equal to 50% to < 80% predicted
	    IIb: FEV_1 greater than or equal to 30% to < 50% predicted
	    With or without chronic symptoms (cough, sputum production, dyspnea)

III: Severe COPD	$FEV_1/FVC < 70\%$ $FEV_1 < 30\%$ predicted or $FEV_1 < 50\%$ predicted plus respiratory failure or clinical signs of right heart failure

GOLD, Global Initiative for Chronic Obstructive Lung Disease; respiratory failure, arterial partial pressure of $O_2 < 60$ mm Hg with or without arterial partial pressure of CO_2 greater than or equal to 50 mm Hg while breathing air at sea level.

Reprinted with permission from Pauwels RA, Buist AS, Calverley PM, Jenkins CR, Hurd SS. Global strategy for the diagnosis, management, and prevention of chronic obstructive pulmonary disease. NHLBI/WHO Global Intiative for Chronic Obstructive Lung Disease (GOLD) Workshop summary. *Am J Respir Crit Care Med.* 2001;163:125-1376.

Incidence and Prevalence of Pathology Affecting Ventilatory Pump Function

Many individuals seen by health professionals are older and also have pathology that affects ventilation. These conditions may alter body homeostasis and may affect function. It is beyond the scope of this chapter to discuss every condition that may affect ventilation. However, the chapter will next discuss the incidence and prevalence of 3 major classifications or health conditions that may affect ventilatory pump function: COPD, neuromuscular disease, and musculoskeletal disorders. Following a discussion of incidence and prevalence of each condition will be an explanation of the pathology and physiological consequences that influence ventilatory pump function.

Chronic Obstructive Pulmonary Disease Pathology Affecting Ventilatory Pump Function

Nearly 14 million adults in the United States (US) have COPD. It is the fourth leading cause of death, responsible for 1 in 20 deaths.[46,47] Those with advanced COPD die from respiratory failure, and these individuals comprise 40% of all cases of chronic respiratory failure.[48,49] According to the Centers for Disease Control and Prevention, approximately 75% of the deaths are due to smoking.[47] COPD is defined as a "disease state characterized by flow limitation that is not fully reversible."[50] The degree of air flow limitation is assessed by FEV_1 and describes disease severity. Individuals are classified as having mild, moderate, severe or very severe based on criteria listed in Table 8-5. As the disease progresses, activity is limited by symptoms of dyspnea, fatigue, and lower extremity (LE) weakness.[51-54] Symptoms do not become overt until the FEV_1 declines substantially ($FEV_1 < 50\%$ predicted) or stage II COPD.[52,55] The prevalence of stage II COPD or higher is approximately 10% worldwide.[56]

Incidence of COPD is increased in those who are older, male, and smoke or have hazardous environmental exposures.[57] Smoking will double the rate of loss of FEV_1 as the individual ages and smoking cessation in smokers will slow this decline.[58,59] The prevalence of COPD is increased in civilized countries where levels of smoking and life expectancy are greater.[60] Countries that are unable to manage the spread of tuberculosis also have an increased prevalence of COPD within the population. Therefore, a variety of socioeconomic and regional factors influence the prevalence of COPD.[60] Genetics appear to play a role in the development of COPD in some individuals.[61] Alpha 1 antitrypsin deficiency is a hereditary condition that results in the loss of an enzyme that protects the lungs. This hereditary condition occurs in 60,000 to 100,000 people with lung disease and comprises approximately 13% of individuals with emphysema.[58,62] In summary, a variety of factors influence the development of COPD, a disease that ends in respiratory failure.[48]

Neuromuscular Conditions Affecting Ventilatory Pump Function

Approximately 1.9% of the US population or 5,596,000 people report some form of paralysis. Distribution of individuals reporting weakness is as follows: stroke 29%, SCI 23%, traumatic brain injury 4%, cerebral palsy 7%, post-polio syndrome (PPS) 5%, and other conditions 9% (amyotrophic lateral sclerosis [ALS], GBS, myasthenia gravis, Parkinson's disease, etc).[63] There are numerous reports of diminished lung capacities and impaired respiratory muscle function that coincides with level of disability in the majority of neuromuscular conditions.[31,64-70] Pulmonary function testing usually reveals a restrictive pattern that is confirmed when $FEV_1/FVC > 85\%$ predicted and FVC falls below 80% predicted.[27,31] Additionally, declines in PI_{max} and PE_{max} values confirm weak respiratory muscles.[3] Most individuals with neuromuscular disease who have impaired breathing mechanics do not notice limitations to activity until measures of FVC and strength (PI_{max} and PE_{max}) drop below 50% predicted.[71] However, these individuals rapidly fall into respiratory failure once these values reach 25% predicted.

Respiratory failure and pneumonia are the major complications leading to increased morbidity and mortality in those with neuromuscular disease.[72-74] Almost all individuals with ALS will die from respiratory failure.[71] Respiratory failure and infection is the cause of death in 75% of individuals who have Duchenne muscular dystrophy (DMD).[31] After a stroke, between 50% and 90% die once they are intubated.[72] The majority of cases resulting in acute respiratory failure from neurological conditions occur in individuals with GBS and myasthenia gravis.[72] Greater than 50% of those with GBS and myasthenia gravis will contract pulmonary conditions and 15% to 30% will requiring mechanical ventilation.[75,76] SCI is the most common cause of chronic ventilatory insufficiency in young adults.[71] Sixty-seven percent of individuals with SCIs (C1 to T12; Grades A, B, or C[77]) have respiratory complications in the initial weeks after injury.[74] Thus, for individuals with neuromuscular conditions, it is critically important to monitor the pulmonary function, specifically FVC and measures of strength (PI_{max} and PE_{max}) to prevent complications and identify interventions to reduce the effects of respiratory compromise.[68,76,78]

Musculoskeletal Disorders Affecting Ventilatory Pump Function

Musculoskeletal disorders may affect ventilatory pump function by restricting the movement of the chest wall. Therefore, these conditions are referred to as *chest wall disorders* (see Table 8-3). Approximately 6% of all individuals with chronic respiratory failure have severe kyphoscoliosis.[49] Kyphosis, scoliosis or kyphoscoliosis are postural deformities that can result from idiopathic causes, osteoporosis or disease (ankylosing spondylitis [AS], arthritis, or neuromuscular conditions). Severe deformity can limit pulmonary function.[79,80] Approximately 32% of individuals with idiopathic scoliosis have pulmonary symptoms either at rest or experience breathlessness that is out of proportion with activity.[81] The frequency of pulmonary complications in those with rheumatoid arthritis has been reported to be as high as 45%.[82] Many of these individuals need surgery, which further impairs breathing mechanics during the postsurgical recovery period.[83,84]

Surgery and traumatic injury to the thorax (rib fractures, flail chest, vertebral and sternal fractures) may make breathing painful. Pain can limit deep breathing for up to 2 weeks post-event and interfere with coughing for up to 6 months.[31] After upper abdominal surgery, the VC may temporarily decrease by 55% in part because of the effects of anesthesia.[85] Anesthesia will depress the central nervous system, decrease diaphragm tone, and increase the FRC.[86] When there is a traumatic injury to the chest wall, lung tissue may be damaged by pneumothorax, pleural effusions, and later empyema if infection occurs. Hemothorax occurs in 70% of individuals having chest trauma.[85] Rib fractures occur in about 10% of patients who have suffered a traumatic injury and are associated with a 35% incidence of pulmonary complications.[87] Risk for mortality after rib fracture is about 12% overall but is much higher in the older individual.[88] Ribs may fracture in 2 or more places and result in a "flail chest." In this case, the chest wall is no longer stable and the injured portion moves paradoxically. Lung contusion is typically associated with this injury.[89] Pneumonia will develop within contused segments in 50% to 70% of individuals, while 35% will develop empyema.[85,90]

PATHOPHYSIOLOGY OF VENTILATORY PUMP DISORDERS

Pathophysiology results when an abnormal condition disrupts the body structure and function of a specific biological system (ie, digestive, respiratory, cardiovascular). The impact of pathology on body structure and function influences activity participation differently in each individual.[91] Contextual factors, such as access to quality rehabilitation, one's adaptability to stress, age, fitness, and existing comorbidities, will further define the eventual level of activity participation for an individual with a ventilatory pump disorder. Therefore, according to the *Guide to Physical Therapist Practice*, pathophysiology is defined as "the interruption of normal processes important to physical functioning and activity participation critical to maintaining or returning to usual self-care, home management, work, community and leisure roles."[92(p 29)] This broad definition goes beyond consideration of the disease state and encompasses the concept of health status. Today's health care environment requires practitioners look at the total well-being and overall health condition as well as the degree to which any disease or injury impacts on participation in expected and desired life roles.

The pathophysiology of ventilatory pump disorders will be described in this section in 2 ways: First, the mechanical and physiologic disruptions that may limit ventilation

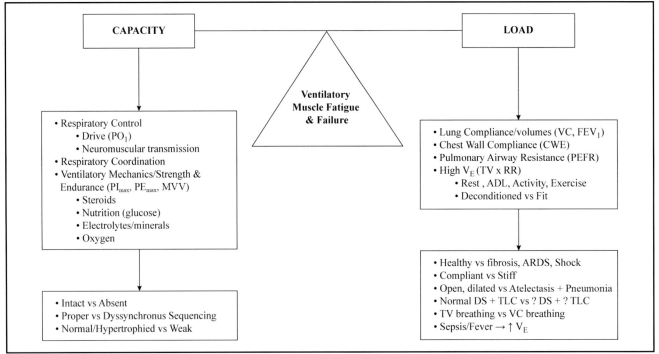

Figure 8-8. Balance of capacity and load for ventilation. ADL, activities of daily living; ARDS, Adult Respiratory Distress Syndrome; CWE, chest wall excursion measurements; DS, dead space; FEV$_1$, forced expiratory volume 1 second; MEP, maximum expiratory pressure; MIP, maximum inspiratory pressure; PEFR, peak expiratory flow rate; PO$_1$, pressure occlusion 1 second; RR, respiratory rate; TLC, total lung capacity; TV, tidal volume; VC, vital capacity; VE, minute ventilation. (Adapted from Vassilakopoulos T, Zakynthinos S, Roussos CH. Respiratory muscles and weaning failure. *Eur Respir J.* 1996;9:2383-2400.)

will be presented. Second, an explanation of the pathophysiology and complications of specific conditions (COPD, neuromuscular conditions, and musculoskeletal disorders) and the factors that affect activity participation will be discussed. Understanding how pathology may affect ventilation should assist the health care professional in identifying which examinations will be important to assist in designing a POC aimed at restoring function. The POC may then be developed to address primary impairments directly resulting from pathology that may lead to ventilatory pump dysfunction (chest wall tightness, respiratory muscle weakness), or the POC may include interventions to assist the individual in compensating for or managing the ventilation disorder (conditioning, breathing control strategies).

Mechanical and Physiologic Limitations to Ventilation

The goal of the ventilatory pump is to create changes in intrathoracic pressure that allow air to move between the lungs and the atmosphere in order to exchange O$_2$ and CO$_2$.[2] Good gas exchange optimizes metabolism and stabilizes blood gases to maintain homeostasis. Pathologic processes may affect ventilation in 2 ways: either the load to the ventilatory muscles is increased or the capacity of the ventilatory muscle is diminished (Figure 8-8).[93] In many individuals both load and capacity are affected by pathology. The actual medical diagnosis may help the clinician identify systems

affected by a disease or condition, but the impact on ventilation is specific to examination of factors related to ventilatory load and capacity.

Factors Related to Ventilatory Load

Ventilatory load is the force that must be overcome to allow movement of gas in and out of the lungs. The factors influencing load include lung tissue and chest wall elasticity (compliance), pulmonary airway resistance, and VE.[93] VE (VE = TV × RR) varies according to activity demands and is lowest at rest (about 6 to 10 L/min) and highest during maximal exercise (over 100 L/min).[1] During quiet breathing at rest about 75% of the breath reaches the gas-exchanging regions (alveolar ventilation) of the lung while 25% is dead-space ventilation and cannot participate in gas exchange.[2] As the need to enhance ventilation increases with activity, VE is elevated by raising both the TV and RR. Eventually, as exercise demands are extended, TV plateaus at about 2 to 2.5 L per breath. To achieve higher levels of activity, RR continues to climb above 40 breaths per minute. The respiratory muscle O$_2$ utilization increases from about 3 mL O$_2$/L at rest to 4.5 mL/L (2% to 4% of total VO$_2$) at peak exercise.[94,95] The respiratory muscles in the healthy individual are strong and well coordinated and can easily meet the increased load imposed by exercise. Individuals with ventilatory pump disorders are unable to increase TV effectively.[1,28] RR increases earlier at lower, submaximal workloads. This pattern of ventilation increases the work of breathing and results in excessive dead-space ventilation.

A variety of pathologies may affect ventilatory load. In pathology the cost of breathing for those with restrictive lung disease (ie, pulmonary fibrosis) may require as much as 25% of the O_2 consumed throughout the body.[95,96] This is because of a higher RR since the rate climbs excessively to compensate for a severely diminished TV. Additionally, chest wall stiffness and decreased lung compliance also require respiratory muscles to generate higher forces to open the lungs. More intercostal and accessory muscles are recruited, adding to energy cost of breathing.[14] The individual with pathology will have an elevated RR, increased dyspnea scores, early onset of accessory muscle use, and possibly oxyhemoglobin desaturation, if there is a ventilation/perfusion (V/Q) mismatch resulting from increased physiologic deadspace.[1]

When dead-space ventilation increases, alveolar ventilation becomes compromised, limiting gas transfer from the alveoli to the pulmonary capillaries. Compared to healthy persons, individuals with a ventilatory pump disorder reach higher VE at a given submaximal workload and require even greater respiratory muscle effort during activity.[1,28,97] Higher VE with submaximal work also occurs because cellular adaptations are underdeveloped, resulting in inefficient oxidative capacity in the peripheral muscle.[28] Mild impairments in ventilatory function (early neuromuscular disease or COPD) are most apparent during exercise.[28] Interventions that reduce chest wall restriction (chest wall mobilization) or offset poor oxidative capacity (energy conservation or aerobic training) may reduce the ventilatory load.[4]

Finally, ventilatory load may be elevated when airway resistance is increased as a result of pathology. This can occur when there is a mechanical torsion and compression of the bronchioles and vasculature (kyphoscoliosis, AS), when there is dynamic airway collapse or bronchospasm (COPD, asthma) or when the individual develops a respiratory complication (pneumonia, pneumothorax, effusion). Infections may produce a fever that can reduce the performance of respiratory muscles.[98] Individuals with infections and poor cough function may have excessive mucus in the airways, and those with lung tumors may have mechanical restrictions obstructing the flow of air. These events all restrict air flow and increase the work of breathing.

Interventions for airway clearance, breathing control or to correct posture may be offered to minimize the pathophysiologic consequences resulting from these conditions.[31] Effective coughing requires high flows to mobilize thick secretions. Individuals with excess mucus who also have excessive compliance and collapsible airways will need to learn alternative strategies, other than vigorous coughing, to clear mucus. High pressures required to generate forceful air flow for coughing (2.7 L/s) contribute to airway collapse and trapping of mucus.[99] Individuals with decreased inspiratory volume (neurological conditions) and poor capacity for forced expiration will need to use cough-assist techniques to create effective expulsion of air to clear mucus.[100]

Factors Related to Ventilatory Capacity

Ventilatory capacity is the potential of the neuromuscular system to work efficiently in a coordinated manner to move the chest wall against the ventilatory load.[93] Inspiratory muscles are recruited repetitively in the most biomechanically efficient manner (see earlier section: Introduction-Inspiration). The VE is adjusted so adequate gas exchange can support activity.[28] Capacity is dependent on respiratory control (drive, neuromuscular transmission), breathing coordination, and ventilatory mechanics (muscular strength and endurance; see Figure 8-8).[93]

Respiratory muscles do not rest and must repetitively contract with enough force to sustain breathing against elastic and resistive loads. The ability to sustain a load without fatigue is called *endurance*. Like all skeletal muscles, the ability to generate and sustain contraction depends on adequate energy supplies (O_2, glucose, fatty acids, blood-borne substrates, etc).[93,101] Respiratory muscles that are well conditioned with good perfusion can extract O_2 and glucose from the blood and also use stored energy (creatine phosphate, adenosine triphosphate, glycogen, etc). However, if the muscle is weak or deconditioned, then capacity is reduced. Abnormal breathing patterns demand higher levels of energy that may not be sustainable. Nutritional support is crucial for individuals using compensatory breathing patterns.[102,103] Respiratory muscle fatigue occurs when either the energy supplies to the muscle are not adequate to meet the energy required for contraction or when neuromuscular transmission is impaired. Either the individual slows activity and becomes less functional or mechanical ventilation is required when TV breathing cannot be managed at rest.

A variety of pathological processes may affect ventilatory capacity. It is important to remember that pathology causes alterations in ventilatory muscle mechanics that increase respiratory muscle demands and limit endurance. This means the inspiratory muscles work longer in the entire respiratory cycle (Ti/T_{TOT}) and they work at a higher percentage of maximum (PI/PI_{max}).[104] This concept is referred to as *tension time index* ($TTI = Ti/T_{TOT} \times PI/PI_{max}$). As TTI increases, so does the energy requirement and the risk for fatigue. Respiratory muscles fatigue when they reach a critical level and work above 40% of the PI_{max}.[101,104] Interventions designed to strengthen the respiratory muscles (ventilatory muscle training [VMT], proprioceptive neuromuscular facilitation [PNF]) or to improve the biomechanics of breathing (abdominal binder, posture alignment) may reduce the TTI and enhance ventilatory capacity.[13,105] In many cases, medical intervention is necessary to eliminate the cause of respiratory muscle failure (sepsis, drug overdose) or to assist the individual through a problem like sleep-induced hypoventilation (by offering noninvasive mechanical ventilation). Clinicians working with the medical team can assist by recognizing and reporting signs and symptoms or respiratory muscle incompetence (Table 8-6). Early intervention with some form of mechanical ventilation improves

TABLE 8-6. SIGNS AND SYMPTOMS OF RESPIRATORY MUSCLE INCOMPETENCE

SIGNS

- RR > 30 at rest
- RPD > 3/10 (Borg Scale) at rest
- VC < 20 mL/kg IBW
- $PI_{max} > -30$ cm H_2O
- $PE_{max} > 40$ cm H_2O
- $PaCO_2 > 50$ mm Hg
- $PaO_2 < 50$ mm Hg (O_2 saturation < 85%)

SYMPTOMS

- ↓ Level of alertness, sleepiness
- Memory loss or change in cognition
- Headache
- Shallow breathing
- Excessive neck/accessory muscle breathing
- Inability to lift head (supine)
- Head bobbing (sitting)
- Respiratory alternans
- Paradoxical breathing
- Dyssynchronous breathing
- Inability to use arms for functional tasks
- Blue/gray appearance

RPD: rating of perceived dyspnea; IBW: ideal body weight.
Reprinted with permission from Mehta S. Neuromuscular disease causing acute respiratory failure. *Respir Care*. 2006;51(9):1016-1021.

long-term survival for most patients who have impending ventilatory pump failure.[68,106]

Pathophysiology and Complications in Ventilatory Pump Disorders

Alveolar hypoventilation, atelectasis, and pneumonia are the primary complications leading to death for individuals with ventilatory disorders.[31,74-76,107] Individuals with severe lung disease or chronic chest wall deformities have high elastic and ventilatory loads that cannot be sustained by the respiratory muscles.[108] Ultimately, breathing becomes shallow, increasing dead-space ventilation. Because the airways are also destroyed or deformed, the lung tissue collapses and foreign matter becomes trapped, setting the stage for pneumonia. Individuals having significant neuromuscular disease will have alveolar hypoventilation due to neuromuscular incompetence (weak respiratory muscles or deficient neurotransmission).[93,108] Dead-space ventilation is increased

and contributes to CO_2 retention, increasing the risk for sleep apnea in those with neurological conditions.[109,110] Bulbar weakness and poor expiratory muscle function lead to aspiration and decreased cough, contributing to onset of pneumonia in those with neuromuscular conditions.[67,75,76,111,112]

Chronic Obstructive Pulmonary Disease: Pathophysiologic Consequences and Complications

COPD arises from an inflammatory process stimulated by foreign matter that enters the lungs. Normal airways are protected by a mucociliary blanket that captures antigens and moves them up and out of the lower airways until they reach the upper airways, where they can be expectorated or coughed up. Foreign particles reaching the alveoli are small but must be managed by the cells of immunity (neutrophils, macrophages, eosinophils, etc). These cells will attract mediators (protease, elastase, and histamine) to the region where an antigen resides and will digest the antigen. Normally, alpha 1-antitrypsin protects the lung by inhibiting the action of the mediators. However, in COPD there are reactive O_2 species (due to smoke, pollution or chemicals from immune cells) that enter the lung compartment and inhibit alpha 1-antitrypsin, leading to a destruction of lung tissue.[113] Thus both oxidative stress and inflammation are partners in a destructive pathophysiologic process in COPD. Some individuals may have a hereditary condition wherein the alpha 1-antitrypsin is not produced in adequate amounts. In those presenting with deficiency, the level of alpha 1-antitrypsin in plasma is only 15% of normal. As a result there is excessive destruction of lung tissue by neutrophil elastase. Normally neutrophil elastase is an immune system mediator designed to eradicate antigens but in excess destroys lung tissue if not controlled by alpha 1-antitrypsin.[61,114]

When there are recurrent inflammatory periods, destruction of alveolar walls becomes significant and damages parts of the pulmonary vasculature. Destruction of alveolar walls decreases the lungs elastic capacity so air will move into the lungs but does not meet a recoiling pressure required for passive expiration. The person with COPD must actively exhale using the respiratory muscles. This raises intrathoracic pressure excessively. Air becomes trapped when high intrathoracic pressure affects fragile collapsible airways, leading to hyperinflation and the development of bullae as disease progresses. Since both the vascular and alveolar walls are destroyed, there is a V/Q mismatch impairing gas transfer and increasing the potential for hypoxemia.[115] Low O_2 results in pulmonary vasoconstriction, which shunts blood away from underventilated areas to patent, well-ventilated airways.[2,116] This event, plus the destruction of portions of the pulmonary vasculature, increase pressure within the vascular system. Hypoxemia stimulates greater red blood cell production and may elevate hematocrit (55% to 60%), increase the risk for thrombosis, and therefore also add to the vascular load on the heart.[114,116] Eventually the individual with COPD develops pulmonary hypertension and cor pulmonale.[115]

TABLE 8-7. COMPLICATIONS ASSOCIATED WITH INCREASED RISK FOR MORTALITY IN CHRONIC OBSTRUCTIVE PULMONARY DISEASE

• Respiratory infections/fever	• Decreased 6MWT (< 350 meters)
• Hypoxemia ($PaO_2 < 50$ mm Hg)	• Decreased VO_{2max}
• Pulmonary hypertension	• Decreased FEV_1 (< 40% pred)
• Cor pulmonale	• Corticosteroid effects
• Hyperinflation (bullae)	○ Osteoporosis
• Spontaneous pneumothorax	○ ↑ Risk of fracture
• Polycythemia/thrombosis/emboli	○ Myopathies
• Sleep apnea ($PaCO_2 > 50$ mm Hg)	• Comorbidities (diabetes, cardiovascular disease)
• Asthma	• Depression
• Decreased body weight	

The inflammatory response also induces hypertrophy of smooth muscle cells and a goblet-cell metaplasia, resulting in hypersecretion and excess mucus production. The risk of infection in the lungs is high and many individuals contract pneumonia. Secondary complications may occur from the medical use of corticosteroids and include myopathies and osteoporosis. These events may lead to poor activity tolerance and back pain. Declining activity impairs exercise capacity and increases the risk for mortality especially when the 6-Minute Walk Test (6MWT) performance falls below 350 meters.[117] Intolerance to activity is one of a variety of factors that affect the risk for mortality in those with COPD (Table 8-7).

Dynamic hyperinflation disrupts the mechanics of breathing during exercise (Figure 8-9).[97] As exercise progresses, more and more air becomes trapped in the lungs, resulting in an increase in end-expiratory lung volume that creates changes in the dimension of thoracic cage. Bucket handle motion is lost when the chest becomes round with alterations in the length tension of the intercostals muscles. The diaphragm becomes flattened and loses its mechanical efficiency as well. Measured changes in chest wall expansion from maximal inspiration to maximal expiration will be diminished. As exercise progresses, individuals with COPD compensate with excessive neck accessory and abdominal muscle contraction. They may also display Hoover's sign, an inward retraction of the rib cage resulting from abnormal alignment of the intercostals muscles.[101,118] De Oca and colleagues demonstrated that PI_{max} and PE_{max} were reduced by 50% to 39% predicted in individuals with severe COPD and found little diaphragmatic contribution during exercise.[119] They reported that in individuals with severe COPD, the ability of accessory muscles to generate good changes in ventilatory pressure was related to exercise capacity.

When TV (or Vt) enhancement is diminished, new air does not reach the alveoli and physiologic dead-space ventilation (Vd) is increased. There is an increase in V/Q mismatch and hypoxemia worsens as activity progresses.[97] Examination of aerobic capacity and physiologic response (heart rate [HR], blood pressure [BP], O_2 saturation, dyspnea scores, etc) to exercise can assist in describing the impact of ventilatory pump dysfunction on activity and define the risk for mortality as well as provide information for development of an exercise prescription. Aerobic training and VMT are known to improve dyspnea scores and PI_{max} (17%) and offer small improvements in FEV_1 (7%), and are therefore important interventions to consider in the POC.[120]

As disease worsens, the hyperinflation leads to an elevation in the pressure load at rest as well as during exercise. The chest wall and lung tissue elastic forces are stiff and work against any respiratory muscle effort to further expand the chest.[51,52] In order to breathe while the lungs are hyperinflated, the individual with COPD must inspire at the end range limits of chest expansion where muscle contraction is inefficient. Thus, the respiratory muscles must work very hard against high restrictive forces, eventually leading to respiratory muscle fatigue. Ventilation cannot be sustained and only small volumes of new air move to areas of the lungs that are viable for gas exchange.[51,121] Dyspnea, the sensation of breathlessness, may be present with activity and may lead to a sedentary lifestyle.[51] Individuals with severe disease and those who have complications may be in respiratory distress at rest. These individuals, with end-stage COPD, will benefit from interventions focused on techniques for breathing control, energy conservation, and relaxation to assist in supporting independence in functioning.

Neuromuscular Conditions: Pathophysiologic Consequences and Complications

Several neurological conditions result in ventilatory pump dysfunction (see Table 8-3). These conditions fall into

Figure 8-9. COPD and exercise limitation. (Adapted from Cerny FW, Zhan S. Chronic obstructive pulmonary disease. In: LeMura L, von Duvillard SP, eds. *Clinical Exercise Physiology Application and Physiologic Principles*. Philadelphia, PA: Lippincott, Williams & Wilkins; 2004:157-168.)

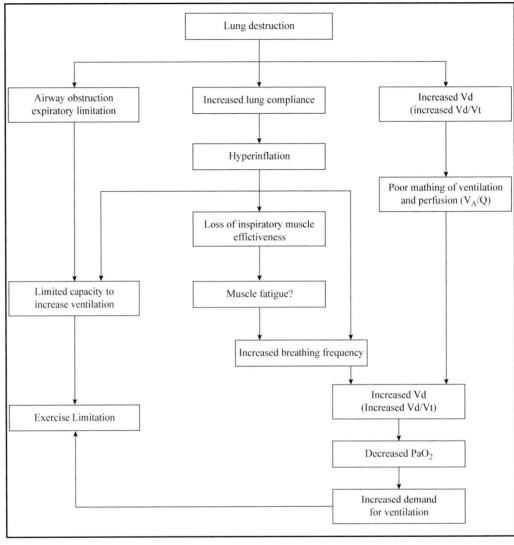

2 categories: progressive and acute injury/illness with recovery. Progressive neuromuscular diseases include; muscular dystrophy, Parkinson's disease, ALS, Huntington's disease, and multiple sclerosis (MS).[92] Neuromuscular disorders arising from an acute event or acute disease include: SCI, GBS, myasthenia gravis, cerebral vascular accident, brain injury, and cerebral palsy. Progressive disease will arise gradually until the ventilatory pump function is significantly impaired while acute events typically require immediate medical intervention to assist ventilation until recovery stabilizes breathing and ventilation support is no longer necessary or is managed with a good respiratory care routine. Despite the time of onset of respiratory dysfunction (early in acute or late in progressive), most individuals with neuromuscular conditions have restrictive disease ($FEV_1/FVC > 0.85\%$ and FVC < 80% predicted) due to limited chest expansion resulting from respiratory muscle weakness and poor breathing mechanics.[122,123] Ventilatory capacity is initially reduced and eventually, over time, ventilatory load is increased with the onset of chest wall restriction and secondary illness (pneumonia).

Acute Conditions

Spinal Cord Injury, Guillain-Barré Syndrome, and Myasthenia Gravis

Ventilatory pump disruption in neuromuscular disease is eminent in those with progressive disease; however, with an acute injury to the nervous system cardiorespiratory recovery is variable and depends on the extent of damage to the nervous system, number of comorbidities, and age.[72,124-126] For example, the incidence of respiratory complications in those with a motor-complete SCI is highest in those with injuries at C1 to C4 (84%) compared to those with injuries at C5 to C8 (60%) or T1 and below (65%).[74] Reduced pulmonary function (FVC), respiratory muscle strength (PI_{max} and PE_{max}) and longer hospitalizations are related to level of injury, with the greatest impairment involving those with the highest levels of injury.[66,127] Pneumonia (25% to 51%) and atelectasis (40% to 42%) are among the most common respiratory complications found in individuals with neurological conditions.[75,128] Secondary conditions or comorbidities that increase the risk for respiratory failure include: obesity, pregnancy, asthma, upper airway obstruction, dysphagia, surgery, cardiovascular disorders (diabetes, atherosclerosis, cor pulmonale), and prior history of smoking.[73,128-131]

GBS is one of the most common causes of acute flaccid tetraplegia. It is an inflammatory demyelinating polyradiculoneuropathy with an incidence of 0.6 to 1.5/100,000 people.[75,76] Myasthenia gravis is an autoimmune disorder of neuromuscular transmission where antibodies are directed against acetylcholine receptors, a condition that affects 0.5 to 14.2 per 100,000 people. Approximately 25% to 50% of patients with GBS[75,78] and 15% to 27% of those with myasthenia gravis will require mechanical ventilation because of rapid progressive weakness involving the respiratory muscles.[78] Factors predicting respiratory failure in GBS are: rapid onset of weakness to hospitalization (< 7 days), an inability to lift the head, and having a VC that is less than 60% predicted when recorded in the supine position.[10,132] Myasthenia crisis is an event related to an exacerbation that produces significant respiratory and oropharyngeal muscle weakness, leading to intubation and will be preceded by infection in 38% of individuals.[73] Some individuals may have autonomic dysfunction, which increases the risk for respiratory failure.[133]

Even when acute neurological injuries are mild, poor cough function increases the risk for pulmonary complications.[74,134] Individuals with tetraplegia or motor-complete SCI between C4 and T4 may demonstrate paradoxical breathing patterns and have poor or even negative chest expansion.[135-139] Once the individual with weak or impaired respiratory mechanics contracts a respiratory illness, the ventilatory load is increased to an already weakened system, predisposing the individual for respiratory muscle fatigue and failure.[75,93] High RR and CO_2 retention are signs of impending failure resulting from an imbalance between ventilatory load and capacity.[110] Monitoring of respiratory status is a priority and intubation is performed in the early stages of the disease when VC < 20 mL/kg ideal body weight, PI_{max} > –30 cm H_2O, PE_{max} < 40 cm H_2O or there is > 30% reduction in VC, PI_{max}, or PE_{max}.[78] Individuals who have RRs > 35 breaths per minute at rest require mechanical ventilation.[140,141]

Most individuals with GBS and myasthenia gravis will be able to recover enough ventilatory capacity to be discontinued from the ventilator and return to normal functioning within 1 year.[76,128] Plasma exchange and immunoglobulin therapy may decrease the time on mechanical ventilation by as much as 50% for those with GBS.[75,133] Individuals with motor complete SCI at C5 and below will recover up to 60% of their VC by the end of the rehabilitation period.[135,137] Regardless of the mechanism of injury, individuals will begin a ventilator discontinuation program when there is a stable medical status if the VC reaches > 10 to 15 mL/kg ideal body weight (≥ 500 to 1000 mL).[142] The person with a neurologic condition will be able to sustain ventilation for activities of daily living (ADL) when the VC reaches 30% predicted (> 1500 mL).[76,140,143] Individuals who are successful in ventilator discontinuation may continue to display signs of respiratory muscle fatigue, bulbar weakness, CO_2 retention, and

present with sleep disturbances.[75,112,144] Most individuals with SCI will have impaired cough function and many will need lifetime respiratory management programs.

Individuals with SCI or intracranial lesions (stroke and brain injury) have acquired nervous system conditions that may result in permanent loss of ventilatory function. Recovery may be incomplete and may range from severe to mild limitations. People living with chronic acquired neurological conditions will need to manage muscle overuse, aging, and comorbidities that may contribute to further weakening of the respiratory muscles later in life.[4] Each individual will need an individualized evaluation and POC for lifetime management of ventilatory pump dysfunction.[4,10] Lifelong management of respiratory impairment may include: recognizing risks associated with respiratory tract infections and respiratory muscle fatigue, incorporating caregiver or self-assisted cough, positioning for optimal V/Q in bed and in upright, using an abdominal binder or positioning to improve breathing mechanics, and respiratory muscle strength training.[4,10,13,86,105,135,137,141]

Stroke

Stroke results from hemorrhage or thrombus leading to infarction of brain tissue. There are approximately 5.4 million stroke survivors in the US.[145] After stroke, presence of an abnormal respiratory pattern (tachypnea and Cheyne-Stokes) increases the risk for mortality.[146] Disruption of cortical inhibition of respiratory drive and increased sensitivity to CO_2 appears to be responsible for producing abnormal respiratory patterns.[71,146,147] About 25% of individuals with acute cerebral infarction require mechanical ventilation because of decreased cognition, poor airway protection or hypoxemia.[71] Approximately 47% of those with a cerebral vascular accident who are admitted to the intensive care unit (ICU) develop pneumonia, with 31% being nosocomial pneumonias.[72] Risk factors associated with an increased risk for pneumonia include abnormal chest radiograph, mechanical ventilation, multiple stroke locations, involvement of the posterior cerebral region, age greater than 60 years, dysphagia, facial muscle weakness, and decreased level of cognition (Glasgow Coma Scale < 10).[72] Turkington and colleagues found 80% of those with acute stroke have some degree of obstructive sleep apnea (OSA).[148] Individuals with sleep apnea are known to have elevations in CO_2 with diminished levels of alertness. CO_2 retention can potentially impair learning for patient education and effective participation in rehabilitation. Thus, respiratory status is critically tied to the success of the rehabilitation program and overall functional outcome for those with stroke.

Hemiparesis disrupts the mechanics of breathing by decreasing the chest wall excursion (CWE) on the paretic side by as much as 50% during voluntary deep breathing.[147,149] TV breathing may, or may not, be significantly lower; however, the diaphragm and intercostals muscle activation is lower on the paretic side.[71,147,150,151] Respiratory muscle strength (PI_{max} and PE_{max}) is 40% to 60% lower in individuals with hemiplegia in comparison to healthy age- and gender-matched controls.[152] Lanini and colleagues reported lower PI_{max} (53.41 ± 21.4 vs 99.4 ± 8.4 cm H_2O) and PE_{max} (61.6 ± 16 vs 121.8 ± 18.1 cm H_2O) in 8 males with hemiplegia at 26 days after onset of initial symptoms.[147] Inability to breathe deeply may decrease lung and chest wall compliance over time.[152] Lower lung volumes and respiratory muscle strength may also limit force-generating capacity for effective coughing, increasing the risk for pneumonia. Fugl-Meyer and colleagues demonstrated that measures of ventilatory function (lung volumes and pressures) were related to the degree of motor impairment and were lower for those with the most severe hemiparesis.[152]

Progressive Conditions

Respiratory muscle weakness often does not produce symptoms in the early stages of progressive neuromuscular disease.[71] Progressive disease results in a gradual loss of limb function and motor control in most muscles throughout the body, including bulbar muscles.[111] As a result people with progressive neuromuscular disease may not complain of dyspnea or difficulty breathing because the loss of motor function to the extremities limits their need to increase ventilation.[67] Respiratory muscle strength deficits result in a corresponding loss of lung volumes but FVC is not significantly affected until the respiratory muscle pressures fall below 50% predicted.[71,153] Chest wall and lung compliance gradually decreases as the individual with neuromuscular disease fails to breathe deeply. Microatelectasis develops, making it harder to expand the chest.[154] Eventually, shallow breathing results in increased dead-space ventilation and CO_2 retention. Sleep disturbances (hypoventilation, insomnia, and decreased rapid eye movement sleep) begin when VC falls below 60% predicted or inspiratory pressure is greater than –34 cm H_2O (less negative) and will precede development of daytime hypercapnia.[155] There are a variety of subtle changes that can be detected by effective monitoring of respiratory status in those with a progressive neurological condition.[131,156]

Duchenne Muscular Dystrophy

DMD is the most common dystrophy in childhood and occurs in 1 of every 3000 male births. It is caused by an X-linked recessive disorder causing a defect in the gene that produces dystrophin, a cytoskeleton protein. Ultimately this defect results in impaired function of the sarcoplasmic reticulum calcium pumps and myosin molecule. Significant respiratory muscle weakness begins between ages 7 and 12 years and leads to progressive lowering of lung functions. Death occurs by age 20 to 23 years. Recently, many individuals with DMD have been offered noninvasive mechanical ventilation when the FVC falls below 40% predicted to help prevent hypercapnia and improve daytime alertness and quality of life.[68] The American Thoracic Society (ATS) has published a consensus statement directing the methods for monitoring respiratory status and the application of ventilation support.[131] Once the individual with DMD is confined to a wheelchair, or has a VC that falls below 80% predicted, the ATS recommends biannual visits to the pulmonologist.

Multiple Sclerosis and Parkinson's Disease

MS is a demyelinating disease of the central nervous system with an initial onset arising in individuals between 15 and 50 years of age; mean 30 years of age. Approximately 400,000 individuals in the US are affected by the disease with about 10,000 new cases each year. Twenty percent of individuals who have MS and die before age 50 will succumb to pneumonia or influenza.[157,158] On average, the first episode of respiratory failure occurs about 6 years after the onset of MS.[71] Factors contributing to onset of respiratory failure include bulbar dysfunction, abnormal motor control (presenting as apneustic breathing or apnea), fever or elevations in temperature that may exacerbate poor nerve conduction and loss of respiratory muscle functions.[71]

Pulmonary impairment and respiratory muscle weakness are present both in mild and advanced stages of MS, with greater loss of expiratory than inspiratory muscle weakness.[65] Respiratory muscle weakness is related to systemic weakness and overall disability.[67] Buyse and colleagues observed individuals with MS who had higher disability scores (Expanded Disability Status Scale) had significant lower VCs.[67] They reported 70% had saturations less than 92% at night. Loss of conditioning, hypoxemia, hypercapnia, steroids, and increases in tumor necrosis factor may lead to further declines in respiratory muscle performance during an exacerbation.[71] Fortunately, there are numerous reports demonstrating that respiratory muscle training can improve lung volume and flows, respiratory muscle strength, respiratory muscle endurance, and cough in those with MS.[158-160]

Less research has been performed on ventilatory function in Parkinson's disease, as a large portion of the population is older than 80 years of age at the time of onset.[161] Pneumonia is a common respiratory complication. Parkinson's disease is a neurodegenerative disorder involving subcortical gray matter in the basal ganglia. The substantia nigra loses its ability to produce dopamine, which is a neurotransmitter that is important in the regulation of motor actions. Coordination is lost throughout the body and affects smooth interaction of inspiratory and expiratory muscle performance. As a result, more than 58% of individuals with Parkinson's disease have a decrease in the PEFR.[162] The PI_{max} declines to about 30% predicted and PE_{max} drops to 35% predicted in advanced stages of the disease.[163] Loss of lung volumes (FVC and FEV_1) and PI_{max} and PE_{max} are correlated to measures of bradykinesia and rigidity.[164]

Early in the disease, inspiratory muscle endurance is decreased despite nearly normal values for PI_{max}. Loss of endurance in the respiratory muscles may be due to the impaired nervous system's ability to sustain repetitive activation during periods of high ventilatory demand as neurotransmitter levels are depleted.[71] Over time as the disease progresses, neck and intercostal muscle activation during inspiration becomes dominant, increasing the energy cost of breathing. Additionally, lack of segmental movement and loss of rotational dissociation between the upper and lower body decreases chest wall movement. The chest wall becomes stiff, and breathing for coughing and deep breathing is poorly coordinated.[71] Reports state anywhere from 12% to 65% of individuals with Parkinson's disease have upper airway obstruction.[163,164] Sabaté and colleagues evaluated[58] individuals with Parkinson's disease and documented postural deformity, vertebral arthrosis, and loss of passive mobility of the cervical column in individuals with ventilatory obstruction.[164] Individuals with Parkinson's disease may benefit from a program of posture correction, chest wall mobilization, and cough assist as well as general conditioning to improve aerobic capacity.[165] PNF approaches to trunk mobilization and cough assist, specifically the counter-rotation and costophrenic assist techniques, are interventions that may help address the ventilatory impairments seen in individuals with Parkinson's disease.[100] Individuals confined to a wheelchair will need good seating and positioning to prevent poor alignment of the cervical column.

Post-Polio Syndrome

PPS is a chronic condition that arises as age and overuse affect muscles initially affected by polio. Technically, it is not progressive in nature but arises and worsens if muscles and joints are not protected from overuse. Approximately 440,000 polio survivors in the US may be at risk for PPS, with 25% to 65% of individuals experiencing muscle weakness in late life.[166,167] Thirty-nine to 42% of individuals with PPS have symptoms of respiratory insufficiency, most commonly in those who required mechanical ventilation during the acute recovery period.[69,166] PPS may result in respiratory compromise if respiratory muscle weakness or bulbar dysfunction goes undetected.[168] Individuals having PPS may be offered surgical options to assist in stabilization of joints or tendon transfers to assist in restoring function. The effects of anesthesia on recovery of respiratory function after an operation can lead to prolonged recovery times and need for mechanical support.[169] Declines in physical function due to new weakness (overuse) and pain are often the primary complaint for individuals with PPS as well as for those living with chronic neurologic conditions. It is important to consider respiratory status prior to proceeding with any elective surgery. A plan for a respiratory care program and conditioning during the rehabilitation period will be important in order to maximize full functional recovery.

Ventilation Limitations to Exercise in Chronic Neuromuscular Disease

Many individuals with neuromuscular conditions survive the acute phase or, in the case of chronic progressive disease, some individuals are able to engage in exercise that postpones the decline in ventilatory pump function.[122] Several reports have demonstrated an increased work of breathing during aerobic activity and suggested there may be ventilation limitations to exercise in those with PPS,[123,170] MS,[171] Parkinson's disease,[165] stroke,[172] and traumatic brain injury.[122,173] Aerobic training programs appear to improve ventilatory capacity in individuals with chronic neurologic conditions.[174,175] Ventilatory limitations to exercise for individuals having neurological conditions are not well documented. In many individuals there is an inability of the peripheral muscle to generate enough force to significantly increase O_2 consumption. In most cases local muscle fatigue occurs prior to reaching near maximal age-predicted HRs. Additionally, overuse of weak muscles may result in poor recovery after exercise and lead to loss of function. Therefore, aerobic capacity assessment and development of an individualized exercise program need to be a carefully monitored component of healthy living for persons with a chronic neuromuscular disorder.

Summary: Pathogenesis and Consequences of Neuromuscular Incompetence

Neuromuscular conditions arise from an inability to transmit nervous system impulses to activate muscle. When there is damage to the nervous system this can affect mechanics of breathing, disrupt sleep, and may decrease the ability to swallow effectively. Respiratory muscle weakness results in a loss of lung volume and capacities leading to alveolar hypoventilation (Figure 8-10).[31] Symptoms appear and interfere with function when the FVC drops below 50% predicted in most cases. Loss of adequate alveolar ventilation limits activity in mild to moderate disease while those with severe neuromuscular incompetence may be unable to breathe without some form of mechanical ventilation. Factors contributing to ventilatory failure and increased risk for mortality in neuromuscular conditions are listed in Table 8-8.

Most individuals with neurological conditions lose the ability to breathe deeply and in some cases the sigh reflex may be absent.[156] The loss of sigh mechanisms or deep breathing capacity can change the alveolar surface tension and increase the potential for atelectasis.[10] When alveoli lose their surface tension, atelectasis develops and the lungs become stiff, increasing the ventilatory load to already weak inspiratory muscles. Because the chest wall does not expand fully, it also becomes stiff over time. Postural deformities (most commonly scoliosis and kyphosis), occurring from muscle imbalances and spasticity, will compromise normal chest wall movement.[176-178] Paradoxical breathing causes a negative chest wall expansion, which will also lead to stiffness of the chest wall.[4,135]

Hypoventilation is the end result of decreased lung volumes and chest wall movement. To enhance VE and respond to increases in ventilatory demand (activity or infection), the individual increases RR. Elevation of RR, as a compensation for small TV, increases dead-space ventilation, reducing alveolar gas exchange. Retention of CO_2 or hypercapnia occurs when there is significant loss of ventilation and respiratory muscle strength drops below 25% predicted.[71,179] Hypercapnia is also associated with sleep apnea and produces changes in mental status and decreased levels of alertness.[68,131,144,180] In progressive diseases, early symptoms such as fatigue and decreased level of alertness are subtle signs that suggest there is difficulty with breathing. These signs appear when there is mild CO_2 retention. Later, as the disease progresses the person with progressive neurological

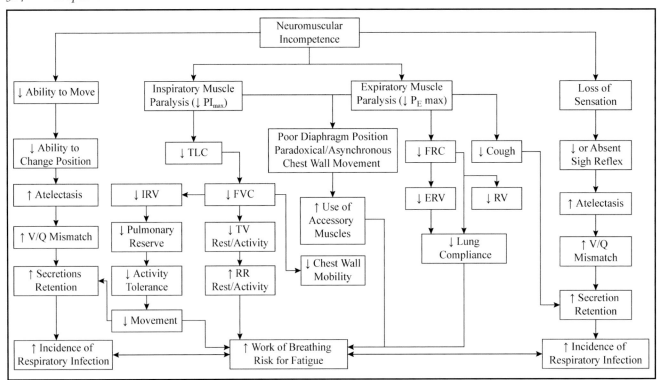

Figure 8-10. Factors contributing to respiratory insufficiency in individuals with neuromuscular conditions. ERV, expiratory reserve volume; FRC, functional residual capacity; FVC, forced vital capacity; IRV, inspiratory reserve volume; RR, respiratory rate; RV, residual volume; TLC, total lung capacity; TV, tidal volume; V/Q, ventilation perfusion. (Adapted from Peat M, ed. *Current Physical Therapy*. Philadelphia, PA: BC Decker; 1988.)

disease becomes severely limited, avoids activity, and uses compensatory breathing strategies at rest. Eventually, severe hypoventilation and CO_2 retention may cause respiratory acidosis and lowers the pH of the body.[181] Respiratory failure is imminent and regular monitoring of respiratory status is recommended.[131]

Those individuals with progressive neuromuscular disease with PI_{max} > –30 cm H_2O (less negative), PE_{max} < 40 cm H_2O or those with a VC below 20 mL/kg body weight are at risk for ventilatory failure and will soon need some mechanical ventilation support.[72,78] Interventions focused on preventing decline in pulmonary status begin with airway clearance and breathing retraining and are recommended when VC drops (45 to 30 mL/kg BW; [FVC = 65% to 40% pred]).[73] Noninvasive mechanical ventilation at night is now being offered early in the disease process to avoid hypercapnia and sleep apnea and should be considered when the FVC falls below 40% predicted.[68] It becomes critical for health professionals to monitor decline in respiratory status as well as loss of function as the disease progresses.[131] Early intervention that includes mobility, wheelchair positioning, cough-assist techniques, and strategies to enhance inspiratory volume and glottis control may postpone the need for full-time mechanical support and prevent life-threatening respiratory complications.

The inability to inspire at least 1500 mL of air may contribute to ineffective flow rate for spontaneous and assisted coughing.[10,24,26,182,183] Coughing is also dependent on good, forceful expulsion of air using contraction of the abdominal

muscles or proper cough-assist technique.[100,184,185] Poor cough limits the ability to clear mucus from the airway and increases the risk for pneumonia. Glottis control is also essential for coughing and for protection of the airway.[186] Bulbar muscle weakness and obligatory supine positioning increase the risk for aspiration of foreign matter into the lungs.[4,10,75,76] Pulmonary infections and atelectasis leads to hypoxemia and fever, increasing the work of breathing and potential for respiratory muscle fatigue.

Musculoskeletal Disorders: Pathophysiologic Consequences and Complications

Musculoskeletal conditions that impact on posture and CWE may result from either primary conditions of the skeleton and its articulating surfaces (osteoporosis, arthritis, AS), or from systemic diseases that destroy connective tissues throughout the body (sarcoidosis, scleroderma). Secondary conditions such as neuromuscular disease, surgical pain, scars (burns, wounds), or obligatory positioning after trauma (management of complex fractures and injuries) may also result in postural deformities, remodeling of skeletal alignment and loss of CWE. Pectus carinatum (pigeon chest) and pectus excavatum funnel chest) may develop as a result of underlying pathology and are associated with long-term conditions (COPD, cystic fibrosis, and neuromuscular disease).[187] These deformities signal muscle imbalance and unequal chest pressures that contribute to inefficient breathing mechanics.

Severe restriction of CWE can result in decreased pulmonary function when the pump handle and bucket handle motions are impaired.[188,189] Additionally, when postural alignment is significantly altered there may be an internal torsion and compression of lung tissue that leads to obstruction of airflow and atelectasis.[190] If the gastrointestinal organs are compressed then aspiration may occur, increasing the risk for pneumonia or pulmonary fibrosis. Distortion of the pulmonary vasculature may restrict blood flow and lead to V/Q mismatch, hypoxemia, and pulmonary hypertension.[191] Exercise-induced pulmonary hypertension may occur before any hypertrophy to the right heart or evidence of right heart failure. Pulmonary pressure increases proportionally when the lateral curvature of the spine is greater than 70 degrees.[187]

Primary conditions of the skeleton include: kyphosis, kyphoscoliosis, and idiopathic scoliosis. Surgery involving the thoracic cage is an acute condition that results in reduced anteroposterior diameter, diminishes lateral costal expansion, and imposes abnormal posturing, which can temporarily compromise ventilation.[31,85] Skeletal deformities occurring in the thoracic region affect CWE and ventilatory capacity as they become severe.[80,192] Postural deformities may arise from an unknown cause (idiopathic scoliosis)[193] or as a secondary disorder associated with osteoporosis (especially vertebral wedge fractures),[189] chronic muscle imbalance or pain syndrome (neurological conditions), postsurgical or traumatic event involving fracture and/or bone repair (eg, rib fractures, pelvic obliquity, cardiothoracic surgery). In the case of idiopathic scoliosis, pulmonary function is compromised as the lateral curvature approaches 60 to 70 degrees and mechanics of inspiratory muscles becomes impaired when the curve is greater than 90 degrees.[31,188,193] Eighty-two percent of deaths in those with clinically significant scoliosis (> 40 degrees curvature) are associated with respiratory complications.[194] Interventions designed to limit the progression of the curvature are applied initially until eventually a surgical correction is necessary.

AS is a chronic inflammatory disease affecting the sacroiliac joint and spine. It is progressive and eventually involves the shoulder, hips, and other LE joints. About one-third of individuals with AS have severe disease with severe kyphosis and spine deformity associated with pathologic fractures of the vertebrae.[188] Approximately 1.2% of those with AS have pulmonary impairment of the upper lobes of the lungs as a result of the mechanical restrictive process and pain that limits anterior CWE.[194] The disease also affects lung parenchyma in addition to decreasing CWE, so there is often pulmonary fibrosis in those with AS. As with other restrictive lung tissue disorders, small lungs are seen on chest X-ray along with pulmonary function tests that confirm a restrictive pattern. Both ventilatory pump dysfunction and noncompliant lung tissue contribute to the overall pattern of restrictive respiratory dysfunction. When lung parenchyma is noncompliant, the patient must work harder for each breath, leading to ventilatory pump fatigue or impaired mechanics appear as a secondary event.[4]

TABLE 8-8. COMPLICATIONS ASSOCIATED WITH INCREASED RISK FOR MORTALITY IN NEUROMUSCULAR CONDITIONS

- Respiratory infections/fever
- Respiratory muscle weakness
  - Impaired mechanics-fatigue
  - ↓ Inspiratory and expiratory capacity
  - Diaphragm paralysis
- Decreased VC
- Ineffective cough
- Increased dead-space ventilation
- Hypoventilation/mechanical ventilation
- Hypercapnia
- Aspiration (bulbar weakness, obligatory positioning)
- Sleep apnea
- Paradoxical breathing
- Postural deformities
- ↑ Atelectasis
- ↓ Residual muscle/deconditioning/↓ CV health
- Immobility
  - Risk of thrombosis/emboli
  - Risk of pressure sores
  - ↓ Stimulus to breathe

Connective tissue disorders may limit ventilation and occur with systemic diseases (scleroderma, sarcoidosis, polymyositis, systemic lupus, rheumatoid arthritis) or as a result of soft tissue destruction (burns, scars) related to trauma or medical interventions.[31,188] In the case of systemic disease, the primary pulmonary involvement occurs in the lung parenchyma and often results in pulmonary fibrosis. In this case, the restrictive pattern of pulmonary function is due to poor lung expansion and increases the work of breathing, especially during activity.[4,94,96,195] For individuals with systemic connective tissue disorders, life-threatening pulmonary complications result from poor lung tissue diffusion, gas transfer impairments, and pneumonia (see Chapter 9).[194,196] Because painful joints, tight skin, or weak respiratory muscles may also limit chest wall movement and increase the work of breathing, it is important to evaluate the extent to which these structures limit ventilation. Specifically addressing pain and tightness may improve the ease of breathing for many. Strengthening weak respiratory muscles and providing aerobic conditioning will be important to maximizing overall functional outcome.

EXAMINATION OF VENTILATORY PUMP DISORDERS

Examination involves history taking, review of systems, and selecting and implementing tests and measures used to determine a physical therapy diagnosis, prognosis, and POC.[92] Although the therapist performs a comprehensive exam and a screen of all major systems, in this chapter we will focus on those examinations that assist in defining the extent of the ventilatory pump disorder and limitations that may be addressed by physical therapy. It is not unusual for individuals with ventilatory pump disorders to be referred to physical therapy with a primary problem other than ventilation (paralysis, immobility due to trauma or postsurgical pain). So often the examination of ventilatory pump function is a component of a larger pathologic process affecting physical functioning. The examination begins with a review of the patient/client history.

Patient/Client History

The history-taking process will review general demographics, including age, gender, and ethnicity, as well as height and weight.[3] All of these factors will influence normal lung and ventilatory muscle functions. Measures of pulmonary impairment (FVC, FEV_1, PEFR, and PCFR) and respiratory muscle performance (PI_{max}, PE_{max}, MVV) are typically compared to expected values reported in the literature.[3,27,36,197-199] The severity of disease and the loss of ventilation will be relative to the age, gender, height, and other demographics. The therapist can use this information to determine whether signs and symptoms are associated with these features or may be explained by other factors (pain, anxiety, deconditioning, etc). Individual characteristics may also influence measures of chest wall expansion,[200] predicted work capacity (6MWT, bike, or treadmill workload),[28,201,202] physiologic responses to activity tolerance testing (HR and BP),[203] and risk for acquiring conditions known to affect ventilation (scoliosis, sarcoidosis).

A review of the family history, lifestyle, and general health status should reveal whether the person is malnourished or obese and overeating, or has ongoing habits, such as smoking or alcohol abuse, that may work against optimal ventilation. The support system (family, caregiver, insurance coverage, access to experts) will influence the person's ability to implement an optimal POC. It will also be important to identify the individual's expected life roles. Does the person have a physically demanding job or participate in leisure activities with high ventilatory requirements? Do the activities include arm work? Many individuals with ventilatory pump dysfunction have symptoms only with activity so it is important to take a good activity history. Ask the client "What activities are hard for you and what makes it difficult?" This kind of questioning can help the therapist determine what type of aerobic capacity test to perform and prioritize functional testing.

Outcome measures such as the Baseline Dyspnea Index (BDI)[204]; Modified Medical Research Council (MMRC) dyspnea scale; and BODE Index (BODE stands for body mass index [BMI], obstruction to airflow [FEV_1], dyspnea [MMRC], and exercise [6MWT distance]),[205,206] St. George's Respiratory Questionnaire (SGRQ),[207] or the Chronic Respiratory Questionnaire (CRQ)[208] are used to quantify the effect of dyspnea on function and health-related quality of life (HRQoL) in individuals with COPD.[209] When a person with a history of repeated admissions has acute ventilatory compromise the therapist should ask "What activities were you able to do after your last hospitalization?" and "What kind of therapy did you have during your last admission?" The answers to these questions and a review of prior functional status can assist in developing realistic goals and POC.

Past medical and surgical history should include prior hospitalizations and procedures with special attention on factors that affect ventilatory capacity. Old scars, fixed postures, and muscle imbalance may be difficult to correct in a new episode of care. The therapeutic plan will may need to be modified if comorbidities (hypertension, heart failure, aberrant conduction, etc) are serious. The current condition and chief complaint is determined by interviewing the individual, family, and medical team to identify the reason for admission, patient/family goals, and desired medical outcomes. During the interview the therapist observes patient status (color, posture, accessory muscle use, phonation etc).

Medical information to review prior to conducting formal tests and measures includes: baseline vital signs, oximetry and arterial blood gases, complete blood count, pulmonary functions tests, sputum and blood cultures, imaging and chest radiographs, cardiac diagnostics, renal/urinary tests, swallowing tests as well as nutritional and hydration status. The therapist will need to be familiar with any contraindications and precautions to activity prior to performing the physical exam.[203,210,211] Medications can alter pain, breathing, ventilatory muscle performance and may introduce symptoms that affect overall functional performance.[212] O_2 and ventilatory support should also be determined. The use of O_2 and mechanical ventilation usually indicates the person with a ventilatory pump disorder also has impaired respiration/gas exchange (see Chapter 9).[115,141] If a person develops a pulmonary infection, acute respiratory failure or has a condition that requires ongoing management of airway clearance, then the primary problem is a gas-exchange problem and not ventilatory pump dysfunction. These conditions are discussed in Chapter 9.

Systems Review

The first thing to consider prior to performing a systems review is to determine whether the reason for breathing difficulty is ongoing or recent and if the symptoms are worse in supine or sitting or with activity. A functional sitting position is preferred when screening vital signs and ventilation. Any support devices (abdominal binders, seating systems, body jackets, O_2) and any use of upper extremity or back support should be noted. Measures may be significantly altered when body position changes or support is removed.

The cardiovascular and pulmonary system should be assessed prior to screening other systems. General screening of the HR, BP, RR and O_2 saturation can quickly define whether there are contraindications to other examinations. These values are compared to recent vitals recorded in the medical record. The RR will be most closely associated with identifying severity of ventilatory pump dysfunction. Rates above 30 breaths per minute at rest suggest low TV and indicate severe loss of ventilatory capacity.[3] Gas-exchange impairments often precede ventilatory pump dysfunction in those with COPD while those with neurological diseases may have gas-exchange deficits well after ventilatory muscle weakness has been identified. Screening for arterial O_2 saturation can identify if there is hypoxemia.

Once the cardiovascular and pulmonary system screening is complete, the other systems are examined grossly. General screening of integumentary system can reveal scars or wounds that may restrict breathing. If wound healing is a problem, this may suggest poor immunity and increased risk for pulmonary infections.[213] Conversely, high ventilatory demands raise metabolic requirements and steal circulation necessary for wound healing.[213,214] Some wounds will confer an obligatory posture and may not support good ventilation to all areas of the lungs. Musculoskeletal and neuromuscular screening may reveal pain or restrictions in range of motion (ROM), weakness, and spasticity that contribute to inefficient movement strategies. Energy cost will be higher for simple tasks. Breathlessness may be related to poor movement patterns or anxiety and not necessarily caused by pulmonary impairments.[215] Communication, affect, cognition, language, and learning style are also part of the systems review. For those with ventilatory pump dysfunction, decreased cognition or poor affect may be an early sign of CO_2 retention.[216] The individual may also have undiagnosed sleep apnea.[180,217]

Tests and Measures

The approach to selecting tests and measures will depend on the underlying cause of impaired ventilation and whether the problem is acute with a sudden onset or progressive. Individuals with COPD can have an acute exacerbation on top of a long history of gradually worsening ventilatory status. People with chronic neuromuscular disease may have no complaints of breathing disorders and may be unaware that the ventilatory reserve is marginal, especially if they are too weak to physically increase O_2 demand. Those with acute conditions may have ventilatory pump dysfunction that can be addressed with early mobility and pain management strategies (postsurgical patients) or they may require prolonged rehabilitation after a severe trauma with muscle paralysis (SCI, brain injury). Therefore, the acuity of the illness and the underlying pathology contributing to impaired ventilation will influence which tests and measure will be important in assisting goal setting and directing the physical therapy POC.

Common categories from which tests and measures are chosen to examine a patient with a ventilatory pump disorder are Posture, Ventilation and Respiration/Gas Exchange, and Aerobic Capacity and Endurance. Testing Cranial Nerve Integrity may be indicated as well as measures of Self-Care and Home Management (including ADL and instrumental ADL [IADL] and/or Environmental, Home, and Work (Job/School/Play) Barriers.

Posture

Posture gives clues to the adaptations the patient may have made over time due to an altered breathing pattern. Individuals with primary pulmonary disease (COPD), as breathing becomes distressed, will appear differently from individuals with ventilatory pump dysfunction arising from secondary disorders (neuromuscular conditions or musculoskeletal conditions). Those with severe COPD will typically lean forward and support their arms on furniture, bed rails, or bedside tables.[218]

Posture is typically observed in a standing or sitting position. The person with muscular weakness from a neurological condition will often be observed in a sitting position and will likely display a posterior pelvic tilt, thoracic kyphosis, and forward head. The position may be fixed or flexible depending on the whether the condition is chronic or acute. The seating system may be adjusted to support ventilation and prevent deformities that work against breathing. Rounded shoulders with kyphosis and severe habitual posterior tilt limit anterior chest wall expansion.[105] Additionally, excessive diaphragm action without good opposition from the intercostals can lead to pectus excavatum (funnel chest). Therefore a posture exam is critical to identify conditions that may be corrected by good seating position and therapeutic interventions to correct chest wall limitations and muscle imbalance.[219] Severe kyphosis in individuals with diseases affecting spine mobility is associated with limitations in lung function.[80]

The position of comfort should be noted at the beginning of the physical exam. The person with severe ventilatory pump dysfunction who has a neuromuscular condition will be more comfortable in supine with the head of bed at about 15 to 30 degrees while the individual with severe COPD will be more comfortable upright and leaning forward with arms supported.

When examining posture, the abnormal postures are documented and the change with and without arm support may be observed. The therapist can rate dyspnea and breathing pattern and measure RR before and after, including arm support, use of abdominal binder, back rest, head rest or with a walker if standing. Counting aloud after maximal inspiration is another method for examining the effects of various postures on ventilation. The higher the number counted in one breath, the greater the ventilation support offered by the specific position or equipment.[4]

Ventilation and Respiration/Gas Exchange

Tests and measures within this category may include examination of chest wall movement, identification of

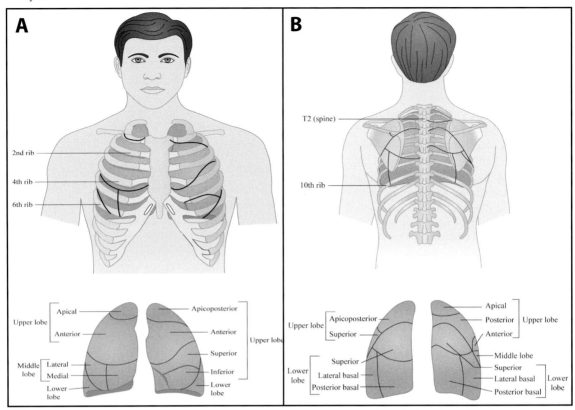

Figure 8-11. Surface markings of the lungs (anterior [A] and posterior [B] aspects). The underlying bronchopulmonary segments are also shown. (Adapted from Cherniak RM, Cherniack L. *Respiration in Health and Disease.* 3rd ed. Philadelphia, PA: WB Saunders; 1983; and Frownfelter D, Dean E, eds. *Cardiovascular and Pulmonary Physical Therapy: Evidence and Practice.* 4th ed. St. Louis, MO: Mosby Elsevier; 2006:695-717.)

breathing patterns, auscultation of breath sounds, and assessment of airway clearance ability.

Chest Wall Movement

Chest wall examination includes palpation, examination of scars, and trigger points as sources of pain, detecting any asymmetrical movement. The purpose of this exam is to identify when more objective assessments may be needed (CWE measures, auscultation, or muscle performance tests). The therapist will examine painful areas by rotating the index finger over critical areas such as the interchondral and sternocostal articulations. Areas that are stressed during a surgical procedure may be painful. The insertion of muscles such as the pectoralis major, serratus anterior, sternocleidomastoid or trapezius may be tender. Any reproducible trigger point can help diagnose the cause of pain and assist in ruling out pain from pulmonary pleurisy or angina.

The therapist uses surface landmarks to identify the region of the lungs for examination (Figure 8-11). The hands are placed over the anterior surface of the upper chest with thumbs aligned over the sternum and manubrium above the fourth rib. Separation of the thumbs is observed as well as upward movement of the chest wall. The upper thoracic cage moves more in the anterior posterior dimension (pump handle) motion and may be diminished if there is pain from surgical incisions (sternotomy). The hands are also placed on the lateral rib cage between ribs 7 and 10 to detect lateral

costal expansion (bucket handle motion). Hand placement between the sixth to fourth rib allows the therapist to note movement in the middle thoracic lung fields (left lingular divisions and the right middle lobes).[218]

Posteriorly, the hands may be placed over the thorax between the inferior angle of the scapula and the tenth rib to palpate expansion of the chest wall under the superior and posterior division of the lower lobes. The posterior upper lobes may be palpated bilaterally on the shoulders and posterior aspect of the scapula above the spine of the scapula (T2). These same surface landmarks may be used to identify the lung fields during auscultation.[12]

A more objective assessment of chest wall movement is to use a tape measure to document the excursion from maximal inspiration to maximal expiration. The 3 regions that should be assessed are upper chest wall expansion (axillary level; second intercostals space or angle of Louis), middle chest wall expansion (xiphoid level) and lower chest wall expansion (half way between xiphoid and umbilicus).[138,220,221] A standard tape measure is used at each site and pulled gently with firm pressure circumferentially around the thoracic cage. The tape should be level all around. The subject is then asked to inspire and expire and the difference in expansion recorded.

Chest wall expansion may be measured with TV breathing (functional excursion) or with VC breathing (maximal excursion). Measures taken during TV breathing indicate resting movement while measures taken during VC breathing will give an indication of the potential for expansion during deep breathing or exercise.[221] Measuring CWE after exercise in those with COPD may demonstrate decreases in movement of the chest wall resulting from dynamic hyperinflation.[222]

Respiratory and Breathing Pattern

Respiratory pattern is a description of the variation between RR, TV, and pause characteristics. Descriptions of respiratory pattern include tachypnea (> 20 breaths/minute), bradypnea (< 10 breaths/minute), hyperventilation, Cheyne-Stokes, Biot's, Kussmaul's, etc.[223]

The examination of breathing pattern is an examination that describes how the individual is moving air in the lungs.[135] The therapist observes ventilation and rates the pattern of breathing by applying a number to 4 regions of the thorax (neck, chest, diaphragm, abdomen) according to the amount of activity observed in the region. Normally, the breathing pattern involves equal expansion of the chest and diaphragm regions. Therefore, a normal breathing pattern is 2 chest and 2 diaphragm with no rating applied to the neck or abdomen. If the person uses neck muscles, diaphragm, and chest then the rating is applied using 4 points according to dominance or respiratory muscle action in the 3 regions. A possible rating would be 1 neck, 1 chest, and 2 diaphragm. This would indicate the individual has begun using neck accessory breathing and the chest wall motion or intercostals action is diminished relative to normal.

Abdominal muscle action is often observed in those with COPD who have hyperinflation. Active contraction of the abdomen is used to move a flattened diaphragm up in the thoracic cage at the end of expiration.[52] In this case, the breathing pattern may be 1 neck, 1 diaphragm, and 2 abdomen. This is because the lungs are hyperinflated, causing the intercostal action and chest component to be minimal.

Auscultation

Auscultation is important for confirming the ventilatory characteristics in the individual with ventilatory pump dysfunction. Lung sounds may be characterized as normal, abnormal or adventitious.[221] For the person with ventilatory pump dysfunction, comparing abnormal auscultatory characteristics to normal is important. Auscultation can be also be useful for determining the region of the lungs where pathology or infectious processes may be affecting ventilation and can assist in the differential diagnosis of specific lung disorders.[221,224] Chapter 9 presents a discussion of adventitious lung sounds related to impaired gas exchange.

When performing auscultation on an individual with ventilatory pump dysfunction who does not yet demonstrate significant gas-exchange deficits, the therapist can listen for inspiratory and expiratory time over bronchial, bronchovesicular, and vesicular regions (Figure 8-12).

Decreased Ti indicates respiratory muscle mechanics are impaired and is common in those with neuromuscular conditions or postsurgical pain. Ventilatory pump dysfunction

BRONCHIAL
loud, high pitched; hollow quality; heard over manubrium; louder on expiration; distinct pause between inspiration (I) and expiration (E)

BRONCHOVESICULAR
mixture of bronchial and vesicular; I:E is 1:1; heard over main-stem bronchi anteriorly, ICS #1 and #2; posteriorly, between scapulae

VESICULAR
soft, low pitched; heard over peripheral lung tissue; no pause between I and E: ratio is 3:1

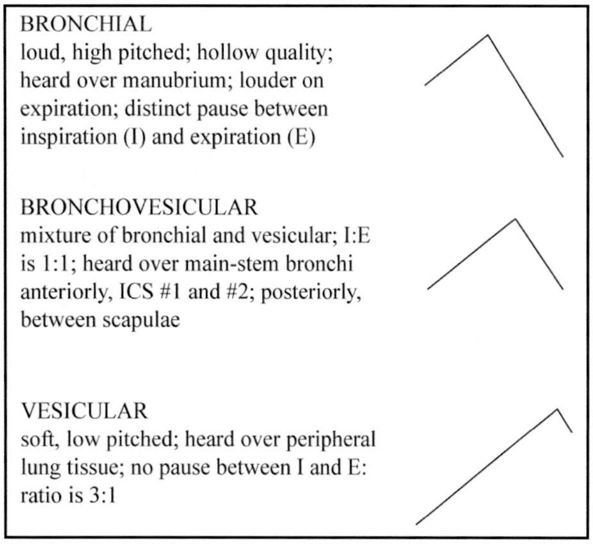

Figure 8-12. Physiology of normal breath sounds. (Adapted from Frownfelter D, Dean E, eds. *Cardiovascular and Pulmonary Physical Therapy: Evidence and Practice.* 4th ed. St. Louis, MO: Mosby Elsevier; 2006.)

will result in decreased breath sounds over the vesicular regions. The individual with asymmetrical weakness due to a neuromuscular condition may have less audible sounds over the vesicular regions on the more involved side. Adventitious sounds such as rhonchi indicate airway narrowing and may be due to secretions or postural torsion in those with severe kyphoscoliosis. Rales may indicate an inflammatory process such as pneumonia is evolving.

The person with COPD may have distant sounds and a more prolonged expiratory phase than heard in the healthy individual. During auscultation bronchial sounds are common if there is lung consolidation (hollow over vesicular areas) or there may be an absence of sound if there is atelectasis.[221] Since lung consolidation and atelectasis may be early signs of respiratory compromise in individuals with ventilatory pump dysfunction, the auscultation session should include an examination of voice-transmitted sounds (egophony, bronchophony, and whispered pectoriloquy).[218] Sounds are transmitted more clearly when there is lung consolidation.

Airway Clearance

An effective cough, which is imperative to efficiently clear pulmonary secretions, is elicited by a deep inspiration followed by closure of the glottis, then a strong contraction of the abdominals causing rapid expulsion of air. Cough can be assessed for effectiveness, control, quality, frequency, and sputum. The therapist should observe the 4 phases of coughing.[225] Phase 1 involves good deep inspiration. Phase 2 is glottis closure prior to forceful contraction of abdominal and intercostals muscles in phase 3. During phase 3 the muscle contractions create a force, putting pressure behind a closed glottis. In phase 4 the glottis opens as air is forcefully expelled.[100]

Cough effectiveness can be quantitated by measuring PCFR. Individuals having a PCFR of less than 160 L/min

TABLE 8-9. EXAMPLES OF AEROBIC CAPACITY TESTING

- Bedside monitor with position changes
- Sitting tolerance testing
- Functional monitor/work-related tasks
- Chair test
- Walking velocity/distance
  - Velocity for over known distance
  - 2-Minute Walk test or 3-Minute Walk test
  - 6MWT
- Modified stress test (arm, bike, or treadmill)
  - Modified protocol (predetermined end point: HR, BP, workload)
  - Endurance test (time at specified RPE, % VO_2 or % HR)
- Formal stress test

RPE: rating of perceived exertion; VO_2: O_2 consumption.

(2.7 L/sec) are below the threshold necessary for secretion clearance.[226] This typically occurs when the FEV_1/FVC is below 60% predicted.[4,99]

Position the person in his or her preferred coughing posture to perform the exam, and ask the individual to inhale deeply and cough forcefully. The cough can be graded as "functional" if the individual is able to cough 2 to 6 times per breath.[100,135] Document the position and any additional trunk or arm motions used to assist the effort. The cough may be "weak functional" if there is some expulsion of air, enough to partially clear secretions. Look to see which phase of coughing is impaired and document what you observe "lacks inspiratory volume" or "poor glottis closure" or "unable to generate adequate abdominal muscle force." The proper treatment can be selected based on these observations. A "nonfunctional" cough will not generate enough force to move secretions.

Cranial Nerve Integrity

Examination of the cranial nerves will detect any problems with swallowing dysfunction that may lead to aspiration and pneumonia. Dysphagia and impaired gag reflex are predictors of the need for mechanical ventilation in individuals with progressive neuromuscular disease.[78] Therefore, examination of the glossopharyngeal, vagus, and hypoglossal nerves (cranial nerves IX, X, and XII) are a priority. Any patient who has been intubated may have acquired damage to the vocal cords and glottis. Examination of these nerves includes listening to voice quality, observing swallowing of a variety of substances, assessing elevation of the soft palate and position of the uvula during vocalization, and checking for a gag reflex. Movement of the tongue is also included in

the exam.[227] For individuals with neurological conditions, swallowing dysfunction may be associated with weakness or tone disorders related to the injury.[228] Examination of the spinal accessory nerves (cranial nerves XI) involves testing muscles (trapezius and sternocleidomastoid) that may act as stabilizers of the head and neck or as accessory muscles to support ventilation. A thorough examination of all the cranial nerves will also assist in identifying visual skills necessary for communication.

Aerobic Capacity

Aerobic capacity may be very low in some individuals with ventilatory pump dysfunction. In some cases the person with a neurological disorder may not be able to use peripheral muscles to perform a formal exercise test. For these individuals time sitting with or without support (binders, chair supports, arm support, mechanical ventilation) may be a method for documenting physiologic response to activity. The therapist can record signs of respiratory muscle fatigue or weakness.

A test of aerobic capacity is performed in a manner that offers an appropriate progressive challenge of the neuromuscular system. The test will introduce an activity level that raises the energy requirement and metabolic need for O_2 and thus ventilation. Examples of aerobic capacity testing are presented in Table 8-9. The goals of the exam are to determine whether the individual can participate safely in activity, to identify the "limiting factor" or the symptom (shortness of breath [SOB], dizziness, leg fatigue) that causes the person to stop activity, and to gather information about how the body adapts to exercise (normal physiologic response or compensatory response).[203] The information provided can help the therapist see whether the ventilatory pump is limiting tolerance to activity and then decide which factors related to ventilatory pump dysfunction (respiratory muscle weakness, stiffness in the chest wall, hyperinflation) can be addressed in the therapeutic POC.

Safety during activity involves analysis of all vital signs (HR, BP, RR, arterial O_2 saturation) and signs and symptoms. In some cases electrocardiogram (EKG) and hemodynamic monitoring may be required (cardiac conditions, history of recent medical instability). Because the individual with a ventilatory pump disorder may have comorbidities, it is important to detect limitations to activity due to other underlying conditions (heart disease, heart failure, peripheral artery disease, extremity pain, etc). Impaired diaphragmatic movement may also limit venous return and preload resulting in poor enhancement of cardiac output during activity.

If the ventilatory pump is limiting activity, the person will display an increase in accessory muscle use and RR that is out of proportion to activity challenge.[29] As exercise progresses and ventilatory pump dysfunction worsens, the individual will complain of increasing SOB. There will be earlier and more dramatic elevations in RR, intercostals muscle retraction, blue-gray appearance, and decreased O_2 saturation. The risks of aerobic capacity testing must be balanced with the purpose of the test and information needed to develop a sound therapeutic program. Therefore, submaximal testing is typically performed in those with ventilatory pump dysfunction. The 6MWT was originally developed for use in those with COPD and is the standard test used today.[201,229]

Recording measures of respiratory demand during activity can assist the medical team in understanding the risk of activity, adjusting medications and help therapist select interventions to improve activity tolerance. The response to exercise can be reexamined after offering support (O_2, ventilator, abdominal binder, chair modifications). Most individuals with ventilatory pump dysfunction will be limited by dyspnea or fatigue. Therefore, a Borg scale may be used to measure rating of perceived dyspnea (RPD) or rating of perceived exertion (RPE).[29,230]

Ergonomics, Environmental, Home, and Work Barriers

Examination of daily tasks performed in the home or work environment will assist in deciding what accommodations may be necessary for successful reintegration back to home and community-life roles. Routine tasks can be simulated in the clinic and measures of dyspnea, RR, RPE, RPD or other physiologic indices limiting performance documented. The therapist can draw on information from the interview and responses to outcome measures to determine which tasks to simulate. An activity log may be used to document routine tasks with a rating of the symptoms and a qualifier defining the importance of the activity to the individual. Reviewing a log can be helpful in identifying which activities are most challenging and a priority for instruction on energy conservation and task simplification strategies.[231]

EVALUATION, DIAGNOSIS, AND PROGNOSIS

Individuals with dyspnea and SOB are either limited by ventilation (ability to move air into the gas-exchanging regions of the lungs) or they may be limited by respiration (the ability to move gas between the pulmonary circulation and alveoli). After a review of the health condition and components of body structure and function, the therapist looks at the physical therapy examination findings to determine whether the person has a problem with ventilation or a problem with gas exchange. In many cases both may be present.

According to *The Guide to Physical Therapist Practice*, a person will have a physical therapy diagnosis of impaired ventilation and respiration associated with ventilatory pump dysfunction or failure (practice pattern 6E) if muscle performance and/or breathing mechanics are the core reason for symptoms of dyspnea or poor tolerance to activity.[92] If the person is experiencing oxyhemoglobin desaturation and/or dyspnea due to destruction of the lung tissue, pulmonary circulation or mucous and inflammation in the bronchioles and lung parenchyma then the primary problem

is respiratory. In this case the physical therapy diagnosis is impaired ventilation and respiration associated with respiratory failure (Practice Pattern 6F will be discussed in Chapter 9). Ventilatory pump dysfunction and failure occur when respiratory muscle performance is affected, which may be evident by diminished percentage predicted FVC, PI_{max}, PE_{max}, poor cough, abnormal breathing strategies or abnormal rise in RR and extreme fatigue with ambulation. Oxyhemoglobin desaturation is rare and elevation in CO_2 more common unless the person has both ventilation and gas-exchange impairments (advanced COPD).

Ventilatory pump dysfunction is distinct from ventilatory pump failure. Ventilatory pump dysfunction occurs when respiratory muscle performance limits exercise training and higher functioning. Ventilatory pump failure results when respiratory muscle function limits routine ADL.[4,141,221]

When determining a POC for the individual with ventilatory pump dysfunction, the therapist must review the examination findings to determine how pathologic processes are impacting on respiration. Specifically, the therapist must decide whether the ventilatory capacity diminished or if the load to the ventilatory muscle increased as a result of pathology. Impaired respiratory muscle performance (low predicted PI_{max}, PE_{max}, MVV, FVC) suggests ventilatory capacity is reduced. Limited chest wall expansion and restriction to passive movement, postural deformities, poor body positioning, dynamic hyperinflation or structural narrowing of airways increase the ventilatory load. The therapist selects interventions to effect body structure and function with the ultimate goal of decreasing the work of breathing. Reducing the work of breathing may be documented by noting lower dyspnea, RR, RPE or RPD values, more efficient breathing patterns, deeper and more controlled breathing for activity. The end result is improved activity tolerance, functional level and decreased dependence in ventilatory support. Examples of goals for individuals with ventilatory pump dysfunction are listed in Table 8-10.

INTERVENTIONS

The therapist will select procedures and techniques to produce changes in ventilatory load or ventilatory capacity. The application of any intervention requires a clinical decision-making process that is ongoing and evaluative. The individual's response to each procedure or technique must be observed, measured, and documented. This process has been referred to as "response dependent care."[232] This process is essential during the acute stage or whenever the prescriptive parameters of treatment are progressed. Responses to monitor and document include RR, dyspnea, RPD or RPE, symptoms of respiratory muscle incompetence (see Table 8-6), O_2 saturation, HR, and BP.

Airway clearance techniques and body positioning are examples of interventions to reduce ventilatory load. Intervention to improve ventilatory capacity may include enhancing respiratory muscle function to wean a patient

TABLE 8-10. SAMPLE THERAPEUTIC GOALS*

COPD	NEUROMUSCULAR
• Increase 6MWD by 50 feet with RPD < 3/10 and O_2 Sat > 90%. • Demonstrate pursed-lipped breathing and efficient coordinated breathing 90% of time when performing dressing, household chores, and work-related tasks (specific to patient goals). • Increase PI_{max} by 10 cc H_2O in order to prevent respiratory muscle fatigue and lower risk for pneumonia (may use FVC or MVV as measures). • Postexercise chest wall expansion will increase by 2 cm (demonstrating less hyperinflation with activity). • Climb 12 steps with railing using proper pacing to allow RPD < 3/10 and O_2 Sat > 90%.	• Apply effective manual cough techniques to clear secretions and prevent pneumonia (include caregiver or self-assist; describe technique used to cough—abdominal thrust, costophrenic assist). • Increase chest wall expansion at xiphoid by one-half inch • Decrease neck breathing and increase diaphragm component of breathing pattern to 1 neck 3 diaphragm (or by 10%) when sitting more than 4 hours. • Increase participation in upper extremity activities by 20% of time in therapy (or routine tasks at home) with RR < 20 with adequate posture support and seating. • Increase efficiency of transfers, bed mobility and ambulation (select task and level) with RPD < 3/10 and decreased time/increased distance. • Demonstrate proper use of coordinated breathing strategies during ADL 90% of the time. • Increase FVC 50 mL to improve reserve for activity (ambulation) and inspiratory volume for coughing to lower risk for pneumonia.

6MWD: 6-Minute Walking Distance; RPD: rating of perceived dyspnea; O_2 Sat: O_2 saturation; PI_{max}: maximal inspiration; RR: respiration rate.

*Specific level of assist, person, goal-oriented tasks, and time frame to be added or modified according to context.

from a ventilator, using an abdominal binder to improve diaphragmatic position during practice of breathing mechanics, and biofeedback to facilitate muscle recruitment for a more efficient breathing pattern. Manual techniques as well as use of diaphragm weights are used in VMT.

Exercise training for endurance requires a prescription that offers a stimulus that is adequate to overload the O_2 transport system without causing overuse of peripheral muscles.[203] A good aerobic conditioning program will increase aerobic reserve for activity and limit the early onset of symptoms. The individual can then participate more comfortably in endurance tasks. The exercise prescription follows the FITT principle and includes 4 components; Frequency, Intensity, Time, and Type.[203]

Therapeutic exercise will also include strength training and flexibility or stretching for the peripheral muscles. Stretching to reduce or prevent contractures provides proper skeletal alignment and mechanics during movement. While strengthening weak muscle increases support for activity. Together these 2 therapeutic interventions allow muscle to be used efficiently, with a lower energy cost.[233] Good economy of movement lowers the ventilatory demand and improves the balance between O_2 supply and demand in the working muscle, resulting in less fatigue and SOB. Activity participation is improves. Use of efficient breathing strategies (coordinated breathing, diaphragmatic breathing and pursed lipped breathing) also improve oxygenation and support good ventilation during activity.[105]

REFERENCES

1. McArdle WD, Katch FI, Katch VL. *The Pulmonary System and Exercise. Essentials of Exercise Physiology.* 3rd ed. New York: Lippincott, Williams & Wilkins; 2005.

2. Widmaier EP, Raff H, Strang KT. *Vander's Human Physiology. The Mechanisms of Body Function.* 11 ed. New York: McGraw Hill Company; 2008.

3. American Thoracic Society/European Respiratory Society. ATS/ERS statement on respiratory muscle testing. *Am J Respir Crit Care Med.* 2002;166:518-624.

4. Massery M, Cahalin L. Physical therapy associated with ventilatory pump dysfunction and failure. In: DeTurk WE, Cahalin LP, eds. *Cardiovascular and Pulmonary Physical Therapy: An Evidence-Based Approach.* New York: McGraw-Hill; 2004:593-646.

5. Cherniack R, Cherniack L. *Respiration in Health and Disease.* 3rd ed. Philadelphia, PA: WB Saunders; 1983.

6. Massery M. Multisystem consequences of impaired breathing mechanics and/or postural control. In: Frownfelter D, Dean E, eds. *Cardiovascular and Pulmonary Physical Therapy: Evidence and Practice.* 4th ed. St. Louis, MO: Mosby Elsevier; 2006:695-717.

7. Frownfelter D, Dean E, Wetzel JL. Primary prevention/risk reduction for cardiovascular/pulmonary disorders (pattern A). In: Moffat M, Frownfelter D, eds. *Cardiovascular/Pulmonary Essentials: Applying the Preferred Physical Therapist Practice Patterns.* Thorofare, NJ: SLACK Incorporated; 2007:1-36.

8. Verschakelen JA, Deschepper K, Demedts M. Relationship between axial motion and volume displacement of the diaphragm during VC maneuvers. *J Appl Physiol (1985).* 1992;72(4):1536-1540.

9. Massery M. The continuum of care for people with lifelong disabilities. Understanding the issues and forging new pathways for physical therapists. Proceedings of the APTA Combined Sections Meeting 2009; Las Vegas, NV 2009.

10. Sciaky A. Impaired ventilation and respiration/gas exchange associated with ventilatory pump dysfunction or failure. In: Moffat M, Frownfelter D, eds. *Cardiovascular/Pulmonary Essentials: Applying the Preferred Physical Therapist Practice Patterns.* Thorofare, NJ: SLACK Incorporated; 2007.

11. Flaminiano LE, Celli BR. Respiratory muscle testing. *Clin Chest Med.* 2001;22(4):661-677.

12. Dean E. Cardiopulmonary anatomy. In: Frownfelter D, Dean E, eds. *Cardiovascular and Pulmonary Physical Therapy: Evidence and Practice.* 4th ed. St. Louis, MO: Mosby Elsevier; 2006:53-72.

13. Massery M. The patient with neuromuscular or musculoskeletal dysfunction. In: Frownfelter D, Dean E, editors. *Principles and Practice of Cardiopulmonary Physical Therapy.* 3rd ed. St. Louis, MO: Mosby-Year Book Inc; 1996:679-702.

14. Derenne J, Macklem PT, Roussos CH. The respiratory muscles: mechanics, control, and pathophysiology. Part I. *Am Rev Respir Dis.* 1978;118:119-133.

15. Reid DW, Dechman G. Considerations when testing and training the respiratory muscles. *Phys Ther.* 1995;75:971-982.

16. Protas EJ. The aging patient. In: Frownfelter D, Dean E, eds. *Cardiovascular and Pulmonary Physical Therapy Evidence and Practice.* 4th ed. St. Louis, MO: Mosby Elsevier; 2006:685-691.

17. Deem JF, Nukker L. *Manual of Voice Therapy.* 2nd ed. Austin, Tex: PRO-ED Inc; 2000.

18. Hodges PW, Gandevia SC. Changes in intra-abdominal pressure during postural and respiratory activation of the human diaphragm. *J Appl Physiol (1985).* 2000(89):967-976.

19. Puckree T, Cerny F, Bishop B. Abdominal motor unit activity during respiratory and nonrespiratory tasks. *J Appl Physiol (1985).* 1998;84(5):1707-1715.

20. Estenne M, Knoop C, Vanvaerenbergh J, Heilporn A, De Troyer A. The effect of pectoralis muscle training in tetraplegic subjects. *Am Rev Respir Dis.* 1989;139(5):1218-1222.

21. Fujiwara T, Hara Y, Chino N. Expiratory function in complete tetraplegics: study of spirometry, maximal expiratory pressure, and muscle activity of pectoralis major and latissimus dorsi muscles. *Am J Phys Med Rehabil.* 1999;78(5):464-469.

22. Dean E. Cardiopulmonary physiology. In: Frownfelter D, Dean E, eds. *Cardiovascular and Pulmonary Physical Therapy: Evidence and Practice.* 4th ed. St. Louis, MO: Mosby Elsevier; 2006.

23. Butler JE. Drive to the human respiratory muscles. *Respir Physiol Neurobiol.* 2007;159(2):115-126.

24. Bach JR. Mechanical insufflation-exsufflation. Comparison of peak expiratory flows with manually assisted and unassisted coughing techniques. *Chest.* 1993;104(5):1553-1562.

25. Leith DE. Cough. In: Brain JD, Proctor D, Reid L, eds. *Lung Biology in Health and Disease: Respiratory Defense Mechanisms.* New York: Marcel Dekker; 1977:545-592.

26. Kang SW, Shin JC, Park CI, Moon JH, Rha DW, Cho DH. Relationship between inspiratory muscle strength and cough capacity in cervical spinal cord injured patients. *Spinal Cord.* 2006;44(4):242-248.

27. American Thoracic Society. Lung function testing: selection of reference values and interpretative strategies. *Am Rev Respir Dis.* 1991;144:1202-1218.

28. Wasserman K, Hansen JE, Sue DY, String WW. *Principles of Exercise Testing and Interpretation.* 4th ed. Philadelphia: Lippincott, Williams & Wilkins; 2004.

29. DeTurk WE, Cahalin L. Evaluation of patient intolerance to exercise. In: DeTurk WE, Cahalin L, eds. *Cardiovascular and Pulmonary Physical Therapy: An Evidenced-Based Approach.* New York: McGraw-Hill Co.; 2004.

30. Janssens JP, Pache JC, Nicod LP. Physiological changes in respiratory function associated with ageing. *Eur Respir J.* 1999;13(1):197-205.

31. Clough P. Restrictive lung dysfunction. In: Hillegass EA, Sadowsky HS, eds. *Essentials of Cardiopulmonary Physical Therapy.* 2nd ed. Philadelphia, PA: W. B. Saunders Company; 2001.

32. McClaran SR, Babcock MA, Pegelow DF, Reddan WG, Dempsey JA. Longitudinal effects of aging on lung function at rest and exercise in healthy active fit elderly adults. *J Appl Physiol (1985).* 1995;78(5):1957-68.

33. Takishima T, Shindoh C, Kikuchi Y, Hida W, Inoue H. Aging effect on oxygen consumption of respiratory muscles in humans. *J Appl Physiol (1985).* 1990;69(1):14-20.

34. Dempsey JA, Seals DR. Aging, exercise, and cardiopulmonary function. In: Holloszy J, ed. *Perspectives in Exercise Science.* New York: Williams & Wilkins; 1995.

35. Enright PL, Kronmal RA, Manolio TA, Schenker MB, Hyatt RE. Respiratory muscle strength in the elderly. Correlates and reference values. Cardiovascular Health Study Research Group. *Am J Respir Crit Care Med.* 1994;149(2 Pt 1):430-438.

36. Black LF, Hyatt RE. Maximal respiratory pressures: normal values and relationship to age and sex. *Am Rev Respir Dis.* 1969;99:696-702.

37. Enright PL, Adams AB, Boyle PJR, Sherrill DL. Spirometry and maximal respiratory pressure references from healthy Minnesota 65- to 85-year-old women and men. *Chest.* 1995;108:663-669.

38. Cardús J, Burgos F, Diaz O, et al. Increase in pulmonary ventilation-perfusion inequality with age in healthy individuals. *Am J Respir Crit Care Med.* 1997;156(2 Pt 1):648-653.

39. Fishman A, Elias J, Fishman J. *Fishman's Pulmonary Diseases and Disorders.* 3rd ed. New York: McGraw Hill; 1998.

40. Peterson DD, Pack AI, Silage DA, Fishman AP. Effects of aging on ventilatory and occlusion pressure responses to hypoxia and hypercapnia. *Am Rev Respir Dis.* 1981;124:387-391.

41. Trappe SW, Costill DL, Vukovich MD, Jones J, Melham T. Aging among elite distance runners: a 22-yr longitudinal study. *J Appl Physiol (1985).* 1996;80(1):285-290.

42. Brischetto MJ, Millman RP, Peterson DD, Silage DA, Pack AI. Effect of aging on ventilatory response to exercise and CO_2. *J Appl Physiol Respir Environ Exerc Physiol.* 1984;56(5):1143-1150.

43. Manning H, Mahler D, Harver A. Dyspnea in the elderly. In: Mahler D, ed. *Pulmonary Disease in the Elderly Patient.* New York: Marcel Dekker; 1993:81-111.

44. De Vito G, Hernández R, Gonzalez V, Felici F, Figura F. Low intensity physical training in older subjects. *J Sports Med Phys Fitness.* 1997;37(1):72-77.

45. Warren BJ, Nieman DC, Dotson RG, et al. Cardiorespiratory response to exercise training in septuagenarian women. *Int J Sports Med.* 1993;14:60-65.

46. Mannino DM, Kiriz VA. Changing the burden of COPD mortality. *Int J Chron Obstruct Pulmon Dis.* 2006;1(3):219-233.

47. Centers for Disease Control and Prevention (CDC). Deaths from chronic obstructive pulmonary disease—United States, 2000-2005. *MMWR Morb Mortal Wkly Rep.* 2008;57(45):1229-1232.

48. Sin DD, Anthonisen NR, Soriano JB, Agusti AG. Mortality in COPD: role of comorbidities. *Eur Respir J.* 2006;28(6):1245-1257.

49. Markou NK, Myrianthefs PM, Baltopoulos GJ. Respiratory failure: an overview. *Crit Care Nurs Q.* 2004;27(4):353-379.

50. Pauwels RA, Buist AS, Calverley PM, Jenkins CR, Hurd SS. Global strategy for the diagnosis, management, and prevention of chronic obstructive pulmonary disease. NHLBI/WHO Global Initiative for Chronic Obstructive Lung Disease (GOLD) Workshop summary. *Am J Respir Crit Care Med.* 2001;163:125-1376.

51. O'Donnell DE, Laveneziana P. Dyspnea and activity limitation in COPD. *COPD.* 2007;4(3):225-2236.

52. O'Donnell DE. Ventilatory limitations in chronic obstructive pulmonary disease. *Med Sci Sports Exerc.* 2001;33(7):S647-S655.

53. Aliverti A, Macklem PT. The major limitation to exercise performance in COPD is inadequate energy supply to the respiratory and locomotor muscles. *J Appl Physiol (1985)*. 2008;105(2):749-751.

54. Simon M, LeBlanc P, Jobin J, Desmeules M, Sullivan MJ, Maltais F. Limitation of lower limb VO(2) during cycling exercise in COPD patients. *J Appl Physiol (1985)*. 2001;90(3):1013-1019.

55. O'Donnell DE, Webb KA. Exertional breathlessness in patients with chronic airflow limitation: the role of hyperinflation. *Am Rev Respir Dis*. 1993;148(5):1351-1357.

56. Buist AS, McBurnie MA, Vollmer WM, et al. International variation in the prevalence of COPD (the BOLD study): a population-based prevalence study. *Lancet*. 2007;370(9589):741-750.

57. de Torres JP, Campo AC, Casanova C, Aguirre-Jaime A, Zulueta J. Gender and chronic obstructive pulmonary disease in high-risk smokers. *Respiration*. 2006;73(3):306-310.

58. Wells CL. Pulmonary pathology. In: DeTurk WE, Cahalin L, eds. *Cardiovascular and Pulmonary Physical Therapy: An Evidence-Based Approach*. New York: McGraw-Hill; 2004: 151-188.

59. Anthonisen NR, Connett JE, Kiley JP, et al. Effects of smoking intervention and the use of an inhaled anticholinergic bronchodilator on the rate of decline of FEV1. The lung health study. *JAMA*. 1994;272(19):1539-1541.

60. Buist AS. COPD: worldwide prevalence. In: Pauwels RA, Postma DS, Weiss ST, eds. *Long-term Intervention in Chronic Obstructive Pulmonary Disease*. 2nd ed. London: Informa Health Care; 2004:15-32.

61. Molfino NA. Genetics of COPD. *Chest*. 2004;125(5):1929-1940.

62. Stoller J. Clinical features and natural history of severe alpha I anti-trypsin deficiency. *Chest*. 1997;111:123S-128S.

63. One degree of separation: paralysis and spinal cord injury in the United States. 2009. http://www.christopherreeve.org. Accessed July 22, 2009.

64. Roth EJ, Nussbaum SB, Berkowitz M, et al. Pulmonary function testing in spinal cord injury: correlation with vital capacity. *Paraplegia*. 1995;33(8):454-457.

65. Smeltzer SC, Utell MJ, Rudick RA, Herndon RM. Pulmonary function and dysfunction in multiple sclerosis. *Arch Neurol*. 1988;45(11):1245-1249.

66. Baydur A, Adkins RH, Milic-Emili J. Lung mechanics in individuals with spinal cord injury: effects of injury level and posture. *J Appl Physiol (1985)*. 2001;90(2):405-411.

67. Buyse B, Demedts M, Meekers J, Vandegaer L, Rochette F, Kerkhofs L. Respiratory dysfunction in multiple sclerosis: a prospective analysis of 60 patients. *Eur Respir J*. 1997;10:139-145.

68. Simonds AK. Recent advances in respiratory care for neuromuscular disease. *Chest*. 2006;130:1879-1886.

69. Dean E, Ross J, Road JD, Courtenay L, Madill KJ. Pulmonary function in individuals with a history of poliomyelitis. **Chest.** 1991;100(1):118-123.

70. McDonald CM, Abresch RT, Carter GT, et al. Profiles of neuromuscular diseases: Duchenne muscular dystrophy. *Am J Phys Med Rehabil*. 1995;74(5):S70-S92.

71. Laghi F, Tobin MJ. Disorders of the respiratory muscles. *Am J Respir Crit Care Med*. 2003;168(1):10-48.

72. Rabinstein AA. Update on respiratory management of critically ill neurologic patients. *Curr Neurol Neurosci Rep*. 2005;5(6):476-482.

73. Bella I, Chad DA. Neuromuscular disorders and acute respiratory failure. *Neurol Clin*. 1998;16(2):391-417.

74. Jackson AB, Groomes TE. Incidence of respiratory complications following spinal cord injury. *Arch Phys Med Rehabil*. 1994;75:270-275.

75. Teitelbaum JS, Borel CO. Respiratory dysfunction in Guillain-Barré syndrome. *Clin Chest Med*. 1994;15:705-714.

76. Orlikowski D, Prigent H, Sharshar T, Lofaso F, Raphael JC. Respiratory dysfunction in Guillain-Barré syndrome. *Neurocrit Care*. 2004;1(4):415-422.

77. American Spinal Injury Association. ASIA classification. *Scientific Spine*. http://www.scientificspine.com/spine-scores/asia-classification.html. Updated July 18, 2011. Accessed June 14, 2014.

78. Mehta S. Neuromuscular disease causing acute respiratory failure. *Respir Care*. 2006;51(9):1016-1021.

79. Newton PO, Faro FD, Gollogly S, Betz RR, Lenke LG, Lowe TG. Results of preoperative pulmonary function testing of adolescents with idiopathic scoliosis. A study of six hundred and thirty-one patients. *J Bone Joint Surg Am*. 2005;87(9):1937-1946.

80. Mellin G, Harjula R. Lung function in relation to thoracic spine mobility and kyphosis. *Scand J Rehabil Med*. 1987;19:89-92.

81. Vedantam R, Crawford AH. The role of preoperative pulmonary function tests in patients with adolescent idiopathic scoliosis undergoing posterior spinal fusion. *Spine*. 1997;22(23):2731-2734.

82. Geddes DM, Brostoff J. Respiratory complications of rheumatoid disease. *BMJ*. 1975;2(5964):175-176.

83. Derenne J, Macklem PT, Roussos CH. The respiratory muscles: mechanics, control and pathophysiology. Part II. *Am Rev Respir Dis*. 1978;118:373-390.

84. Mohamad F, Parent S, Pawelek J, et al. Perioperative complications after surgical correction in neuromuscular scoliosis. *J Pediatr Orthop*. 2007;27(4):392-397.

85. George RB, Light RW, Matthay MA, Matthay RA. *Chest Medicine: Essentials of Pulmonary and Critical Care Medicine*. 3rd ed. Baltimore, MD: Williams & Wilkins; 1995.

86. Dean E. Body positioning. In: Frownfelter D, Dean E, eds. *Cardiovascular and Pulmonary Physical Therapy: Evidence and Practice*. 4th ed. St. Louis, MO: Mosby Elsevier; 2006:307-324.

87. Ziegler DW, Agarwal NN. Morbidity and mortality of rib fractures. *J Trauma*. 1995;37(6):975-979.

88. Battistella FD, Din AM, Perez L. Trauma patients 75 years and older: long-term follow-up results justify aggressive management. *J Trauma*. 1998;44(4):618-623.

89. Jones M, Moffatt F. Chest wall deformity or disruption. In: Watts A, ed. *Cardiopulmonary Physiotherapy*. Oxford, U.K.: BIOS Scientific Publishers Ltd; 2002:26-29.

90. Clough P, Lindenauer D, Hayes M, Zekany B. Guidelines for routine respiratory care of patients with spinal cord injury. A clinical report. *Phys Ther*. 1986;66(9):1395-1402.

91. World Health Organization. *International Classification of Functioning, Disability and Health*. Geneva: Author; 2001.

92. American Physical Therapy Association. *Guide to Physical Therapist Practice*. 2nd ed. Alexandria, VA: Author; 2003.

93. Vassilakopoulos T, Zakynthinos S, Roussos CH. Respiratory muscles and weaning failure. *Eur Respir J*. 1996;9:2383-2400.

94. Gonzalez J, Coast JR, Lawler JM, Welch HG. A chest wall restrictor to study effects on pulmonary function and exercise. *Respiration*. 1999;66:188-194.

95. Field S, Kelly SM, Macklem PT. The oxygen cost of breathing in patients with cardiorespiratory disease. *Am Rev Respir Dis*. 1982;126(1):9-13.

96. Coast JR, Cline CC. The effect of chest wall restriction on exercise capacity. *Respirology*. 2004;9(2):197-203.

97. Cerny FW, Zhan S. Chronic obstructive pulmonary disease. In: LeMura L, von Duvillard SP, eds. *Clinical Exercise Physiology Application and Physiologic Principles*. Philadelphia, PA: Lippincott, Williams & Wilkins; 2004:157-168.

98. Poponick JM, Jacobs I, Supinski G, DiMarco AF. Effect of upper respiratory tract infection in patients with neuromuscular disease. *Am J Respir Crit Care Med*. 1997;156(2 Pt 1):659-664.

99. Downs AM, Lindsay KLB. Physical therapy associated with airway clearance dysfunction. In: DeTurk WE, Cahalin L, eds. *Cardiovascular and Pulmonary Physical Therapy: An Evidence-Based Approach*. New York: McGraw-Hill Co.; 2004.

100. Frownfelter D, Massery M. Facilitating airway clearance with coughing techniques. In: Frownfelter D, Dean E, eds. *Cardiovascular and Pulmonary Physical Therapy Evidence and Practice*. 4th ed. St. Louis, MO: Mosby Elsevier; 2006:363-376.

101. Derenne J, Macklem PT, Roussos CH. The respiratory muscles: Mechanics, control and pathophysiology. Part III. *Am Rev Respir Dis.* 1978;118:581-601.

102. Blissitt PA. Nutrition in acute spinal cord injury. *Crit Care Nurs Clin North Am.* 1990;2(3):375-384.

103. Rochester DF, Arora NS. Respiratory muscle failure. *Med Clin North Am.* 1983;67(3):573-597.

104. Bellemare F, Grassino A. Effect of pressure and timing of contraction on human diaphragm fatigue. *J Appl Physiol Respir Environ Exerc Physiol.* 1982;53(5):1190-1195.

105. Frownfelter D, Massery M. Facilitating ventilation patterns and breathing strategies. In: Frownfelter D, Dean E, eds. *Cardiovascular and Pulmonary Physical Therapy Evidence and Practice.* 4th ed. New York: Mosby Elsevier; 2006:377-403.

106. Bach JR, Rajaraman R, Ballanger F, et al. Neuromuscular ventilatory insufficiency: effect of home mechanical ventilator use v oxygen therapy on pneumonia and hospitalization rates. *Am J Phys Med Rehabil.* 1998;77(1):8-19.

107. Islam T, Brar NK, Hage JE, et al. Respiratory complications and outcomes in a neuro-intensive care unit. *Chest.* 2008;134(4):p123002.

108. Shaffer TH, Wolfson MR, Bhutani VK. Respiratory muscle function, assessment, and training. *Phys Ther.* 1981;61(12):1711-1723.

109. Roussos C, Zakynthinos S. Ventilatory failure and respiratory muscles. In: Roussos C, ed. *The Thorax.* 2nd ed. New York: Marcel Dekker; 1995:2071-2199.

110. Misuri G, Lanini B, Gigliotti F, et al. Mechanism of CO(2) retention in patients with neuromuscular disease. *Chest.* 2000;117(2):447-453.

111. Hadjikoutis S, Pickersgill TP, Dawson K, Wiles CM. Abnormal patterns of breathing during swallowing in neurological disorders. *Brain.* 2000;123(9):1863-1873.

112. Wolf C, Meiners TH. Dysphagia in patients with acute cervical spinal cord injury. *Spinal Cord.* 2003;41(6):347-353.

113. Maestrelli P, Saetta M, Mapp CE, Fabbri LM. Remodeling in response to infection and injury. Airway inflammation and hypersecretion of mucus in smoking subjects with chronic obstructive pulmonary disease. *Am J Respir Crit Care Med.* 2001;164(10):S76-S80.

114. Garritan S. Chronic obstructive pulmonary diseases. In: Hillegass EA, Sadowsky HS, eds. *Essentials of Cardiopulmonary Physical Therapy.* 2nd ed. Philadelphia, PA: W.B. Saunders Co.; 2001:257-284.

115. Sadowsky HS, Frownfelter D, Moffat M. Impaired ventilation and respiration/gas exchange associated with respiratory failure (pattern F). In: Moffat M, Frownfelter D, eds. *Cardiovascular/Pulmonary Essentials: Applying the Preferred Physical Therapist Practice Patterns.* Thorofare, NJ: SLACK Incorporated; 2007:193-236.

116. Dean E. Individuals with acute medical conditions. In: Frownfelter D, Dean E, eds. *Cardiovascular and Pulmonary Physical Therapy Evidence and Practice.* 4th ed. St. Louis, MO: Mosby Elsevier; 2006:507-528.

117. Cote CG, Casanova C, Marín JM, et al. Validation and comparison of reference equations for the 6-min walk distance test. *Eur Respir J.* 2008;31(3):571-578.

118. Clanton TL, Diaz PT. Clinical assessment of the respiratory muscles. *Phys Ther.* 1995;75:983-995.

119. de Oca MM, Rassulo J, Celli BR. Respiratory muscle and cardiopulmonary function during exercise in very severe COPD. *Am J Respir Crit Care Med.* 1996;154:1284-1289.

120. Ramirez-Venegas A, Ward JL, Olmstead EM, Tosteson AN, Mahler DA. Effect of exercise training on dyspnea measures in patients with chronic obstructive pulmonary disease. *J Cardiopulm Rehabil.* 1997;17(2):103-109.

121. O'Donnell DE, Webb KA. Mechanisms of dyspnea in COPD. In: Mahler D, O'Donnell DE, eds. *Dyspnea: Mechanisms, Measurement, and Management.* 2nd ed. New York: Taylor & Francis Group; 2005:29-58.

122. Sisto SA. Cardiopulmonary concerns in the patient with neurological deficits: an evidence-based approach. In: DeTurk WE, Cahalin LP, eds. *Cardiovascular and Pulmonary Physical Therapy: An Evidence-Based Approach.* New York: McGraw-Hill; 2004:395-422.

123. Stanghelle JK, Festvag L, Aksnes AK. Pulmonary function and symptom-limited exercise stress testing in subjects with late sequelae of poliomyelitis. *Scand J Rehabil Med.* 1993;25(3):125-129.

124. Bernard PL, Mercier J, Varray A, Prefaut C. Influence of lesion level on the cardioventilatory adaptations in paraplegic wheelchair athletes during muscular exercise. *Spinal Cord.* 2000;38(1):16-25.

125. Marinelli WA, Leatherman JW. Neuromuscular disorders in the intensive care unit. *Crit Care Clin.* 2002;18(4):915-929.

126. Cohen IL, Lambrinos J. Investigating the impact of age on outcome of mechanical ventilation using a population of 41,848 patients from a statewide database. *Chest.* 1995;107:1673-1680.

127. Arima T, Noguchi T, Mochida J, Toh E, Konagai A, Nishimura K. Problems of long-term hospitalised cervical spinal cord injury patients in university hospitals. *Paraplegia.* 1994;32(1):19-24.

128. Thomas CE, Mayer SA, Gungor Y, et al. Myasthenia crisis: clinical features, mortality, complications and risk factors for prolonged intubation. *Neurology.* 1997;48(5):1253-1260.

129. Linn WS, Spungen AM, Gong H Jr, Bauman WA, Adkins RH, Waters RL. Smoking and obstructive lung dysfunction in persons with chronic spinal cord injury. *J Spinal Cord Med.* 2003;26(1):28-35.

130. Burns SP, Kapur V, Yin KS, Buhrer R. Factors associated with sleep apnea in men with spinal cord injury: a population-based case-control study. *Spinal Cord.* 2001;39(1):15-22.

131. American Thoracic Society. Respiratory care of the patient with Duchenne muscular dystrophy. ATS consensus statement. *Am J Respir Crit Care Med.* 2004;170:456-465.

132. Sharshar T, Chevret S, Bourdain F, et al. Early predictors of mechanical ventilation in Guillain-Barré syndrome. *Crit Care Med.* 2003;31(1):278-283.

133. Sundar U, Abraham E, Gharat A, Yeolekar ME, Trivedi T, Dwivedi N. Neuromuscular respiratory failure in Guillain-Barré syndrome: evaluation of clinical and electrodiagnostic predictors. *J Assoc Physicians India.* 2005;53:264-268.

134. Kocan MJ. Pulmonary considerations in the critical care phase. *Crit Care Nurs Clin North Am.* 1990;2(3):369-374.

135. Alvarez SE, Peterson M, Lunsford BR. Respiratory treatment of the adult patient with spinal cord injury. *Phys Ther.* 1981;61(12):1737-1745.

136. Wetzel JL, Lunsford BR, Peterson MJ, Alvarez SE. Respiratory rehabilitation of the patient with a spinal cord injury. In: Irwin S, Techlin JS, eds. *Cardiopulmonary Physical Therapy.* 3rd ed. St. Louis, MO: Mosby; 1995:579-603.

137. Wetzel JL. Management of respiratory dysfunction. In: Field-Fote EC, ed. *Spinal Cord Injury Rehabilitation.* Philadelphia, PA: F.A. Davis; 2009:337-392.

138. Feldman D, Ouellette M, Villamez A, Massery M, Cahalin LP. The relationship of ventilatory muscle strength to chest wall excursion in normal subjects and persons with cervical spinal cord injury. Abstract. *Cardiopulm Phys Ther J.* 1998;9(4):20.

139. Massery MP, Dreyer HE, Bjornson AS, Cahalin LP. Chest wall excursion and tidal volume change during passive positioning in cervical spinal cord injury. (Abstract). *Cardiopulm Phys Ther J.* 1997;8(4):27.

140. Gerold K. Physical therapists' guide to the principles of mechanical ventilation. *Cardiopulm Phys Ther J.* 1992;3:8-13.

141. Ciesla N. Physical therapy associated with respiratory failure. In: DeTurk WE, Cahalin LP, eds. *Cardiovascular and Pulmonary Physical Therapy: An Evidence-Based Approach.* New York: McGraw-Hill; 2004:541-592.

142. Make BJ, Hill NS, Goldberg AI, et al. Mechanical ventilation beyond the intensive care unit. Report of a consensus conference of the American College of Chest Physicians. *Chest.* 1998;113(5):259S-344S.

143. MacIntyre NR, Cook DJ, Ely EW Jr, et al. Evidence-based guidelines for weaning and discontinuing ventilatory support: a collective task force facilitated by the American College of Chest Physicians; the American Association for Respiratory Care; and the American College of Critical Care Medicine. *Chest.* 2001;120(6 Suppl):375S-395S.

144. Burns SP, Rad MY, Bryant S, Kapur V. Long-term sleep apnea in persons with spinal cord injury. *Am J Phys Med Rehab.* 2005;84(8):620-626.

145. American Heart Association: Heart and stroke statistical-2005 update. Dallas: American Heart Association; 2005.

146. Vingerhoets F, Bogousslavsky J. Respiratory dysfunction in stroke. *Clin Chest Med.* 1994;15(4):729-737.

147. Lanini B, Blanchi R, Romagnoli I, et al. Chest wall kinematics in patients with hemiplegia. *Am J Respir Crit Care Med.* 2003;168:109-113.

148. Turkington PM, Bamford J, Wanklyn P, Elliott MW. Prevalence and predictors of upper airway obstruction in the first 24 hours after acute stroke. *Stroke.* 2002;33:2037-2042.

149. Cohen E, Mier A. Diaphragmatic movement in hemiplegic patients measured by ultrasonography. *Thorax.* 1994;49:890-895.

150. Fluck DC. Chest movements in hemiplegia. *Clin Sci.* 1966;31:383-388.

151. De Troyer A, Zegers De Beyl D, Thirion M. Function of respiratory muscles in acute hemiplegia. *Am Rev Respir Dis.* 1981;123(6):631-632.

152. Fugl-Meyer AR, Linderholm H, Wilson AF. Restrictive ventilatory dysfunction in stroke: its relation to locomotor function. *Scand J Rehabil Med Suppl.* 1983;9:118-124.

153. De Troyer A, Borenstein S, Cordier R. Analysis of lung volume restriction in patients with respiratory muscle weakness. *Thorax.* 1980;35:603-10.

154. Estenne M, Gevenois PA, Kinnear W, Soudon P, Heilporn A, De Troyer A. Lung volume restriction in patients with chronic respiratory muscle weakness: the role of microatelectasis. *Thorax.* 1993;48(7):698-701.

155. Ragette R, Mellies U, Schwake C, Voit T, Teschler H. Patterns and predictors of sleep disordered breathing in primary myopathies. *Thorax.* 2002;57(8):724-728.

156. Ropper AH, Kennedy SF. Critical care of Guillain-Barré syndrome. In: Ropper AH, ed. *Neurological and Neurosurgical Intensive Care.* New York: Raven Press Inc; 1993:363-382.

157. Redelings MD, McCoy L, Sorvillo F. Multiple sclerosis mortality and patterns of comorbidity in the United States from 1990 to 2001. *Neuroepidemiology.* 2006;26:102-107.

158. Fry DK, Pfalzer LA, Chokshi AR, Wagner MT, Jackson ES. Randomized control trial of effects of a 10-week inspiratory muscle training program on measures of pulmonary function in persons with multiple sclerosis. *J Neurol Phys Ther.* 2007;31(4):162-172.

159. Gosselink R, Kovacs L, Ketelaer P, Carton H, Decramer M. Respiratory muscle weakness and respiratory muscle training in severely disabled multiple sclerosis patients. *Arch Phys Med Rehabil.* 2000;81(6):747-751.

160. Chiara T, Martin D, Davenport PW, Bolser DC. Expiratory muscle strength training in persons with multiple sclerosis having mild to moderate disability: effect on maximal expiratory pressure, pulmonary function, and maximal voluntary cough. *Arch Phys Med Rehabil.* 2006;87(4):468-473.

161. O'Sullivan SB. Parkinson's disease. In: O'Sullivan SB, Schmitz TJ, eds. *Physical Rehabilitation: Assessment and Treatment.* 5th ed. Philadelphia, PA: F.A. Davis; 2007:853-892.

162. Bogaard JM, Hovestadt A, Meerwaldt J, vd Meché FG, Stigt J. Maximal expiratory and inspiratory flow-volume curves in Parkinson's disease. *Am Rev Respir Dis.* 1989;139(3):610-614.

163. de Bruin PF, de Bruin VM, Lees AJ, Pride NB. Effects of treatment on airway dynamics and respiratory muscle strength in Parkinson's disease. *Am Rev Respir Dis.* 1993;148(6 Pt 1):1576-1580.

164. Sabaté M, González I, Ruperez F, Rodríguez M. Obstructive and restrictive pulmonary dysfunction in Parkinson's disease. *J Neurol Sci.* 1996;138(1-2):114-119.

165. Protas EJ, Stanley RK, Jankovic J, MacNeill B. Cardiovascular and metabolic responses to upper- and lower-extremity exercise in men with idiopathic Parkinson's disease. *Phys Ther.* 1996;76(1):34-40.

166. Matheson MJ. Practical tips on postpolio syndrome. *Can Fam Physician.* 1995;41:669-672.

167. Ramlow J, Alexander M, LaPorte R, Kaufmann C, Kuller L. Epidemiology of the post-polio syndrome. *Am J Epidemiol.* 1992;136(7):769-786.

168. Jubelt B. Post-polio syndrome. *Curr Treat Options Neurol.* 2004;6(2):87-93.

169. Lambert DA, Giannouli E, Schmidt BJ. Postpolio syndrome and anesthesia. *Anesthesiology.* 2005;103(3):638-644.

170. Weinberg J, Borg j, Bevengard S. Respiratory response to exercise in post-polio patients with severe inspiratory muscle dysfunction. *Arch Phys Med Rehabil.* 1999;80(9):1095-1100.

171. Foglio K, Cini E, Facchetti D, et al. Respiratory muscle function and exercise capacity in multiple sclerosis. *Eur Respir J.* 1994;7(1):23-28.

172. Del Bigio MR, Deck JH, MacDonald JK. Syrinx extending from conus medullaris to basal ganglia: a clinical, radiological, and pathological correlation. *Can J Neurol Sci.* 1993;20(3):240-246.

173. Mossberg KA, Ayala D, Baker T, Heard J, Masel B. Aerobic capacity after traumatic brain injury: comparison with a nondisabled cohort. *Arch Phys Med Rehabil.* 2007;88(3):315-320.

174. Mossberg KA, Orlander EE, Norcross JL. Cardiorespiratory capacity after weight-supported treadmill training in patients with traumatic brain injury. *Phys Ther.* 2008;88:77-87.

175. Köseoglu F, Inan L, Ozel S, et al. The effects of a pulmonary rehabilitation program on pulmonary function tests and exercise tolerance in patients with Parkinson's disease. *Funct Neurol.* 1997;12(6):319-325.

176. Balmer GA, MacEven GD. The incidence and treatment of scoliosis in cerebral palsy. *J Bone Joint Surg Br.* 1970;52:134-137.

177. Cambridge W, Drennan JC. Scoliosis associated with Duchenne muscular dystrophy. *J Pediatr Orthop.* 1987;7(4):436-440.

178. Bridwell KH, Baldus C, Iffriq TM, Lenke LG, Blanke K. Progress measures and patients/parents evaluation of surgical management of spinal deformities in patients with progressive flaccid neuromuscular scoliosis. (Duchenne's muscular dystrophy and spinal muscular atrophy). *Spine.* 1999;24:1300-1309.

179. Braun NM, Arora NS, Rochester DF. Respiratory muscle and pulmonary function in polymyositis and other proximal myopathies. *Thorax.* 1983;38:616-623.

180. Berlowitz DJ, Brown DJ. Sleep-disordered breathing. *Arch Phys Med Rehabil.* 2002; 83(9):1325.

181. Epstein SK, Singh N. Respiratory acidosis. *Respir Care.* 2001;46(4):366-383.

182. Kang SW, Bach JR. Maximum insufflation capacity. *Chest.* 2000;118:61-65.

183. Bach JR, Kang SW. Disorders of ventilation. *Chest.* 2000;117:301-303.

184. Chatwin M, Ross E, Hart N, et al. Cough augmentation with mechanical insufflation/exsufflation in patients with neuromuscular weakness. *Eur Respir J.* 2003;21(3):502-508.

185. Bach JR. Cough in SCI patients. *Arch Phys Med Rehabil.* 1994;75(5):610.

186. Bach JR. Prevention of respiratory complications of spinal cord injury: a challenge to "model" spinal cord injury units. *J Spinal Cord Med.* 2006;29(1):3-4.

187. Pozzi E, Gulotta C. Classification of chest wall diseases. *Monaldi Arch Chest Dis.* 1993;48:65-68.

188. Leard JS, Wells CL. Cardiopulmonary concerns in the patient with musculoskeletal and integumentary deficits: an evidenced-based approach. In DeTurk WE, Cahalin L, eds. *Cardiovascular and Pulmonary Physical Therapy: An Evidenced-Based Approach.* New York: McGraw-Hill Co.; 2004.

189. Culham EG, Jimenez HA, King CE. Thoracic kyphosis, rib cage mobility and lung volumes in normal women and women with osteoporosis. *Spine (Phila Pa 1976)*. 1994;1(11):1250-1255.

190. Al-Katten K, Simonds AK, Chung KF, Kaplan DK. Kyphoscoliosis and bronchial torsion. *Chest*. 1997;111(4):1134-1137.

191. Krachman S, Criner G. Hypoventilation syndrome. *Clin Chest Med*. 1998;19(1):139-157.

192. Leong JC, Lu WW, Luk KD, Karlberg EM. Kinematics of the chest cage and spine during breathing in healthy individuals and in patients with adolescent idiopathic scoliosis. *Spine (Phila Pa 1976)*. 1999;24(13):1310-1315.

193. Grissom LE, Harcke HT. Thoracic deformities and the growing lung. *Semin Roentgenol*. 1998;33(2):199-208.

194. Wiedemann HP, Matthay RA. Pulmonary manifestations of the collagen vascular diseases. *Clin Chest Med*. 1989;10(4):677-715.

195. Miller JD, Beck KC, Joyner MJ, Brice AG, Johnson BD. Cardiorespiratory effects of inelastic chest wall restriction. *J Appl Physiol (1985)*. 2002;92(6):2419-2428.

196. Murin S, Weidemann H, Matthay RA. Pulmonary manifestations of systemic lupus erythematosus. *Clin Chest Med*. 1998;19(4):641-665.

197. American Thoracic Society. Standardization of spirometry, 1994 update. *Am J Respir Crit Care Med*. 1995;152:1107-1136.

198. Cherniak RM, Rabner MD. Normal standards for ventilatory function using an automated wedge spirometer. *Am Rev Respir Dis*. 1972;106:38.

199. Knudson RJ, Slatin RC, Lebowitz MD, Burrows B. The maximal expiratory flow volume curve normal standards variability and effects of age. *Am Rev Respir Dis*. 1976;113(5):587-600.

200. Oatis CA. Structure and function of the bones and joints of the thoracic spine. Chap 29. In: Oatis CA, ed. *Kinesiology: The Mechanics and Pathomechanics of Human Movement*. Philadelphia: Lippincott, Williams & Wilkins; 2004:488-514.

201. American Thoracic Society. ATS statement: Guidelines for the six-minute walk test. *Am J Respir Crit Care Med*. 2002;166:111-117.

202. Enright PL, Sherrill DL. Reference equations for six-minute walk in healthy adults. *Am J Respir Crit Care Med*. 1998;158:1384-1387.

203. American College of Sports Medicine. *ACSM's Guidelines for Exercise Testing and Prescription*. 8th ed. Philadelphia, PA: Wolters Kluwer Health/Lippincott Williams & Wilkins; 2010.

204. Mahler DA, Weinberg DH, Wells CK, Feinstein AR. The measurement of dyspnea. Contents, interobserver agreement, and physiologic correlates of two new clinical indexes. *Chest*. 1984;85(6):751-758.

205. Brooks SM. Surveillance for respiratory hazards. *ATS News*. 1982;8:12-16.

206. Celli BR, Cote CG, Marin JM, et al. The body-mass index, airflow obstruction, dyspnea, and exercise capacity index in chronic obstructive pulmonary disease. *N Engl J Med*. 2004;350(10):1005-1012.

207. Jones PW, Quirk FH, Baveystock CM, Littlejohns P. A self-complete measure of health status for chronic airflow limitation: The St. George's Respiratory Questionnaire. *Am Rev Respir Dis*. 1992;145(6):1321-1327.

208. Guyatt GH, Berman LB, Townsend M, Pugsley SO, Chambers LW. A measure of quality of life for clinical trials in chronic lung disease. *Thorax*. 1987;42(10):773-778.

209. Hajiro T, Nishimura K, Tsukino M, Ikeda A, Koyama H, Izumi T. Analysis of clinical methods to evaluate dyspnea in patients with chronic obstructive pulmonary disease. *Am J Respir Crit Care Med*. 1998;158(4):1185-1189.

210. Ciesla ND, Murdock KR. Lines, tubes, catheters, and physiologic monitoring in the ICU. *Cardiopulmon Phys Ther J*. 2000;11(1):16-25.

211. Hergenroeder AL. Implementation of a competency-based assessment of interpretation of laboratory values. *Acute Care Perspectives*. 2006;15(1):7-15.

212. Ciccone CD. *Pharmacology in Rehabilitation*. 4th ed. Philadelphia, PA: F.A. Davis; 2007.

213. Sussman C. Introduction to wound diagnosis. In: Sussman C, Bates-Jensen B, eds. *Wound Care: A Collaborative Practice Manual for Health Professionals*. 3rd ed. Baltimore, MD: Wolters Kluwer: Lippincott, Williams & Wilkins; 2007.

214. Harms CA, Babcock MA, McClaran SR, et al. Respiratory muscle work compromises leg blood flow during maximal exercise. J Appl Physiol 1997;82(5):1573-83.

215. Wien MF, Garshick E, Tun CG, Lieberman SL, Kelley A, Brown R. Breathlessness and exercise in spinal cord injury. *J Spinal Cord Med*. 1999;22(4):297-302.

216. Dodd JW, Getov SV, Jones PW. Cognitive function in COPD. *Eur Respir J*. 2010;35(4):913-922.

217. Dhand UK, Dhand R. Sleep disorders in neuromuscular diseases. *Curr Opin Pulm Med*. 2006;12(6):402-408.

218. Butler SM. Clinical assessment of the cardiopulmonary system. In: Frownfelter D, Dean E, eds. *Cardiovascular and Pulmonary Physical Therapy Evidence and Practice*. 4th ed. St. Louis, MO: Mosby; 2006.

219. Frownfelter D, Massery M. Body mechanics: the art of positioning and moving patients. In: Frownfelter D, Dean E, eds. *Cardiovascular and Pulmonary Physical Therapy Evidence and Practice*. 4th ed. St. Louis, MO: Mosby Elsevier; 2006:749-758.

220. Harris J, Johansen J, Pedersen S, LaPier T. Site of measurement and subject position affect chest excursion measurements. *Cardiopulm Phys Ther J*. 1997;8(4):12-17.

221. Cahalin LP. Pulmonary evaluation. Chap 9. In: DeTurk WE, Cahalin LP, eds. *Cardiovascular and Pulmonary Physical Therapy: An Evidence-Based Approach*. New York: McGraw-Hill; 2004:221-269.

222. Dias KJ, Collins S. A systematic evaluation of endurance impairments: the reversible and irreversible components. Proceedings of the APTA Combined Sections Meeting 2010; San Diego, CA; 2010.

223. Schmitz TJ. Vital signs. Chap 4. In: O'Sullivan SB, Schmitz TJ, eds. *Physical Rehabilitation: Assessment and Treatment*. 4th ed. Philadelphia, PA: F. A. Davis; 2001:77-100.

224. Bettencourt PE, Del Bono EA, Spiegelman D, Hertzmark E, Murphy RL Jr. Clinical utility of chest auscultation in common pulmonary diseases. *Am J Respir Crit Care Med*. 1994;150(5 Pt 1):1291-1297.

225. Linder SH. Functional electrical stimulation to enhance cough in quadriplegia. Chest 1993;103(1):166-9.

226. Bach JR. Indications for tracheostomy and decannulation of tracheostomized ventilator users. Monaldi Arch Chest Dis 1995;50(3):223-7.

227. O'Sullivan SB. Examination of motor function: motor control and motor learning. In: O'Sullivan SB, Schmitz TJ, eds. *Physical Rehabilitation*. Philadelphia, PA: F.A. Davis; 2007.

228. Zablotny C. Evaluation and management of swallowing dysfunction. In: Montgomery J, editor. *Clinics in Physical Therapy Physical Therapy for Traumatic Brain Injury*. New York: Churchill Livingstone; 1995:99-115.

229. Enright PL. The six-minute walk test. *Respir Care*. 2003;48(8):783-785.

230. Borg GA. Psychophysical bases of perceived exertion. *Med Sci Sports Exerc*. 1982;14:377-381.

231. Watchie J. Cardiovascular and pulmonary physical therapy treatment. In: Watchie J, ed. *Cardiovascular and Pulmonary Physical Therapy: A Clinical Manual*. 2nd ed. St. Louis, MO: Saunders Elsevier; 2010:298-341.

232. Perme C, Dean E. An Evidence-Based Approach to Weaning ICU Patients From Mechanical Ventilation. Proceedings of the World Confederation of Physical Therapy; Vancouver, Canada; 2007.

233. Hartman MJ, Fields DA, Byrne NM, Hunter GR. Resistance training improves metabolic economy during functional tasks in older adults. *J Strength Cond Res*. 2007;21(1):91-95.

CASE STUDY 8-1

Jane L. Wetzel, PT, PhD

EXAMINATION

History

Current Condition/Chief Complaint

Mr. Fortnight was a 64-year-old obese, White, English-speaking male referred to home physical therapy services after a recent 3-week hospitalization for pneumonia and acute exacerbation of COPD. At the time of the initial physical therapy visit, Mr. Fortnight complained of "trouble breathing and having no energy" for most household activities. He reported a new onset of neck pain since using his continuous positive airway pressure (CPAP) machine and couldn't seem to keep the CPAP mask on all night.

History of Current Complaint

He was hospitalized after multiple visits to his physician for a chronic cough and fever. A bronchoalveolar lavage was performed on day 2 of his admission. He was placed on broad-spectrum antibiotics initially while awaiting the results of a sputum culture. The culture indicated he had bacterial *Streptococcus pneumonia*. Chest radiographs revealed an enlarged heart and consolidation in the right lower lobes (posterior basal division and lateral basal division).

During the admission, Mr. Fortnight was also diagnosed with OSA and placed on CPAP ventilation via a mask with O_2 to assist his breathing. At the time of the initial physical therapy appointment he used the CPAP machine at night.

A review of his medical record showed the following results from the pulmonary function tests performed during his admission: FVC (2.8 liters; 60% predicted); FEV_1 (1.5 liters; 43% predicted; post-bronchodilator 2.0 liters; 57% predicted); FEV_1/FVC (0.53; 70% predicted) with diffusion capacity (DLCO) (20.50 mL/min/mm Hg; 61% predicted).

Clinician Comment *COPD is a term applied to a variety of lung disorders. Specific tests and measures were reviewed in the medical record to determine the severity of lung disease and type of impairment. Both FVC and FEV_1 were reduced; however, FEV_1 was decreased more than FVC and the ratio of FEV_1/FVC was less than 0.70, suggesting obstructive disease.[1] Therefore, the tissues were the primary component affected.*

Mr. Fortnight also had impaired ventilatory pump dysfunction as well since his FVC was decreased. Mr. Fortnight's tests indicated that he had stage II COPD (FEV_1/FVC = 0.53 [70% predicted] and FEV_1 = 43% predicted).[2] See Table 8-5 earlier in the chapter.

Prior to visiting Mr. Fortnight, the therapist reviewed the results of pulmonary function and the classification according to the Global Initiative for Chronic Obstructive Lung Disease GOLD criteria (see Table 8-5).[2] The therapist also referred to the Respiratory Impairment Classification to project potential function limited by dyspnea.[3,4]

RESPIRATORY IMPAIRMENT CLASSIFICATION[3,4]

Test/Observation	Class 1 0% Impaired	Class 2 20% to 30% Impaired	Class 3 40% to 50% Impaired	Class 4 60% to 90% Impaired
Dyspnea	Consistent with activity demands	None at rest; occurs during routine ADL. Person can ambulate and keep pace on level without SOB. Slow pace for stairs/hills	None at rest; occurs during routing ADL. Person can walk 1 mile at his own pace but cannot keep pace with others on level	Dyspnea present at rest and with activities such as climbing stairs or walking 100 yards on level
FEV_1	Not < 85% predicted	70% to 85% predicted	55% to 70% predicted	< 55% predicted
FVC	Not < 85% predicted	70% to 85% predicted	55% to 70% predicted	< 55% predicted
O_2 saturation	Not applicable	Not applicable	Usually ≥ 88% at rest and after exercise	Usually < 88% at rest and after exercise

Social History/Environment

Mr. Fortnight lived alone in a 2-story house with 4 steps to enter. There was a railing on both sides of the entrance steps to enter the home and a railing to assist with the ascent of the interior staircase. There were 3 bedrooms, including his bedroom, on the second floor with full bath. There was a small bathroom with sink and toilet downstairs on the ground floor.

He reported he was unable to climb the stairs to his bedroom as he had done prior to his hospitalization. He had been sleeping on a couch located on the ground floor since he returned home from the hospital.

He had 2 daughters who lived out of state, and a son and 2 close friends who lived nearby. He liked to bowl and golf. Prior to the hospital admission, he was able to ride a golf cart and play 9 holes of golf. He golfed every other weekend. He noted that 5 years prior he was able to walk and play 18 holes of golf. On most weekends, he spent time watching sports on television.

Employment/Work (Job/School/Play)

He was anxious about his recovery, especially with regard to his job. Mr. Fortnight worked as a salesman in charge of marketing and advertisement for a large corporation. He reported that he needed to return to work as soon as possible; he was concerned that his sales region might be changed during his absence to one with a lower potential for commissions. Further, the company had not been performing as well lately but he reported that he could not consider a career change at the moment. As part of his job duties, Mr. Fortnight needed to entertain clients during golf and dinner events. He was also expected to participate in fundraising activities sponsored by his corporation.

Social/Health Habits

Mr. Fortnight smoked 2 packs of cigarettes per day, and had for 25 years. He tried smoking cessation classes without much success. He drank beer and smoked cigars with his coworkers when golfing and bowling. He thought cigar smoking was less harmful than cigarette smoking. He reported he would drink several martinis when out for dinner.

Medical/Surgical History

Mr. Fortnight was recovering from bacterial pneumonia (streptococcus) complicated by atelectasis and asthma. He had 2 prior admissions for coronary artery disease (CAD) and COPD exacerbations and progressive worsening of dyspnea. The first admission, 7 years prior to the physical therapy appointment, was for an episode of respiratory acidosis and severe SOB. During that admission, he received instruction in management strategies for asthma and a referral to a smoking cessation program.

On a subsequent admission, 4 years prior to this physical therapy appointment, Mr. Fortnight was diagnosed with dilated cardiomyopathy due to significant CAD. A 3-vessel bypass was performed. After his recovery, his cardiac ejection fraction improved from 35% to 50%.

Two years prior to the physical therapy appointment, he developed hemoptysis. A fiber optic bronchoscopy revealed significantly inflamed hemorrhagic mucosa in left upper lobe.

Mr. Fortnight had previous diagnoses of hyperuricemia and gouty arthritis at age 44 years, hypertension and hyperlipidemia at 52 years, low back pain 54 years, Type II diabetes at age 56 years, and renal insufficiency. Past surgical history also included surgical repair of hernia at age 49 and tonsillectomy age 12.

Reported Functional Status

His house was messy, including a pile of dirty dishes are in the sink. He reported he had been unable to get upstairs to the bathroom to bathe. He reported he could walk only 40 to 50 feet around his home at a time. He leaned on furniture as he walked from one room to another. Mr. Fortnight reported that, prior to his last exacerbation, he was able to manage stairs but needed increased time for ascending the flight of stairs in his home, including one rest break when part way up and the use of the right railing. Prior to his last admission, he reported he could walk 5 to 6 blocks before becoming SOB.

Medications

Mr. Fortnight's medical record showed the following medications[5]:

- Low-flow O_2 (2LPM) via nasal cannula
- Cefuroxime and erythromycin
- Spiriva (tiotropium)
- Ventolin (albuterol)
- Glucophage (metformin)
- Zyloprim (allopurinol)
- Zocor (simvastatin)
- Diovan (valsartan)
- Cordarone (amiodarone)

Clinician Comment *Spiriva is a muscarinic receptor antagonist or anticholinergic agent. It primarily acts on receptors located on smooth muscle cells and submucosal glands to inhibit smooth muscle contraction and mucus secretion, thereby causing vasodilation and secretion management. Sore throat and dry mouth are common side effects.*

Ventolin is a short-acting beta2 agonist that works specifically on beta2 receptors in smooth muscle to cause relaxation. Because it is a beta2 specific drug it has little effect on the heart. Ventolin is provided as an inhaler to Mr. Fortnight to control wheezing, SOB and chest tightness. Using the inhaler 15 minutes prior to vigorous activity such as climbing stairs may assist breathing.[6] The therapist should observe the respiratory response to exercise and note if there is increased distress in the period immediately post exercise. Side effects of Ventolin are tremors, dizziness, and headaches.

Glucophage is a biguanide that acts to decreases hepatic glucose production and absorption from the gastrointestinal system. It also increases insulin sensitivity and glucose uptake in peripheral cells. Hypoglycemia is a side effect that may be triggered by exercise.[7,8] Prior to activity the therapist should review when the individual last took his medication and when the medication peaks as well as food intake to avoid hypoglycemia with Mr. Fortnight. Mr. Fortnight should be asked to check his blood glucose with a glucometer before performing an exercise tolerance test or activity on stairs. Values below 100 mg/dL fasting would suggest Mr. Fortnight may need carbohydrate supplementation prior to exercise.[8] Observing for signs and symptoms of hypoglycemia during all treatment sessions, keeping a source of carbohydrates available, and encouraging good hydration would be critical for safe and effect treatment of Mr. Fortnight.

Zyloprim is a xanthine oxidase inhibitor that is used to reduce the production of uric acid in the body. Elevated levels of uric acid may cause gout attacks. Side effects include gastrointestinal distress and drowsiness.

Zocor is an inactive lactone that is hydrolyzed after ingestion to a β-hydroxyacid form. The biosynthesis of cholesterol is limited by interfering with enzymatic actions. Side effects include rhabdomyolysis, which is a process where skeletal muscle is damaged and myoglobin is released into the bloodstream. The myoglobin load can lead kidney damage. Statin dosage is also related to respiratory muscle strength due to induced muscle myopathy.[9] Renal insufficiency may be due to rhabdomyolysis, hyperglycemia or dehydration. The therapist must be cognizant of fragile kidney function and avoid muscle-damaging exercise. Symptoms of muscle soreness may be due to rhabdomyolysis or eccentric myofibrillar damage.[10]

Diovan is an angiotensin II receptor antagonist that blocks the action of hormones that act to constrict blood vessels. Vasodilation occurs and increases blood flow to organs and muscles while lowering BP. Side effects include headaches, dizziness, back and joint pain, and excessive fatigue.

Cordarone is an antiarrhythmic that works by relaxing overactive heart muscle. It is may prevent serious, life-threatening ventricular arrhythmias. Side effects include constipation, headache, loss of appetite, and sleeplessness.

Other Clinical Tests Identified in Chart Review

Complete Pulmonary Function Testing

Lung Volume/ Compartment	Predicted	PRE-BRONCHO-DILATOR		POST-BRONCHO-DILATOR	
		Actual	%	Actual	%
FVC (L)	4.67	2.80	60%		
SVC (L)	4.67	3.10	66%		
FEV$_1$	3.48	1.5	43%	2.0	57%
FEV$_1$/FVC	.75	.53	705		
PEFR (L/s)	7.40	3.84	52%	4.19	56%
TLC (L)	7.21	8.43	110%		
FRC (L)	4.07	4.97	1225		
RV (L)	2.41	3.46	135%		
IC (L)	3.08	1.97	64%		
RV/TLC ratio (%)	33	41	124%		
Diffusion					
DLCO mL/min/ mm Hg	33.60	20.50	61%		
Respiratory Pressures					
MIP (– cc H$_2$O)	–108	–88	81%		
MEP (+ cc H$_2$O)	227	140	61%		

MIP: maximal inspiratory pressure; MEP: maximal expiratory pressure; SVC: slow vital capacity.

Clinician Comment *Prior to visiting Mr. Fortnight, the therapist reviewed the results of pulmonary function and the classification according to GOLD criteria (see Table 8-5).[2] The therapist also referred to the Respiratory Impairment Classification to project potential function limited by dyspnea.[3,4] Mr. Fortnight's FEV$_1$ (43%) was below 55% predicted but moved to 57% after using his bronchodilator. His FVC was 60% predicted. The pulmonary function tests indicated that Mr. Fortnight had the potential to achieve Respiratory Impairment Classification level 3 functionally if he used his bronchodilator. The FEV$_1$ improved from 43% to 57% after bronchodilator use. The DLCO was 61% predicted and indicated supplemental O$_2$ might be needed to maintain a safe level of O$_2$ saturation during activity.[11]*

Sleep Study

Apnea is defined as a complete cessation of airflow for at least 10 seconds. Mr. Fortnight's sleep study identified that he had 28 events in an hour. This placed him in the moderate sleep apnea category, as determined by the apnea hypoventilation index.[12] Further, there were 18 episodes of oxyhemoglobin desaturation of greater than 4% lower than baseline.

Clinician Comment *Sleep apnea was a new diagnosis for Mr. Fortnight. He most likely had OSA resulting from obesity, having a short wide neck, and poor sleeping position. The number of apnea episodes are reduced when the individual loses weight[12] and learns to sleeps on his side with the head slightly elevated rather than supine with head flat.[13] Mr. Fortnight will need education in the importance of weight loss and proper sleeping position. Sleeping position or mask position may also be contributing to his neck pain.*

Chest X-Rays

A chest X-ray taken at discharge revealed an enlarged heart, elevated aortic arch, flattened diaphragms with 7 ribs showing above the right hemidiaphragm. Ribs were horizontal in appearance. The right lower lobes (lateral and posterior divisions) were clear without infiltrates.

Clinician Comment *The pulmonary function tests results identified in the chart review indicated increased FRC, RV, and TLC typically seen with an individual with obstructive airways disease. These lung volume measures and the flattening of the diaphragm with horizontal ribs on the chest X-ray indicate hyperinflation at rest.[14] The RV/TLC ratio indicates that air trapping is worsening when the increase in RV is greater than the increase in the TLC. As FRC and RV increase, the IC decreases. The IC decrease is due in part to the changes in length tension of the intercostals muscles and diaphragm, resulting in a loss of contractile force.[15,16] The respiratory muscle pressures (MIP = 81% predicted and MEP = 61%) confirm weakness to both the inspiratory and expiratory muscles.[17]*

Lab Values

ARTERIAL BLOOD GASES	ADMISSION	D/C
FIO_2	Room Air	24%
PaO_2 (mm Hg)	56	65
$PaCO_2$ (mm Hg)	68	55
pH	7.32	7.40
HCO_3^- (mEq/L)	32	29
O_2 Saturation (%)	87	93

BLOOD CHEMISTRY	ADMISSION	D/C
Hemoglobin (g/dL)	20	19
Hematocrit (%)	56	54
Platelet (cells/μL)	460,000	300,000
White blood cells (cells/ccm)	12500	8500
Glucose (g/dL random)	220	150
Creatinine (mg/dL)	1.5	1.3
Blood urea nitrogen (mg/dL)	22	20

Clinician Comment *Laboratory values indicated that Mr. Fortnight was in partially compensated ($HCO_3^- = 32$ mEq/L) respiratory acidosis (pH = 7.32; $PaCO_2 = 68$ mm Hg), and had hypoxemia ($PaO_2 = 56$ mm Hg; O_2 Sat = 87%).[14] His white blood cells were elevated, signaling an infection was likely. Elevated creatinine and blood urea nitrogen indicated the possibility of mild renal insufficiency, but may also have indicated that Mr. Fortnight was dehydrated.[18] His hematocrit and hemoglobin were elevated, suggesting mild polycythemia. Individuals with Type II diabetes mellitus have impaired fibrinolysis so Mr. Fortnight may have had an increased risk for clot development.*

Cardiac Studies

A heart catheterization study completed 4 years prior to the physical therapy appointment indicated Mr. Fortnight had diffuse CAD in most coronary arteries with major stenosis in the left main (75%), left diagonal (80%), and left circumflex (84%) and an ejection fraction of 35% post-coronary artery bypass grafting (CABG), which improved to 50% by discharge. During the most recent hospital admission, an echocardiogram was performed and revealed an ejection fraction of 55%. Electrocardiogram (EKG) showed normal sinus rhythm with right ventricular hypertrophy and no evidence of myocardial infarction.

Clinician Comment *Cardiac pump failure or pulmonary hypertension could have been contraindications to exercise. There were no comments in the medical record history about pulmonary hypertension and no comments about blood-streaked sputum. The ejection fraction was 55% and the EKG demonstrated normal sinus rhythm, indicating good cardiac function. Exercise can improve the fibrinolytic process, augment the immune system, improve glucose uptake, and reverse deconditioning for Mr. Fortnight.[8] Activity and endurance training are important for Mr. Fortnight to return to his social and occupation roles.*

At discharge the oxyhemoglobin saturation was acceptable at rest when Mr. Fortnight was placed on supplemental O_2 (2LPM). The blood gas values were compensated (pH = 7.40) and PaO_2 increased as the lung consolidation resolved. Any gas-exchange problems at rest are related to obesity and poor ventilatory pump mechanics. During activity, there is a risk for worsening of gas exchange due to dynamic hyperinflation, ventilation perfusion mismatch, and respiratory muscle fatigue. Mr. Fortnight would need to be told to keep hydrated because his creatinine and blood urea nitrogen were still elevated. Hematocrit and hemoglobin were still elevated so fatigue was less related to O_2-carrying capacity or blood quality. The white blood cells were in the normal range by discharge and he no longer had a fever, indicating the infection was controlled. At discharge, Mr. Fortnight was instructed to establish a regular time for taking glucophage, to eat regular meals, and to monitor his glucose intake prior to activity. He was placed on a low-salt and low-calorie diet. Weight loss may reduce sleep apnea events and decrease the work of breathing.[12]

Mr. Fortnight would likely be limited in activity because of reduced expiratory airflow caused by poor elastic recoil that could lead to dynamic hyperinflation. The airway resistance due to asthma could be managed by proper use of an inhaler prior to activity. Obesity and deconditioning may also contribute to the dyspnea limited exercise.

The interview and the chart review had not identified any contraindications to exercise and physical therapy for Mr. Fortnight. Next in the examination was the systems review.

Systems Review

Cardiovascular/Pulmonary (Resting Values)

- HR = 88
- BP = 138/86
- RR = 18
- Dyspnea rating = 0/10 (CR 10 Borg scale for dyspnea)[19]
- Fatigue rating = 1/10 (CR 10 Borg scale for RPE)
- O_2 saturation = 93% on 2LPM
- Edema = 1+ pitting edema bilateral ankles
- Change in weight = 277 pounds (279 pounds at discharge); loss of 2 pounds

Clinician Comment *Bilateral ankle edema can occur with obesity, heart failure or renal insufficiency. Fluid shifts may occur because of positional changes when standing upright for prolonged period of time or with immobility. Mr. Fortnight did not move around much so muscle contraction did less to assist venous return. Additionally, impaired diaphragmatic mechanics could*

have limited venous return and increased the vascular load in the venous system. Increased capillary hydrostatic pressure can cause a shift to extracellular compartments. Monitoring Mr. Fortnight's weight should be included in the POC to note any increase in extracellular fluid, which could occur with heart failure. Routine auscultation before and after exercise may help the clinician detect earlier signs of heart failure (rales, S3 heart sounds) that contraindicate exercise. This activity may induce cardiac decompensation.

Mr. Fortnight's high resting HR may have been due to anxiety, poor O_2 use, or deconditioning. The BP was normal for his age[20] but was controlled by Diovan. The therapist confirmed Mr. Fortnight had taken his medication on the day of the initial physical therapy visit. Mr. Fortnight's report of his typical BP matched the measured BP as well as the measures recorded in his medical record.

Dyspnea ratings were added to his systems review to document the impact of impaired respiratory mechanics on the ventilatory pump at rest. Although dyspnea would likely limit Mr. Fortnight's activity, it was important to recognize that each person differs in ability to cope with symptoms of dyspnea and fatigue. Ultimately, the use of breathing control, pacing and coping with symptoms may override Mr. Fortnight's pulmonary impairments and permit increased physical functioning.

Fatigue ratings at rest were also included to document baseline effects of O_2 uptake in the periphery. These symptoms were likely limitations to activity for Mr. Fortnight. and resulted from impaired O_2 transport. It was important to gather baseline symptoms reflecting cardiopulmonary status prior to performing tests and measures to avoid causing excessive fatigue.

Integumentary

- Old scar over the anterior chest wall from prior sternotomy
- Foot calluses medially over first toe and metatarsal
- Flaky skin around heels and longitudinal arch

Clinician Comment *Calluses and dry skin are common in individuals with Type 2 diabetes.*

Musculoskeletal

- Height = 71 inches (5 feet, 11 inches)
- Weight = 277 pounds
- Gross ROM = within functional limits except mild hip flexion contractures bilaterally
- Gross strength = generalized weakness throughout bilateral upper and LEs

Neuromuscular

Gait

Short steps, waddling with lateral weight shifting, occasional reaching for furniture.

Balance

- Intact static and dynamic sitting balance
- Dynamic standing balance impaired.

Locomotion, Transfers, and Transitions

- Preferred to sit on chairs with high seat height and armrests.
- Moved in a routine path from living room through the dining room to the kitchen holding furniture.

Communication, Affect, Cognition, Language, and Learning Style

Mr. Fortnight was anxious about returning to work. He was alert during 80% of the physical therapy visit but had occasional lapses in attention. Mr. Fortnight had a sense of humor. He demonstrated interest in managing his recovery by asking questions about diet, energy for activity, and use of O_2.

Clinician Comment *Mr. Fortnight had difficulty remaining attentive during the interview and systems review. In planning the Tests and Measures portion of the examination, his arousal, attention, and cognition needed to be assessed.*

Obesity may impose an increased ventilatory load to the respiratory muscles, adding a restrictive component to the disorder.[21] Obesity also increased his risk for comorbidities such as diabetes and atherosclerosis, as well as increased the overall demand to working muscles raising the metabolic requirement for activity. Since obesity can be a contributing factor to sleep apnea as well as breathing disorders, anthropometric measures were indicated. Additionally, his posture and his level of pain needed to be assessed.

The systems review indicated additional tests and measures of integument, ROM, and muscle performance were indicated. Further tests and measures of his ventilation and gait were indicated from the systems review but were also factors to consider prior to any aerobic capacity testing. The therapist planned an exercise tolerance test as part of the examination, expecting the performance to be limited by dyspnea and fatigue since cardiac dysfunction, pulmonary hypertension, and anemia were ruled out as potential activity limitations during the chart review and no red flags for testing were revealed in the review of systems. Given that regaining function was a prime consideration for Mr. Fortnight, a more thorough baseline needed to be defined for self-care and home management as well as work, community, and leisure reintegration.

Tests and Measures

Arousal, Attention and Cognition

Mini-Mental Exam: Score 24; Difficulty with serial 7s and spelling "world" backward and complex commands.[22]

Trails A = 35 seconds; Trails B = 78 seconds (low average for both).[23]

Clinician Comment *Individuals with OSA and hypoxia may have attention and learning deficits. The most consistently affected cognitive functions in those with sleep apnea are vigilance, sustained attention, controlled attention, efficiency of information processing, and response time.[24] Learning and memory may also be affected. Mr. Fortnight demonstrated low average functioning for attention. This finding suggested that a component of the POC would need to include monitoring of Mr. Fortnight's ability to remember exercises and recall important facts about disease management (eg, proper use of inhaler).*

Anthropometric Characteristics

BMI = 38.5; falls in the "obese" category.[25]

Clinician Comment *Obesity imposes mechanical effects whereby fat mass makes the chest wall stiffer and less compliant. Obesity also reduces lung compliance and increases airway resistance, especially in the supine position.[26] The person who is obese adjusts to increased elastic and resistive loads by decreasing TV and increasing RR.[27] The therapist noticed Mr. Fortnight had shallow breaths with a relatively high RR at rest. In severe obesity hypoventilation syndrome individuals have hypoxemia and hypercapnia, resulting in abnormal ventilatory control and an inability to compensate for low TV with high RR.[28] Mr. Fortnight was still compensating while awake and sitting upright.*

Pain

Mr. Fortnight rated his neck pain at rest as 4/10 on the numeric rating scale. Pain increased to 6/10 with cervical flexion, rotation, and lateral flexion (right [R] > left [L]).

Posture

Mr. Fortnight had a barrel chest appearance, slightly rounded shoulders, forward head, and mild thoracic kyphosis.

Clinician Comment *Kyphosis of the thoracic spine is correlated with FVC and FEV_1.[29] The therapist also examined the mobility of the spine and shortened muscle groups that may be contributing to rounded shoulders.*

In addition, decreased chest expansion can occur after CABG. Mr. Fortnight strictly followed sternal precautions that caused abnormal habitual postures that could still be correctable. Although only preliminary evidence exists, exercises directed toward correcting these deformities may improve respiratory pressures and efficiency of breathing.[30]

Integumentary

Mr. Fortnight's skin color had a gray tinge. There were no skin abrasions from the CPAP mask. Upon further inspection of Mr. Fortnight's feet, additional calluses laterally over the fifth toe and middle of the transverse arch were noted. Mr. Fortnight wore gym shoes with a firm heel counter, undercut heel, and a rubber insole he purchased from the pharmacy. Inside the shoes the toe box was worn on the lateral and medial sides. Aside from callused areas, peripheral sensation was intact.

Circulation

Radial pulse was regular with strong upstroke at a rate of 88 beats per minute (bpm). Dorsalis pedis pulse was weak but palpable bilaterally. Auscultation of the heart revealed no pathological sounds.

Ventilation

Auscultation of the lungs identified clear lung fields with diminished sounds in the right lower lobes; lateral and posterior divisions. There were no wheezes heard since Mr. Fortnight used his inhaler prior to the therapy session. Respiratory pattern was shallow. The breathing pattern demonstrated excessive movement of the upper chest and shoulders and decreased lower costal expansion. The chest wall was over-expanded with little movement in the lower costal region. His cough was functional and Mr. Fortnight reported he produced about 2 tablespoons of white/yellow mucous a day. Mr. Fortnight could count aloud to 20 in one breath.

Clinician Comment *Examination of pain, integumentary, circulation, and ventilation are prioritized early in the set of tests and measures and always before activity. It is important to establish a good baseline for vitals, to screen for signs and symptoms of heart failure (S_3 heart sounds, rales, increased body weight or 1 to 2 pounds overnight) and identify any contraindications to exercise (abnormal pulse rate or rhythm). ROM, muscle performance, and activity examinations may need to be modified to protect the skin and minimize pain. An aerobic capacity test should be pain free in order to fully examine the status of the cardiovascular and pulmonary systems. The selection of exercise mode for activity tolerance testing may be influenced by pain or skin breakdown, especially if the extremities are involved. Since Mr. Fortnight has neck pain, the therapist prioritized this cervical ROM exam prior to extremity exam for this measure.*

Range of Motion (Including Muscle Length)

Cervical Range of Motion

MOTION	ACTIVE RANGE	PASSIVE RANGE—SLIGHT OVERPRESSURE
Flexion	Full	Full
Extension	35 degrees	40 degrees
Right lateral flexion	30 degrees*	NT
Left lateral flexion	40 degrees	45 degrees
Rotation right	50 degrees*	NT
Rotation left	55 degrees	60 degrees
*= painful 6/10.		

Upper and Lower Extremity Range of Motion

Mr. Fortnight had AROM that was within normal limits bilaterally except for the measurements indicated here.

MOTION (BILATERAL)	ACTIVE RANGE	PASSIVE RANGE
Shoulder flexion	165 degrees	170 degrees
Shoulder abduction	160 degrees	165 degrees
Shoulder external rotation	75 degrees	80 degrees
Hip extension	–15 degrees	–15 degrees
Ankle dorsiflexion*	0	0
*Same ROM with knee flexion and fully extended.		

Muscle length tests indicated shortening in bilateral sternocleidomastoids, scalenes, upper trapezius R > L, levator scapulae R > L, pectoralis major, hip flexors and gastroc-soleus muscles. Pain was reproduced with palpation at the origin of the sternocleidomastoid muscle and with lengthening of the upper trapezius. Since Mr. Fortnight sleeps on his left side, the right lateral flexors and trapezius were shortened.

Chest Wall Expansion

- Axillary: 1.20 inches (3.0 cm; 3.3 cm = age-based norm)[31] change with VC breathing
- Xiphoid: 1.15 inches (2.9 cm; 4.1 cm = age-based norm) change with VC breathing

Muscle Performance (Including Strength, Power, and Endurance)

All manual muscle tests were within functional limits except bilateral:

- Hip abductors = 4/5
- Dorsiflexors = 4/5
- Plantar flexors = 3/5

Five times sit to stand (STS) = 14.2 seconds (age-based performance >11.4 seconds indicates below average in LE power).[32,33]

Clinician Comment *The 5 times STS test exhibits moderately high correlations with 1-repetition maximum isotonic leg press strength in older adults and is thus used as a functional test of strength.[34] Bohannon performed a meta-analysis (13 papers meeting inclusion criteria) and reported that individuals with times exceeding the following have worse than average performance: 11.4 seconds (60 to 69 years), 12.6 seconds (70 to 79 years), and 14.8 seconds (80 to 89 years).[33] The STS is reliable, valid, and able to identify individuals with balance deficits.[35] In this case the STS test was selected to assist in quantifying LE power since the manual muscle tests were 5/5 for most muscle groups. Manual muscle testing had reached a ceiling and would not show incremental improvement. The therapist also wanted to measure functional performance and would include the STS results in the Short Performance Physical Battery (SPPB) test.[36] The score on the SPPB would be used to document risk for mobility disability. General muscle weakness may be a side effect of Zocor.*

Gait, Locomotion, and Balance

Gait

- 4-meter walk = 6 seconds (67 m/sec)

- Ambulated independently 40 feet without device. Mr. Fortnight used a wide-based gait, short step length, and occasional foot slap. He was limited by dyspnea and fatigue (RPD = 4/10; RPE = 6/10; O_2 saturation = 92% [O_2 2 LPM]). He said he didn't think he could walk any more that session.

- He reported he used a cane in his right hand when walking from the house to the garage to get to the car.

- He reported that prior to his more recent hospitalization, his walking distance capacity was limited to 4 to 5 blocks because of SOB.

Locomotion, Transfers, and Transitions

- Independent supine to sit; STS using armrests.

- He reported that he needed the cane to help when lowering himself onto the low seat of his car and again when rising from the low car seat.

- He managed stepping up and down curbs with assist from the cane or by leaning on objects or companions. As during the interview, he reported that he was unable to climb flight of stairs.

Balance

- Sitting balance: Intact static and dynamic.

- Standing balance: Static held semi-tandem posture for 12 seconds, full tandem for 8 seconds (>10 seconds = normal).

- Timed Up and Go (TUG) test = 8 seconds (low risk for falls)[37]

Short Performance Physical Battery

Score = 8 (mild limitations)[38]

Clinician Comment *One of the goals of physical therapy for Mr. Fortnight would be to prevent mobility disability and future hospitalizations. Individuals with a gait speed below 0.6 m/s are known to have 3 times greater risk than those who walk 1.0 m/s or faster.[39] Mr. Fortnight was approaching a risk threshold that would greatly increase his chances of a future hospitalization. Mr. Fortnight has an SPPB score of 8. Guralnik et al reported that individuals with SPPB scores of 7 to 9 had a relative risk of 1.6 for developing ADL disability over a 4-year period when compared to scores of 10 to 12.[38] A 1-point change in SPPB score represents a meaningful difference in the risk for future mortality and nursing home admissions.[40] Recently, the SPPB was selected as an outcome measure to justify the impact of physical therapy as a cost-effective measure for managing physical performance and preventing long-term disability in individuals with COPD.[41]*

Aerobic Capacity/Endurance Conditioning

Seated Step Test

Results were as follows[42]:

WORKLOAD AND TIME	HR	BP	O₂ SAT	DYSPNEA	RPE
Rest	88	138/86	93% (2L)	0/10	1/10
6 inch step/ 7 min (2.3 METs)	96	144/84	92%	.5/10	2/10
12 inch step/7 min (2.9 METs)	115	150/84	92%	2/10	4/10
18 inch/2 min (3.5 METs)	130	156/88	90%	5/10	6/10
18 c arms (3.9 METs)	NT				
Postexercise 2 minutes	92	136/84	93%	0/10	2/10
METs: metabolic equivalents; O₂ Sat: O₂ saturation; RPE: rating of perceived exertion.					

Interpretation: Adaptive HR and BP throughout with mild oxyhemoglobin desaturation from 93% to 90% while using 2 LPM O_2. Mr. Fortnight was limited by LE fatigue (RPE 6/10). Test terminated because of fatigue. Postexercise recovery 90% complete in 2 minutes with lungs clear and without wheezes or rales. No S3 noted.

Two-Minute Walk Test

Results with cane on R (conducted on second visit).

Distance 63 meters with 3 standing pauses (Norm = 130 mean for 70-year-olds)[43]

ACTIVITY	HR	BP	O₂ SAT (2 LPM)	DYSPNEA	RPE
Rest	84	134/86	94%	0/10	1/10
Peak 2 minutes	112	NT	92%	3/10	6/10
Post-1 minute	96	145/88	92%	2/10	4/10
Post-5 minutes	82	132/84	94%	0/10	1/10
O₂ Sat: O₂ saturation; RPE: rating of perceived exertion.					

Interpretation: Adaptive HR response to exercise with mild oxyhemoglobin desaturation. The test was limited by fatigue. Recovery was complete within 5 minutes. There were no adverse physiologic responses. The below average distance covered by Mr. Fortnight was below threshold for community functioning.

Clinician Comment *The therapist chose the seated step test to examine the cardiovascular and pulmonary response to exercise. A graded exercise test (seated step test) was used in addition to endurance walking (2-Minute Walk Test [2MWT] conducted on second visit, session 2). Physiological responses from the graded exercise tolerance testing were reliable and results compare well with self-reported measures of functional status.[44] Because Mr. Fortnight had balance deficits and the exam was being conducted in the home setting, this test was feasible and allowed an accurate examination of BP response to activity. It is easier to measure BP during this test than during a walking activity. Monitoring of BP during a walk test may invalidate the results and interpretation of walk distance. The limiting factor for Mr. Fortnight was fatigue. The presentation of fatigue supported the hypothesis of deconditioning and generalized weakness as major findings. Dyspnea and oxyhemoglobin desaturation likely contributed to fatigue since less than optimal blood quality was delivered to the muscles. The HR and BP were adaptive and suggested that activities at 3.5 metabolic equivalents (METs) would be safe and that his medications were appropriate for controlling BP during activity. Fatigue may also be a side effect of Diovan.*

Since Mr. Fortnight could manage only 40 feet during the initial exam, a 2MWT was selected as an outcome measure. The test was conducted on the second visit to allow Mr. Fortnight to be well rested for the test. Recently the 2MWT was found to be significantly correlated with the 6MWT (r = 0.937, p < 0.01) and VO$_{2max}$ (r = 0.555, p < 0.01) in individuals with COPD.[43] The 2MWT also demonstrated responsiveness to rehabilitation as significant improvements are reported after rehabilitation for 2MWT distance (17.2 ± 13.8; moderate effect size 0.61) and change in 2MWT are significantly correlated with change in 6MWT (r = 0.70, p < 0.05).

Self-Care and Home Management

A more specific survey of his self-care and home management further showed Mr. Fortnight was limited by fatigue and dyspnea for most household chores. He could not wash dishes to clean up after eating. His son helped with laundry and general household cleaning duties (vacuuming and dusting). Mr. Fortnight sat on a chair to shave and wash up. He could not reach his feet to dry them after bathing. He was unable to don socks and so walked barefoot or wore only slip-on shoes.

Work, Community, and Leisure Reintegration

Mr. Fortnight was dependent on his son to take him grocery shopping and to medical appointments. He had little energy for carrying shopping bags or emptying trash. His memory was sometimes "foggy" so he depended on his son to help him remember what the health care professionals recommended. He did not perform any outdoor maintenance to his home. Mr. Fortnight was unable to return to work or participate in golf outings.

Clinician Comment *Mr. Fortnight's report of activities limited by fatigue matches the results of aerobic capacity testing. His activity level was limited by fatigue to 3.5 METs. He had decreased walking endurance (63 meters with 3 pauses). MMRC dyspnea rating = 3 (stops for breath after about 100 m or after a few minutes on the level).[45]*

The MMRC Dyspnea Scale is a 5-point self-report scale that examines SOB with routine activity. The MMRC is reliable and has concurrent validity with the Oxygen Cost Diagram, the BDI, and the SGRQ in persons with COPD.[45] The MMRC requires less than 2 minutes to complete and is therefore easier for clinicians to administer. Additionally, the results of the MMRC are useful in applying the BODE Index score.[46,47] The BODE Index is used widely to predict risk for mortality in persons with COPD by classifying the individual according to FEV$_1$ % predicted, 6MWT distance, MMRC dyspnea scale, and BMI. The higher the BODE Index score, the greater the risk for mortality and hospitalization.[47,48] Mr. Fortnight had an estimated BODE Index of 6 out of 10. His risk for hospitalization was about twice that of someone with a BODE score of 0 to 2.[48]

BODE Index

VARIABLE	POINTS ON BODE INDEX			
	0	1	2	3
FEV_1 (% predicted)	≥65	50 to 64	36 to 49	≤35
6MWT (meters)	≥350	250 to 349	150 to 249	≤149
MMRC Dyspnea Scale	0 to 1	2	3	4
BMI	>21	≤21		

Mr. Fortnight was at risk for rehospitalization and had a moderate risk for long-term mobility disability (BODE Index = 6, SPPB Score = 6, Gait Speed = 0.67 m/sec). He had stage II COPD with an FEV_1 of 43% predicted, which improved to 57% predicted with appropriate bronchodilator use. He required education on sources of infection (dirty dishes), fall prevention (foot wear, wet feet), proper use of inhaler, and functional/aerobic training in order to return to independence in ambulation of 5 blocks and stair climbing.

EVALUATION

Diagnosis

Practice Pattern

Mr. Fortnight was post-hospitalization for pneumonia and acute exacerbation of his COPD. He was newly diagnosed with sleep apnea, had a new onset of neck pain, and was deconditioned. He had several comorbidities (hypertension, gout, renal insufficiency, diabetes, and obesity) that required monitoring and modification of therapeutic sessions. Mr. Fortnight had no contraindications to activity but was at risk for mobility disability and rehospitalization.

Mr. Fortnight had poor posture, obesity, and hyperinflation restricting air flow into the lungs. There was also some lung tissue impairment and V/Q mismatch resulting mild gas-exchange dysfunction at rest and with activity. Ventilation and gas exchange was worse at night as obstructed airways caused apnea and severe arterial O_2 desaturation. CPAP was required to prevent CO_2 retention and hypoxia.

These findings are consistent with Practice Pattern 6E: Impaired Ventilation and Respiration/Gas Exchange Associated With Ventilatory Pump Dysfunction or Failure.[49] Since his lungs became clear and pneumonia resolved, the remaining gas-exchange problems were primarily resulting from hypoventilation. Although the lungs were hyperinflated, the airways collapsed easily and the abnormal mechanics of breathing limited the volume of new air reaching the alveoli which caused hypoventilation. Mr. Fortnight also fit in

Practice Patterns 6B: Impaired Aerobic Capacity/Endurance Associated With Deconditioning; 4B: Impaired Posture; 4C: Impaired Muscle Performance; and 5G: Impaired Motor Function and Sensory Integrity Associated With Acute or Chronic Polyneuropathies.[49]

International Classification of Functioning, Disability, and Health Model

See ICF Model on p 328.[50]

Prognosis

Mr. Fortnight had a good prognosis for reversing his deconditioning and improving his functional abilities from household level to limited community ambulation including stair climbing.

Mr. Fortnight's goal of returning to work was dependent on consistent follow through with therapeutic exercise program as well as disease management and risk-prevention strategies.

Plan of Care

Intervention

Mr. Fortnight required a detailed therapeutic plan to return to limited community ambulation, manage stair ambulation, and implement strategies to prevent falls, infection, and mobility disability. The therapeutic plan would include gait, locomotion, and balance training, assistive device training, aerobic conditioning, respiratory muscle training, resistive exercise (hip abductors, dorsiflexors, plantar flexors), flexibility and stretching (anterior chest wall, cervical muscles), posture exercises, energy conservation strategies, breathing control techniques, sleep position, and environmental reorganization. Further, Mr. Fortnight would need to learn to incorporate energy conservation and breathing control during his ADL and instrumental ADL (IADL) training. Education was indicated on proper use of inhaler prior to exercise, importance of using assistive devices to prevent falls, modification of environment (removing dirty dishes, throw rugs, unstable furniture) and home exercise program.

Proposed Frequency and Duration of Physical Therapy Visits

Mr. Fortnight would be scheduled for physical therapy, 3 times per week for 4 weeks, in his home. Each session length would be 45 minutes.

Anticipated Goals

1. Mr. Fortnight will correctly perform flexibility exercises to increase anterior chest wall motion and improve posture (1 week).

2. He will use pursed lip breathing, pacing and coping strategies with verbal cuing during exercise sessions 60% of the time (1 week).

ICF Model of Disablement for Mr. Fortnight

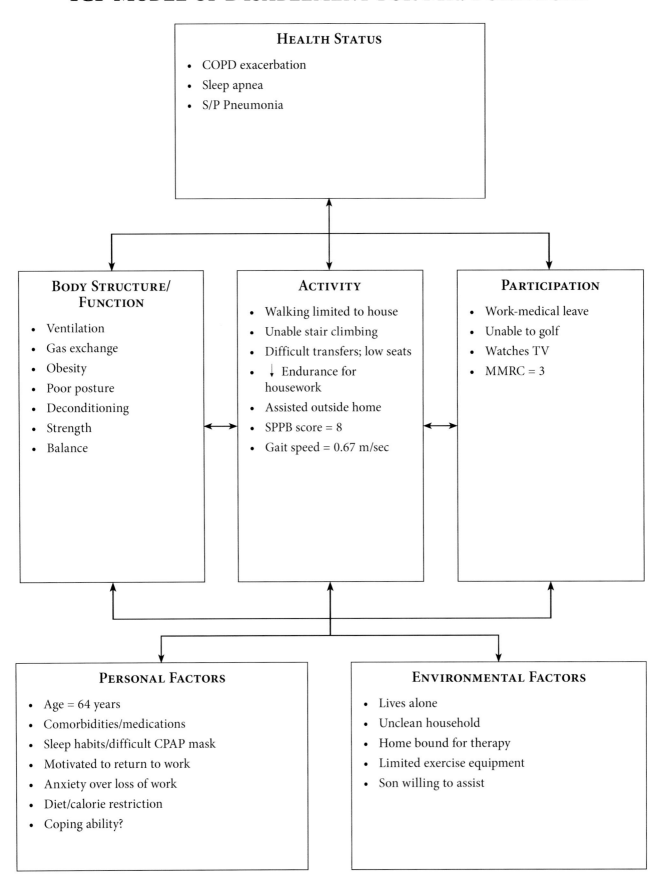

HEALTH STATUS

- COPD exacerbation
- Sleep apnea
- S/P Pneumonia

BODY STRUCTURE/ FUNCTION

- Ventilation
- Gas exchange
- Obesity
- Poor posture
- Deconditioning
- Strength
- Balance

ACTIVITY

- Walking limited to house
- Unable stair climbing
- Difficult transfers; low seats
- ↓ Endurance for housework
- Assisted outside home
- SPPB score = 8
- Gait speed = 0.67 m/sec

PARTICIPATION

- Work-medical leave
- Unable to golf
- Watches TV
- MMRC = 3

PERSONAL FACTORS

- Age = 64 years
- Comorbidities/medications
- Sleep habits/difficult CPAP mask
- Motivated to return to work
- Anxiety over loss of work
- Diet/calorie restriction
- Coping ability?

ENVIRONMENTAL FACTORS

- Lives alone
- Unclean household
- Home bound for therapy
- Limited exercise equipment
- Son willing to assist

3. Mr. Fortnight will be able to repeat preliminary instructions for home safety and his own health management follow through with the instructions >90% of the time (1 week).

4. He will lift 5 pounds against gravity weight-training exercises for hip abduction, red Theraband against gravity for dorsiflexion, and perform 5 unilateral toe raises through full ROM (2 weeks).

5. His neck movements will be symmetrical, without symptoms (3 weeks).

6. He will be able to walk 90 meters with RPD $\leq 2/10$ and RPE $\leq 4/10$ during the 2MWT with only one rest break (3 weeks).

7. He will be able to climb 12 stairs with 2 rests and RPD <3/10 (3 weeks).

8. Mr. Fortnight will achieve a time of < 12.5 seconds on the 5 times STS test (3 weeks).

9. He will have no loss of balance when walking around obstacles or when bending forward to retrieve items from the floor (4 weeks).

10. Mr. Fortnight will be independent in IADL ≤ 3 METS performed slowly while incorporating breathing control techniques >90% of the time (4 weeks).

11. Mr. Fortnight will demonstrate an SPPB score of ≥ 10 and gait speed of ≥ 80 m/sec in order to decrease the risk of mobility disability and rehospitalization.

12. Mr. Fortnight will increase the TUG to ≤ 6 sec to decrease the risk for falls.

Expected Outcomes (4 Weeks)

1. Mr. Fortnight will be independent in all ADL with RPD < 3/10 including stair climbing to the second floor bathroom in his home.

2. He will be independent with moderate distance community ambulation with an assistive device and have a lower risk for falls, mobility disability, and rehospitalization.

3. Mr. Fortnight will be modified independent in return to work for 4 hour sessions, 20 hours per week.

4. Mr. Fortnight will be minimally assisted with IADL for grocery shopping, household management (gardening and lawn care) and supervised for activities that are ≤ 4 METs applying energy conservation and breathing control strategies 100% of the time.

5. Mr. Fortnight will use safe practices when transporting O_2 and apply self-monitoring of breathlessness and O_2 saturation 100% of the time.

Discharge Plan

It was anticipated that Mr. Fortnight would be able to meet or exceed the anticipated goals and expected outcomes in 4 weeks. With the anticipated improved function after 4 weeks of physical therapy in his home, Mr. Fortnight would be able to successfully transition to an outpatient pulmonary rehabilitation program. Mr. Fortnight understood, and agreed with, the POC.

INTERVENTION

Coordination, Communication, and Documentation

Prior to the initial physical therapy visit in Mr. Fortnight's home, the therapist coordinated with the home health agency for a complete review of Mr. Fortnight's medical record. The schedule of Mr. Fortnight's treatment sessions were set-up to best manage his fatigue as well as to not interfere with the visits by his home health nurse.

Communication with the referring physician, Mr. Fortnight's home health nurse and Mr. Fortnight's family highlighted his primary limiting factor of fatigue and potential hypertensive response with activity. Consequently, consistent vital signs monitoring occurred, especially during activity. The therapist's concerns regarding Mr. Fortnight's fatigue and his Diovan medication were communicated to his referring physician in a phone call and his physician adjusted the dose. The therapist planned to follow-up with Mr. Fortnight's physician by phone to report Mr. Fortnight's responses to exercise after the medication adjustment at the reexamination.

Any patient-related instructions would be provided in writing to address Mr. Fortnight's mild cognitive impairment. Mr. Fortnight and his son were informed of the importance of cleanliness in the house, creation of a fall risk-free home environment and Mr. Fortnight's consistent participation in the therapeutic recommendations. Specifically these were: use of an assistive device for ambulation, adjustment of Mr. Fortnight's sleep position, and his compliance with the home exercise program. The therapist communicated with the nutritionist to ensure that Mr. Fortnight's weight loss plan would still offer calories required for exercise and overall energy. The adjusted nutritional supplements were adequate to support his anticipated increased activity level without increasing sugar or offering excessive protein load to his kidneys.

Documentation included the initial evaluation, treatment sessions and reexamination using the home health agency forms and in accordance with professional standards.

Patient-/Client-Related Instruction

Mr. Fortnight and his son were educated on the risk of infection including the importance of regular hand washing and keeping away from individuals with colds or viral infections. Mr. Fortnight was educated in energy-conservation techniques, signs and symptoms of infection as well as the benefits of exercise for improving immunity[51] and oxidative capacity for function.[52] Safety in bathing (drying the feet), footwear and proper foot inspection was reviewed.

Additionally, Mr. Fortnight was taught proper timing and use of the inhaler, how to use breathing control and coordinated breathing strategies with routine activities, and how to manage a sudden attack of SOB. Although Mr. Fortnight continued to use a cane in his right hand for ambulation, instruction on the use of a wheeled walker to manage fall risk and to increase walking distance and physiologic tolerance for community ambulation was also provided.[53]

Procedural Interventions

Therapeutic Exercise Prescription

Flexibility Exercises/Warm-up Exercises

Mode
Seated LE exercises

Intensity
Performance to the point of moderate tension

Duration
Hold for 5 seconds and release.

Frequency
Perform 5 reps to each muscle group daily and especially prior to aerobic exercise.

Description of the Intervention
Seated hurdle position, one leg out straight and the other bent with heel down and under the chair slightly. Stretching to the hamstring on outstretch leg and stretching to the soleus on bent leg. Lean forward with flat back.

Progression
In standing at countertop resting hands lightly for balance, stand in stride position to apply stretch to gastroc-soleus with knee extended while bending knee to stretch soleus on contralateral LE. Heels should remain in contact with the ground. Hold as above and switch leg position. The sets were progressed from 1 set to 2 sets.

Clinician Comment *Seated position provides stability when balance deficits are present. The therapist asked Mr. Fortnight to extend the position further at the end of the fourth repetition and hold a new position during the fifth repetition. Mr. Fortnight should exhale as he flexes forward and inhale as he returns to upright to begin to build energy efficient coordinated breathing with activity.*

Mode
Head and neck mobility exercises

Intensity
Moved to the point of moderate tension with each muscle group with pain scale < 3/10.

Duration
Hold for 5 seconds and release

Frequency
Perform 5 repetitions in each direction, daily.

Description of the Intervention
Seated position, AROM Chin tucks (capital flexion); chin lifts (capital extension), cervical rotation, lateral neck flexion.

Mode
Trunk mobility exercises

Intensity
Moved to point of moderate tension on opposite (uppermost) side with lateral trunk leaning.

Duration
Hold for 5 seconds and release

Frequency
Perform 5 repetitions for each exercise, daily, and prior to aerobic exercise.

Description of the Intervention
Seated position, AROM lateral trunk lean, flexion and extension, trunk rotation with flexion/extension reaching with arms to the floor with flexion and up into shoulder flexion and abduction with trunk extension.

Progression
Added coordinated breathing so Mr. Fortnight exhaled on flexion and inhaled on extension. During lateral trunk flexion hold, a pause with deep inspiration was added to actively recruit intercostals and further open the rib cage.

Mode
Upper extremity and anterior chest mobility exercises_

Intensity
Move to the point of moderate tension in pectoralis major and soft tissues of the anterior chest.

Duration
Hold for 5 seconds

Frequency
Perform 5 repetitions each during treatment session.

Description of the Intervention
Anterior chest mobility using AROM, passive positioning and PNF. While seated and performing trunk flexion and rotation, Mr. Fortnight incorporated the butterfly position of the arms (shoulders abducted, scapula retracted, elbows flexed with hand behind head). He inhaled with shoulder abduction and with trunk extension and exhaled with shoulder adduction and trunk flexion. Rotation was added as Mr. Fortnight began to understand the motion. Breathing actions assisted in mobilizing soft tissues around costosternal, costochondral, and costovertebral articulations.

When Mr. Fortnight was erect and seated with arms in the open butterfly position the therapist resisted adduction and closing of the butterfly position near the end of range abducted position. Contract-relax commands were offered to assist in reeducation to the scapular retractors and shoulder abductors while inhibiting the pectoralis major and anterior deltoid.[54]

Mr. Fortnight also had a positioning program using supine lying over a towel roll which was positioned longitudinally along his spine.[55] Mr. Fortnight lay in this position in bed in the morning to apply a stretch to the anterior chest.

The positional stretch was progressed by moving the arms into shoulder abduction and flexion above the head.

Posture Training

Posture awareness training in sitting followed the flexibility and AROM exercises for the spine and upper extremity/anterior chest. A mirror was used to assist Mr. Fortnight in self-correction of poor positioning of the upper thorax.

> **Clinician Comment** *Seated stretching allows muscles to warm up prior to strength and endurance exercise and minimize the risk of injury.[25] Individuals with diabetes have shortening of the connective tissue.[56] Aging, immobility and medications may also contribute to loss of elasticity in muscle groups.[20,57] Cervical and trunk stretching may help lengthen the accessory muscles and increase AROM to the thoracic cage to decrease work of breathing. Mobility of the spine preceded flexibility and strengthening exercises to muscles of the scapula and shoulder. Alignment of the thoracic spine improved kinematics for posture exercises.*

Strength, Power, and Endurance Training

Mode

Active exercise against gravity, lifting body weight for resistance, using light cuff weights and extremity positioning to challenge stronger muscles.

Intensity

Moving and holding position; light weight without losing proper form.

Duration

Hold for 5 seconds

Frequency

Mr. Fortnight performed 5 to 10 repetitions of resistance exercise 2 to 3 days per week.

Description of the Intervention

In the sitting position Mr. Fortnight performed scapular retraction exercises with chin tucks and moving naval toward spine to actively engage postural muscles. In supine, Mr. Fortnight was taught pelvic tilt exercise and progressed to bridging and to bridging with heel taps and then with one leg extended. In the side-lying position Mr. Fortnight was taught proper technique for active hip abduction to strengthen the hip abductors. Abductors were also trained eccentrically in a standing position, with one leg flexed and resting on padded dining room chair he contracted and released the abductors to shift body weight onto the bent LE.

Quadriceps strengthening for leg power was performed using seated squats. The seat height was gradually lowered as Mr. Fortnight improved. Toe raises were performed while standing at the counter, with light upper extremity contact for balance. Toe raises were performed first bilaterally, then shifting body weight toward one side and eventually progressing toward unilateral toe raises over the course of 12 visits. Standing anterior/posterior weight shifting was used to strengthen the dorsiflexors. Ventilatory muscle strengthening was performed using a threshold loading device and using higher loads as BP permitted. Mr. Fortnight was instructed to exhale with effort and lifting to avoid the effects of a Valsalva maneuver. Physiological monitoring of HR, BP, RPE, RPD, and O_2 saturation occurred throughout during therapeutic visits.

Progression

Once Mr. Fortnight demonstrated proper form for each exercise the weights were increased to low repetition and high intensity (as long as resting BP was below 160/105). The reps will be 6 reps each using a daily adjusted progressive resistive exercise protocol.[58]

Aerobic Capacity/Endurance Conditioning or Reconditioning

Mode

Walking program for exercise using wheeled walker.

Intensity

RPE < 4/10

Duration

Twenty minutes performed in 2 10-minute bouts with rests as needed. Mr. Fortnight ambulated a distance of 900 meters total while using the wheeled walker.

Frequency

Two times daily; 5 days per week.

Description of the Intervention

Exercise walking with a wheel walker was selected to permit a natural movement pattern in a safe manner so that a higher intensity challenge could be imposed on the cardiovascular system. A wheeled walker also permitted the use of accessory muscles for ventilation support.[53] He performed pursed-lipped breathing with diaphragmatic control during ambulation and continued to use 2 LPM O_2, which could be transported on the walker. Mr. Fortnight walked in a long pathway from the kitchen, through the dining room to the living room and back. The therapist spoke to Mr. Fortnight and his son about the feasibility of buying an exercise bike.

Progression

Decreased number of rests and bouts until Mr. Fortnight could ambulate for 400 meters without a rest break. Walking was then performed daily with a focus on increasing the total distance and number of minutes of ambulation.

Mode

Upper extremity repetitive lifting task

Intensity

RPE = 3/10

Duration

10 minutes

Frequency

Once daily

Description of the Intervention

From the sitting position, place hands on either side of a cane. Raising arms from lap above shoulder height to predetermined heights marked on a poster mounted on the wall. The activity simulates the upper limb exercise test.[59] All physiologic measures were monitored to assure the activity was a safe cardiovascular challenge.

Progression

Increased number of repetitions, height of lift and lifting time. Light weights were added to increase the challenge.

Clinician Comment *The therapeutic program was established using ATS evidence-based guidelines for pulmonary rehabilitation.[60] These guidelines recommend using high intensity (>60% VO$_2$ peak) to achieve optimal benefits to enhance peripheral oxidative capacity. Upper extremity aerobic training is recommended by the guidelines. Repetitive cane lifting was designed to decrease dependence on the accessory muscles for breathing and improve diaphragm action.[61] The goal was to improve Mr. Fortnight's ability to carry packages with less dyspnea. Additionally, individuals with COPD have low muscle mass in the muscles of ambulation. Changes in strength and aerobic capacity can be achieved through participation a program lasting 8 to 12 weeks, 2 to 3 times per week for 40 to 90 minutes.*

Gait and Locomotion Training

Mode

Walking program using cane for community function, including stairs.

Intensity

RPE <3/10; RPD <2/10 and O2 saturation >90%

Duration

10 minute; 60 to 80 feet

Frequency

Twice daily.

Description of the Intervention

Mr. Fortnight used a straight cane in his right hand during functional ambulation training. He practiced pacing and breathing control while keeping physiological measures below threshold intensity levels. The goal was to increase walking distance without regard to speed. Stair climbing using a railing with the right hand, and cane transferred to the left hand, and incorporating breathing control was also practiced. Mr. Fortnight practiced breathing control and coordinated breathing with all transfers.

Balance, Coordination, and Agility Training

Mode

Body positioning, moving outside base of support: static and dynamic

Intensity

RPE <3/10

Duration

5 minutes: hold position up to 30 seconds for static balance.

Frequency

4 times per week.

Description of the Intervention

On examination Mr. Fortnight could hold a semi-tandem standing posture for 12 seconds and a full tandem for 8 seconds. Mr. Fortnight practiced holding the full tandem stance and alternating which foot was forward. He ambulated in a heel-to-toe manner for as many steps as possible both forward and backward and eventually around obstacles. To increase the challenge, the therapist would place objects on chairs or the floor for Mr. Fortnight to reach down and pick up. Breathing control without breath holding and proper use of a cane as necessary was used during this activity.

Functional Training in Self-Care and Home Management Activities of Daily Living and Instrumental Activities of Daily Living

Self-Care

Mr. Fortnight practiced getting into and out of the tub using proper set-up, towel placement, prechecking water temperature, drying feet, and donning shoes. He practiced dressing while seated and transferring in and out of bed. In the bedroom the therapist made suggestions for placement of a chair to sit while reaching for clothing, reviewed methods for using the dressing stick and donning shoes. A light was placed next to the bed, as was automated motion-activated timed on-off lighting in the halls and bathroom. His son installed grab bars near the toilet and tub and a bath bench was added.

Home Management

Mr. Fortnight used a stool and sat while washing dishes and modified the shelves in the kitchen, improving the ease of putting dishes away. He practiced carrying bags of groceries from the kitchen to the dining room in preparation for future shopping trips. Breathing control (diaphragmatic, pursed-lip breathing) and coordinated breathing were incorporated into each task. Mr. Fortnight used a 1:2 (inhalation to exhalation) ratio and energy conservation strategies to pace activities.

Functional Training in Work (Job/School/Play), Community, and Leisure Integration or Reintegration, Including Instrumental Activities of Daily Living, Work Hardening, and Work Conditioning

Job Reintegration

Task simulation was implemented and modifications for efficient energy conserving movements at work. Mr. Fortnight practiced correct posture. A wireless earpiece for phone calls, ergonomically designed seat height, desk, and computer, full-length armrests to the office chair, and moving file drawers were recommended. Timing of meals and preparing a quick supply of glucose in the desk drawer were discussed.

Community Reintegration

A wheeled walker was kept in the car and used when walking distances for shopping, restaurants with poor lighting, and for exercise ambulation outside the home. Because Mr. Fortnight preferred using a cane, safety education was provided. It is expected that Mr. Fortnight will continue to improve strength, balance, and walking endurance as he progresses in an outpatient pulmonary rehabilitation program.

Leisure Reintegration

Mr. Fortnight was encouraged to continue golfing and would take a motorized golf cart. He used pursed-lipped breathing and pacing strategies to improve oxygenation and decrease fatigue. Mr. Fortnight learned to avoid riding in the cart with a friend who was a heavy smoker and placed his O_2 in a small rolling cart along with 1 or 2 clubs as needed when moving from motorized cart to the green.

Prescription, Application, and, as Appropriate, Fabrication of Devices and Equipment (Assistive, Adaptive, Orthotic, Protective, Supportive, or Prosthetic)

Adaptive Devices

- Automatic motion-sensitive lighting
- Wireless earpiece for phone calls
- Bath bench
- Grab bars

Assistive Devices

- Cane
- Wheeled walker
- Rollator for O_2
- Long-handled reacher

Orthotic Devices

- Selection of shoes with extra depth, undercut heels
- Evaluation for foot orthotics vs inserts in extra-depth shoe

Support Devices

- CPAP at 10 cm H_2O at night
- Supplemental O_2, 2 LPM pulsed at rest; continuous for exercise and walking

REEXAMINATION

Mr. Fortnight's program was progressed regularly and a formal reexamination occurred after 4 weeks of treatment and discharge was anticipated.

Subjective

"I feel I know how to control my breathing and I have more energy for most of my day."

Objective

Pain

Mr. Fortnight reported that his neck pain improved from 4/10 to 0/10.

Posture

His posture was aligned with scapulas retracted over a more erect thoracic spine.

Ventilation

Respiratory muscle strength (MIP and MEP) improved. Chest expansion measures improved 1 cm in the xiphoid region.

Range of Motion

His neck ROM was within normal limits for all motions.

Muscle Performance

His LE muscle grades have improved to 5/5 throughout except for plantar flexion 4/5. He could perform the STS test in 11.6 seconds.

Aerobic Capacity/Endurance Conditioning

Mr. Fortnight's 2MWT distance improved to 105 meters without rest breaks. The test was performed with a cane in his right hand as at the initial evaluation. Mr. Fortnight was limited only by dyspnea.

ACTIVITY	HR	BP	O_2 SAT (2 LPM)	DYSPNEA	RPE
Rest	78	132/82	96%	0/10	0/10
Peak 2 min	118	NT	94%	3/10	2/10
Post-1 minute	94	138/80	94%	2/10	1/10
Post-5 minutes	76	132/84	96%	0/10	0/10
O_2 Sat: O_2 saturation; RPE: rate of perceived exertion; NT: not tested.					

Clinician Comment *Mr. Fortnight's symptoms of fatigue were decreased through medication adjustment and aerobic training that may have reversed deconditioning. The dyspnea-limiting symptoms were likely due to dynamic hyperinflation, which shortened the inspiratory muscles limiting the enhancement of TV necessary for ventilation during exercise.[62]*

Self-Care and Home Management

Mr. Fortnight was independent in climbing 12 steps with railing on the R side with RPD <3/10 and O_2 saturation >90%. He incorporated breathing control and pacing strategies during ambulation, transfers, and for all bathing, dressing, and household tasks. Mr. Fortnight can sleep in his bed upstairs and wear the CPAP mask through the night. He could reach down and dry his feet after bathing and put on socks and shoes. His energy level improved and the household environment was free from risk for infection and falls. There was less dependence on his son for many tasks. Mr. Fortnight could attend medical appointments independently.

Work, Community, and Leisure Reintegration

He could walk 400 meters when using a walker and was ready to complete a 6MWT. He was also prepared to enter pulmonary rehabilitation as an outpatient. His SPPB score increased to 10 points and the 4 meter walk was 5 seconds (.80 m/sec), demonstrating a reduced risk for mobility disability and rehospitalization.

Assessment

Mr. Fortnight improved self-care and household level functioning. His gait was safe, he could walk for 150 feet (about 100 meters) with a cane, and he was able to ascend 12 steps with <3/10 dyspnea and O_2 saturation >90% on 2LPM. His physiologic responses indicated that he was no longer limited by LE fatigue but still experienced dyspnea.

The 2MWT distance with the cane and overall walking distance with the walker indicate he had good endurance for community functioning. Over the course of 12 weeks, Mr. Fortnight's risk for mortality (BODE Index), falls (TUG now 6 secs), and rehospitalization (SPPB and gait speed) all decreased.

Plan/Discharge

Mr. Fortnight was discharged from home health physical therapy. Suggestions for progression of the home exercise program for strength, balance, and endurance training were offered. He planned to return to work 4 hours, 3 days a week, using ergonomically efficient devices and energy-cost techniques.

He was referred for a driving evaluation with vocation rehabilitation and to outpatient pulmonary rehabilitation. It was anticipated he would require twice-a-week sessions of pulmonary rehabilitation for 9 to 18 weeks to increase endurance to allow return to full-time work and full IADL management.

Clinician Comment *The ATS guidelines[60] state that extending the exercise training program beyond 12 weeks offers greater improvement in aerobic capacity.*

Therefore, Mr. Fortnight was encouraged to attend formal exercise at a community center program once he completed his pulmonary rehabilitation program.

OUTCOMES

Five months after discharge and having participated in pulmonary rehabilitation, Mr. Fortnight was able to return to work for 30 hours a week, manage household chores, and ambulate, safely and independently, with a cane for 300 meters during a 6MWT.

REFERENCES

1. Reid DW, Chung F. *Clinical Management Notes and Case Histories in Cardiopulmonary Physical Therapy.* Thorofare, NJ: SLACK Incorporated; 2004.
2. Pauwels RA, Buist AS, Calverley PM, Jenkins CR, Hurd SS. Global strategy for the diagnosis, management, and prevention of chronic obstructive pulmonary disease. NHLBI/WHO Global Initiative for Chronic Obstructive Lung Disease (GOLD) Workshop summary. *Am J Respir Crit Care Med.* 2001;163:125-1376.
3. Pulmonary anatomy and pulmonary therapy. In: Rothstein JM, Roy SH, Wolf SL, eds. *The Rehabilitation Specialist's Handbook.* 3rd ed. Philadelphia, PA: F.A. Davis; 2005.
4. Mckeown RM, Gsell GF, Kessler HH, et al. The respiratory system. *JAMA.* 1965;194(8):919-932.
5. National Center for Biotechnology Information. http://www.ncbi.nlm.nih.gov/guide. Accessed December 19, 2010.
6. O'Donnell DE, Banzett RB, Carrieri-Kohlman V, et al. Pathophysiology of dyspnea in chronic obstructive pulmonary disease. *Proc Am Thorac Soc.* 2007;4:145-168.
7. American Diabetes Association. Standards of medical care in diabetes-2009. Position statement. *Diabetes Care.* 2009;32(Suppl 1):S13-S61.
8. Gulve EA. Exercise and glycemic control in diabetes: benefits, challenges and adjustments to pharmacotherapy. *Phys Ther.* 2008;88:1297-1321.
9. Chatham K, Gelder CM, Lines TA, Cahalin LP. Suspected statin-induced respiratory muscle myopathy during long-term inspiratory muscle training in a patient with diaphragmatic paralysis. *Phys Ther.* 2009;89(3):257-266.
10. Friden J, Sjostrom M, Ekblom B. Myofibrillar damage following intense eccentric exercise in man. *Int J Sports Med.* 1983;4(3):170-176.
11. Pulmonary assessment. In: Brannon FJ, Foley MW, Starr JA, Saul LM, eds. *Cardiopulmonary Rehabilitation: Basic Theory and Application.* 3rd ed. Philadelphia, PA: F.A. Davis; 1998.
12. Johansson K, Neovius M, Lagerros YT, et al. Effect of a very low energy diet on moderate and severe obstructive sleep apnoea in obese men: a randomised controlled trial. *BMJ.* 2009;339:b4609.
13. Neill AM, Angus SM, Sajkov D, McEvoy RD. Effects of sleep posture on upper airway stability in patients with obstructive sleep apnea. *Am J Respir Crit Care Med.* 1997;155(1):199-204.
14. Cahalin LP. Pulmonary evaluation. In: DeTurk WE, Cahalin LP, eds. *Cardiovascular and Pulmonary Physical Therapy: An Evidence-Based Approach.* New York, NY: McGraw-Hill; 2004:221-269.
15. American Thoracic Society/European Respiratory Society. ATS/ERS statement on respiratory muscle testing. *Am J Respir Crit Care Med.* 2002;166:518-624.
16. O'Donnell DE. Ventilatory limitations in chronic obstructive pulmonary disease. *Med Sci Sports Exerc.* 2001;33(7):S647-S655.

17. Enright PL, Kronmal RA, Manolio TA, Schenker MB, Hyatt RE. Respiratory muscle strength in the elderly. Correlates and reference values. Cardiovascular Health Study Research Group. *Am J Respir Crit Care Med.* 1994;149(2 Pt 1):430-438.

18. Hergenroeder AL. Implementation of a competency-based assessment of interpretation of laboratory values. *Acute Care Perspectives.* 2006;15(1):7-15.

19. Borg GA. Psychophysical bases of perceived exertion. *Med Sci Sports Exerc.* 1982;14:377-381.

20. Protas EJ. The aging patient. In: Frownfelter D, Dean E, eds. *Cardiovascular and Pulmonary Physical Therapy Evidence and Practice.* 4th ed. St. Louis, MO: Mosby Elsevier; 2006:685-691.

21. Clough P. Restrictive lung dysfunction. In: Hillegass EA, Sadowsky HS, eds. *Essentials of Cardiopulmonary Physical Therapy.* 2nd ed. Philadelphia, PA: W. B. Saunders Company; 2001.

22. Folstein MF, Folstein SE, McHugh PR. "Mini-mental state". A practical method for grading the cognitive state of patients for the clinician. *J Psychiatr Res.* 1975;12(3):189-198.

23. Ashendorf L, Jefferson AL, O'Connor MK, Chaisson C, Green RC, Stern RA. Trail making test errors in normal aging, mild cognitive impairment, and dementia. *Arch Clin Neuropsychol.* 2008;23:129-137.

24. Bruce AS, Aloia MS, Ancoli-Israel S. Neuropsychological effects of hypoxia in medical disorders. In: Grant I, Adams KM, editors. *Neuropsychological Assessment of Neuropsychiatric and Neuromedical Disorders.* 3rd ed. Cary, NC: Oxford University Press; 2009:336-349.

25. American College of Sports Medicine. *ACSM's Guidelines for Exercise Testing and Prescription.* 8th ed. Philadelphia, PA: Wolters Kluwer Health/Lippincott Williams & Wilkins; 2010.

26. Zerah F, Harf A, Perlemuter L, Lorino H, Lorino AM, Atlan G. Effects of obesity on respiratory resistance. *Chest.* 1993;103:1470-1476.

27. Koenig SM. Pulmonary complications of obesity. *Am J Med Sci.* 2001;321(4):249-279.

28. Mokhlesi B, Kryger MH, Grunstein RR. Assessment and management of patients with obesity hypoventilation syndrome. *Proc Am Thorac Soc.* 2008;5:218-225.

29. Mellin G, Harjula R. Lung function in relation to thoracic spine mobility and kyphosis. *Scand J Rehabil Med.* 1987;19:89-92.

30. Renno ACM, Granito RN, Driusso P, Costa D, Oishi J. Effects of an exercise program on respiratory function, posture and on quality of life in osteoporotic women: a pilot study. *Physiotherapy.* 2005;91(2):113-118.

31. LaPier TK, Cook A, Droege K, et al. Intertester and intratester reliability of chest excursion measurements in subjects without impairment. *Cardiopulmonary Phys Ther J.* 2000;11(3):95-98.

32. Bean JF, Kiely DK, Herman S, et al. The relationship between leg power and physical performance in mobility-limited older people. *J Am Geriatr Soc.* 2002;50:461-467.

33. Bohannon RW. Reference values for the five-repetition sit-to-stand test: a descriptive meta-analysis of data from elders. *Percept Mot Skills.* 2006;103:215-222.

34. Jones CJ, Rikkli RE, Beam WC. A 30-S chair-stand test as a measure of lower body strength in community-residing older adults. *Res Q Exerc Sport.* 1999;70(2):113-119.

35. Whitney SL, Wrisley DM, Marchetti GF, Gee MA, Redfern MS, Furman JM. Clinical measurement of sit-to-stand performance in people with balance disorders: validity of data for the five-times-sit-to-stand-test. *Phys Ther.* 2005;85(10):1034-1045.

36. Guralnik JM, Ferrucci L, Pieper CF, et al. Lower extremity function and subsequent disability: consistency across studies, predictive models, and value of gait speed alone compared with the short physical performance battery. *J Gerontol A Biol Sci Med Sci.* 2000;55(4):M221-M231.

37. Shumway-Cook A, Brauer S, Woollacott M. Predicting the probability for falls in community dwelling older adults using the timed up and go test. *Phys Ther.* 2000;80(9):896-903.

38. Guralnik JM, Ferrucci L, Simonsick EM, Salive ME, Wallace RB. Lower-extremity function in persons over the age of 70 years as a predictor of subsequent disability. *N Engl J Med.* 1995;332:556-561.

39. Studenski S, Perera S, Wallace D, et al. Physical performance measures in the clinical setting. *J Am Geriatr Soc.* 2003;51:314-322.

40. Guralnik JM, Simonsick EM, Ferrucci L, et al. A short physical performance battery assessing lower extremity function: association with self-reported disability and prediction of mortality and nursing home admission. *J Gerontol A Biol Sci Med Sci.* 1994;49:M85-M94.

41. Eisner MD, Iribarren C, Blanc PD, et al. Development of disability in chronic obstructive pulmonary disease: beyond lung function. *Thorax.* 2011;66:108-114.

42. Smith EL, Gilligan C. Physical activity for the older adult. *Phys Sports Med.* 1983;11(8):91-101.

43. Leung ASY, Chan KK, Sykes K, Chan KS. Reliability, validity and responsiveness of a 2-min walk test to assess exercise capacity of COPD patients. *Chest.* 2006;130:119-125.

44. Simonsick EM, Fried LP. Exercise tolerance and body composition. In: Guralnik JM, Fried LP, Simonsick EM, eds. *The Women's Health and Aging Study: Health and Social Characteristics of Older Women With Disability.* Bethesda, MD: NIH Publication No. 95-4009; 1995:106-117.

45. Darbee JC, Ohtake PJ. Outcome measures in cardiopulmonary physical therapy: medical research council (MRC) dyspnea scale. *Cardiopulmonary Phys Ther J.* 2006;17(1):29-37.

46. Brooks SM. Surveillance for respiratory hazards. *ATS News.* 1982;8:12-16.

47. Celli BR, Cote CG, Marin JM, et al. The body-mass index, airflow obstruction, dyspnea, and exercise capacity index in chronic obstructive pulmonary disease. *N Engl J Med.* 2004;350:1005-1012.

48. Ong K, Earnest A, Lu S. A multidimensional grading system (BODE index) as predictor of hospitalization for COPD. *Chest.* 2005;128:3810-3816.

49. American Physical Therapy Association. *Guide to Physical Therapist Practice.* 2nd ed. Alexandria, VA: Author; 2003.

50. O'Shea SD, Taylor NF, Paratz J. Peripheral muscle strength training in COPD: a systematic review. *Chest.* 2004;126(3):903-914.

51. Nieman DC. Does exercise alter immune function and respiratory infections? *Research Digest.* 2001;3(13):1-8.

52. Wasserman K, Hansen JE, Sue DY, String WW. *Principles of Exercise Testing and Interpretation.* 4th ed. Philadelphia, PA: Lippincott, Williams & Wilkins; 2004.

53. Wesmiller SW, Hoffman LA. Evaluation of an assistive device for ambulation in oxygen dependent patients with COPD. *J Cardiopulmonary Rehab.* 1994;14(12):122-126.

54. Kisner C, Colby LA. Management of pulmonary conditions. In: Kisner C, Colby LA, eds. *Therapeutic Exercise: Foundation and Techniques.* 4th ed. Philadelphia: F.A. Davis Co; 2002.

55. Frownfelter D, Massery M. Facilitating ventilation patterns and breathing strategies. In: Frownfelter D, Dean E, eds. *Cardiovascular and Pulmonary Physical Therapy Evidence and Practice.* 4th ed. New York, NY: Mosby Elsevier; 2006:377-403.

56. Smith LL, Burnet SP, McNeil JD. Musculoskeletal manifestations of diabetes mellitus. *Br J Sports Med.* 2003;37:30-35.

57. Ciccone CD. *Pharmacology in Rehabilitation.* 4th ed. Philadelphia, PA: F.A. Davis; 2007.

58. Kisner C, Colby LA. Resistive exercise for impaired muscle performance. In: Kisner C, Colby LA, eds. *Therapeutic Exercise: Foundations and Techniques.* 5th ed. Philadelphia, PA: F.A. Davis; 2007.

59. Takahashi T, Jenkins SC, Strauss GR, Watxon CP, Lake FR. A new unsupported upper limb exercise test for patients with chronic obstructive pulmonary disease. *J Cardiopulmonary Rehab.* 2003;23:430-437.

60. Ries AL, Bauldoff GS, Carlin BW, et al. Pulmonary rehabilitation: joint ACCP/AACVPR evidenced-based clinical practice guidelines. *Chest.* 2007;131:4S-42S.

61. Breslin EH. Dyspnea-limied response in chronic obstructive pulmonary disease. *Rehabilitation Nursing.* 1992;17(1):12-20.

62. O'Donnell DE, Webb KA. Mechanisms of dyspnea in COPD. In: Mahler D, O'Donnell DE, eds. *Dyspnea: Mechanisms, Measurement, and Management.* 2nd ed. New York, NY: Taylor & Francis Group; 2005:29-58.

9

Individuals With Gas-Exchange Disorders

Jane L. Wetzel, PT, PhD and Brian D. Roy, PT, DPT, MS, CCS

CHAPTER OBJECTIVES

- Describe the path of an oxygen (O_2) molecule from air in the lungs to its binding on a hemoglobin (Hgb) molecule.

- Discuss the factors in ventilation perfusion matching.

- Answer the question: What effect does air quality have on gas exchange?

- Compare and contrast the contributing factors in altered alveolar gas exchange for a patient with an acute disorder, such as pneumonia, and a patient with a chronic disorder, such as asthma.

- In the first learning objective, now categorize the type of gas-exchange disorder that could occur in each step in the process as the O_2 molecule moves from the lung air space to the Hgb molecule.

- Identify the factors that can impair the ability of a patient to have an effective cough.

- Discuss breathing exercise techniques that can be implemented to improve lung volume and gas distribution.

CHAPTER OUTLINE

- Physiologic Requirements for Normal Gas Exchange
  - Ventilation and Airway Opening
  - Gas Exchange
  - Perfusion and Blood Quality
  - Ventilation Perfusion Matching
- Factors Influencing Gas Transfer
  - Exercise

- Air Quality: Environment and Oxygen
- Epidemiology
  - Age-Related Changes and Gas Exchange
  - Incidence and Prevalence of Pathology Affecting Gas Exchange
    - Pneumonia
    - Atelectasis
    - Chronic Obstructive Pulmonary Disease
    - Asthma
    - Cystic Fibrosis
    - Pulmonary Edema and Pulmonary Emboli
- Pathophysiology of Gas-Exchange Disorders
  - Acute Disorders
    - Pneumonia
    - Atelectasis
    - Pulmonary Edema
    - Acute Respiratory Distress Syndrome
    - Pleural Effusions and Empyema
    - Pneumothorax
    - Pulmonary Vascular Disorders
  - Chronic Disorders
    - Chronic Obstructive Pulmonary Disease
    - Emphysema
    - Chronic Bronchitis
    - Asthma
    - Cystic Fibrosis
    - Interstitial Lung Diseases

Coglianese D, ed. *Clinical Exercise Pathophysiology for Physical Therapy: Examination, Testing, and Exercise Prescription for Movement-Related Disorders (pp 337-383).*
© 2015 Taylor & Francis Group.

Gas exchange is the ability to move O_2 and carbon dioxide (CO_2) to and from the pulmonary circulation. The gas-exchange process is called *respiration* and is distinct from *ventilation*, which involves changes in the dimensions of the lung and chest wall to create movement of air in and out of the atmosphere.[1] The primary role of the cardiovascular and pulmonary system is to move O_2 to the working muscle to support metabolic processes providing energy for movement.[2,3] Therefore, evaluation of all movement-related disorders must first consider the patient's ability to breathe and transport O_2 to organs and tissues in order for metabolism to take place. A patient who cannot breathe adequately cannot move or move efficiently. This chapter will describe the cellular, tissue, and organ changes associated with the pathophysiology of acute and chronic gas-exchange disorders and the role of physical therapy in evaluation and treatment of individuals who have problems with gas exchange. Abbreviations and terminology related to pulmonary function and respiratory muscle performance are listed in Table 8-2.

PHYSIOLOGIC REQUIREMENTS FOR NORMAL GAS EXCHANGE

Ventilation and Airway Opening

An adequate ventilatory pump is needed to keep blood O_2 content in inspired air elevated and to clear CO_2 from the lungs. Gas exchange and ventilation are interdependent as CO_2 and O_2 stimulate central and peripheral chemoreceptors signaling ventilation.[2] A negative pressure is created in the lungs when the muscles of inspiration contract. This causes air to move from the atmosphere to the alveoli. Pulmonary function (forced vital capacity [FVC], forced expiratory volume in 1 second [FEV_1], FEV_1/FVC) and respiratory muscle performance tests (maximal inspiration [PI_{max}], maximal expiration [PE_{max}], maximum voluntary ventilation [MVV]) are conducted to determine loss of ventilation. If ventilation is poor and respiratory pattern is shallow, the air will not reach the gas-exchanging regions of the lungs and the alveoli will not receive an adequate volume of good oxygenated air. When breathing is shallow there is increased dead-space ventilation and a majority of the inspired volume reaches only the conducting zone in the lungs, where gas exchange does not occur.[2] A simple act like deep breathing can improve the volume and quality of the air in the alveoli and thereby enhance gas exchange.

In addition to ventilation, airways must be kept clear to allow the volume of air to move unobstructed to the alveoli. In healthy individuals, the airways are kept clear by capturing foreign pathogens as air passes over mucosal tissues, nose hairs and over cilia supporting a layer of mucus.[4] Forceful

Box 9-1. Equation Used to Calculate Diffusion (D$_L$CO)

The volume of gas (V$_{gas}$) moved per minute is represented by:

$$V_{gas} = (A/T)D(P_1 - P_2)$$

A = Surface area (clinically; the entire lungs [L])
T = Thickness of the membrane
D = Diffusion constant for the gas
P = Pressure of gas on either side of the membrane

Normal D$_L$CO = 25 mL/min/mm Hg

Carbon monoxide (CO) testing is performed as this gas equilibrates rapidly.

expiratory muscle contraction or coughing can generate a high flow, expelling any trapped particles. In this way, infection is prevented and inflammation in the tissue is kept low, allowing for optimal gas exchange.[5] Airways must also be stable enough during coughing and deep breathing to remain open. In individuals with lung disease, high flow rates occurring with coughing and exercise can cause dynamic airway collapse of alveoli and bronchioles, obstructing the flow of air.[6]

Gas Exchange

Once the air reaches the alveoli, gas transfer depends on diffusion. Diffusion of O_2 from the alveolar sacs to the pulmonary circulation depends on; the surface area (A) of the alveolar capillary membrane; the thickness of the alveolar/capillary interface (T); the driving pressure of gas (D).[2,5,7] Diffusion of the lung (DL) is usually examined with a tracer gas, carbon monoxide (CO), and the test is abbreviated DLCO in the medical record (Box 9-1). The test indicates how well all these factors are working together. If any or all of these factors are impaired, then gas exchange is altered.

The surface area of the lungs is approximately the size of a tennis court in the healthy individual. If the lung surface is decreased by disease or hypoventilation, then less gas is transferred into the blood leading to lower arterial saturation of oxyhemoglobin (SaO$_2$). To reach the Hgb molecule in the pulmonary circulation, the O_2 must transfer across the surfactant lining on the interior of the alveoli, move through the epithelial membrane, through the interstitium, then across the endothelial membrane of the capillary, across the blood plasma and into the red blood cell (RBC) to the Hgb molecule (Figure 9-1).[5]

The partial pressures of O_2 and CO_2 in the alveoli and in the blood plasma are different. The partial pressure in the alveoli is represented by PA while the partial pressure in the arterial blood plasma is represented by Pa. Venous blood also carries gas, and the partial pressure in venous blood is represented by Pv. The difference between partial pressure of

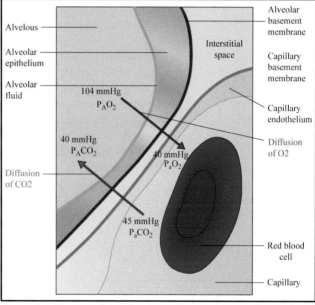

Figure 9-1. Diagram of the alveolar capillary membrane. Venous blood returning to be oxygenated.

gases is called a pressure gradient, which is a force that favors gas movement in a specific direction. CO_2 in venous blood has a PvCO$_2$ of 45 mm Hg and the PaCO$_2$ is 40 mm Hg, creating a difference that favors elimination of CO_2 from the blood. O_2 in the venous blood has a PvO$_2$ of 40 mm Hg while the partial pressure of alveolar O_2 (PaO$_2$) is about 104 mm Hg, creating a wide gradient favoring movement of O_2 into the blood as it passes through the lungs.[2]

Once the O_2 passes across the alveolar capillary membrane, the plasma in oxygenated arterial blood has a PaO$_2$ of 100 mm Hg. This level of PaO$_2$ is important for Hgb affinity and saturation. Saturation refers to having O_2 occupy each of the 4 Hgb molecule-binding sites. If PaO$_2$ decreases then the affinity of Hgb for O_2 also decreases and some of the sites on the Hgb do not accept O_2, resulting in desaturation.[8] SaO$_2$ is expressed as a percentage based on the ratio of the amount of

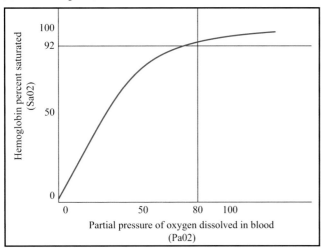

Figure 9-2. Oxyhemoglobin dissociation curve. (Reprinted with permission from Carroll RG. *Integrated Physiology.* Philadelphia, PA: Mosby Elsevier; 2007.)

O_2 bound to Hgb relative to the O_2-carrying capacity of the Hgb. The relationship between PaO_2 in blood plasma and SaO_2 is represented by the oxyhemoglobin dissociation curve (Figure 9-2). It is clear that a PaO_2 of 60 mm Hg results in SaO_2 of 90% and then the curve drops off steeply. Hgb has a high affinity for O_2 at high PaO_2 levels (ie, 60 to 100 mm Hg or higher) but is less likely to combine with O_2 at lower levels (ie, <60 mm Hg) and therefore less saturated. Therefore, as the oxyhemoglobin molecule moves to the peripheral circulation near the cells where partial pressure of O_2 is low, the Hgb affinity for O_2 decreases and O_2 is released to the cells favoring energy production. The O_2 saturation of Hgb in venous blood (SvO_2 is about 70% to 75%).[9]

Perfusion and Blood Quality

The pulmonary capillary blood volume and flow must be adequate as it passes by the alveoli. In addition there must be sufficient RBCs with available Hgb to carry O_2. The O_2-carrying capacity is determined by the amount of Hgb present in the blood.[5] Hematocrit (Hct) and Hgb must be within normal ranges. If the O_2-carrying ability of the blood is hindered then gas transfer at the tissue level is altered or inhibited. Individuals with anemia may have fully saturated Hgb but poor O_2-carrying capacity. The person with anemia may be tired and have activity intolerance due to poor blood quality and not necessarily poor tissue oxygenation due to gas-exchange problems.

The content of O_2 in the arterial blood (CaO_2) is the sum of oxyhemoglobin and dissolved O_2.[2] Approximately 1.34 mL of O_2 can bind to 1 gram of Hgb to create oxyhemoglobin. Oxyhemoglobin binding depends on its saturation level (oxyhemoglobin $= Hgb \times 1.34 \times SaO_2$). The PaO_2 in plasma is important because it affects Hgb saturation. Only 0.003 mL of O_2 are dissolved in plasma per mm Hg PaO_2 (dissolved $O_2 = 0.003 \times PaO_2$). This means the majority of O_2 is transported to the working muscle as oxyhemoglobin. Therefore, $CaO_2 = (Hgb \times 1.34 \times SaO_2) + (0.003 \times PaO_2)$.[2,8] If

Hgb is 15 g/dL and is 97% saturated at a PaO_2 of 100 mm Hg, then the $CaO_2 = 19.7$ mL O_2 per 100 mL of blood. Normally the CaO_2 ranges from 17 to 20 mL/dL.[8]

Good cardiac output (CO) and CaO_2 are required for delivery of adequate O_2 to be available to tissues. Ultimately, the volume of O_2 consumed (VO_2) is equal to CO times the difference between CaO_2 and CvO_2 (called the aVO_2 difference). Therefore, $VO_2 = CO \times aVO_2$ diff ($CaO_2 - CvO_2$).[8] In this way the quality of the blood and good gas transfer determines the amount of O_2 available to the working muscle and the amount of work that can be performed. The content of O_2 returning in the venous (CvO_2) blood is much lower than CaO_2 and diminishes according to the amount of O_2 extracted for metabolism.

The mechanisms regulating blood flow through the pulmonary circulation determine perfusion. If there is poor alveolar oxygenation in a region of the lung, then the pulmonary blood vessels respond by vasoconstriction to shunt blood to more viable areas for gas exchange.[5] The vasoconstriction may be well tolerated in healthy individuals but may increase pressure in the pulmonary vasculature in those with lung pathologies. The increased pressure creates a stress to the right heart and cor pulmonale may develop. Gravity also influences perfusion and increases hydrostatic pressure in the lower lung fields (in the most downward position). Thus body positioning changes affect blood flow and can be used as a therapeutic intervention.[1,5]

Ventilation Perfusion Matching

Ventilation is also influenced by gravity, causing upper alveoli to be more fully distended, or stiffer, than lower airways. Because lower airways are more compliant they can more readily accept new air. This new air in combination with increased perfusion in the most gravity-dependent position of the lung results in improved opportunity for gas exchange. Therefore, the best matching of ventilation to perfusion (V/Q) is near the most gravity-dependent positions.[5] In the upright person the most gravity-dependent region would be the base of the lungs. The ratio of V/Q across the lungs is 0.8 and allows gas exchange to provide normal PaO_2 to the blood.[10] When ventilation is in excess of perfusion (blood clot) in a region of the lung, the ratio is high. If the perfusion is in excess of ventilation (dead space) in a region of the lung, then the ratio is low. As V/Q ratios move further apart from the norm, then low PaO_2 (hypoxemia) develops.[5]

FACTORS INFLUENCING GAS TRANSFER

Exercise

Changes in DL will have a large affect on PaO_2 and cause a decrease in gas transfer. Normally there is a long and sufficient time course of blood flow through the pulmonary circulation, approximately 0.75 seconds with the PaO_2 of 100 mm Hg being achieved in 0.25 seconds (Figure 9-3).[8]

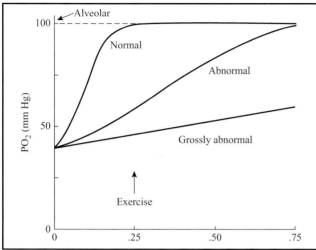

Figure 9-3. O_2 time courses in the pulmonary capillary when diffusion is normal and abnormal. Under normal conditions, blood reaches a partial pressure of O_2 (PO_2) of 100 mm Hg within 0.25 seconds even though the time course of travel through the capillary is 0.75 seconds. When there is a limitation in diffusion, the time to reach a PO_2 of 100 mm Hg is prolonged, as noted by the "abnormal" line. When diffusion is severely limited, blood exiting the pulmonary capillary will not achieve a normal PO_2 level, as indicated by the "grossly abnormal" line. The time course is shortened during exercise (as noted by the arrow) and may result in below-normal PO_2 levels when limitations in diffusion are present. (Reprinted with permission from West JB. *Respiratory Physiology.* 4th ed. Baltimore, MD: Williams & Wilkins Co; 1990.)

This time is necessary for O_2 to move from the alveoli into the capillary and for CO_2 to move into the alveoli from the blood. The pulmonary transit time is reduced during exercise, resulting in O_2 desaturation of arterial blood when pathology is present.[8,10,11]

TABLE 9-1. ESTIMATED FRACTION OF INSPIRED OXYGEN (FIO_2) WITH LOW FLOW DEVICES AND CORRESPONDING PARTIAL PRESSURE OF ARTERIAL OXYGEN (PaO_2)		
OXYGEN DELIVERY DEVICE	ESTIMATED FIO_2	AVAILABLE PaO_2 (MM HG)
Room Air	0.21	104
Nasal Cannula (L/min)		
1	0.24	119
2	0.28	140
3	0.32	158
4	0.36	182
5	0.40	239
Mask (L/min)		
5 to 6	0.40	239
6 to 7	0.50	311
7 to 8	0.60	384
Mask With Reservoir (L/min)		
7	0.70	456
8	0.80	528
9	0.90	601
10	1.00	673

AIR QUALITY: ENVIRONMENT AND OXYGEN

The air arriving in the alveoli in the healthy individual is a mixture of gases (nitrogen [N_2], O_2 and CO_2). Seventy-eight percent of the inspired air is N_2, which is inert, while 21% is O_2 and .04% is CO_2. Thus the fraction of inspired O_2 (FiO_2) is 21% in room air and is adequate to offer a PaO_2 of about 104 mm Hg. Individuals with gas-exchange deficits will often require increases in the FiO_2 to raise the PaO_2 in order to widen the O_2 pressure gradient between the alveoli and the arterial blood. Supplemental O_2 increases the PaO_2 and ultimately the PaO_2. Since supplemental O_2 is delivered by nasal cannula, mask or the ventilator, the liter flow or FiO_2 may be documented. Table 9-1 offers a guide to the amount of O_2 delivered with low-flow devices seen in practice. Increasing the FiO_2 increases the PaO_2, which will improve the gradient to aid in overcoming the impaired diffusion due to thickened membranes or to improve V/Q matching.

The environment also affects air quality and therefore gas exchange. The PaO_2 decreases when an individual moves to high altitude. This can produce hypoxic vasoconstriction and pulmonary edema and may be the cause of death in competitive mountain climbers. An older individual with marginal gas exchange may find they need supplemental O_2 with sudden acute changes in altitude. Those with pulmonary pathology will need special arrangements for O_2 support when flying on airplanes. Air pollution, occupational atmosphere (hay, animal dander, coal dust) can also change the composition of inspired air and stimulate an immune reaction in the lungs. Over time the lung tissues become scarred or develop fibrosis, impairing gas-exchanging processes. Exercise in cold, dry air is known to trigger bronchospasms or asthmatic events.[8]

EPIDEMIOLOGY

Gas-exchange deficits ultimately result in hypoxemia and may also produce hypercapnia. There are 4 major causes of hypoxemia: hypoventilation, diffusion, shunt, and V/Q inequality.[12] Hypoventilation occurs with severe ventilatory pump dysfunction and failure and is discussed in detail in Chapter 8. Diffusion deficits result when the blood-gas barrier is thickened as seen in disorders such as asbestosis, sarcoidosis, pneumoconiosis, alveolar cell carcinoma or collagen disease. Shunts are the result of a significant portion of pulmonary circulation not passing through ventilated regions of the lung. The arterial blood in shunt disorders lacks normal SaO_2 either because of an anatomical shunt (congenital heart diseases) or physiologic shunt (inflammatory processes). The shunt fraction is the percentage of deoxygenated blood in the arterial system and is normally 3% to 4% in healthy individuals but increases with disease. Finally, V/Q inequalities may cause hypoxemia and result from disorders that affect lung tissues or vascular conditions or both. Chronic obstructive pulmonary disease (COPD) is a primary disorder whereby V/Q mismatch is the cause of hypoxemia. Vascular and respiratory systems are impaired in individuals with severe COPD. Individuals with pulmonary hypertension, emboli, or pulmonary edema may also lose good equality of gas exchange in some regions of the lungs.[13]

Many diseases and disorders may present with more than 1 of the 4 causes of hypoxemia. A few of the most common conditions leading to gas-exchange deficits are pneumonia, atelectasis, COPD, asthma, cystic fibrosis (CF), pulmonary edema, and pulmonary emboli (PE). Neuromuscular and chest wall disorders may have gas-exchange deficits due to hypoventilation and are discussed in Chapter 8. There are also age-related changes in gas exchange that may contribute to earlier impairment when pathology is present.

Age-Related Changes and Gas Exchange

There is a loss of elastic recoil in the lungs of the older individual. In addition the chest wall stiffens as costal cartilage calcifies and the vertebral discs narrow. Movement of air is limited, especially during exercise, resulting in lower absolute tidal volume (TV) and minute ventilation (VE) at peak exercise.[14] Submaximal exercise requires greater respiratory muscle effort in order to sustain ventilation. Thus the older individual will have a higher submaximal respiratory rate (RR) than younger individuals performing similar work. Residual volume (RV) increases as airways do not recoil and unstable airways trap air. In the older individual, the alveolar-capillary surface area and total gas-exchanging surface area of the lung is reduced, increasing the physiologic dead space. Compared to younger counterparts, the older individual has a reduced DL, decreased pulmonary capillary blood volume, and a wider V/Q mismatch.[15] The resting PaO_2 declines 5 to 10 mm Hg by age 75 but does not affect SaO_2 or CaO_2.[14] During exercise, only a small number of older individuals have arterial hypoxemia. In the vascular system, some may experience increased pulmonary artery pressures and mild pulmonary edema that could lead to V/Q mismatch and DL deficits.[14] Exercise in older individuals is limited more by decreased CO than by mild differences in gas exchange. The slight changes in PaO_2 may place older individuals at increased risk for hypoxemia when medical conditions (anesthesia, surgery) or lung pathology are also present.

Incidence and Prevalence of Pathology Affecting Gas Exchange

Pneumonia

Pneumonia is an acute pulmonary disorder that continues to be a major cause of morbidity and mortality. In the United States pneumonia and influenza combined are the eighth leading cause of death.[16,17] Pneumonia has been attributed to an overwhelming majority of deaths despite the widespread availability and use of antibiotics. More than 56,000 people died from complications of pneumonia in 2008.[17] Approximately 50% of pneumonia cases are believed to be caused by viruses and tend to result in less severe illness than bacteria-caused pneumonia. Mycoplasmas are the smallest free-living agents of disease in man, with characteristics of both bacteria and viruses. The agents generally cause a mild and widespread pneumonia. The most prominent symptom of mycoplasma pneumonia is a cough that tends to come in violent attacks, but produces only sparse whitish mucus. Mycoplasmas are responsible for approximately 15% to 50% of all adult cases of pneumonia and an even higher rate in school-aged children.[18] An estimated 40,000 deaths occur yearly from pneumococcal pneumonia. The mortality rate is highest among children, elderly, and the black race. There are approximately 7.4 deaths per 100,000 for older individuals aged 65 to 79 years and 17.4 deaths per 100,000 for those over 80 years of age.[19]

Atelectasis

Atelectasis occurs when all or part of the lung collapses. Atelectasis can occur in a wide variety of acute and chronic conditions and may lead to pneumonia. Acute respiratory distress syndrome (ARDS) is a severe form of atelectasis caused by extensive lung inflammation resulting from pulmonary infections, pulmonary edema, trauma, and/or sepsis. There are approximately 1.5 to 75 cases of ARDS per 100,000 persons and an estimated 150,000 to 190,000 adults in the United States are affected.[20,21] The mortality rate in individuals with ARDS is 25% to 70%.[21-23] Mortality rate is higher in older individuals and may approach 90% if sepsis is present.[21]

Postoperative conditions have the greatest risk for atelectasis. The effects of anesthesia, procedural effects and pain lead to an increased V/Q mismatch, decreased functional residual capacity (FRC) and a decreased diaphragmatic excursion.[24,25] On average the FRC is decreased 20% after most postsurgical conditions and drops as much as 30% with upper abdominal surgeries.[25] The SaO_2 is 90% or less is in 35% of postoperative conditions.[25]

Chronic Obstructive Pulmonary Disease

COPD is increasing. The term *COPD* is a concept referring to flow-obstructing diseases. The 2 common disease states in this category, which frequently coexist, are emphysema and chronic bronchitis. The United States morbidity rate of COPD is 4% and it is exceeded only by myocardial infarction (MI), cancer, and cerebrovascular accident.[26] Variations in death rates from COPD may be related to smoking (type and manufacturing), pollutants, occupational exposures, childhood respiratory infections, climate, and genetics. Deaths due to COPD have been on the rise in the United States overall, but while the death rate of men has stabilized, the rate of death due to COPD for women is rising.[27] COPD is the second leading cause of hospitalization for adults in the United States.[16] Almost 2% of all hospitalizations in 1998 were attributed to COPD.[28] The cost to the United States in 2009 was approximately $109 billion in care for those affected by COPD.[16]

Female smokers are nearly 13 times as likely to die from COPD as women who have never smoked. Male smokers are nearly 12 times as likely to die from COPD as men who have never smoked.[29] Smoking-related diseases, including cancers, premature births due to maternal smoking, second-hand exposure as well as COPD, claim approximately 438,000 United States lives each year.[30] Tobacco use is the cause of 87% of deaths from lung cancer and approximately 171,000 deaths from lung cancer in the United States in 2010.[31]

Asthma

Asthma, a reversible obstructive lung disease, was estimated to affect 23 million United States citizens in 2008.[32] Acute attacks of asthma leading to emergency room visits and hospital admissions affect 12.7 million United States citizens, of whom 4.1 million are children.[32,33] Children under age 15 years accounted for approximately 32.7% of all hospital discharges that were asthma related in 2006. Overall, asthma is the third leading cause of hospitalization among children, leading to total health care costs of approximately $20.7 billion.[16] In adults, there were more than 3600 deaths attributed to asthma in 2006 or a rate of 1.2 per 100,000 after adjusting for age. Approximately 64% of the deaths were women.[34]

Cystic Fibrosis

CF is an inherited, multisystem condition that primarily affects the lungs. Among inherited disorders, it is the second leading cause of death in children in the United States, behind only sickle cell anemia.[35] A mutation of ΔF508 accounts for two-thirds of all CF alleles worldwide and occurs primarily in Caucasian individuals of European descent. The result is impaired structure, function or production of cyclic adenosine 5'-monophosphate–dependent transmembrane chloride channel protein, also called *CF transmembrane conductance regulator* (CFTR) protein.[35] There is impaired chloride ion transmission across epithelial cells and excessive sodium reabsorption, resulting in thick mucus that blocks ducts and tubes throughout the body.

An estimated 30,000 people have CF in the United States and in 2004, 41% were adults.[36] The mean age of survival is now about 37 years.[36] Mortality is associated with complications from the obstructive airways disease, with respiratory failure as the primary cause of death in 90% of those with CF.[35] Risk for mortality is highest in people infected with *Pseudomonas aeruginosa*, *Pseudomonas cepacia*, and in those with a VO$_2$ peak of less than 28% predicted.[35,37] An estimated 50% of cases with bronchiectasis in the United States result from CF.[38]

Pulmonary Edema and Pulmonary Emboli

Because the pulmonary circulation participates in gas exchange, it is important to recognize that pulmonary edema and PE contribute to gas-exchange impairments. Pulmonary edema occurs when exudates build up in the interstitial space because of heart failure or organ system failure, resulting in high volumes and pressures in the circulation around the lungs. As the pressure builds in the pulmonary circulation, proteins and other particulates seep out of the vascular system and into the interstitial space. The oncotic force draws fluid into the space, increasing the distance between vascular circulation and alveoli for gas exchange.[2] O$_2$ desaturation of Hgb is common in severe heart failure.[39] In the United States there are about 5.7 million people with heart failure, resulting in 300,000 deaths per year.

PE create dead-space ventilation where alveoli filled with air are not seen by the pulmonary circulation and cannot participate in gas exchange. There are approximately 650,000 cases of PE per year. It is estimated there are about 9 postoperative PE per 1000 surgical discharges.[40] There are about 200,000 deaths per year in the United States, and 10% of adults who present with an acute massive PE die within 1 hour of onset.[41-43] Massive PE account for 4% to 5% of all cases and nonmassive PE 95% to 96%. Nonmassive PE are more stable, with a systolic arterial pressure above 90 mm Hg, so the death rate is less than 5% in the first 3 to 6 months of anticoagulant therapy.[43,44] Anticoagulation therapy, preventive devices (pneumatic devices, stockings), lower extremity (LE), exercise and an appropriate activity regimen are critical to prevent deep vein thrombosis (DVT), a primary cause of PE.

PATHOPHYSIOLOGY OF GAS-EXCHANGE DISORDERS

The major causes of hypoxemia—hypoventilation, diffusion, shunt, and V/Q inequality—are present in a variety of cardiovascular and pulmonary disorders.[12] In many cases there will also be hypercapnia as poor oxygenation of tissues leads to increased anaerobic metabolism and excess production of CO$_2$. *The Guide to Physical Therapist Practice* refers to impaired respiration/gas exchange as being associated with airway clearance dysfunction (Pattern 6C), ventilatory pump dysfunction or failure (Pattern 6E), and respiratory failure (adults and neonate; Pattern 6F and 6G).[45] However, as mentioned previously, there can be impaired gas exchange in severe cardiovascular pump failure (Pattern 6D). Mechanisms of hypoventilation that cause hypoxemia and poor gas exchange are primarily associated with ventilatory

TABLE 9-2. STAGES OF INFLAMMATION	
INFLAMMATORY RESPONSE TO INJURY	
Stage 1	Increased blood flow to the area including blood and plasma volume bringing the essential cells and proteins to the site
Stage 2	Increased permeability of blood vessels allowing fluid and cells into tissues, (acute inflammatory exudate)
Stage 3	Release of cells, proteins, macrophages, T lymphocytes, neutrophils, and inflammatory mediators to break down damaged tissue to liquefy and remove and then repair/reconstruct the damaged tissue.

Reprinted with permission from Porth CM. Inflammation and healing. Chapter 20. In: Porth CM, ed. *Pathophysiology: Concepts of Altered Health States.* 7th ed. Philadelphia: Lippincott, Williams & Wilkins; 2005.

pump disorders (Pattern 6E). The focus of this chapter will be directed toward the pathophysiology of acute and chronic conditions leading to gas-exchange impairments associated with airway clearance (Pattern 6C) dysfunction and respiratory failure (Pattern 6F).

Acute Disorders

The hallmark of an acute process begins with inflammation. Inflammation is defined as "a local response to cellular injury that is marked by capillary dilatation, leukocytic infiltration, redness, heat, and pain and that serves as a mechanism initiating the elimination of noxious agents and of damaged tissue."[46] This local response is similar whether the local area is the lung, the kidney or the dermis. The inflammatory response is mediated by a variety of factors that are influenced by the specific tissues and structures affected.[47] In the pulmonary system the site of inflammation is most commonly the large airways, the smaller airways, and bronchioles or the lung parenchyma. Additionally, the response differs to some degree depending on the precipitant.

There are 3 major stages of cellular and systemic activity associated with inflammation (Table 9-2).[47] These stages allow the body to defend itself against all types of noxious stimuli including allergens such as pollen or cigarette smoke and infecting organisms such as bacteria, viruses, and fungi.[47,48] In the pulmonary system these defenses occur and are mediated on both a short-term basis, such as in response to an acute allergen or infection, or on a long-term basis, such as in individuals who have chronic diseases like emphysema or chronic bronchitis.[48]

Acute inflammation is the result of a stimulus that activates an immune response sending chemical mediators to move to the site. As exudates and cell products are released at the site, swelling appears. Once the injury or infection resolves, the acute process subsides. If there is extensive necrosis and little to no regeneration of tissue or the inflammatory process is repeated over and over, then the process becomes chronic inflammation. During chronic inflammation macrophages, lymphocytes, and plasma cells promote the growth of endothelial cells and fibroblasts.[48] This process stiffens lung tissues, creating noncompliance and cellular dysfunction.

Pulmonary inflammation has been studied for years and only recently has there been recognition of the central role that inflammation plays in most pulmonary-related disorders (Figure 9-4). The complexity of the processes involved in the inflammatory response and similar clinical manifestations observed in individuals affected by pulmonary disease have made recognition, diagnosis, and subsequent management of individual pulmonary disease pathologies challenging.[7] Next, the pathophysiology of common conditions are described to clarify how the inflammatory processes contribute to pulmonary disorders and to assist therapists in differential diagnosis for sound clinical decision making.

Pneumonia

Pneumonia is an inflammatory reaction in the lungs in response to foreign substances that pass through the upper airways and reach the bronchioles and alveoli. Antigens may also arrive via the pulmonary circulation, with protein and chemical mediators leaking into the interstitial fluid between the alveoli and pulmonary capillaries. These foreign substances may be bacterial, viral, fungal, or mechanical.[21] Bacterial or typical pneumonia occurs when the inflammatory response exists extracellularly in the alveoli, outside the interstitial space, leading to mucus production that may obstruct airways.[49] Viral or atypical pneumonia exist in the alveolar septum and interstitial space and, therefore, patients produce limited sputum. The elderly, immunocompromised, pediatric and postsurgical populations are most at risk.[49] An airway clearance program may be efficacious for bacterial pneumonia where mucus exists extracellularly but would not be effective for viral pneumonia. The role of the physical therapist should be focused on preventing all types of pneumonia (encouraging immunization and avoiding treating immunocompromised individuals when the therapist is ill).

Bacterial pneumonia results in an inadequate white blood cell (WBC) response to the area of infection. When an organism enters the lung, alveolar macrophages isolate the material and then phagocytosis occurs.[50] Normal mucociliary transport of mucus and exudates may be altered or slowed, contributing to the pneumonia or infection. The small bronchioles and alveoli become clogged with exudate and infection sets in. The 4 stages of pneumonia are listed in Table 9-3.[50]

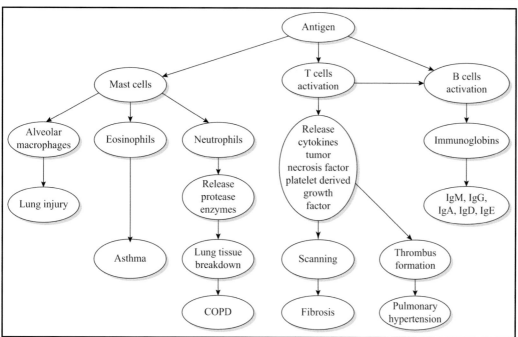

Figure 9-4. Immune response and pulmonary disease. (Adapted from Wells CL. Pulmonary pathology. In: DeTurk WE, Cahalin L, eds. *Cardiovascular and Pulmonary Physical Therapy: An Evidence-Based Approach.* New York: McGraw-Hill; 2004.)

TABLE 9-3. PATHOGENIC STAGES OF PNEUMONIA[50]	
PATHOGENESIS OF PNEUMONIA	
Stage 1	Edematous: vascular enlargement and alveolar exudate
Stage 2	Red hepatization: erythrocytes, fibrin, and inflammatory cells move into the alveoli
Stage 3	Gray hepatization: large numbers of macrophages move into the alveoli
Stage 4	Resolution: destruction and removal of exudate and rebuilding of normal lung begins

The major determinant of abnormal pulmonary gas exchange in patients with pneumonia is illustrated by increases in intrapulmonary shunt along with mild to moderate V/Q mismatch.[51] Hypoxia may or may not be evident, depending on the health of the remaining lung tissue. Treatment with specific antibiotics depends on the organism found in cultures, whether the pneumonia is community, hospital or nursing home acquired, and the overall health of the individual.[21] In some people the cough may be diminished or weakened. Individuals with dysphagia may aspirate fluid into the lungs.[21] A speech therapy evaluation, determination of oral management of food consistency, positioning during eating, and bulbar exercises to improve swallowing control are important strategies to prevent aspiration pneumonia.[52]

Atelectasis

Atelectasis is a collapse of the lung parenchyma, which can be localized to specific alveoli, patches of alveoli, lung segment(s) or can involve a complete lobe(s). It is usually caused by gradual and progressive loss of lung volume leading to inadequate intra-alveolar stretch tension, which reduces the production of surfactant.[49] The decrease in surfactant reduces the surface tension among alveoli, resulting in collapsing of alveoli and bronchioles, obstruction of airflow,

and progressive loss of lung volumes. Atelectasis is usually a symptom of some other condition involved either directly or indirectly in the lung.[21]

Acquired atelectasis is usually due to airway obstruction and lung compression.[21] Obstruction may be due to a mucus plug, external compression from fluid (pleural effusion), tumor mass, exudates or deficient transpulmonary pressure (loss of surfactant, imbalance or pleural pressures within the thorax due to respiratory muscle weakness, pain or deformity).[53] Primary atelectasis occurs in premature infants in whom there is insufficient surfactant production in underdeveloped lungs. Insufficient surfactant can also occur with the aspiration of gastric contents, use of anesthesia, high concentrations of O_2, smoke inhalation, and interstitial fibrosis.

The primary complication of atelectasis is hypoxia since the surface area available for gas exchange is reduced. The degree of hypoxia depends on the amount of lung tissue affected and the health of the remaining lung. Hypoxia also stimulates vasoconstriction of the pulmonary vessels.[5] As vasoconstriction occurs in hypoxic areas, other portions of the pulmonary circulation develop an increase in circulation that causes a rise in hydrostatic pressure. The hydrostatic pressure in the circulation around marginal but viable regions of the lung may lead to further alveolar collapse and

Figure 9-5. Mechanisms involved in development of ARDS. (Adapted from Porth CM. Disorders of ventilation and gas exchange. In: Porth CM, ed. *Pathophysiology: Concepts of Altered Health States.* 7th ed. Philadelphia, PA: Lippincott, Williams & Wilkins; 2005:689-724.)

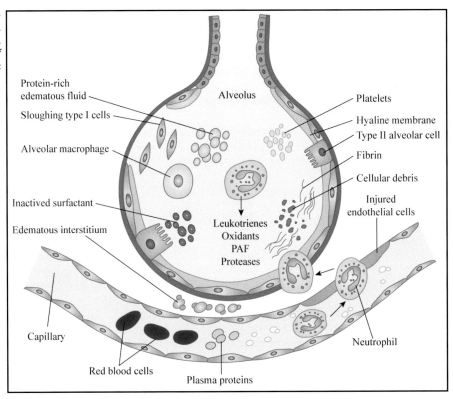

extension of atelectatic condition. A right to left shunt occurs within 24 to 48 hours if atelectasis is massive enough as pulmonary edema and ARDS develop.[21] Therefore it is critical to find strategies to recruit more alveoli and improve ventilation in postsurgical or infectious conditions. Changes in position, deep breathing, ventilation support, postural drainage, and mobility programs may improve alveolar ventilation and are good preventive strategies.

Pulmonary Edema

Pulmonary edema is a reaction where extravascular fluid is drawn into either the interstitial tissue or the alveoli or both.[21] The factors that can contribute to keeping the interstitium and alveolus dry are a pulmonary circulation plasma oncotic pressure (25 mm Hg) that is greater than hydrostatic pressure (7 to 12 mm Hg), connective tissue and cellular barriers that are somewhat impermeable to plasma proteins, and an adequate lymphatic system.[54] Normally when fluid builds in the interstitium, the lymphatic flow increases. Pulmonary edema appears when the lymphatics are overwhelmed and the interstitial fluid and pressures back up until eventually the alveolar capillary membranes leak and flood the alveoli.

The causes of pulmonary edema may be cardiogenic or noncardiogenic. Cardiogenic pulmonary edema is the result of elevated filling pressures on the left side of the heart from cardiovascular disorders (valve impairment, MI, cardiomyopathy, congestive heart failure [CHF], etc). Noncardiogenic causes may include excess fluid retention resulting from impaired sodium and water excretion in renal disorders or by decreased serum and albumin associated with liver disease, lymphatic obstruction or tissue injury (acute lung injury or

ARDS).[21] Medical management is focused on optimizing cardiac performance, electrolyte regulation, treating the cause of the primary illness, and improving gas exchange and transport of O_2 to the tissues. Severe hypoxia can lead to respiratory distress and failure.

Acute Respiratory Distress Syndrome

Adult ARDS is characterized by diffuse pulmonary microvascular injury. The initial site of damage may be the alveolar-capillary units, alveolar spaces, alveolar walls or neighboring lung tissue.[21] Injury to the cell inactivates surfactant and causes fluids, proteins, and blood cells to leak into the interstitium creating pulmonary edema (Figure 9-5). In ARDS, the alveolar epithelial barrier breaks, allowing flooding of the alveolar space and making it difficult or impossible for O_2 to diffuse into the capillaries. Hypoxia is largely related to intrapulmonary shunting.[55,56]

Mechanical ventilation is usually required to maintain ventilation and gas exchange during the healing process while the medical team works on treating the underlying condition causing the ARDS. Underlying causes may include: chest trauma, sepsis of the lung or other organs, complications of cardiopulmonary bypass, aspiration, drowning, smoke/chemical inhalation, drug overdose, and emboli.[21] Massive atelectasis and severe pulmonary edema (described previously) may result in ARDS. The earliest sign of ARDS is an elevated RR and shortness of breath (SOB) appearing within 12 to 48 hours. Physical therapists can assist the medical management team by offering positioning programs and intervening early to encourage deep breathing and mobility when feasible.

Pleural Effusions and Empyema

Normally there is approximately 5 mL of pleural fluid distributed throughout the intrapleural space. The fluid helps to decrease the work of breathing by promoting the sliding of the visceral pleura against the parietal fluid.[7] If the fluid in the pleural space increases or decreases the lungs cannot expand as effectively. When lung movement is altered, atelectasis and its own ramifications may occur. In its extreme, pleural effusions can cause shunting of blood from hypoventilated areas and hypoxia may result.

Pleural effusions are classified into 2 groups: transudates and exudates. Transudate is a water fluid that leaks out of the pulmonary circulation when there is an elevation in microvascular hydrostatic pressure or decrease in oncotic pressure (ascites, CHF, renal disorders).[25] High pressures force fluid out of the pulmonary capillaries.[21] Exudates are due to pleural inflammation, in which there exists an increased permeability of the pleural surface to proteinaceous fluid (infection, malignancy or trauma). Exudate is a fluid with a high concentration of protein and cellular debris that escapes from the pulmonary vasculature.[21] Lymphatic blockage may also contribute to a build-up of pleural fluid. Both transudates and exudates will alter lung compliance.[25]

Positioning changes, breathing exercises, and increased activity can assist in preventing further complications.[25] A pleural effusion can compress lung tissue if it is large, causing atelectasis. If the fluid becomes infected the pleural effusion evolves into an empyema or pus in the pleural space.[53] It may be inappropriate to place the good lung in a dependent position because of the need to avoid fluid shifts and spread of infection. Fever may be present with empyema and the individual develops fatigue, weakness, and malaise. A thoracocentesis may be performed using a needle to remove the exudate, or a thoracoscopic procedure may be required to remove tissue, sample or remove fluid. Sometimes a chest tube or pigtail catheter is inserted into the pleural space to drain large amounts of fluid.[25,57]

Pneumothorax

A pneumothorax (PTX) is free air between the visceral and parietal pleurae. There are different types of PTX including traumatic, spontaneous, and tension.[53] When air leaks into the pleural space, the change from a normally negative pressure to a more positive pressure causes pulmonary collapse. The collapse, like in atelectasis, can lead to shunting of blood from nonventilated regions because of hypoxic vasoconstriction. Symptoms may include dyspnea, shock, life-threatening respiratory failure, and circulatory collapse.

In trauma, the lung collapse may be due to an open PTX, a condition where a penetrating chest wound allows air from the atmosphere to enter the pleural space yet some air can still escape to the atmosphere. Lung collapse may also be due to tension PTX. A tension PTX allows air to enter the pleural space but not leave (Figure 9-6).[53] The air increases in the pleural space with each breath, causing ipsilateral collapse, mediastinal shift to the opposite side, collapse to the contralateral lung, and cardiac compromise. This is a

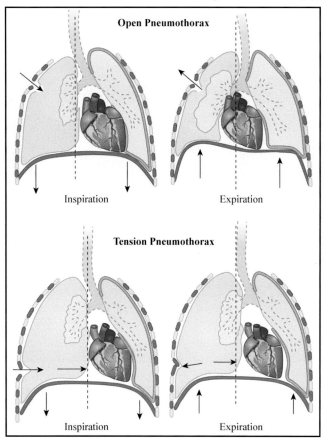

Figure 9-6. Open PTX and tension PTX. (Adapted from Porth CM. Disorders of ventilation and gas exchange. In: Porth CM, ed. *Pathophysiology: Concepts of Altered Health States.* 7th ed. Philadelphia, PA: Lippincott, Williams & Wilkins; 2005:689-724; figure p.692.)

life-threatening situation if not reversed with a chest tube immediately.[53,57]

For individuals who require high-pressure mechanical ventilation to maintain open airways, there is a risk of a closed PTX. An example of this would be a patient with ARDS who receives high-pressure ventilation (>70 cm H_2O) to open stiff, collapsed airways.[58] Pressure ventilation can induce barotraumas to the compliant portions of the lung, creating a closed PTX.[59]

Iatrogenic PTX is a traumatic complication often caused by some medical procedure.[57] Spontaneous PTX is a condition where air enters the pleural space and collapses the lung with no apparent trauma. This can occur in high altitudes or in deep sea diving. Spontaneous PTX can also occur in disease states where weakened lung tissues, like bullae in patients with emphysema, are easily subject to changes in pressures.[57] Physical therapists should respond quickly and report any signs and symptoms of severe SOB with high RRs in people who are admitted with traumatic injuries, who are on high-pressure ventilation or who may have had significant cardiothoracic surgery. It will be important to check chest tube placement is secure and sutured in prior to mobility and changes in position.[59] Once the PTX is resolved segmental breathing and prescriptive body positioning may be employed.[1,25]

TABLE 9-4. WELL'S CLINICAL PREDICTION RULE FOR DEEP VEIN THROMBOSIS[61]

CLINICAL PRESENTATION	SCORE
• Active cancer [within 6 months of Dx or receiving palliative care]	1
• Paralysis, paresis, or recent immobilization of lower extremities	1
• Bedridden for more than 3 days or major surgery in the last 4 weeks	1
• Localized tenderness in the center of the posterior calf, popliteal space, or along the femoral vein in the anterior thigh, groin	1
• Entire lower extremity swelling	1
• Unilateral calf swelling [more than 3 mm larger than uninvolved side]	1
• Unilateral pitting edema	1
• Collateral superficial veins [nonvaricose]	1
• An alternative diagnosis is as likely [or more likely] than DVT	–2

Interpretation	Total Points	Probability of DVT
	–2 to 0	Low probability of DVT [3%]
	1 to 2	Moderate probability of DVT [17%]
	3 or more	High probability of DVT [75%]

BOX 9-2. PHYSIOLOGIC FACTORS CONTRIBUTING TO DEEP VEIN THROMBOSIS[53]

- • Venous stasis
- • Venous endothelial injury
- • Hypercoagulability

Pulmonary Vascular Disorders

A pulmonary embolism is a blood clot, emboli or thrombus that has lodged itself in the pulmonary vasculature. It prevents blood flow to the lung tissue distal to the blockage, mechanically obstructing the pulmonary circulation and stimulating neurohumoral reflexes leading to vasoconstriction.[53] The size of the clot determines the amount of lung parenchyma affected. Obstruction of the vasculature may produce dead-space ventilation, V/Q, shunting, and systemic hypoxia. This may cause a fall in O_2 content of the coronary blood supply. If the affected area is large enough, there may be a sudden increase in pulmonary artery pressure (pulmonary hypertension), leading to right ventricular strain and heart failure.[53] This increased right ventricular pressure may shift leftward causing pressure within the left ventricle and a decreased CO. Reflex bronchospasm may increase the work of breathing and diminishes pulmonary compliance.[53] Almost all PE arise from DVT in the LEs and are due to a variety of physiologic causes (Box 9-2).

Thrombosis in the veins is triggered by venostasis, hypercoagulability, and vessel wall inflammation, known as *Virchow's triad*. All clinical risk factors for DVT and PE have their basis in one or more of the three. PE can arise from DVT anywhere in the body. LE venous thrombosis usually starts in the calf veins. Fatty emboli can form after fractures but are rare. Fatal PE can result from a thrombus originating in the axillary or subclavian veins, veins of the pelvis, or from around indwelling central venous catheters. Individuals who have a diagnosis of cancer, CHF, paralysis, or are status post-LE surgery are at increased risk for developing thrombosis. The role of the physical therapist is preventing PE by identifying the signs of DVT early using prediction rules (Table 9-4) and good observation skills.[60,61] Checking the prothrombin time, platelet, and international normalization ratios in the medical chart can also assist the physical therapist in identifying individuals at risk for blood clots or bleeding disorders.[62]

Chronic Disorders

Chronic respiratory system disorders may follow acute conditions when there is destruction of alveolar tissue and/or the pulmonary circulation, fibrosis, chronic inflammation of the bronchial wall leading to hypertrophy and hypersecretion of mucus.[53] Common chronic conditions include COPD, asthma, CF, and bronchiectasis and interstitial lung diseases. Individuals with chronic CHF may also have impairments in gas exchange.

Chronic Obstructive Pulmonary Disease

According to the Global Initiative on Obstructive Lung Disease (GOLD), "COPD is a disease characterized by airflow limitation that is not fully reversible.[63] The airflow limitation is usually progressive and is associated with an abnormal inflammatory response of the lungs to noxious particles and gases." COPD includes several pathological subsets (chronic bronchitis, asthma, and emphysema) that often are found coexisting in individuals with respiratory symptoms.[64] Yet, obstruction to airflow is a problem that reaches beyond COPD and shifts among conditions that differ in pathogenesis and reversibility. For example, airflow obstruction in asthma is reversible, and the degree of airflow obstruction in emphysema and chronic bronchitis may be diminished resulting in fluctuations in gas-exchange impairment with each condition (Figure 9-7).

Asthma is commonly described as reversible, yet some individuals with COPD have some asthma and may show partial reversibility of airway obstruction when bronchodilator medication is employed. Thus the 2 conditions coexist.[64] Chronic bronchitis is defined as the presence of a productive cough for 3 months over 2 successive years.[64] Part of the year these individuals may be free of symptoms. Emphysema is defined as abnormal permanent enlargement of air spaces distal to the terminal bronchioles.[64] The enlargement can progress to actual holes in the lung parenchyma with loss of lung elasticity and collapse of small airways. When diagnosing people with respiratory system disorders, the physician uses the most common clinical characteristics to label the disease process knowing that there may be more than one subset of conditions involved and differences in the airflow limitation.

Emphysema

Emphysema is the anatomic destruction of alveolar walls and elastic parenchymal tissue distal to the terminal bronchioles.[65] It can be caused by either the lack of proteolytic enzyme inhibitor or too much proteolytic enzyme, leading to enzymatic destruction of lobule support structures.[50,65] Smoking and α1-antitrypsin deficiency are 2 factors that are known to contribute to enzymatic destruction in the lung.[53] The destruction of alveolar lung tissue and evolution of large air spaces result in a decrease in surface area for gas exchange. There is V/Q mismatching and shunting of blood. There is a decreased elastic recoil and loss of alveolar surface tension that results in a loss of the radial traction forces that hold open the distal bronchioles.[53,57] Imbalances in transpulmonary pressures and bronchiole closure cause early airway collapse on expiration.[2] The loss of alveolar tissue elasticity, air trapping, and collapse all contribute to pulmonary function deficits that may be measured with spirometry. The FEV_1 should be about 80% of the FVC. Airflow obstruction is significant when FEV_1/FVC falls below 0.70 post-bronchodilator.[21,63] Hyperinflation of lung develops and there is an increased in RV. During activity or exercise the air trapping worsens, causing dynamic hyperinflation, further increasing the RV, impaired breathing mechanics, and dyspnea.[66]

Hypoxemia is imminent because of the loss of surface area in poorly ventilated regions of the lung. Hypoxic vasoconstriction and damage to the pulmonary circulation impair perfusion. Thus, both impaired perfusion and ventilation result in V/Q mismatch and shunting.[53] Pulmonary hypertension and cor pulmonale appear when capillaries are damaged and the vessel intima thickens.[21] As air trapping progresses

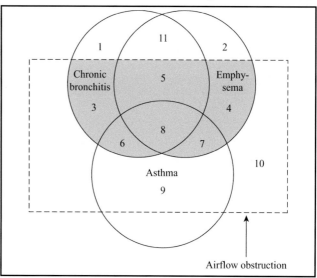

Figure 9-7. Schema of COPD. (Reprinted with permission from Celli BR, Snider GL, Heffner J, et al. Standards for the diagnosis and care of patients with chronic obstructive pulmonary disease. *Am J Respir Crit Care Med.* 1995;152:S77-S120.)

the mechanics of ventilation are disturbed, causing alveolar hypoventilation and poor gas exchange. Hypercarbia may be seen as CO_2 accumulates within the poorly ventilated areas of the lung. If the emphysema is severe, bullous formations can occur and the individual has an increased risk for spontaneous or ventilator-induced PTX.[65] Peripheral muscle wasting is also seen in individuals with emphysema, and COPD is related to corticosteroid dosage and increased tumor necrosis factor production.[21,67]

Chronic Bronchitis

Chronic bronchitis is defined by the clinical signs and symptoms of an excessive productive cough lasting for 3 months and for 2 consecutive years.[21,64] Cigarette smoking, pollution, and industrial fumes are closely linked to this disease. Inflammation in the airways causes edema and hyperplasia of submucosal glands and epithelial goblet cells.[53] The glands enlarge and the cells increase contributing to over-production of mucus. Initially, hypersecretion begins in the large airways and later progresses to involvement of small airways.[68] Chronic bronchitis is confirmed when expiratory flow decreases and FEV_1/FVC ratio <75%.[21] Hypoxia can result if the obstruction is severe enough and exudate begins to occlude small airways. Infection occurs when there is impaired ciliary function and retention of mucous in the lungs causing an inability to clear foreign particles adequately.[53] Patients with chronic bronchitis develop higher levels of CO_2 retention, have a barrel chest, a blue-gray appearance, and often rely on the hypoxic signals in peripheral chemoreceptors to signal breathing during end stages of the disease.[53]

Asthma

Asthma is a chronic disorder of the airways that is characterized by reversible airflow obstruction and airway inflammation, persistent airway hyperactivity, and airway

BOX 9-3. TYPES OF ASTHMA[21]

- Extrinsic: IgE mediated external allergens, foods, pollutants, pollen, dust, animal dander.

- Intrinsic: Nonallergic, no known trigger, associated with chronic and recurrent infection. Hypersensitivity to a bacteria or virus.

- Occupational: Work exposures to dust, gases, acids, molds, vapors, etc.

remodeling.[69] Cellular infiltration occurs along with epithelial disruption, mucosal edema, and mucus plugging.[21] There is typically an event that triggers an immune system response sending many cells and cell mediators to the airways (mast cells, neutrophils, T cells, eosinophils, and epithelial cells).[53] The response may be stimulated by extrinsic, intrinsic or occupational irritants (Box 9-3).[21] Clinical manifestations of asthma are recurrent episodes of bronchospasm, dyspnea, and wheezing.[53,68] During an episode the individual struggles to breathe and hyperventilates, causing excess removal of CO_2. This causes hypocapnia and respiratory alkalosis because excess CO_2 is removed from the blood. Later during the attack the respiratory muscles fatigue and the individual hypoventilates and develops hypercapnia and a respiratory acidosis as CO_2 accumulates in the blood.[68] Hypoxia occurs because of V/Q mismatch and widening of the diffusion gradient. It is important for the physical therapist to recognize early signs of an attack and encourage proper use of inhalers and timing of medications. Patients with asthma should be tested for allergens and educated in avoiding environmental triggers. Monitoring the peak expiratory flow rate (PEFR) and knowing baseline reactivity prior to exercise is critical to ensure a safe and efficacious therapeutic session.[68]

Exercise-induced asthma (EIA) is a condition that physical therapists may encounter in practice. This condition occurs when there is exposure to cold, dry air during rapid ventilation (as in exercise). EIA is confirmed when there is a drop of 10% of FEV_1 or PEFR from baseline during the first 5 minutes after an 8- to 10-minute bout of moderately intense (VO_2 70% to 85% max) aerobic exercise.[70] The therapist can suggest using a scarf around the mouth and nose to warm the air, premedicating with bronchodilators 30 minutes prior to exercise, avoiding activities that are higher in ventilation flow (soccer, sprinting, hockey, etc) or trying to use bronchoprovocation strategies during warm-up periods for individuals with refractory EIA.[21,71]

Cystic Fibrosis

CF is an inherited chronic disease of the exocrine glands that affects the respiratory, hepatic, digestive, and reproductive systems.[53] Exocrine gland dysfunction leads to abnormal mucus secretion and obstruction in the bronchi, bile ducts, pancreatic ducts, small intestine, cervix, and vas deferens.[72] In the lungs the chloride ion is secreted into the airway through CFTR protein-modulated channels.[68] There is increased sodium absorption and water movement from the

airways into the blood. The water content of the mucociliary blanket is decreased and viscous mucus begins to obstruct the airways.[53] Lung infections are prevalent and over time result in structural changes in the bronchial wall leading to bronchiectasis. More than 50% of individuals with bronchiectasis have CF.[21]

Over-secretion of mucus in the bronchioles will cause dyspnea and eventual hypoxia. During exercise individuals with severe CF lung disease develop increased end expiratory lung volume due to air trapping from dynamic hyperinflation.[73] Thus impaired breathing mechanics may explain the increased dyspnea with aerobic exercise. Exercise intolerance may also be related to skeletal muscle dysfunction caused by hypoxia, corticosteroids or abnormal CFTR function or genotype in skeletal muscles.[74,75] More than 90% of individuals with CF have pancreatic insufficiency and develop diabetes as adults. Thus, glucose monitoring will be necessary prior to exercise and throughout the therapeutic exercise program for many adult individuals with CF.[68] Diabetes and malabsorption syndrome result in poor nutrition status that can impair exercise tolerance in individuals with advanced CF.[76]

Interstitial Lung Diseases

Interstitial lung diseases are the result of long-term inflammatory conditions that produce fibrosis and stiffening of the interalveolar structures of the lungs. Interstitial lung diseases may be due to occupational and environmental exposures, sarcoidosis, hypersensitivity pneumonitis, radiation or pulmonary fibrosis.[53] Approximately two-thirds of the cases of pulmonary fibrosis are idiopathic (arising from an unknown cause) while the remaining one-third arise from healing after active conditions (ARDS, systemic sclerosis, tuberculosis).[21] Hypoxemia is common across all interstitial disease as fibrosis leads to a loss of compliance, and decreased ventilation and surface area for diffusion and severe dyspnea with activity.[21] Severe arterial O_2 desaturation limits safe activity. Supplemental O_2 is effective as long as the DLCO is above 40% predicted.[77]

As the disease progresses, there is fibroblast proliferation, deposition of collagen, and destruction of elastic tissue in the capillaries within the pulmonary vasculature.[21,53] The individual presents with a dry cough, fatigue, and severe dyspnea that is out of proportion to activity. The lungs are small on x-ray because of reduced volumes.[25] The pulmonary function examination reveals significant restrictive disease (FEV_1/FVC ratio > 85).[10] Energy conservation strategies become necessary when DLCO falls below 40% predicted and supplemental O_2 becomes less effective during activity.[77] Individuals with significant interstitial disease may require a lung transplant.

EXAMINATION OF GAS-EXCHANGE DISORDERS

The physical therapy examination is a process that involves a screen of all major systems. Many individuals with gas-exchange disorders have multisystem involvement either from the disease process (CF, CHF, sarcoidosis) or from the medical management required (radiation, corticosteroids). This section of the chapter will focus on physical therapy examinations directly related to gas-exchange disorders. An example of the entire physical therapy examination process across all systems is presented in the case at the end of the chapter.

Patient/Client History

History taking begins with a review of the general demographics such as age, gender, height, weight, language, race, culture, and education.[45] These factors are used to interpret respiratory function[63,78] and tests of physical work capacity (ie, 6-Minute Walk Test [6MWT]).[79] Measures of pulmonary impairment (FVC, FEV_1, PEFR), respiratory muscle performance (PI_{max}, PE_{max}, MVV) and diffusing capacity (DLCO) are compared to expected values reported in the literature.[63,78,80-84] Gathering facts related to growth and development is especially important in children who may have gas-exchange disorders related to CF,[6,76] asthma,[85] or prematurity (respiratory distress syndrome or bronchopulmonary dysplasia).[25] Body weight records may reveal trends that a child is undernourished. Although adults are fully grown, it is important to check and see whether changes in body weight have occurred since admission.

The therapist should review the known social and work history as well as the individual's living environment prior to the personal interview.[45] It is critical to avoid exhaustive questioning during the physical exam. The overall goal of history taking is to determine which activities are included in the person's everyday work and leisure routine and identify any signs, symptoms or medical limitations that may interfere with activity participation. Family history can also be reviewed to help identify familial diseases, lifestyle patterns,[86] and the quality of the support system for the person with a gas-exchange disorder. Educating and recruiting support to assist the family in implementing strategies to help reduce risk factors is important for management of diabetes, smoking cessation, obesity, and other modifiable conditions. The therapist should also learn if there are environmental exposures (dust, animals or occupational inhalants) that may be compromising the long-term health of the individual.

History of present illness will include a review of the medical chart and the recent course of the disease. The therapist should determine the reason for the present hospitalization and the chief complaint. Is the hospitalization or reason for referral because of severe dyspnea or infection, or related comorbidities such as heart failure? What medical management procedures have been offered to manage the signs and symptoms or to stabilize the current medical condition? If a surgery was performed, postoperative protocols are noted. Are there any contraindications to activity or conditions that would require a modification of the physical therapy examination?[59,62,86,87] Additionally, questions about sleep pattern are important for detecting early signs of CO_2 retention (snoring, apnea) or heart failure (orthopnea or paroxysmal nocturnal dyspnea).[88]

Medical information to review prior to performing the physical examination should include reports of baseline vital signs (including oximetry), arterial blood gases, complete blood count, pulmonary functions tests (including DLCO), sputum cultures, imaging and chest radiographs, cardiac diagnostics (echocardiography, electrocardiogram [EKG], catheterization reports) nutritional support, and renal/urinary tests.[89] The therapist should note the type of mechanical ventilation support as well as O_2-delivery devices (mask, nasal cannula, etc), method of O_2 delivery (pulsed or continuous flow), and prescription (liters/min). All medications need to be reviewed for their purpose, potential side effects, and the time course for effectiveness. Does the individual have postsurgical pain after lung transplantation or bullectomy? How is this pain being managed? Is there an asthmatic component to the lung disorder? Will the individual need to have a rescue inhaler available or premedicate prior to participating in an activity examination? The therapist should note whether medications influence the cardiac response as this can influence the interpretation of physiologic responses.

Clinical outcome tools are important for individuals with gas-exchange impairments. Disease-specific tools (St. George's Respiratory Questionnaire[90] or Chronic Respiratory Questionnaire[91]) may be necessary because many functional outcome measures (Functional Independence Measure,[92] SF-36[93,94]) may have ceiling effects in higher-functioning individuals with gas-exchange problems. Presently, methods used to examine outcomes depend on physiological tests and questionnaires.[95] Physiological tests include testing lung function, exercise capacity, and physical activity. Questionnaires typically focus on symptoms that limit activity and factors known to influence health status and quality of life. Many elements included in the questionnaire portion of the outcome tools need to be documented prior to developing a bias about the individual and should be considered prior to the physical examination.[95] Therefore, outcome tools are selected early in the history-taking portion of the exam. Several outcome tools for individuals with gas-exchange disorders are listed in Table 9-5.

Systems Review

The systems review is a brief examination designed to screen all major systems that may affect the ability of the individual to participate in purposeful movement.[45] Once cognition and communication are established, measures may be taken to examine each system. The first major system to screen is the cardiovascular/pulmonary system. The heart rate (HR), blood pressure (BP), RR, SaO_2, and presence of edema should all be measured at rest. Any contraindications to physical therapy examinations must be identified immediately, and individuals who are not appropriate for testing referred back to the physician. The therapist should be familiar with normal and abnormal values for each measure and use appropriate terminology to document resting data.

TABLE 9-5. OUTCOME ASSESSMENT TOOLS FOR INDIVIDUALS WITH GAS-EXCHANGE DISORDERS

	OUTCOME TOOL	DESCRIPTION AND PURPOSE	ADMINISTRATION
Dyspnea	BDI/TDI[96]	Eight of 9 items describing routine activities. Individual is asked to describe the amount of breathlessness at baseline and change in breathlessness over time.	Interview
	MRC-Scale[97,98]	Individual selects a grade from a list of descriptors indicating activities that cause dyspnea	Self-administered
	Borg-Scale (CR10)[99]	The individual rates the amount of perceived dyspnea at rest and during activity	Self-administered
Symptom Measure— Pneumonia	CAP-Sym[100]	An 18-item measure that assesses the annoying symptoms of pneumonia during the past 24 hours using a 6-point Likert scale.	Self-administered
Health Status and Quality of Life	SGRQ[90]	A disease-specific questionnaire that examines the frequency and severity of symptoms, activity impact, and psychosocial impact (76 items)	Self-administered
	CRQ[91]	A disease-specific measure of physical-functional and emotional limitations due to chronic lung diseases. Individual is asked to recall the 5 most important activities that caused breathlessness in the last 2 weeks.	Interview
	SOLQ[101]	Disease-specific questionnaire designed to measure physical function, emotional function, coping skills, and treatment satisfaction of individuals with COPD. May be used to predict hospitalization and mortality.[102]	Self-administered
	QWB[103,104]	This scale measures well-being based on social preferences for mobility, physical activity and social activity. There are 4 levels to measure physical activity and 5 levels to measure social activity and mobility. Symptoms that impair function are scored. Validated in COPD[103] and CF.[104]	Interview
	SF-36[93]	Generic health survey. There are 36 items requiring the individual to self-assess psychological, physical, and social aspects of their quality of life.	Self-administered
Multi-Dimensional Tools	BODE[105,106]	Prognostic indicator for individuals with COPD. Utilizes 4 components (BMI, FEV_1, MMRC, 6MWT) to describe severity of disease and function.	Scores from physical exams and questionnaires.

6MWT: 6-Minute Walk Test; BDI: Baseline Dyspnea Indexes; BMI: body mass index; BODE: body mass index, airflow obstruction, dyspnea, exercise capacity; CAP-Sym: Community-Acquired Pneumonia Symptom Questionnaire; CRQ: Chronic Respiratory Questionnaire; MMRC: Modified Medical Research Council; MRC-Scale: Medical Research Council Scale; QWB: Quality of Well-Being Scale; SGRQ: St. George's Respiratory Questionnaire; SOLQ: Seattle Obstructive Lung Disease Questionnaire; TDI: Transition Dyspnea Indexes.

The integumentary system screen may be performed prior to the musculoskeletal or neuromuscular systems review. It is important to identify wounds or incisions that should not be stressed during examination of range of motion (ROM) or functional movement. The therapist should note the presence and quality of scar formation and document the location and size of any incision or wound. The color, temperature, and integrity of the skin should be noted. The musculoskeletal system screen includes a gross examination of ROM, strength, postural symmetry, height, and weight. This is followed by a screen of the neuromuscular system.

During the neuromuscular screen the therapist examines gross movement involving balance, gait, locomotion, transfers, transitional movements, and motor control or motor learning considerations.[45] The systems review may conclude with more detailed testing of cognition, affect, language and communication, and overall appraisal of learning style.

Information from the interview and the system review begins to direct the physical therapist to the categories of tests and measures indicated. Even before the exact test and measures are selected, the physical therapist has started to gather information just by observing the patient (Table 9-6).

TABLE 9-6. CLINICAL OBSERVATIONS	
General appearance	Observe the level of mentation and note any presence of confusion or disorientation. Also look for facial characteristics that may suggest psychological distress or anxiety. The therapist should notice the use of any accessory muscles, nasal flaring, and self initiated pursed-lip breathing, which may be signs of air hunger.
Color	Observe the skin, lip, and gum color for signs of cyanosis (blue-gray coloration)
Chest wall and posture	Note the initial body position, any RR and TV abnormalities (hyper/hypoventilation); chest wall motion and deformity. Observe any abnormal movement or lack of movement of the chest wall. Check for abnormal diaphragm motion (belly breathing), paradoxical chest movement, and presence of any asymmetrical head and trunk positions during breathing (see Chapter 8).
Neck	The therapist should observe the neck for excessive accessory muscle use (see Chapter 8). While the person is lying supine with the head and neck at a 45-degree angle, the therapist can observe jugular venous distention.[107] The presence of jugular venous distention signifies CHF or pulmonary vascular fluid overload.[89,107]
Phonation	Listen to the voice and note whether it is loud or quiet. How many words can the person speak before taking a breath? Are there audible secretions in the airway during speech?
Nail beds	Look for clubbing of the fingers, a broadening of the distal finger tips with an increased Lovibond angle (Figure 9-8) may indicate chronic hypoxia and Mees' lines, a white discoloration of the nail with transverse lines, may be seen in renal failure, heart disease, and pneumonia.[108]

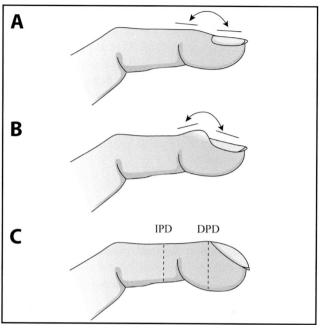

Figure 9-8. Normal digit configuration (A) and digital clubbing (B). Note that the angle between the nail and the proximal skin exceeds 180 degrees. (C) Also note that the distal phalangeal depth (DPD) is greater than the interphalangeal depth (IPD). (Adapted from Wilkins RL, Krider SJ. *Clinical Assessment in Respiratory Care.* St. Louis, MO: Mosby; 1985.)

individual with gas-exchange disorders is generated. Specific tests and measures may be similar to those selected for ventilatory pump dysfunction (chest wall excursion, posture, respiratory muscle strength, and cough). This is especially true if gas-exchange impairment is due to hypoventilation. If the ventilatory pump is failing then gas exchange worsens and the problem may progress to respiratory failure (Practice Pattern 6F).[45]

Gas-exchange impairment can also occur in conditions such as pulmonary edema, pulmonary fibrosis or lung tissue diseases where respiratory muscle is strong but the lung condition increases the ventilatory demand. The selection of tests and measures from the category of Ventilation and Respiration/Gas Exchange will figure prominently. Additional tests and measures may also be indicated from the categories of: Arousal, Attention and Cognition, Posture, and Aerobic Capacity/Endurance. Other measures may be indicated from the categories of Circulation, Range of Motion, and Muscle Performance.

Arousal, Attention, and Cognition

Elevations in CO_2 are often associated with decreased attention and cognitive processing.[109] Therefore, the clinician should include such examinations as the Mini-mental exam[110] and the Trails Making test to further exam cognitive functioning.[111] Arousal may be decreased and result in slower responses to stimuli. Attention can be tested by asking the individual to perform the Digit Span Test where a series of numbers is repeated forward and backward. Walking while talking (or locating objects) is a means of testing divided attention.[112]

Tests and Measures

Observation

After completion of the systems review screening and observation period, a list of specific tests and measures for the

Posture

Posture should be assessed for the presence of increased anterior-posterior diameter of the chest, kyphosis, and scoliosis. These abnormal postures can often be the result of long-term pulmonary disease. A more rigid chest wall will also contribute to restrictive disease. Chest wall expansion measures are reliable and can be taken at a xiphoid and axillary sites and compared to norms in the literature.[113-116] Impaired posture may contribute to loss of ROM in the cervical spine and shoulders.

Ventilation and Gas Exchange

For individuals with gas-exchange impairments, the examination ventilation and gas exchange is performed early in the physical exam. Examination of ventilation includes assessment of posture and chest wall assessment (see Chapter 8), which will be followed by a detailed examination of ventilatory mechanics and breathing pattern (see Chapter 8), respiration, and auscultation. Baseline measures for breathing pattern, RR and pattern, dyspnea, SaO_2, and auscultation are taken in the initial position and may be repeated with changes in positions. Aerobic capacity examination is performed after all baseline measures are completed so the therapist may screen findings for any contraindication to exercise.

Chest Wall Exam

Palpation is used to examine the chest wall. The purpose of this manual examination is to detect abnormalities in the chest wall movement or lung parenchyma and identify specific locations where more detail examination (auscultation) is required. The hands are placed on the chest over the upper lobes, middle lobes, and lower lobes as the person inhales and exhales maximally (Figure 9-9).[107] The individual is also asked to speak. Normal vibrations from the voice may be felt and these are called vocal fremitus. If vocal fremitus or vibration is not felt then this could indicate consolidation, effusion, or lung collapse. If pulmonary secretions are present in the airways, stronger vibrations may be felt. This is called tactile fremitus. More detailed examinations of vocal sounds may be examined with a stethoscope.

Tracheal position is palpated to determine any deviations. If the trachea is not midline this could indicate PTX or collapse. The trachea would shift toward the collapsed lung.[107] Many times with PTX or chest wall trauma air can leak under the subcutaneous tissues of the chest and neck. If the therapist finds bubbling and crackling felt under the skin this may be subcutaneous emphysema. The condition should be immediately reported to the physician. A chest tube may need to be surgically inserted to reverse the air leak.

Pain is easily assessed during palpation. If pain is elicited during gentle palpation of the ribs, sternum, clavicle, scapula, or spine it should be assessed using a visual analog scale (VAS), numerical pain scale or other pain scale.[72,117,118] Fractures may be felt if the chest wall is displaced or flail chest is present.[25]

Mediate Percussion

Mediate percussion is another screening tool used to differentiate between solid or fluid- and air-filled spaces in the thorax. Percussion is performed by tapping the dominant middle finger onto the opposite distal middle finger while over an intercostal space.[7,88,107] Normal resonant sound and vibration is heard and felt over the first to eleventh intercostal spaces and should be the same bilaterally.[7] When hyper-resonance is noted, this may indicate fluid or increased air, as with a large pleural effusion or a tension PTX. When a dull or flat sound is noted, it may indicate consolidation, collapse, or solid tissue and may suggest a dense pneumonia, atelectasis, or tumor.[88,107,119] When abnormalities are noted, this indicates a need for further examination to confirm a diagnosis. The sensitivity of chest percussion is very low and therefore the inter- and intra-rater errors are high.[120]

Respiratory Rate and Pattern

RR is normally 12 to 18 breaths per minute. Respiratory pattern describes the variation between RR, TV, and pause characteristics. Descriptions of respiratory pattern include tachypnea (> 20 breaths/minute), bradypnea (< 10 breaths per minute), hyperventilation, Cheyne-Stokes, biots, Kussmaul's, etc.[121] Tachypnea or rapid RR can be caused by exertion, fever, pain or hypoxia, and ventilatory pump disorders. Bradypnea or slow RR can be caused by medications, especially narcotics, hypothermia or injuries to the brain stem. When the RR at rest is below 8 or above 30 at rest, this is a sign of medical instability and a contraindication to treatment.[59,122]

Dyspnea

Dyspnea is the sensation of feeling breathless and may be examined using the Borg scale (ratio or ordinal),[99,123] VAS,[88,124] numeric rating scale,[125] ventilatory response index,[126] or as part of a survey examining perception of dyspnea during routine activity (Modified Medical Research Council [MMRC] Dyspnea Scale[97] or Baseline Dyspnea Index[96]). Dyspnea is typically measured at rest and again during functional activity or aerobic capacity examinations. The Modified Borg scale of dyspnea has been widely used clinically in a variety of respiratory conditions to quantify the sensation of breathlessness at rest and during activity.[86,123,127]

Oximetry

Gas-exchange deficits are routinely examined by measuring the SaO_2 using a pulse oximeter at rest, with changes in position and during activity. SaO_2 monitors or pulse oximeters are hand-held devices that indirectly measure SaO_2 of the arterial blood by reading the pulsatile change in light absorption of the blood (SpO_2 = refers to the indirect pulsatile estimation of SaO_2). The monitoring unit displays a digital percentage readout of a calculated estimate of the amount of Hgb that is saturated with O_2. For adults without lung disease the normal SpO_2 is greater than 95%. Normative values may vary according to age and race.[87] The accuracy of SaO_2 may be limited by motion artifact, nail polish, poor perfusion, and will be less precise as SaO_2 decreases (Box 9-4).[128]

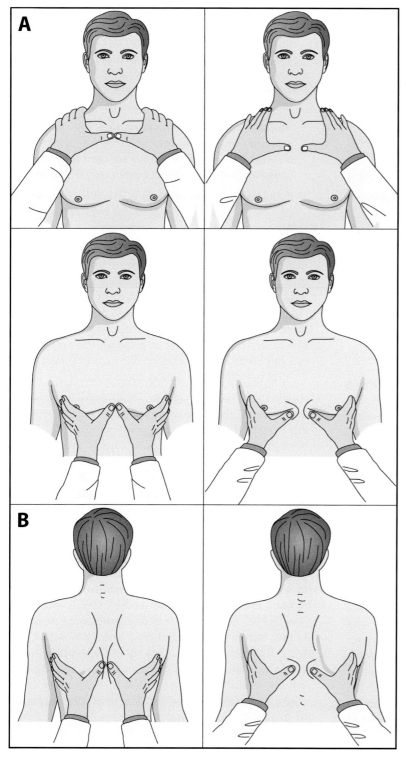

Figure 9-9. Manual screening examination of the chest wall. (A) Anterior aspect. (B) Posterior aspect. (Adapted from Cherniack RM, Cherniack L. *Respiration in Health and Disease.* 2nd ed. Philadelphia, PA: WB Saunders, 1972, in Hillegass E. *Essentials of Cardiopulmonary Physical Therapy.* 3rd Ed. W.B. Saunders Company; 2010.)

The physical therapist will need to review the quality of the oximeter with respect to motion artifact. Perfusion may be affected by changes in temperature, vasospasm, and gripping actions (using a walker, handrails or arm crank handles). Alternative placement of the oximeter sensor (forehead, earlobe) may help improve readings.

Medicare guidelines for reimbursement of supplemental O_2 at home are: PaO_2 less than or equal to 55 mm Hg, SaO_2 less than or equal to 88% or SpO_2 less than or equal to 88%.

Individuals may qualify for supplemental O_2 if the PaO_2 is greater than 55 mm Hg and the SaO_2 or SpO_2 is greater than 88% if one of the following conditions is met[129]:

- Peripheral edema secondary to CHF

- Cor pulmonale documented on an EKG or by an echocardiogram, gated blood pool scan, or direct pulmonary artery pressure measurement

- Hct greater than 56%

Box 9-4. Limitations to Accurate Pulse Oximetry[116,121,130]

- Excessive motion at the probe placement
- Abnormal hemoglobins
- Ambient light exposure to the probe
- Intravascular dyes
- Low vascular perfusion
- Skin pigmentation
- Nail polish or nail coverings with finger probe used
- Inability to detect saturations below 83% with the same degree of accuracy and precision seen at higher saturations
- Inability to quantitate the degree of hyperoxemia present

Auscultation

Auscultation is one of the most important examinations for patients with gas-exchange disorders and is more reliable when performed by an experienced therapist.[131] Recent chest x-ray results should be reviewed prior to auscultation to determine potential areas of compromise. Lung auscultation may provide important information regarding the type and location of various lung pathologies when interpreted with information from medical diagnostics (chest x-ray reports).[132]

A stethoscope is used over the chest wall areas that correspond to anatomical structures in the pulmonary system (see Chapter 8; Figure 8-11). Normal breath sound characteristics vary according to the anatomical region and are labeled "bronchial" (heard over the trachea; manubrium), "bronchovesicular" (heard over the main stem bronchi; first and second intercostals spaces), or "vesicular" (heard over peripheral lung tissues).[107] The inspiratory time is shorter and expiratory time longer when auscultation is over proximal structures and inspiratory time longer and expiratory shorter for distal structures (see Chapter 8, Figure 8-12). In addition to appreciating normal sound quality, timing, and pause characteristics, the examination also includes an assessment of voice-transmitted sounds, abnormal breath sounds, and adventitious sounds.

- Voice sounds: Spoken words are muffled and indistinct and whispered words are usually not heard at all during auscultation in the healthy individual. However, the spoken sounds become clear or more distinct when heard over abnormal lung tissue. These abnormal voice sounds may indicate increased densities due to fluid or solid masses.[107] The presence of pathologies typically cause consolidation of lung tissue so sounds are transmitted easily, becoming more distinct and audible.[7,88,89,119] The voice sounds included in the examination are:

  - Whispered pectoriloquy: The person is instructed to whisper the words "one, two, three" while the examiner listens through the diaphragm of the stethoscope over areas of suspected tissue abnormality. The sounds will be clearly and distinctly auscultated over areas of lung consolidation or will sound faint or muffled over normal healthy tissues.

  - Bronchophony: The individual says "99" while the examiner auscultates over areas of suspected tissue abnormality. The voice sounds are clear over areas of consolidation and indistinct over normal lung tissue.

  - Egophony: Here the person is asked to say "E" (as in "sweet") and "A" (as in sway) over consolidated regions.

- Abnormal breath sounds: Sounds are considered abnormal if bronchial or bronchovesicular sounds are heard over peripheral lung tissue. Normally, there would be quiet air movement over the majority of the lung parenchyma but these sounds become loud and tubular when there is lung consolidation or pathology.[88] There may also be decreased or absent lung sounds that could indicate hypoventilation in a region due to muscle weakness, PTX, hyperinflation or airway obstruction.[107]

- Adventitious breath sounds: Additional extraneous sounds heard throughout inspiration or expiration usually described in the following ways may be continuous or discontinuous.[133] Continuous sounds may be high pitched (wheezes or sibilant rhonchi) or low pitched (wheeze or sonorous rhonchi) and usually indicate a narrowing of the airway due to either bronchospasm, inflammation or mucus. Discontinuous sounds may be moist sounding (coarse rales) or dry sounding (fine rales). The discontinuous sound arises from a "snapping open" of alveoli. Differences exist in terminology when describing lung sounds but can be summarized in simple terms by applying the term *wheezes* to continuous sounds and *rales* or *crackles* to discontinuous sounds.[89,133] Moist rales typically indicate the presence of pneumonia or interstitial fluid associated with CHF while fine rales are typically a sign of interstitial fibrosis. When documenting the presence of adventitious sounds, describe the phase within the respiratory cycle where the sound is heard (eg, late inspiratory crackles or inspiratory and expiratory wheezes).[88] Adventitious lung sounds and their interpretation are summarized in Table 9-7.

Although auscultation and interpretation of breath sounds may appear to be subjective, this examination procedure has met the rules of Evidence-Based Medicine with success.[134,135] The accuracy of using lung sounds in determining a diagnosis has revealed that wheezes can predict asthma (likelihood ratio [LR] +6). Fine inspiratory crackles are common in pulmonary fibrosis (LR + 5.9) and fine or coarse inspiratory crackles are consistently identified in chronic bronchitis (LR + 14 to 20). Voice-transmitted sounds (bronchophony, egophony, and pectoriloquy) are consistently

TABLE 9-7. ADVENTITIOUS LUNG SOUNDS

ATS TERMINOLOGY	ACCP TERMINOLOGY	DEFINITION AND SOUND CHARACTERISTICS	CLINICAL INTERPRETATION
Coarse crackle	Coarse rales	Discontinuous bursts of popping bubbles heard on inspiration; moist low pitch sounds that are interrupted	Pulmonary edema Resolving pneumonia
Fine crackle	Fine rales	Discontinuous brief bursts of high pitched sounds (softer and shorter); dry crackling of cellophane wrap	Alveoli snapping open Interstitial fibrosis
Wheeze "high-pitched wheeze"	Sibilant rhonchi	Continuous high-pitched musical sounds varying in duration; whistling	Airway narrowing Asthma
Rhonchus "low-pitched wheeze"	Sonorous rhonchi	Continuous low-pitched musical snoring sound	Sputum obstruction in airways
Stridor	Stridor	High-pitched monophasic sound heard during inspiration	Upper airway mechanical obstruction or stenosis
Pleural rub	Pleural rub	Squeaking or grating sound; can be either inspiratory or expiratory. Sounds like 2 pieces of leather rubbing together	Rubbing of pleural surfaces due to scar tissue or fibrosis

ACCP: American College of Chest Physicians; ATS: American Thoracic Society.

Data adapted from Cahalin LP. Pulmonary evaluation. In: DeTurk WE, Cahalin LP, eds. *Cardiovascular and Pulmonary Physical Therapy: An Evidence-Based Approach.* 2nd ed. New York: McGraw-Hill; 2004:221-269; Hillegass EA. Examination and assessment procedures. In: Hillegass EA, ed. *Essentials of Cardiopulmonary Physical Therapy.* 3rd ed. St. Louis, MO: Elsevier; 2011:534-567; Butler SM. Clinical assessment of the cardiopulmonary system. In: Frownfelter D, Dean E, eds. *Cardiovascular and Pulmonary Physical Therapy: Evidence and Practice.* 4th ed. St. Louis, MO: Mosby Elsevier; 2006; Watchie J. Cardiopulmonary assessment. In: Watchie J, ed. *Cardiovascular and Pulmonary Physical Therapy: A Clinical Manual.* 2nd ed. St. Louis, MO: Saunders Elsevier; 2010:273-297; and Pulmonary terms and symbols. A report of the ACCP-ATS Joint Committee on Pulmonary Nomenclature. *Chest.* 1975;67:5-10.)

associated with lung consolidation and pneumonia (LR + 4.1) if fever and cough are also present.[134,136,137]

Cough

The cough should be examined for ability to clear secretions. Detailed examination of all 4 phases of coughing (see Chapter 8) should be performed.[138] Glottis control and ability to close the nasal passages should be present to allow the individual to build pressure before releasing a forceful exhalation. The cough should be characterized as "strong functional" (able to effectively clear moderately thick secretions), "weak functional" (requires several less forceful efforts to clear thin secretions) or "nonfunctional" (unable to clear secretions; requires suctioning or specific inspiratory and expiratory assist). Any sputum expectorated should be captured and the quantity, consistency, and color of the sputum should be recorded (Table 9-8).

Ventilatory Flow, Forces and Volume

The ability to ventilate well is examined with spirometry and tests of respiratory muscle performance (see Chapter 8). The physical therapist may wish to examination ventilatory capacity in individuals with gas-exchange impairments. It is especially important to review the percentage predicted FEV_1 to determine the degree of disease severity in individuals with COPD (GOLD classification; see Chapter 8,

Table 8-5).[63] The individual with a low percentage predicted FEV_1 (stage 4 GOLD criteria) will have less reserve for activity and is at greater risk for gas-exchange impairments. The FEV_1 measure is considered the most important value in the diagnosis of airway obstruction.[129,139] The FEV_1 decreases as obstruction increases and improves as obstruction is successfully treated.[139] Measures of PEFR can help monitor the onset of bronchospasm in individuals with asthma.

Restrictive diseases such as obesity, scoliosis, chest trauma, neuromuscular disorders including spinal cord injuries and pain can reduce FVC. Pneumonias and disorders where fluid or excessive secretions fill the alveoli and inhibit air entry may reduce the FVC as can interstitial lung diseases, pulmonary fibrosis, and CHF.[139] The low FVC is nonspecific, but can be used as a measurement pre- and then postintervention. If a therapist plans to implement a respiratory care program, the FVC and measures of PI_{max} and PE_{max} may help monitor progress.

Circulation

Normal temperature is 98.6°F or 37°C.[121] Elevation of temperature generally indicates infection. The 3 Ws are used when considering the source of infection: Wind: suspecting infection in the respiratory system. Wound: suspecting infection in integumentary integrity. Water: suspecting infection in the urinary system.[140-143]

TABLE 9-8. EXAMINATION OF SPUTUM

COLOR	CAUSES
Red	Blood (hemoptysis)
Rusty	Lobular pneumonia, pneumococcus, mycoplasma
Green	Pseudomonas infection
Brown	Anaerobic infection/lung abscess
Yellow	Infection, *Haemophilus*
Pink frothy	Pulmonary edema
Black	Specks from smoke inhalation, coal dust
CHARACTERISTIC	
Thin (mucoid)	Moves easily, not infectious
Mildly thickened (mucopurulent)	Slightly discolored, suspicion of infection
Thick (purulent)	Difficult to mobilize; needs hydration
Foul-smelling, copious	Long-term infection; *Pseudomonas*
QUANTITY	
Indicate the volume of sputum expectorated in mL over 24 hours	
Airway clearance techniques may be indicated when sputum volume > 20 to 30 mL/day	

Data adapted from McCool FD, Rosen MJ. Nonpharmacologic airway clearance therapies: ACCP evidence-based clinical practice guidelines. *Chest*. 2006;129:250S-259S; Middleton S, Middleton PG. Assessment and investigation of patients' problems. In: Pryor JA, Prasad SA, eds. *Physiotherapy for Respiratory and Cardiac Problems Adults and Paediatrics*. 4th ed. London: Churchill Livingstone Elsevier; 2008.

Many individuals with gas-exchange disorders have abnormalities in the heart and systemic circulation. Therefore, the pulse quality and characteristics are examined. Individuals who smoke may have damaged the peripheral circulation and may have decreased or absent peripheral pulses. When palpating the pulse quality the therapist should determine if the pulse is regular or irregular and observe for pulsus alternans (variation between strong and weak pulse) and pulsus paradoxus (decreased pulse strength during inspiration or drop in systolic BP with inspiration).[39] These may be signs of cardiac muscle dysfunction. Individuals with heart failure may have changes in fluid volume. Daily body weight must be examined to detect early signs of cardiac decompensation, which may result in pulmonary edema.[144] Patients, after open heart surgery, can gain substantial weight because of intraoperative fluids given. Excessive fluid overload can greatly affect the cardiopulmonary system and result in hypoxia due to impaired-gas exchange. Unexplained weight loss or gain could be a serious sign and would need referral for further medical workup.[145-149]

Auscultation of the heart is an examination that is recorded under the circulation section of the physical therapy examination.[45] When fluid accumulates it may result in incomplete closure of the heart valves or it may cause pressure changes in the heart that result in abnormal heart sounds. Individuals with gas-exchange disorders often develop cor pulmonale, which may cause an S3 heart sound or murmurs.[89,150] A loud S2 sound that may be split with an accent on the P2 component will be present with pulmonary hypertension.[150] In some cases, individuals with cardiac disorders will develop pulmonary edema, which results in a gas-exchange disorder as a secondary condition.[39]

Range of Motion

Upper extremity (UE) ROM may be limited by changes in posture (kyphosis).[151] Additionally, the habitual use of a forward lean with weightbearing on the UEs may result in hip flexion contractures. Cervical and trunk ROM in all directions (rotation, lateral bending as well as flexion and extension) should be examined in detail. In addition to examining ROM in the extremities, chest wall expansion measurements are taken at 3 sites and the difference recorded and compared to norms in the literature.[114,115,152]

Muscle Performance

Many individuals with gas-exchange deficits are prescribed steroids to reduce inflammation. The literature has identified that the dosage of steroids may introduce a myopathy that can be at least partially reversed with strength training.[67,153] Stability muscles (quadriceps, calf) and respiratory muscles are known to have the greatest loss of strength.[67] Yet the strength deficits may not be detectable by manual muscle testing. Hand-held dynamometer or isokinetic devices may assist in quantifying peripheral muscle strength.[154,155] Respiratory muscle performance should also be quantified using PI_{max} and PE_{max} and MVV testing according to ATS standards.[81,156,157]

Gait, Locomotion, and Balance

Walking ability can be examined for gait quality as well as endurance. The therapist will note posture, use of any breathing and pacing strategies and assistive device, assess loss of balance or instability, and determine the individual's capacity to safely manage household and community distances. The walk distance over 2, 3 or 6 minutes may be used to quantify baseline endurance and risk for mobility disability.[79,158-161] Formal testing of balance and mobility using such tools as the Timed Up and Go,[162] Berg Balance Test,[163] and the Stair Climb Power Test[164] can be helpful for defining functional impairments in patients with COPD.[164,165,166]

Aerobic Capacity/Endurance

Exercise testing stresses the systems involved in O_2 delivery and consumption required for human movement.[3] The exercise test may examine aerobic capacity using a maximal effort or a submaximal effort. A maximal graded exercise test (GXT) is designed to evaluate the maximal ability of an individual to deliver and consume O_2. It is called a test of maximal aerobic capacity or VO_{2max}.[3,8] The therapist should determine if there are any contraindications to exercise prior to testing aerobic capacity. The endpoint of a VO_2 max test will either be symptom limited (fatigue, SOB) or physiologically limited (EKG abnormality, undesirable BP, O_2 desaturation). O_2 consumption (VO_2) is either measured or estimated.[86] Individuals with gas-exchange disorders will typically be limited by poor oxygenation resulting in a decrease in SaO_2 (physiologic limitation) or extreme SOB and cyanosis (symptom limited).[66,167] Individuals with pulmonary hypertension may also be limited by a drop in systolic BP (physiologic limitation) and dizziness (symptom limitation).[167]

A submaximal test, such as the 6MWT, examines the cardiorespiratory responses using a workload that is well beneath a maximum effort and is often used clinically to safely estimate aerobic capacity in people with known disease.[168,169] Most daily activities are performed at submaximal levels of exertion and therefore submaximal functional tests appear to translate to physical ability required for daily functioning.[168,170] The goal of any exercise test is to measure the symptomatic and physiologic response to movement and determine overall limitations to performance so they may be treated with therapeutic interventions or medication.[167]

In clinics offering pulmonary rehabilitation, the 6MWT and the shuttle-walking test are submaximal tests used to examine aerobic capacity and endurance.[79,168,171,172] The 6MWT is recognized as a valid and reliable test that may be used to estimate VO_2 ($r = 0.81$, $p < 0.0001$)[173] in persons with end-stage pulmonary disease.[168,169,174-177] The 6MWT distance and estimated VO_2 may be used clinically to describe functional capacity, evaluate the benefits of medication, make decisions for transplantation, and offer prognostic value.[3,37,79,169,178] The minimal clinically important difference is approximately 86 meters.[179] A regression equation for estimating VO_2 peak from the 6MWT distance is as follows[180]:

Mean peak $VO_2 = 4.948 + (0.023 \times 6MWT \text{ distance})$

(Standard error of estimate 1.1 mL/kg/min)

GXT protocols commonly used in persons with gas-exchange disorders include the Godfrey protocol (CF)[181] and the Massachusetts Respiratory Hospital.[182] These protocols, designed for persons with gas-exchange deficits, use the FEV_1 to assist in setting the workload stages.[183] The Godfrey protocol also considers the child's growth stage and age.[181] GXT offers greater cardiovascular challenge since a maximal effort is provoked. Yet, individuals with gas-exchange disorders are typically limited by ventilation (VE) or serious declines in SaO_2 prior to reaching the limits of CO during the GXT.[3,8]

In the acute stage, after a pulmonary exacerbation, the aerobic capacity is measured by examining responses to changes in position, functional training, and walking.[184,185] A 2-Minute Walk Test (2MWT) may be more feasible at this stage but does not adequately measure endurance required to manage community-level distances.[160,168,172] Recording physiologic responses during activity can assist the medical team in adjusting medications and help the therapist select interventions to improve activity tolerance. The response to exercise can be reexamined after offering support (O_2, ventilator) or educating the patient in breathing strategies (pursed-lip breathing [PLB], breathing control, pacing).[186] Energy-conserving techniques and breathing strategies may lower the physiologic work during functional activities.[119] It is important to assess tasks typically included in the individual's daily routine and then document strategies used to manage symptoms. The MET level can be documented and a progressive set of more demanding tasks examined with a functional monitor. The therapist records the manifestation of symptoms (rate of perceived exertion (RPE), rate of perceived dyspnea (RPD), color, accessory muscle use or chest discomfort) and records the physiologic responses (HR, SaO_2, RR, BP, EKG) for each stage of work.

Assistive and Adaptive Devices

Many individuals with gas-exchange deficits will require supplemental O_2. It will be important for the therapist to examine the effectiveness of O_2 support equipment and devices (see Table 9-1). Additionally, the method of transporting O_2 delivery devices should be examined and recorded as part of any functional assessment. Does the person use the O_2 device properly? Are there changes in the physiologic responses with different carrying devices (supported on walker vs carrying over shoulder)?[187]

Orthotic, Protective, and Supportive Devices

Some individuals will require a form of mechanical ventilation. The therapist should note the mode of ventilation and whether there will be good ventilatory support for ambulation. Because many individuals with gas-exchange deficits are being mobilized while they are receiving mechanical ventilation[188,189] the therapist should note the TV, RR, VE, FiO$_2$ and number and method of ventilator-supported breaths.[190] Familiarization with alarms and interdisciplinary communication will also be important so the therapy session is offered safely with confidence and assurance. Tolerance to activity for individuals who are receiving mechanical ventilation is examined by noting the SaO2, VE, and BP. The VE is usually 4 to 5 L/min with a RR of 18 breaths/minute or less.[191] If the VE rises above 20 L/min then early mobility is not being tolerated. Pressure support ventilation can affect cardiac output and may cause variations in BP.[59] Pneumatic compression devices and stockings may be required to prevent DVTs and to control edema.

Ergonomics, Environmental, Home, and Work Barriers

The ability to work efficiently at a low energy cost is an important part of the physical therapy examination. Therefore, routine tasks may be simulated during the physical therapy examination and evaluated for the physiologic stress imposed, breathing strategies employed, and efficiency of performance. The therapist can then identify items to include in the educational session that may improve self-management of symptoms and improve safety and efficiency for returning to work and participation in activities in and around the home.

EVALUATION, DIAGNOSIS, AND PROGNOSIS

Individuals with gas-exchange disorders may have impairments in aerobic capacity/endurance,[66,192] posture, BMI,[193] balance deficits,[165,166] decrease muscle performance (respiratory muscle and peripheral muscle),[153,194,195] poor chest wall and spine mobility,[115,196] impaired airway clearance,[6,197] abnormal breathing strategies,[186] knowledge deficits regarding disease management (pacing, breathing strategies, energy conservation)[186,198] and education on safe and effective use of supplemental O$_2$.[199] The physical therapy diagnosis may be "Impaired Ventilation, Respiration/Gas Exchange, and Aerobic Capacity/Endurance Associated with Airway Clearance Dysfunction" (Practice Pattern 6C) or "Impaired Ventilation and Respiration/Gas Exchange Associated with Respiratory Failure" (Practice Pattern 6F).[45] Individuals with ventilatory pump failure will spiral down from Practice Pattern 6E (Chapter 8) to Practice Pattern 6F. Dyssynchronous or paradoxical breathing, RR >35 at rest and O$_2$ desaturation are signs that the individual with ventilatory pump failure (Practice Pattern 6E) has moved to respiratory failure (Practice Pattern 6F).[45,59] Many individuals with pulmonary exacerbations will also fall under Practice Pattern 6B: Impaired Aerobic Capacity/Endurance Associated With Deconditioning.

Determining the physical therapy prognosis will require the therapist to consider the medical history (exacerbations) and severity of lung disease (FEV$_1$ and DLCO). Prognosis in individuals with CF is affected by low aerobic capacity (28%, 8-year survival with VO$_2$ peak $\leq$ 58% pred) and presence of *Pseudomonas cepacia*.[37] The BODE score utilizes the 6MWT distance, FEV$_1$, MMRC, and the BMI to provide a measure of risk for mortality and risk of hospitalization.[193,200] The physical therapy program may improve these risks if the individual can comply with recommendations to lose weight, participate in a conditioning program, and learn strategies to manage dyspnea.

The severity of lung disease (FEV$_1$) is not expected to change with physical therapy. However, the proper use of medications may partially reverse airway obstruction in some individuals. The 6MWT should be performed after bronchodilation medications are taken.[79] The physical therapist may consider the level of functioning prior to the last exacerbation as a guide to determining functional prognosis for most individuals with gas-exchange deficits. A person with poor lung function who has already participated in pulmonary rehabilitation will be less likely to achieve substantial functional improvement. Outpatient pulmonary rehabilitation is typically approved for 18 to 36 visits. Sample goals are presented in Table 9-9.

INTERVENTIONS

Mobilization and exercise are the most efficacious interventions to offer individuals with gas-exchange disorders because these interventions enhance all steps in the O$_2$ transport system.[201] Recent evidence suggests early mobilization in critically ill persons can reduce hospitalization and decrease the length of stay.[188] A physiologic treatment hierarchy of interventions to enhance the O$_2$ transport system in individuals having gas exchange deficits is listed in Table 9-10.[105] Body positioning, breathing control and coughing maneuvers (active airway clearance strategies) are among the most effective treatments. Suctioning and postural drainage are less effective in enhancing O$_2$ transport but may be the best option for individuals who are extremely weak, medically paralyzed or cognitive unable to participate.

Many interventions discussed in Chapter 8 are appropriate for individuals with gas exchange disorders. There is an increased ventilatory load when airway clearance problems exist. The respiratory muscles may or may not be weak depending on the chronicity of the illness and ability of the muscle to adapt to a load. Individuals with cystic fibrosis with mild to moderate disease may actually have higher than normal MIP values.[202] The respiratory muscles have adapted to the excessive demands required for removing secretions, yet the FEV$_1$ may be reduced due to obstruction. FEV$_1$ is highly related to peak work capacity (r = 0.79; p < .001) for people with cystic fibrosis.[202] Interventions that remove airway obstruction (bronchodilators, breathing control, and

TABLE 9-9. EXAMPLES OF PHYSICAL THERAPY GOALS

EXAMPLES OF GOALS*

- Increase ventilation of _____ lobes as measured by air entry upon auscultation (no adventitious sounds) and improved chest x-ray.
- Vital capacity will increase to ___ mL as measured on incentive spirometer.
- Demonstrate effective cough to independently clear pulmonary secretions.
- Demonstrate proper technique for airway clearance (active cycle breathing, positive expiratory pressure, flutter, etc).
- Demonstrate proper breathing retraining strategies (deep breathing, diaphragmatic breathing, pursed-lip breathing).
- Recite and demonstrate correct application of energy-conservation techniques, home exercise program, and self-monitoring.
- Independent and safe with bed mobility and transfers with dyspnea < 3/10 and SpO_2 > 90%.
- Increase 6MWT by ___ feet with RPD < 3/10 and SpO_2 > 90%.
- Demonstrate pursed-lipped breathing and efficient coordinated breathing 90% of the time when performing dressing, household chores, and work-related tasks (specific to individual goals).
- Independently climb 12 steps with railing using proper pacing to allow RPD < 3/10 and O_2 Sat > 90%.

POSTSURGICAL CONDITIONS

- Adhere to all sternal/postsurgical precautions during mobility
- Utilize pillow correctly during coughing.
- Demonstrate proper posture in sitting/standing independently.
- Independently perform deep/segmental breathing with pain < 2/10.

*Each goal will include "The patient will…" and a time frame.

TABLE 9-10. INTERVENTIONS TO IMPROVE OXYGEN TRANSPORT

- Mobilization and exercise
- Body positioning
- Breathing control maneuvers
- Coughing maneuvers/active airway clearance
- Relaxation and energy conservation
- ROM exercises (cardiopulmonary indications)
- Postural drainage positioning
- Manual techniques for airway clearance
- Suctioning for airway clearance

Reprinted with permission from Frownfelter D, Dean E, eds, *Cardiovascular and Pulmonary Physical Therapy Evidence and Practice.* 4th ed, Dean E, Optimizing outcomes: relating interventions to an individual's needs, 247-261, Copyright Elsevier 2006.

airway clearance) are likely to improve exercise capacity and therefore participation in the therapeutic program.

Positioning

Position changes can have a significant impact on the gas exchange capability in the individual with a pulmonary impairment. When positioning is used as an intervention, the therapist identifies the causes of hypoxemia (hypoventilation, diffusion, shunt, and V/Q inequality) and determines the physiology imposed by therapeutic changes in position.[1,12,203-205] Prescriptive body positioning may improve the mechanics of breathing in hypoventilation, V/Q matching and may improve the pressure and flow of the pulmonary circulation and lymphatic circulation.[1,10,206] Positioning is also used in postural drainage to allow gravity assistance in mobilizing secretions.[6,207,208]

Gravity has an impact on perfusion since blood tends to flow most easily toward the dependent position.[5] Ventilation is also influenced by gravity as the pleural pressure is most negative in the uppermost region of the lung.[5] Negative intrapleural pressure causes alveoli to become distended and air enters the area of least resistance.[10] Therefore, the resting volume is greatest in the uppermost portions of the lung. For example, if an individual is left side-lying for a prolonged period, the air volume will be best in the right lung. The open airways allow gravity to work to drain mucous from bronchopulmonary segments.[209] Areas of atelectasis may open if present in the right lung.

Bronchial (Postural) Drainage

In accordance to bronchopulmonary anatomy and the physiology of body positioning, each lung segment can be positioned optimally to against gravity. This may maximize ventilation to that lung segment and drain secretions with the help of gravity (Table 9-11 and Figure 9-10).[207]

Positioning to Decrease the Work of Breathing

Several positions can assist in reducing the work of breathing, including leaning against a wall between distances walked or part way up the stairs as well as forward leaning while on a walker; sitting with hands on knees; or standing or sitting with arms resting on a table, countertop, or bench.[210]

TABLE 9-11. CONTRAINDICATIONS/PRECAUTIONS FOR POSTURAL DRAINAGE[6,194]

CONTRAINDICATIONS/PRECAUTIONS FOR POSTURAL DRAINAGE	CONTRAINDICATIONS/PRECAUTIONS FOR TRENDELENBURG POSITION (HEAD DOWN POSITION)
• Intracranial pressure (ICP) > 20 mmHg: ask for clearance before changing positioning • Head and neck injuries that are not stabilized or recent spine surgery • Acute untreated pneumothorax • Active hemorrhage: watch risk of bleeding • Empyema: pus in the pleural cavity • Bronchopleural fistula • 48 hours post-renal transplant: must lay on surgical side • Pulmonary edema with CHF • Large pleural effusion: you may compress the heart excessively in some positions • Pulmonary embolism: watch coagulation status/clots • Rib fracture/stress fracture with osteoporosis history: consult physician with osteoporosis • Surgical wound or healing issues	Avoid Trendelenburg in the following situations. • If ICP increases are to be avoided (such as after eye surgery) • Uncontrolled hypertension • Distended abdomen (may be present with a shunt) • Esophageal surgery • Hemoptysis 20 to surgery or lung carcinoma • Uncontrolled aspiration • Acute CHF • Recent food consumption (meal or stomach tube feeding within 30 min) • Postoperative craniotomy

These positions can conserve energy and enhance the use of accessory muscle breathing and may increase diaphragmatic excursion.[211] In people with chronic obstructive diseases, the diaphragm becomes flattened because of the continual air trapping and increased anterior-posterior chest wall diameter. The diaphragm loses its contractile efficiency.[212] The forward leaning position causes the abdominal contents to move up into the thoracic region placing the diaphragm into a more responsive position to contract, allowing better ventilation to occur.[211]

Airway Clearance Techniques

Over-production of goblet cell and mucus gland secretions may be the result of pulmonary disorders like chronic bronchitis, asthma, bronchiectasis, and CF.[213] Pulmonary infections such as pneumonia increase WBC formation and pus, which then accumulate in the alveolar spaces.[53] Impaired mucociliary transport of normal as well as abnormal pulmonary secretions can occur most markedly in smokers but also with individuals who have had general anesthesia.[1] In smokers, the cilia are chronically slowed or altered. In patients undergoing general anesthesia, the mucociliary transport is temporarily altered. The longer the anesthesia time is, than the greater the risk for postoperative pulmonary complications.[184]

Cough

Common causes of an ineffective cough include weakness, paralysis or lack of motor control/performance, pain, sedation, or depression of the central nervous system. Cough is assessed for strength, quality, frequency, and sputum production. If the cough is not effective enough to clear secretions, alternate types of assisted coughing should be utilized. Postsurgically, pain may interfere with coughing. Increasing inspiratory volume with breath stacking and segmental breathing may be followed by pillow-splint coughing.[211] Huff coughing (Table 9-12) may be used when glottis closure and Valsalva is contraindicated.

Individuals with muscle weakness will need to use a cough-assist technique (abdominal thrust, costophrenic assist, counter-rotation assist).[138,214,215] Selection of cough-assist technique may be determined by examining the effectiveness of cough performance (peak flow cough rate) and reviewing contraindications that may exclude abdominal pressure (vena cava filters, incisions, internal bleeding) or costal pressure (rib fractures). The peak cough flow rate normally ranges from 6 to 20 L/s and will need to reach a minimum of 2.7 L/s to be minimally effective.[138,216,217] To improve cough effectiveness, the therapist will emphasize development of each of the stages of cough when teaching coughing.[215] Glottis control exercises are important for people who have dysphagia or recurring pneumonia.[52] Inspiratory volume enhancement with breath stacking is more effective when glottal control is adequate.[218,219]

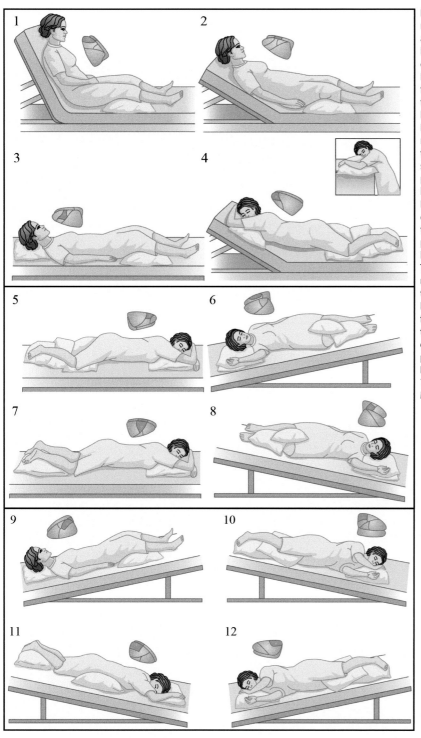

Figure 9-10. Postural drainage positions. (1) Left and right anterior apical segments of the upper lobes: in a semifowler's position, with a 45-degree trunk tilt backward. (2) Left and right posterior apical segments of the upper lobes: trunk forward lean 45 degrees. (3) Left and right anterior segments of the upper lobes: full supine lying, with the head of the bed (HOB) flat. (4) Posterior segment of the right upper lobe: left side-lying, one-quarter turn from prone with the HOB flat. (5) Posterior segment of the left upper lobe: right side-lying, one-quarter turn from prone, with the HOB the elevated 30 degrees. (6) Left and right superior (apical) segments of the lower lobes: full prone lying with the HOB flat. (7) Right middle lobe: left side-lying, one-quarter turn from supine, with the HOB in Trendelenburg position 15 degrees. (8) Lingula of the left upper lobe: right side-lying, one-quarter turn from supine, with the HOB in Trendelenburg position 15 degrees. (9) Lateral segment of the left lower lobe: full right side-lying with the HOB in Trendelenburg position 30 degrees. (10) Lateral segment of the right lower lobe: full left side-lying with the HOB in Trendelenburg position 30 degrees. (11) Left and right anterior segments of the lower lobes: full supine lying with the HOB in Trendelenburg position 30 degrees. (12) Left and right posterior segments of the lower lobes: full prone lying in Trendelenburg position 30 degrees. (Adapted from Frownfelter D, Dean E, eds. *Cardiovascular and Pulmonary Physical Therapy: Evidence and Practice.* 4th ed. St. Louis, MO: Mosby Elsevier; 2006.)

Manual Techniques

Percussion

Percussion is applied to the chest wall using cupped hands and a rhythmic striking of the chest wall directly over the involved lung segment. It can be 1-handed or 2 depending on the segment. Percussion can be performed for up to 5 minutes or longer but usually for 1 to 2 minutes or until secretions are mobilized and coughing occurs spontaneously. Hand-held plastic percussors can be used if the therapist is not effective with his or her hands. Mechanical percussors (air compression and electrical devices) are also available. The evidence describing the best rate and force of percussion is equivocal and therefore the application of percussion is individualized. Percussion is credited for releasing secretions from the bronchial walls and into the airway. It is most beneficial when combined with bronchial drainage and breathing control techniques. Contraindications and precautions are listed in Table 9-13.[207,209,220]

TABLE 9-12. SECRETION MOBILIZATION TECHNIQUES

SECRETION MOBILIZATION TECHNIQUE	DESCRIPTION
FET, also called "huff" coughing. Performed to mobilize secretions without prematurely collapsing airways.[221] • Low volume • High volume	The individual inhales deeply and then releases air through an open glottis. The air is released slowly for low-volume and quickly for high-volume huffing. Low-volume huffing occurs from deep inspiration to TV and mobilizes secretions in peripheral airways. High-volume huffing is quick and forceful and mobilizes secretions in upper airways. After breathing at low to mid-lung volumes or tidal breaths, the patient is instructed to take a mid-to-large deep breath from the diaphragm followed by a forceful expulsion of air through an open mouth, inhibiting glottis closure (huff).
Active cycle breathing	The individual is instructed in a sequence of breathing designed to alternate rest phase diaphragmatic breathing with deep lateral costal breathing and diaphragmatic breathing. Deep breathing is facilitated to encourage inspiration to different levels or volumes prior to using a low-volume huff. A 3- to 4-second pause occurs at the top of each deep inspiration. After several low-volume huffs are performed (mobilizing secretions from peripheral airways) from a position of deep inspiration, then 1 to 2 larger, more forceful high-volume huffs are used for expulsion of mucus. The technique may be performed in a variety of positions.
Autogenic drainage[222] Breathing control occurs in stages to mobilize secretions from peripheral airways to upper airways. The goal is to use air flow and intrapulmonary pressure to mobilize secretions without collapsing airways that are fragile, resulting in trapping mucous.	The technique begins with several breaths moving air from the bottom of TV and exhaling deep into ERV. Each inspiration is below normal TV levels. As mucous is felt in the peripheral airways the individual inhales using slightly larger breaths from above TV exhaling through TV into the ERV using a mid-volume breath with pauses at the top of inspiration. As secretions are felt, after several mid-volume breaths, the person takes large-volume breaths, gradually increasing the inspiratory volume into the IRV. Expiration is performed with and open glottis using an FET that gradually increase the volume and peak flow on expiration. Cough is suppressed as long as possible to avoid trapping mucus.
PEP Exhaling against resistance during the expiratory phase slows breathing, controls pressure and introduces a back pressure to keep small airways open longer increasing time for oxygenation.	The individual inhales deeply and then exhales slowly into a mask or mouthpiece. Valves releasing the expired air are under pressure. Usually low pressure is 10 to 20 cm H_2O. The person inhales a full TV followed by an inspiratory hold (3 to 4 seconds) and exhales slowly. After about 10 breaths or to tolerance, the individual is asked to perform an FET. This sequence can be repeated about 5 times for up to 20 minutes. The device can be used with bronchodilator therapies and is portable.
Flutter valve PEP[223]	The individual inhales deeply and then exhales slowly into a pipe-like device housing a metal ball. As exhaled air moves forward, the ball moves and sends a vibration down the airways to assist in loosening of mucus. This is repeated for 5 to 10 breaths until secretion are mobilized. The patient then performs a high-volume huff followed by a cough to clear the airway. This can be performed for 10 minutes or to tolerance.
Oscillatory PEP (Acapella, Smiths Medical)[223] The device combines the resistive capability of a PEP device with the vibrating capability of a Flutter valve.	The individual inhales deeply and then exhales slowly into a small plastic football-shaped device. As expired air enters the device, a magnetic system opens and closes, creating vibrations in the pulmonary airways to assist in loosening of mucus. The technique is applied in the same manner as the PEP and Flutter devices. A valve may be adjusted to change pressure and 2 sizes are available (child and adult).

ERV: expiratory reserve volume; FET, forced expiratory technique; IRV: inspiratory reserve volume; PEP, positive expiratory pressure.

Data adapted from Downs AM. Clinical application of airway clearance techniques. In: Frownfelter D, Dean E, eds. *Cardiovascular and Pulmonary Physical Therapy Evidence and Practice*. 4th ed. St. Louis, MO: Mosby Elsevier; 2006:341-376; Pryor JA. Physiotherapy for airway clearance in adults. *Eur Respir J*. 1999;14:1418-1424; and Wetzel JL. Management of respiratory dysfunction. In: Field-Fote EC, ed. *Spinal Cord Injury Rehabilitation*. Philadelphia, PA: F.A. Davis; 2009:337-392.

TABLE 9-13. CONTRAINDICATIONS AND PRECAUTIONS FOR PERCUSSION, VIBRATION, AND SHAKING	
• Osteoporosis	• Subcutaneous emphysema
• Osteomyelitis	• Coagulopathy
• Long-term steroid use	• Frank hemoptysis
• Rib fractures or flail chest	• Bony metastases to the ribs
• Recent epidural spinal infusion or spinal anesthesia	• Reactive airways (unable to modify with breathing control techniques)
• Compromised integumentary on the chest wall (burns, grafts, open wounds)	• Elevated intracranial pressure (ICP)
• Pain	• Tuberculosis

Data adapted from Downs AM, Bishop KL. Physical therapy associated with airway clearance dysfunction. In: DeTurk WE, Cahalin L, eds. *Cardiovascular and Pulmonary Physical Therapy: An Evidence-Based Approach.* 2nd ed. New York: McGraw-Hill Co.; 2011:499-527; Downs AM. Clinical application of airway clearance techniques. In: Frownfelter D, Dean E, eds. *Cardiovascular and Pulmonary Physical Therapy Evidence and Practice.* 4th ed. St. Louis, MO: Mosby Elsevier; 2006:341-376; and Downs AM. Physiological basis for airway clearance techniques. In: Frownfelter D, Dean E, eds. *Cardiovascular and Pulmonary Physical Therapy: Evidence and Practice.* 4th ed. St. Louis, MO: Mosby Elsevier; 2006:325-339.

Vibration

The therapist applies vibration-generating movement from the shoulders through the UEs to the hands, which are placed over the region of the thorax approximating the lung segment involved. The vibratory oscillations from the hands are transmitted onto the person's rib cage and ultimately to the airways to move secretions to where they can be more easily be coughed out or retrieved.

The maneuver is used with deep breathing and the vibrations are applied upon exhalation. It is the air movement along with the vibrations that mobilize secretions. The best frequency of the oscillations to actually move secretions is unknown and may vary with the individual. People with asthma tolerate it quite well but may need to be instructed to control exhalations in order to manage airway reactivity. The technique should be performed for 6 to 10 breaths, to tolerance or when secretions are mobilized and coughing occurs. It is usually performed after percussion and enhanced with bronchial drainage. Contraindications and precautions for vibration are listed in Table 9-13.

Suctioning

Suctioning techniques are a necessary intervention to remove abnormal pulmonary secretions and maintain optimum ventilation and oxygenation in patients who are unable to clear these secretions independently. The person performing this technique should be competent in assessing the need for suction.[59] The decision to perform this procedure should be based on clinical signs and symptoms and review of contraindications and should not be undertaken as a matter of routine.[59] Suctioning should take no longer than 10 to 15 seconds. Before suctioning the individual is encouraged to take deep breaths, either actively or passively through artificial means. Susceptibility to hypoxemia should be monitored for episodes of bradycardia, desaturation, and/or hypotension. Indications and complications for suctioning are presented in Table 9-14.

Breathing Control Maneuvers and Breathing Retraining

The purpose of any breathing exercise is primarily to increase lung volume, redistribute ventilation, and therefore affect gas exchange. Breathing control can help in normalizing RR and breathing pattern to decrease the work of breathing and minimize dyspnea. Some techniques are also used to assist in managing pain.[224] The entire respiratory care program is progressed in a logical sequence. It is critically important to provide airway clearance and pain reduction strategies before initiating chest mobilization and breathing retraining.[225] This approach will optimize results for session.

Breathing Exercises to Improve Lung Volume and Gas Distribution

Breathing exercises begin with subtle changes in position that may challenge the respiratory muscles to become more active. Typically a position supine with the head of bed elevated 15 to 30 degrees allows the diaphragm to move freely.[186,226] The therapist can offer active assistance and manual cues to the diaphragm by placing one hand over the epigastric region at the costophrenic angle opposite ribs 6 through 8.[186] At the end of expiration the therapist applies a "squeeze" and lifts the diaphragm slightly higher in the thoracic cavity before asking the individual to inhale. This improves the length tension and active contraction of the diaphragm. Active contraction of the diaphragm may be improved by asking the individual to "sniff" as he or she inhales.[210] Breath stacking is used to increase the inspiratory volume with each sniff or inspiratory effort. Two to 3 breaths are taken on top of the initial breath to increase chest wall expansion and inspiratory volume. As the individual gains control and begins deep breathing on his or her own, maximal inspiratory hold maneuvers are included. The individual inhales slowly and deeply through the nose to total lung capacity and holds this volume for 2 to 3 seconds.

| TABLE 9-14. INDICATIONS AND COMPLICATIONS FOR SUCTIONING ||
INDICATIONS FOR SUCTIONING	COMPLICATIONS FOR SUCTIONING
<ul><li>Altered hemodynamics</li><li>Artificial ventilation patients with increased airway pressures, adventitious breath sounds, and reduced oxygen saturation</li><li>Change of color (cyanosis, pallor)</li><li>Copious, retained secretions in people who cannot cough effectively</li><li>Deteriorating arterial blood gas values or SaO_2</li><li>Diminished/absent breath sounds on auscultation</li><li>For assessing airway patency, cough reflex stimulation, and sputum specimen</li><li>Individuals with feelings of secretions in the chest</li><li>Paradoxical chest movement</li><li>Preset TV on the ventilator not being delivered</li><li>Secretions in artificial airways</li><li>Tachypnea</li></ul>	<ul><li>Apnea, laryngospasm, bronchospasm</li><li>Atelectasis</li><li>Elevated intracranial pressure</li><li>Hypoxemia with suctioning</li><li>Mechanical trauma</li><li>Pathogens/contamination</li><li>Vasovagal response causing cardiac arrhythmias</li></ul>

Adapted from Ciesla ND, Kuramoto JD. Physical therapy associated with respiratory failure. In: DeTurk WE, Cahalin LP, eds. *Cardiovascular and Pulmonary Physical Therapy: An Evidence-Based Approach.* 2nd ed. New York: McGraw-Hill; 2011:585-642.

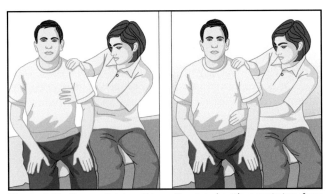

Figure 9-11. Segmental breathing. (Reprinted with permission from Frownfelter D, Dean E, eds. *Cardiovascular and Pulmonary Physical Therapy: Evidence and Practice.* 4th ed. St. Louis, MO: Mosby Elsevier; 2006.)

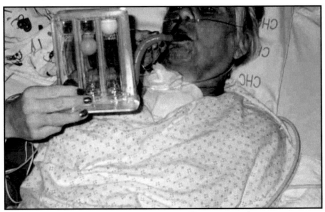

Figure 9-12. Incentive spirometry using a flow-oriented spirometer.

As the individual breathes the therapist notes areas of chest expansion and decides which areas are not expanding well and why, such as when the respiratory muscles are weak and unable to offer adequate force. Facilitation is then applied. Positioning, quick stretch, tapping, and tactile cues can be applied to segmental muscles (intercostals) and accessory muscles (pectorals, serratus anterior, latissimus dorsi and neck accessories). Lateral costal expansion exercises work well to facilitate the intercostals muscles and encourage expansion of the lower lobes.

If the therapist decides that pain is limiting chest wall expansion and inhibiting the respiratory muscles, then different breathing techniques are offered. The session begins by finding a comfortable position for the individual. The incision may need to be supported with a pillow or layers of towels. The person is taught to hold the pillow firmly but not forcefully over the incision. The level of pressure should be maintained as the person inhales. Initially, small to moderate breath sizes are used. The therapist should check the incision for drainage or stress to the skin before asking for deeper breathing.

Areas that are not expanding well can be facilitated with segmental breathing (Figure 9-11). During segmental breathing the therapist uses specific positioning to maximize ventilation to the affected lung segment, while using tactile stimulation over that affected segment with cues for PI_{max} (Figure 9-12). Stretch may or may not be used on end expiration.

Incentive spirometry uses a hand-held device with a mouth piece attached to a closed chamber with balls or a disc that rises as flow or volume is increased. The person is asked to exhale fully then inhale maximally while a disc or ball rises within the spirometer cylinder (see Figure 9-12). The disc/ball rises to the measured maximal lung volume achieved. The maneuver is performed for 10 repetitions, followed by a huff/forced exhalation technique or cough. The individual is instructed to repeat this hourly while awake. There is no evidence that incentive spirometry will reduce postoperative complications in individuals with cardiac and upper abdominal surgeries.[227] Incentive spirometry may still be effective in providing feedback for teaching deep breathing and for individuals who are not able to routinely ambulate or transfer bed to chair.[228]

Breathing Exercises to Decrease the Work of Breathing and Dyspnea

- PLB: The individual expires passively through pursed (almost closed) lips. This creates a back pressure or positive pressure, preventing premature alveolar collapse. This may maximize O_2 distribution and help to reduce dyspnea. PLB decreases air trapping and reduces breathlessness by lengthening the time of expiration and total respiratory cycle time.[198,229] There is little evidence to suggest incorporating diaphragmatic breathing during activity improves dyspnea in people with COPD and may actually cause dyssynchronous breathing.[198]

- Paced breathing: Low-frequency breathing is performed with activity to normalize the inspiratory/expiratory ratio. Normal breathing ratio is 2/4. With activity such as walking, a patient is asked to inhale to a count of 2 while taking 2 steps, then exhale to a count of 4 while taking 4 steps. This can be translated to other activities.

- Exhalation with activity: Movement occurs only during exhalation. Individuals who have contraindications to breath holding or Valsalva are taught to "exhale on effort" to avoid fluctuations in BP.[210]

- Coordinated breathing: The individual is instructed to exhale when flexing the trunk or reaching down to tie shoes, pick up an object from the floor or bending down to place dishes in a dishwasher. During trunk extension and reaching overhead, the person is instructed to inspire. In this way the chest wall mobility assists in expanding the chest for inspiration or compressing the abdominal contents for expiration. Breathing is more efficient and tasks are easier to accomplish.[186]

Techniques to Conserve Energy and Decrease the Work of Breathing

Activities of daily living (ADL) alone can cause dyspnea during gas-exchange impairment. Specific tasks related to self-care, home management, and community functions that increase dyspnea level are modified to minimize demands for O_2. Energy conservation techniques can include the following:

- The use of adaptive equipment such as the following: use a rolling walker during ambulation to aid in balance, decrease accessory muscle breathing and decrease the work of the posture musculature; use a shower/tub chair to sit on rather than standing during shower time; use a reacher to pick up things on the floor rather than bending forward.

- Planning and preparing activities such as the following: establish a routine; schedule and organize the day; prioritize tasks and eliminate unnecessary ones; organize the work area and avoid lifting overhead; adjust work height and avoid sustained positions.

- Pacing and breathing strategies with all activities; utilization of aforementioned breathing exercises to decrease the work of breathing with ADL and instrumental ADL (IADL); pacing activities throughout the day; taking rest in-between activities, such as stopping half way up a flight of stairs to rest; avoid Valsalva with movement and utilization of the exhalation during movement technique.

- Relaxation techniques: Jacobson's progressive relaxation exercise,[186] Benson's relaxation response,[230] imagery, biofeedback,[130,138] yoga, meditation, hypnosis, massage, and chest wall mobilization.[186]

Therapeutic Exercise

Pulmonary rehabilitation guidelines recommend strength training, aerobic training, unsupported UE endurance training, and education to improve health-related quality of life and decreased hospitalizations for people with COPD.[231,232] LE exercise training that is high intensity (60% to 80% VO_2 peak) will lead to greater physiologic improvements than exercise that is lower in intensity.[233,234] Clinical benefits are possible with both low- and high-intensity aerobic exercise.[199,231,235] Components of an exercise prescription to improve cardiorespiratory fitness follows the FITT principle (Frequency, Intensity, Time, and Type)[86]:

- Frequency: 3 to 5 times per week

- Intensity: 60% VO_2 peak or may be guided by SpO_2 ≥90% with RPD = 4/10 to 6/10

- Time: 20 to 60 minutes

- Type: activities that exercise large muscle groups in continuous repetitive movement (bike, treadmill [TM], corridor walking). Include unsupported UE endurance exercise.[236]

- Progression: increase intensity and/or time slowly over a number of weeks. Initially time is increased using moderate intensity 50% to 60% VO_2 peak to encourage compliance.[231,232,235] Begin to increase intensity using an interval training strategy.[237] Interval training can help avoid limitations due to dynamic hyperinflation.[238] A minimum of 20 sessions at least 3 times per week is necessary.

Aerobic exercise training programs are initiated and the prescription adjusted according to physiological responses and symptoms presented Any contraindications to exercise or criteria suggesting termination of activity may indicate medical instability.[86] Symptoms of fatigue or dyspnea are monitored and kept between 4/10 and 6/10 on the Borg scale to arrive at a safe and effective training intensity.[232] The therapist will periodically reexamine the aerobic capacity using a formal test (6MWT or GXT) to adjust the prescription.

While the conditioning phase of formal exercise is typically 20 to 30 minutes of activity at 50% to 85% of VO_2 peak, very unfit or critically ill individuals may benefit from shorter and/or more frequent periods of exercise initially.[239] The patient in the intensive care unit may tolerate only 5 minutes of exercise activity at a time. Also, because of monitoring or supportive equipment, the exercise sessions may include: bed exercises, transfer training, marching in place, and seated restorator pedaling. Monitoring of exercise sessions is ongoing and reexamination occurs each visit. The response of HR, RR, RPE, BP, lung auscultation, and mentation should be carefully observed and documented. Therapeutic sessions are provided using a "response-dependent" doseage.[184,185]

Strength training should be combined with aerobic exercise training to improve overall functional capacity.[191] The individual performs 50% to 85% of a 1-repetition maximum (1 RM) for 6 to 12 repetitions for 2 to 4 sets.[153] Stability muscle groups are emphasized (gluteus maximus, quadriceps, hamstrings, abductors, calf) as well as UE muscles (serratus, latissimus, pectoralis major, triceps, biceps). About 8 to 10 groups are included in resistive training at least 2 days per week.[86] Stair ambulation is related to LE power.[164] Additionally, balance deficits and fall risk are increased in patients with COPD and need to be addressed in the therapeutic exercise program.[165,166]

Education

Education is now integral to all comprehensive pulmonary rehabilitation programs. It leads to a better understanding of the physical and psychological changes that occur with pulmonary illness, and helps individuals and their families explore ways to cope with those changes.[240] Self-management and adherence to the treatment plan improves through formal instruction. Education can be provided in small groups or on an individual basis, depending on the needs of the person, the site, the resources, and the design of the physical therapy program. The educational needs of the pulmonary-impaired patient are determined at the initial examination and are reassessed during the therapy. Topics frequently incorporated into education programs are airway clearance, breathing strategies, benefits of exercise, energy conservation, self-monitoring, symptom recognition, and proper use of medications (including supplemental O_2). The importance of using breathing strategies, supplemental O_2 or assistive devices for ambulation is carried over during functional training to improve self-care, home management, work-related tasks, and community roles.

REFERENCES

1. Dean E. Body positioning. In: Frownfelter D, Dean E, eds. *Cardiovascular and Pulmonary Physical Therapy: Evidence and Practice.* 4th ed. St. Louis, MO: Mosby Elsevier; 2006:307-324.
2. Widmaier EP, Raff H, Strang KT. *Vander's Human Physiology. The Mechanisms of Body Function.* 11th ed. New York: McGraw Hill Company; 2008.
3. Wasserman K, Hansen JE, Sue DY, String WW. *Principles of Exercise Testing and Interpretation.* 4th ed. Philadelphia: Lippincott, Williams & Wilkins; 2004.
4. Dean E. Cardiopulmonary anatomy. In: Frownfelter D, Dean E, eds. *Cardiovascular and Pulmonary Physical Therapy: Evidence and Practice.* 4th ed. St. Louis, MO: Mosby Elsevier; 2006:53-72.
5. Dean E. Cardiopulmonary physiology. In: Frownfelter D, Dean E, eds. *Cardiovascular and Pulmonary Physical Therapy: Evidence and Practice.* 4th ed. St. Louis, MO: Mosby Elsevier; 2006.
6. Downs AM, Bishop KL. Physical therapy associated with airway clearance dysfunction. In: DeTurk WE, Cahalin L, eds. *Cardiovascular and Pulmonary Physical Therapy: An Evidence-Based Approach.* 2nd ed. New York: McGraw-Hill Co.; 2011:499-527.
7. Zadai CC. *Pulmonary Management in Physical Therapy.* New York: Churchill Livingston, Inc; 1992.
8. McArdle WD, Katch FI and Katch VL. The pulmonary system and exercise. In: *Essentials of Exercise Physiology.* 3rd ed. New York: Lippincott, Williams & Wilkins; 2005.
9. Marino PL, Sutin KM. Oximetry and capnography. In: Marino PL, Sutin KM, eds. *The ICU Book.* 3rd ed. Philadelphia: Lippincott, Williams & Wilkins; 2007:385-402.
10. West JB. *Respiratory Physiology: The Essentials.* 8th ed. Baltimore, MD: Lippincott, Williams & Wilkins; 2008.
11. Peel C. The cardiopulmonary system and movement dysfunction. *Phys Ther.* 1996;76:448-455.
12. Pulmonary anatomy and pulmonary therapy. In: Rothstein JM, Roy SH, Wolf SL, eds. *The Rehabilitation Specialist's Handbook.* 3rd ed. Philadelphia, PA: F.A. Davis; 2005.
13. Au VW, Jones DN, Slavotinek JP. Pulmonary hypertension secondary to left-sided heart disease: a cause for ventilation-perfusion mismatch mimicking pulmonary embolism. *Br J Radiol.* 2001;74:86-88.
14. Protas EJ. The aging patient. In: Frownfelter D, Dean E, eds. *Cardiovascular and Pulmonary Physical Therapy: Evidence and Practice.* 4th ed. St. Louis, MO: Mosby Elsevier; 2006: 685-691.
15. Cardus J, Burgos F, Diaz O, et al. Increase in pulmonary ventilation-perfusion inequality with age in healthy individuals. *Am J Respir Crit Care Med.* 1997;156(2):648-653.
16. National Heart, Lung, and Blood Institute. *Morbidity & Mortality: 2009 Chart Book On Cardiovascular, Lung And Blood Diseases.* U.S. Department of Health and Human Services: National Institute of Health; 2009.
17. Minino AM, Xu J, Kochanek KD. National Vital Statistics Reports. Deaths: Preliminary Data, 2008. Hyattsville, MD: National Center for Health Statistics; 2010:1-71.
18. American Lung Association. Pneumonia fact sheet. http://www.lung.org/lung-disease/influenza/in-depth-resources/pneumonia-fact-sheet.html. Accessed June 6, 2014.
19. Robinson KA, Baughman W, Rothrock G, et al. Epidemiology of invasive streptococcus pneumoniae infections in the United States, 1995-1998: opportunities for prevention in the conjugate vaccine era. *JAMA.* 2001;285(13):1729-1735.
20. Wheeler AP, Bernard GR. Acute lung injury and acute respiratory distress syndrome: a clinical review. *Lancet.* 2007;369:1553-1565.
21. Ikeda B, Goodman CC. The respiratory system. In: Goodman CC, Fuller KS, eds. *Pathology Implications for Physical Therapists.* 3rd ed. St. Louis, MO: Saunders Elsevier; 2009:742-827.
22. Centers for Disease Control and Prevention. Compressed Mortality File: Years 1968-1978 with ICD-8 Codes, 1979-1998 with ICD-9 Codes and 1999-2010 with ICD-10 Codes. *CDC WONDER.* http://wonder.cdc.gov/wonder/help/cmf.html. Accessed February 1, 2011.

23. Acute respiratory distress syndrome. American Lung Association. Washington, DC. 2010. http://www.lungusa.org/lung-disease/acute-respiratory-distress-syndrome. Accessed February 1, 2011.

24. George RB, Light RW, Matthay MA, Matthay RA. *Chest Medicine: Essentials of Pulmonary and Critical Care Medicine.* 3rd ed. Baltimore: Williams & Wilkins; 1995.

25. Hillegass E, Clough P. Restrictive lung dysfunction. In: Hillegass EA, ed. *Essentials of Cardiopulmonary Physical Therapy.* 3rd ed. St. Louis, MO: Elsevier Saunders; 2011:137-200.

26. Hurd S. The impact of COPD on lung health worldwide. *Chest.* 2000;117:1S-4S.

27. American Lung Association. Washington, DC. 2010. COPD. http://www.lungusa.org/lung-disease/copd/. Accessed February 1, 2011.

28. Popovic JR, Kozak LJ. National hospital discharge survey: annual summary, 1998. *Vital Health Stat 13.* 2000;148:1-194.

29. U.S. Department of Health and Human Services. *The Health Consequences of Smoking: A Report of the Surgeon General.* Atlanta, GA: U.S. Department of Health and Human Services, Centers for Disease Control and Prevention, National Center for Chronic Disease Prevention and Health Promotion, Office on Smoking and Health; 2004. http://www.cdc.gov/tobacco/data_statistics/sgr/2004. Accessed February 2, 2011.

30. Centers for Disease Control and Prevention (CDC). Annual smoking-attributable mortality, years of potential life lost, and productivity losses—United States, 1997-2001. *MMWR Morb Mortal Wkly Rep.* 2005;54:625-628.

31. American Cancer Society. Cancer facts and figures 2010. Atlanta: American Cancer Society; 2010.

32. Summary Health Statistics For U.S. Adults: National Health Interview Survey, 2008. U.S. Department of Health and Human Services, Centers for Disease Control and Prevention, and National Center for Health Statistics. 2009. http://www.cdc.gov/nchs/data/series/sr_10/sr10_242.pdf. Accessed February 3, 2011.

33. Centers for Disease Control and Prevention: National Center for Health Statistics, National Health Interview Survey Raw Data, 2009. Analysis by the American Lung Association Research and Program Services Division using SPSS and SUDAAN software.

34. American Lung Association. Asthma in adults fact sheet. 2010. http://www.lungusa.org/lung-disease/asthma/resources/facts-and-figures/asthma-in-adults.html. Accessed February 3, 2011.

35. Grosse SD, Boyle CA, Botkin JR. Newborn screening for cystic fibrosis: evaluation of benefits and risks and recommendations for state newborn screening programs. *MMWR Recomm Rep.* 2004;53(RR-13):1-36.

36. Cystic Fibrosis Foundation. Patient Registry 2006 Annual Report. Bethesda, MD: Cystic Fibrosis Foundation; 2008. http://www.cff.org/UploadedFiles/research/ClinicalResearch/2006%20Patient%20Registry%20Report.pdf. Accessed June 6, 2014.

37. Nixon PA, Orenstein DM, Kelsey SF, Doershuk CF. The prognostic value of exercise testing in patients with cystic fibrosis. *N Engl J Med.* 1992;327:1785-1788.

38. American Lung Association. Bronchiectasis fact sheet. January 2005. http://copd.about.com/od/bronchiectasis/a/bronchiectasis.htm. Accessed February 5, 2011.

39. Hillegass EA, Cahalin L. Cardiac muscle dysfunction and failure. In: Hillegass EA, ed. *Essentials of Cardiopulmonary Physical Therapy.* 3rd ed. St. Louis, MO: Elsevier Saunders; 2011:84-135.

40. Agency for Healthcare Research and Quality. National Health Quality Report 2003. U.S. Dept. of Health and Human Services. Rockville, MD: AHRQ.

41. Dalen JE, Alpert JS. Natural history of pulmonary embolism. *Prog Cardiovasc Dis.* 1975;17(14):259-270.

42. Anderson FA Jr, Wheeler HB, Goldberg RJ, et al. A population-based perspective of the hospital incidence and case-fatality rates of deep vein thrombosis and pulmonary embolism. The Worcester DVT Study. *Arch Intern Med.* 1991;151(5):933-938.

43. Goldhaber SZ, Visani L, De Rosa M. Acute pulmonary embolism: clinical outcomes in the International Cooperative Pulmonary Embolism Registry (ICOPER). *Lancet.* 1999;353(9162):1386-1389.

44. Kucher N, Rossi E, De Rosa M, Goldhaber SZ. Massive pulmonary embolism. *Circulation.* 2006;113(4):577-582.

45. American Physical Therapy Association. Guide to Physical Therapist Practice. 2nd ed. Alexandria, VA: American Physical Therapy Association; 2003.

46. Merriam-Webster Unabridged Dictionary. http://www.merriam-webster.com/dictionary/inflammation. Accessed February 6, 2011.

47. Porth CM. Inflammation and healing. Chapter 20. In: Porth CM, ed. *Pathophysiology: Concepts of Altered Health States.* 7th ed. Philadelphia: Lippincott, Williams & Wilkins; 2005.

48. Goodman CC. Injury, inflammation and healing. In: Goodman CC, Fuller KS, eds. *Pathology Implications for the Physical Therapist.* 3rd ed. St. Louis, MO: Saunders Elsevier; 2009:197-240.

49. Porth CM. Respiratory tract infections, neoplasms and childhood disorders. Chapter 30. In: Porth CM, ed. *Pathophysiology: Concepts of Altered Health States.* 7th ed. Philadelphia, PA: Lippincott, Williams & Wilkins; 2005.

50. Irwin SC, Techlin JS. *Cardiopulmonary Physical Therapy: A Guide To Clinical Practice.* 4th ed. St. Louis, MO: Mosby; 2004.

51. Rodriguez-Rosin R, Roca J. Update '96 on pulmonary gas exchange pathophysiology in pneumonia. *Semin Respir Infect.* 1996;11(1):3-12.

52. Zablotny C. Evaluation and management of swallowing dysfunction. In: Montgomery J, ed. *Clinics in Physical Therapy Physical Therapy for Traumatic Brain Injury.* New York: Churchill Livingstone; 1995:99-115.

53. Porth CM. Disorders of ventilation and gas exchange. In: Porth CM, ed. *Pathophysiology: Concepts of Altered Health States.* 7th ed. Philadelphia, PA: Lippincott, Williams & Wilkins; 2005:689-724.

54. Nowakowski JF. Acute alveolar edema. *Emergency Medicine Clinics of North America.* 1983;1(2):313-343.

55. Tomashefski JFJ. Pulmonary pathology of acute respiratory distress syndrome. *Clinics in Chest Medicine.* 2000;21(3):435-466.

56. Lechin AE, Varon J. Adult respiratory distress syndrome (ARDS): the basics. *J Emerg Med.* 1994;12:63-68.

57. Wells CL. Pulmonary pathology. In: DeTurk WE, Cahalin L, eds. *Cardiovascular and Pulmonary Physical Therapy: An Evidence-Based Approach.* 2nd ed. New York: McGraw-Hill; 2011:165-208.

58. Hall J, Schmidt G, Wood I. Principles of critical care for the patient with respiratory failure. In: Murray J, Nadel J, eds. Textbook of Respiratory Medicine. 2nd ed. Philadelphia, PA: Saunders; 1994:2575.

59. Ciesla ND, Kuramoto JD. Physical therapy associated with respiratory failure. In: DeTurk WE, Cahalin LP, eds. *Cardiovascular and Pulmonary Physical Therapy: An Evidence-Based Approach.* 2nd ed. New York: McGraw-Hill; 2011:585-642.

60. Riddle DL, Wells PS. Diagnosis of lower-extremity deep vein thrombosis in outpatients. *Phys Ther.* 2004;84:729-735.

61. Wells PS, Andersen DR, Bormanis J, et al. Value of assessment of pretest probability of deep-vein thrombosis in clinical management. *Lancet.* 1997;350:1795-1798.

62. Hergenroeder AL. Implementation of a competency-based assessment for interpretation of laboratory values. *Acute Care Perspectives.* 2006;15(1):7-15.

63. Pauwels RA, Buist AS, Calverley PM, Jenkins CR, Hurd SS. Global strategy for the diagnosis, management, and prevention of chronic obstructive pulmonary disease. NHLBI/WHO Global Intiative for Chronic Obstructive Lung Disease (GOLD) Workshop summary. *Am J Respir Crit Care Med.* 2001;163(5):1256-1376.

64. Celli BR, Snider GL, Heffner J, et al. Standards for the diagnosis and care of patients with chronic obstructive pulmonary disease. *Am J Respir Crit Care Med.* 1995;152:S77-S120.

65. Gurney J. Pathophysiology of obstructive airways disease. *Radiologic Clin North Am.* 1998;36(1):15-27.

66. Dias KJ, Collins S. A systematic evaluation of endurance impairments: the reversible and irreversible components. Proceedings of the APTA Combined Sections Meeting 2010; San Diego, CA; 2010.

67. Decramer M, Lacquet LM, Fagard R, Rogiers P. Corticosteroids contribute to muscle weakness in chronic airflow obstruction. *Am J Respir Crit Care Med.* 1994;150(1):11-16.

68. Garritan S. Chronic obstructive pulmonary diseases. In: Hillegass EA, ed. *Essentials of Cardipulmonary Physical Therapy.* 3rd ed. St. Louis, MO: Elsevier Saunders; 2001:257-284.

69. Maddox L, Schwartz DA. The pathophysiology of asthma. *Ann Rev Med.* 2002;53:477-498.

70. Kaplan TA. Exercise challenge for exercise-induced bronchospasm: confirming presence, evaluating control. *Phys Sports Med.* 1995;23(8):47-57.

71. Storms WW. Review of exercise-induced asthma. *Med Sci Sports Exerc.* 2003;35(9):1464-1470.

72. Wong DL, Hockenberry-Eaton M, Wilson D, Winkelstein ML, Schwartz P. *Wong's Essentials of Pediatric Nursing.* 6th ed. St. Louis, MO: Mosby Inc; 2001.

73. Regnis JA, Donnelly PM, Robinson M, Alison JA, Bye PTP. Ventilatory mechanics at rest and during exercise in patients with cystic fibrosis. *Am J Respir Crit Care Med.* 1996;154:418-425.

74. Troosters T, Langer D, Vrijesen B, et al. Skeletal muscle weakness, exercise tolerance and physical activity in adults with cystic fibrosis. *Eur Respir J.* 2009;33:99-106.

75. Selvadurai HC, McKay KO, Blimkie CJ, Cooper PJ, Mellis CM, Van Asperen PP. The Relationship between genotype and exercise tolerance in children with cystic fibrosis. *Am J Respir Crit Care Med.* 2002;165(6):762-765.

76. Marcotte JE, Canny GJ, Grisdale R, et al. Effects of nutritional status on exercise performance in advanced cystic fibrosis. *Chest.* 1986;90(3):375-379.

77. Pulmonary assessment. In: Brannon FJ, Foley MW, Starr JA, Saul LM, eds. *Cardiopulmonary Rehabilitation: Basic Theory and Application.* 3rd ed. Philadelphia, PA: F.A. Davis; 1998.

78. American Thoracic Society. Standardization of spirometry, 1994 update. *Am J Respir Crit Care Med.* 1995;152:1107-1136.

79. ATS Committee on Proficiency Standards for Clinical Pulmonary Function Laboratories. ATS statement: guidelines for the six-minute walk test. *Am J Respir Crit Care Med.* 2002;166(1):111-117.

80. American Thoracic Society. Lung function testing: selection of reference values and interpretative strategies. *Am Rev Respir Dis.* 1991;144(5):1202-1218.

81. American Thoracic Society/European Respiratory Society. ATS/ERS statement on respiratory muscle testing. *Am J Respir Crit Care Med.* 2002;166:518-624.

82. Black LF, Hyatt RE. Maximal respiratory pressures: normal values and relationship to age and sex. *Am Rev Respir Dis.* 1969;99:696-702.

83. Cherniak RM, Rabner MD. Normal standards for ventilatory function using an automated wedge spirometer. *Am Rev Respir Dis.* 1972;106:38.

84. Knudson RJ, Slatin RC, Lebowitz MD, Burrows B. The maximal expiratory flow volume curve normal standards variability and effects of age. *Am Rev Respir Dis.* 1976;113:587-600.

85. Wohl MEB, Majzoub JA. Asthma, steroids, and growth. *N Engl J Med.* 2000;343(15):1113-1114.

86. *ACSM's Guidelines for Exercise Testing and Prescription.* 8th ed. Philadelphia, PA: Wolters Kluwer Health/Lippincott Williams & Wilkins; 2010.

87. Ciesla ND, Murdock KR. Lines, tubes, catheters, and physiologic monitoring in the ICU. *Cardiopulm Phys Ther J.* 2000;11(1):16-25.

88. Cahalin LP. Pulmonary evaluation. Chapter 9. In: DeTurk WE, Cahalin LP, eds. *Cardiovascular and Pulmonary Physical Therapy: An Evidence-Based Approach.* 2nd ed. New York: McGraw-Hill; 2004:221-269.

89. Hillegass EA. Examination and assessment procedures. In: Hillegass EA, ed. *Essentials of Cardiopulmonary Physical Therapy.* 3rd ed. St. Louis, MO: Elsevier 2011:534-567.

90. Jones PW, Quirk FH, Baveystock CM, Littlejohns P. A self-complete measure of health status for chronic airflow limitation: the St. George's Respiratory Questionnaire. *Am Rev Respir Dis.* 1992;145:1321-1327.

91. Guyatt GH, Berman LB, Townsend M, Pugsley SO, Chambers LW. A measure of quality of life for clinical trials in chronic lung disease. *Thorax.* 1987;42:773-778.

92. Pashkow P. Outcomes in cardiopulmonary rehabilitation. *Phys Ther.* 1996;76(6):643-656.

93. Ware JE Jr, Gandek B. Overview of the SF-36 Health Survey and the International Quality of Life Assessment (IQOLA) project. *J Clin Epidemiol.* 1998;51(11):903-921.

94. Moorer P, Suurmeijer ThP, Foets M, Molenaar IW. Psychometric properties of the RAND-36 among three chronic disease (multiple sclerosis, rheumatic diseases and COPD) in the Netherlands. *Qual Life Res.* 2001;10(7):637-645.

95. Glaab T, Vogelmeier C, Buhl R. Outcome measures in chronic obstructive pulmonary disease (COPD): strengths and limitations. *Respir Res.* 2010;11:79.

96. Mahler DA, Weinberg DH, Wells CK, Feinstein AR. The measurement of dyspnea: contents, interobserver agreement, and physiologic correlates of two new clinical indexes. *Chest.* 1984;85:751-758.

97. Darbee JC, Ohtake PJ. Outcome measures in cardiopulmonary physical therapy: medical research council (MRC) dyspnea scale. *Cardiopulm Phys Ther J.* 2006;17(1):29-37.

98. Cassola M, MacNee W, Martinez FJ, et al. American Thoracic Society/European Respiratory Society Task Force on outcomes of COPD: outcomes for COPD pharmacological trials: from lung function to biomarkers. *Eur Respir J.* 2008;31(2):416-469.

99. Borg GA. Psychophysical bases of perceived exertion. *Med Sci Sports Exerc.* 1982;14:377-381.

100. Lamping DL, Schroter S, Marquis P, Marrel A, Suprat-Lomon I, Sagnier PP. The community-acquired pneumonia symptom questionnaire: a new patient-based outcome measure to evaluate symptoms in patients with community acquired pneumonia. *Chest.* 2002;122(3):920-929.

101. Tu SP, McDonell MB, Spertus JA, Steele BG, Fihn SD. A new self-administered questionnaire to monitor health-related quality of life in patients with COPD. *Chest.* 1997;112:614-622.

102. Fan VS, Curtis JR, Tu SP, McDonell MB, Fihn SD. Using quality of life to predict hospitalization and mortality in patients with obstructive lung diseases. *Chest.* 2002;122:429-436.

103. Kaplan RM, Atkins CJ, Timms R. Validity of a quality of well-being scale as an outcome measure in chronic obstructive pulmonary disease. *J Chronic Dis.* 1984;37:85-95.

104. Orenstein DM, Nixon PA, Ross EA, Kaplan RM. The quality of well-being in cystic fibrosis. *Chest.* 1989;95:344-347.

105. Dean E. Optimizing outcomes: relating interventions to an individual's needs. In: Frownfelter D, Dean E, eds. *Cardiovascular and Pulmonary Physical Therapy Evidence and Practice.* 4th ed. St. Louis, MO: Mosby Elsevier; 2006:247-261.

106. Celli BR, Cote CG, Marin JM, et al. The body-mass index, airflow obstruction, dyspnea, and exercise capacity index in chronic obstructive pulmonary disease. *N Engl J Med.* 2004;350:1005-1012.

107. Butler SM. Clinical assessment of the cardiopulmonary system. In: Frownfelter D, Dean E, eds. *Cardiovascular and Pulmonary Physical Therapy: Evidence and Practice.* 4th ed. St. Louis, MO: Mosby Elsevier; 2006.

108. Boissonnault WG. *Examination in Physical Therapy Practice: Screening for Medical Disease.* 2nd ed. Philadelphia, PA: Churchill Livingstone Inc; 1995.

109. Dodd JW, Getov SV, Jones PW. Cognitive function in COPD. *Eur Respir J.* 2010;35(4):913-922.

110. Folstein MF, Folstein SE, McHugh PR. "Mini-mental state". A practical method for grading the cognitive state of patients for the clinician. *J Psychiatr Res.* 1975;12(3):189-198.

111. Ashendorf L, Jefferson AL, O'Connor MK, Chaisson C, Green RC, Stern RA. Trail Making Test errors in normal aging, mild cognitive impairment, and dementia. *Arch Clin Neuropsychol.* 2008;23(2):129-137.

112. O'Sullivan SB. Examination of motor function: motor control and motor learning. In: O'Sullivan SB, Schmitz TJ, eds. *Physical Rehabilitation.* 5th ed. Philadelphia, PA: F.A. Davis; 2007:239-242.

113. Harris J, Johansen J, Pedersen S, LaPier TK. Site of measurement and subject position affect chest excursion measurements. *Cardiopulmon Phys Ther J.* 1997;8(4):12-17.

114. LaPier TK, Cook A, Droege K, et al. Intertester and intratester reliability of chest excursion measurements in subjects without impairment. *Cardiopulmon Phys Ther J.* 2000;11(3):95-98.

115. Oatis CA. Structure and function of the bones and joints of the thoracic spine. Chapter 29. In: Oatis CA, ed. *Kinesiology: The Mechanics and Pathomechanics of Human Movement.* Philadelphia, PA: Lippincott, Williams & Wilkins; 2004:488-514.

116. Carlson B. Normal chest expansion. *Phys Ther.* 1973;53:10-14.

117. McCaffery M, Pasero C. *Pain Clinical Manual.* 2nd ed. St. Louis, MO: Mosby; 1999.

118. Herr KA, Mobily PR, Kohout FJ, Wagenaar D. Evaluation of the faces pain scale for use with the elderly. *Clin J Pain.* 1998;14(1):29-38.

119. Watchie J. Cardiopulmonary assessment. In: Watchie J, ed. *Cardiovascular and Pulmonary Physical Therapy A Clinical Manual.* 2nd ed. St. Louis, MO: Saunders Elsevier; 2010:273-297.

120. Vos PJ, van Herwaarden CL. Physical examination—percussion of the thorax. *Ned Tijdschr Geneeskd.* 1999;143(36):1812-1815.

121. Schmitz TJ. Vital signs. Chapter 4. In: O'Sullivan SB, Schmitz TJ, eds. *Physical Rehabilitation: Assessment and Treatment.* 5th ed. Philadelphia, PA: F. A. Davis; 2007:81-120.

122. Gerold K. Physical therapists' guide to the principles of mechanical ventilation. *Cardiopulmon Phys Ther J.* 1992;3:8-13.

123. Burdon JG, Juniper EF, Killian KJ, Hargreave FE, Campbell EJ. The perception of breathlessness in asthma. *Am Rev Respir Dis.* 1982;126(5):825-828.

124. Gift AG. Validation of a vertical visual analogue scale as a measure of clinical dyspnea. *Rehabil Nurs.* 1989;14(6):323-325.

125. Gift AG, Narsavage G. Validity of the numeric rating scale as a measure of dyspnea. *Am J Crit Care.* 1998;7(3):200-204.

126. Frownfelter D, Ryan J. Dyspnea: measurement and evaluation. *Cardiopulmon Phys Ther J.* 2000;11(1):7-15.

127. Bausewein C, Farquhar M, Booth S, Gysels M, Higginson IJ. Measurement of breathlessness in advanced disease: a systematic review. *Respir Med.* 2007;101:399-410.

128. Mengelkoch LJ, Martin D, Lawler J. A review of the principles of pulse oximetry and accuracy of pulse oximeter estimates during exercise. *Phys Ther.* 1994;74:40-49.

129. Dweik RA. Pulmonary function testing. eMedicine. 2004. www.emedicine.com/med/topic2972.htm. Accessed April 6, 2011.

130. Morrison SA. Biofeedback to facilitate unassisted ventilation in individuals with high-level quadriplegia. A case report. *Phys Ther.* 1988;68(9):1378-1380.

131. Brooks D, Thomas J. Interrater reliability of auscultation of breath sounds among physical therapists. *Phys Ther.* 1995;75(12):1082-1088.

132. Weitz HH, Mangione S. In defense of the stethoscope at the bedside. *Am J Med.* 2000;108:669-671.

133. Pulmonary terms and symbols. A report of the ACCP-ATS Joint Committee on Pulmonary Nomenclature. *Chest.* 1975;67:5-10.

134. Delaunois LM. Lung auscultation: back to basic medicine. *Swiss Med Wkly.* 2005;135:511-512.

135. Sackett DL, Richardson WS, Rosenberg W, Haynes RB. *Evidence-Based Medicine: How To Practice And Teach EBM.* New York: Churchill Livingstone; 1997.

136. Mangione S. *Physical Diagnosis Secrets.* Philadelphia, PA: Hanley & Belfus; 2000.

137. McGee S. *Evidence-Based Physical Diagnosis.* Philadelphia, PA: Saunders; 2001.

138. Massery M, Cahalin L. Physical therapy associated with ventilatory pump dysfunction and failure. In: DeTurk WE, Cahalin LP, eds. *Cardiovascular and Pulmonary Physical Therapy: An Evidence-Based Approach.* New York: McGraw-Hill; 2004:643-684.

139. Petty TL, Enright PL. Simple office spirometry for primary care practitioners. NLHEP and AlphaMedica Inc; 2003. http://www.thepcrj.org/journ/vol12_3/090_093vanschayck.pdf; Accessed April 12, 2011.

140. Cline D, Stead L. *Stead Abdominal Emergencies.* New York: McGraw Hill Professional; 2007:146.

141. Staffel JG, Denny JC, Eibling DE, Johnson JT, Kenna MA, Piman KT. Postoperative fevers. In: Wax MK, ed. *Primary Care Otolaryngology.* Alexandria, VA: American Academy of Otolaryngology—Head and Neck Surgery Foundation; 2005:1-7.

142. Marik PE. Fever in the ICU. *Chest.* 2000;117(3):855-869.

143. Green RJ, Clarke DE, Fishman RS, Raffin TA. Techniques for evaluating fever in the ICU. A stepwise approach for detecting infectious and noninfectious causes. *J Crit Illn.* 1995;10(1):67-71.

144. Braunwald E. Clinical manifestations of heart failure. In: Braunwald E, ed. *Heart Disease: A Textbook of Cardiovascular Medicine.* Philadelphia, PA: Saunders; 1988.

145. Cagini L, Capozzi R, Tassi V, et al. Fluid and electrolyte balance after major thoracic surgery by bioimpedance and endocrine evaluation. *Eur J Cardiothorac Surg.* 2011;40(2):e71-e76.

146. White MM, Howie-Esquivel J, Caldwell MA. Improving heart failure symptom recognition: a diary analysis. *J Cardiovasc Nurs.* 2010;25(1):7-12.

147. Lobo DN, Macafee DA, Allison SP. How perioperative fluid balance influences postoperative outcomes. *Best Pract Res Clin Anaesthesiol.* 2006;20(3):439-455.

148. Eastwood GM. Evaluating the reliability of recorded fluid balance to approximate body weight change in patients undergoing cardiac surgery. *Heart Lung.* 2006;35(1):27-33.

149. Shawgo T, York N. Preoperative versus postoperative weights: which one should be used for cardiac surgery patients' drug and hemodynamic calculations? *Crit Care Nurse.* 1999;19(5):57-60.

150. Cahalin LP. Cardiovascular evaluation. In: DeTurk WE, Cahalin LP, eds. *Cardiovascular and Pulmonary Physical Therapy: An Evidence-Based Approach.* 2nd ed. New York: McGraw-Hill; 2011:293-340.

151. Leard JS, Wells CL. Cardiopulmonary concerns in the patient with musculoskeletal and integumentary deficits: an evidence-based approach. In: DeTurk WE, Cahalin L, eds. *Cardiovascular and Pulmonary Physical Therapy: An Evidenced-Based Approach.* 2nd ed. New York: McGraw-Hill Co.; 2011:395-407.

152. Dueker JA, Gabriel RJ, Tretter SM, Gordon EM, Sahrmann SA. Intra- and interrater reliability of a method of measuring chest expansion. *Phys Ther.* 1995;65(5):720.

153. O'Shea SD, Taylor NF, Paratz J. Peripheral muscle strength training in COPD: a systematic review. *Chest.* 2004;126(3):903-914.

154. Frese E, Brown M, Norton BJ. Clinical reliability of manual muscle testing. *Phys Ther.* 1987;67(7):1072-1076.

155. Bohannon RW. Manual muscle testing overlooks many knee extension strength deficits among older adults. *Isokin Exerc Sci.* 2010;18(4):185-187.

156. Troosters T, Gosselink R, Decramer M. Respiratory muscle assessment. *Eur Respir Mon.* 2005;31:51-71.

157. Flaminiano LE, Celli BR. Respiratory muscle testing. *Clin Chest Med.* 2001;22(4):661-677.

158. Enright PL. The six-minute walk test. *Respir Care.* 2003;48:783-785.

159. Enright PL, Sherrill DL. Reference equations for six-minute walk in healthy adults. *Am J Respir Crit Care Med.* 1998;158:1384-1387.

160. Leung ASY, Chan KK, Sykes K, Chan KS. Reliability, validity and responsiveness of a 2-min walk test to assess exercise capacity of COPD patients. *Chest.* 2006;130:119-125.

161. Iriberri M, Gáldiz JB, Gorostiza A, Ansola P, Jaca C. Comparison of the distances covered during 3 and 6 min walking test. *Respir Med.* 2002;96(10):812-816.

162. Shumway-Cook A, Brauer S, Woollacott M. Predicting the probability for falls in community dwelling older adults using the Timed Up & Go Test. *Phys Ther.* 2000;80(9):896-903.

163. Berg KO, Wood-Dauphinee SL, Williams JI, Gayton D. Measuring balance in elderly: preliminary development of an instrument. *Physiother Can.* 1989;41:304-311.

164. Roig M, Eng JJ, MacIntyre DL, Road JD, Reid WD. Associations of the Stair Climb Power Test with muscle strength and functional performance in people with chronic obstructive pulmonary disease: a cross-sectional study. *Phys Ther.* 2010;90(12):1774-1782.

165. Butcher SJ, Meshke JM, Sheppard S. Reductions in functional balance, coordination, and mobility measures among patients with chronic obstructive pulmonary disease. *J Cardiopulm Rehabil.* 2004;24(4):274-280.

166. Beauchamp MK, Hill K, Goldstein RS, Janaudis-Ferreira T, Brooks D. Impairments in balance discriminate fallers from non-fallers in COPD. *Respir Med.* 2009;103(12):1885-1891.

167. DeTurk WE, Cahalin L. Evaluation of patient intolerance to exercise. In: DeTurk WE, Cahalin L, eds. *Cardiovascular and Pulmonary Physical Therapy: An Evidenced-Based Approach.* 2nd ed. New York: McGraw-Hill Co.; 2011:377-394.

168. Solway S, Brooks D, Lacasse Y, Thomas S. A qualitative overview of the measurement properties of functional walk tests used in the cardiorespiratory domain. *Chest.* 2001;(119):256-270.

169. Knox AJ, Morrison JFJ, Muers MF. Reproducibility of walking test results in chronic obstructive disease. *Thorax.* 1988;43:388-392.

170. Noonan V, Dean E. Submaximal exercise testing: clinical application and interpretation. *Phys Ther.* 2000;80(8):782-807.

171. Singh SJ, Morgan MDL, Scott S, Walters D, Hardman AE. Development of a shuttle walking test of disability in patients with chronic airways obstruction. *Thorax.* 1992;47:1019-1024.

172. Butland RJ, Pang J, Cross ER, Woodcock AA, Geddes DM. Two-, six-, 12-minute walking tests in respiratory disease. *Br Med J (Clin Res Ed).* 1982;284(6329):1607-1608.

173. Carter R, Holiday DB, Stocks J, Grothues C, Tiep B. Predicting oxygen uptake for men and women with moderate to severe chronic obstructive pulmonary disease. *Arch Phys Med Rehab.* 2003;84(8):1158-1164.

174. Cahalin L, Pappagianopoulos P, Prevost S, Wain J, Ginns L. The relationship of the 6-minute walk test to maximal oxygen consumption in transplant candidates with end-stage lung disease. *Chest.* 1995;108:452-459.

175. Gulmans VA, van Veldhoven NH, deMeer K, Helders PJ. The six-minute walking test in children with cystic fibrosis: reliability and validity. *Pediatr Pulmonol.* 1996;22(2):85-89.

176. Nixon PA, Joswiak ML, Fricker FJ. A six-minute walk test for assessing exercise tolerance in severely ill children. *J Pediatr.* 1996;129(3):362-366.

177. Elpern EH, Stevens D, Kesten S. Variability in performance of timed walk tests in pulmonary rehabilitation programs. *Chest.* 2000;118:98-105.

178. Redelmier DA, Bayoumi AM, Goldstein RS, Guyatt GH. Interpreting small differences in functional status: the Six Minute Walk Test in chronic lung disease patients. *Am J Respir Crit Care Med.* 1997;155:1278-82.

179. Wise RA, Brown CD. Minimal clinically important differences in the six-minute walk test and the incremental shuttle test. *COPD.* 2005;2(1):125-129.

180. Ross RM, Murthy JN, Wollak ID, Jackson AS. The six minute walk test accurately estimates mean peak oxygen uptake. *BMC Pulm Med.* 2010;10(31):1-9.

181. Godfrey S, Mearns M. Pulmonary function and response to exercise in cystic fibrosis. *Arch Dis Child.* 1971;46:144-151.

182. Massachusetts Respiratory Hospital. Exercise Testing Protocol. Braintree, MA. As cited in: Brannon FJ, Foley MW, Starr JA, Black MG. *Cardiopulmonary Rehabilitation: Basic Theory and Application.* 2nd ed. Philadelphia, PA: F. A. Davis Company; 1992.

183. Berman L, Sutton J. Exercise for the pulmonary patient. *J Cardiopulm Rehab.* 1986;6(2):55-59.

184. Dean E. Individuals with acute medical conditions. In: Frownfelter D, Dean E, eds. *Cardiovascular and Pulmonary Physical Therapy Evidence and Practice.* 4th ed. St. Louis, MO: Mosby Elsevier; 2006:507-528.

185. Perme C, Dean E. An Evidence-Based Approach to Weaning ICU Patients from Mechanical Ventilation. Proceedings of the World Confederation of Physical Therapy; Vancouver, Canada; 2007.

186. Frownfelter D, Massery M. Facilitating ventilation patterns and breathing strategies. In: Frownfelter D, Dean E, eds. *Cardiovascular and Pulmonary Physical Therapy: Evidence and Practice.* 4th ed. New York: Mosby Elsevier; 2006:377-403.

187. Wesmiller SW, Hoffman LA. Evaluation of an assistive device for ambulation in oxygen dependent patients with COPD. *J Cardiopulm Rehabil.* 1994;14(12):122-126.

188. Bailey P, Thomsen GE, Spuhler VJ, et al. Early activity is feasible and safe in respiratory failure patients. *Crit Care Med.* 2007;35(1):139-145.

189. Hopkins RO, Spuhler VJ, Thomsen GE. Transforming ICU culture to facilitate early mobility. *Crit Care Clin.* 2007;23:81-96.

190. Thomsen GE, Snow GL, Rodriguez G, Hopkins RO. Patients with respiratory failure increase ambulation after transfer to an intensive care unit where early activity is a priority. *Crit Care Med.* 2008;36:1119-1124.

191. Sadowsky HS, Frownfelter D, Moffat M. Impaired ventilation and respiration/gas exchange associated with respiratory failure (pattern F). In: Moffat M, Frownfelter D, eds. *Cardiovascular/Pulmonary Essentials: Applying the Preferred Physical Therapist Practice Patterns.* Thorofare, NJ: SLACK Incorporated; 2007:193-236.

192. Simon M, LeBlanc P, Jobin J, Desmeules M, Sullivan MJ, Maltais F. Limitation of lower limb VO(2) during cycling exercise in COPD patients. *J Appl Physiol (1985).* 2001;90(3):1013-1019.

193. Ong K, Earnest A, Lu S. A multidimensional grading system (BODE index) as predictor of hospitalization for COPD. *Chest.* 2005;128:3810-386.

194. Enright PL, Kronmal RA, Manolio TA, Schenker MB, Hyatt RE. Respiratory muscle strength in the elderly. Correlates and reference values. *Am J Respir Crit Care Med.* 1994;149:430-438.

195. de Oca MM, Rassulo J, Celli BR. Respiratory muscle and cardiopulmonary function during exercise in very severe COPD. *Am J Respir Crit Care Med.* 1996;154:1284-1289.

196. Mellin G, Harjula R. Lung function in relation to thoracic spine mobility and kyphosis. *Scand J Rehabil Med.* 1987;19:89-92.

197. McCool FD, Rosen MJ. Nonpharmacologic airway clearance therapies: ACCP evidence-based clinical practice guidelines. *Chest.* 2006;129:250S-259S.

198. Dechman G, Wilson CR. Evidence underlying breathing retraining in people with stable chronic obstructive pulmonary disease. *Phys Ther.* 2004;84:1189-1197.

199. American Association of Cardiovascular and Pulmonary Rehabiliation. *Guidelines for Pulmonary Rehabilitation Programs.* 4th ed. Champaign, IL: Human Kinetics; 2011.

200. Sin DD, Anthonisen NR, Soriano JB, Agusti AG. Mortality in COPD: role of comorbidities. *Eur Respir J.* 2006;28(6):1245-1257.

201. Dean E. Mobilization and exercise. In: Frownfelter D, Dean E, eds. *Cardiovascular and Pulmonary Physical Therapy: Evidence and Practice.* 4th ed. St. Louis, MO: Mosby Elselvier; 2006:263-306.

202. Alison JA, Donnelly PM, Lennon M, et al. The effect of a comprehensive, intensive inpatient treatment program on lung function and exercise capacity in patients with cystic fibrosis. *Phys Ther.* 1994;74:583-593.

203. Watchie J. Cardiovascular and pulmonary physical therapy treatment. In: Watchie J, ed. *Cardiovascular and Pulmonary Physical Therapy: A Clinical Manual.* 2nd ed. St. Louis, MO: Saunders Elsevier; 2010:298-341.

204. Dean E. Effect of body position on pulmonary function. *Phys Ther.* 1985;65(5):613-618.

205. Ross J, Dean E. Body positioning. In: Zadai CC, ed. *Clinics in Physical Therapy, Pulmonary Management in Physical Therapy.* New York: Churchill Livingstone Inc; 1992.

206. Browse NL. The physiology and pathology of bed rest. Springfield, IL: C.C. Thomas; 1965.

207. Downs AM. Clinical application of airway clearance techniques. In: Frownfelter D, Dean E, eds. *Cardiovascular and Pulmonary Physical Therapy Evidence and Practice.* 4th ed. St. Louis, MO: Mosby Elsevier; 2006:341-376.

208. Pryor JA. Physiotherapy for airway clearance in adults. *Eur Respir J.* 1999;14:1418-1424.

209. Downs AM. Physiological basis for airway clearance techniques. In: Frownfelter D, Dean E, eds. *Cardiovascular and Pulmonary Physical Therapy: Evidence and Practice.* 4th ed. St. Louis, MO: Mosby Elsevier; 2006:325-339.

210. Kisner C, Colby LA. Management of pulmonary conditions. In: Kisner C, Colby LA, eds. *Therapeutic Exercise: Foundation and Techniques.* 4th ed. Philadelphia, PA: F.A. Davis Co.; 2002.

211. Sciaky A, Pawlik A. Interventions for acute cardiopulmonary conditions. In: Hillegass EA, ed. *Essentials of Cardiopulmonary Physical Therapy.* 3rd ed. St. Louis, MO: Elsevier Saunders; 2011.

212. Derenne J, Macklem PT, Roussos CH. The respiratory muscles: mechanics, control, and pathophysiology. Part I. *Am Rev Respir Dis.* 1978;118:119-133.

213. Additional components of pulmonary rehabilitation. In: Brannon FJ, Foley MW, Starr JA, Saul LM, eds. *Cardiopulmonary Rehabilitation: Basic Theory and Application.* 3rd ed. Philadelphia, PA: F.A. Davis; 1998.

214. Massery M. The patient with neuromuscular or musculoskeletal dysfunction. In: Frownfelter D, Dean E, eds. *Principles and Practice of Cardiopulmonary Physical Therapy.* 3rd ed. St. Louis: Mosby-Year Book Inc; 1996:679-702.

215. Frownfelter D, Massery M. Facilitating airway clearance with coughing techniques. In: Frownfelter D, Dean E, eds. *Cardiovascular and Pulmonary Physical Therapy Evidence and Practice.* 4th ed. St. Louis, MO: Mosby Elsevier; 2006:363-376.

216. Bach JR, Saporito L. Criteria for extubation and tracheostomy tube removal for patients with ventilatory failure: a different approach to weaning. *Chest.* 1996;110:1566-1571.

217. Bach JR. Mechanical insufflation-exsufflation: comparison of peak expiratory flows with manually assisted and unassisted coughing techniques. *Chest.* 1993;104:1553-1562.

218. Bach JR. Prevention of respiratory complications of spinal cord injury: a challenge to "model" spinal cord injury units. *J Spinal Cord Med.* 2006;29(1):3-4.

219. Kang SW, Bach JR. Maximum insufflation capacity: vital capacity and cough flows in neuromuscular disease. *Am J Phys Med Rehabil.* 2000;79(3):222-227.

220. AARC (American Association for Respiratory Care) clinical practice guideline. Postural drainage therapy. *Respir Care.* 1991;36(12):1418-1426.

221. Hietpas B, Roth R, Jensen W. Huff coughing and airway patency. *Respir Care.* 1979;24:710.

222. Schöni MH. Autogenic drainage: a modern approach to physiotherapy in cystic fibrosis. *J R Soc Med.* 1989;82(Suppl 16):32-37.

223. Volsko TA, DiFiore JM, Chatburn RL. Performance comparison of two oscillating positive pressure devices: Acapella versus Flutter. *Respir Care.* 2003;48(2):124-130.

224. Levenson CR. Breathing exercises. In: Zadai CC, ed. *Pulmonary Management in Physical Therapy.* New York: Churchill Livingstone Inc; 1992.

225. Wetzel JL. Management of respiratory dysfunction. In: Field-Fote EC, ed. *Spinal Cord Injury Rehabilitation.* Philadelphia, PA: F.A. Davis; 2009:337-392.

226. Wetzel JL, Lunsford BR, Peterson MJ, Alvarez SE. Respiratory rehabilitation of the patient with a spinal cord injury. In: Irwin S, Techlin JS, eds. *Cardiopulmonary Physical Therapy.* 3rd ed. St. Louis, MO: Mosby; 1995:579-603.

227. Overend TJ, Anderson CM, Lucy SD, Bhatia C, Jonsson BI, Timmermans C. The effect of incentive spirometry on postoperative pulmonary complications: a systematic review. *Chest.* 2001;120(3):971-978.

228. Smith CM, Cotter V. Age-related changes in health. In: Capezuti E, Zwicker D, Mezey M, Fulmer T, eds. *Evidence-Based Geriatric Nursing Protocols for Best Practice.* 3rd ed. New York: Springer Publishing Co; 2008:431-458.

229. Bianchi R, Gigliotti F, Romagnoli I, et al. Chest wall kinematics and breathlessness during pursed-lip breathing in patients with COPD. *Am J Respir Crit Care Med.* 1999;159(5):1666-1682.

230. Benson H, Beary JF, Carol MP. The relaxation response. *Psychiatry.* 1974;37:37-46.

231. Ries AL, Bauldoff GS, Carlin BW, et al. Pulmonary rehabilitation: joint ACCP/AACVPR evidence-based clinical practice guidelines. *Chest.* 2007;131(5 Suppl):4S-42S.

232. Nici L, Donner C, Wouters E, et al. American Thoracic Society/European Respiratory Society statement on pulmonary rehabilitation. *Am J Respir Crit Care Med.* 2006;173(12):1390-1413.

233. Maltais F, LeBlanc P, Jobin J, et al. Intensity of training and physiologic adaptation in patients with chronic obstructive pulmonary disease. *Am J Respir Crit Care Med.* 1997;155(2):555-561.

234. Casaburi R, Patessio A, Ioli F, Zanaboni S, Donner CF, Wasserman K. Reductions in exercise lactic acidosis and ventilation as a result of exercise training in patients with obstructive lung disease. *Am Rev Respir Dis.* 1991;143(1):9-18.

235. Dattal D, ZuWallack R. High versus low intensity exercise training in pulmonary rehabilitation: is more better? *Chron Respir Dis.* 2004;1(3):143-149.

236. Breslin EH. Dyspnea-limited response in chronic obstructive pulmonary disease. *Rehabil Nurs.* 1992;17(1):12-20.

237. Vogiatzis I. Prescription of exercise training in patients with COPD. *Curr Respir Med Rev.* 2008;4(4):288-294.

238. Vogiatzis I, Nanas S, Kastanakis E, Georgiadou O, Papzahou O, Roussos C. Dynamic hyperinflation and tolerance to interval exercise in patients with advanced COPD. *Eur Respir J.* 2004;24:385-390.

239. Pate RR, Pratt M, Blair SN, et al. Physical activity and public health. a recommendation from the Centers for Disease Control and Prevention and the American College of Sports Medicine. *JAMA.* 1995;273:402-407.

240. Sciaky A. Patient education. In: Frownfelter D, Dean E, editors. *Cardiovascular and Pulmonary Physical Therapy: Evidence and Practice.* 4th ed. St. Louis, MO: Mosby, Elsevier; 2006:495-504.

CASE STUDY 9-1

Brian D. Roy, PT, DPT, MS, CCS

EXAMINATION

History

Current Condition/Chief Complaint

Ms. Garden was an 80-year-old female who was referred for physical therapy evaluation and intervention by inpatient physical therapy on her first postoperative day following emergency coronary artery bypass surgery.

History of Current Complaint

Ms. Garden came to the emergency room the day prior complaining of dizziness, sweating, and profound weakness of 1 week's duration. She could not recall any episodes of palpitations, chest pain, or dyspnea. Two days prior she had a colonoscopy and polypectomy and reported she had not taken any of her medications for 4 days. In the emergency room, she was diagnosed with a probable subendocardial MI.

A cardiac catheterization showed 80% occlusion of the stent in her left anterior descending artery, 90% occlusion of the circumflex artery, and 60% occlusion of the right coronary artery (RCA). Her unstable angina and severe hypotension were treated with an intra-aortic balloon pump (IABP) by way of the left femoral artery while she was prepared for surgery.

She underwent surgery to place 4 coronary artery bypass grafts (CABGs) using the left internal mammary artery (LIMA) and the right saphenous vein. At the time of the referral for physical therapy on postoperative day 1, she had been weaned and extubated from the ventilator. The IABP had been discontinued in the operating room 8 hours prior.

Social History/Environment

Ms. Garden was married and lived with her husband in a ground-floor condominium. She had worked as a secretary before her retirement. She attended bingo 3 times per week. She enjoyed shopping and cooking.

Social/Health Habits

She smoked 4 cigarettes a day. Until the recent past, she had smoked one pack of cigarettes per day and had done so since the age of 18. She reported that she would drink alcohol at social events.

Family History

She had 4 living siblings who were without significant medical history. Ms. Garden's mother had been healthy all her life and died in her 90s. A brother and Ms. Garden's father died at a young age of cardiac disease. Ms. Garden's 2 grown children were healthy.

Medical/Surgical History

Ms. Garden had been diagnosed previously with peripheral vascular disease. Three years prior she had an anterior MI that was treated with angioplasty and stent placement in her left anterior descending artery. A thallium stress test performed 4 months prior was unremarkable. She was managed medically for anemia, hyperlipidemia, and hypertension. Three months prior to this admission, an abdominal aneurysm, with a diameter of 3.8 cm, was documented on computed tomography (CT) scan. She had chronic bronchitis for 10 years.

Clinician Comment *Even prior to this recent cardiac event, Ms. Garden had significant risk factors for cardiac disease.[1-3] In addition to a 62 pack-year history of smoking, she had a positive family history. She had a*

previous MI. Active diagnoses of hyperlipidemia, peripheral vascular disease, and hypertension were present. At 80 years old, she was postmenopausal.

In all likelihood, her abdominal aneurysm was being monitored. Surgery is considered when the diameter becomes greater than 5 cm.

Reported Functional Status

She reported that during the week prior to going to the emergency room, she had experienced increasing fatigue and inability to do her usual daily chores. Her usual activities included daily housework, grocery shopping, and cooking. At 80 years old, she still drove herself to run errands.

Medications

Preoperative medications: atenolol, aspirin, Zocor (simvastatin), Plavix (clopidogrel bisulfate), Altace (ramipril)

Postoperative medications: atenolol, Altace, aspirin, Losartan, Zocor, morphine, oxycodone, Colace (docusate), intravenous (IV) nitroglycerin, IV vancomycin

Other Clinical Tests

A review of her medical record showed the following postoperative lab values:

- WBCs 12.06 K/cmm
- RBCs 3.32 m/cmm
- Hgb 10.3 gm/dL
- Hct 29.9%
- Electrolytes
  - Sodium 141; chloride 108
  - Potassium 4.2; CO_2 27

Clinician Comment *What had been learned from the interview and chart review was that Ms. Garden had a recent decline in function, but she did not participate in regular exercise. Given her advanced age, she was fully independent with ADL and IADL, including all mobility. She wanted to continue with her independence, which included driving. Ms. Garden had a supportive husband who was willing and able to help her once she returned home. She had 2 adult children who lived close by. She lived on the ground floor, so she did not have stairs as a physical barrier.*

Her preoperative medications were mostly cardiac in nature. She had an extensive history of smoking and chronic bronchitis, yet she was not currently being followed by a pulmonologist. Her lab values were all within normal limits (WNL) except for a low Hct and Hgb. These low values likely reflect a normal loss of blood products during surgery. They were not critical but did need daily monitoring with respect to interpreting her BP and blood O_2 levels. Namely, a low Hct could contribute to a low BP measure and a low Hgb value could lead to poor blood O_2-carrying capability.

Her medical history, again, was mainly cardiovascular in nature, given her ongoing coronary artery disease, MIs, stents, peripheral vascular disease, aneurysm, and hypertension. With the sternotomy for the CABG surgery, she was at high risk for postoperative pulmonary complications, especially given her previous tobacco use.[4]

The systems review in acute care, and especially in critical care, often is the initial physical therapy examination. In these settings, the systems review may be as much as can be accomplished in the first session. In acute and critical care, the patient evaluation can be ongoing and may evolve daily. Goals may need to be added or even dropped when there is a clearer understanding of the patient's status.

Systems Review

The findings in the review of systems appear as follows:

REVIEW OF SYSTEMS	Height: 5 feet, 3 inches; Weight: 135 pounds preop; 148 pounds postop	
CARDIOVASCULAR/ PULMONARY	Resting HR: 81; BP: 129/54; RR: 20, on 5l/min nasal cannula	
	NOT IMPAIRED	**IMPAIRED**
MUSCULOSKELETAL		
Gross ROM	☐	☒ 90 degrees flexion at right knee o/w WNL
General strength	☐	☒ Left hip flexion 3–/5; o/w 3+/5 UE and LE
Gross symmetry/posture	☐	☒ Head and trunk flexed forward
INTEGUMENTARY		
Continuity of color	☐	☒ Pale
Skin integrity	☐	☒ Median sternotomy incision; saphenous vein incision from right medial thigh from groin to medial malleolus; chest tube insertion sites (inferior and left lateral to the xiphoid)
Pliability	☐	☒ Taut at LEs due to 1 to 2+ edema
Presence of scar	☒	☐
NEUROMUSCULAR		
Gait	☐	☒
Locomotion/transfers/transitions	☐	☒
Balance	☐	☒
Motor function (motor control, motor learning)	☒	☐
COMMUNICATION/LEARNING		
Communication	☐	☒ Lethargic and sleepy likely due to pain medication recently given
Orientation	☒	☐
BARRIERS TO LEARNING	☐ None ☐ Language ☐ Vision ☒ Other: hard of hearing	
READINESS FOR LEARNING	☒ Accepting ☐ No interest ☐ Denying ☐ Refuses	
PREFERRED LEARNING STYLE	☐ Pictures ☒ Read ☒ Listen ☒ Demonstrate	
EDUCATION NEEDS	☒ Disease process ☒ Safety ☒ Assistive devices ☒ ADL	
	☒ Exercise program ☒ Other: sternal precautions; smoking ☒ Other: energy conservation; safety; pain ☒ Other: symptom recognition	

Clinician Comment *Patients having cardiac surgery can gain as much as 30 pounds of extra water weight after being on cardiopulmonary bypass depending on the length of the surgery and bypass time. This process often leads to increased postoperative pulmonary complications.[5,6] Surgeons may opt to perform surgery off the bypass pump if the vessels that are occluded are minimal and more anterior. Though Ms. Garden gained only 13 pounds, the additional fluid could still be significant.*

The IV nitroglycerin needed to be considered with regard to interpreting her vital signs. Nitroglycerin is a potent medication for BP and arrhythmia control. In addition, she would need to be closely monitored for orthostatic hypotension since she was also on beta blockade. This intervention would reduce her BP and lower her HR. Beta blockade used in combination with pain medications, especially morphine, can have a vasodilatory effect and further reduce BP.

This systems review revealed impairments of gas exchange, given she requires 5 L/minute (40% FiO$_2$) of supplemental O$_2$ via nasal cannula, which may be purely because of pulmonary volume overload common after heart surgery and/or postoperative pulmonary complications; ROM, which

is likely due to incisions and edema and less likely to joint impairment; strength, which should resolve rapidly once she mobilizes and is most likely due to bed rest and recent immobilization; integument due to incision sites and edema common after heart surgery; cognition, which is presumed due to anesthetic effects and sedation for incision pain. Cognition deficits should resolve in time, but directions, instructions, and questions would likely need to be repeated. She had specific learning needs that would need to be addressed. Her hearing loss needed to be considered when giving verbal instructions.

Her gait, locomotion, and balance were presumed to be impaired in the systems review. Before assisting Ms. Garden out of bed, however, to more thoroughly examine her functional mobility, her circulation and respiration/gas-exchange status needed to be examined. Pain and impaired ROM and muscle performance noted in the systems review also needed further examination. Her need for supplemental O$_2$ and her hemodynamic response would then be monitored during any functional mobility testing. The decision to test her aerobic capacity would be made after judging her response to the tests and measures noted previously.

Tests and Measures

The tests measures categories that needed to be addressed are summarized in the following chart.

	IMPAIRED	NOT IMPAIRED	NOT EXAMINED		IMPAIRED	NOT IMPAIRED	NOT EXAMINED
Aerobic capacity and endurance	☒	☐	☐	Motor function	☐	☒	☐
Arousal, attention and cognition	☒	☐	☐	Muscle performance	☒	☐	☐
Assistive and adaptive devices	☒	☐	☐	Orthotic, protective and supportive devices	☐	☐	☒
Circulation	☒	☐	☐	Pain	☒	☐	☐
Community and work integration	☒	☐	☐	Posture	☒	☐	☐
Cranial nerve integrity	☐	☐	☒	Range of motion	☒	☐	☐
Environmental, home, work	☐	☐	☒	Reflex integrity	☐	☐	☒
Ergonomics and body mechanics	☐	☐	☒	Self-care and home management	☒	☐	☐
Gait, locomotion and balance	☒	☐	☐	Sensory integrity	☐	☒	☐
Integumentary integrity	☒	☐	☐	Ventilation, respiration and circulation	☒	☐	☐
Joint integrity and mobility	☐	☒	☐				

Circulation

- HR/rhythm: 81 normal sinus on EKG

- Heart sounds: Normal S_1 and S_2; possible S_4 noted but inconsistent

- BP via right radial arterial line: 129/54 (while on IV nitroglycerin)

- Anginal equivalent: extreme fatigue and diaphoresis

- Body temperature: 100.2 degrees F

- Cardiac output (CO): 3.2 liters/min via continual monitor through pulmonary arterial monitor

Clinician's Comment *Initial low-grade temperatures immediately postoperative may be indicative of postoperative pulmonary complications. Her anginal equivalent was not the classic substernal chest, jaw or arm pain. Her reported symptoms would need to be monitored closely since she may experience angina postoperatively without ischemic events. An S_4 heart sound can commonly be heard with patients having chronic coronary artery disease and hypertension. It would be important to monitor her heart sounds especially after exercise. If an S_3 were to be noted, then Ms. Garden might be showing signs of heart failure, of which she was at risk during the acutely postoperative period.*

Ventilation and Respiration/Gas Exchange

Her RR was 20 to 28 breaths per minute.

Breath sounds were absent at the left lower lobe at all segments and bronchial above this area. A few crackles were noted at the right lung base. Otherwise, breath sounds were diminished throughout all lung fields. Upper airway rhonchi were also noted.

Mediate percussion over the left lower lobe region was hyperresonant.

Her breathing pattern was shallow with obvious splinting. She showed decreased chest wall excursion at her lower lung fields with left more limited than right. Excursion of mid- and upper lung fields were grossly normal.

Arterial blood gases analysis showed 90/45/7.38/26. SaO_2 was 94% on 5 liters/min flow of O_2 via nasal cannula (40% $FiO2$), as was her SpO_2. Her SpO_2 dropped to 87% when the supplemental O_2 was removed for 1 minute while at rest.

Ms. Garden's cough was weak, throaty, and nonproductive but congested sounding.

Her chest x-ray showed a left lower lobe collapse and right lower lobe atelectasis; as well as left pleural effusion with pulmonary vascular congestion.

Her maximal inspiratory volume with the incentive spirometer was 500 mL.

Clinician's Comment *Ms. Garden showed adequate oxygenation but only with high amounts of supplemental O_2 to maintain it. Her CO_2 was high normal,* which may have been a result of the following: secretion retention, pain that limited adequate ventilatory pump, chronic bronchitis, and tobacco use (possible CO_2 retention), pain medication-induced decreased ventilatory pump, or all in combination.

The decrease in her left chest wall excursion might have been due to atelectasis/collapse and pleural effusion. Left pleural effusions are very common in patients having CABG, especially those who received a LIMA graft. LIMA grafts can disrupt the lymphatics in the chest and can cause increased pain often elicited in the shoulder and/or scapular region.[7] Pleural effusions can lead to further lobar collapse due to compression of the alveolar spaces. Increased resonance is often felt with mediate percussion over large areas of fluid such as a pleural effusion.

Integumentary Integrity

Wound sites: all incisions were attended to by nursing. Ms. Garden had minimal serous drainage from her sternotomy incision. For the saphenous vein harvest incision in her right LE, there was minimal serous drainage in the region of her knee. Her left groin incision site for the IABP access was sutured closed but showed reddening with 1 to 2+ edema present.

The entry sites for the mediastinal chest tubes sites were clean, dry, and intact as was the single left pleural chest tube site. The insertion of the temporary pacing wires into the mid-diaphragm region was also clean, dry, and intact. The right radial arterial line was sutured in place. The placement site for the Swan-Ganz catheter to the pulmonary artery through the right jugular vein was clean, dry, and intact.

Clinician's Comment *Chest tubes used for drainage of surgical sites can lead to further splinting of the chest because of pain and increase the incidence of atelectasis. Patients can ambulate with chest tubes off suction as long as there is no evidence of PTX or air leak seen on the Pleur-Evac container. Otherwise, extension tubing or portable suction devices attached to the Pleur-Evac are indicated.*

A Swan-Ganz catheter, however, is an invasive line into the heart and ends in the pulmonary artery. Ambulation away from the bedside may not be recommended when a Swan-Ganz catheter is in place because the line would need to be clamped and disconnected from the monitor. More important, a tensioned line could cause the catheter to be pulled from within the pulmonary artery back into the right ventricle—a displacement that could cause life-threatening ventricular arrhythmias. Arterial lines are invasive to an artery and if dislodged can result in rapid blood loss. Again, ambulation away from the bedside may not be recommended in most instances. Care with all invasive lines and tubes is crucial in the care of the patient who is critically ill.

Pain

Using the 0 through 10 faces pain scale, Ms. Garden rated her premedicated pain level from her chest and LE incisions as 8/10. After taking 2 Percocets (oxycodone and acetaminophen), she rated her pain in the same regions as 3/10.

Range of Motion

No changes in her ROM examination were seen compared to the systems review. Only her right knee flexion was symptom-limited to 100 degrees. All other joints showed WNL movements. She also had a decrease in chest wall excursion as noted earlier.

Muscle Performance

Her left hip flexion strength was 3/5. All other UE and LE manual muscle tests were 3+ to 4/5. She showed limited cough strength resulting in ineffective airway clearance.

Clinician's Comment *Her right groin was likely inflamed and sore from the IABP placement previously. She showed signs of deconditioning due to bed rest.*

Gait, Locomotion, and Balance

Ms. Garden was able to roll to the left using her LE to help and with minimal assist of 1. To roll to her right, she required moderate assist of 1. To move from right side-lying to a sitting position, she needed minimal/moderate assist of 1 but with maximal cues to avoid use of her UEs. The limitation of UE use was required in order to maintain sternal precautions of less than 10 pounds of resistance with the UEs as in pushing, pulling, or lifting. She was able to move from sitting to standing, and then complete a step transfer to a chair with moderate assist of 1.

She showed independent head and trunk control to maintain her sitting balance. Her standing balance was fair. She required moderate assist of 1 to maintain her standing balance while moving. She was able to maintain static standing balance with only minimal assist of 1.

With the use of a rolling walker, Ms. Garden ambulated 5 feet to bedside chair with moderate assist of 1. She was breathing supplemental O_2 with a flow of 5 liters/minute using a nasal cannula and maintained an SpO_2 of 93%.

Clinician's Comment *Her need for moderate assistance when rolling right was consistent with her left hip flexor weakness and impaired ability to use the left LE to assist with turning. Her ambulation away from the bedside was limited by the invasive right radial arterial line and right jugular Swan-Ganz catheter, not her hemodynamic response.*

Since she tolerated moving from the bed to the bedside chair, it was decided to let her rest a few minutes and then assess her aerobic capacity.

Aerobic Capacity/Endurance

Ms. Garden was able to stand in the walker with a moderate assist of 1, march in place 20 times, rest, and then march in place another 20 times. Her CO remained steady at 2.8 to 3.2 L/min throughout the activity. She continued to use supplemental 5 L/min flow of O_2 by nasal cannula. She rated her RPE using the Borg scale, 6 to 20, at rest, while marching, and during a seated recovery. The results are shown as follows.

	HR	BP	SpO$_2$	RPE	RR
Rest (seated)	88	123/52	94%	7/20	20
Peak (standing)	105	113/55	92%	15/20	28
Recovery (seated)	86	132/64	96%	8/20	23

Clinician's Comment *The drop in BP with exercise may have been orthostatic. It may have been due to the IV presser and pain medication, or a combination. CO remained at 2.8 to 3.2 L/min, most likely due to the increase in HR with activity to compensate for a lower BP.*

EVALUATION

Diagnosis

Practice Pattern

Ms. Garden was an 80-year-old female in intensive care following emergent CABG ×4 after an acute MI. The primary, and most acute impairments, that needed to be addressed were her postoperative pulmonary complications of atelectasis and lobar collapse. If not resolved quickly, she might develop pneumonia. Her cardiovascular issues would be addressed concurrently. Based on her history, systems review, and tests and measures, Ms. Garden was classified into 2 preferred practice patterns using the American Physical Therapy Association *Guide to Physical Therapy Practice*. Once the major pulmonary impairments were resolved then the cardiovascular pump dysfunction would become the primary diagnosis.

- Impaired Ventilation, Respiration/Gas Exchange, and Aerobic Capacity/Endurance Associated With Airway Clearance Dysfunction (6C)
- Impaired Aerobic Capacity/Endurance Associated With Cardiovascular Pump Dysfunction (6D)

Clinician's Comment *Her impaired gas exchange may have been also compounded by inadequate ventilatory pump due to the sternotomy.*

International Classification of Functioning, Disability and Health Model of Disability

See the ICF model on p 380.

Prognosis

Ms. Garden had a good inpatient physical therapy prognosis. She could be expected to improve her pulmonary function, decrease her work of breathing, and eliminate the need for supplemental O_2. She could be expected to regain sufficient functional mobility to safely return home with her husband.

Plan of Care

Intervention

Proposed Frequency and Duration of Physical Therapy Visits

Ms. Garden would be scheduled daily to twice daily physical therapy for the anticipated 5 days of continued inpatient care.

Anticipated Goals

1. Effective cough to independently clear her own pulmonary secretions (2 days).
2. Afebrile (3 days).
3. No need for supplemental O_2 (4 days).
4. Active ROM (AROM) of right LE: WNL with pain < 3/10; all strength > 3+/5 (4 days).
5. Left lower lobe without collapse as measured by improved air entry upon auscultation and improved chest x-ray (4 to 5 days).
6. Vital capacity to at least 1500 mL as measured on incentive spirometer (4 to 5 days).
7. Independent with self-care (4 to 5 days).

Expected Outcomes (5 days)

1. Independent and safe with bed mobility and transfers with pain < 3/10 (5 days).
2. Independent and safe with ambulation > 500 feet or 5 minutes, 3 times per day (TID) while maintaining: RPE < 15; SpO_2 > 92%; RR < 30 bpm; HR and systolic BP rise no greater than 30 points from resting values (5 days).
3. Independent with all deep breathing, airway clearance and coughing techniques; all sternal precautions; symptom recognition; energy conservation techniques; home exercise program and self-monitoring (5 days).

Discharge Plan

It was anticipated that Ms. Garden would achieve the anticipated goals and expected outcomes on or before her sixth postoperative day and be discharged to home.

INTERVENTION

Coordination, Communication, and Documentation

- Coordinate care with nursing, respiratory, and nutrition services
- Coordinate pain medication with nursing
- Communicate and document O_2 needs at rest and with activity to nursing, respiratory therapy, case manager, and physicians
- Document progression toward goals and communicate discharge needs to physicians, nursing, and case manager
- Coordination and communication of care are acceptable to the patient
- Patient and family have a full understanding of goals and expected outcomes
- Documentation occurs regarding the patient's response to and progression of therapy
- Discharge needs are met (home with husband)

Patient-/Client-Related Instruction

Ms. Garden would be instructed in the following:
- Use of an incentive spirometer and flutter device
- Diaphragmatic breathing, PLB, paced breathing
- Effective coughing and huffing techniques
- Posture awareness
- Sternal precautions for 6 to 8 weeks: No lifting > 10 pounds; limit pushing and pulling with UEs; no driving; avoid sitting behind airbags while a passenger in a car; use lap seat belt only; no prone lying
- Symptom recognition
- Disease process/progression
- Energy conservation with all activities
- Pain control and medication timing
- Initiation of smoking cessation
- Independent AROM UE and LE exercises for warm-up prior to ambulation
- Functional mobility with a sternal incision
- Progressive home walking/endurance program using the RPE scale as a guide

Procedural Interventions

Ms. Garden would receive direct intervention in the following:
- Therapeutic exercise
- Functional training in self-care and home management

ICF Model of Disablement for Ms. Garden

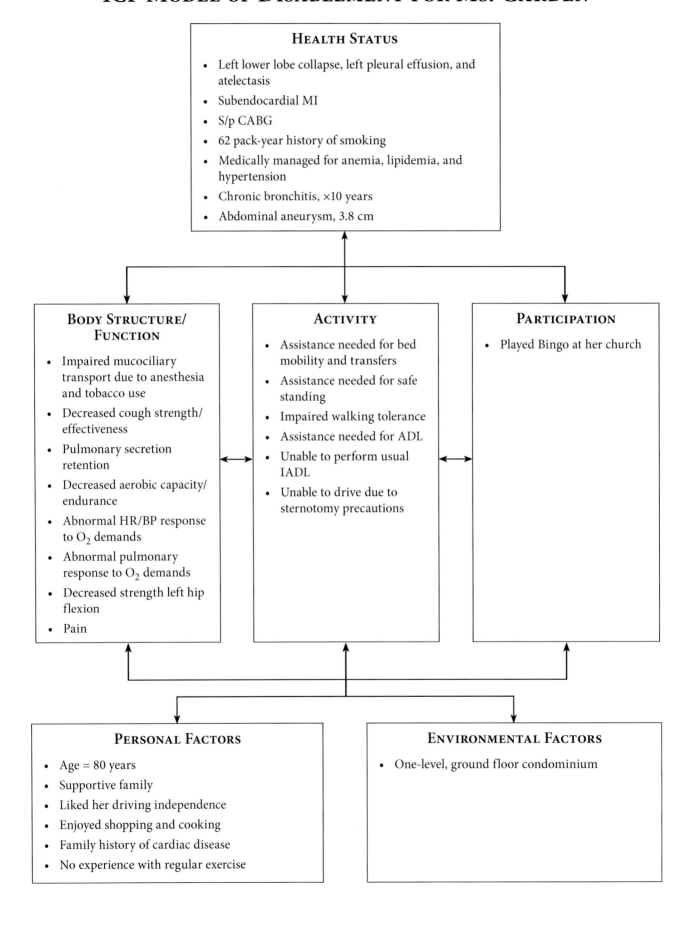

HEALTH STATUS

- Left lower lobe collapse, left pleural effusion, and atelectasis
- Subendocardial MI
- S/p CABG
- 62 pack-year history of smoking
- Medically managed for anemia, lipidemia, and hypertension
- Chronic bronchitis, ×10 years
- Abdominal aneurysm, 3.8 cm

BODY STRUCTURE/ FUNCTION

- Impaired mucociliary transport due to anesthesia and tobacco use
- Decreased cough strength/ effectiveness
- Pulmonary secretion retention
- Decreased aerobic capacity/ endurance
- Abnormal HR/BP response to O_2 demands
- Abnormal pulmonary response to O_2 demands
- Decreased strength left hip flexion
- Pain

ACTIVITY

- Assistance needed for bed mobility and transfers
- Assistance needed for safe standing
- Impaired walking tolerance
- Assistance needed for ADL
- Unable to perform usual IADL
- Unable to drive due to sternotomy precautions

PARTICIPATION

- Played Bingo at her church

PERSONAL FACTORS

- Age = 80 years
- Supportive family
- Liked her driving independence
- Enjoyed shopping and cooking
- Family history of cardiac disease
- No experience with regular exercise

ENVIRONMENTAL FACTORS

- One-level, ground floor condominium

- Airway clearance
- Aerobic capacity/endurance training
- Prescription/application/fabrication of assistive devices and equipment

Therapeutic Exercise

Flexibility and Strength Exercises:

Mode
AROM

Intensity
RPE < 15/20

Duration
3 sets of 10 to 20 repetitions

Frequency
Daily to twice daily by PT, but encouraged to do independently 3 times per day, prior to ambulation

Description of the Intervention
Ms. Garden would be shown and would practice the following exercises while seated: knee flexion/extension, hip flexion, ankle pumps, shoulder flexion, and horizontal abduction/adduction without extension.

Clinician's Comment *Shoulder ROM/chest wall mobility exercises should be initiated to prevent pectoralis tightness, promote inspiratory effort, and improve posture. Patients with sternal incisions tend to flex forward and limit the mobility of the UEs, which further contributes to improper spinal alignment and restriction of the chest wall.*

Functional Training

Mode
Bed mobility and transfer training to bathroom.

Intensity
With assistance progressing to independence

Duration
N/A

Frequency
Daily to twice daily by PT, with reinforcement by nursing.

Injury Prevention

- Education of sternal precautions with bed mobility, transfers, self-care, and home management;
- Safety awareness

Airway Clearance Techniques and Breathing Maneuvers

Mode
Maximal inspiratory hold maneuvers with lateral costal and/or segmental expansion.

Intensity
Maximal inspiratory effort by patient with a 2- to 3-second breath hold.

Duration
10 breaths

Frequency
Daily to twice daily by PT for 5 days and as needed.

Mode
Incentive spirometry device.

Intensity
Maximal inspiratory effort by patient.

Duration
10 breaths.

Frequency
Independently once an hour while awake (with reinforcement by PT, nursing, and respiratory therapy) for 1 week and as needed.

Mode
Oscillatory positive expiratory pressure device.

Intensity
Maximal inspiratory effort and exhalation for 3 to 4 seconds by patient.

Duration
10 breaths.

Frequency
Daily to twice daily by PT and independently every hour while awake (with reinforcement by nursing and respiratory therapy) for 1 week and as needed.

Mode
Modified postural drainage and chest percussion and/or vibration as indicated to left lower lobe region, in right side-lying, head of bed flat if tolerated.

Intensity
To patient's tolerance; keep SpO_2 > 92%; RR < 30.

Duration
~2 minutes of percussion followed by 6 to 10 maximal breaths with vibration upon exhalation.

Frequency
Daily to twice daily by PT for 5 days as needed (with reinforcement by nursing and respiratory therapy as indicated).

Clinician's Comment *All techniques may be used individually or in combination depending on the specific need. Examination is ongoing during an episode of care. Focus of the interventions can change during each interaction with the patient. Many techniques are adjunct to hands-on skilled therapy. Patient and caregiver education is key to the improvement of pulmonary function.*

Mode
Coughing/huffing techniques.

Intensity
Forceful enough to mobilize secretions.

Duration
1 to 3 efforts or until secretions are mobilized.

Frequency
Daily to twice daily by PT and independently once an hour while awake for 1 week and/or after all airway clearance techniques and breathing maneuvers are performed.

Clinician's Comment *Nasotracheal suctioning may be indicated if her cough remains ineffective; her temperature and WBC count continue to rise, her SpO$_2$ drops < 90% on same FiO$_2$, or she exhibits increased respiratory distress. Suctioning techniques may be indicated if pulmonary secretions are not cleared by: airway clearance, breathing maneuvers, effective coughing/huffing, and functional mobility.*

Positioning may be used to maximize ventilation and perfusion as able. Many patients with cardiac disease may not tolerate bed flat side-lying because of dyspnea and the increased workload on the cardiopulmonary system. Sitting for airway clearance techniques of deep breathing maneuvers and coughing may be the optimum position for Ms. Garden. Alternate side-lying and modified positioning with emphasis on the left lower lobe should be encouraged every 2 hours when she is in bed.[8,9]

Aerobic Capacity/Endurance Training

Mode
Progressive ambulation with breathing maneuvers.
Intensity
With RPE < 15/20; SpO2 > 92%; RR < 30; HR and systolic BP rise < 30 from resting values.
Duration
Up to 10 minutes of walking.
Frequency
Daily to twice daily by PT for 5 to 10 days (3 to 4 times per day total with nursing and family reinforcement), then reexamination once home by Home Health physical therapist.
Description of the Intervention
Ms. Garden will progress from marching in place, to gait training with a rolling walker and assistance as indicated for balance, safety, and energy conservation, and further progression to complete independence on level surfaces if able. The following strategies will be incorporated into this intervention:

- Posture awareness reinforced during gait and functional mobility
- Paced and PLB maneuvers with energy expenditure
- Diaphragmatic breathing during all activity

Prescription/Application of Devices and Equipment

Assistive Devices

A rolling walker will be prescribed for home use if she cannot achieve functional independence by the time she is medically cleared from the hospital.

Supportive Devices

Supplemental O$_2$—titrate O$_2$ to keep SpO$_2$ > 92%.

Clinician comment *If Ms. Garden could not achieve SpO$_2$ > 88% on room air at rest, then supplemental O$_2$ would likely be indicated for home. If she had a room air SpO$_2$ > 88% at rest but desaturated below 88% with activity, then supplemental O$_2$ would be added and titrated to the least amount to keep her > 88%. With this information, her physician would then be able to prescribe the correct type and amount of home O$_2$. Evaluation of her supplemental O$_2$ needs would be ongoing during each intervention and finalized at discharge to home.*

REEXAMINATION

Subjective

"I'm ready to go home."

Objective

Ms. Garden was seen twice a day for physical therapy during her hospital stay. She was reassessed on postoperative day 6 just prior to her discharge to home.

Circulation

HR/rhythm: 76 bpm, normal sinus rhythm
Heart sounds: Normal S$_1$ and S$_2$
BP: 132/65 mm Hg
Afebrile

Ventilation and Respiration/Gas Exchange

Her chest x-ray was markedly improved. All lung fields were clear to auscultation, including the left lower lobe. Ms. Garden had been breathing room air without supplemental O$_2$ for 24 hours. She was able to maintain SpO$_2$ levels at 96% at rest. Her RR was 18 to 20 breaths/minute at rest. She was close to achieving 1500 mL with her incentive spirometer.

Integumentary Integrity

Mediastinal staples were removed on postoperative day 3. All incisions were healing without signs of redness or swelling.

Pain

Ms. Garden reported that she was aware of her chest incisions with deep breathing. Her hip symptoms were less than 3/10 with transfers and bed mobility. She reported she was able to complete most of her self-care without symptoms.

Range of Motion

She was able to complete all exercises with normal ROM, including right hip flexion.

Muscle Performance

Right LE was able to demonstrate > 3+/5 strength throughout.

Gait, Locomotion and Balance

Ms. Garden was able to walk on a level surface without gait deviations. She also demonstrated that she was able to ascend and descend a flight of stairs with 2 to 3 rests on the stairs to avoid fatigue.

Aerobic Capacity/Endurance

Ms. Garden was able to walk 625 feet in 6 minutes in the hospital hallway while keeping a pace to allow RPE < 15. Her SpO_2 remained above 92%. Her HR rose to 92 bpm but returned to her resting rate of 76 bpm after 8 minutes of sitting rest.

Assessment

Ms. Garden was able to achieve all the anticipated goals established at the time of her initial evaluation. She also had good understanding of the educational items identified in her treatment plan. She was aware of the sternal precautions to follow for the next 6 to 8 weeks.

Plan

Ms. Garden would be discharged from inpatient physical therapy in anticipation of her discharge to home.

OUTCOMES

Upon discharge to home, Ms. Garden had a program of exercise and activity to follow on her own. It would be anticipated that by 4 weeks after her surgery and before outpatient cardiac rehabilitation would be recommended to begin, the following outcomes would be expected:

- Independent at home with ADL and minimal assist with IADL (shopping, groceries, laundry)
- Independently ambulating > 30 minutes daily on level surface at her normal/comfortable pace without dyspnea and RPE < 13

- Incentive spirometer to 2000 mL
- Pain free
- Smoking cessation
- Bingo, as tolerated

REFERENCES

1. Hillegass EA. Examination and assessment procedures. In: Hillegass EA, ed. *Essentials of Cardiopulmonary Physical Therapy.* 3rd ed. St. Louis, MO: Elsevier; 2011:534-567.
2. U.S. Department of Health and Human Services. *The Health Consequences of Smoking: A Report of the Surgeon General.* Atlanta, GA: U.S. Department of Health and Human Services, Centers for Disease Control and Prevention, National Center for Chronic Disease Prevention and Health Promotion, Office on Smoking and Health; 2004. http://www.cdc.gov/tobacco/data_statistics/sgr/2004. Accessed February 2, 2011.
3. Centers for Disease Control and Prevention (CDC). Annual smoking-attributable mortality, years of potential life lost, and productivity losses—United States, 1997-2001. *MMWR Morb Mortal Wkly Rep.* 2005;54:625-628.
4. Hulzebos EHJ, Van Meeteren NLU, De Bie RA, Dagnelie PC, Helders PJM. Prediction of postoperative pulmonary complications on the basis of preoperative risk factors in patients who had undergone coronary artery bypass graft surgery. *Phys Ther.* 2003;83(1):8-16.
5. Clark SC. Lung injury after cardiopulmonary bypass. *Perfusion.* 2006;21(4):225-228.
6. Conti VR. Pulmonary injury after cardiopulmonary bypass. *Chest.* 2001;119:2-4.
7. Berrizbeitia LD, Tessler S, Jacobwitz IJ, et al. Effects of sternotomy and coronary bypass on postoperative pulmonary mechanics. Comparison of internal mammary and saphenous vein bypass grafts. *Chest.* 1989;96:873-876.
8. Ross J, Dean E. Body positioning. In: Zadai CC, ed. *Pulmonary Management in Physical Therapy.* New York, NY: Churchill Livingston Inc; 1992:79-98.
9. Dean E. Body positioning. In: Frownfelter D, Dean E, eds. *Cardiovascular and Pulmonary Physical Therapy: Evidence and Practice.* 4th ed. St. Louis, MO: Mosby Elsevier; 2006:307-324.

10

Individuals With Localized Musculoskeletal and Connective Tissue Disorders

Debra Coglianese, PT, DPT, OCS, ATC

CHAPTER OBJECTIVES

- Compare and contrast the connective tissue characteristics in fibrous connective tissues, cartilage, and bone.

- Identify the general water holding function of proteoglycan structure and how differences in proteoglycan concentration can affect tissue properties.

- Summarize the effect of physical stress on tissues using the physical stress theory.

- Identify muscle adaptation to lengthening or shortening loads.

- Define the tissue pathology distinctions between tendonitis and tendinopathy.

- Summarize how the differences in vascularity impact healing for each component of a joint: capsule, ligaments, synovium, articular cartilage, tendon, muscle, and bone.

- Identify nerve structure characteristics that allow nerves to glide with body movements and factors that can compromise neural mobility.

- Discuss the information that can be gathered on a first encounter with a patient in an out-patient setting before the formal interview begins.

CHAPTER OUTLINE

- Epidemiology

- Basic Tissues
  - Epithelial Tissue
  - Connective Tissue
    - Extracellular Matrix
    - Fibrous Connective Tissue
    - Cartilage
    - Bone
  - Nervous Tissue
  - Muscle Tissue
  - Tissue Damage and Healing
    - Basic Tissues' Shared Events
    - Immediate Response
    - Inflammation
    - Tissue Repair/Regeneration
    - Maturation/Remodeling
    - Tissue Health
  - Physical Stress Theory
- Muscles
  - Morphology (Gross Anatomy and Histology) and Physiology
    - Muscle Response to Loading
      - Lengthening and Shortening Loads
      - Resistive Loads
    - Muscle Nutrition and Healing

Coglianese D, ed. *Clinical Exercise Pathophysiology for Physical Therapy: Examination, Testing, and Exercise Prescription for Movement-Related Disorders* (pp 385-442).
© 2015 Taylor & Francis Group.

- ○ Muscle Disorders
  - ▪ Contusion
  - ▪ Strain
  - ▪ Tear/Rupture
  - ▪ Overuse Injuries
  - ▪ Stretch Weakness
- Tendons
  - ○ Morphology and Physiology
    - ▪ Tendon Response to Loading
    - ▪ Tendon Nutrition and Healing
  - ○ Tendon Disorders
    - ▪ Tendonitis
    - ▪ Tendinopathy
    - ▪ Tear/Rupture
- Bone
  - ○ Morphology and Physiology
    - ▪ Bone Response to Loading
    - ▪ Nutrition and Healing
  - ○ Bone Disorders (Nonsystemic)
    - ▪ Fractures
    - ▪ Stress Fractures
    - ▪ Skeletal Alignment
      - □ Spinal
        - - Kyphosis
        - - Scoliosis
      - □ Extremity
        - - Valgus/Varus
- Joints
  - ○ Joint Morphology and Physiology
    - ▪ Ligaments
    - ▪ Synovium
    - ▪ Articular Cartilage
    - ▪ Joint Response to Loading
    - ▪ Joint Nutrition and Healing
  - ○ Joint Disorders
    - ▪ Joint Effusion
    - ▪ Adhesive Capsulitis
    - ▪ Ligament Sprain/Rupture
    - ▪ Osteoarthritis
- Peripheral Nerves
  - ○ Morphology and Physiology
    - ▪ Nerve Responses to Loading
    - ▪ Nerve Nutrition and Healing
  - ○ Peripheral Nerve Disorders
    - ▪ Compression
    - ▪ Traction
    - ▪ Neural Immobility
    - ▪ Hypersensitivity
- Musculoskeletal Examination
  - ○ Examination
    - ▪ History
      - □ Patient Interview
    - ▪ Systems Review
    - ▪ Tests and Measures
    - ▪ Summary
- References

There are those who might think that the inclusion of a chapter on musculoskeletal disorders is an odd choice for a text that presents a view of patients from a largely cardiovascular and pulmonary perspective. Admittedly, a thorough examination to identify muscle imbalances, joint dysfunctions or altered alignment in the spine and extremities may seem beyond what is required for care when a patient is referred to physical therapy during a hospital admission for a cardiac pump dysfunction. But what happens when that patient's status improves and is referred later to outpatient cardiac rehab? Mr. Cedar, one of the patient cases in Chapter 5, is an example of someone who was not able to succeed with traditional cardiac rehab because of an orthopedic disorder. It is not known how many patients don't bother to pursue, or fail to succeed in, cardiovascular or pulmonary rehabilitation because of musculoskeletal disorders.

On the other hand, any perplexity regarding a musculoskeletal chapter inclusion in this text is exceeded only by the bewilderment of physical therapists guided to take vital signs on patients with musculoskeletal disorders. Noting vital signs is the standard for the examination of the cardiac and pulmonary systems in the systems review from the Patient/Client Management Model.[1] The need to take vital signs can be opinioned by therapists treating patients with musculoskeletal disorders as being a big waste of time.[2] But what about Mrs. Mason from the introduction in Chapter 1? She was referred to an outpatient physical therapy facility because of a pelvic fracture. Her challenged pulmonary status from sarcoidosis absolutely needed to be considered during her examination and the establishment of her treatment plan.

So despite the diversity of specialty settings within physical therapy, each therapist is responsible for the basic competencies required to examine all the systems within the scope of the Patient/Client Management Model. The process of completing the full evaluation also requires an understanding of how the systems overlap and influence the patient's ability to achieve the expected outcomes.

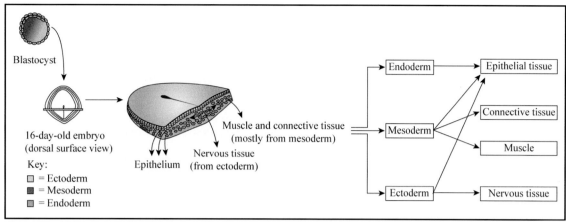

Figure 10-1. Embryonic and fetal development of tissues. Primary germ layer formation is one of the first events of embryonic development. Ectoderm is the most superficial of the layers. Mesoderm is the middle layer. Endoderm is the deepest layer. The primary germ layers specialize to form the 4 primary tissues. (Adapted from http://classes.midlandstech.edu.carterp/Courses/bio210/chap04/chap04.html and Kørbling M, Estove Z. Adult stem cells for tissue repair—a new therapeutic concept? *New Engl J Med.* 2003;349(6):570-582.)

This chapter will present the essential pathophysiology for local musculoskeletal and connective tissue disorders. The physiology of the structures involved and the basic tissues that comprise them will begin the chapter. How these structures respond when injured as well as how they are affected by compromised cardiovascular and pulmonary status will also be discussed. Special considerations for the examination of local musculoskeletal and connective tissue dysfunction will be outlined. The chapter will conclude with a patient case.

EPIDEMIOLOGY

How unusual is the situation for Mr. Cedar, Mrs. Mason, and others to be in a more-than-one medical diagnosis situation? That is difficult to quantify from the dizzyingly array of statistics for health status in the United States. The sheer numbers for 2 separate categories of diagnoses—chronic obstructive pulmonary diseases (COPD) and musculoskeletal disorders—suggest a significant overlap could easily exist. In Chapter 8 it is noted that nearly 14 million adults in the United States have a pulmonary pump dysfunction in the form of COPD. What are the chances that all these patients have perfectly functioning joints, optimal alignment, and normal strength? Certainly some will have musculoskeletal complaints that will lead to referrals for physical therapy.

Conversely, in the latest available statistics from the National Ambulatory Medical Care Survey, musculoskeletal complaints were the number 2 reason for physician office visits in a survey of all office visits.[3] It is estimated that 1 in 4 Americans have a musculoskeletal disorder according to a report on the United States Bone and Joint Decade.[4] It could reasonably be assumed that many of these musculoskeletal disorders will occur in individuals with a cardiovascular or pulmonary dysfunction.

BASIC TISSUES

Before the significance that an injured joint, or altered alignment, can have on functional endurance, or performance, the features of the musculoskeletal structures involved need to be understood. The joints, musculotendinous units, and peripheral nerves are grouped together only because of their basic commonality as structures of the musculoskeletal system. In fact, each structure is quite different from the others. Basic to them all, however, are the body's basic 4 tissues. And, even though it will be shown later in the chapter that each of the structures in the musculoskeletal system actually contains more than one of the basic tissues, knowledge about the organization and physiology of basic tissues will aid in the understanding of the physiology and pathophysiology of the musculoskeletal system.

Specialized cells and tissues in the human body develop from the germ layers of the embryo. These layers in the embryo are derived from the germ cells (ova and sperm). The outer germ layer (ectoderm) contributes to the formation of nervous tissues, most glands and the epidermis. The middle layer (mesoderm) develops into connective tissues. The inner layer (endoderm) contributes to the tissues of the intestinal tract.[5]

In the distribution of characteristics from the germ layers, 4 basic tissues develop. They are epithelial tissue, connective tissue, nervous tissue, and muscle. Each of these basic tissues has a distinctive cell type. In addition, the tissue characteristics are further defined by the substances, or structure, between the cells as well as by the fluids that nourish the tissue and carry off waste products (Figure 10-1).[5]

Epithelial Tissue

Epithelial tissue forms into continuous cellular sheets that cover the outside of the body as well as line most internal body regions.[5,6] Any of the germ layers of the embryo gives

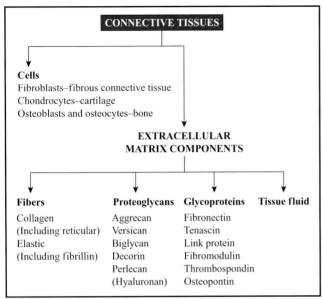

Figure 10-2. Principal components of connective tissues. (Adapted from Culav EM, Clark CH, Merriless MG. Connective tissues: matrix composition and its relevance to physical therapy. *Phys Ther.* 1999;79:310.)

rise to this simple tissue. For example, the membranes of the heart, blood vessels, and lymphatic vessels are called endothelium but these linings actually arose from mesoderm.[5] Simple epithelial membranes of contiguous cells have near absence of intercellular substances. Glands can develop from epithelium; secretory cells can be situated within the tissue. Epithelium can be categorized by cell shape, the number and arrangement of cell layers, and the type of dominant cell. Epithelial tissue is avascular. These tissues rely on nutrition from underlying connective tissue to which the epithelial tissue is attached by tightly bonding with an intervening basement membrane.

The discussion of integument disorders treated by physical therapists is beyond the scope of this chapter. It should be noted, however, that in the treatment of musculoskeletal disorders consideration is given to skin mobility. As well, the mobility of tissues below the basement membrane—the dermis, subcutaneous tissue/superficial fascia, and deep fascia—is assessed. As will be shown later in the chapter, musculoskeletal tissues need to adapt to mechanical loads. Skin as an epithelial tissue, along with the underlying tissues, needs to adapt to mechanical loads as well.[7]

Connective Tissue

Connective tissues arise from the embryonic mesoderm and constitute a large portion of total body mass. Their general role is connecting and nourishing other tissues. Connective tissue can range from ordinary loose or dense tissues to the highly specialized tissues of cartilage and bone.[5] Most connective tissues are "strong, resilient and capable of repairing themselves."[8]

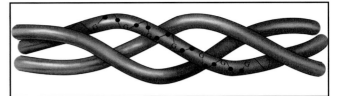

Figure 10-3. Portion of a collagen molecule showing individual alpha chains coiled to form a triple helix. Within each chain, the amino acids are similarly arranged in a helix, with glycine (G) facing the center of the triple helix. The other amino acids are represented by the dots. (Adapted from Culav EM, Clark CH, Merriless MG. Connective tissues: matrix composition and its relevance to physical therapy. *Phys Ther.* 1999;79:311.)

Extracellular Matrix

The properties of epithelial, nervous, and muscle tissues are distinctive because of what lies within the cells of these tissues as well as how the cells are arranged. Connective tissue differs. The properties of connective tissues are determined by the amount, type, and arrangement of the large quantities of intercellular substances manufactured by the discrete connective tissue cells.[9] These intercellular substances, called the extracellular matrix, surround the cells. The "blast" version of the cell produces the extracellular matrix until it is surrounded. Then it becomes somewhat trapped when the matrix matures. For example, fibroblasts, chondroblasts, and osteoblasts—types of connective tissue cells—produce the extracellular matrix that will mature to become fibrous connective tissue, cartilage, and bone, respectively (Figure 10-2). In mature connective tissue, the "blast" version of the cell, now trapped within the matrix, matures to the "cyte" version. The fibrocyte, chondrocyte, or osteocyte remains within the extracellular matrix to maintain its respective tissue as well as aid in repair if the tissue becomes damaged because of injury or disease.

Fibrous Connective Tissue

In connective tissues where fibroblasts are the dominant cell type, the 3 major components of the extracellular matrix are the fibers themselves along with proteoglycans and glycoproteins. Collagen and elastin are the major protein fibers produced by fibroblasts.

Collagen is formed from triple chains of amino acids where every third acid in each chain is glycine. The smaller glycine molecule allows a bend in each chain wherever the glycine appears, which leads to the characteristic helix shape. Intermolecular bonds between 3 helix chains, wound together, create collagen's ability to resist tensile loads (Figure 10-3). The assembly of triple helix chains into fibrils, and then fibers with more crosslinks, further aids collagen's resilience to elongation (Figure 10-4). The 19 distinct types of collagen are defined by the amino acids used to make the chains and whether the triple chains in the helix are all alike or differ in 1 or 2 of the chains.[9]

Elastin fibers are also made from fibroblasts. These fibers, as the name suggests, are highly extensible to tension forces.

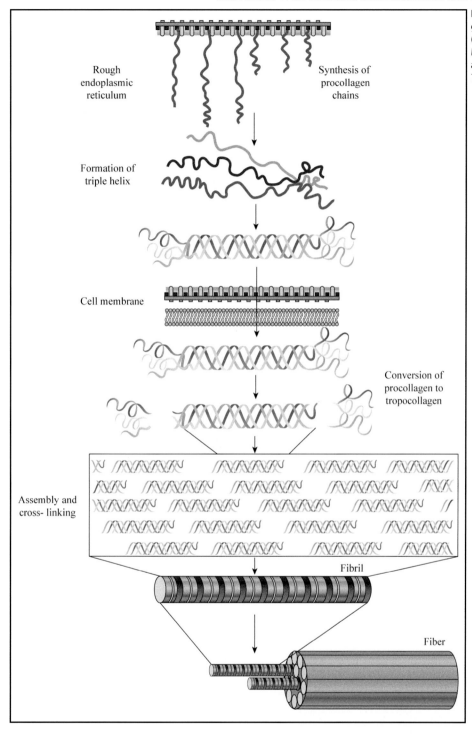

Rough endoplasmic reticulum

Synthesis of procollagen chains

Formation of triple helix

Cell membrane

Conversion of procollagen to tropocollagen

Assembly and cross-linking

Fibril

Fiber

Figure 10-4. Representation of collagen synthesis, secretion, and assembly. (Adapted from Culav EM, Clark CH, Merriless MG. Connective tissues: matrix composition and its relevance to physical therapy. *Phys Ther.* 1999;79:312.)

Generally, they will recoil to their original length when tension is released. For these properties, connective tissue with elastin has a large distribution throughout the body. Elastin can be organized in concentric sheets to accommodate pressure changes, as in the aorta, or as individual fibers to allow stretching in multi-directions, as in skin. The amount of elastin fibers, and their orientation, will depend on the amount of stretch to be withstood, and the direction, respectively.[9,10]

The ratio of collagen to elastin within a fibrous connective tissue can vary. Tendons connecting muscles to bone, and ligaments in high stress regions, need to withstand high-tension forces. These fibrous connective tissues will, therefore, have a higher proportion of collagen fibers to elastin. Other ligaments that need to be more flexible will have greater amounts of elastin (Figure 10-5).

A proteoglycan in the extracellular matrix of fibrous connective tissue consists of a strand of protein—the protein core (PC)—on which repeating side chains of disaccharides attach—the glycosaminoglycan chains (GAG chains). The PC can vary in type and size but specific proteoglycans have

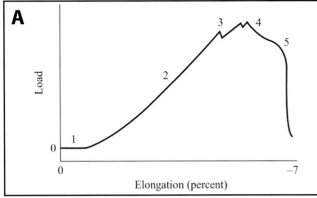

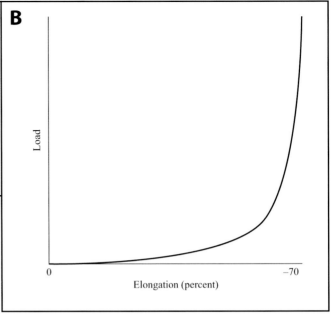

Figure 10-5. Mechanical behavior of 2 ligaments experimentally tested in tension to failure: one with a high percentage of collagen fibers and the other with a high percentage of elastic fibers. (A) Load-elongation curve for a human anterior cruciate ligament (90% collagen fibers) tested in tension to failure. (B) Load-elongation curve for human ligamentum flavum (60% to 70% elastic fibers) testing in tension to failure. At 70% elongation the ligament failed abruptly. (Reprinted with permission from Frankel VH, Nordin M. *Basic Biomechanics of the Skeletal System*. Philadelphia, PA: Lea & Febiger; 1980.)

Figure 10-6. Representation of an aggrecan monomer with keratan sulfate (KS) and chondroitin sulfate (CS) GAG side chains attached to the PC. The monomer is attached to hyaluronan and is stabilized at this binding region by link protein. Numerous monomers attach to hyaluronan to form the large proteoglycan aggregate. (Adapted from *Phys Ther*. 1999;79:308-319, with permission of the American Physical Therapy Association. Copyright © 1999 American Physical Therapy Association.)

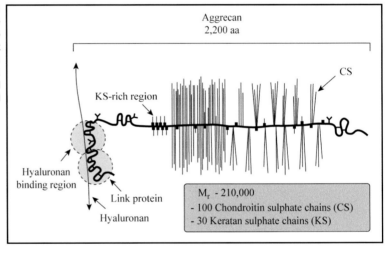

specific PCs. The properties of a proteoglycan are largely defined, however, by the number and type of the GAG side chains. Of note is the water-holding capacity of the side chains. The review article on connective tissue matrix by Culav et al explains:

> All GAGs are negatively charged and have a propensity to attract ions, creating an osmotic imbalance that results in the PG-GAG absorbing water from surrounding areas. This absorption helps maintain the hydration of the matrix; the degree of hydration depends on the number of GAG chain and on the restriction placed on the PG swelling by the surrounding collagen fibers...[9(pp313-314)]

Proteoglycans can aggregate onto single strands of hyaluronan to form large molecule complexes. The best known of these is aggrecan (Figure 10-6). A glycoprotein—link protein—aids in the stability of aggrecan. Other glycoproteins help stabilize the components of the extracellular matrix.

The function of the fibrous connective tissue will dictate the proportion of fiber to proteoglycan concentration as well as the orientation of the fibers. In general, ligaments and tendons, which are dense regular connective tissues, have lower proportions of proteoglycans to fibers because the need to withstand compression forces is less. The presence of proteoglycans in these tissues helps to keep the fibers apart to limit undesired crosslinks (Table 10-1). In some instances, the underside of a tendon may have a bit more proteoglycans in its tissue to withstand the compression that occurs as the tendon comes in contact with underlying bone.[9,11]

Nonconnective tissue cells can be found within the connective tissue matrix. Mast cells containing heparin and histamine, macrophages, white blood cells [WBCs]), and lymphocytes are located within the matrix and are ready for activation if the tissue is damaged by injury or disease.[8]

TABLE 10-1. CLASSIFICATION OF FIBROUS CONNECTIVE TISSUE

DENSE		
Dense Regular	Characteristics	Dense parallel arrangement of collagen fibers Higher collagen to proteoglycan ratio Compactness of tissue leads to limited vascular supply
	Properties	High tensile strength Withstands unidirectional stress Little extensibility Increased healing time after trauma
	Tissue examples	Tendons, ligaments
Dense Irregular	Characteristics	Dense but multidirectional arrangement of collagen fibers Higher collagen to proteoglycan ratio but lower than dense regular tissue Improved vascularity compared with dense regular tissue
	Properties	Withstands multidirectional stress Improved healing time compared to that of dense regular tissue
	Tissue examples	Aponeuroses, joint capsules, periosteum, dermis of skin, fascial sheaths (under high degree of mechanical stress)
LOOSE		
Loose Irregular	Characteristics	Sparse, multidirectional framework of collagen and elastin fibers Higher proteoglycan to fiber ratio Greater vascularity compared with the other connective tissue types
	Properties	Lowest ability to resist stress Designed to withstand multidirectional low stress Best ability to heal of the fibrous connective tissue types
	Tissue examples	Superficial and some deep fascia, nerve and muscle sheaths, endomysium, supportive framework of the lymph system and internal organs

Adapted from Grodin JA, Cantu RI. *Myofascial Manipulation: Theory and Clinical Management*. Berryville, VA: Forum Medicum Inc; 1989.

Cartilage

As noted previously, a greater proportion of proteoglycans to fibers is found in connective tissue that is subjected to high compressive forces. The second portion of the quote noted previously from Culav et al describes cartilage as, "[the] limited expansion [due to the constraint of surrounding collagen fibers] provides rigidity of the matrix and, where PG content is high, endows the tissue with the ability to resist compressive forces."[9(p314)] Cartilage is structured to withstand high compressive forces.

There are variations of cartilage types. Cartilage is a semirigid tissue but it can also be flexible where needed as in the elastic cartilage of the ear and the epiglottis of the throat. Tendon insertions and the intervertebral discs are reinforced with collagen fibers in a tough form of cartilage identified as fibrocartilage. The long bones of the body began as cartilage that was gradually replaced by bone. Hyaline cartilage

remained at the bone ends. Children have cartilaginous growth plates between the bone ends and the long bone shaft (Figure 10-7).

Cartilage can grow by expanding from within. This interstitial growth occurs by division of young chondral cells within the matrix. Each newly divided cell will secrete more matrix around itself. This swelling-from-within growth that cartilage can do does not occur in bone.

Appositional growth used by cartilage and bone simply adds another layer of tissue to the outside of what has already formed. Appositional growth creates an interesting contrast for tendons and ligaments inserting into cartilage and those into bone. Tendons and ligaments inserting into cartilage continue the blending of collagen fibers into fibrocartilage as the cartilage grows outwardly. Tendons or ligaments attaching to bone, on the other hand, become gradually embedded in the ever increasing outer rings of bone. These embedded collagen fibers are called Sharpey's fibers (Figure 10-8).[5]

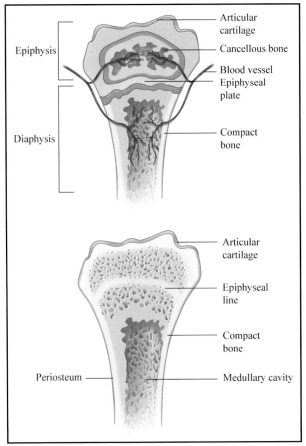

Figure 10-7. Comparison of the cartilaginous epiphyseal growth plate in still lengthening childhood bone with the no longer lengthening epiphyseal line in adult bone.

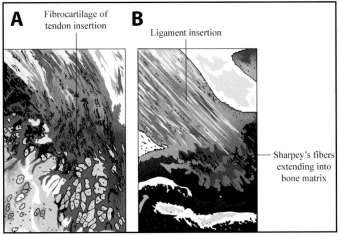

Figure 10-8. (A) Tendon insertion (patellar tendon of rat). (B) Ligament insertion (anterior cruciate of rat). (Reprinted with permission from Cormack DH. *Introduction to Histology.* 2nd ed. Philadelphia, PA: Lippincott Williams & Wilkins; 2001.)

Cartilage is avascular. It relies on nutrients from capillaries outside the cartilage to diffuse throughout the cartilage, a relatively long distance of travel for such essential components to cartilage health. Another nutrition challenge for cartilage occurs when deposits of insoluble calcium salts cause calcification of the matrix. When this calcification occurs, it interferes with diffusion and, thus, the nutrition of the entire cartilage. Bone, on the other hand, is able to calcify without disruption of its tissue nutrition.

Bone

Aside from the commonalities as connective tissue, bone shares additional characteristics with cartilage. First, once osteocytes, like chondrocytes, become embedded in the encasing extracellular matrix, each resides within a small space called a lacuna. And, despite the obvious difference in the composition of the extracellular matrix between cartilage and bone, discussed next, the extracellular matrix of both are reinforced by collagen fibrils. Second, bone's outer surface is covered by a fibrous layer called periosteum that is similar to the perichondrium for cartilage. The highly vascularized periosteum, however, becomes incorporated into bone, which creates an essential difference in the overall nutrition of bone compared to cartilage.

Bone, however, is clearly different from cartilage in that bone has a highly calcified and unyielding extracellular matrix. As a specialized connective tissue, bone arises from embryonic mesoderm. The formation of bone, osteogenesis, occurs in 1 of 2 ways. The flat bones of the skull are formed by bone tissue developing directly in the mesenchyme membrane in a process called intramembranous osteogenesis. The majority of bone tissue, including long bones, grows on an intervening and temporary model of cartilage. This process of bone formation is called endochondral osteogenesis.[5] The final bone tissues, regardless of the osteogenesis process followed, are the same.

As noted previously, a less obvious difference between cartilage and bone is that bone has a better structure in place for its nutritional needs. Osteocyte lacunae are interconnected by tiny canals called canaliculi (Figure 10-9). Tissue fluids rich in nutrients and oxygen travel through the canaliculi. These interconnecting canals may serve also as a network for transmitting signals with changes in bone loading and unloading. The fluids of the canaliculi are refreshed by nearby capillaries which were incorporated into the bone structure during development. Osteocytes, with surrounding calcified matrix, grow appositionally around a vascular supply to eventually form Haversian systems (Figure 10-10). All bone, therefore, is not far from a vascular supply, which further ensures the delivery of adequate available nutrition from capillaries via the canaliculi.

Nervous Tissue

The cells and tissue of the nervous system arise from the mid-dorsal embryonic ectoderm. Specifically, a flat and elongated neural plate forms that then folds and connects dorsally to become the neural tube. The brain and spinal cord develop from the neural tube and become the central nervous system (CNS). The peripheral nervous system (PNS), which innervates the trunk, limbs, and head arises from the

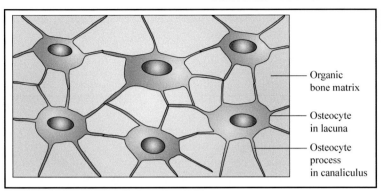

Figure 10-9. Osteocytes in lacuna with canaliculi. (Adapted from Cormack DH. *Introduction to Histology.* Philadelphia, PA: J.B. Lippincott Co; 1984.)

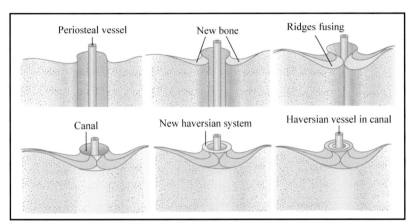

Figure 10-10. Bone widening occurs when new Haversian systems are added to the periphery diaphysis. Periosteal vessels become incorporated in the new Haversian canals. (Adapted from Cormack DH. *Introduction to Histology.* Philadelphia, PA: J.B. Lippincott Co; 1984.)

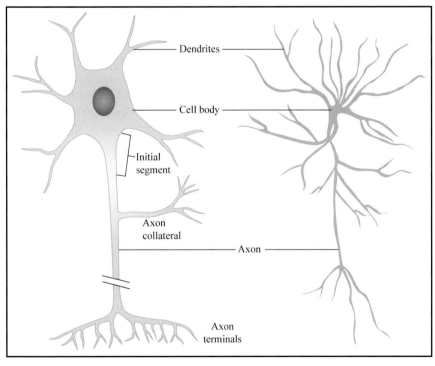

Figure 10-11. A representation of a neuron. The long length of the axon, compared to that of the cell body, defines its function to connect with other neurons—even in other parts of the body. (Adapted from Widmaier EP, Hershel R, Strang KT. *Vander, Sherman, Luciano's Human Physiology: The Mechanism of Body Function.* 9th ed. New York: McGraw-Hill; 2004.)

neural crest, an extension of nervous tissue that appears along both sides of the neural tube.

The basic structure of nerve cells reflects their specialized function to carry excitatory signals along nervous system pathways that interconnect all parts of the body. Branching dendrites, at one end of the nerve cell, transmit electrical signals along the outer membrane of the cell toward the cell body. The signal continues along the outer membrane of the cell body and then the long extension of the cell, the axon, until branching at the axon end connects with dendrites of other nerve cells (Figure 10-11). The transmission of current from one nerve cell to another, the synapse, can lead to the

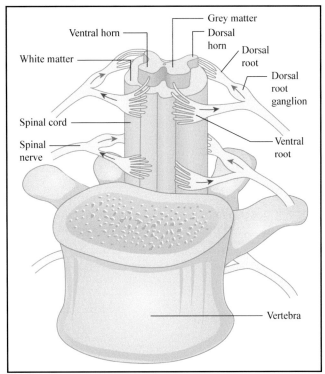

Figure 10-12. Section of the spinal cord, ventral view. The arrows indicate the direction of transmission of neural activity. (Adapted from Widmaier EP, Hershel R, Strang KT. *Vander, Sherman, Luciano's Human Physiology: The Mechanism of Body Function.* 9th ed. New York: McGraw-Hill; 2004.)

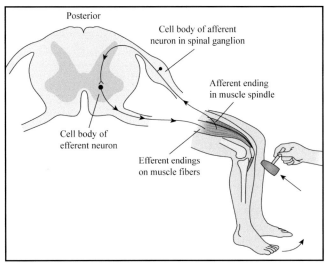

Figure 10-13. The neural structure of the stretch reflex. (Adapted from Cormack DH. *Introduction to Histology.* Philadelphia, PA: J.B. Lippincott Co; 1984.)

Muscle Tissue

The fourth basic tissue formed from germ layers is muscle. The fetal muscle cells arise from the mesoderm layer. The predominant characteristic of muscle tissue is the ability to use energy to contract. Aiding in this function is the formation of long multinucleated muscle fibers from small nucleated muscle cells during fetal development. In addition, fetal muscle cells differentiate along 3 pathways to form striated cardiac and skeletal muscle, and nonstriated smooth muscle (see Figure 1-10).

All 3 muscle types rely on actin and myosin filaments for contractile properties though how the filaments are arranged differ. Each muscle type has a network structure to disperse a depolarizing signal to all fibers to initiate a contraction. Each has a structure for the wide release, and reabsorption, of calcium ions.

In skeletal muscle, the myofilaments within the muscle fiber, the myofibril, are arranged in a repeating pattern. Within the unit of the repeating pattern, the sarcomere, the myosin molecules bundle to form thick filaments. A myosin filament bundle is surrounded by an arrangement of nonbundled lighter actin filaments. One end of the actin filaments are attached to interconnecting proteins, the Z-line (Figure 10-14).

A single actin filament is encircled by end-to-end chains of tropomyosin that block the myosin-binding sites on the actin filament. When calcium ions are released, the calcium binds with the troponin molecules on the tropomyosin chains. This causes the tropomyosin chain to reconfigure, which then moves the chain off the binding sites on the actin filament. A myosin cross-bridge binds with the now available site on the actin filament, causing the energized cross-bridge to rotate and the myofilaments to slide past each other.

The presence of adenosine triphosphate (ATP) energizes the cross-bridge for rotation and force generation. ATP then

electrical charge continuing along the second nerve or inhibiting the nerve to accept other charges.

In the brain and spinal cord, cell bodies will cluster together. These areas were labeled gray matter because of their gray appearance in tissue cross sections. White matter are areas with predominately dendrites and axons. The outer edge of the brain, called the cortex, is largely gray matter with white matter seen in the central regions of the brain. The reverse arrangement occurs in the spinal cord, with gray matter central and white matter on the periphery (Figure 10-12).

A characteristic common both to gray and white matter is that there is very little connective tissue present. Without the supporting structure of an extracellular matrix and connective tissue layers, the tissues of the CNS are soft. The nerve tissue of the PNS differs from that of the CNS by the incorporation of connective tissue layers into the structure of peripheral nerves that provide resilience.

Afferent nerves transmit electrical impulses generated by sensory receptors, afferent endings, to the spinal cord and brain. Cell bodies for afferent nerves cluster in the cranial ganglia for cranial nerves and the posterior dorsal root ganglia for peripheral nerves.

Efferent nerve cell bodies are located in the motor cortex of the brain and anterior horn of the spinal cord. Efferent nerves transmit signals from the brain and spinal cord largely to muscle fibers (Figure 10-13).

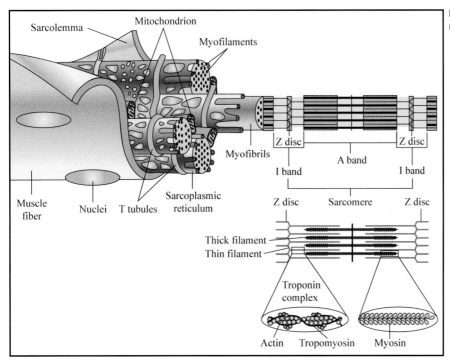

Figure 10-14. Organization of muscle monofilaments and Z-line/disc.

enables the myosin cross-bridge to release from the bond and re-energize. This prepares the myosin cross-bridge to bond again on the actin filament with more sliding of the myofilaments past each other (Figure 10-15).

The calcium ions are released from, and reabsorbed back into, the sarcoplasmic reticulum. Corresponding to the endoplasmic reticulum within most other cells in the body, the sarcoplasmic reticulum creates a sleeve-like network of tubes outside each myofibril. Two pairs of tubes, the terminal cisternae, surround the muscle fiber at the level of the junction of the A bands and the I bands on the sarcomere. Anastomosing tubes, the sacrotubules, span the region corresponding to the A band (Figure 10-16).

The connective tissue outer layer of the myofibril, the sarcolemma, sends projections of tissue, the T-tubules, to nestle between a pair of terminal cisternae. When the sarcolemma is depolarized, the signal is carried along the T-tubules, which then activates the release of calcium ions from the sarcoplasmic reticulum (Box 10-1).

Tissue Damage and Healing

Basic Tissues' Shared Events

The differences in the structure of the basic tissues also lead to differences in the specific events that occur when each tissue is damaged by injury or disease. Variations in the paths and rates of healing also exist. There are, however, considerable commonalities. Since, the basic tissues migrated during fetal development and layered to form the components of the musculoskeletal system—the joints, musculotendinous units, and peripheral nerves—an understanding of those basic commonalities is useful. Important variations to note will appear in later sections of the chapter.

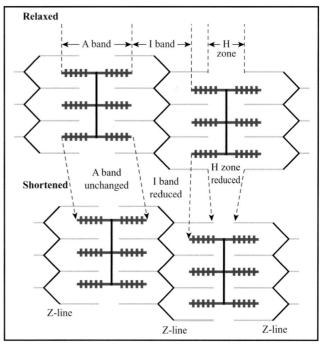

Figure 10-15. The I-Band and H-Band regions narrow as thick filaments slide past thin filaments. The actual fibers don't shorten but the sarcomere length does. (Adapted from Widmaier EP, Hershel R, Strang KT. *Vander, Sherman, Luciano's Human Physiology: The Mechanism of Body Function.* 9th ed. New York, NY: McGraw-Hill; 2004.)

Damage to tissues from an injury or disease will trigger a series of overlapping events within the first hours and days. The healing and recovery sequences that follow will proceed over weeks and months. The multilayered process can be roughly defined as occurring with an immediate response and the 3 phases of inflammation, tissue repair/regeneration, and maturation/remodeling.

Figure 10-16. A drawing showing the myofibrillar striations in relation to the sarcoplasmic reticulum and transverse tubules location on a muscle fiber. (Adapted from Cormack DH. *Introduction to Histology.* Philadelphia, PA: J.B. Lippincott Co; 1984.)

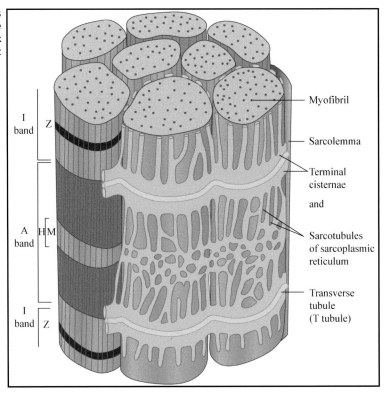

I band — Z

A band — H M

I band — Z

Myofibril

Sarcolemma

Terminal cisternae and

Sarcotubules of sarcoplasmic reticulum

Transverse tubule (T tubule)

BOX 10-1. THE SLIDING FILAMENT THEORY OF MUSCLE CONTRACTION

1. Local currents depolarize the adjacent muscle cell plasma membrane to its threshold potential, generating an action potential that propagates over the muscle fiber surface and into the fiber along the T-tubules.

2. Action potential in the T-tubules triggers release of Ca2+ from terminal cisternae of the sarcoplasmic reticulum.

3. Ca2+ binds to troponin on the thin filaments, causing tropomyosin to move away from its blocking position, thereby uncovering cross-bridge binding sites on actin.

4. Energized myosin cross-bridges on the thick filaments bind to actin.

5. Cross-bridge binding triggers release of adenosine triphosphate (ATP) hydrolysis products from myosin, producing an angular movement of each cross-bridge.

6. ATP binds to myosin, breaking linkage between actin and myosin and thereby allowing cross-bridges to dissociate from actin.

7. ATP bound to myosin is split, energizing the myosin cross-bridge.

8. Cross-bridges repeat steps 4 to 7, producing movement (sliding) of thin filaments past thick filaments. Cycles of cross-bridge movement continue as long as Ca2+ remains bound to troponin.

9. Cytosolic Ca2+ concentration decreases as Ca2+ is actively transported into sarcoplasmic reticulum by Ca2+-ATPase.

10. Removal of Ca2+ from troponin restores blocking action of tropomyosin, the cross-bridge cycle ceases, and the muscle fiber relaxes.

Sequence of events in skeletal muscle fiber contraction.

Reprinted with permission from Widmaier EP, Hershel R, Strang KT. *Vander, Sherman, Luciano's Human Physiology: The Mechanism of Body Function.* 9th ed. New York: McGraw-Hill; 2004. Copyright McGraw-Hill Education.

Immediate Response

When an injury occurs, the crushed cells spill their contents into the area of injury along with blood and lymphatic fluids leaking from damaged vessels. Nearby cells with a lost blood supply due to damaged capillaries will also lose the ability to survive and maintain their outer cell walls, thus more cellular debris is added. A disease process in tissues can begin with lyzing of otherwise healthy cells creating a similar "pool" of cellular debris. One immediate damage control response, actually signaled by the presence of cellular debris, begins with the conversion of prothrombin, in the leaked blood and lymph exudate, into thrombin. Fibrinogen, also in the cellular debris, will be activated by the thrombin to form fibrin-based clots. The clot formation ensures that any continued bleeding into the area not already curtailed by vasoconstriction, another immediate damage control response, is stopped. The fibrin and the cellular debris create a gel-like seal over the area.[12] The region of tissues damaged by invading disease will undergo a similar effort at containment by fibrin clots.[13]

Inflammation

A chemical signal, chemotaxis, from the cellular debris and the process of clot formation sets off local and system reactions that lead to inflammation. Bradykinin, a vasodilator, is activated locally. It, in turn, stimulates the release of potent prostaglandins, which improve the ability of arriving neutrophils and monocytes to enter interstitial spaces by increasing the permeability of capillary walls. The characteristic signs of inflammation—tissue redness, swelling, and tenderness—result from the vasodilation, increased presence of fluids in the interstitial spaces, and the stimulation of nociceptors by bradykinin and prostaglandins.

In an example of the overlapping of events, the clearing of cellular debris as a step preceding tissue repair is underway even while the inflammatory phase is just developing. Macrophages located in the extracellular matrix of the injured tissues begin digesting the cellular debris within an hour of the injury.[13] Within a few hours after injury, and with the phase of inflammation now well underway, these macrophages will be joined by neutrophils and monocytes that have followed the chemotaxis signal to the area. The mature neutrophils will begin phagocytosis immediately on arrival at the periphery of the debris. The monocytes, on the other hand, arrive but then need a period of 8 to 12 hours to change into mature macrophages. The ability of the neutrophils to begin phagocytosis immediately is advantageous to control bacteria, which may be present when inflammation is associated with a disease process, in a timely manner. When time is not as critical, macrophages have the advantage of greater capacity for phagocytosis as well as the ability to phagocytize larger particles—including spent neutrophils. Macrophages can also phagocytize necrotic tissues.[13] The effects of inflammation may last nearly a week. Gradually, however, the symptoms fade as a transition occurs from the task of cleaning up cellular debris to one of tissue rebuilding.

Tissue Repair/Regeneration

Clearing of the cellular debris stimulates vascular growth. During angiogenesis capillary buds form on the edge of cleared debris and become vessels. This in turn provides a blood supply for the tissue rebuilding work of tenocytes, osteocytes, and myocytes. Tissue regeneration efforts can be challenged, however, by the body's need to quickly restore mechanical integrity to the injured tissues to allow a gradual resumption of function.

The distinction between tissue repair and tissue regeneration is an important one. Tissue regeneration means that the damaged tissue is replaced by tissue that eventually will be indistinguishable, or nearly so, from that which was damaged. Repair tissue is the creation of a scar tissue patch that is unlikely to be an exact match to the mechanical properties of the original tissue.[12] So, time, along with the size of the injury area and the tissue type, will determine the extent to whether tissue repair will dominate. Tissue regeneration may be progressing well but simply becomes overrun by the faster repair offered by collagen-producing fibroblasts.

The phase of regeneration and repair continues for 4 to 6 weeks, until the entire area of injury has a stabilizing structure in place, whether regeneration tissue or scar tissue. The structural organization and overall strength of the new tissue can be enhanced by the gradual introduction of mechanical forces in the form of controlled movements.[14-17]

Maturation/Remodeling

The final stage of healing allows the new tissues to mature and strengthen. The initial collagen fibers in repaired tissues are gradually replaced by a stronger form. Bone, a regenerated tissue, undergoes remodeling to achieve its final optimum structure. The process of maturation and remodeling can go on for more than 1 year depending on the tissue.

The final tissue properties that are restored will vary. Largely collagen-based tissues may recover only about 75% of their original strength.[18] Regenerated fractured bone, on the other hand, can become indistinguishable in appearance or structural properties from the original bone. All of the basic tissues have shown enhanced recovery of structural properties with gradually increasing mechanical loads.[7,14-17]

Tissue Health

A number of factors can impede the recovery of injured tissues. A compromised cardiovascular or pulmonary status may diminish the adequate delivery of essential oxygen and nutrients to the tissue rebuilding site. Disruption of early capillary formation will delay the stages of healing.[12] Medications useful for controlling inflammatory processes in one part of the body may interfere with the tissue building in another.[19] Smoking adversely affects bone and wound healing as well as increase rates of postoperative complications with surgeries requiring microvascular repair.[20,21] The information on tissue injury and healing gives rise to several questions: Can the causes of tissue injury be identified? What can be done to aid injured tissues? Is there any way to help tissues resist physical stress and avoid injury? A theoretical framework for the answers to these questions can be found in the Physical Stress Theory (PST).

Physical Stress Theory

Mueller and Maluf theorized that an adaptive response could be predicted in all biological tissues relative to the

BOX 10-2. SUMMARY OF FUNDAMENTAL PRINCIPLES FOR PHYSICAL STRESS THEORY

BASIC PREMISE: CHANGES IN THE RELATIVE LEVEL OF PHYSICAL STRESS CAUSE A PREDICTABLE ADAPTIVE RESPONSE IN ALL BIOLOGICAL TISSUE

Fundamental Principles:

A. Changes in the relative level of physical stress cause a predictable response in all biological tissues.

B. Biological tissues exhibit 5 characteristic responses to physical stress [Figure 10-17]. Each response is predicted to occur within a defined range along a continuum of stress levels. Specific thresholds define the upper and lower stress levels for each characteristic tissue response. Qualitatively, the 5 tissue responses to physical stress are decreased stress tolerance (eg, atrophy), maintenance, increased stress tolerance (eg, hypertrophy), injury, and death.

C. Physical stress levels that are lower than the maintenance range result in decreased tolerance of tissues to subsequent stresses (eg, atrophy).

D. Physical stress levels that are in the maintenance range result in no apparent tissue change.

E. Physical stress levels that exceed the maintenance range (ie, overload) result in increased tolerance of tissues to subsequent stresses (eg, hypertrophy).

F. Excessively high levels of physical stress result in tissue injury.

G. Extreme deviations from the maintenance stress range that exceed the adaptive capacity of tissues result in tissue death.

H. The level of exposure to physical stress is a composite value, defined by the magnitude, time, and direction of stress application.

I. Individual stresses combine in complex ways to contribute to the overall level of stress exposure. Tissues are affected by the history of recent stresses.

J. Excessive physical stress that causes injury can occur from 1 or more of the following 3 mechanisms: (1) a high-magnitude stress applied for a brief period, (2) a low-magnitude stress applied for a long duration, and (3) a moderate-magnitude stress applied to the tissue many times.

K. Inflammation occurs immediately following tissue injury and renders the injured tissue less tolerant of stress than it was prior to injury. Injured and inflamed tissues must be protected from subsequent excessive stress until acute inflammation subsides.

L. The stress thresholds required to achieve a given tissue response may vary among individuals depending on the presence or absence of several modulating variables. Factors that can influence thresholds for tissue adaptation and injury are summarized in Box 10-3 and include movement and alignment, extrinsic, behavioral, and physiological factors.

level of physical stress to which the tissues were exposed.[19] The authors of the PST offer an overview of the fundamental principles of tissue adaptations for the tissues, and the organ systems composed of those tissues, most relevant to the scope of practice for physical therapists. The evidence-based shared reactions of the tissues and organ systems have been identified (Box 10-2).

Also integral to the PST are those factors that will further affect tissue adaptation (Box 10-3). Systemic pathology, poor control of alignment of fractured bone ends, and medications are consistent with the impediments to tissue healing mentioned previously.

As physical stress levels increase or decrease from a level that maintains tissue integrity level, predictable outcomes can be outlined (Figure 10-17). Chapter 4 discussed the tissue adaptations—decreased tissue tolerance—that occur with decreased physical stress. Similarly, effects of training on tissues presented in Chapter 5 illustrate the specific increased tissue tolerances that develop as a result of graded increased physical stress.

The overview offered by the PST can be used as the vantage point from which to view the effect that compromised cardiovascular and pulmonary systems have on musculoskeletal structures. From the perspective of the PST, any compromise of the cardiovascular and pulmonary systems has the potential to affect tissue physical stress tolerance, and thus, contribute to the development of a musculoskeletal disorder. In addition, systemic pathology, along with the other factors listed in Box 10-3, can affect the recovery from a musculoskeletal disorder.

BOX 10-3. FACTORS AFFECTING THE LEVEL OF PHYSICAL STRESS ON TISSUES OR THE ADAPTIVE RESPONSE OF TISSUES TO PHYSICAL STRESS

- Movement and alignment factors
  - Muscle performance (force generation, length)
  - Motor control
  - Posture and alignment
  - Physical activity
  - Occupational, leisure, and self-care activities
- Extrinsic factors
  - Orthotic devices, taping, assistive devices
  - Footwear
  - Ergonomic environment
  - Modalities
  - Gravity

- Psychosocial factors
- Physiological factors
  - Medication
  - Age
  - Systemic pathology
  - Obesity

Reprinted from *Phys Ther.* 2002;82:383-403, with permission of the American Physical Therapy Association. Copyright © 2012 American Physical Therapy Association.

MUSCLES

Morphology (Gross Anatomy and Histology) and Physiology

Observations on skeletal muscle morphology (gross anatomy and histology) and physiology (including biochemistry) provide insight into muscle function. The long fibers of skeletal muscle can be arranged to run along the entire length of a muscle and parallel with the tendon line of pull. This strap-like arrangement of fibers allows for an increased range of action. It does so, however, at the expense of power.[22] Conversely, a muscle can consist of shorter fibers aligned obliquely to the line of pull, as in a triangular or pennate arrangement. This muscle would be found where the required degree of shortening through the tendon is lower but muscle power higher.[23] Multiple variations in skeletal muscle fiber arrangements occur between these 2 extremes to reflect the myriad of action, power, and stabilization functions required of skeletal muscle.

Initially, whole muscles in animals were classified by appearance. The "slow" muscles of endurance appeared darker because of the greater concentration of myoglobin and capillaries than in the observed "fast" white muscles.[24] Later fibers within muscle were identified as slow-twitch or fast-twitch fibers. Muscle cross sections were stained to highlight the increased number of mitochondria in, or capillaries around, the Type I slow-twitch fibers. The fast-twitch Type II fibers were seen to have greater cross-sectional diameters, high concentrations of glycolytic enzymes, and large glycogen stores (Figure 10-18).[25]

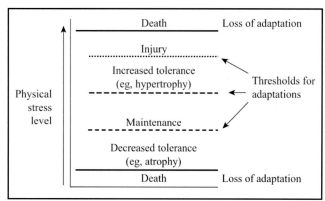

Figure 10-17. The effect of physical stress on tissue adaptation. Biological tissues exhibit 5 adaptive responses to physical stress. Each response is predicted to occur within a defined range along a continuum of stress levels. Specific thresholds define the upper and lower stress levels for each characteristic tissue response. The relative relationship between these thresholds is fairly consistent between people, whereas the absolute values for thresholds vary greatly. (Reprinted from *Phys Ther.* 2002; 82(4):383-403, with permission of the American Physical Therapy Association. Copyright © 2002 American Physical Therapy Association.)

Three current methods of muscle fiber typing differentiate by identifying myosin ATPase hydrolysis rates, myosin heavy chain isoforms or metabolism enzymes.[24] There are variable correlations, however, between the fiber types identified in each typing method (Figure 10-19).[24] Given the 7 human fiber types identified with analyzing myosin ATPase hydrolysis rates, and the variable correlations with the fibers identified in the other methods of fiber typing, what can be said about human muscle fiber types that would be accurate?

Figure 10-18. Drawings of muscle cross sections. (A) Appearance of a muscle cross section if the capillaries had been stained. The small-diameter oxidative fibers are surrounded by capillaries. (B) Staining the mitochondria highlights the large numbers of mitochondria in the small-diameter oxidative fibers. (Adapted from Widmaier EP, Hershel R, Strang KT. *Vander, Sherman, Luciano's Human Physiology: The Mechanism of Body Function.* 9th ed. New York: McGraw-Hill; 2004.)

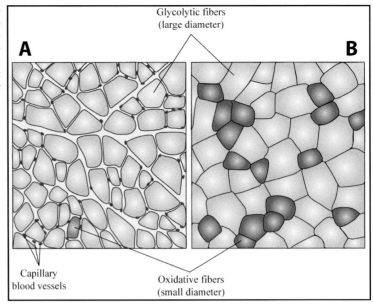

Figure 10-19. Comparison of 3 different skeletal muscle fiber type classification: histochemical staining for myosin adenosine triphosphatase (mATPase), myosin heavy chain identification, and biochemical identification of metabolic enzymes. Note: in humans, MHCIIb are now more accurately referred to as MHCIIx/d. The question marks indicate the poor correlation between biochemical and myosin heavy chain or mATPase fiber type classification schemes. (Reprinted from *Phys Ther.* 2001;81:1810-1816, with permission of the American Physical Therapy Association. Copyright © 2001 American Physical Therapy Association.)

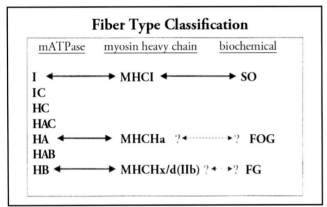

It would be safe to say that there are Type I fibers that rely on aerobic/oxidative pathways for energy metabolism. And that, on the other side of the fiber type spectrum, there are fibers, Type II, that use anaerobic/glycolytic metabolism. Then there appears to be muscle fiber types to cover the spectrum in between.[24]

A muscle with an even distribution of aerobic/oxidative fibers and anaerobic/glycolytic fibers would yield a muscle of average performance ability. Skewing the distribution of these fibers types in either direction would produce a muscle more prepared for endurance events or one for speed and power. But what determines the distribution? Can the distribution be altered? What role do the fibers in the middle of the spectrum play?

The heterogeneity of fiber types within a skeletal muscle contrasts with the homogeneity of motor units.[26] Multiple motor neurons, of various activation thresholds and transmission speeds, are situated to deliver electrical activation signals to a muscle. A motor unit consists of one motor neuron and the multiple muscle fibers its branches innervate. All the fibers within one motor unit are the same fiber type. The neuron of the motor unit appears to determine the muscle fiber type of the motor unit.[27]

Muscles contract and offer resistance under 3 different loading conditions.

> If the force developed by the muscle is greater than the load on the muscle, a shortening (concentric) contraction occurs. When the force developed by the muscle and the load are equivalent, or the load is immovable, a fixed length, or isometric contraction, results. The third type of contraction occurs when the load on the muscle is greater than the force developed by the muscle and the muscle is stretched, producing a lengthening (eccentric) contraction.[28(p93)]

Muscle fiber lengths are variable in these 3 muscle contraction scenarios. What is consistent about the physiology of a contraction is the sarcomeres' attempt to shorten with cyclic cross-bridge formation noted earlier (see Box 10-1).[28]

With an established human muscle morphology, and the number of muscle fibers essentially fixed at birth, how can muscle performance in patients be altered? What are the effects of different types of loading on a muscle? And, how is muscle performance changed by altered cardiovascular and pulmonary function?

Muscle Response to Loading

Lengthening and Shortening Loads

Much of what is known about muscle lengthening comes from animal studies. The consistency of results across animal species encourages the tendency to extrapolate the findings to human muscle. Adult animal muscles immobilized in a lengthened position—defined as longer than resting length but not beyond normal muscle range of length—adapted by adding serial sarcomeres.[29] This stretch-induced myofibrillogenesis has also been reported in animal models when muscles were indirectly lengthened during distraction osteogenesis procedures.[30] These results suggest that the increase in tissue tension, when the muscle is held beyond its resting length, is relieved by the addition of the sarcomeres.[31]

When adult animal muscles are immobilized in a shortened length, serial sarcomeres numbers decrease. Again, this may be an adjustment to maintain an optimal tension. When immobilization ends, lengthened and shortened muscles can return to preimmobilized conditions. Animal studies have shown that immobilized shortened muscles may recover normal peak tension values after 120 days of resumed unrestricted movements.[32]

The theory of optimal tension also seems to explain the difference that occurs in the same lengthening experiment with young animals. The musculoskeletal unit in young animals immobilized in a lengthened position adapted by lengthening the tendon. This adaptation occurred to such an extent that, in the first 5 days, the muscle belly decreased the rate of sarcomere addition compared to what would have been expected by animals' normal growth. By 2 weeks, the continued tendon lengthening resulted in a decrease in the number of sarcomeres in the lengthening muscle.[31]

In the young animal, therefore, the disparity between the tendon and muscle length adaptation becomes part of the developmental experience and may not be reversed. There is not a lot of opportunity to study the same effect in humans. It might not be unrealistic, however, to note any disparities in the symmetry of muscle to tendon length in an adult who reports a prolonged immobilization in childhood for an orthopedic condition or injury.

With the exception of serial casting and splinting, the passive stretching exercise treatments performed by physical therapists and physical therapist assistants use an intermittent lengthening to muscles. What is known about the effects of intermittent passive stretching? It is believed that light to moderate passive stretch in passive range of motion exercises primarily affects muscle fibers and not the perimuscular connective tissues. It has been proposed that stretch-induced myofibrillogenesis is still the result of therapeutic intermittent passive stretching even though the calculated sarcomere lengthening is less than that used in the animal muscle lengthening studies noted previously.[30]

What are the effects of moderate or greater intermittent passive stretching? Animal studies have shown that cyclic stretching of muscle at 50% of failure length resulted in muscle more resilient to lengthening before failure.[33] Greater length before failure has been attributed to the increase in muscle length from serial sarcomeres. The viscoelastic properties of muscle and the perimuscular connective tissues are also a factor. Viscoelastic tissues will return from a stretched position a little more relaxed. In repeated cycles of stretching the muscle will be less stiff to the stretching load and, again,

a little more relaxed on release. This effect of less stiffness and more relaxation with cyclic load and release, called hysteresis, will be seen for about 5 to 6 cycles in a session before reaching a plateau.[34]

Passive stretching of innervated muscles also offers a mild training effect. Initiation of the muscle spindle can occur, which increases tension in the muscle with subsequent mild hypertrophy.[27]

In adult animals, immobilization of muscles in the shortened position had a fiber-type effect as well. Acknowledging the challenge of comparing animal to human fiber typing and the variations in typing that exist, a decrease in Type I fibers was seen and an increase in Type II fibers noted.[31] Again, this is difficult to study to the same degree in humans. It may be safe to say, however, that the possibility exists that Type I fibers may be more affected by disuse or shortening. As cited in Chapter 4, animal research has added the observation that anti-gravity muscles are even more affected by disuse.

Resistive Loads

Motor unit recruitment for muscle concentric contractions is dependent on the force required, the size of the motor unit, and the threshold for activation. For low-intensity activities, and the lower threshold required for activation, slow-twitch/oxidative motor units, type I, are activated first. As the muscle force required for a task increases, the larger-sized motor units with greater activation thresholds—those of fast-twitch/oxidative/glycolytic fibers—will be activated and added to the contraction force. With the highest force activity, activation of all motor units is required, including fast-twitch/glycolytic fibers (Figure 10-20). A muscle task requiring the highest levels of motor unit activation will also be a task for which fatigue occurs more quickly because of the reliance on Type II fibers.

Muscles can adapt to gradually increasing loads. Exercise training to improve Type I fiber endurance will need to use activities of relatively low intensity that can reasonable be increased in duration, over time, to intervals longer than 5 to 6 minutes. For many patients, this would be accomplished with a progressive ambulation program. The training effect at the muscle level would be seen by the increased presence of mitochondria, increased myoglobin content, and increased capillary network in Type I muscle cells. Strength gains seen in an improved ability to step up a stair or climb a flight of stairs suggest that Type II fibers have been recruited.

Activation of Type II fibers with the goal of strengthening can occur with repeated functional tasks, movements against gravity or resisted motion against increasing loads. Initial strength gains in a resistance exercise program of 2 to 6 weeks' duration will occur because of improved effectiveness in neural coordination of the motor unit activation in the exercising muscle as well as the improved relaxation in the antagonists.[26] Continued training, greater than 6 to 10 weeks, can lead to hypertrophy of the exercising muscle fibers. This largely anaerobic work stimulates the addition of increased parallel sarcomeres, contractile proteins of actin and myosin and, as a result, increased cross-sectional area.

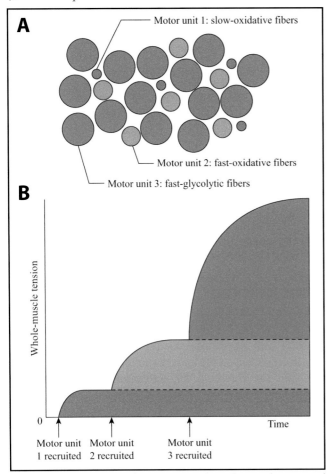

A

Motor unit 1: slow-oxidative fibers

Motor unit 2: fast-oxidative fibers

Motor unit 3: fast-glycolytic fibers

B

Whole-muscle tension

0

Time

Motor unit 1 recruited   Motor unit 2 recruited   Motor unit 3 recruited

Figure 10-20. (A) Diagram of a cross section through a muscle composed of 3 types of motor units. (B) Tetanic muscle tension resulting from the successive recruitment of the 3 types of motor units. Note that motor unit 3, composed of fast glycolytic fibers, produces the greatest rise in tension because it is composed of the largest-diameter fibers and contains the largest number of fibers per motor unit. (Reprinted with permission from Widmaier EP, Hershel R, Strang KT. *Vander, Sherman, Luciano's Human Physiology: The Mechanism of Body Function.* 9th ed. New York: McGraw-Hill; 2004. Copyright McGraw-Hill Education.)

High-performance training can influence fibers in the middle of the metabolic spectrum to show adaptive changes. Longer intervals of heavy resistance training have shown a transition of Type IIx fibers to Type IIa fibers, which are more resistant to fatigue.[35,36] In high-performance training, some Type I fibers can shift from a slow to a fast version of myosin to become faster in order to deliver the force required.[24] At the extremes of performance muscle training, however, muscles make a more thorough adaptation when the specificity of training is for high aerobic or high anaerobic performance, but not both.[26]

There is an element of tissue injury with strengthening. The entire resistive training program relies on the body's ability to build itself back stronger when confronted with a proportional challenge.

The length of time required to recover muscle strength from immobilization or disuse atrophy is dependent on the length of time the limb was unloaded.

The recovery of muscle function following short-duration unloading appears to be completed in a shorter time span than the duration of unloading, whereas unloading periods of 4 to 6 weeks result in a recovery period lasting as long as the unloading period or longer.[37(p771)]

In comparisons of injured limbs, the rate of strength recovery has been shown to be determined by the length of disuse regardless of the retraining exercise mode selected. Despite the evidence that strength gains can be made with retraining, surveyed patients have reported continued function deficits in the injured limb compared with the uninjured limb for significant periods postinjury.[37]

Muscle Nutrition and Healing

Skeletal muscles have a good system of nutrient delivery. In addition, the extensive capillary network will meet the increase in oxygen demand required by exercising trained muscles. Adequate vascularization is a factor in muscle recovery from exercise as well. Patients with a diminished capacity to deliver adequate amounts of oxygenated blood to exercising muscle will have limited exercise tolerance as well as decreased ability to recover from an exercise session.

Similarly, a healthy, trained muscle is less likely to be injured. When an injury does occur a conditioned muscle has a better support network in place to aid healing than does an injured deconditioned muscle. Even in healthy muscles, however, there is a challenge to healing. Muscle tissue has the healing situation where despite effective attempts by satellite cells to regenerate muscle cells the process is overrun by fibroblastic repair.

Satellite cells regenerative efforts have been shown to be enhanced with injections of growth factors. High concentrations of growth factors have been required, however, to detect any significantly improved regeneration. Researchers will continue to explore the use of gene therapy to deliver regenerative enhancing growth factors to improve the extent of regenerative healing in injured muscle tissues.[38]

Muscle Disorders

Contusion

A muscle contusion occurs when a blunt force into a muscle belly crushes the muscle fibers between the force and the underlying bone. The scenarios of a hit from a tackle in football, or someone being hit by a forcefully thrown firm ball, come to mind. But this is also the injury that can occur to muscle when someone falls against a piece of furniture or onto the ground.

The force of the impact crushes muscle fibers, and their supporting structures, resulting in torn cell membranes in the region of the direct impact. A lighter force may damage more superficial tissue and, perhaps, outer layer muscle cells with the result of little more than a colorful but tender bruise on the skin surface and mild impairment of muscle contraction. Greater forces will also yield ecchymosis, which might have a delayed appearance of a few days to reflect the injury to deeper muscle fibers closer to the underlying bone. Depending on the extent of the contusion, injured muscle fibers are unable to contract or will contract weakly. Disrupted capillaries bleed and nociceptors on nerves still intact on the periphery of injured region are stimulated by chemicals released by damaged cells.

Along with the neutrophils and macrophages that come into the area to clean up the cellular debris, muscle satellite cells are activated. Regeneration of damaged myofilaments by the satellite cells will have time to occur where there has been limited damage to a muscle fiber. Satellite cells are capable of regenerating areas of more extensive damage to an area of muscle fibers but succumb to the area being more quickly patched by fibrous scar tissue. This patch will become more of a pulley to the still intact contracting sarcomeres adjacent to the region of injury. Depending on the extent of the damage, the overall potential for muscle tension may be diminished.

Following a brief period of rest that corresponds to the initial inflammatory phase, the introduction of controlled motion will aid muscle recovery. Graded movements "produces more rapid disappearance of the hematoma and inflammatory cells; more extensive, rapid, and organized myofiber regeneration; and more rapid increase in tensile strength and stiffness."[39]

Gentle stretching assists with maintaining previous sarcomere numbers.[40] Pliability of perimuscular connective tissues is enhanced along with the same for the fibrous connective tissue patch. A progression of submaximal isometrics then active movements initiates a restoration of muscle strength.

> Minimum loading, such as would be achieved by normal weightbearing activity, appears necessary for unimpaired muscle fiber repair and/or regeneration and is particularly important to the maturation of newly formed myofibers.[41(p1407)]

Resistance exercise will assist with the restoration of strength toward the recovery of functional activities.

Strain

A simplified definition of a muscle strain could be illuminated by a standard stress-strain graph of muscle's material properties. But muscle is unique for a material property test because it can generate its own internal tension by muscle contraction. Contracting muscle is able to resist the lengthening force, the stress, applied. A better method of displaying muscle's material properties might be to consider the passive elements to strain with the active resistance to strain muscle can provide (Figure 10-21).

What happens when the resisting and actively contracting muscle becomes the unyielding object that then meets an irresistible force in the form of a stress beyond the muscle's ability to resist? A laboratory study that subjected an electrically stimulated maintained muscle contraction to a lengthening stress to failure showed that the tissue failure occurred initially in the muscle fibers, not the connective tissue layers.[42] Fortunately, functioning muscles have protective

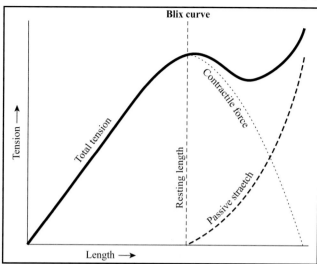

Figure 10-21. The Blix curve depicting muscle length-tension relationship. Note that the greatest contractile force is developed when the muscle is at its resting length, about halfway between its extremes of length. As the muscle is passively stretched beyond its resting length, its contractile force gradually diminishes, but the passive resistance of the connective tissue components gradually develop more tension so that the total tension in the muscle increases. (Reprinted with permission from Salter RB. *Textbook of Disorders and Injuries of the Musculoskeletal System.* 2nd ed. Baltimore, MD: Williams & Wilkins; 1983.)

mechanisms that help to avoid a sustained contraction to this degree of failure. Muscle fiber strains will occur, however, when the resisting or passive muscle is overwhelmed just enough to cause mild to moderate muscle tissue injury. A strain doesn't happen only with attempted feats requiring incredible strength—or with repeated contractions in a fatiguing muscle. A strain can occur with the simple task of tightening a quadriceps muscle while attempting to slowly control the lowering of the body's center of gravity so that the other foot can reach down 8 inches to a stair.

Muscles subjected to a single exercise session of repetitive eccentric loads for which the muscles have not been trained can experience delayed onset muscle soreness (DOMS). Symptoms will include muscle discomfort that increases in the first 24 hours following the exercise session, "peaks between 24 and 72 hours, subsides and eventually disappears by 5-7 days postexercise."[43] Range of motion deficits and alterations in muscle recruitment and sequencing have been reported. No one theory adequately explains DOMS. The cause may be a collection of factors including muscle or perimuscular connective tissue damage. Gentle exercise to aid the break-up of forming adhesions, remove noxious waste, and trigger an endorphin release has been proposed for treatment. Recommended to avoid DOMS would be a gradual introduction of an activity requiring eccentric loading.[43]

Muscle tissues injured by strain will improve along the course described in healing of muscle contusions. There are areas in the body where muscle inserts into a fascial sheet of tissue. Strain at these muscle and connective tissue junctions, such as abdominal muscle layers, may take longer to heal because of the relative decrease in fascial blood supply compared with muscle.

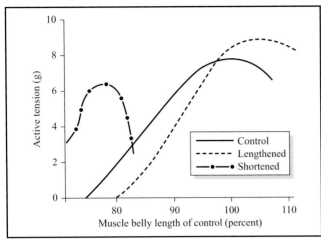

Figure 10-22. Anatomic muscle length adaptation. Lengthened muscle develops greater peak tension at longer length. The same muscle in a shortened position develops less tension than the control muscle in a normal position. (Adapted from *Phys Ther.* 1982;62(12):1799-1808, with permission of the American Physical Therapy Association. Copyright © 2001 American Physical Therapy Association.)

Tear/Rupture

As noted previously, muscles have protective mechanisms to prevent extensive muscle fiber damage from excessive loads. Even with these protective organs, however, muscles can sustain severe strains and tears.

The descriptors of "partial thickness tear" and "full thickness tear" are more frequently heard to describe tendon injuries but apply to muscle tears as well. The torn muscle fibers will retract. A reparative connective tissue patch heals over the area. The restoration of the previous optimal muscle tension will be diminished. This defect in the preinjury muscle morphology may, or may not, affect general functioning of the involved limb depending on the extent of the tear.

A complete muscle rupture will affect function. The extent to which function is impaired will be a factor whether a surgical repair is attempted. In addition, the muscle's health and the tear location are factors affecting whether a successful surgical outcome is possible.

Overuse Injuries

Muscle overuse injuries occur when the force required of a muscle might be adequate for the task but not for an increased duration of the task. Muscle fatigue occurs with the repetition of the task over a longer duration. The muscle fatigue can lead to a slight, or not so slight, erosion of optimal joint position. Decreased muscle control due to fatigue can also lead to inappropriate loading of other structures not prepared, or designed, for the load.

Researchers have identified inadequate hip stabilization and control of the femur as contributors to altered hip and patellofemoral biomechanics.[44,45] Decreased strength in scapular stabilizing musculature has been linked to shoulder impingement during simulated work tasks with arms overhead.[46]

Stretch Weakness

Each muscle has a defined length that allows the muscle to generate optimal tension. Generally, this optimal tension-generating length is near the muscle's resting length. What happens in muscles that adapt to a longer resting length as the result of altered posture combined with the effect of gravity's pull? Or in muscles otherwise utilized for sustained periods of time at a length beyond resting length?

Muscles in a prolonged position of lengthening can be presumed to adapt with the addition of serial sarcomeres. The muscle is now longer and its length tension curve has shifted to the right (Figure 10-22). What happens when this muscle is now asked to generate force in the position of its previous resting length? The muscle tests weaker, and is actually weaker, for activities in this position. The muscle, in its adaptation to the lengthening load, is now weaker when asked to work in a more anatomically aligned position. This observed phenomena, called muscle stretch weakness, was described by the Kendalls in their work with post-polio patients[47] and reinforced by researchers since.[31]

Asking the lengthened muscle to spend more time in a more appropriate anatomical position will require it to contract in a less strong and shortened position. Over time, as was shown in animal studies, it is theorized that the muscle adjusts to this new length with removal of serial sarcomeres. The optimal muscle strength is restored at a more anatomically appropriate resting length and the muscle can now generate its optimal tension in the range required for the task.[44]

There is a metabolic energy requirement when attempting to maintain optimal postural alignment such as correct shoulder girdle alignment when involved in a sustained arms forward task (driving or keyboarding) or arms forward movement task (bell ringing, choir conducting, scrubbing walls). Impaired cardiovascular and pulmonary status may make this adjustment in largely postural and stabilizing muscle difficult. Further, a severely deconditioned patient may be challenged to activate and maintain postural muscles for the simple tasks of sitting or standing with erect posture.

TENDONS

Morphology and Physiology

Tendons connect skeletal muscle to bone. They serve as the pulleys that transmit the force from contracting muscle to the bone with the intent to move, or stabilize, the bone. Tendons are made of tough, dense connective tissue.

In a simple description, the connective tissue layers surrounding muscle fibers, and bundles of muscle fibers, continue on past the end of the contractile portion of the muscle and converge at the musculotendinous junction to form the tendon. The actual structure of the musculotendinous junction, however, shows an overlapping of the tendon tissues with the myofilaments to spread out the concentration of tensile forces.[48] The tendon, short or long, continues on in a strap configuration—rounded cord or flattened band—to anchor onto bone. At the bone insertion site, the tendon can move through zones of the dense tendon tissue to fibrocartilage then mineralized fibrocartilage to bone.[49,50] Or, the tendon can insert into concentric layers of bones by Sharpey's fibers mentioned earlier in the chapter.[5,50] Generally, the structure of the tendon to bone junction minimizes fiber stress and failure.[49]

Tendon Response to Loading

In a musculotendinous unit, the tendon needs to withstand tensile loads whether the muscle is contracting or lengthening. While the tensile load may be low when a muscle undergoes a gentle passive stretch, the load on the tendon increases dramatically with muscle contraction. Strain analysis shows that tendon tissue begins to undergo microscopic failure at lengths greater than 4% of resting length (Figure 10-23).

Tendons vary in their ability to transmit loads from the contracting muscle to the bony attachment related to the differences that exist in tendon thickness and collagen content. A gradual increase in loading will result in an increased cross sectional area due to an increase in collagen fiber size. Tendon stiffness, thus the ability to resist lengthening strain, also improves.

As would be predicted by the PST, under-loading of tendons will have the opposite effect. Cross-sectional area decreases. Collagen fiber size and content declines. Cyclic load testing will show a hysteresis pattern that reflects softening of tendon tissue that will reduce its ability to avoid microinjury due to tissue fatigue.[51]

Tendon Nutrition and Healing

Blood supply to tendons is a somewhat patched network. The extensive capillary system of the contractile muscle will supply, at best, the third of the tendon close to the myotendinous junction. At the other end of the tendon, some blood supply is available just for the distinct portion of the tendon inserting into the bone. Modest vascularity is available from synovial sheaths and paratendons.[49] Regions of hypovascularity have been identified in tendons at 1 cm or a range of 2 to 7 cm from the bone attachment.[49] With one source of blood supply at one end, another at the other end, and a third for the area in between, it may not be surprising that areas of tendon hypovascularity have been identified. Tendon and ligaments insertions through a zone of fibrocartilage have an additional challenge to vascularity.[50]

The metabolism for tendons is an adaptation to the less than direct or effusive blood supply. It also reflects the pulley function tendons perform. Tenocytes have oxidative and glycolytic ability. The anaerobic pathways are well developed; tendons consume 7.5 less oxygen than skeletal muscle. The advantage of a low metabolic rate—lower oxygen requirement—in the tendon means that there is a reduced possibility of tissue ischemia when the tendon is under sustained loads with accompanying poor profusion. The lower metabolic rate of tendons unfortunately also means that there is a slower rate of healing.[49]

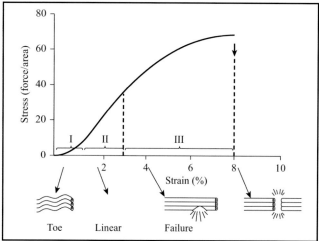

Figure 10-23. The crimped configuration of the collagen fibers and fibrils at rest begins to flatten with strains up to 2%. With continued lengthening, intramolecular sliding of collagen triple helices allows tendons to lengthen linearly with the strain. If the increased length remains less than 4%, the tendon will show an elastic property and will return to its starting length when the load is removed. Strains greater than 4% will lead to microscopic failure. Lengthenings greater than 8% to 10% result in macroscopic failure from the damage to fibrils by collagen molecule slippage. (Reprinted with permission from Sharma P, Maffulli N. Tendon injury and tendinopathy: healing and repair. *J Bone Joint Surg Am.* 2005;87:187-202.)

Tendon Disorders

Tendonitis

Though the term *tendonitis* is conventionally used for any tendon reactivity, the term is appropriate in limited situations. A tendon that experiences a low increase in the regular load required of it may experience a discrete episode of inflammation that would be appropriately called tendonitis. This might be a single session of repetitive movement or, perhaps, the rubbing of a tendon. With these limited scenarios, the inflammatory process would ensue. It might reasonably be assumed that a complaint of decreased function or pain was due to inflammation of the tendon when the recovery of the tendon corresponded to the expected time frame for healing from an inflammatory event, 3 to 7 days. The only way to be absolutely certain that the complaint was due to tendonitis would be to analyze the actual tendon tissues and identify the increased presence of neutrophils, monocytes, and macrophages that accompany the inflammatory process.

After the inflammatory phase, controlled stretching of the tendon will promote increased collagen synthesis and improve fiber alignment. This aids in the restoration of tendon resistance to tensile loading.[52]

Tendinopathy

The accurate term to describe the more common presentation of a painful and poorly functioning tendon would be tendinopathy. Rather than the inflammatory process seen in tendonitis, tendinopathy appears to be a process of tendon degeneration. What are the possible factors that might cause a tendon to begin a degenerative process? The patient may describe a series of events that resulted in repetitive excessive loading of the tendon. Tendons can also be used in positions that are less than optimal, leading to uneven loading.

What is known about tendinopathy has come from studies of tendon ruptures. It has been shown that long before the tendon ruptured, the tissues of the tendon had changed. The tendon tissues are observed to have "lost their normal glistening-white appearance and to have become gray-brown and amorphous."[49(p191)] The histology of tendinopathic tissues show an absence of inflammatory cells but the presence of disordered and haphazard healing along with fiber thinning and disorientation. The histology suggests that the tendon may not have had enough time to heal adequately.[49]

The exact intrinsic cause of tendinopathy is not yet known but there are several theories. It is possible that tissue-damaging oxygen-free radicals are formed in the tendon when a muscle relaxes and the tendon is reperfused with oxygenated blood after a period of relative hypovascularity during tensile loading. This oxidative stress theory appears supported by the increased concentration of antioxidant enzymes found in examined tendinopathic tendons.[53] Oxidative stress has also been linked with an increased presence of spontaneous cell death in tendinopathic tendons.[54] Hypoxia and localized cell hyperthermia have also been proposed as explanations for degeneration. An increase in prostaglandins with cyclic load is another avenue of investigation.[55]

Initially, tendinopathy might not be painful. Patients can also make unconscious adjustments in how activities are performed to avoid any symptoms. For some patients, the first indication that degenerative tissue changes have occurred in a tendon may be when the tendon finally ruptures. With this possibility of not identifying the tendinopathy until after the fact, patients with pain and decreased function who are referred to physical therapy with suspected tendinopathy are fortunate. What is the best method to treat tendinopathy?

Curwin and Stanish described an eccentric exercise protocol to address tendinopathy.[56] Once the contributing factors are addressed, an exercise is identified that produces an eccentric load to the ailing tendon.[48] The amount of load needs to be gauged so the patient can complete 3 sets of 10 repetitions. The goal is to have manageable symptoms reported during the performance of the third set but not during the first 2 sets. When mild symptoms are no longer reported during the third set, then the load in the exercise needs to increase.[57] This symptom-to-load criteria leads to a tendon load that is adequate to ensure a gradually improved tendon status with performance of functional tasks in 6 to 8 weeks.[48] This approach has had successful outcomes in the treatment of Achilles and patellar tendinopathy as well as with lateral epicondylitis in the forearm.[48,56,58] Success with a similar eccentric protocol has been reported.[59]

Tear/Rupture

Though tendons are designed to withstand high tensile loads, a tendon can rupture. A greater risk for rupture occurs with a quickly, or unevenly, applied load.[49] And, as mentioned earlier, it is believed that tendon ruptures can be precipitated by undetected degenerative tendinopathy.[60]

The presence of tendon degenerative changes was found in 100% of 74 patients with an Achilles tendon rupture.[61] Degenerative changes were found in 97% of 891 spontaneously ruptured tendons compared with 33% of control tendons.[62] More degenerative changes are found in tendons that rupture than those simply painful because of overuse.[60] These histological studies suggest that significant tissue degeneration can precede a tendon rupture.

As with muscles, tendons can sustain tears that range from partial thickness tears, full thickness tears to full tendon ruptures. The decision whether to repair a tendon tear or rupture surgically will be dependent on how much of the tendon is torn, where the tear is located within the tendon, and the extent to which function would be affected without a surgical repair. Postsurgical management of repaired tendons requires a balance between maintenance of joint mobility with the need for repaired tendons to progress well through the repair stage of healing before any significant tensile loads are applied.

With either a partial thickness tear left to heal with some acceptance of a diminished pulley force or with a surgical repair, both are dependent on the adequate perfusion of tissues and delivery of nutrients. Healing occurs from cell proliferation by local tenocytes within the tendon. For tendons within a synovial sheath, fibroblasts from the sheath and synovium can take over. Better tendon healing and more normal gliding results from the former, for tendons in a synovial sheath, while disruption of gliding can occur with the latter. Tendon-dependent variations in these healing patterns exist.[49]

Strategic mechanical loading during the maturation/remodeling phase of healing in animal studies is credited with improving "the tensile strength, elastic stiffness, weight and cross-sectional area of tendons…by an increase in collagen extracellular matrix synthesis by tenocytes."[49(p191)] Postoperative protocols with early introduction of controlled movements have been shown to be beneficial.[63-66]

BONE

Morphology and Physiology

The calcified extracellular matrix of bone tissue makes it uniquely suited to provide the skeletal framework for the body. In this role, however, skeletal bone needs to find a balance between the competing needs of the adequate rigidity required to withstand loading and the lightness to aid energy-efficient movement. Bone finds the balance through the integration of 2 bone types.

In osteogenesis, small spicules of bone called trabeculae connect to form a somewhat porous network of bone called *cancellous bone*. As the trabeculae continue appositional growth, a less porous and denser bone develops called *cortical bone* (Figure 10-24). Though the bones of the skeleton do begin with a genetic blueprint,[67] bone physiology attempts to

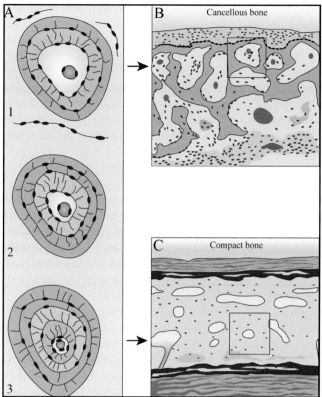

Figure 10-24. Key stages in the process of conversion of cancellous bone to compact bone (developing skull). (A) Soft tissue spaces fill in with concentric lamellae that accumulate and become a Haversian system. (B) Developing cranial bone (stage 1 in A). (C) Growing cranial bone (stage 3 in A). (Adapted from Cormack DH. *Introduction to Histology*. Philadelphia, PA: J.B. Lippincott Co; 1984.)

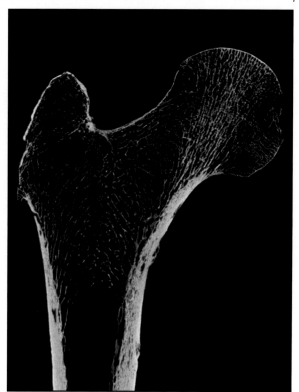

Figure 10-25. An image of trabecular bone structure in the proximal femur scanned on a GE Nanotom5 system (NanoCT System). (Reprinted with permission from Dr. Karl Jepsen and Erin Bigelow, Orthopaedic Research Laboratories, University of Michigan.)

keep the skeleton light by creating the compact cortical bone only where required.

Cortical layers at bone ends and the perimeter of long bones resist torsion and bending forces. The porous but resilient scaffolding of cancellous bone can shock-absorb to accommodate compressive loading.[68] The architecture of the trabeculae in cancellous bone offers an observable blueprint of loading stress (Figure 10-25). Further, the extensive vascularity in the regions of cancellous bone assists the body's use of skeletal bone as a mineral repository. The calcium, phosphorus, sodium, and magnesium stored in bone can be withdrawn to maintain extracellular fluid concentrations for nerve conduction and muscle contraction.[68]

Even with the excellent network of canaliculi and the proximity of blood vessels around which the Haversian systems form, the extracellular matrix of bone can weaken over time.[5] Bone remodeling is the process by which bone maintains itself by removing weakening sections of matrix and replacing it with new bone. Within the structure of the Haversian system, osteoclasts will absorb layers of bone and osteoblasts will rebuild new bone. In this mode of remodeling, both cell types work nearby on the same layer of bone, leaving behind only a cement line marking the outer wall of the replaced bone layer. Bone remodeling can also take the form of reshaping bones to accommodate growth as with the widening curve needed in cranial bones to accommodate brain growth. In this situation, osteoclasts work on one side of the bone to remove the narrow curve while osteoblasts work on the other side to widen the curve.

Bone Responses to Loading

Bone needs to adapt to a variety of loads placed on it. Musculotendinous attachments place a traction stress during muscle contraction, weightbearing activities cause compression stress, and weightbearing with direction changes can create compression combined with torsional stress, to name a few. The bone's adaptation is also a form of bone remodeling but one that accommodates a changing mechanical stress. The adaptation can reflect the magnitude and as well as the direction of the mechanical load.

Bone may be the musculoskeletal tissue that has received the greatest research scrutiny over the longest period of time. Long before the PST was proposed, biomechanical research on bone was based on the understanding from Wolff's Law that bone grows according to the stresses and strains placed on it. Numerous animal experimental models have been pursued to define bone's mechanical properties. To summarize the commonalities found from these animal research models, as well as state concepts of bone adaptation that could be expressed in mathematical terms, Turner[67] proposed the following 3 rules for bone adaptation to mechanical loads:

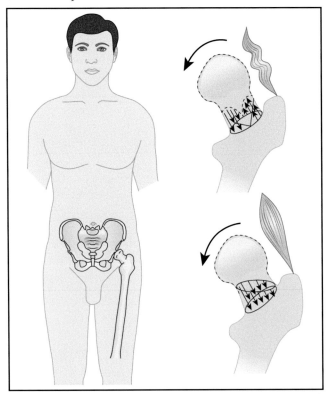

Figure 10-26. Stress distribution in a femoral neck subjected to bending. When the gluteus medius muscle is relaxed (top), tensile stress acts on the superior cortex and compressive stress acts on the inferior cortex. Contraction of this muscle (bottom) neutralizes the tensile stress. (Adapted from Frankel VH, Nordin M. Biomechanics of bone. In: Nordin M, Frankel VH, eds. *Basic Biomechanics of the Musculoskeletal System.* 3rd ed. Philadelphia, PA: Lippincott Williams & Wilkins; 2001.)

1. Bone adaptation is driven by dynamic, rather than static, loading.

2. Only a short duration of mechanical loading is necessary to initiate an adaptive response. Extending the loading duration has a diminishing effect on further bone adaptation.

3. Bone cells accommodate to a customary mechanical loading environment, making them less responsive to routine loading signals.

The application of these rules to patient situations does require a bit of extrapolation, but the rules are still useful. First, there are probably no patient situations that would correspond to the static loading of bone used in animal research models—with the possible exception of spinal cord-injured patients weightbearing in a standing table. In patients without paralysis, however, even static standing is actually a dynamic process. Maintaining static standing balance is a control of the normal occurrence of side-to-side and forward-to-back perturbations. Each slight shift in body position reloads bone and meets the definition described in Turner's rules of dynamic loading.

With the initial loading of bone, it is believed that an electronic potential, a piezoelectric signal, is induced. If the load doesn't change, and in other word remains a static load,

the initial induced electronic potential will fade. But if the load is lifted and repeated, and lifted and repeated again and again, as in dynamic loading, then the electronic potential will be induced with each repeated loading. The generation of piezoelectric signals that then travel along the network of canaliculi is believed to be a factor in the stimulation of bone formation. The absence of loading signals may favor bone absorption over formation as noted in the deconditioning effects on bone with immobilization and bed rest surveyed in Chapter 4.

Second, once a sufficient level of loading occurs in either magnitude or frequency, or both, bone is stimulated to adapt. The second rule suggests that past a certain point more loading or exercise within a period of time does not lead to more bone formation.[67] The notion that more may not be better in terms of duration or within a period of time is consistent with the PST. Even an initially tolerable load can pass a point of tolerance if continued for too long a duration. An increased but tolerable load that is repeated within an insufficient time to for the tissue to adapt may lead to injury.[19] Insufficient time for bone to adapt to an increased load will be explored again in the section on stress fractures later in the chapter.

As with other body tissues, once bone tissue adapts to a routine level of loading no further adaptation is stimulated. This isn't to suggest that bone remodeling isn't continuing because it does. Even without a change in the load the bone remodeling process that replaces areas of declining matrix continues. In terms of an unchanging routine load, however, an equilibrium in the bone can be reached. Increasing bone formation requires the unusual load event to occur.

The amount and orientation of collagen fibers within bone will adapt to the mechanical loading environment. The area between concentric rings in an osteon (aka Haversian system) will contain collagen fibers. The space between the layers of bone in cancellous bone allows a greater the area for collagen fibers than in compact bone (see Figure 10-24). The orientation of fibers can assist the resistance to mechanical loads.[69] Even within a single bone the orientation of fibers can adjust to the loading forces. Strain gauge data in equine radius were compared to the collagen fiber orientation. Fibers were oriented obliquely in areas of compression located in the distal segment, and longitudinally in areas of tensile loading found in the proximal.[69-71]

In humans the loading forces can vary with the same bone also. In the proximal femur during weightbearing activities, the superior aspect of the femoral neck undergoes tension loading while the underside, the inferior aspect, compression (Figure 10-26). In adult humans the tension side of bone undergoes the greater stress because adult bone is less resilient to tensile loading. Fortunately, contracting muscle can counter the tensile stress placed on bone. In the example of the proximal femur, a stabilizing contraction of the gluteus medius reduces the tensile loading on the superior aspect of the femoral neck.[72]

Bone needs to keep a balance between having adequate stiffness to resist loading forces but with an accommodating resilience to those same forces. In other words, bone needs to

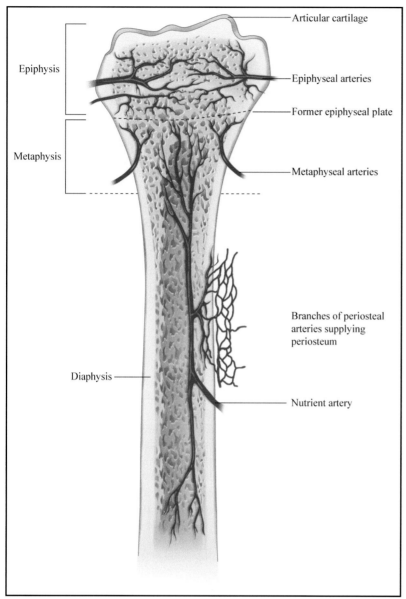

Figure 10-27. Blood supply of an adult long bone (tibia). (Adapted from Cormack DH. *Introduction to Histology.* Philadelphia, PA: J.B. Lippincott Co; 1984.)

Articular cartilage

Epiphysis

Epiphyseal arteries

Former epiphyseal plate

Metaphysis

Metaphyseal arteries

Branches of periosteal arteries supplying periosteum

Diaphysis

Nutrient artery

give a little. In certain circumstances bone shows an amazing ability to accommodate a distraction force.

Strategic application of traction on a growing jaw is a standard procedure in successful orthodontia. Gymnasts who accentuate lumbar hyperextension during major bone growth years have an unintended lengthening of posterior vertebral structures leading to spondylolisthesis.[73,74] Orthopedists are able to induce distraction osteogenesis by scoring through the periosteum and cortex of bone and gradually lengthening the fracture callus.[75-78]

Nutrition and Healing

Bone is not as challenged as other connective tissues for nutrition. Integral to its structure is the incorporation of a rich blood supply. Bones are vascularized by a main nutrient artery and by metaphyseal and epiphyseal arteries at bone ends. The terminal branches of all 3 artery types will create an anastomosing network. This ensures that most parts of

bone will continue to have a blood supply even if the supply from a main artery is disrupted. The superficial periosteum is supplied by periosteal arteries. "The metaphyseal arteries are former periosteal arteries that became incorporated into bone tissue" when the bone ends widened (Figure 10-27).[5]

Incorporated periosteal vessels in Haversian systems, now Haversian vessels, run longitudinally through bone and are supplied by the main arteries via blood vessels running through obliquely angled canals in bone called Volkmann canals (Figure 10-28). Osteocytes within lacunae, and working osteoblasts and osteoclasts, receive oxygen and nutrients from the Haversian vessels via the tissue fluid running through the interconnecting canaliculi.

Bone may patch defects with woven bone in the regenerative phase of healing. This is a mineralized bone that has a less organized pattern. It has less mechanical strength than the more organized bone that replaces it in the remodeling phase.

Figure 10-28. A longitudinal and transverse section through secondary Haversian bone. Note the orientation of the vascular channels (Haversian and Volkmann's canals) relative to the secondary osteons. Cement lines demarcate the boundary of each secondary osteon. (Adapted from Loitz-Ramage BJ, Zernicki RF. Bone biology and mechanics. In: Magee DJ, Zachazewski JE, Quillen WS, eds. *Scientific Foundations and Principles of Practice in Musculoskeletal Rehabilitation.* St. Louis, MO: Saunders Elsevier Inc; 2007.)

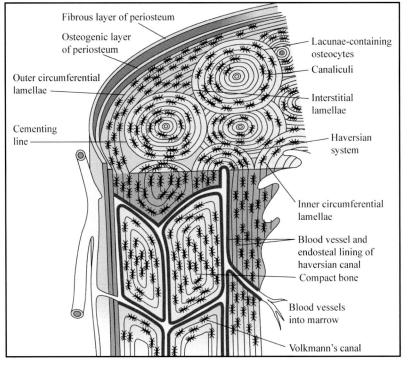

Bone Disorders (Nonsystemic)

Fractures

Fractures happen. Even the strongest of bone can be placed in a challenging situation where the forces being absorbed exceed the bone's ability to resist. From a high-velocity, high impact of a knee into a car dashboard during a motor vehicle accident to a more slowly evolving fall to the floor onto an outstretch hand, fractures occur.

In adult long bones a fracture generally begins on the tension side rather than the compression side. Younger bones may have greater ability to withstand tension but less compression.[72] But what really happens to bone tissue when it fractures?

Under tension forces, the bone segment lengthens and then fails when osteons separate at the cement lines.[72] With compression loads, the bone fails because of "oblique cracking of the osteons."[72]

The speed with which the load is applied to the bone is a factor in the type of fracture and the extent to which the surrounding soft tissues are injured. A misstep that leads to a fall but allows the person enough time to reach for support slows the fall. The slower speed of loading creates an outcome different from one from a motor vehicle accident. In the former, the lower loading speed allows some of the energy building in the bone while under load to dissipate through the initial crack created in the bone. The more slowly loaded bone to failure will have bone ends with little displacement and little soft tissue damage. In the latter scenario—the motor vehicle accident—the quick loading allows greater energy to build up in the bone under load that is then released abruptly when the bone fails. The bone may break into pieces and cause extensive damage to the soft tissues in the region of the fracture.[72]

Bone fractures can be classified by descriptions of the fracture line, location within the bone, and whether the fracture was open or closed to name a few. More highly specified fracture patterns observed for distinct bone segments have been described in more elaborate classification systems.[79-81] Fracture classification schemes aid in communication about the fracture as well as facilitate comparison of interventions and outcomes.

Bone fracture healing follows the general shared pattern for the 4 basic tissues with a few key differences. The major task the fracture bone needs to accomplish is to span the fracture gap, ultimately with bone.

The immediate ends of fractured bone suffer a disruption in blood supply and die. Once inflammation develops, the processes begin to span the gap. Trabecular bone just past the dead bone begins to send columns of bone along the medullary canal across the gap. From the rich vascularity of the endosteum of the medullary canal on the inner surface of bone and the periosteum on the outer surface of bone, osteoprogenitor cells arrive and proliferate. In the region behind the fracture with vascularity, the osteoprogenitor cells differentiate to osteoblasts. On the superficial outer region where vascularity is lower, chondroblasts are formed. A chondral sleeve forms around the fracture area and offers modest structural support. The osteoblasts aid the efforts of the trabecular bone on the inner and outer surfaces of fractured bone as well as assist with the remodeling of the chondral sleeve (Figure 10-29).[5]

Through endochondral ossification, the chondral sleeve is replaced with cancellous bone. Remodeling continues until the thickening of the cancellous bone creates cortical bone around the bone's perimeter. In an example of tissue regeneration, a healed bone segment previously fractured generally becomes indistinguishable from the bone tissue adjacent to it.

Effective fracture healing requires stabilization in the early stages of tissue rebuilding to span the fracture gap. If the initial efforts of trabecular bone to span the gap or if the process of angiogenesis to revascularize the area are disrupted by excessive movement or delayed by poor nutrition or cardiovascular pulmonary status, then the avascular chondral sleeve may begin to dominate.

The chondral sleeve formation in the regions of relatively decreased vascularity may extend deep into the fracture area and across the gap. If continued disruption occurs, the cartilage may mature over the bone ends rather than serving as a scaffolding for ossification.

External fixation and surgical internal fixation have been utilized by orthopedists to ensure fracture fixation.[82] In an effect to allow modest load sharing to enhance woven bone callus formation, however, a shift toward less rigid fixation has been proposed.[83] This might take the form of an unlocked intramedullary nail.

In addition, efforts have been made to keep much of the overlying soft tissue intact, which augments the blood supply for the periosteum (see Figure 10-27).

During the remodeling/maturation stage, intermittent bone loading may be introduced to enhance bone healing. The rationale is explained in the 3 rules for bone growth discussed earlier. Intermittent bone loading has been shown to be beneficial in animal models.[84,85]

Stress Fractures

Bone stimulated by an abrupt increase in physical activity or the initiation of a new activity will undergo remodeling to meet the new demand. In the initiation of the remodeling process, bone can become caught in the situation where the osteoclastic resorption of bone outstrips the osteoclastic formation of new bone. This results in a weakened bone that is vulnerable to injury, which describes the bone pathophysiology that can lead to a stress fracture.[86] New terms would describe the remodeling imbalance noted previously as the "stress reaction" with the "stress fracture" as the resultant structural failure of bone.[69] Though more stress fractures have been reported in lower extremities, most bones of the extremities have had reported stress fractures as well as ribs and the spine.[86]

The bone pathophysiology can manifest as pain with activity that is relieved with rest. Tenderness to palpation over the bone is noted. A history of a recently started new activity or activity increase accompanies the complaint. Prevention of a stress reaction from leading to a stress fracture is challenged by the difficulty to confirm the diagnosis with an effective time period.

Radiographs can show bone changes of early lucent zones but generally the complaint occurs before radiographic bone changes are detected.[86] Bone scans are very sensitive to areas of increased bone activity. Increased activity, however, is not

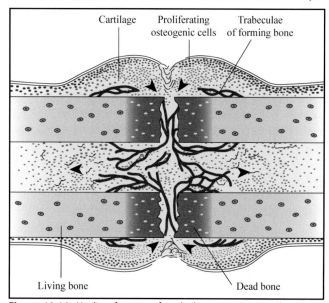

Figure 10-29. Healing fracture of a rib (later stage). Cancellous bone is indicated in black; cartilage is shown lightly stippled. Arrowheads indicate direction of trabecular growth in internal and external callus. (Adapted from Cormack DH. *Introduction to Histology.* Philadelphia, PA: J.B. Lippincott Co; 1984.)

specific for an imminent stress fracture. A fracture may be detected on magnetic resonance imaging (MRI) sooner than will show up on radiographs.[69]

Most studies tracked participants who had engaged in weightbearing activities of running, jumping or dancing. Those subjects with initially lower fitness levels were more vulnerable to stress fractures. Though not directly applicable to the sudden initiation of weightbearing with a walking program for a deconditioned patient, a few observations from these studies are worth noting.

The tibia accounted for 41% to 55% of stress fractures. For the same level of activity, women sustained stress fractures at a rate 2 to 10 times higher than men. Older participants or white participants had higher rates of fractures. High arches, greater varus and valgus angulation at the knee, or leg length differences were each significant risk factors.[86] These observations suggest that patients beginning new repetitive weightbearing activities should be started gradually and with supportive shoes to reduce foot and lower extremity alignment variations.

Skeletal Alignment

Altered skeletal alignment can affect a person's ability to move efficiently. The energy expenditure required for movement may increase in cases of severe malalignment. Increased muscle control needed to optimize efficient movements may lead to muscle fatigue sooner than expected in routine activities. The potential for development of muscle imbalances may increase. The PST notes that movement and alignment are factors in the level of physical stress experienced by tissues.[19] For a patient with any cardiovascular or pulmonary compromises, alignment-impaired movement offers yet another stressor to optimum performance. What may seem an inconsequential alignment variation for a patient during a critical event requiring hospitalization may need to be considered as the patient works to recover function.

Spinal

In normal development of the spine, balanced curves form in the cervical, thoracic, and lumbar spines as viewed from the side. Viewed from behind, the spine should be straight and in midline from the base of the skull to the sacral base. In forward bending, the right and left contours of the thorax—the rib cage—will be symmetrical. Spinal alignment may be altered by degenerative tissue, paralysis, congenital disorders or trauma.[87]

Kyphosis

Kyphosis is the exaggeration of the curve in the thoracic spine. Postural kyphosis may be observed in a patient challenged to stand erect against gravity. The weakness in postural muscles is an aftereffect of prolonged bed rest or deconditioning. Restoration of adequate postural strength will reduce a postural kyphosis and related potential for ventilatory pump compromise. Even in able-bodied subjects, standing with increased trunk flexion, measured at 25 and 50 degrees from the vertical, increased metabolic energy expenditure from that required in erect standing.[88]

Though a less flexed trunk posture may be more energy efficient, it may not be possible when the kyphosis reflects structural changes in the spinal segments of the thoracic spine. Structural kyphosis may be present due to "degenerative diseases (such as arthritis), developmental problems (the most common example being Scheuermann's disease), osteoporosis with compression fractures of the vertebrae, and/or trauma."[89]

Scoliosis

Scoliosis is a lateral curvature of the spine in one direction accompanied by rotation in the opposite direction. To clarify, a spine will side bend to the left if the left side height of the vertebral body, or bodies at several spinal levels, is less than that of the right. The involved vertebral segments will rotate right. The right rib cage, if the curve is located in the thoracic spine, will show a rib projection (a rib hump) posteriorly during forward bending. Ribs on the left project anteriorly and may crowd together depending on the severity of the curve.

A congenitally malformed vertebral level or multiple levels can be diagnosed in infancy, especially when the child begins to move against gravity. The most common form of scoliosis, however, appears during adolescent bone growth and is termed "idiopathic" because no single cause has been identified. Evidence links adolescent idiopathic scoliosis with a genetic sex-linked trait that does not appear every generation or is expressed variably.[87] Calcium transport deficits, variations in platelet morphology and physiology, and altered special orientation have each been correlated with idiopathic scoliosis.[90]

With idiopathic scoliosis, 90% of the curves are right rotated. When a left-rotated curve is first diagnosed, it can prompt radiograph and MRI studies to rule out other pathology. Idiopathic scoliosis curves are not painful. Neurological signs are negative. It is not normal for one of these curves to progress radically after skeletal maturity.

Assertions by Kendall et al[91] decades ago for prescriptive exercises to address scoliosis and recent advocacy for other exercise interventions have not yet proven the case for exercise as a sole intervention. Bracing for moderate curves and surgical correction for fast progressing curves are the current interventions standards.[87,92]

The extent of the curve at spinal maturity will predict the curve progression.

> Curves less than 30 degrees at bone maturity are unlikely to progress, whereas curves measuring from 30 degrees to 50 degrees progress an average of 10 to 15 degrees over a lifetime. Curves greater than 50 degrees at maturity progress steadily at a rate of 1 degree per year. In most patients, life-threatening effects on pulmonary function do not occur until the scoliotic curve is 100 degrees or greater.[93]

In the adult, altered alignment of the scapula "high" on an upper thoracic curve means the stabilizing musculature is at a biomechanical disadvantage. Generally, when there is a postural fault of a downwardly rotated scapula, scapular stabilizers are weaker.[46] When this altered position occurs along with underlying altered spinal alignment, the scapula does not have the option of becoming correctly aligned. A scapular position can be improved with strengthening of scapular stabilizers but may always have a "built-in" disadvantage due to the variation in position atop the spinal curve and rotated ribs.

Extremity

Valgus/Varus

In the lower extremities, varus and valgus angulation at the knee can appear mild while the patient is in a stance position. In the single-leg stance position or in walking, however, an increased varus angulation can appear because of degenerative changes in the medial compartment of the knee. The same could occur for increased valgus with lateral compartments involved. Inadequate hip stabilization strength may also manifest as increased knee valgus due to the femur's tendency to medially rotate with the decreased control. This situation is further challenged by increased hip anteversion and/or ankle valgus/foot varum. Increased knee valgus angulation in military recruits had a strong correlation with increased stress fracture rates during basic training.[86]

No studies were identified with measures of the energy expenditure of gait in subjects with increased varus or valgus angulation at the knee, ankle or foot. Less than optimal alignment of the lower extremity, which may lead to less stability of the foot at propulsion, can be analogous to the additional effort required to walk in loose sand. Improving the lower extremity biomechanics might require improving muscle strength at the hip. An intervention could also be as simple as having the patient wear supportive shoes with weightbearing tasks such as standing transfers at bedside or walking in hospital corridors.

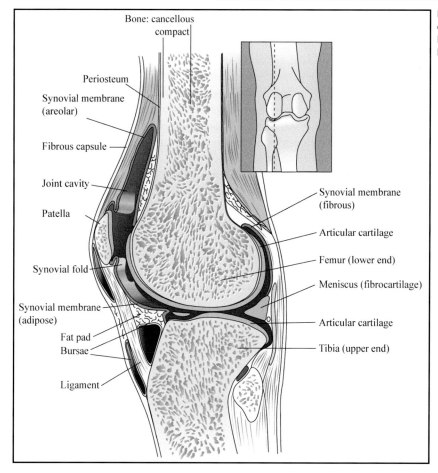

Figure 10-30. Cross section of a knee joint as an example of a synovial joint. (Adapted from Cormack DH: *Introduction to Histology.* Philadelphia, PA: J.B. Lippincott Co; 1984.)

JOINTS

Joint Morphology and Physiology

In the skeleton, joints hold articulating bone ends together and allow varying amounts of movement. Joints can be classified by the degree of movement permitted, as in the following:

- Synarthrosis (little or no movement)
- Amphiarthrosis (slight mobility)
- Diarthrosis (variety of movements)

They may also be classified by the structure of how the joint is held together—fibrous, cartilaginous or synovial. Most joints of the human adult musculoskeletal system are diarthrodial synovial joints.[22]

A synovial joint can be viewed as a functioning unit of components derived from nearly all the possible variations of connective tissue. A cross section of a representative synovial joint, the knee, allows identification of the essential components (Figure 10-30).

The bones at the distal femur and at the proximal tibia are constructed of mostly cancellous bone with cortical bone just along the bone ends and the perimeters. The trabecular architecture of the femur and the tibia will mirror the pattern of compression, tensile, and torsion loading of these bones

near the knee joint. Articular cartilage covers the bone ends along the complete length of the articulating surfaces. A fibrous joint capsule completely surrounds and encases the articulating bone ends. The capsule is lined with a specialized connective tissue membrane, the synovium. Ligaments are reinforcing thickened bands of the fibrous joint capsule or may appear separately within the joint.

Joint Capsule

The joint capsule consists of dense ordinary connective tissue (see Table 10-1). The multidirectional arrangement of fibers helps the capsule withstand the equally multidirectional stresses that occur with functional movements. The presence of elastin-like fibers in the joint capsule aids the capsule's need to stretch and accommodate the full amplitude of joint movement. Further, the ability of the joint capsule to expand also allows for "enlargement of the joint space in the effused joint."[94]

The thickness of the joint capsule varies from the thick dense capsule of the knee to the thinner capsule of the glenohumeral joint, at the shoulder, with redundant folds.[94] The fibers of the capsule continue in a cross-hatched or random pattern as the fibers blend with the fibrous periosteum of the articulating bones. Joint capsules are well innervated.[50] Myelinated and unmyelinated fibers connect with pressure-sensitive mechanoreceptors in the form of free nerve endings and pacinian corpuscles.[5]

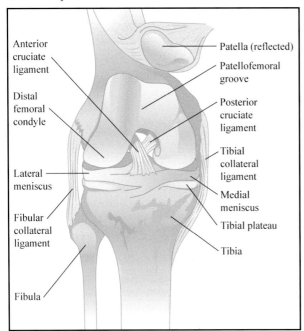

Anterior cruciate ligament

Distal femoral condyle

Lateral meniscus

Fibular collateral ligament

Fibula

Patella (reflected)

Patellofemoral groove

Posterior cruciate ligament

Tibial collateral ligament

Medial meniscus

Tibial plateau

Tibia

Figure 10-31. Ligaments of the knee. (Adapted from Johnson MW. Acute knee effusions: a systemic approach to diagnosis. *Am Fam Physician*. 2000;61(8):2391-2400.)

Ligaments

Within the multidirectional fiber architecture of the joint capsule there are areas of more dense fibers aligned in a more parallel pattern. These cord-like thickenings within the joint capsule are the joint ligaments. Other ligamentous straps of dense regular connective tissue can exist outside of the capsule but are also considered joint ligaments.

In a simplified view of their function, ligaments connect bone to bone. The medial and lateral collateral ligaments in the knee are examples of ligaments that exist within the structure of the joint capsule. Others, such as the anterior and posterior cruciate ligaments of the knee, do truly connect from one bone to another across the joint space without being a part of the joint capsule (Figure 10-31). Ligaments can be named "by their points of bone attachment (coracoacromial), their shape (deltoid), their gross functions (capsular), their relationships to a joint (collateral) or their relationships to each other (cruciates)."[95]

Ligaments provide stability to the joint by serving as checks against unwanted directions of movements and, thus, reinforce the intended planes of movement. The medial and lateral collateral ligaments of the knee limit the varus and valgus movements of the tibia on the femur in open chain movements and the femur on the tibia in closed. The collaterals do not limit flexion and extension except at extreme end ranges for the knee.

Movements that can be described, and measured, by the joint angles created when 2 bones move in a joint such as flexion and extension are termed osteokinematic movements. Another type of movement describes the movements of the joint surfaces to one another within the joint. These are rocking, sliding, and rotation movements and are termed

arthrokinematics. Ligaments separate from the joint capsule, such as the anterior and posterior cruciates, also check unwanted movements of the joint. They also play a role to guide the desired arthrokinematic movements required for knee osteokinematic movements.

The role of ligaments to provide joint stabilization is reflected in the stronger structure for ligament insertion into bone. As with tendons, ligaments can have direct or indirect insertions into bone. The insertion type varies between ligaments and can also vary between the proximal and distal attachments in the same ligament.[50]

The fibers of the superficial layer in direct insertions will become continuous with the fibers of the periosteum. Over the span of 1 mm, the deep fibers transition through 4 zones. The first zone consists of the ligament, or tendon, fibers. In the second zone, the fibers become continuous with those in a fibrocartilaginous layer. The third zone is mineralized fibrocartilage where minerals appear between the collagen fibrils. Even though chondrocytes in this zone are surrounded by mineralized matrix, the lacunae are intact, which allows continuous activity by the chondrocytes.[50] The fourth zone is bone where the fibers from the ligament become the collagen fibers between bone layers. The distinct tissue line that marks the nonmineralized layer from the mineralized, the tidemark, is located between the second and the third zones.[50]

Indirect insertions have a larger superficial layer that runs parallel with, and blends into, the fibers of the periosteum. The deeper fibers, Sharpey's fibers, insert obliquely into bone without a transition layer. There is still a tidemark between nonmineralized and mineralized tissue.

Ligaments are innervated with mechanoreceptive afferent nerve endings to detect tensile forces and pressure. There are also ligamentous equivalent of Golgi tendon-like organs to detect when a ligament is approaching its length limit during tensile loading.[96]

Synovium

The joint capsule is lined with a richly vascularized layer of connective tissue, the synovial membrane. The synovium is not strictly continuous and has different consistencies depending on the location in the joint cavity.[5,97]

This generally soft tissue has an outer layer, the intima, that faces the joint cavity. The intima lies on top of the underlying supporting layer of fibrous, alveolar or adipose tissue. Irregular dense fibrous tissue covers tendons, ligaments, and other areas subject to pressure. Loose connective tissue, alveolar, lies in regions of the joint cavity that have synovial folds and villi. The areas of the synovium with alveolar tissue have some ability to move independent of the fibrous capsule.[5] Intra-articular fat pads are covered with synovial adipose tissue. These tissues of the supporting layer then merge with those of the fibrous capsule.

The fluid secreted by the synovium provides lubrication for joint surfaces and a method of transport for nutrients to the articular cartilage. The cells of the synovium, the synoviocytes, secrete the additional hyaluronic acid and glycoproteins that give the synovial fluid its excellent friction reducing quality. The highly viscous fluid fills the joint cavity. Usually the joint cavity has a narrow intra-articular space and only a thin film of synovial fluid is required between articulating surfaces.

The generally loose arrangement of tissues allows the fluid of the joint cavity to infiltrate into the deeper layers of the synovium. As well, the nutrients and fluids delivered by capillaries within the supportive layer are able to disperse through the interstitial spaces in the loose tissues and move into the joint cavity.

Innervation of the synovium appears to be with slowly conducting fibers without specialized endings. This means that the synovial membrane may be able to transmit only diffuse sensation that may be interpreted, in turn, as diffuse pain in situations of increased pressure or nociceptive chemicals.

Articular Cartilage

Articular cartilage covers the surfaces of articulating bone ends in synovial joints. Anyone who has ever cut up a whole roasted chicken has observed the pearlized smooth coverings on the surfaces of bone ends that appear after cutting through the thick and tough fibrous capsule. This pristine white coating on articulating bone ends is the articular cartilage. The smoothness of the articular cartilage surface, along with a thin film of synovial fluid, aids the ease of joint movements.

The chondrocytes in articular cartilage are arranged in 4 layers. These layers appear between a most superficial layer, the lamina splendens, and the underlying subchondral bone. The lamina splendens, so named for its bright appearance in phase-contrast studies, is a clear film layer of fine fibrils with chondrocytes. It is believed that the lamina splendens can be sheared off with joint trauma.

The 4 zones begin with the tangential zone. Here the chondrocytes are flattened and, along with the collagen fibers in the zone, are arranged parallel with the subchondral bone. Collagen fibers and proteoglycans have a stronger association than usual in this zone, which may aid in resisting shearing forces.[50]

The chondrocytes in the next zone, the transitional zone, are a full rounded shape and are dispersed, along with collagen fibers, throughout this large volume layer. In the next layer, the radial zone, the chondrocytes stay rounded but are larger and tend to align themselves in vertical columns 4 to 8 cells high. The fourth layer, the calcified layer, the chondrocytes are surrounded by mineralized matrix.

As the zones move from superficial to deep, the density of chondrocytes will decrease. The reverse occurs with regard to collagen fiber size showing greater fiber thickness as fibers move deeper in the zones. The proteoglycan concentration also increases. The aggregates of proteoglycans are compressed and held somewhat contained by the surrounding collagen fibers. The water-holding capacity of proteoglycans enhances the articular cartilage's ability to resist compression even though the overall water content has decreased in the deeper layers. The aggregates of proteoglycans help to prevent displacement of proteoglycans during tissue deformation with loading.[98]

> It is tempting to believe that the differences in matrix composition and organization among zones reflect differences in mechanical function. That is, the superficial zone may primarily resist shearing forces, the transitional zone may allow the change in orientation of collagen fibrils from the superficial zone to the radial zone, and the radial zone may primarily help to resist and distribute compressive loads. The zone of calcified cartilage would then provide a transition in material properties between hyaline (articular) cartilage and bone, as well as anchor the hyaline cartilage to the bone.[99(p419)]

In addition to the belief that the properties of the chondrocytes and the content of the surrounding matrix are different for each layer, it is believed that it is also important to consider the properties of the matrix relative to its proximity to chondrocytes within layers. So within each layer the matrix regions have been identified. Pericellular matrix surrounds a chondrocyte. A wider layer around a single chondrocyte or small clusters of 2 to 3 chondrocytes is the territorial matrix. Fibers here form a fibrillar basket around chondrocytes that may provide protection from mechanical loads. The remaining matrix, the interterritorial matrix, is the largest matrix region within zones. Fiber alignment in the interterritorial zone is consistent with that of the chondrocyte alignment: parallel at the superficial layer and perpendicular to the joint surface at the redial zone.[99]

So though articular cartilage could be summed up as "aneural, largely avascular and acellular,"[94] it is also a uniquely complex tissue with amazing ability to resist mechanical loads.

Joint Response to Loading

Joint capsules are designed to accommodate multidirectional stresses. The configuration of the fibers of the capsule insertion to bone, however, is consistent with a relatively low need to withstand tensile loading. This is no doubt because of the greater load being borne by the stronger arrangement of fibers in the reinforcing ligaments within the capsule. As presented earlier, the fiber-bone insertion structure for ligaments also reflects this. Ligaments, therefore, were designed to withstand tensile loads.

Ligaments, and tendons, show characteristics of a viscoelastic substance with the ability to have an initial reaction to a load but then gradually accommodate to the load over time. The extent to which ligaments can withstand tensile loads, and under varying circumstances, has been widely studied.[18,100-102] We owe a lot of our current understanding of ligament properties under loading to these early studies. And, we need to extrapolate from these studies what needs to be considered for interventions moving forward because it is not likely that any of these studies will be repeated.

A summary of what has been learned about ligaments and exercise is depicted in Figure 10-32. Ligaments exposed to

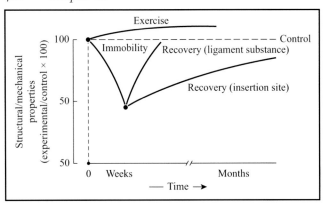

Figure 10-32. Summary of the homeostasis responses of the components of the bone-ligament-bone complex when subjected to different levels of physical activity. (Reprinted with permission from Woo SLY, Maynard J, Butler D, et al. Ligament, tendon and joint capsule insertions to bone. In: Woo SL-Y, Buckwalter JA, eds. *Injury and Repair of the Musculoskeletal Soft Tissues*. Rosemont, IL: American Academy of Orthopaedic Surgeons; 1988.)

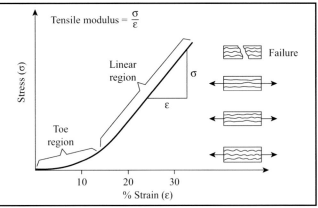

Figure 10-33. Typical tensile stress-strain curve for connective tissues and articular cartilage. The drawings at the right of the curve show the configuration of the collagen fibrils at various stages of loading and stretch. (Reprinted with permission from Mow V, Rosenwasser M. Articular cartilage biomechanics. In: Woo SL-Y, Buckwalter JA, eds. *Injury and Repair of the Musculoskeletal Soft Tissues*. Rosemont, IL: American Academy of Orthopaedic Surgeons; 1988.)

gradual increases in exercise show increased structure—size and weight—and mechanical load when evaluated in load to failure testing. Immobilization on the other hand results in greater than 50% loss within weeks when the same load to failure property is assessed. Recovery from the structural and mechanical property losses has been seen to occur in the ligament structure to near control levels. Recovery of strength at the insertion site takes longer and has not yet been seen to return to control levels.

The other component in the joint closely linked with the fibrous capsule and reinforcing ligaments is the synovial lining. The loose tissue of the synovium is not thought of as providing much resistance to tensile loading. It is, however, responsive to greater than usual loading of the joint as will be seen in the section on joint disorders, specifically, joint effusion and synovitis.

Articular cartilage also shows viscoelastic properties (Figure 10-33). While tendons and ligaments are able to show tensile stress-relaxation and creep because of loading of collagen and elastin fibers, articular cartilage shows these same viscoelastic properties in compression because of movement of interstitial fluid.[103]

Under compression loading, deformation occurs at the top elastic layers to improve joint congruency with the result that fluid is pushed out of the tissues, weeps, onto the joint surface. As soon as the load is released, the fluid is reabsorbed back into the cartilage layers. Under larger compressive loads for longer duration, the articular cartilage top layers again deform with fluid movement out of the tissues. A slower deformation occurs slowly over time at the lower zones. If the duration of loading continues but there is not a change in the size of the load, however, the amount of deformation—greater at the top layers, less at the deeper—redistributes to be shared among all the zone layers.

Despite the forces pressing joint surfaces together during loading, the slipperiness between the surfaces means the sliding and gliding of joint arthrokinematic movements

occurs with a low coefficient of friction (COF) that is even lower than a skate gliding on ice.[94] "The lower the COF, the lower the resistance to sliding…[M]ore force is needed to produce motion when the COF is high."[94] And similar to pressure of the skate blade on ice creating a fluid layer just in front of the blade, articular cartilage will also extrude a film of fluid to decrease friction under loading conditions.[94]

The articular cartilage further assists keeping friction forces low by providing a softer rather than a harder surface. The elasticity of articular cartilage on both ends of the articulating bones allows accommodation to the shape of joint surfaces. The surfaces become more congruent.[94,98,103]

Joint Nutrition and Healing

As has been discussed previously, access to adequate vascularity affects a tissue's ability to heal. In general, joint structures have good access to blood and nutrients with a few notable exceptions, though it should be noted that variations in vascularity do exist between joints.[94]

The simple fact that cartilage is avascular starts to highlight the disparities within joint structures with regard to nutrition. With this reminder of tissue physiology, the difficulty for articular cartilage to have adequate oxygen and nutrients is apparent. Nutritional components are released by capillaries into the supportive layer of the synovium. By diffusion the oxygen and nutrients move through the synovial layers, combine with the synovial fluid, and float across the joint space to the articular cartilage where, by continued diffusion, the nutrients move through the articular cartilage. The process of mechanical loading—the pushing out and then pulling back in of fluid—may improve the flow of nutrients and metabolites into the cartilage.[98] Even with this possible enhancement to simple diffusion, articular cartilage's relative avascularity impairs its ability to repair itself.

Less obvious is the avascularity for ligaments, or tendons, that have attachments to bone through a zone of fibrocartilage. Short distance vascularity may exist for the portion of

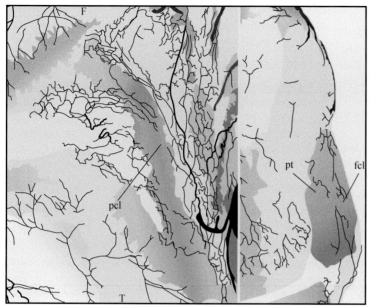

Figure 10-34. Side view of the posterior cruciate ligament (pcl) in a 33-year-old man. A number of vessels penetrate at various levels in the ligament, where they split upward and downward, but not into the osseous attachments. F: femur; T: tibia. (Adapted from Scapinelli R. Studies on the vasculature of the human knee joint. *Acta Anat (Basel).* 1968,70(3):305-331.)

the attachment on the bone side from blood vessels in the bone. Surrounding tissues may provide access to a capillary network for the mid-sections of ligaments, or tendons, on the other side of the fibrocartilage. The region of fibrocartilage remains avascular (Figure 10-34). Though healing of ligaments injured in the fibrocartilage layer is still theoretically possible, surgical repair of ligaments tears in or near the fibrocartilage zone have proved frustrating. Despite initial success with healing restoration of the insertion site structure, the measured strength after 1 year was, at most, 50% of that measured on the uninjured side.[102]

In contrast, the synovium has a rich vascular and lymphatic supply.[5] The areas of the synovial lining with fibrous tissue have slightly less vascularity than the portions of the lining with alveolar or fatty tissues.[94] Injured areas of the synovium regenerate easily.[5]

Joint Disorders

Joint Effusion

The amount of lubricating synovial fluid contained within the fibrous joint capsules of synovial joints is generally small. In certain circumstances, however, the fluid volume can increase, and increase dramatically. Faced with traumatic injury to joint structures, overuse conditions, or the presence of systemic disease, a rise in synovial fluid volume will be seen, and seen literally since the previous small joint space expands markedly to accommodate the increase in fluid.

The marked expansion of the joint space, now overfilled with synovial fluid, is termed a *joint effusion*. The discussion here will be limited to joint effusion due to an increase in synovial fluid. Note, however, that joint effusions also occur with bleeding into the joint space as with traumatic injury, a hemophilia event or the result of oral anticoagulant therapy.[104]

The presence of cell injury within the joint will stimulate events that lead to an increase in synovial fluid. The exact mechanisms for this response in the joint to inflammation are not completely understood.[105] It has been suggested that synoviocytes increase production of synovial fluid.[106] Fluid from the blood capillaries in the synovium are another identified source.[97]

A general characteristic of inflammatory chemotaxis is the increased permeability of capillary walls to plasma proteins, which then move from the capillaries into the tissue interstitial spaces. The presence of these proteins in the tissues disrupts the osmotic balance, prompting fluid from the capillaries to flow into the tissues to dilute the now protein-rich region and restore osmotic balance. An increase of fluid within the loose cellular structure of the synovium would then flow into the joint space.

These events with inflammation support the proposal that the source of increased synovial fluid is fluid from the capillary network in the synovium. In addition, however, increased synoviocyte production of proteins with inflammation may also add to an osmotic imbalance that, in turn, increases fluid flow from the capillaries in the synovium and adds to the fluid volume in the joint space. With prolonged inflammation the synovium can undergo hypertrophic and proliferative changes.[105]

The filling of the joint space with synovial fluid expands redundant folds of the capsule. Since fluid does not compress, the usual amplitude of joint movements are reduced. Any movements of the joint that meets the fluid-resisted capacity of the capsule will further stretch an already distended capsule and be painful. Joint effusions can be characterized by the joint position the joint assumes when maximally effused such as the around –20 degrees of extension seen in the knee joint.[104] Even before maximum effusion levels are reached, it has been shown that a joint effusion also has the capacity to prompt an inhibitory effect on supportive joint musculature.[107,108]

Adhesive Capsulitis

Adhesive capsulitis is characterized by painful and limited passive and active range of motion of a joint. Generally thought to be a disorder of the glenohumeral joint, it has been reported to occur at the hip, wrist, and ankle.[109] Whether a spontaneous onset or linked with joint injury, the actual mechanism of tissue disorder of adhesive capsulitis is not well understood.

In a stark contrast with the development of a distended effused joint in reaction to inflammation, the joint capsule in adhesive capsulitis becomes thickened with the loss of redundant folds and joint space recesses. A "proliferation of inflammatory infiltrate may precede the initiation and progression of the fibrous thickening process."[109] Phases of the process have been identified.

> For the glenohumeral joint, 3 distinct phases have been described in staging this condition. The first is an early painful phase, or "freezing stage," with a duration of 2 to 9 months. This is followed by an intermediate stiffening or adhesive phase, which has a duration of 4 to 12 months. In this phase, patients typically experience increasing stiffness, but less pronounced pain. The final phase is known as the recovery, or "thawing" phase, which lasts anywhere from 5 to 24 months. Here, patients display a gradual return of movement.[109]

The return of movement reverses the observed capsular pattern of movement loss. In the glenohumeral joint, lateral rotation is limited most, followed by abduction then medial rotation.[109,110] In the ankle, dorsiflexion has near full restriction while plantarflexion is decreased by almost 50%.[109]

Arthrokinematic movements are the generally unobserved movements that occur between joint surfaces that are, nevertheless, essential for the observed osteokinematic movements to occur. A hypomobile glenohumeral capsule will restrict the ability of the humeral head to glide inferiorly in the glenoid fossa thus thwarting an important assist by the rotator cuff muscles to shoulder movements. A hypomobile ankle capsule will show a decrease in an anterior-to-posterior gliding movement of the talus within the ankle mortise, which results in a limitation of ankle dorsiflexion.

Joint mobilization techniques follow these arthrokinematic movements, also called accessory movements, to restore joint movement. Small repeated oscillations are applied at mid-range or end range of the available capsular mobility for the restricted accessory movement in the joint.[111,112] The property of tissue hysteresis explains the treated tissue's response to become less stiff, and more relaxed, as a result of the application, and release, of the tensile load for the specific mobilization performed.

Use of mobilization techniques and exercises in the treatment of patients with glenohumeral adhesive capsulitis who also undergo one intraarticular corticosteroid injection, lead to range of motion gains being made more quickly when compared to patients who also receive the injection and follow a home program of the exercise.[113] A significant difference in trend was found with the use of high-grade mobilization techniques compared with low-grade mobilization in the treatment of glenohumeral adhesive capsulitis.[114]

Ligament Sprain/Rupture

Ligaments can be subjected to joint movements or outside forces that result in a tensile stress to the ligamentous tissues. The amount of injury will depend on the direction of the force as well as the position of the joint at the time. Ligament sprain can range from the following[115]:

- Grade I (mild, no increased laxity)
- Grade II (moderate, slight but not significant laxity)
- Grade III (severe, significant laxity to complete disruption)

Depending on the direction, magnitude, and rate of the applied load, the tension on the ligamentous arrangement around a joint will occur in a load-sharing pattern.[116] The result may be that more than one ligament in the joint may be injured.

Since some ligaments are structures within the joint fibrous capsule, the applied load may generate tissue reactions in the joint capsule as well as the synovium. In addition, collagen fibers in the ligamentous tissue can sustain a tensile load to the extent that some fibers fail. Even after healing, the ligament may offer less resistance to loading. Clinical testing of ligament resilience may show that less force is required to lengthen the ligament. The result is greater movement of the joint in the direction tested. A hypermobile joint may lead to altered within-the-joint biomechanics during loading situations. The resultant unwanted movement(s) challenge joint stability and create further irritation of joint structures. An effused joint adopts a loose-pack position rendering the joint less stable when functioning in what was once its more stable closed-pack position.[97]

Because of the fibrocartilage layer for some tendon insertions, surgical repair may not be attempted. Reconstructive surgery to replace an excessively hypermobile or ruptured ligament, such as the anterior cruciate ligament of the knee, can restore stable joint biomechanics.

Osteoarthritis

What is the long-term effect of repeated episodes of joint effusion, inhibited protective muscular support or altered biomechanics in a joint due to ligamentous laxity? Add to that the effect of increased compression loading such as occurs to the weightbearing joint in workers who stand for job tasks on cement floors.

The degenerative process in osteoarthritis has several components. Radin described that excessive compression loading in weightbearing joints is shock-absorbed not by the articular cartilage but by the underlying trabecular bone on both sides of the joint.[117] The bone responds during remodeling to heal the trabecular microfractures in addition to refortifying the bone. The result is a stiffer trabecular bone structure. Now the articular cartilage is subjected to higher stress due to the stiffer-than-before subchondral bone. As the

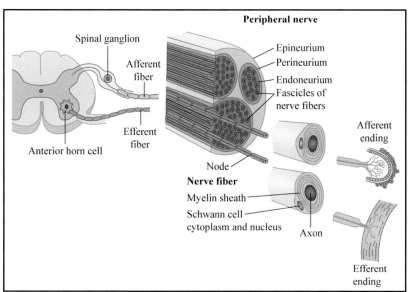

Figure 10-35. PNS organization. (Adapted from Cormack DH. *Introduction to Histology.* Philadelphia, PA: J.B. Lippincott Co; 1984.)

PST predicts, the articular cartilage begins to show degenerative changes though the total impact may not be clinically apparent for years.

"The harder the surface, the higher the friction."[97] The superficial layer on articular cartilage, the lamina splendens, may shear off with increased surface friction. This exposes the top zone of articular cartilage to the increased friction, which in turn begins to erode the surface. The previously smooth articulating surfaces will not be able to maintain the protective lubricating layer of fluid with joint movements, which further increases the surface to erosion.

Incongruity of joints can contribute to the development of osteoarthritis. Joints with greater contact area are less likely to develop arthritis.[117] A function of articular cartilage is to provide a more congruous surface. Changes in the exposed outer surface of the articular cartilage alter its ability to conform. The decreased contact surface becomes another contributor to increased surface loading.

Graduated loading of articular cartilage after it has undergone changes with immobilization may restore loading tolerance.[97] "Therapists should recognize that after immobilization or unloading (rest), articular cartilage is less stiff and less capable of tolerating high loads, loads normally within the physiological capacity of healthy cartilage."[97]

Degenerative changes in articular cartilage have little ability to reverse. The avascularity of articular cartilage deprives it of the ability to produce an inflammatory response and subsequent repair.[97]

PERIPHERAL NERVES

Morphology and Physiology

The nervous tissue of the PNS differs in 2 ways from that of the CNS. First, when nerve axons in the PNS bundle together, a connective tissue layer surrounds the bundle. This layer, as well as the extracellular matrix between axons within the bundle, provides strength. The bundle, called a *fascicle*, will organize with other fascicles to form nerves with further resilience-enhancing connective tissue layers and the extracellular matrix (Figure 10-35).

Second, most axons in the PNS will be wrapped with segmental, concentric, layered sheaths of myelin formed by individual Schwann cells. The spaces between the segments, the nodes of Ranvier, allow axons to branch as well as allow an electrical impulse to skip from node to node for faster transmission (Figure 10-36).

The connective tissue layers around nerve units offer other advantages. Loose connective tissue—the extracellular matrix with fibers mentioned previously—extend to the surrounding layers to fill in the spaces within fascicles and between fascicles in a nerve. This offers a little biological padding, thus, protection from compression. This loose lattice of elastin and collagen fibers also allows axons and fascicles to slide independently of each other within one nerve to accommodate varying tensions.

Bilateral nerve roots branch off from the spinal cord at every vertebral segment. At cervical and lumbar/sacral levels, the nerve roots divide and regroup with nerve roots from adjacent levels. The dividing and recombining occurs in several more stages until the pattern of brachial and lumbar/sacral plexuses is formed (Figure 10-37). This structural pattern of dividing and regrouping of nerve axons continues on past the plexus.

A single nerve axon does not stay in just one peripheral nerve fascicle throughout the axon's length.[118] Instead, there is repeated dividing and regrouping of axons (Figure 10-38). Despite all the regrouping, however, axons intended for the same nerve branch will be sorted to end up in the same fascicle just before the fascicle branches off the larger nerve.[119] This variable path for each axon may minimize the overall effect from a partial nerve injury but may also complicate a nerve's effort to repair itself.[118]

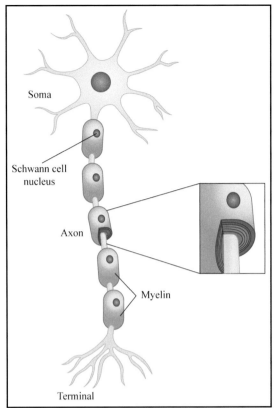

Figure 10-36. Myelin formed by Schwann cells. (Adapted from Widmaier EP, Hershel R, Strang KT. *Vander, Sherman, Luciano's Human Physiology: The Mechanism Of Body Function.* 9th ed. New York: McGraw-Hill; 2004.)

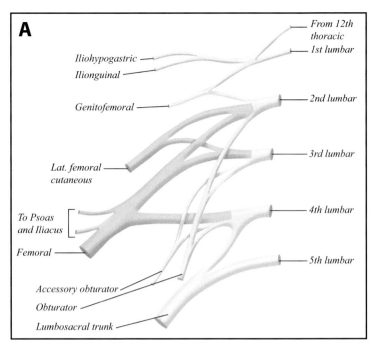

Figure 10-37. (A) Brachial plexus. *(continued)*

Along with the structural pattern of dividing and regrouping seen in the plexus and the fascicles, neural tissues share another pattern.

> A nerve trunk runs an undulating course in its bed, the fasciculi run an undulating course in the epineurium, and the nerve fibers run an undulating course in the inside the fasciculi. This means that the length of a nerve trunk, and its contained nerve fibers between any 2 fixed points on the limb, is greater than a straight line joining those points.[119]

The gradual straightening of these waves when a nerve is slowly tensioned minimizes overstretching of peripheral nerve tissues.

Axonal transport within a neuron and impulse propagation along a neuron share an energy source but their mechanisms for energy access differ. This makes it possible to block the action potential without affecting axoplasmic flow. A nerve under the inhibiting effect of a blocking agent, such as procaine, cannot conduct impulses but the axonal transport function is maintained.[120]

Ion channels are located along nerve axons. These channels can open or close to ions that may excite the neuron. An even distribution of separate ion channels for electrical, chemical, mechanical or temperature stimuli could be altered in only a few days to reflect a change in the local nerve tissue environment.[121]

When a soft tissue injury occurs, the nerve tissue in the region would have increased exposure to bradykinins and prostaglandins during the immediate response and inflammatory phase. In the natural turnover of ion channels every few days, exposed axons might then reflect accommodation to the new environment, with a greater percentage of ion channels to detect nociceptive chemicals.[121] The greater number of ion channels for nociception on the nerve would change the balance of the types of stimuli being relayed to the dorsal root ganglion. The dorsal root ganglion, in turn, would reconfigure its receptors to accommodate this change in input.

Nerve Responses to Loading

Peripheral nerves are able to slide within fascicles and have undulations to allow accommodation to length changes. How adequate are these properties to prevent overstretching in everyday activities? Sunderland, a pioneer and esteemed nerve researcher, believed that generally the tensile forces generated with normal limb movements would not be likely to compromise nerve fibers within the fasciculi.[119] From his mechanical properties' view of overstretching, perhaps his view is accurate. More has been learned since about the changes in peripheral nerves as a result of lower stresses. The answer to the question may now be, "Well, it depends."

First, the extent to which a fascicle can slide within a nerve structure is variable. Tissue of the interfascicular epineurium with loose connections to the outer perineurium does allow sliding of one fascicle independent of others within a nerve.[118] Areas of perineural tissue with greater amounts of adipose tissue also aid gliding. In areas where the nerve branches or vessels exit or enter the nerve, however, the epineurium has greater attachment to the perineurium. The result is that less nerve sliding is available at these points.[122]

B

Figure 10-37 (continued). (B) Lumbar plexus.

Cords   Divisions   Trunks   Roots

Dorsal scapular nerve

Suprascapular nerve

Nerve to subclavius

Lateral pectoral nerve

Lateral cord

Musculocutaneous
nerve

Posterior cord

Axillary
nerve

Medial cord

Median
nerve

Ulnar
nerve

Radial
nerve

Medial cutaneous nerve of the arm

Medial cutaneous nerve
of the forearm

Medial pectoral
nerve

Upper subscapular nerve

Thoracodorsal nerve

Lower subscapular nerve

Long thoracic
nerve

C5

C6

C7

C8

T1

Second, there are areas in the body where peripheral nerves are more challenged to slide to accommodate tensile forces. Nerves are held more adherent by the adjacent tissues at sites where nerves must pass over, thus closely, to bony structures. Movement of the radial nerve is diminished as it passes at the elbow. The common peroneal nerve has less mobility at the head of the fibula.[121,118]

Third, combinations of movements can challenge the nerves' ability to accommodate length requirements. The median nerve bed has to adapt to a length 20% longer when the shoulder is abducted 90 degrees and the elbow and wrist move from fully flexed positions to fully extended.[121] This is the same movement as reaching sideways from a low car to retrieve a ticket from the machine at a parking structure. The tingle one can feel at the ventral aspect of the wrist and hand is the median nerve registering the effects of a tensile load.

Generally, peripheral nerves will glide, when able, to reduce tensile stress. In the example of reaching for the parking garage ticket, imagine the person reaching is also wearing mittens connected by a string. As he reaches out for the ticket, the string needs to slide toward the reaching side to enable the elbow and wrist to extend. Similarly, the median nerve glides toward the elbow—convergence—from the "slack" at the shoulder and neck. When the arm is brought back into the car, the median nerve glides proximally—divergence.[118]

In those areas where attachments may limit the extent of convergence and divergence for the nerve, or for a task that

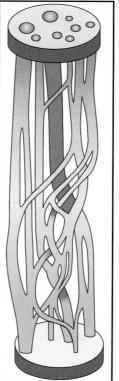

Figure 10-38. Fascicular plexus formations in a 3 cm length of the musculocutaneous nerve reconstructed from a serially sectioned specimen. (Adapted from Sunderland S. The anatomy and physiology of nerve injury. *Muscle Nerve.* 1990:13:771-784.)

challenges nerve length, peripheral nerves do have the ability to adjust to modest change in length demands. Because

Figure 10-39. Physical stresses placed on peripheral nerve. Tensile stress applied longitudinally to peripheral nerve creates an elongation of the nerve (an increase in strain). The transverse contraction that occurs during this elongation is greatest at the middle of the section undergoing tensile stress. (Adapted from Topp KS, Boyd FS. Structures and biomechanics of peripheral nerves: nerve responses to physical stresses and implications for physical therapist practice. *Phys Ther.* 2006;86(1):92-109.)

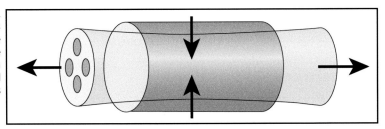

nervous tissue has viscoelastic properties, along with the connective tissue layers, it can adjust to small increments of elongation with creep and stress-reduction.

When a peripheral nerve is elongated, a transverse contraction occurs that narrows the diameter in the middle of the section undergoing the tensile load (Figure 10-39). The decrease in cross-sectional area increases pressure within the nerve and intrafascicular microcirculation is compromised.[119] In the example of reaching for the ticket at a parking garage, the tingle felt in the wrist and hand at the extreme end of the reach is likely due to microcirculation compromise from pressure within the median nerve with elongation. Nerves are extraordinarily sensitive to ischemia.[118,119,121]

Nerve Nutrition and Healing

Nerves rely on, and have, a robust blood supply. The vas nervorum is a complex system of arteries with anastomosing arterioles running longitudinally in the epineurium. Blood flows through this network to supply capillaries to the axons within the fascicules. The vas nervorum keeps all nerve components adequately oxygenated even if some of the feeder arteries are damaged.[118,121] Further, the arteries that enter segmentally along the nerve are coiled to better accommodate the mobility required of peripheral nerves.[118,121]

Special features of the blood supply create a barrier at the perineurium to bacteria. This allows nerves to pass through areas of infection without impairment of nerve function.[121] The barrier at the perineurium, however, does not allow lymphatic vessels to cross. This means that any edema within a nerve will take longer to resolve.[120]

The rich blood supply is required for effective nerve function because nerves are extremely sensitive to ischemia. Microvascular ischemia can occur with the increased transverse contraction pressure from nerve elongation as well as with nerve compression. As with other tissues, increasing the duration of small elongation or compression loads will have more of an ischemic effect as would increasing the amount of elongation or pressure.

Classification of severe nerve injuries has long been established. Stages of healing have been well defined for these injuries (Figure 10-40). Severely injured nerves degenerate from the point of injury and distally. Nerve healing takes the form of nerve regeneration from the point of injury after the stage of degeneration is completed. Simply having the nerve regenerate along its complete length is a daunting task but it is not the only challenge. The new nerve needs to be able to conduct electric signals as well as tolerate gliding to accommodate to tensile stress.

Less widely considered have been nerve injuries within the category of preneurapraxias. In a number of injury scenarios involving other tissues, it is reasonable to surmise that portions of a fascicle might also have been injured or exposed to inflammatory agents. The change in ion channels, leading to adjustments made at the dorsal root ganglion, are not always considered.

A mantra-like guideline to direct interventions has been identified based on nerve physiology and the environment required for nerve healing.

- Nerves want space.
- Nerves want movement.
- Nerves want oxygen.[123]

The need for space is based on the notion that an ailing nerve is less tolerant of conditions of possible compression or elongation. The space is the absence of compression or elongation. Because of the ion channel changes, the nerve is even more sensitive to mechanical stress than before the injury.

Nerves conduct signals but, as has been discussed previously, nerves also move. They are designed to move. Not moving, especially in injured nerves, may contribute to additional nerve changes. Alterations in axoplasmic flow due to injury may gradually resume with gentle nerve gliding movement. Nerve glides can be identified that gently allow the involved nerve to move. These glides can even be performed without disturbing adjacent tissues if indicated for the healing of those other tissues.

Nerves are highly sensitive to ischemic situations. "The action potential and the axoplasmic flow both require a source of energy; they access a common pool of an ATP. In an anoxic nerve, both axoplasmic flow and the action potential will stop within 15 minutes."[121] Any compromise of cardiovascular or pulmonary status will affect nerve healing.

Peripheral Nerve Disorders

Compression

Nerves face compression forces in everyday activities. From arms leaning on chair armrests to sitting on hard surfaces, nerves encounter pressure. Further, some nerves are subject to greater compression exposure because of their location such as the median nerve in the carpel tunnel. The organization of fascicles with a nerve can minimize or increase the effect of compression. Nerves with several small fascicles surrounded by a large amount of epineurium padding are less vulnerable to compression than are nerves

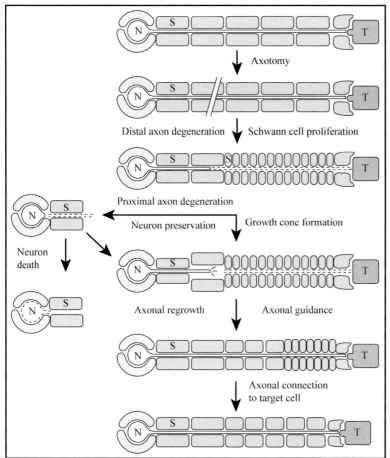

Figure 10-40. Sequence of events with peripheral nerve damage. An injury across an axon will disrupt the connection between the neuron (N) and its target cell (T). Distal to the injury site, the axon degenerates and Schwann cells (S) proliferate. If the neuron cell body survives the degeneration, the proximal portion of the axon will regenerate to span the injury site and be guided to the target cell. As the regeneration occurs, the Schwann cells reestablish their supporting association with the new axon. (Adapted from Lundborg G, Rydevik B, Manthorpe. Peripheral nerve: the physiology of injury and repair. In: Woo SL-Y, Buckwalter JA, eds. *Injury and Repair of the Musculoskeletal Soft Tissues.* Park Ridge, IL: American Academy of Orthopaedic Surgeons; 1988.)

with 1 or 2 large fascicles with only a small relative volume of connective tissue matrix.[120,121] Most nerves, however, are able to tolerate low compression forces for brief durations and recover.

The exact parameters of safe nerve compression are difficult to define. The functional positions noted previously, and others, can approach or exceed the limit of 20 to 30 mm Hg, which is known to impair nerve blood flow.[118]

> Simply placing the hand on a computer mouse was shown to increase the tunnel pressure from the resting 5 mm Hg to 16 to 21 mm Hg, and actively using the mouse to point and click increased the tunnel pressure to 28 to 33 mm Hg, a pressure high enough to reduce nerve blood flow.[118]

At the compression level of 20 to 30 mm Hg, the first sign of impaired microvascularity is seen in a reduced blood flow to endoneurial tissues. The impaired capillary flow reduces the oxygen supply for the endothelial cells of the capillaries. As noted in the events of inflammation for the basic tissues, this anoxic situation leads to increased capillary permeability. Fluid and proteins leak from the capillary into the endoneurial tissues causing edema in the endoneurial tissues. After 2 to 4 hours of low pressure conditions, the fluid pressure of the endoneurium can increase more than 3 times the baseline level.[120] A local metabolic conduction block occurs.[120]

Held briefly the nerve tissue recovers without irreversible changes. It will take longer for the edema to resolve than with other tissues because of the lack of lymphatic vessels within the nerve. Compression pressures that are enough to block axonal transport may produce a deficit that lasts for days after. Compressive position held longer, or in situations of repetitive compression, neurapraxia—a demyelinating conduction block—can occur.[120] High-compression forces can sever axons.

Traction

Elongated nerves initially suffer the effects of compression with the increased pressure from transverse contraction. The resultant impaired microvascularity leads to endoneurial edema as described previously. A nerve held for a short duration at a length 6% to 8% greater than its resting length will experience transient changes in blood flow.[118] Healthy adults have reported intolerance to positions identified in cadaver studies as being only 8% greater than resting lengths. "Common positions used to assess the neurodynamics of the upper limb may result in nerve strain that approaches or exceeds the 11% strain that is known to result in long-term damage."[118] Neural mobility will be compromised in nerves that have had an impedance of blood flow from a previous episode, or episodes, of elongation stress.

The electrophysiology properties of nerve can be affected even with gradually increasing tensile loads. Extreme

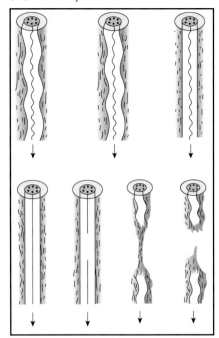

Figure 10-41. Changes occurring in the various components of a nerve trunk as it is stretch to structural failure. Only one fasciculus in the nerve is represented. (Adapted from Sunderland S. The anatomy and physiology of nerve injury. *Muscle Nerve.* 1990:13:771-784; and Sunderland S. *Nerves and Nerve Injuries.* Edinburgh, Churchill Livingston: 1979.)

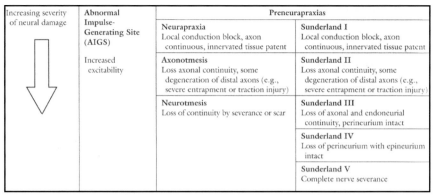

Increasing severity of neural damage	Abnormal Impulse-Generating Site (AIGS) Increased excitability	Preneurapraxias	
		Neurapraxia Local conduction block, axon continuous, innervated tissue patent	**Sunderland I** Local conduction block, axon continuous, innervated tissue patent
		Axonotmesis Loss axonal continuity, some degeneration of distal axons (e.g., severe entrapment or traction injury)	**Sunderland II** Loss axonal continuity, some degeneration of distal axons (e.g., severe entrapment or traction injury)
		Neurotmesis Loss of continuity by severance or scar	**Sunderland III** Loss of axonal and endoneurial continuity, perineurium intact
			Sunderland IV Loss of perineurium with epineurium intact
			Sunderland V Complete nerve severance

Figure 10-42. Categories of nerve injuries. (Reprinted with permission from Butler DS, Tomberlin JP. Peripheral nerve: structure, function, and physiology. In: *Scientific Foundations and Principles of Practice in Musculoskeletal Rehabilitation*, Magee DJ, Zachazewski JE, Quillen WS, eds, Copyright Saunders Elsevier Inc 2007.)

elongation stress can lead to axonal injury and functional impairment. The classic studies by Sunderland depict the sequence of events as a nerve continues to experience an increasing tensile load (Figure 10-41). The nerve undergoes layer by layer failure of its structure: axon, endoneurium, perineurium, epineurium. Beginning with the loss of axonal continuity, the neuron(s) will need to undergo degeneration and regeneration to recover. Each additional layer of failure within the nerve adds to the nerve's recovery challenge (Figure 10-42).

Neural Immobility

The mechanical property of nerve mobility can be impaired with exposure to mechanical stresses. Repetitive episodes of prolonged elongation or compression, even at low loads, can cause edema in nerves. Chronic edema from inflammation leads to fibrotic changes in the connective tissues located within and between nerve fascicles. The loss of this loose tissue will lead to a decreased ability for fascicles to slide independently of each other within a nerve when encountering varying tensile loads.

A single episode of increased compression or elongation will also result in an inflammatory episode within the injured neural connective tissue layers. The resulting decreased nerve mobility can occur whether or not it was apparent that other tissues in the region were also injured in the episode. The probability that nerve mobility could become impaired increases when a regional musculoskeletal injury is immobilized. The opportunity for the development of fiber crosslinks in connective tissues is enhanced when fibers are held static.[34] The crosslinks will further stiffen the connective tissues in and around fascicles. Instructions to move fingers, or toes, when a patient is in an arm, or leg, cast can assist with the maintenance of neural mobility even when the joint movements seem far removed from the immobilized region.

A sciatic nerve with inadequate ability to slide to accommodate the length flexibility of the surrounding hamstring muscle fibers can be subject to intolerable elongation with "normal" stretches. The same situation can occur for recovering fascicles or partial fascicles within a nerve with "normal" movements.

Consider the impact on nerve mobility for a critically ill patient who spent days lying in bed in a state of relative immobility. The simple act of sitting up on the side of the bed could require more ease of mobility from the sciatic nerve than it may be ready to provide. Sitting on the side of the bed and performing ankle pumps with an extended knee could further challenge nerve mobility.

What would be the impact on a patient's movements over the few days following a surgical or medical procedure during which a fascicle or partial fascicle was held inadvertently in an elongated or compressed position? Well into the inflammatory phase, the swollen tissues of the fascicle might not allow the usual ease of gliding. The symptoms from nerve ischemia might not be the first possibility that comes to mind when the patient reports pain. Making this link to what might be occurring at the tissue level is challenged further because with a gentle tug on the fascicle the ischemia might take a few minutes to develop. There can be a delay between the brain's interpretation of the incoming stimuli and the patient's report of pain.

How is the concept of neural mobility best incorporated into patient care? Recognizing that a neural mobility deficit is possible is the first step. For the sciatic nerve scenario mentioned previously, the remedy could be as simple as an intervening range of motion exercise in supine to check the ease and comfort of hip flexion before asking the patient to sit up for the first time. The guideline of testing the ease of the movement with passive then active-assistive exercise has served physical therapists, and their patients, well even before the effects of decreased neural mobility were identified. There are identified patterns in limbs where nerves have more or less ability to be compliant with mobility demands. Guidelines for careful mobility testing and interventions are available.[124] The ability of a fascicle or nerve to recover from a single episode of increased load, or repetitive loads, is affected by the patient's cardiovascular and pulmonary status. Further, systemic pathologies of note for impaired neuronal function are diabetes mellitus, hypothyroidism, alcoholism, immune deficiency syndromes, and rheumatoid arthritis.[121]

Hypersensitivity

Many physical therapists have a biomedical perspective regarding pain and will search for a cause of the pain when pain is reported. The focus is on anatomical and biomechanical principles to explain the causes of pain. This perspective has been effective for many patients but not all. There is a growing awareness that hypersensitivity of the nervous system offers an explanation for the examination and treatment of patients with pain complaints that persist long after any sign of other tissue injury is evident. This may also offer assistance for the management of patients whose reported symptom intensities far outweigh noted tissue injury. Further, research has established a link between altered pain beliefs and altered movement performance in patients with increased and prolonged reports of pain.[125]

An evolving biopsychosocial perspective on pain strongly acknowledges interactions between the brain and the body, specifically with regard to the nervous system. Pain is an output. David Butler has offered the following insights to go along with the notion that pain is an output:

- Pain is a critical protective device.
- Pain depends on how much danger your brain thinks you are in, not how much you are really in.
- Pain is one of many systems designed to get you out of trouble.
- Tissue damage and pain often do not relate.
- As pain persists the nervous system becomes better at producing pain.[126]

Pain as an output can take a bit of getting used to for clinicians. In a study that assessed the pain knowledge of clinicians and patients, untrained clinicians fared no better than patients in accurately answering a questionnaire (Figure 10-43).[127]

Axons in the region of a musculoskeletal injury can begin the process of ion channel changes to respond to environment of inflammation. Over the days and weeks of recovery, perhaps with restoration of normal movements including neural mobility, the ion channel balance reverts back to the baseline state. What will happen if a neuron does not return

	QUESTIONS	before			after		
		T	F	U	T	F	U
1	When part of your body is injured, special pain receptors convey the pain message to your brain						
2	Pain only occurs when you are injured						
3	The intensity of pain matches the severity of the injury						
4	Nerves have to connect a body part to the brain in order for that part to be in pain						
5	In chronic pain, the central nervous system becomes more sensitive to nociception (danger messages from tissues)						
6	The body tells the brain when it is in pain						
7	The brain can sends messages down your spinal cord that can increase the nociception (danger messages) going up the spinal cord						
8	Peripheral nerves can adapt by increasing their resting level of excitement						
9	Chronic pain means an injury hasn't healed properly						
10	The brain decides when you will experience pain						
11	The pain you feel is the same pain your grandparents felt						
12	Worse injuries always result in worse pain						
13	When you are injured, the environment that you are in will not have an effect on the amount of pain that you experience						
14	It is possible to have pain and not know about it						
15	Stress can make a peripheral nerve fire						
16	Your internal pain control system is more powerful than any drug taken by mouth or injected.						
17	The immune system has nothing to do with a pain experience						
18	Pinched nerves always hurt						
19	It is possible to treat pain by causing pain						
20	Chronic pain is more common in wealthier countries than poorer countries.						

Figure 10-43. Adapted Moseley's Pain Sciences Quiz (2003). (Reprinted from *J Pain*, 4(4), Moseley L, Unraveling the barriers to reconceptualization of the problem in chronic pain: the actual and perceived ability of patients and health professional to understand the neurophysiology, pp 184-189, Copyright 2003, with permission from Elsevier.)

to baseline but instead continues getting better and better at responding to any stimulus? What if it doesn't even need a stimulus but just fires on its own? Abnormal impulse-generating sites can form on a neuron, producing ectopic discharges (Figure 10-44).[121] With increased messages coming in from the periphery, other parts of the nervous system—the dorsal root ganglion and the brain—reconfigure and the nervous system can become hypersensitive.[128] What has been effective to turn down this hypersensitivity?

The use of functional MRIs to plot the areas of the brain with increased activity has helped evaluate the effectiveness of interventions. Of most significance is the improvement in functional movements that are matched with decreased brain neurotag activity in patients after the patients participate in an education session about the physiology of pain.[129]

Further, patients have shown improvements in understanding and managing their chronic low back pain that were greater after an educational session on the physiology of pain and nociception than after a session on anatomy and physiology of the lumbar spine.[130] Simple drawings can assist the explanation of pain physiology (Figures 10-45 and 10-46).[131]

Figure 10-44. Possible abnormal impulse-generating sites represented on one neuron. (Reprinted from Butler DS. *The Sensitive Nervous System.* Adelaide, Australia: Noigroup; 2000, with permission from Noigroup Publications.)

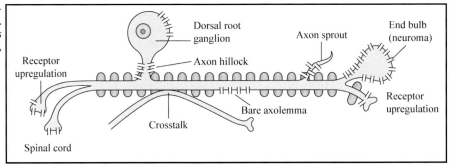

Figure 10-45. The alarm message meets the spinal cord. Alarm messages coming to the spinal cord from tissue nerves are dampened when met by inhibiting chemicals activated by descending pathways from the brain. (Reprinted from Butler D, Moseley L. *Explain Pain.* Adelaide, Australia: Noigroup; 2003, with permission from Noigroup Publications.)

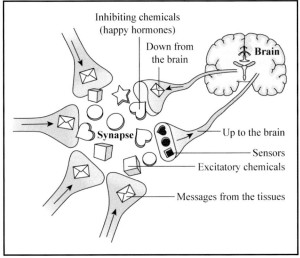

Figure 10-46. Altered CNS at the spinal cord. Enhanced sensitivity of the alarm system is nearly always a main feature in persistent pain. (Reprinted from Butler D, Moseley L. *Explain Pain.* Adelaide, Australia: Noigroup; 2003, with permission from Noigroup Publications.)

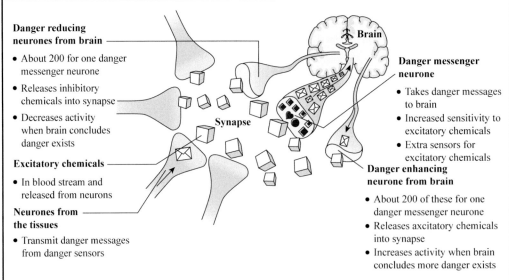

Musculoskeletal Examination

The Guide to Physical Therapist Practice identifies the elements of the patient/client management model. Whether in an inpatient or outpatient setting, the examination of patients begins with gathering information about the current complaint. This may also require identifying past medical history related to the presenting complaint. In the inpatient setting, a chart review, and discussions with nurses, the patient's family, and attending physician may precede interviewing the patient. There are patient cases in this text to identify the process with a hospitalized patient. This chapter will highlight examination considerations for a patient seeking outpatient physical therapy services for a musculoskeletal complaint.

Examination

History

Patient Interview

Therapists in an outpatient clinic who are able to greet a new patient in the waiting area, walk with the patient back to a private treatment room, and get the patient settled comfortably for the interview, start the examination with several advantages. The physical therapist is able to offer a welcoming greeting using the patient's surname and then establish, right from the start, how the patient would prefer to be addressed. It is always worth asking, "Would you like for me to call you Mr. Halo?"

The therapist is able to observe the patient's ability to stand from sitting, navigate through doorways/corridors and walk the distance to the treatment room. Walking with the patient allows an initial impression of the patient's gait to be made. Asking a question such as, "Did you have any trouble finding us?" and observing whether the patient's gait changes as he answers introduces whether difficulty with dual tasking might need to be considered. The availability of a private treatment room enhances the patient's experience right away since respect for the patient's privacy has been identified as an important consideration in patient satisfaction.[132] Another transfer is observed as the patient sits in the treatment room chair. Small treatment rooms exist where the process of just getting to the chair provides insight into whether the patient is proficient with maneuvering in very tight spaces.

Offer to have the patient sit in a comfortable chair with armrests but also mention that if standing or walking in the room would make the patient more comfortable during the interview, he is free to do so. After asking what brings the patient to physical therapy, let the patient have an opportunity to talk for a few minutes without interruption. The conversation can be redirected as needed in a few minutes. Letting the patient talk can lead to the successful gathering of needed information even if the order in which the information is reported seems random.

At the end of the interview, it is important to have learned the nature of the complaint including the body part involved, what functions are impaired, and for how long. Identifying past medical history, medications, and general health helps to establish what other factors may be affecting the physical stress of tissues.

Since functional activities will be one standard against which to judge patient progress, the use of functional surveys and outcome measures are useful. As well a series of specific questions can be asked with the format of, "If 100% was the level where you are able to perform dressing, bathing and generally taking care of just yourself in your home independently—and performing those tasks in the manner you think you should be able to perform them—what percentage are you able to do now?" Note what aspects of those tasks are difficult for the patient and why, as well as what tasks can't be done to reach the 100% level.

The same question can be repeated with the substitution of instrumental activities of daily living (IADL) or work tasks. As well the actual physical demands of the patient's job tasks should be surveyed, including what is required for the patient to commute to work. Commutes can vary markedly. One patient may describe his commute as walking from his house to a car parked in the driveway, driving to work, and parking close to the work building. Another has a commute consisting of walking several blocks to a bus stop, descending a flight of steps to a train, balancing while standing in a full commuter train, ascending a flight of stairs, and walking several more blocks to the work building.

If the patient has a regular fitness program, the same question outlined before can be used again to assist gathering a clear picture of the patient's functional status.

Then establish what the patient's functional status was before the recent complaint started. It should not be assumed that the patient was 100% before the injury.

Technically a thorough pain survey belongs in the tests and measures portion of the examination. Many patients referred to outpatient physical therapy with a musculoskeletal complaint report pain so a detailed survey of symptoms, including aspects of pain behavior, will generally be an indicated measure to be completed. Knowing that, it makes sense to complete this survey during the interview. As well, the pain survey at this point will identify whether modifications need to be made during examination testing to avoid aggravating tissues with reported high irritability.[133]

An evaluation form that has the topics to be covered during the interview ordered in a manner that makes the interaction flow smoothly is invaluable. Being familiar with the evaluation form, to know exactly the best place to record each piece of information, also makes the entire examination process easier. Whether a student in the clinic for the first time, or an experienced clinician confronted with a brand new form format, taking time to learn the form, so that where to record findings is automatic, is recommended.

Systems Review

The process of the interview, along with the systems review, helps determine whether the patient is a candidate for physical therapy. The information gathered will help identify which tests and measures will be required in the examination to best establish the patient's status. In an outpatient setting the systems review may not look to be an actual separate section of the examination. The systems review is, however, a distinct critical thinking step.

Several components of the systems review are already established by the time the patient interview is completed. Generally it has already been established by the patient's report that range of motion and strength are impaired. The creation of a mental checklist begins that will include range of motion and muscle performance measures of the affected limb in the next step of the examination. A screen of the gross range of motion and strength of the uninvolved limbs can be completed.

Gross screening of deficits in balance, gait, transfers, and transitions has also occurred with observation of the patient in the waiting room, walk to the treatment room, and in the treatment room. The patient may be judged to be cleared of neuromuscular deficits or tests and measures in these areas are added to the mental list.

Decisions on whether further testing is required to establish deficits in the patient's communication, affect, cognition, and language have also been made based on the interview. Again, "cleared" or "need for further testing" will be decided. The patient's preferred learning style can be a simple question to complete this component of the systems review at this point.

Questions whether the patient has any scars or open sores can be asked and screened if present. Additional notation of scars or altered integument not screened from the patient report can be noted throughout the examination.

The patient has been resting during the interview, so taking resting vital signs then completes the systems review. Vital signs measured with activity can be recorded during the next aspect of the examination.

Tests and Measures

Most outpatient physical therapy departments have an array of initial evaluation forms for each body part. In essence, the next step in the critical-thinking process—which tests and measures are indicated for this patient—can be usurped by these forms. Sometimes not all the tests listed on the form are appropriate for a particular patient examination. Or there is a list of special tests that do not make a distinction in whether range of motion, muscle performance or joint mobility are being examined. It is important to have a clear plan for which tests and measures are absolutely indicated. Therapists need to create and then follow an examination plan that has been based on the interview and systems review and individualized for the patient. Once these critical thinking decisions are made then using a predesigned form can make recording findings easier.

Tests and measures categories often used to examine patients with musculoskeletal complaints include: pain, posture, gait, range of motion, muscle performance, joint integrity and mobility, and peripheral nerve integrity. Depending on the extent of functional limitations, functional measures categories for work or ADL may be included.

The patient's experience during the process needs to be kept in mind. Good judgment should to be used on how much of the examination is attempted on the first visit. Ordering of the tests and measures can make the difference between gathering adequate information before the patient's symptoms become aggravated or he has to stop too soon.

Similarly, if a patient has a symptom-limited ability to lift an arm against gravity but the same limb can be taken through a full range of motion passively then it can be determined that strength is impaired. The testing to establish the extent of the strength deficit and assign a manual muscle testing grade can be postponed to the next visit.

Wise strategies make musculoskeletal examinations successful. When a patient reports symptoms during the interview that suggest neural mobility might be a possible contributing impairment, plan the examination accordingly. If the testing of neural mobility initially appears to be negative, build in a little time between neural mobility tests to allow a delay of symptoms to be noted.

When it is possible for the patient to tolerate more specific testing, completing the critical thinking process will make establishing the treatment plan more specific. Deciding impingement is present for a shoulder complaint is only part of the equation. Is there impingement because the glenohumeral capsule lacks ease of movement to allow unrestricted inferior gliding or is the supraspinatus too weak to adequately depress the humeral head? If it is a combination of both, do findings suggest one is a larger contributor to the altered glenohumeral biomechanics than the other? The answers to these questions determine whether the intervention will have a main emphasis on improving glenohumeral accessory movement or strengthening the supraspinatus.

Summary

A thorough examination guides the evaluation to establish the diagnosis and prognosis including the plan of care. Using these to develop the indicated intervention ensures the best opportunity for a good outcome. The following case will demonstrate how the elements of the patient/client management model are used along with an understanding of musculoskeletal tissue pathophysiology to provide a successful outcome for a patient referred to physical therapy with a musculoskeletal complaint.

REFERENCES

1. American Physical Therapy Association. Guide to Physical Therapist Practice. 2nd ed. *Phys Ther.* 2001;81:9-746.
2. Online class discussion. Diagnostic Screening for Physical Therapists. Institute of Health Professions. Summer 2003.
3. National Ambulatory Medical Care Survey 1998-2006. Data obtained from: U.S. Department of Health and Human Services; Centers for Disease Control and Prevention; National Center for Health Statistics. https://www.orthopedicsmagazine.com/foundation/tco_bones.html. Accessed July 23, 2010.
4. *United States Bone and Joint Decade: The Burden of Musculoskeletal Diseases in the United States.* Rosemont, IL: American Academy of Orthopaedic Surgeons; 2008.
5. Cormack DH. *Introduction to Histology.* Philadelphia, PA: J.B. Lippincott Co.; 1984.
6. Moran DT, Rowley JC. Epithelia. In: *Visual Histology.* Philadelphia, PA: Lea & Febenger; 1988. http://www.visualhistology.com/products/atlas/VHA_Chpt2_Epithelia.html. Accessed August 11, 2010.
7. Sanders JF, Goldstein BS, Leotta DF. Skin response to mechanical stress: adaptation rather than breakdown—a review of the literature. *J Rehabil Res Dev.* 1995;32(3):214-226.
8. Moran DT, Rowley JC. Connective tissue. In: *Visual Histology.* Philadelphia, PA: Lea & Febenger; 1988. http://www.visualhistology.com/products/atlas/VHA_Chpt3_Connective_Tissue.html. Accessed August 11, 2010.

9. Culav EM, Clark CH, Merriless MG. Connective tissues: matrix composition and its relevance to physical therapy. *Phys Ther.* 1999;79:308-319.

10. Nordin M, Frankel VH. Biomechanics of collagenous tissues. In: Frankel VH, Nordin M, eds. *Basic Biomechanics of the Skeletal System.* Philadelphia, PA: Lea & Febiger; 1980.

11. Gelberman R, Goldberg V, An K-N, Banes A. Tendon. In: Woo SL-Y, Buckwalter JA, eds. *Injury and Repair of the Musculoskeletal Soft Tissues.* Park Ridge, IL: American Academy of Orthopedic Surgeons; 1988.

12. Lee AC, Quillen WS, Magee DJ, Zachazewski JE. Injury, inflammation, and repair: tissue mechanics, the healing process, and their impact on the musculoskeletal system. In: Magee DJ, Zachazewski JE, Quillen WS, eds. *Scientific Foundations and Principles of Practice in Musculoskeletal Rehabilitation.* St. Louis, MO: Saunders Elsevier Inc; 2007.

13. Guyton AC. *Textbook of Medical Physiology.* Philadelphia, PA: W.B. Saunders Co.; 1981.

14. Brown CR, Boden SD. Fracture repair and bone grafting. In: Fischgrund JS, ed. *Orthopaedic Knowledge Update 9.* Rosemont, IL: American Academy of Orthopaedic Surgeons; 2008.

15. Jung H-J, Fisher MB, Woo SL-Y. Role of biomechanics in the understanding of normal, injured and healing ligaments and tendons. *Sports Med Arthrosc Rehabil Ther Technol.* 2009;1(1):9.

16. Smith HK, Maxwell L, Rodgers CD, McKee NH, Plyley MJ. Exercise-enhanced satellite cell proliferation and new myonuclear accretion in rat skeletal muscle. *J Appl Physiol (1985).* 2001;90(4):1407-1414.

17. Wren TA, Beaupré GS, Carter DR. A model of load-dependent growth, development, and adaptation of tendons and ligaments. *J Biomech.* 1998;31(2):107-114.

18. Noyes FR. Functional properties of knee ligaments and alterations induced by immobilization: a correlative biomechanical and histological study in primates. *Clin Orthop.* 1977;123:210-242.

19. Mueller MJ, Maluf KS. Tissue adaptation to physical stress: a proposed "Physical Stress Theory" to guide physical therapist practice, education, and research. *Phys Ther.* 2002;82(4):383-403.

20. Hoogendoorn JM, Simmermacher RK, Schellekens, van der Werken C. Adverse effects of smoking on healing of bones and soft tissues [article in German]. *Unfallchirurg.* 2002;105(1):76-81.

21. Porter SE, Hanley EN Jr. The musculoskeletal effects of smoking. *J Am Acad Orthop Surg.* 2001;9(1):9-17.

22. Williams PL, Warwick R, eds. *Gray's Anatomy.* 36th ed. Philadelphia, PA: W.B. Saunders Company; 1980.

23. Lieber RL, Bodine-Fowler SC. Skeletal muscle mechanics: implications for rehabilitation. *Phys Ther.* 1993;73(12):844-856.

24. Scott W, Stevens J, Binder-Macleod SA. Human skeletal muscle fiber type classifications. *Phys Ther.* 2001;81:1810-1816.

25. Widmaier EP, Hershel R, Strang KT. *Vander, Sherman, Luciano's Human Physiology: The Mechanism of Body Function.* 9th ed. New York: McGraw-Hill; 2004.

26. Kraemer WJ, Spiering BA, Vescovi JD. Adaptability of skeletal muscle: responses to increased and decreased use. In: Magee DJ, Zachazewski JE, Quillen WS, eds. *Scientific Foundations and Principles of Practice in Musculoskeletal Rehabilitation.* St. Louis, MO: Saunders Elsevier Inc; 2007.

27. Caplan A, Carlson B, Faulkner J, et al. Skeletal muscle. In: Woo SL-Y, Buckwalter JA, eds. *Injury and Repair of the Musculoskeletal Soft Tissues.* Park Ridge, IL: American Academy of Orthopaedic Surgeons; 1988.

28. Faulkner JA, Brooks SV, Opiteck JA. Injury to skeletal muscle fiber during contractions: conditions of occurrence and prevention. *Phys Ther.* 1993;73(12):911-921.

29. Williams PE, Goldspink G. Changes in sarcomere length and physiologic properties in immobilized muscle. *J Anat.* 1978;127(3):459-466.

30. De Deyne PG. Application of passive stretch and its implications for muscle fibers. *Phys Ther.* 2001;81(2):819-827.

31. Gossman MR, Sahrmann SA, Rose SJ. Review of length-associated changes in muscle. *Phys Ther.* 1982;62(12):1799-1808.

32. Booth FW, Seider MJ. Recovery of skeletal muscle after 3 mo of hindlimb immobilization in rats. *J Appl Physiol Respir Environ Exerc Physiol.* 1979;47(2):435-439.

33. Garrett WE Jr. Muscle strain injuries. *Am J Sports Med.* 1996;24(6 Suppl):S2-S8.

34. AkesonWH, Woo SLY, Amiel D, Matthews JV. Biomechanical and biochemical changes in the periarticular connective tissue during contracture development in immobilized rabbit knee. *Connect Tissue Res.* 1974;2(4):315-323.

35. Adams GR, Hather BM, Baldwin KM, Dudley GA. Skeletal muscle myosin heavy chain composition and resistance training. *J Appl Physiol (1985).* 1993;74(2):911-915.

36. Kraemer WJ, Fleck SJ, Evans WJ. Strength and power training: physiological mechanisms of adaptation. *Exerc Sport Sci Rev.* 1996;24:363-397.

37. Shaffer MA, Okerike E, Esterhai JL Jr, et al. Effects of immobilization on plantar-flexion torque, fatigue resistance, and functional ability following an ankle fracture. *Phys Ther.* 2000;80(8):769-780.

38. Huard J, Li Y, Fu FH. Muscle injuries and repair: current trends in research. J Bone Joint Surg Am. 2002;84-A(5):822-832.

39. Buckwalter JA. Effects of early motion on healing of musculoskeletal tissues. *Hand Clin.* 1996;12(1):13-24.

40. Williams PE. Use of intermittent stretch in the prevention of serial sarcomere loss in immobilized muscle. *Ann Rheum Dis.* 1990;49(5):316-317.

41. Smith HK, Maxwell L, Rodgers CD, et al. Exercise-enhanced satellite cell proliferation and new myonuclear accretion in rat skeletal muscle. *Am J of Sports Med.* 1995;23(1):65-73.

42. Hasselmann C, Bets TM, Seaber AV, Garrett WE Jr. A threshold and continuum of injury during active stretch of rabbit skeletal muscle. *Am J Sports Med.* 1995;23(1):65-73.

43. Cheung K, Hume PA, Maxwell L. Delayed onset muscle soreness. *Sports Med.* 2003;33(2):145-164.

44. Sahrmann SA. *Diagnosis and Treatment of Movement Impairment Syndromes.* St. Louis, MO: Mosby; 2002.

45. Powers CM. The influence of altered lower-extremity kinematics on patellofemoral joint dysfunction: a theoretical perspective. *J Ortho Sport Phys Ther.* 2003;33(11):639-646.

46. Ludewig PM, Cook TM. Alterations in shoulder kinematics and associated muscle activity in people with symptoms of shoulder impingement. *Phys Ther.* 2000;80(3):276-291.

47. Kendall HO, Kendall FP. Reprint from *Physiotherap Rev.* 1947;3:27. In: Kendall FP, McCreary EK, Provance PG, et al. *Muscles: Testing and Function with Posture and Pain.* 5th ed. Philadelphia, PA: Lippincott Williams & Wilkins; 2005.

48. Curwin SL. Tendon pathology and injuries: Pathophysiology, healing, and treatment considerations. In: Magee DJ, Zachazewski JE, Quillen WS, eds. *Scientific Foundations and Principles of Practice in Musculoskeletal Rehabilitation.* St. Louis, MO: Saunders Elsevier Inc; 2007.

49. Sharma P, Maffulli N. Tendon injury and tendinopathy: healing and repair. *J Bone Joint Surg Am.* 2005;87:187-202.

50. Woo SLY, Maynard J, Butler D, et al. Ligament, tendon and joint capsule insertions to bone. In: Woo SLY, Buckwalter JA, eds. *Injury and Repair of the Musculoskeletal Soft Tissues.* Park Ridge, IL: American Academy of Orthopaedic Surgeons; 1988.

51. Moore H, Nichols C, Engles M. Tissue response. In: Donatelli RA, Wooden MJ, eds. *Orthopaedic Physical Therapy.* 4th ed. St. Louis, MO: Churchill Livingstone Elsevier Inc; 2010.

52. Kellett J. Acute soft tissue injuries—a review of the literature. *Med Sci Sport Exerc.* 1995;18(5):489-500.

53. Wang MX, Wei A, Yuan J, et al. Antioxidant enzyme peroxiredoxin 5 is upregulated in degenerative human tendon. *Biochem Biophys Res Commun.* 2001;284(3):667-673.

54. Yuan J, Murrell Ga, Trickett A, Wang MX. Involvement of cytochrome c release and caspace-3 activation in the oxidative stress-induced apoptosis in human tendon fibroblasts. *Biochim Biophys Acta*. 2003;1641(1):35-41.

55. Wang JH, Jia F, Yang G, et al. Cyclic mechanical stretching of human tendon fibroblasts increases the production of prostaglandin E2 and levels of cyclooxygenase expression: a novel in vitro model study. *Connect Tissue Res*. 2003;44(3-4):128-133.

56. Curwin S, Stanish WD. *Tendinitis: Its Etiology and Treatment*. Lexington, MA: Collamore Press; 1984.

57. Stanish WD, Curwin S, Mandell S. *Tendinitis: Its Etiology and Treatment*. 2nd. Oxford, England: Oxford University Press; 2000.

58. Stanish WD, Rubinovich RM, Curwin S. Eccentric exercise in chronic tendonitis. *Clin Orthop Rel Res*. 1986;208:65-68.

59. Alfredson H, Peitila T, Jonsson P, Lorentzon R. Heavy-load eccentric calf muscle training for the treatment of chronic Achilles tendinosis. *Am J Sports Med*. 1998;26:360-366.

60. Tallon C, Maffulli N, Ewen SW. Ruptured Achilles tendons are significantly more degenerated than tendinopathic tendons. *Med Sci Sports Exerc*. 2001;33:1983-1990.

61. Arner O, Lindholm A, Orell SR. Histologic changes in subcutaneous rupture of the Achilles tendon: a study of 74 cases. *Acta Chir Scand*. 1959;116:484-490.

62. Kannus P, Józsa L. Histopathological changes preceding spontaneous rupture of a tendon: a controlled study of 891 patients. *J Bone Joint Surg Am*. 1991;73(10):1507-1525.

63. Gelberman RH, Woo SL, Lothringer K, Akeson WH, Amiel D. Effects of early intermittent passive mobilization on healing canine flexor tendons. *J Hand Surg Am*. 1982;7(2):170-175.

64. Pneumaticos SG, McGarvey WC, Mody DR, Trevino SG. The effects of early mobilization in the healing of Achilles tendon repair. *Foot Ankle Int*. 2000;21(7):551-557.

65. Woo SL, Gelberman RH, Cobb NG, Amiel D, Lothringer K, Akeson WH. The importance of controlled passive mobilization on flexor tendon healing. *Acta Orthop Scand*. 1981;52(6):615-622.

66. Kangas J, Pajala A, Ohtonen P, Leppilahti J. Achilles tendon elongation after rupture repair: a randomized comparison of 2 postoperative regimens. *Am J Sports Med*. 2007;35(1):59-64.

67. Turner CH. Three rules for bone adaptation to mechanical stimuli. *Bone*. 1998;23(5):399-407.

68. Downey PA, Siegel MI. Bone biology and the clinical implications for osteoporosis. *Phys Ther*. 2006;86(1):77-91.

69. Loitz-Ramage BJ, Zernicki RF. Bone biology and mechanics. In: Magee DJ, Zachazewski JE, Quillen WS, eds. *Scientific Foundations and Principles of Practice in Musculoskeletal Rehabilitation*. St. Louis, MO: Saunders Elsevier Inc; 2007.

70. Riggs CM, Vaughan LC, Evans GP, Lanyon LE, Boyde A. Mechanical implications of collagen fibre orientation in cortical bone of the equine radius. *Anat Embryol (Berl)*. 1993;187(3):239-248.

71. Riggs CM, Lanyon LE, Boyde A. Functional associations between collagen fibre orientation and locomotor strain direction in cortical bone of the equine radius. *Anat Embryol (Berl)*. 1993;187(3):231-238.

72. Frankel VH, Nordin M. Biomechanics of bone. In: Nordin M, Frankel VH, eds. *Basic Biomechanics of the Musculoskeletal System*. 3rd ed. Philadelphia, PA: Lippincott Williams & Wilkins; 2001.

73. Bennett DL, Nassar L, Delano MC. Lumbar spine MRI in the elite-level female gymnast with low back pain. *Skeletal Radiol*. 2006;35(7):503-509.

74. Ciullo JV, Jackson DW. Pars interarticularis stress reaction, spondylolysis and spondylolisthesis in gymnasts. *Clin Sports Med*. 1985;4(1):95-110.

75. Ilizarov GA. Clinical applications of the tension-stress effect for limb lengthening. *Clin Orthop Relat Res*. 1990;250:8-26.

76. Cattaneo R, Villa A, Catagni MA, Bell D. Lengthening of the humerus using the Ilizarov technique. Description of the method and report of 43 cases. *Clin Orthop Relat Res*. 1990;250:117-124.

77. Renzi-Brivio L, Lavini F, De Bastiani G. Lengthening in the congenital short femur. *Clin Orthop Relat Res*. 1990;250:112-116.

78. Coglianese DB, Herzenberg JE, Goulet JA. Physical therapy management of patients undergoing limb lengthening by distraction osteogenesis. *J Ortho Sports Phys Ther*. 1993;17(3):124-132.

79. Salter RB, Harris WR. Injuries involving the epiphyseal plate. *J Bone Joint Surg Am*. 1963;45(3):587-622.

80. Marsh JL, Slongo RF, Agel J, et al. Fracture and dislocation classification compendium-2007: Orthopaedic Trauma Association classification, database and outcomes committee. *J Orthop Trauma*. 2007;21(10 Suppl):S1-S133.

81. Wheeless CR III. Seinsheimers classification of subtrochanteric fractures. Wheeless' *Textbook of Orthopaedics*. www.wheelessonline.com. Updated August 20, 2011. Accessed January 30, 2012.

82. Chao EY, Aro HT, Lewallen DG, Kelly PJ. The effect of rigidity on fracture healing in external fixation. *Clin Orthop Relat Res*. 1989;241:24-35.

83. Brown CR, Boden SD. Fracture repair and bone grafting. In: Fischgrund JS, ed. *Orthopaedic Knowledge Update 9*. Rosemont, IL: American Academy of Orthopaedic Surgeons; 2008.

84. Punjabi MM, White AA, Wolf JW. A biomechanical comparison of the effects of constant and cyclic compression of fracture healing in rabbit long bones. *Acta Orthop Scand*. 1979;50:653-661.

85. Wolf JW, White AA 3rd, Punjabi MM, Southwick WO. A comparison of cyclic loading versus compression in the treatment of long bone fractures in rabbits. *J Bone Joint Surg Am*. 1981;63(5):805-810.

86. Jones BH, Thacker SB, Gilchrist J, Kimsey CD Jr, Sosin DM. Prevention of lower extremity stress fractures in athletes and soldiers: a systemic review. *Epidemiol Rev*. 2002;24(2):228-247.

87. Heim HA, Hensinger RN. Spinal deformities: scoliosis and kyphosis. *Clin Symp*. 1989;41(4):3-32.

88. Saha D, Gard S, Fatone S, Ondra S. The effect of trunk-flexed postures on balance and metabolic energy expenditure during standing. *Spine (Phila Pa 1976)*. 2007;32(15):1605-1611.

89. Kyphosis. Wikipedia. Updated January 9, 2012. Accessed January 9, 2012.

90. Burwell RG. Aetiology of idiopathic scoliosis: current concepts. *Pediatr Rehabil*. 2003;6(3-4):137-170.

91. Kendall FP, McCreary EK, Provance PG, Rodgers MM, Romani WA. *Muscles: Testing and Function with Posture and Pain*. 5th ed. Philadelphia, PA: Lippincott Williams & Wilkins; 2005.

92. Wagner TA. Scoliosis—A patient primer. http://www.orthop.washington.edu/PatientCare/OurServices/Spine/Articles/ScoliosisAPatientPrimer.aspx.Updated December 31,2009. Accessed February 5, 2012.

93. Reamy BV, Slakey JB. Adolescent idiopathic scoliosis: review and current concepts. *Am Fam Physician*. 2001;64(1):111-117.

94. Lundon K, Walker JM. Cartilage of human joints and related structures. In: Magee DJ, Zachazewski JE, Quillen WS, eds. *Scientific Foundations and Principles of Practice in Musculoskeletal Rehabilitation*. St. Louis, MO: Saunders Elsevier Inc., 2007.

95. Frank C, Woo S, Andriacchi T. Normal ligament: structure, function, and composition. In: Woo SL-Y, Buckwalter JA, eds. *Injury and Repair of the Musculoskeletal Soft Tissues*. Park Ridge, IL: American Academy of Orthopaedic Surgeons; 1988.

96. Williams GN, Krishnan C. Articular neurophysiology and sensorimotor control. In: Magee DJ, Zachazewski JE, Quillen WS, editors. *Scientific Foundations and Principles of Practice in Musculoskeletal Rehabilitation*. St. Louis: Saunders, an imprint of Elsevier Inc; 2007.

97. Walker JM. Pathophysiology of inflammation, repair and immobility. In: Walker JM, Helewa A. *Physical Rehabilitation in Arthritis*. 2nd ed. St. Louis, MO: Saunders Elsevier; 2004.

98. Buckwalter JA, Mankin HJ. Articular cartilage: Part I. Tissue design and chondrocyte-matrix interactions. *J Bone Joint Surg Am*. 1997;74(4):600-611.

99. Buckwalter J, Hunziker E, Rosenberg L. Articular cartilage: composition and structures. In: Woo SL-Y, Buckwalter JA, eds. *Injury and Repair of the Musculoskeletal Soft Tissues*. Park Ridge, IL: American Academy of Orthopedic Surgeons; 1988.

100. Noyes FR, DeLucas JL, Torvik PJ. Biomechanics of anterior cruciate ligament failure. An analysis of strain-rate sensitivity and mechanisms of failure in primates. *J Bone Joint Surg Am*. 1974;56(2):236-253.

101. Woo SL, Gomez MA, Sites TJ, Newton PO, Orlando CA, Akeson WH. The biomechanical and morphological changes in the medial collateral ligament of the rabbit after immobilization and remobilization. *J Bone Joint Surg Am*. 1987;69(8):1200-1211.

102. O'Donoghue DH, Rockwood CA Jr, Frank GR, Jack SC, Kenyon R. Repair of the anterior cruciate ligament in dogs. *J Bone Joint Surg Am*. 1966;48(3):503-519.

103. Mow V, Rosenwasser M. Articular cartilage biomechanics. In: Woo SL-Y, Buckwalter JA, eds. *Injury and Repair of the Musculoskeletal Soft Tissues*. Park Ridge, IL: American Academy of Orthopaedic Surgeons, 1988.

104. Johnson MW. Acute knee effusions: a systemic approach to diagnosis. *Am Fam Physician*. 2000;61(8):2391-2400.

105. Bucala R, Ritchlin C, Winchester R, Cerami A. Constitutive production of inflammatory and mitogenic cytokines by rheumatoid synovial fibroblasts. *J Exp Med*. 1991;173(3):569-574.

106. Iwanaga T, Skikichi M, Kitamura H, Yanase H, Nozawa-Inoue K. Morphology and functional roles of synoviocytes in the joint. *Arch Histol Cytol*. 2000;63(1):17-31.

107. Jensen K, Graf BK. The effects of knee effusion on quadriceps strength and knee intraarticular pressure. *Arthroscopy*. 1993;9(1):52-56.

108. Spencer JD, Hayes KC, Alexander IJ. Knee joint effusion and quadriceps reflex inhibition in man. *Arch Phys Med Rehabil*. 1984;65(4):171-177.

109. Shamsi B, Falk J-N, Pettineo SJ, Ali S. Clinical review of adhesive capsulitis of the ankle: An introductory article and clinical review. *The Foot and Ankle Online Journal*. 2011;4:10. DOI: 10.3827/faoj.2011.0410.0002.

110. Chepeha JC. Shoulder trauma and hypomobility. In: Magee DJ, Zachazewskit JE, Quillen WS, eds. *Pathology and Intervention in Musculoskeletal Rehabilitation*. St. Louis, MO: Saunders Elsevier; 2009.

111. Vermeulen HM, Obermann WR, Burger BJ, Kok GJ, Rozing PM, van Den Ende CH. End-range mobilization techniques in adhesive capsulitis of the shoulder joint: a multiple-subject case report. *Phys Ther*. 2000;80(12):1204-1213.

112. Yang JL, Chang CW, Chen SY, Wang SF, Lin JJ. Mobilization techniques in subjects with frozen shoulder syndrome: randomized multiple-treatment trial. *Phys Ther*. 2007;87(10):1307-1315.

113. Carette S, Moffet H, Tardif J, et al. Intraarticular corticosteroids, supervised physiotherapy, or a combination of the two in the treatment of adhesive capsulitis of the shoulder. *Arthritis Rheuma*. 2003;48(3):829-838.

114. Vermeulen HM, Rozing PM, Obermann WR, le Cessie S, Vliet Vlieland TP. Comparison of high-grade and low-grade mobilization techniques in the management of adhesive capsulitis of the shoulder: randomized controlled trial. *Phys Ther*. 2006;86(3):355-368.

115. Andriacchi T, Sabiston P, DeHaven K, et al. Ligament: Injury and repair. In: Woo SL-Y, Buckwalter JA, eds. *Injury and Repair of the Musculoskeletal Soft Tissues*. Park Ridge, IL: American Academy of Orthopaedic Surgeons; 1988.

116. Hildebrand KA, Hart DA, Rattner JB, et al. Ligament injuries: Pathology, healing, and treatment considerations. In: Magee DJ, Zachazewski JE, Quillen WS, eds. *Scientific Foundations and Principles of Practice in Musculoskeletal Rehabilitation*. St. Louis, MO: Saunders Elsevier Inc; 2007.

117. Radin EL. The physiology and degeneration of joints. *Semin Arthritis Rheum*. 1972-1973;2(3):245-257.

118. Topp KS, Boyd FS. Structures and biomechanics of peripheral nerves: nerve responses to physical stresses and implications for physical therapist practice. *Phys Ther*. 2006;86(1):92-109.

119. Sunderland S. The anatomy and physiology of nerve injury. *Muscle Nerve*. 1990;13(9):771-784.

120. Lundborg G, Rydevik B, Manthorpe. Peripheral nerve: The physiology of injury and repair. In: Woo SL-Y, Buckwalter JA, eds. *Injury and Repair of the Musculoskeletal Soft Tissues*. Park Ridge, IL: American Academy of Orthopaedic Surgeons; 1988.

121. Butler DS, Tomberlin JP. Peripheral nerve: Structure, function, and physiology. In: Magee DJ, Zachazewski JE, Quillen WS, eds. *Scientific Foundations and Principles of Practice in Musculoskeletal Rehabilitation*. St. Louis, MO: Saunders Elsevier Inc; 2007. Millesi H, Zöch G, Reihsner R. Mechanical properties of peripheral nerves. *Clin Orthop Relat Res*. 1995;314:76-83.

122. Millesi H, Zock G, Reihsner R. Mechanical properties of peripheral nerves. *Clin Orthop Relat Res*. 1995;314:76-83.

123. Louw A. *Course Notes—Mobilization of the Nervous System*. Baltimore, MD: The Neuro Orthopaedic Institute; 2010.

124. Butler DS. *The Sensitive Nervous System*. Adelaide, Australia: Noigroup; 2000.

125. Moseley GL. Joining forces—combining cognition-targeted motor control training with group or individual pain physiology education: a successful treatment for chronic low back pain. *J Man Manip Ther*. 2003;11(2):88-94.

126. Butler D. Presentation notes—It's in your brain—get used to it: The delicate art of conceptual change. Annual Conference and Exposition of the American Physical Therapy Association. National Harbor, MD. June 19, 2011.

127. Moseley L. Unraveling the barriers to reconceptualization of the problem in chronic pain: The actual and perceived ability of patients and health professional to understand the neurophysiology. *J Pain*. 2003;4(4):184-189.

128. Moseley GL. A pain neuromatrix approach to patients with chronic pain. *Man Ther*. 2003;8(3):130-140.

129. Moseley GL. Widespread brain activity during an abdominal task markedly reduced after pain physiology education; fMRI evaluation of a single patient with chronic low back pain. *Aust J Physiother*. 2005;51(1):49-52.

130. Moseley GL. Evidence for a direct relationship between cognitive and physical change during an education intervention in people with chronic low back pain. *Eur J Pain*. 2004;8(1):39-45.

131. Butler D, Moseley L. *Explain Pain*. Adelaide, Australia: Noigroup Publications; 2003.

132. Goldstein MS, Elliott SD, Guccione AA. The development of an instrument to measure satisfaction with physical therapy. *Phys Ther*. 2000;80(9):853-863.

133. Maitland GD. *Peripheral Manipulation*. 3rd ed. London, UK: Butterworth-Heinemann; 1991.

CASE STUDY 10-1

Debra Coglianese, PT, DPT, OCS, ATC

EXAMINATION

History

Current Condition/Chief Complaint

Mr. Halo was a 51-year-old White male who was referred to physical therapy by his primary care physician with a chief complaint of bilateral shoulder pain, left greater than right. He also noted left elbow and wrist symptoms. Mr. Halo associated the onset of symptoms with the increased lifting required to move his daughter home from college. He has had similar symptoms, however, with regular ringing of large hand bells as a member of a hand bell choir.

Social History/Environment

Mr. Halo was employed as a software consultant. He worked from an office in his home. The majority of his work tasks occurred at a computer station. He was active with the hand bell choir at his church. He lived with his wife and 2 daughters.

He reported that he lived in a 2-story home with a basement. Both flights of stairs had sturdy rails. He reported stairs posed no barrier for him.

Social/Health Habits and Family History

Mr. Halo rated his health as good despite his reported complaint. He had no smoking history and consumed only an occasional glass of wine.

He completed a 1-hour workout at his gym 2 times per week. His workout included use of aerobic equipment as well as an upper and lower extremity resistance training program. In good weather he liked to ride his bike for fitness.

His father was 83 years old and had coronary artery disease (CAD) and Type II diabetes. His mother was diagnosed with Crohn's disease at 79 but was stable.

Clinician Comment *Already the interview has gathered a good amount of information to help understand Mr. Halo's situation. He had an acute complaint that might be superimposed on a more chronic musculoskeletal complaint. It was possible that he had an acute tendonitis but it was also possible that there was an underlying tendinopathy. He had a largely sedentary job that he offset with a regular exercise program.*

What risks did he have for his health because of his family medical history? He had a higher risk of CAD due to the presence of a family history of CAD.[1] Though his father has Type II diabetes, Mr. Halo may not be at more risk.

Family history of diabetes is less of a predictor for progression from impaired glucose tolerance to Type II.[2] There was no evidence of glucose tolerance testing in Mr. Halo's online medical record.

Crohn's disease is an inflammatory bowel disease characterized by diseased sections of bowel through all layers of the bowel wall in the involved sections. Healthy sections of bowel will exist between the diseased ones. A family history of Crohn's occurs in 20% to 25% of the cases.[3]

Medical/Surgical History

Mr. Halo reported he was diagnosed with Crohn's disease when he was 36 years old. He reported that his status with regard to his Crohn's disease was stable and controlled with medications. He was diagnosed with associated osteopenia 2 years prior to his initial physical therapy evaluation.

Mr. Halo reported episodes of left wrist pain associated with bell ringing for several years "off and on."

He noted that he had seasonal allergies.

Clinician Comment *The strongest risk factor for Crohn's disease development is having a relative with the disease.[4] Mr. Halo's mother was diagnosed at age 79 years, whereas his diagnosis occurred when he was 36 years old. This is consistent with the findings that the age of diagnosis of the child is younger than the age of diagnosis of the parent.[4]*

His more recent diagnosis of osteopenia was not surprising. Reduced bone mineral density is prevalent in patients with Crohn's disease.[5] Risk factors identified are the altered intestinal absorption characteristic of Crohn's disease that, in turn, affects all aspects of adequate nutrition. The usual prolonged use of corticosteroids to medically manage Crohn's may have been a factor also in his decreased bone density.

Reported Functional Status

He reported unrestricted ADL, IADL, and work tasks. Mr. Halo followed a regular exercise program, noted earlier.

Medications

Mr. Halo reported the following medications:

- Sulfasalazine, 1 gram, 2 times per day, along with folic acid
- Calcium supplement
- Allegra (fexofenadine HCL), 60 mg, 1 to 2 times per day
- Flonase (fluticasone propionate), 2 times per day
- Multivitamins

Clinician Comment *Sulfasalazine is a pro-drug and breaks down in the colon to 2 active metabolites, sulfapyridine and 5-aminosalicylic acid. Mr. Halo was receiving a standard dose.[6]*

Disease-modifying anti-rheumatic drugs, such as sulfasalazine, can be folic acid antagonists and supplemental folic acid, 1 mg once daily, may be prescribed.

Mr. Halo took a calcium supplement to improve calcium absorption related to his osteopenia.

Allegra is an antihistamine prescribed to treat seasonal allergies. Mr. Halo was taking a standard dose.[6]

Flonase is a corticosteroid used in a nasal spray to relieve the discomfort of hay fever and other nasal allergies. Mr. Halo was using a standard dose.[6]

Other Clinical Tests

A review of Mr. Halo's online medical record listed the following information within the year prior to his initial physical therapy evaluation.

LAB VALUES	
WBC	6.2
Red blood cell	4.49 m/uL
Hemoglobin	12.7
Hematocrit	40.1%
Mean corpuscular volume, mean corpuscular hemoglobin, mean corpuscular hemoglobin concentration, red blood cell distribution width	WNL
Cholesterol	179 mg/dL
High-density lipoprotein	40
Low-density lipoprotein	90
Prostate-specific antigen	0.8 ng/mL
Colonic mucosal biopsies (10)	all WNL

Clinician Comment *Mr. Halo's WBC was within the normal range for adults, 4.5 to 11.0.[3] With the normal range of red blood cells for adult males as 4.5 to 5.3 106/mm[3], Mr. Halo was slightly below the normal range.[3] Similarly, his hemoglobin was measured as slightly low since, for adult males, < 4 mL is considered significant.[3] Anemia is defined as a hematocrit of < 41% in males, though a range of 37% to 49% is suggested as within normal limits (WNL). Mr. Halo was slightly anemic.[3]*

The size (mean corpuscular volume) and the distribution (red blood cell distribution width) of his red blood cells were WNL as were the amount (mean corpuscular hemoglobin)

and concentration (mean corpuscular hemoglobin concentration) of hemoglobin in his red blood cells.

Mr. Halo met the desirable range of < 200 mg/dL for cholesterol, greater than or equal to 40 mg/dL for high-density lipoprotein, and optimal < 100 mg/dL for low-density lipoprotein.[7]

Prostate antigen assay is considered normal at 4 ng/mL and less but a range of 4 to 10 ng/ml can also be normal. The prostate-specific antigen should not rise more than 0.75 ng/mL per year.[3]

Mr. Halo had 10 colonic mucosal biopsies taken during his colonoscopy and all 10 were assessed as WNL.

Thus far there were no red flags that would indicate Mr. Halo might not be a candidate for physical therapy. The review of systems was completed next.

Systems Review

Cardiovascular/Pulmonary

Seated, resting:
HR: 60 beats per minute
Respiration rate: 12 breaths per minute
Blood pressure: 138/78 mm Hg
Edema: None noted.

Clinician Comment *The normal range for heart rate in adults is 60 to 100 bpm. Conditioned adults may have heart rates 50 to 60 bpm.[3] Mr. Halo's heart rate was in the low portion of the normal range and may have reflected his conditioning from regular aerobic exercise.*

The normal breathing rate for adults is 10 to 20 breaths per minute. A ratio of 4:1 is suggested for pulse rate to respiration rate.[3] Using this ratio, a predicted respiration rate for Mr. Halo would be 15 breaths per minute. Again, he was at the lower portion of normal range and, again, might be due to his fitness.

His systolic blood pressure measure was in the prehypertension range, 120 to 139, while his diastolic measure was in the normal range.[8] With these blood pressure values, Mr. Halo had only a 5% risk of developing CHD.[7]

Mr. Halo had no signs of peripheral edema.

Integumentary

Mr. Halo showed no sign of skin disruption, areas of altered skin color or presence of scar formation.

Musculoskeletal

Gross Symmetry/Posture

- Mr. Halo sat and stood with mildly slumped posture and asymmetrical positioning of shoulder girdle.

- Mild anterior translation in lower cervical segments occurred when he was seated but not in standing.

Gross Range of Motion

- Bilateral shoulders showed WNL active range of motion except for a slight decrease in combined movements on the left.
- Bilateral elbow and wrist showed WNL active range of motion.

Gross Strength

- Five of 5 strength in manual muscle testing screen of bilateral upper extremities without reproduction of symptoms during testing.
- Patient noted "awareness" of left shoulder symptoms 2 minutes after gross strength screen completed.
- Height: 6 feet; Weight: 174 pounds

Neuromuscular

Mr. Halo showed no deficits in balance, gait, transfers or transitions.

Communication, Affect, Cognition, Language, and Learning Style

- Mr. Halo was alert and oriented to person/place/time.
- He wished to continue with his activities including hand bell ringing.
- He reported no learning barriers. He preferred to have exercises written out after demonstration and practice.

Clinician Comment *Mr. Halo's cardiovascular/pulmonary status, at rest, was unimpaired. He showed no sign of integumentary or neuromuscular deficits. His body mass index was 23.6, which placed him in the normal weight range.[9] There seemed to be no impairments in his ability to communicate, or comprehend instructions, in physical therapy treatments.*

One effective upper extremity screening tool uses the active ranges of shoulder flexion, then abduction followed by a combined movement of shoulder adduction, medial rotation, and extension.[10] The combined shoulder movement, performed with a bent elbow, has the patient reach up and behind on his posterior thorax along the spine, as high as is comfortable. Combining each of the movements of shoulder adduction, extension and medial rotation as described individually[11] allows, when combined, the hand of the upper extremity being tested to reach to the mid- to lower thoracic spine.

Mr. Halo's left shoulder showed modestly decreased range compared to the right with the screening tool described previously. And, though he was able to complete the manual muscle testing[12] without complaint at the time of applied resistance, his symptoms in the left shoulder were mildly reproduced after testing.

The next step in the examination was to select the indicated tests and measures. A survey of Mr. Halo's pain was needed

to determine what positions or activities were associated with his symptoms. Findings in the system review suggested that his posture needed to be evaluated further. He may have had altered biomechanics in his shoulder and shoulder girdle due to faulty movement patterns adopted with sustained arms-forward tasks such as keyboarding.

His active range of motion for the left shoulder from the systems review needed to be compared to the available passive range of motion. It was possible that a contribution to symptoms might be cervical movement restrictions or altered upper extremity neural mobility. Additional muscle performance measures needed to consider scapular position with manual muscle testing. Finally, joint integrity and mobility for the left glenohumeral joint needed to be determined.

Mr. Halo had resting cardiovascular and pulmonary measures that were mostly normal. He reported that he followed a regular aerobic exercise program without complaint. He probably did not have an aerobic capacity deficit but his response to exercise needed to be measured. There was not time at the initial evaluation to complete this test.

At the first follow-up visit, his resting vital signs were taken and matched those noted previously. He rode the stationary bicycle at a moderate pace for 5 minutes as a warm-up prior to treatment. His reported a rate of perceived exertion that was ~13/20. His postexercise vital signs showed a heart rate of 84 bpm and blood measure of 140/80 mm Hg. His response to increased aerobic demand was documented as normal with no further aerobic capacity testing indicated.

Tests and Measures

Pain

Mr. Halo reported:

- P_1: "ache but not a sharp pain" at anterolateral left humerus, with occasional symptoms on the right. He noted this symptom always occurred on the left the morning after ringing bells or any lifting tasks. Symptom intensity was a 2 to 3/10.
- P_2: "tenderness" was reported at left lateral epicondyle and associated with bell ringing.
- P_3: "nagging ache" at the left posterior shoulder girdle that he reported had occurred "off and on for years." These symptoms would also occur with long hours of keyboarding.

Clinician Comment *This is an example of a thorough pain survey. The location, type, and behavior of each pain complaint is listed. Each individual pain complaint is recorded and "named." Having a designation for each pain is useful during the physical examination.[10] When a symptom is reproduced, the P_1, P_2, or P_3*

designation can be recorded rather than writing out "reproduced the-ache-but-not-sharp-pain at...."

The patient rates the pain intensity on an 11-point scale where "0/10" represents no pain and "10/10" is the worst pain one can imagine, pain so bad no movement is possible. An 11-point, 0 to 10 pain scale is as valid and reliable as the much-studied Visual Analog Scale.[13]

An association has been showed between upper extremity musculoskeletal complaints and keyboarding, especially in situations when spending increased time keyboarding against a deadline.[14] No study could be located that defined the musculoskeletal complaints associated with hand bell ringing. Similar complaints to those reported by Mr. Halo, however, have been reported by music teachers whose upper extremities also maintain sustained arms-forward positions as well as arms-forward movement positions.[15]

Posture (Standing)

- Right shoulder girdle dropped greater than expected for right handedness.

- Left scapula mildly abducted and elevated compared to right.

- Mild thoracic spine scoliotic curve, left, with trace lumbar compensatory curve, right with forward bend.

- When asked to demonstrate posture for bell ringing tasks using a 5-pound weight as the bell, his left scapula downwardly rotated.

- When asked to demonstrate posture with keyboard tasks, his shoulder girdle moved into a greater protracted position.

Clinician Comment *In right-handed persons the right shoulder girdle tends to be slightly dropped compared to the left. Mr. Halo showed this asymmetry but with a greater magnitude than expected for only a handedness pattern.[12] The finding noted previously with corresponding asymmetry of scapular positions suggested to the evaluating physical therapist to rule out, or in, the presence of an underlying spinal curvature. The Adam's forward bend test confirmed the presence of spinal curvature.[16]*

Altered scapular positions are important to note with the report of shoulder pain.[12] Subjects with kyphosis and rounded shoulders have reported increased incidence of interscapular pain.[17] Forward head posture is associated with increased incidence of cervical, interscapular, and headache pain.[17]

Mr. Halo's altered scapular position could be considered abnormal when compared to a research sample.[18] The inability to maintain the scapula in upward rotation with upper extremity forward and overhead has been shown to be greater in subjects with 3 or more of 6 identified impingement signs.[19]

Range of Motion (Including Muscle Length)

- Passive range of motion for bilateral shoulders, elbows, and wrists were all WNL except medial rotation for left shoulder.

- Muscle length tests showed that the left supraspinatus length was 50% of right on medial rotation length test. Mild symptoms were reproduced on the left during the muscle length test.

- Bilateral wrist extensors showed WNL length and without symptoms.

- Active range of motion, cervical spine was pain free, symmetrical, and patient's optimum (mild limit at extension, moderate limits for bilateral side bending).

Muscle Performance (Including Strength, Power, and Endurance)

Despite the ability to hold against resistance at a 5/5 manual muscle testing level, Mr. Halo had difficulty maintaining his left scapular position during movement testing of left shoulder medial rotation.

Clinician Comment *The results of the passive range of motion testing and closer observation of left scapular control gave more information. Decreased shoulder medial rotation due to decreased length of supraspinatus and presence of reactivity has been described by Sahrmann.[20] Further, altered scapular control has been identified as a sign of a faulty timing or movement pattern between scapulohumeral muscles and scapuloaxial muscles.[20]*

Joint Integrity and Mobility

Accessory movement testing in bilateral glenohumeral joints showed 3/6 mobility. Trace resistance was noted in the left glenohumeral joint for lateral glides and posterolateral glides. The left humeral head had a slight decrease in anterior-posterior vs posterior-anterior glide with shoulder assessed in neutral.

Clinician Comment *Joint mobility can be graded on a 0 to 6 scale where 3/6 is normal mobility. Grade of 0, 1, and 2 are grades of hypomobility with "0/6" indicating no movement as in an ankylosed joint. Grades 4, 5, and 6 are grades of hypermobility with 6/6 representing the mobility of a grossing unstable joint.[21]*

Cranial and Peripheral Nerve Integrity

Upper extremity neural provocation and mobility testing were negative.

Clinician Comment *The neural mobility testing used with Mr. Halo were patterns for the median, radial, and ulnar nerves.[22] They did not reproduce his symptoms and so it was fair to conclude that he did not have a neural immobility component to his complaint.*

That said, however, the quality of the testing used then compared with the more specific technique the evaluating therapist has learned since is great. Based on the groans heard around the room during the lab sessions in a continuing education course, Mobilization of the Nervous System, one wonders if anyone can be taken to the ends of the refined patterns without any neural elongation and ischemic symptoms.[23,24] In a study of asymptomatic men, evoked sensory responses were monitored and increased with each component addition during neural mobility testing for the median nerve.[25] The point to remember is not whether any symptoms are produced with neural mobility testing but whether the reported symptoms are reproduced.

EVALUATION

Diagnosis

Practice Pattern

Mr. Halo showed signs and reported symptoms consistent with supraspinatus reactivity in his left shoulder. He also had altered spinal and shoulder girdle mechanics for sustained arms forward tasks, such as keyboarding, and forward-movement tasks, such as bell ringing with heavy bells. The altered mechanics probably led to mild impingement of his left supraspinatus.

These findings placed him in the musculoskeletal practice pattern 4D—Impaired joint mobility, motor function, muscle performance, range of motion associated with connective tissue dysfunction.

International Classification of Functioning, Disability, and Health Model of Disability

See ICF model on p 437.

Prognosis

Mr. Halo had an excellent physical therapy prognosis. He could expect improved awareness and control of his shoulder girdle posture. His improved posture along with decreased reactivity in his left supraspinatus should allow him to continue with his current activities with symptoms controlled.

Plan of Care

Intervention

Mr. Halo would benefit from instruction in management strategies to reduce the reactivity in his left supraspinatus. These would include identification and practice with symptom-relieving positions and postures as well as regular use of ice packs. He needed education regarding how to position himself in his work space to reduce the postural strain from keyboarding. He needed practice with posture corrections required to provide a stable scapula for upper extremity movement tasks.

He would benefit from therapeutic exercise to lengthen shortened postural musculature and strengthen supporting musculature. Gradual length stretching of his left supraspinatus would assist with tissue healing along with pulsed ultrasound for 1 to 2 sessions. Once the tendon was able to begin tolerating mild overpressure, he could then progress to strengthening of the supraspinatus with attention to scapular stabilization. Ultimately, he would need to practice simulated bell ringing with his scapular position controlled.

Clinician Comment *It was still not clear whether he had a tendonitis or a tendinopathy. There was a pattern of increased symptoms after activity rather than symptoms preventing activity. The use of ice packs and positioning were to reinforce self-management strategies in the event a component of his symptoms was due to activities that irritated his supraspinatus tendon.*

A Cochrane Systematic Review of shoulder pain interventions was not able to support or refute the efficacy of common interventions for shoulder pain, including undefined physical therapy.[26] Further, a clinical science review for tendonitis was unable to locate retrospective randomized controlled trials, or in sufficient number, to provide evidence for diagnosis, etiology or treatment of tendonitis.[27]

Attention to shoulder positioning to aid healing is based on identified microvascularity changes in rotator cuff with shoulder in different positions.[28] The use of ice packs to reduce inflammation and aid healing is a recommended management strategy for Mr. Halo's shoulder tendon reactivity.[29] There is poor evidence to include, or exclude, pulsed ultrasound as an intervention for nonspecific shoulder tendonitis.[30]

The exercise chosen for lengthening of the supraspinatus actually provided small eccentric loading of the tendon. The exercise was not specifically chosen to provide the eccentric load since the therapist had not been aware of Curwin and Stanish's work with tendinopathy at the time of Mr. Halo's treatment. The therapist had noticed patients with supraspinatus reactivity were able to move on to mild strengthening once symptoms resolved with performance of this exercise and mild overpressure was tolerated. The next step in the lengthening series added a 1-pound weight that, again, provided a small increase in the eccentric load.

ICF Model of Disablement for Mr. Halo

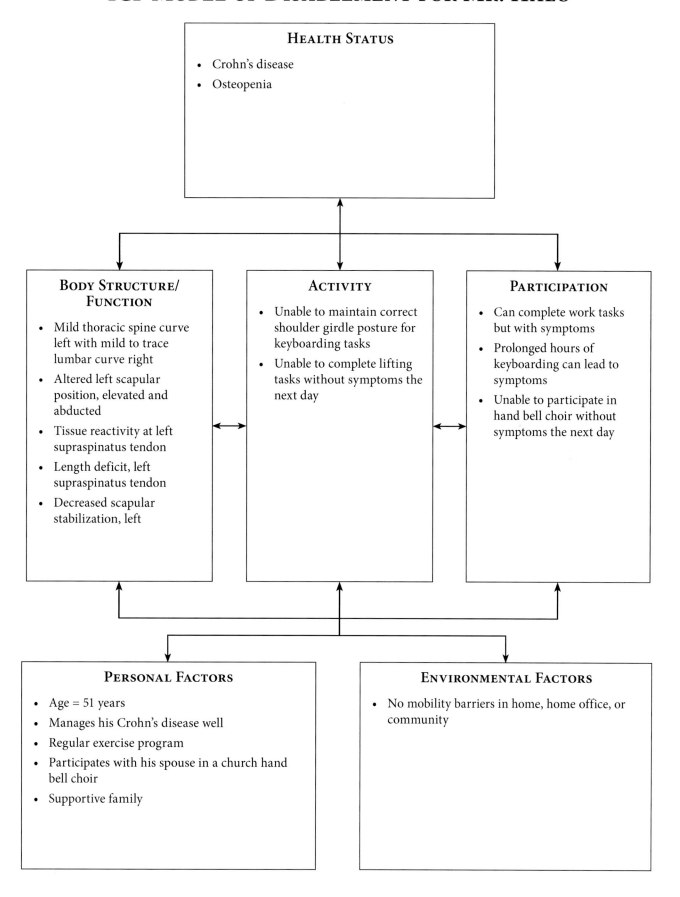

Health Status

- Crohn's disease
- Osteopenia

Body Structure/ Function

- Mild thoracic spine curve left with mild to trace lumbar curve right
- Altered left scapular position, elevated and abducted
- Tissue reactivity at left supraspinatus tendon
- Length deficit, left supraspinatus tendon
- Decreased scapular stabilization, left

Activity

- Unable to maintain correct shoulder girdle posture for keyboarding tasks
- Unable to complete lifting tasks without symptoms the next day

Participation

- Can complete work tasks but with symptoms
- Prolonged hours of keyboarding can lead to symptoms
- Unable to participate in hand bell choir without symptoms the next day

Personal Factors

- Age = 51 years
- Manages his Crohn's disease well
- Regular exercise program
- Participates with his spouse in a church hand bell choir
- Supportive family

Environmental Factors

- No mobility barriers in home, home office, or community

Raising the height of the terminal is not enough to correct spinal posture and head position.[31] To ensure improved head and neck position, patients must be shown the associated lumbar and pelvic positioning required for best seated posture.[32]

Because fatigue in scapular stabilizers can decrease shoulder strength by 50% with 2 minutes of upper extremity arm-forward work, Mr. Halo needed attention to his scapular position with any strengthening exercises identified.[33] Further, since fatigue can alter scapulohumeral rhythm he needed instruction, and practice, with self-monitoring of his posture with keyboarding and bell ringing tasks.[33]

Stretching needed to include posterior shoulder musculature[34] and pectoralis minor,[20,35] as well as relaxation of upper trapezius with upper extremity movement.[20,34] Strengthening of supporting scapular musculature was indicated to prevent the shoulder impingement.[18,20,29,34]

Proposed Frequency and Duration of Physical Therapy Visits

Mr. Halo would be scheduled for 4 appointments over a 4-week time span. Specifically, he would be seen 2 times for the first week and then once the second week. During the third week, Mr. Halo would follow his exercise program at home. He would be scheduled to return for one follow-up visit, and probable discharge, during the fourth week.

Anticipated Goals

1. Mr. Halo would be knowledgeable regarding use of symptom-relieving postures and use of ice packs to decrease tendon reactivity (1 week).

2. Mr. Halo would report changes in his work station, and awareness of his body in it, to allow correct posture with performance of his job tasks (1 week).

3. Left supraspinatus would tolerate length stretching without an increase in symptoms afterward (1 week).

4. Mr. Halo would be independent in length stretch to left supraspinatus (1 week).

5. Mr. Halo would self-correct his posture during treatment sessions (2 weeks).

6. Left supraspinatus would show full length, without symptoms, and be tolerant of over-pressure (2 weeks).

7. Mr. Halo would be independent in a program of general upper extremity mobility exercises (2 weeks).

8. Mr. Halo would tolerate initial supraspinatus strengthening exercises with scapular position controlled (2 weeks).

9. Mr. Halo would be able to demonstrate sustained arms-forward activity—keyboarding—with optimal posture maintained (4 weeks).

10. Mr. Halo would be able to demonstrate simulated heavy hand bell ringing with left scapular position controlled (4 weeks).

Expected Outcomes (4 weeks)

Mr. Halo would report unrestricted, and pain free, participation in sustained arms-forward activities of keyboarding and driving, as well as with the arms-forward movement activity of bell ringing.

Discharge Plan

It was anticipated that Mr. Halo would achieve the anticipated goals and expected outcomes defined in the plan of care. He could expect to be discharged to a home exercise and management program.

INTERVENTION

Coordination, Communication, and Documentation

The findings from the examination and the proposed treatment plan were discussed with Mr. Halo. An initial evaluation summary was entered into the Mr. Halo's online medical record and forwarded to his primary care physician. All aspects of his physical therapy treatment were recorded in his paper outpatient physical therapy record.

Patient-/Client-Related Instruction

Mr. Halo received verbal instruction on, and had the opportunity to practice, symptom-relieving positions for his left shoulder. He was instructed in the use of ice packs. The management instructions, as well as those for identified exercises for his home program, were written out for him and accompanied by hand-drawn illustrations. Prepared handouts illustrating recommended guidelines for computer station set-up were reviewed with, and given to, Mr. Halo.

Procedural Interventions

Therapeutic Exercise

Posture Training

Mode
Posture correction practiced at mirrors.
Intensity
Correction to position of mild tension.
Duration
5 to 10 minutes.
Frequency
During the first 3 physical therapy follow-up sessions.
Description of the Intervention
Mirrors were arranged around Mr. Halo, seated on a stool, so that he was able to look forward into one mirror and see his reflection from the side from the second mirror. Initially, he held the corrected posture position for a slow count to 5 in sets of 3 to 4 repetitions and then gradually increased to

holding for 30 to 60 seconds. Then he practiced the corrected posture with simulated work tasks, driving, and bell ringing.

> **Clinician Comment** *This strategy of holding a corrected posture position allowed elongated muscles with probable stretch weakness to practice the new "shortened" length. Mr. Halo needed to expend an increase in muscular work to hold the "shortened" position and then gain endurance as well as awareness to be able to apply to functional situations.*

Flexibility Exercises

Mode
Muscle length exercise

Intensity
To a position of mild discomfort only, <2 to 3/10

Duration
One set of 8 repetitions with 5-count hold at muscle length end range.

Frequency
During treatment sessions and then 1 to 2 times per day with home exercise program.

Description of the Intervention
The lengthening exercises began with a mild length stretch to the left supraspinatus. With Mr. Halo in supine and arm abducted to 90 degrees with elbow bent and on a pillow, he was prompted to maintain his shoulder girdle position in the corrected position and then let his hand fall forward into medial rotation.

Once the reactivity in the left supraspinatus allowed a full length stretch and was tolerant of mild overpressure, then a full program of shoulder stretches were identified and practiced for his home program. Included were alternate shoulder flexion, leading with thumb and then repeated leading with back of hand, quadrant, lateral rotation, and medial rotation, each with a 1-pound weight to apply mild overpressure at end range. Also included were a posterior shoulder stretch (supine) and inferior shoulder stretch (seated), each using the right hand to provide mild overpressure.

Strengthening Exercise

Mode
Supine strengthening exercise with Theraband.

Intensity
Limited to ensure symptom intensity held < 2/10.

Duration
10 minutes

Frequency
Once daily

Description of the Intervention
Mr. Halo was positioned in supine hook-lying with padding under each elbow so that the elbow was slightly abducted from the side of his body and elevated off the table slightly higher than his shoulder. Elbows were bent 90 degrees and hands slightly more abducted over the elbows.

Initially he was taught an exercise progression of isometric lateral rotation. With these exercises, he held a piece of latex band, tensioned without slack, between his hands with forearms supinated. In the first set of 6 repetitions, he was instructed to position his shoulder girdle in the corrected position and hold his left hand still while the right hand moved into lateral rotation—a distance of about 1 inch. He needed to watch his left hand to ensure it did not move with the increase in load being applied through the band. Then he did the opposite for 6 repetitions—hold the right and move the left. Then he laterally moved both for 6 repetitions. When he was able to complete this progression 2 times and experienced no symptoms, he was progressed to a different exercise.

In this exercise, the hand position changed so that he was holding the band as if he were holding onto a bar, forearms pronated. He corrected his shoulder girdle, began to supinate his forearms "as if the thumbs were moving to the outside position" and applied mild stretch to the band. With this position maintained, he was to reach for the ceiling with hands aligned over his upper chest and slowly lower. This exercise was performed for 2 sets of 4 repetitions. This exercise would serve as the warm-up exercise.

Then "Arms Overhead with Theraband" had him begin as with the now warm-up exercise, "Reach for the Ceiling with Theraband," movement but then maintain the tension in the band while moving his arms over his head to the point of tightness with special attention to maintaining the arm position. Once back over his head, he would hold this position for 5 counts, and return to the ceiling position before bringing arms back over his head again for another 5 counts. Then he returned to the reach for the ceiling position before bending his elbows and bringing his arm back to the starting position. He was to perform 6 to 8 sets of 2 repetitions of this exercise.

> **Clinician Comment** *The reasoning for these last 2 exercises is that the position of arms, hands, and Theraband require activation of the rotator cuff muscles. Rather than the possibility of these muscles firing ineffectively or stopping a contraction, the exercise ensures—as long as the correct position is maintained and the band has some tension—that through the available range of motion, the humeral head will be controlled. Sometimes, at the point where the rotator cuff muscles might have shut off if left to their own choice, the upper extremity will begin to shake to indicate fatigue in the muscles at that point in the range. Patients are cautioned not to progress too far into "the shake zone."*

Manual Therapy Techniques, Including Mobilization/Manipulation

Description of the Intervention
Mr. Halo's right shoulder was mobilized with small amplitude movements toward the end, and to the end (Grade III

to IV–) of the available capsular mobility in the following movements and positions:

- Inferior glide with glenohumeral joint flexed 5 degrees less than pain-free flexion range.
- Lateral glide with glenohumeral joint flexed to 90 degrees.
- Posterior-lateral glides with glenohumeral joint positioned at end range of pain free flexion.

Small oscillations were delivered 2 every seconds until 20 were completed. Two sets of 20 oscillations were completed in each of the 3 positions noted previously. Following each mobilization set, the "after" mobilization range was compared with the "before" to ensure joint mobility had improved.

Functional Training in Work (Job/School/Play), Community, and Leisure Integration or Reintegration, Including Instrumental Activities of Daily Living, Work Hardening, and Work Conditioning

Description of the Intervention
See Patient-/Client-Related Instruction.

REEXAMINATION

Subjective

"I participated in a week-long program of bell ringing without any pain in my shoulder."

Objective

Pain

- Reactivity to palpation of left supraspinatus tendon decreased to absent.
- Symptoms, left shoulder, controlled, 1 to 2/10, after lifting tasks or hand bell choir practice/performance including recent 1-week hand bell conference/workshop.
- "Awareness" level symptoms only, 1/10, at left wrist and elbow after week-long workshop.

Posture

- Able to maintain optimum shoulder girdle posture for identified supine and seated postural and shoulder-strengthening exercises.
- Mr. Halo is able to correct his posture to optimum and maintain keyboarding tasks for 20 minutes by patient report.
- He is able to ring hand bells, including lower note heavy bells, and maintain corrected posture for an entire piece, 2 to 5 minutes, by his report.

Range of Motion

- Left supraspinatus length now WNL and without symptoms
- Mr. Halo was independent with identified range of motion exercises.

Muscle Performance

- Left scapular stabilization improved in upper extremity movements
- Manual muscle testing of left supraspinatus at 5/5 strength without symptoms afterward.
- Mr. Halo was independent with identified upper extremity strengthening exercises.

Assessment

The tissue reactivity in Mr. Halo's left supraspinatus tendon decreased to absent with palpation as well as with length and strength testing. He reported he was able to complete work tasks and participate in hand bell ringing with symptoms in control. He was independent in his home exercise and management programs. All the anticipated goals and expected outcomes established at the initial evaluation were met.

Plan

Mr. Halo was discharged to the identified home exercise and management program.

OUTCOMES

Mr. Halo was not asked to complete any formal outcome measures.

Clinician Comment *A review of the evidence supports the use of a general health status questionnaire and a shoulder-specific questionnaire for Mr. Halo.[36]*

The Functional Status Questionnaire (FSQ) is an example of a general health status questionnaire.[37,38] Using Mr. Halo's report to score the section of the FSQ on Intermediate ADL, his score at the initial evaluation would have been 93, whereas at discharge, he had a score of 100. These are estimated scores and reflect a change only in the items directly related to Mr. Halo's report of increased control of symptoms with bell ringing and lifting activities. All of the other scales within the FSQ would have been scored as 100 at the initial and discharge appointments based on his report.

- *General Health Status Questionnaire*
- *FSQ*

- *Intermediate ADL*
  - *Initial = 93*
  - *Discharge = 100*

The Disabilities of the Arm, Shoulder, and Hand (DASH) is a shoulder-specific questionnaire.[39] In a systematic review of the literature for shoulder questionnaires the DASH received the best ratings for its clinimetric properties.[40] Further, it showed reliability and validity with a broad spectrum of upper extremity disorders.[41] Again, using Mr. Halo's report to score the standard questionnaire as well as the Sports and Performing Arts supplement to the DASH, he showed full recovery.

Shoulder-Specific Questionnaire: DASH.

	INITIAL	DISCHARGE
Standard	22.5	0
Sports/Performing Arts Module	12.5	0

Did Mr. Halo have tendonitis or tendinopathy? The short time period required to show improvement in his symptoms suggested that he had tendonitis. On the other hand, the eccentric component of the initial exercises may have assisted with a tendon that might have been headed toward a more tendinopathy situation.

REFERENCES

1. Grech ED, Ramsdale DR, Bray CL, Faragher EB. Family history an independent risk factor of coronary artery disease. *Eur Heart J.* 1992;13(10):1311-1315.

2. Edelstein SL, Knowler, Bain RP, et al. Predictors of progression from impaired glucose tolerance to NIDDM: an analysis of six prospective studies. *Diabetes.* 1997;46(4):701-710.

3. Goodman CC, Boissonnault WG, Fuller KS. *Pathology: Implications for the Physical Therapist.* 2nd ed. Philadelphia, PA: Saunders; 2003.

4. Freeman HJ. Familial Crohn's disease in single or multiple first-degree relatives. *J Clin Gastroenterol.* 2002;35(1):9-13.

5. Habtezion A, Silverberg MS, Parkes R, Mikolainis S, Steinhart AH. Risk factors for low bone density in Crohn's disease. *Inflamm Bowel Dis.* 2002;8(2):87-92.

6. Medline Plus. U.S. National Library of Medicine and National Institutes of Health. http://www.nlm.nih.gov/medlineplus/druginformation.html. Updated January 25,2012. Accessed February 5, 2012.

7. National Cholesterol Education Program. Detection, Evaluation and treatment of High Blood Cholesterol in Adults (Adult Treatment Panel III). National Institutes of Health, NIH Publication No. 01-3670, May 2001.

8. The Joint National Committee (JNC) on Prevention, Detection, Evaluation and Treatment of High Blood Pressure – JNC VII (released May 21, 2003).

9. Obesity Education Initiative. Body Mass Index Calculator. National Heart, Lungs and Blood Institute. 1991.

10. Maitland GD. *Peripheral Manipulation.* 3rd ed. London, UK: Butterworth-Heinemann; 1991.

11. American Academy of Orthopaedic Surgeons. *Joint Motion: Method of Measuring and Recording.* Edinburgh, UK: Churchill Livingstone; 1965.

12. Kendall FP, McCreary EK, Provance PG, Rodgers MM, Romani WA. *Muscles: Testing and Function with Posture and Pain.* 5th ed. Philadelphia, PA: Lippincott Williams & Wilkins; 2005.

13. Bijur PE, Latimer CT, Gallagher EJ. Validation of a verbally administered numerical rating scale of acute pain for use in the emergency department. *Acad Emerg Med.* 2003;10(4):390-392.

14. Bernard B, Sauter S, Fine L, Petersen M, Hales T. Job task and psychosocial risk factors for work-related musculoskeletal disorders among newspaper employees. *Scan J Work Environ Health.* 1994;20(6):417-426.

15. Fjellman-Wiklund A, Sundelin G. Musculoskeletal discomfort of music teachers: an eight-year perspective and psychosocial work factors. *Int J Occup Environ Health.* 1998;4(2):89-98.

16. Côté P, Kreitz BG, Cassidy JD, Dzus AK, Martel J. A study of the diagnostic accuracy and reliability of the Scoliometer and Adam's forward bend test. *Spine (Phila Pa 1976).* 1998;23(7):796-802.

17. Griegel-Morris P, Larson K, Mueller-Klaus K, Oatis CA. Incidence of common postural abnormalities I the cervical, shoulder and thoracic regions and their association with pain in two age groups of healthy subjects. *Phys Ther.* 1992;72(6):425-431.

18. Ludewig PM, Cook TM. Alterations in shoulder kinematics and associated muscle activity in people with symptoms of shoulder impingement. *Phys Ther.* 2000;80(3):276-291.

19. Lukasiewicz AC, McClure P, Michener L, Pratt N, Sennett B. Comparison of 2-dimensional scapular position and orientation between subjects with and without shoulder impingement. *J Orthop Sports Phys Ther.* 1999;29(10):574-583.

20. Sahrmann SA. *Diagnosis and Treatment of Movement Impairment Syndromes.* St. Louis, MO: Mosby; 2002.

21. Paris S, Loubert P. *Foundations of Clinical Orthopedics.* 3rd ed. St. Augustine, FL: Institute Press; 1999.

22. Magee DJ. *Orthopedic Physical Assessment.* 5th ed. St. Louis, MO: Saunders Elsevier; 2008.

23. Louw A. *Course Notes—Mobilization of the Nervous System.* Baltimore, MD: The Neuro Orthopaedic Institute; 2010.

24. Butler DS. *The Sensitive Nervous System.* Adelaide, Australia: Noigroup; 2000.

25. Coppieters P, Stappaerts KH, Everaert DG, Staes FF. Addition of test components during neurodynamic testing: effect on range of motion and sensory responses. *J Orthop Sports Phys Ther.* 2001;31(5):226-235; discussion 236-237.

26. Green S, Buchbinder R, Glazier R, Forbes A. Interventions for shoulder pain. *Cochrane Database Syst Rev.* 2000;2:CD001156.

27. Almekinders LC, Temple JD. Etiology, diagnosis, and treatment of tendonitis: an analysis of the literature. *Med Sci Sports Exerc.* 1998;30(8):1183-1190.

28. Gross MT. Chronic tendonitis: pathomechanics of injury, factors affecting the healing response, and treatment. *J Orthop Sports Phys Ther.* 1992;16(6):248-261.

29. Kamkar A, Irrgang JJ. Whitney SL. Nonoperative management of secondary shoulder impingement syndrome. *J Orthop Sport Phys Ther.* 1993;17(5):212-224.

30. Philadelphia Panel. Philadelphia Panel evidence-based clinical practice guidelines on selected rehabilitation interventions for shoulder pain. *Phys Ther.* 2001;81(10):1719-1730.

31. Kietrys DM, McClure PW, Fitzgerald GK. The relationship between head and neck posture and VDT screen height in keyboard operators. *Phys Ther.* 1998;78(4):395-403.

32. Black KM, McClure P, Polansky M. The influence of different sitting positions on cervical and lumbar posture. *Spine (Phila Pa 1976).* 1996;21(1):65-70.

33. McQuade KJ, Dawson J, Smidt GL. Scapulothoracic muscle fatigue associated with alterations in scapulohumeral rhythm kinematics during maximum resistive shoulder elevation. *J Orthop Sports Phys Ther.* 1998;28(2):74-80.

34. Ludwig PM, Borstad JD. Effects of a home exercise programme on shoulder pain and functional status in construction workers. *Occup Environ Med.* 2003;60(11):841-849.

35. Roddey TS, Olson SL, Grant SE. The effect of pectoralis muscle stretching on the resting position of the scapula in persons with varying degrees of forward head/rounded shoulder posture. *J Man Manip Ther.* 2002;10(3):124-128.

36. Beaton DE, Richards RR. Measuring function of the shoulder: a cross-sectional comparison of five questionnaires. *J Bone Joint Surg Am.* 1996;78(6):882-890.

37. Medical Outcomes Trust. SF-36. www.SF-36.org. Accessed April 16, 2004.

38. Jette AM, Davies AR, Cleary PD, et al. The Functional Status Questionnaire: reliability and validity when used in primary care. *J Gen Intern Med.* 1986;1(3):143-149.

39. American Academy of Orthopaedic Surgeons. Disabilities of the arm, shoulder, and hand (DASH). http://www.dash.iwh.on.ca. Accessed February 5, 2012.

40. Bot SD, Terwee CB, van der Windt DA, Bouter LM, Dekker J, de Vet HC. Clinimetric evaluation of shoulder disability questionnaires: a systematic review of the literature. *Ann Rheum Dis.* 2004;63(4):335-341.

41. McClure P, Michener L. Measures of adult shoulder function. *Arthritis Rheum.* 2003;49(5S):S50-S58.

11

Individuals With Systemic Musculoskeletal and Connective Tissue Disorders

Susan L. Edmond, PT, DSc, OCS

CHAPTER OBJECTIVES

- List the factors that place women at greater risk for osteoporotic fractures than men.

- Outline the ratio of osteoblastic activity to osteoclastic before the age of 25 years and after age 30.

- Discuss the various roles exercise can play in osteoporosis management.

- Outline the progression of events that occur with rheumatoid arthritis in an involved joint.

- Identify body organs—other than joints—that can be involved in rheumatoid arthritis.

- Identify 4 subcategories of rheumatoid arthritis and the disease process for each.

- Discuss the evidence that changed the perception of the role of exercise in managing patients with rheumatoid arthritis.

CHAPTER OUTLINE

Coglianese D, ed. *Clinical Exercise Pathophysiology for Physical Therapy: Examination, Testing, and Exercise Prescription for Movement-Related Disorders (pp 443-464).*
© 2015 Taylor & Francis Group.

Systemic musculoskeletal diseases are those that affect connective tissue throughout multiple organ systems, including the musculoskeletal system. Many of the consequences of musculoskeletal and connective tissue symptoms, which include limitations in functional activity performance, loss of independence, social isolation, depression, and a decrease in the ability to work and generate income occur among individuals with systemic musculoskeletal diseases. Two of the most common systemic musculoskeletal diseases seen in physical therapy clinics are discussed below. A third common musculoskeletal disease is discussed in the context of a case. Together, they exemplify the thought processes required of a physical therapist to manage patients with these complex, multi-organ disorders.

OSTEOPOROSIS

Overview and Epidemiology

Osteoporosis is defined as a condition characterized by a decrease in bone mass and micro-architectural deterioration of bone leading to bone fragility and greater risk of bone fracture.[1,2] Approximately 10 million Americans over the age of 50 have osteoporosis, and an additional 34 million have low bone mineral density.[3] In 2005, an estimated $17 billion was spent on health care costs for osteoporotic fractures alone.[3]

After achieving peak bone mass between the ages of 25 and 30 years, men lose approximately 0.5% to 1% of total bone mass per year.[4,5] Before undergoing menopause, women have similar rates of bone loss. However, this loss is accelerated immediately following menopause because of a decrease in the production of estrogen. During the 6 years after undergoing menopause, bone loss can occur at a rate 3 to 10 times greater than what occurs during the premenopausal years.[6] By the age of 65 to 70, men and women once again lose bone mass at a similar rate.[7] Men, however, are protected from osteoporosis by their larger bones and increase in bone mass at peak bone age, even when taking body size into account.[7]

Women are therefore at greater risk for osteoporotic fractures than men. It has been estimated that up to 60% of women over the age of 50 will sustain at least one osteoporotic fracture in their lifetime.[8] For a man, this lifetime risk is estimated to be 20%.[9] While the incidence of osteoporotic fractures is difficult to determine directly, in one model it was determined that at least 90% of all hip and spine fractures among elderly White women are attributable to osteoporosis. Smaller percentages of fractures attributable to osteoporosis occur among other populations, and among fractures in other bones.[10]

Osteoporotic fractures occur most often in the hip, vertebral body, and wrist. In relation to hip fractures, incidence increases exponentially after age 70. In contrast, the incidence of vertebral body fractures increases beginning around age 60, but at a much less dramatic rate than that of hip fractures; and the incidence of wrist fractures increases until around age 70 and then decreases slightly.[11] Whereas osteoporotic vertebral body fractures are most prevalent, hip fractures are associated with the greatest mortality and morbidity. Mortality following a hip fracture has been reported to be as high as 33% in the first year following fracture.[12] Among those who survive a hip fracture, only 25% regain their previous level of function.[13]

Pathophysiology

Normal bone tissue is continuously remodeling. This process occurs as osteoblasts produce new bone tissue by creating a protein matrix that later calcifies, and osteoclasts reabsorb bone tissue by stimulating production of acids and enzymes that dissolves older bone.

Peak bone mass occurs between the ages of 25 and 30 years. Prior to achieving peak bone mass, net osteoblastic activity exceeds net osteoclastic activity. After achieving peak bone mass, anatomic and physiologic aging cause osteoclastic activity to exceed osteoblastic activity, thus there is greater bone removal than replacement. This disequilibrium eventually leads to osteoporosis. The presence of specific medical conditions can also cause the balance between osteoblastic and osteoclastic activity to be disrupted in favor of osteoclastic activity. Trabecular, or cancellous, bone has a greater turnover rate than cortical bone. Areas such as the vertebral body, hip, and wrist, which have relatively higher percentages of trabecular bone than other bones, are therefore most susceptible to osteoporotic fractures.[1]

The disequilibrium between osteoblastic and osteoclastic activity is accentuated in postmenopausal women, since the onset of menopause is associated with a reduction in estrogen, and estrogen is responsible for the inhibition of bone reabsorption.[14] In some medical conditions, such as those that are treated pharmacologically with glucocorticoids, this disequilibrium is compounded by a disruption of the micro-architectural integrity of bone tissue, resulting in a reduction in the quality and quantity of the bone tissue that is formed.[2]

Osteoporosis is classified by etiology as either primary or secondary. Primary osteoporosis is associated with biological changes that take place throughout the life span, and includes Type I and Type II forms. Type I primary osteoporosis occurs in postmenopausal women in conjunction with a decrease in estrogen, whereas Type II primary osteoporosis is associated with the aging process. Secondary osteoporosis is characterized by bone loss caused by medical conditions including certain metabolic and nutritional disorders, the intake of some medications, and immobilization with resultant loss of muscle function. Primary osteoporosis is therefore far more prevalent than secondary osteoporosis. The common risk factors for osteoporosis are numerous, and are listed in Table 11-1. Specific causes for many of these risk factors are unknown.

Diagnosis

The presence of osteoporosis alone is not associated with pain or functional limitations. The primary pathologic concern with osteoporosis is that the associated bone loss increases the likelihood of sustaining a fracture, which

TABLE 11-1. COMMON RISK FACTORS FOR OSTEOPOROSIS

FACTOR CATEGORIES	RISK FACTORS
Demographic risk factors	• Female sex • Age • Low body weight (less than 127 pounds) • Family history of osteoporosis • Caucasian or Asian race
Medical risk factors	• Long term use of corticosteroids • Antiseizure medication • Gonadotropin hormone medication • Immunosuppression medication • Excessive use of aluminum-containing antacids • Medication to treat some gastrointestinal diseases, such as Cushing's syndrome • Excessive thyroid hormone medication • Certain anticancer medications • Treatments that decrease estrogen levels • Paralysis • Prolonged immobilization • Chronic kidney, liver, lung or gastrointestinal disorders • Hypogonadism • Turner's or Klinefelter syndrome • Myeloma • Postmenopause, amenorrhea • Anorexia Nervosa • Low testosterone levels in men
Lifestyle risk factors	• Inadequate physical activity • Low calcium/vitamin D intake • Excessive use of alcohol • Current cigarette smoking

frequently does result in significant pain and loss of function. The diagnosis of osteoporosis is often not made until a pathological fracture occurs, as the occurrence of the pathological fracture prompts an investigation of the underlying cause. Osteoporosis is therefore referred to as the "silent disease" because it is asymptomatic until a fracture occurs.

Osteoporosis can be identified through the quantification of bone loss. Bone loss is detected by evaluating bone mineral density, or bone mass using radiography. The gold standard for determining bone mass is a dual-energy X-ray absorptiometry (DXA) scan of the hip and spine. Results are reported using T-scores. T-scores are reported in standard deviations, and represent the amount to which the individual deviates from an average 30-year-old of similar sex and race/ethnicity. A 1 standard deviation reduction in the T-score is equivalent to a 10% to 20% decrease in bone mineral density.[2] In relation to osteoporosis of the hip, for every 1-point reduction in the T-score, the risk of hip fracture increases approximately 2.6 times.[8]

T-scores of between –1 and –2.5 identify an individual as being osteopenic, or "preosteoporotic." Osteoporosis is diagnosed when an individual has a T-score of –2.5 or less. An individual with a T-score of –2.5 or less who has sustained a fracture is considered to have "established" osteoporosis.

All patients with known risk factors for osteoporosis should be screened for bone loss. DXA scans are therefore recommended for the following individuals:

• All women aged 65 years or older

• Women considering medication for osteoporosis

• Postmenopausal women under age 65 with one or more additional risk factors

• Postmenopausal women who present with a fracture[2,11]

Medical Intervention

One key to preventing osteoporosis is to build bone mass during the skeletal growth years and early adulthood.[15-17] At-risk individuals include those who did not achieve sufficient levels of exercise at this key stage in bone development, as well as those with nutritional deficiencies, including eating disorders.

An adequate intake of nutrients, especially calcium and vitamin D, is fundamental to preventing and treating osteoporosis. For older adults, who are at a higher risk of osteoporosis, current recommendations include between 1000 and 1500 mg of calcium, and between 800 and 1000 international units (IU) of vitamin D per day.[2] Many older adults, especially those who are institutionalized, do not get sufficient amounts of calcium and vitamin D to maintain bone health.[9] If a physical therapist suspects that a patient with osteoporosis has a dietary deficiency, a consultation with a nutritionist is recommended.

Among women, the extent to which bone mass can be maintained or increased depends on the individual's menopausal status: premenopausal women are more likely to demonstrate gains in bone mass with exercise than postmenopausal women.[18] While exercise remains a component of the medical management of postmenopausal women and all other patients with osteoporosis, once significant bone loss has been identified in postmenopausal women, the focus of the medical management is on pharmaceutics while also maintaining an appropriate intake of calcium and vitamin D.[19]

Many patients with osteoporosis are managed pharmacologically with bisphosphonates (alendronate, ibandronate, risedronate, zoledronate). Those patients who do not tolerate bisphosphonates can often manage their bone loss with selective estrogen receptor modulators (raloxifene) or with calcitonin. Short-term treatment with parathyroid hormone (teriparatide) can be an option for patients with severe disease.[2,9] One other option for patients with severe disease is Denosumab, which is typically administered at 6-month intervals by injection.[20]

Once a fracture has occurred, treatment is similar to that provided to a patient who does not have osteoporosis. Since bone stock is compromised in patients with osteoporosis, these patients present with an increased risk of delayed healing, and in the case of surgical intervention, a decrease in the ability of the bone stock to support the surgical procedure that was performed.

Osteoporosis and Exercise

Bone responds to alterations in mechanical stress in a manner similar to that of other connective tissue. Inactivity decreases bone strength, whereas muscle contraction and the gravitational force involved with weightbearing act as a stimulus to increase bone strength. Loss of bone mass can therefore theoretically be reversed with exercise; however, with advancing age, the restoration of bone mass becomes increasingly more difficult. Irrespective of age, premenopausal women respond more favorable to exercises directed at addressing osteoporosis than postmenopausal women.[18]

Most clinical studies addressing the effect of exercise on osteoporosis measured outcomes related to bone density. While measures of low bone density are strongly predictive of fractures, bone density changes per se do not change levels of pain or functional limitations.

To stimulate osteogenesis through exercise, workloads must exceed the daily strains experienced when performing usual activities.[21] Some types of exercises have a greater effect on maintaining or increasing bone mineral density than others; however, the exact type and intensity of exercise that is required to optimize net bone reabsorption has not yet been determined. Most of the studies that were performed on humans included only women as subjects; therefore the generalizability of these study results to men is questionable. In those studies that did include men, results suggested that outcomes from exercise were equivocal[22] if not better for men than for women.[23]

Some broad exercise considerations are especially applicable to individuals who have or are at-risk for developing osteoporosis. Patients must first recognize that they need to perform specific exercises, because simply increasing activity level is not sufficient to increase, maintain or minimize loss of bone mass.[21] Furthermore, to maintain the benefits of exercise, an exercise program must be performed on an ongoing basis throughout the lifespan, because improvements in bone density are reversed when the exercise program is discontinued.[24,25] It is therefore important to consider motivational factors when prescribing an exercise program for treatment of osteoporosis. A patient is more likely to adhere to an exercise regimen if it is enjoyable or meets that patient's recreational goals. Finally, the effects of exercise on bone mass can occur only if the individual ingests adequate amounts of calcium and vitamin D.

The evidence supports the implementation of exercise for the treatment and prevention of osteoporosis. In a 1999 meta-analysis, the authors concluded that there is a small improvement of approximately 1% with either endurance or strengthening exercises on hip and spine bone density in pre- and postmenopausal, nonosteoporotic women.[26] In 2 more recent critical reviews, the authors concluded that exercise results in a slight improvement in bone mineral density in postmenopausal women[27] and a small reduction in fracture risk in older adults.[28]

Specific exercise recommendations have been outlined in 2 separate position papers. The Canadian Academy of Sports and Exercise Medicine recommend performing weightbearing endurance exercises for 30 to 60 minutes 3 to 5 days per week, and strength training 3 days per week.[29] Similarly, the Belgium Bone Club recommends 15 to 60 minutes of weightbearing endurance exercises and a series of strength training exercises performed 2 to 3 times per week. The exercise program should be performed at an intensity of 70% to 80% functional capacity or maximum strength. All strengthening exercises should be site-specific.[30]

One additional concern for patients with osteoporosis involves the increase in the kyphotic curvature of the spine that accompanies vertebral body fractures. Thoracic kyphosis has been shown to have an adverse effect on functional activities, especially those activities that involve mobility tasks.[31] In one study, exercise, consisting of stretching, posture retraining, respiratory muscle strengthening, and walking was effective in reducing the kyphotic curvature in subjects with demonstrated osteoporosis of the spine.[32]

Outcomes

Depending on the age and sex of the patient, the etiology/type and extent of osteoporosis, and the drug regimen, it is possible to increase bone mass. Nevertheless, for many postmenopausal women, exercise-related treatment goals focus on preventing or minimizing further bone loss and subsequent fracture, and countering the effects of prior fractures. In most cases, drug therapy is required to reverse bone loss in this population.[19] For males, females who are premenopausal, and those who have developed osteoporosis because they were immobilized, reversal of bone loss by performing strenuous exercises and increasing activity levels is a more realistic goal.[33] Outcomes for individuals with osteoporosis from other causes have not been studied.

Physical Therapy Management

Examination

The physical therapy examination procedures performed on a specific patient vary from patient to patient, depending on the specific goals, symptoms, and physical presentation of each individual. For example, for an older female patient with a known lumbar vertebral body osteoporotic fracture, the history would focus on the presence and nature of lumbar pain and changes in lumbar curvature, and subsequent functional limitations. The physical examination would focus on the physical properties of the lumbar spine and lower extremities, such as posture, range of motion and strength, and the results of pain-provocation tests. Nevertheless, the physical therapy examination and evaluation of a patient with a diagnosis of osteoporosis follow the same history taking, systems review, and testing procedures as for most musculoskeletal conditions, with several additional considerations described next.

During the history portion of the examination, the therapist obtains information regarding the severity of the osteoporosis, to determine the patient's risk for fracture during activities of daily living (ADL) as well as during a prescribed exercise program. The therapist also solicits medical and musculoskeletal information that would affect the patient's strengthening and weightbearing exercise program. For example, a known cardiac history would potentially modify the prescription for load in a strengthening exercise program.

The physical examination includes specific tests, such as anthropometric measures, ergonomics and body mechanics, gait, locomotion and balance, muscle performance, range of motion, and posture. Emphasis is placed on alignment, joint, and muscle impairments that affect pain and/or function.

The examination of posture is especially important if the patient is female and over 50 years of age, since osteoporotic vertebral fractures are often asymptomatic[34] and therefore undiagnosed. Undiagnosed patients who have experienced a loss of height or an increase in their kyphotic curvature might benefit from a medical referral for a work-up for possible osteoporosis, since these changes are often associated with vertebral body osteoporotic fractures in older adults.

Since patients with osteoporosis are at increased risk of fracture following a fall, fall risk is also often evaluated during the physical examination. Several assessment tools, such as the Tinetti Balance Test, the Berg Balance Scale, and the Timed Up-and-Go Test are commonly used by physical therapists to assess risk for falls. Nevertheless, none of these aforementioned tools have been shown to be highly predictive of falls in at-risk patients.[35] Test results might be better used to identify areas requiring intervention than simply to identify those at high risk for subsequent falls.

Finally, any examination procedure that could potentially cause a fracture must not be performed. For example, the examination of joint accessory motion in joints composed of bones with osteoporotic changes is not routinely recommended in patients with osteoporosis.[36]

Physical Therapy Intervention Considerations

As with any other patient with a musculoskeletal condition, interventions for the patient with osteoporosis are determined through a process of integrating examination findings and patient goals. There are several issues, however, listed below, that are directly related to the management of the patient with osteoporosis.

Since fractures often result from falls,[11] ensuring a safe environment and monitoring the patient during exercise to prevent falls is an important component of injury prevention. This includes guarding and providing balance support when indicated. The physical therapist also considers implementing an intervention consisting of fall reduction strategies. If balance is impaired, exercises to improve balance and proprioception are a component of the patient's program, even though these exercises are not likely to have a direct impact on bone mass. The therapist also considers other strategies to reduce the number and impact of falls, such as providing the patient with gait assistive devices and hip pads.

Patients with osteoporosis are at risk of fracture from resistive and aerobic exercises. Nevertheless, resistive and/or aerobic exercises are necessary for bone loss to be minimized or reversed. There is currently no protocol for determining safe exercise parameters from the perspective of avoiding fractures in osteoporotic individuals. Physical therapists therefore evaluate the medical and physical status of the patient, including the extent of bone loss, and make a judgment regarding the maximal amount of exercise that the patient can safely tolerate. For example, patients with severe osteoporosis should not engage in high-impact exercises.

When uncertain as to whether the patient can tolerate a specific exercise, the therapist does not prescribe that exercise to the patient.

Certain spinal movements increase compressive forces on the vertebral bodies, increasing the likelihood of compression fractures. To prevent vertebral body fractures, the therapist instructs the patient to avoid positioning in spinal flexion, as well as resisted rotation, while exercising.[37] For similar reasons, the therapist discourages flexed posture positions and twisting while lifting during ADL with patients with known osteoporosis.

RHEUMATOID ARTHRITIS

Overview and Epidemiology

Rheumatoid arthritis (RA) is a chronic, multi-systemic disease affecting almost 1% of the population of North America.[38] It is nearly 3 times more common among women than men.[38] Researchers have estimated that there is a 50% probability of work disability within 4.5 to 22 years following diagnosis.[39] The most apparent manifestation of RA is the gradual destruction of articular cartilage and bone. Joints that are most often affected include the hands, wrists, shoulders, elbows, cervical spine, and hips; and to a lesser extent, the knees, and ankles and feet.[38]

RA is characterized as an autoimmune disease. Autoimmune diseases are those in which the body's immune system responds to a "false alarm," inappropriately triggering an inflammatory response and fighting the body's own proteins when there is no foreign substance to fight off. In the case of RA, the targeted structure is the joint. The exact cause(s) of RA is unknown. Genetic factors have been implicated, since RA is more likely to occur among family members of individuals with RA. Environmental triggers that have yet to be identified may also play a role in the etiology of RA.[38]

Onset can begin at any age, but RA most often becomes symptomatic in individuals between the ages of 35 to 50 years. During this range in age, many patients are raising families and making significant career inroads. The impact of this disease on functional activity performance and quality of life therefore can be severe.

Pathophysiology

The primary target of the autoimmune process associated with RA is the synovium, resulting in a joint capsule that is thickened and inflamed.[40] As synovial fluid levels increase, the joint swells. This inflammation also causes contractile tissue surrounding the joint to spasm, shorten, and lose strength, eventually causing the corresponding joint to sublux. Over time, the synovial tissue becomes weakened from the enzymatic action of inflammation on collagen tissue. Pannus, a flap consisting of granulation tissue, forms within the joint and eventually attacks adjacent bone and cartilage, causing these structures to erode.[40] Fibrous tissue gradually invades the pannus and forms scar tissue within the joint space. This fibrous tissue eventually calcifies, resulting in bony ankylosis. The end result of these processes is a joint that is stiff, weak, painful, and deformed.

Since the primary tissue affected by RA is the joint synovium, the hallmark finding in RA is joint redness, swelling, stiffness, and pain. Nevertheless, other organs are commonly affected. Anemia is prevalent among individuals with RA. Rheumatoid nodules and dermal vasculitic lesions often form in the skin. The eyes can become affected by keratoconjunctivitis sicca, episcleritis, and scleritis. As ligaments become weakened, cervical spine instability, as well as peripheral nerve entrapment, is a common occurrence. Interstitial lung disease and pericardial effusion is present in many individuals with RA, although these latter 2 conditions are often asymptomatic.[38,40]

Muscle is also targeted in patients with RA. From a metabolic perspective, the disease process associated with RA results in a catabolic state. Therefore, generalized muscle weakness is a common finding.[41,42] Other conditions contributing to muscle weakness in patients with RA include side effects of the medications used to treat the condition, and deconditioning secondary to pain and fatigue.

Diagnosis

In 1987, the American Rheumatism Association published a list of 7 specific criteria that identifies the presence of RA.[43] This diagnostic classification system was in common usage until recently. In response to the finding that patients who are diagnosed and treated early have better outcomes, new criteria for diagnosing RA were developed in 2010.[44] These criteria are provided in Table 11-2.

RA is therefore a medical diagnosis that is determined by the presence of a combination of signs, symptoms, and medical tests. Nevertheless, clusters of signs and symptoms indicating the presence of RA are identifiable by physical therapists during the evaluation of musculoskeletal pain. It is therefore imperative that when a physical therapist identifies some of these signs and symptoms that indicate that the patient might have RA, the therapist refers that patient to a rheumatologist for diagnosis and medical management. In the case of the aforementioned RA diagnostic criteria, categories A and D can be observed by a physical therapist (see Table 11-2).

Subclassification of Rheumatoid Arthritis by Pathology

There are more than 100 different types of diseases classified as RA, each with a different pattern of targeted organ damage, and resultant differences in signs and symptoms. An accurate diagnosis within these subcategories is often difficult, since many patients do not present with typical symptoms for a particular sub-category of RA, and most subcategories are characterized by joint swelling and destruction. It is also unclear from a physiological perspective how these different subcategories differ from one another. Several of these rheumatoid subcategories are described next.

TABLE 11-2. THE 2010 ACR/EULAR CLASSIFICATION CRITERIA FOR RHEUMATOID ARTHRITIS

CLASSIFICATION CRITERIA FOR RHEUMATOID ARTHRITIS (RA)	SCORE
A. Joint Involvement	
1 large joint	0
2 to 10 large joints	1
1 to 3 small joints (with or without involvement of large joints)	2
4 to 10 small joints (with or without involvement of large joints)	3
> 10 joints (at least 1 small joint)	5
B. Serology (At least 1 test result is needed for classification)	
Negative RF and negative ACPA	0
Low-positive RF or high-positive ACPA	2
High-positive RF or high-positive ACPA	3
C. Acute-Phase Reactants (at least 1 test result is needed for classification)	
Normal CRP and normal ESR	0
Abnormal CRP or abnormal ESR	1
D. Duration of Symptoms	
<6 weeks	0
>6 weeks	1

Target population: Patients who have at least one joint with definitive clinical synovitis and in whom the synovitis is not better explained by another disease. Add the score of categories A to D; a score of >6 (out of possible 10) is needed for classification of a patient as having definite RA. ACR: American College of Rheumatology; EULAR: European League Against Rheumatism; RF: rheumatoid factor; ACPA: anti-citrullinated peptide antibody; CRP: C-reactive protein; ESR: erythrocyte sedimentation rate.

Adapted from Aletaha D, Neogi T, Silman AJ, et al. 2010 Rheumatoid arthritis classification criteria: an American College of Rheumatology/European League Against Rheumatism collaborative initiative. *Arthritis Rheum.* 2010;62(9):2569-2581.

Lupus

Lupus is a sub-category of RA characterized by a red, butterfly-shaped rash that appears across the nose and cheeks. In addition to its effects on joints and skin, lupus also affects the kidneys, heart, and blood-forming organs, nervous system, eye, mucous membranes, lungs and, to a lesser extent, the gastrointestinal and peripheral vascular systems. Patients with lupus are especially susceptible to infection, and have increased risk for kidney failure and greater sun sensitivity.[45]

Lupus is 10 times more common in women than men. It is also more prevalent among people of African ancestry. Symptoms generally begin to appear between the ages of 15 and 45 years.

Scleroderma

Scleroderma is an autoimmune disease that is characterized by the production of excessive collagen. Signs and symptoms of this condition are caused by inflammation and resultant fibrosis of multiple tissues, including the skin, blood vessels, synovium, skeletal muscle, and certain internal organs such as the kidneys, lungs, heart, and gastrointestinal system. The finding most characteristic of this rheumatic condition is skin thickening and tightening, beginning at the distal extremities and progressing proximally. As with other rheumatic diseases, symptoms of scleroderma vary from individual to individual, and can cause symptoms ranging from mild to severe.[45]

In the more mild form, termed *localized scleroderma*, symptoms are usually limited to the skin, although muscles and bones also can be affected. Skin symptoms consist of whitish, hard, oval-shaped patches that sometimes are accompanied by a purple ring (morphea-type lesions), or lines of thickened skin (linear-type lesions). Both of these skin lesions limit joint motion, since they produce scarring that infiltrates bone and muscular tissue.[46]

The more severe form of scleroderma is called *systematic scleroderma*. In some cases of systematic scleroderma, skin lesions are limited to the face, hands, and fingers. In other cases, onset is rapid, skin thickening occurs throughout the body, and arthritic symptoms resembling those of RA are present. Reduced function can occur in joints, muscles and hands. Other organs, including the gastrointestinal track, lungs, heart, and kidneys are often targeted.[46] Pulmonary hypertension is especially prevalent in this population, and is a common cause of mortality.[47]

Gout

Gout is a form of inflammatory arthritis caused by an increase in serum uric acid or a decrease in the ability to excrete uric acid from the blood secondary to an abnormality in purine metabolism.[48] This increase in uric acid in the blood causes urate crystals to form in joint synovium and surrounding tissues.[48,49] The lifetime prevalence of gout is estimated to be approximately 2%[48]; affecting primarily older men.[48,49]

Gout is characterized by a sudden onset of excruciating joint pain accompanied by joint swelling, warmth, and rubor. The joint most commonly affected by gout is the first metatarsophalangeal joint.[48,49] About 50% of patients with initial onset of gout have recurring symptoms. Recurrent gout can result in chronic arthritis with associated pain and joint stiffness.[49] Acute gout is most often treated with anti-inflammatory medication. With individuals who have recurrent flares, management consists of medications to reduce the levels of serum uric acid, such as allopurinol or febuxostat.[48] With proper medical management, an individual with chronic gout can live a normal life.[49]

Ankylosing Spondylitis

Ankylosing spondylitis is characterized by back pain and stiffness, beginning in the lower lumbar and pelvic regions, and progressing up the spine. In addition to spinal pain and stiffness, patients with ankylosing spondylitis often experience eye symptoms, fever, and fatigue. At the end stages of the disease, the shoulders, hips, and knees become affected. Ankylosing spondylitis is more common in men than women,[50] with symptoms usually beginning before the age of 40. Unlike most other rheumatic conditions, patients with ankylosing spondylitis are negative for rheumatoid factor (RF), one of the blood markers that help diagnose RA.

With ankylosing spondylitis, the vertebrae gradually ossify as the disease progresses, resulting in a characteristic bamboo-like appearance to spinal structures on radiographs. The spine also becomes progressively more osteoporotic, and therefore is more susceptible to fracture. Frequently, as with many other forms of RA, the ligaments of the atlantoaxial joint become lax, potentially resulting in spinal cord or brain stem compression.

In the early stages, ankylosing spondylitis often is misdiagnosed as mechanical low back or sacroiliac joint pain. It therefore should be suspected in any patient who is less than 40 years of age and reports pain and stiffness in the mid- or low back for longer than 3 months, especially if the patient is male.

Medical Intervention

There is currently no cure for RA. Pharmacological management is the primary treatment for this condition. The main goal of pharmacological management is to control intra-articular swelling, thereby minimizing the progressive destruction of articular structures. Once the joint has been destroyed, the only recourse is joint surgery. Early pharmacological treatment is therefore crucial to minimize pain and loss of function.

Several classes of medications are used to control the inflammatory component of RA. The most often prescribed class of medications is commonly known as nonsteroidal anti-inflammatory drugs (NSAIDs). These drugs often are used in the early stages of the disease. If RA symptoms are mild, these medications can be used throughout the patient's lifespan. Steroids have traditionally been used in more severe cases to control joint inflammation; however, the side effects of long-term steroid use can be severe. More recently, a different class of medication, called disease modifying antirheumatic drugs (DMARDs), has been developed. These medications interrupt the autoimmune reaction, thus reducing many of the symptoms of RA. Often, different patients react differently to the same medication. Finding an effective drug regimen therefore often involves a series of medication trial and error.

Rheumatoid Arthritis and Exercise

For many years, most therapists believed that patients with RA should perform only exercises that place small amounts of stress on joints, such as active range of motion and isometric strengthening. The goal was to minimize the loss of range of motion and muscle strength that commonly occurs with disease progression. Therapists were reluctant to prescribe more aggressive exercises, such as resistance training, for patients with RA because they believed that these exercises would increase pain, accelerate joint destruction, or exacerbate the disease process. Unfortunately, for patients with RA, as with most other chronic conditions, more aggressive exercises often are required to improve functional levels and quality of life. This incongruity was the catalyst for a number of recent studies evaluating outcomes of exercise for patients with RA have been performed.

The results of these studies have been synthesized in several recent literature reviews addressing the safety and effectiveness of exercise in patients with RA.[41,51-59] One of the early reviews[51] addressed the efficacy of all types of therapeutic exercise. Based on a review of 17 studies, the authors concluded that there was good evidence that therapeutic exercise benefits patients with RA by reducing pain, increasing muscle strength, and improving functional status. They further concluded that the exercise program should include functional training and either high- or low-intensity exercise.

This critical review was helpful in dispelling the belief that exercise can be detrimental to patients with RA, as it demonstrated that exercise does not increase pain or exacerbate joint destruction. Nevertheless, it was not useful in pinpointing the specific effects of high- vs low-intensity exercise, or in determining which type of exercise is most beneficial. As a reaction to these concerns, 3 additional critical reviews were performed, specifically addressing moderate- and/or high-intensity exercise programs.

In a literature review performed by Hakkinen,[54] only moderate- or high-intensity strengthening exercises were studied. These exercises were effective in increasing muscle strength, and did not cause adverse effects on pain or disease progression in the short term. Only one study in this review followed subjects for a relatively long period of time. The authors therefore could not draw firm conclusions regarding long-term effects on function or disease progression.[54]

A landmark critical review[53] included only studies in which a randomized controlled trial was performed, the exercise program was performed at an intensity of more than 60% of the identified maximal heart rate for at least 20 minutes, exercises were performed at least twice a week, and the exercise program lasted 6 weeks or longer. Six studies met these criteria. The authors concluded that these exercise programs increased aerobic capacity and muscle strength. There were no adverse effects on pain or disease activity; however, the effects on function and radiologic changes were unclear.

A 2005 review[52] included those studies that evaluated the effects of long-term moderate- or high-intensity exercises, and therefore provided greater insight into the effects of these exercises on function and disease progression. The authors concluded that moderate- or high-intensity exercises improve aerobic capacity, muscle strength, functional ability, and psychological well-being. Furthermore, these exercises did not appear to have an adverse effect on disease activity or radiologic evidence of progression of joint damage of the small joints such as the hands and feet. However, damage to large weightbearing joints with preexisting joint damage, especially the joints of the shoulder and subtalar region, could not be ruled out. This issue was addressed in a subsequent clinical trial, in which investigators studied high-intensity exercises with respect to progression of damage in large joints. These investigators concluded that high-intensity exercises were safe, except for a subpopulation of subjects with preexisting extensive joint damage.[55] These conclusions related to the efficacy of aerobic and/or strengthening exercises have been confirmed in several subsequent systematic reviews of exercise and RA. In each of these reviews, the authors concluded that exercise has no adverse effects.[56-60]

For many patients, RA is characterized by flares and remissions. Flares are characterized by an increase in symptoms, usually accompanied by joint inflammation, and can be confirmed with blood tests. Traditionally, the management of a patient with RA who is in a flare has been different from when that patient is in remission. The goals of exercise during a flare were to maintain range of motion and minimize loss of strength without incurring additional damage to joint structures. Most often, this entailed an exercise program consisting of active range of motion exercises, pacing of daily activities, and advice to remain relative sedentary. In a 2000 randomized clinical trial, these assumptions were challenged. In this study, the effects of an intensive exercise program consisting of isokinetic and isometric strength training were evaluated among subjects experiencing a flare. Subjects assigned to the exercise group received strengthening exercises performed at 70% maximum voluntary contraction. They also exercised on a stationary bicycle at 60% maximum heart rate. Exercises were adjusted based on pain tolerance and fatigue. Disease activity over the 24-week follow-up period was similar in both groups, indicating that high-intensity exercise did not have a short-term adverse effect on patients with RA experiencing a flare.[61] Long-term effects, including those on articular structures, were not evaluated.

Several recommendations can be extrapolated from combining our knowledge of exercise physiology with the information acquired from these publications:

- Regular physical activity is not detrimental to patients with RA, and should be incorporated into their lifestyle.

- An individually tailored supervised program of high-intensity exercises can be beneficial to patients with RA, unless there is extensive joint damage in large joints.

- The specific type of high-intensity exercise program that will produce optimal gains in function and pain reduction is unknown; however, it is likely that patients will obtain different benefits from different types of exercises. The optimal exercise program therefore includes both strengthening and endurance type of exercises, and is based on the functional goals and the motivational level of the individual patient.

- While the specific benefits of aquatic exercises for patients with RA are not known, this method of exercising might provide the patient with joint impairments a means of performing high-intensity exercise without unduly affecting pain levels.

- Pain often is increased during or after exercise. Physical therapy interventions to manage pain can improve the patient's tolerance to exercise.

- The exercise program should be modified, based on changes in the medical status and the functional goals of the individual patient, but the intensity of exercise should not be decreased simply because the patient is experiencing a flare.

- When joint damage and/or structural impairments are present, the involved joints should be provided with external support when exercising muscles surrounding these joints. External support can be provided through the use of equipment such as braces, tape, assistive devices, and parallel bars. Changes in the manner in which the specific exercise is being performed to provide more protection to the joint can also be implemented.

- Moderate- or high-intensity exercises involving joints with preexisting extensive joint damage should be avoided.

To investigate the possibility that the optimal type of exercise program varies across patients with different subcategories of RA, a number of studies restricted subjects to a specific RA type. In a 2007 critical review,[62] the authors concluded that exercise is recommended for patients with Sjögren's RA and mild to moderate lupus; however, there was insufficient evidence to recommend a specific type of exercise. Several studies have addressed this issue specifically in relation to ankylosing spondylitis. These studies were performed despite the wide acceptance of the belief that exercise is a key intervention for patients with ankylosing spondylitis. For the most part, these studies focused on different practice settings for administering exercises (home vs clinic) and the addition of other interventions to an exercise program. Three recent papers have been published that critically analyzed this literature.[50,63,64] In the 2 earlier literature reviews, the authors concluded that exercise was effective in reducing pain,[65] improving spinal mobility[50,63] and/or improving overall well-being.[50] In the most recent critical review,[64] the authors simply recommended home exercises and posture training for patients with ankylosing spondylitis. None of the 3 reviews could provide information about the optimal type of exercise, although in the one good-quality randomized controlled trial that was included in these reviews, positive outcomes were experienced among subjects who received functionally based exercises, and exercises designed to address range of motion, strength, and endurance impairments using normal movement patterns and proprioceptive neuromuscular facilitation (PNF) techniques. In this study, subjects were also provided with patient education, including instructions in home-based exercises.[65] Studies published after these 2 earlier critical reviews also reported improvements in spinal mobility,[65,66] function,[66] and work capacity[67] with a comprehensive exercise program.

Outcomes

The clinical course for individuals with RA has been categorized as follows: Irrespective of treatment, approximately 5% to 10% of patients will experience remissions for relatively long lengths of time. Approximately 15% will experience a slow progressive course, with short episodes of flares. For the remaining majority, the disease is unrelenting and progressive, resulting in significant joint deformity.[68]

Historically, for patients who fall into these last 2 categories, long-term outcomes were dismal. The disease process eroded joints and soft tissue, and the reduction in functional levels were marked. Recently, major inroads in the pharmacological management of RA have changed this scenario by preventing disease progression and subsequent joint destruction. As a result, for patients who are successfully managed pharmacologically, daily pain levels are more tolerable, and functional levels decline more slowly. Outcomes from exercise are far less dramatic, but they complement the effects of medication to improve quality of life for patients with RA beyond the levels attained in the absence of an exercise regimen.

Physical Therapy Management

Examination

RA is a systemic disease requiring a detailed physical therapy history and systems review. Interview questions focus on prior medical, surgical, and physical therapy interventions involving the patient's rheumatic condition, and the current status of all aspects of the patient's medical management. Within the review of symptoms, the physical therapist addresses the potential medical comorbidities associated with RA, including cardiac and gastrointestinal conditions, and considers how these conditions might affect physical therapy interventions. A detailed review of the current signs and symptoms, and functional limitations, is also essential.

Radiographs are viewed to determine the extent and nature of joint destruction.

RA is a chronic condition. Most patients with RA become accustomed to living with a certain amount of pain, discomfort, and limitations in functional activities. Therefore, they are most likely to seek help from a physical therapist when they experience a change in status, either from a medical or a psychosocial perspective. In the subjective component of the examination, the therapist therefore identifies the reason the patient is currently seeking physical therapy services and the functional goals that the patient would like to achieve as a result of this episode of care.

The physical therapy inspection includes an evaluation of the patient's posture, joint alignment, and joint appearance. During the palpation examination, swelling, soft tissue tenderness, and muscle spasm are assessed. Passive range of motion, strength, and neurological integrity of all relevant joints also are evaluated. In most cases, this physical examination is conducted from more of a global and functional perspective than that which occurs with many other musculoskeletal conditions. For example, since multiple joints are often involved with patients with RA, and since attaining normal joint range of motion often is not a feasible goal unless there is a specific reason to do otherwise, a range of motion examination of a swollen and painful knee would be described in functional terms rather than with quantitative goniometric measurements. Similarly, since muscle weakness is usually pervasive, it is often impractical to test and describe the results of a manual muscle test for specific muscles or muscle groups. Strength is therefore also often described in functional terms, rather than designating specific grades of muscle strength to each muscle or muscle group.

Additional Considerations

RA is often accompanied by numerous medical conditions in addition to those associated with joint swelling that can be addressed within the context of a physical therapy episode of care. Patients with RA often experience increased levels of fatigue, general malaise, and anemia. It is unclear the extent to which these conditions are a consequence of the effect of pain on activity level, a direct effect of the disease process, or a combination of both. Nevertheless, the physical therapy evaluation addresses endurance and aerobic capacity, and the effects of these evaluation findings on function. Furthermore, patients with RA also often develop osteoporosis.[7,69-73] If risk factors for osteoporosis are present, bone loss can be determined by a physician, and if present, identified by the physical therapist as a condition that affects the physical therapy plan of care. Finally, cardiac conditions are common among patients with RA.[74-76] A detailed history of the patient's cardiac status is performed to identify any known preexisting cardiac conditions

Focus on Function

During the evaluation process, impairments identified during the history and physical examination process are integrated with the patient's functional goals. For example, if a patient reports ankle pain producing difficulty ambulating more than 2 blocks, then the evaluation focuses on identifying the lower extremity impairments that contribute to pain and functional limitations. An intervention program is then designed to address the specific impairments and functional limitations identified, taking into consideration any medical precautions. In the above example, if the ankle pain is caused by joint instability secondary to RA, then the intervention options include strengthening and stabilization exercises, as well as the provision of assistive devices to improve function, patient education addressing self-management of the patient's condition, and bracing to control joint laxity.

Exercise Prescription

The long-term goal of physical therapy for patients with RA is to decrease pain and minimize loss of function throughout the course of the patient's life. Physical therapy intervention often includes patient education, use of physical agents, provision and instruction in the use of assistive and protective devices, and specific prescription of therapeutic exercise. Exercise is a key component to the physical therapy management of the patient with RA. The exercise prescription most often targets joint pain and stiffness through range of motion exercises, muscle weakness through strengthening exercises, and decreased endurance through aerobic conditioning exercises.

Several concerns must be considered before prescribing an exercise program for a patient with RA. The most important of these considerations has to do with the possibility that the disease process produced laxity in the upper cervical ligaments. An estimated 40% to 80% of individuals with RA have radiographic evidence of instability, and 7% to 13% experience signs of neurological deficits.[77] If upper cervical ligament instability is present, then anterior dislocation of the atlas or superior migration of the odontoid process of the axis into the foramen magnum could occur with exercises that produce movement at the upper cervical joints. Movement at these joints is therefore minimized during exercise, as well as with daily activities. For example, exercises involving cervical rotation range of motion, and positions such as prone lying, must be avoided. Often, the use of assistive devices such as bracing can be used to stabilize hypermobile joints during exercise, including those of the upper cervical spine.

Other precautions are specific to the medical status of the individual. Patients with RA are more likely to experience cardiac, pulmonary, gastrointestinal, and kidney complications as a result of this condition. Heart rate, blood pressure, and respiratory rate are therefore monitored before, during, and after exercise. Since many cardiac conditions are not symptomatic, monitoring occurs irrespective of cardiac history. In the presence of known medical comorbidities, such as pulmonary hypertension or heart failure, physical therapy interventions are modified to reflect the medical condition. Exercises are prescribed at an intensity that will not cause harm to the patient; rather the exercise program is administered at a level that addresses both the RA and the comorbid condition. Additionally, many patients with RA have undergone joint replacement surgery. If so, then the precautions specific to that surgery are adhered to. Finally, if there is loss of bone mass consistent with osteoporosis, then strengthening and weightbearing exercises might also be appropriate, depending on the extent to which the patient is at risk for a pathological fracture and the amount of joint destruction.

Often, the patient will experience soreness after performing an intensive exercise program. While there is no research to help determine whether or how postexercise pain or soreness can be used to modify the intensity of the exercise program for a particular patient, one common guideline is that the patient's pain should return to the preexercise level within 2 hours of exercising for the exercise program to be considered safe.[41]

It is important to recognize that an intensive exercise program will be effective only if it is performed on an ongoing basis. After cessation of active training, the improvements in physical function have been shown to disappear.[41,54] To optimize adherence, the exercise regimen is determined taking into consideration the patient's interests and motivational levels. To improve motivation, the patient, with guidance from the physical therapist, might benefit from identifying an optimal time of day to exercise. Ideally, the exercise program is performed after morning stiffness has subsided, but before fatigue has set in. The exercise program is modified based on patient feedback regarding the intensity and duration of soreness following past exercise sessions. Since many of these concerns require ongoing input from a physical therapist, patients with RA who are performing intensive exercises should receive ongoing supervision at a level appropriate for that particular patient. Given adherence to a well-designed home exercise regimen, the patient with RA should benefit with gains in functional levels and a reduction in pain levels.

REFERENCES

1. Bonaiuti D, Shea B, Iovine R, et al. Exercise for preventing and treating osteoporosis in postmenopausal women. *Cochrane Database Syst Rev.* 2002;3:CD000333.
2. National Osteoporosis Foundation. About Osteoporosis. http://www.nof.org/node/51. Accessed February 26, 2012.
3. Burge R, Dawson-Hughes B, Solomon DH, Wong JB, King A, Tosteson A. Incidence and economic burden of osteoporosis related fractures in United States, 2005-2025. *J Bone Miner Res.* 2007;22(3):465-475.
4. Glynn NW, Meilahn EN, Charron M, Anderson SJ, Kuller LH, Cauley JA. Determinants of bone mineral density in older men. *J Bone Miner Res.* 1995;10:1769-1777.
5. Jones G, Nguyen T, Sambrook P, Kelly PJ, Eisman JA. Progressive loss of bone in the femoral neck in elderly people: longitudinal findings from the Dubbo osteoporosis epidemiology study. *BMJ.* 1994;309(6956):691-695.
6. Hedlund LR, Gallagher JC. The effect of age and menopause on bone mineral density of the proximal femur. *J Bone Miner Res.* 1989;4:639-642.
7. Iacono MV. Osteoporosis: a national public health priority. *J Perianesth Nurs.* 2007;22(3):175-183.
8. Cummings SR, Black DM, Nevitt MC, et al. Bone density at various sites for prediction of hip fractures. *Lancet.* 1993;341(8837):72-75.
9. Keen R. Osteoporosis: strategies for prevention and management. *Best Pract Res Clin Rheumatol.* 2007;2:109-122.
10. Melton LJ 3rd, Thamer M, Ray NF, et al. Fractures attributable to osteoporosis: report from the National Osteoporosis Foundation. *J Bone Miner Res.* 1997;12(1):16-23.

11. Wilkins CH, Birge SJ. Prevention of osteoporotic fractures in the elderly. *Am J Med.* 2005;118(11):1190-1195.

12. Kahn R, Fernandez C, Kashifi F, Shedden R, Diggory P. Combined orthogeriatric care in the management of hip fractures: a prospective study. *Ann R Coll Surg Engl.* 2002;84(2):122-124.

13. Birge SJ, Morrow-Howell N, Proctor EK. Hip fracture. *Clin Geriatr Med.* 1994;10:589-609.

14. Cleveland Clinic. Menopause and osteoporosis. http://my.clevelandclinic.org/disorders/Menopause/hic_Menopause_and_Osteoporosis.aspx. Accessed March 1, 2012.

15. MacKelvie KJ, Khan KM, Petit MA Janssen PA, McKay HA. A school-based exercise intervention elicits substantial bone health benefits: a 2-year randomized controlled trial in girls. *Pediatrics.* 2003;112(6 Pt 1):e447.

16. MacKelvie KJ, Petit MA, Khan KM, Beck TJ, McKay HA. Bone mass and structure are enhanced following a 2-year randomized controlled trial of exercise in prepubescent boys. *Bone.* 2004;34:755-764.

17. Nichols DL, Sanborn CF, Love AM. Resistance training and bone mineral density in adolescent females. *J Pediatr.* 2001;139:494-500.

18. Bassey EJ, Rothwell MC, Littlewood JJ, Pye DW. Pre- and post-menopausal women have different bone mineral density responses to the same high-impact exercise. *J Bone Miner Res.* 1998;13:1793-1796.

19. Kaplan B, Hirsch M. Current approach to fracture prevention in postmenopausal osteoporosis. *Clin Exp Obstet Gynecol.* 2004;31(4):251-255.

20. Gallacher SJ, Dixon T. Impact of treatments for postmenopausal osteoporosis (biophosphonates, parathyroid hormone, strontium ranelate, and denosumab) on bone quality: a systematic review. *Calcif Tissue Int.* 2010;87(6):469-484.

21. Kemmler W, Weineck J, Kalender WA, Engelke K. The effect of habitual physical activity, non-athletic exercise, muscle strength, and VO_{2max} on bone mineral density is rather low in early postmenopausal osteopenic women. *J Musculoskel Neuron Interact.* 2004;4:325-334.

22. Welsh L, Rutherford OM. Hip bone mineral density is improved by high-impact aerobic exercise in postmenopausal women and men over 50 years. *Eur J Appl Physiol Occup Physiol.* 1996;74:511-517.

23. Madalozzo GF, Snow CM. High intensity resistance training: effects on bone in older men and women. *Calcif Tissue Int.* 2000;66(6):399-404.

24. Dalsky GP, Stocke KS, Ehsani AA, Slatopolsky E, Lee WC, Birge SJ Jr. Weight-bearing exercise training and lumbar bone mineral content in postmenopausal women. *Ann Intern Med.* 1988;108:824-828.

25. Winters KM, Snow CM. Detraining reverses positive effects of exercise on the musculoskeletal system in premenopausal women. *J Bone Miner Res.* 2000;15:2495-2503.

26. Wolff I, van Croonenborg JJ, Kemper HC, Kostense PJ, Twisk JW. The effect of exercise training programs on bone mass: a meta-analysis of published controlled trials in pre- and postmenopausal women. *Osteoporosis Int.* 1999;9:1-12.

27. Howe TE, Shea B, Dawson LJ, et al. Exercise for preventing and treating osteoporosis in postmenopausal women. *Cochrane Database of Syst Rev.* 2011;7.:CD000333.

28. Kemmler W, Haberle L, von Stengal S. Effects of exercise on fracture reduction in older adults: a systematic review and meta-analysis. *Osteoporosis Int.* 2013;24(7):1937-1950.

29. Fletcher JA. Canadian Academy of Sport and Exercise Medicine Position Statement: Osteoporosis and exercise. *Clin J Sport Med.* 2013;23(5):333-338.

30. Body J-J, Bergmann P, Boonen S, et al. Non-pharmacological management of osteoporosis: a consensus of the Belgian Bone Club. *Osteoporosis Int.* 2011;22:2769-2788.

31. Ryan SD, Fried LP. The impact of kyphosis on daily functioning. *J Am Geriatr Soc.* 1997;45(12):1479-1486.

32. Renno ACM. Effects of an exercise program on respiratory function, posture and on quality of life in osteoporotic women: a pilot study. *Physiotherapy.* 2005;91(2):113-118.

33. Sinaki M, Brey RH, Hughes CA, Larson DR, Kaufman KR. Significant reduction in risk of falls and back pain in osteoporotic-kyphotic women through a spinal proprioceptive extension exercise dynamic (SPEED) program. *Mayo Clin Proc.* 2005;80:849-855.

34. Edmond SL, Kiel DP, Samelson EJ, Kelly-Hayes M, Felson DT. Vertebral deformity, back symptoms, and functional limitations among older women: the Framingham Study. *Osteoporosis Int.* 2005;16:1086-1095.

35. Yelnik A, Bonan I. Clinical tools for assessing balance disorders. *Neurophysiol Clin.* 2008;38(6):439-445.

36. Edmond SL. *Joint Mobilization/Manipulation Extremity and Spinal Techniques.* 2nd ed. St. Louis, MO: Mosby Elsevier; 2006.

37. Chilibeck PD, Vatanparast H, Cornish SM, et al. Evidence-based risk assessment and recommendations for physical activity: arthritis, osteoporosis, and low back pain. *Appcl Physio Nutr Metab.* 2011;36 Suppl 1:S49-79.

38. Arthritis Foundation. Who gets rheumatoid arthritis? http://www.arthritis.org/who-gets-rheumatoid-arthritis.php. Accessed February 26, 2012.

39. Burton W, Morrison A, Maclean R, Ruderman E. Systematic review of studies of productivity loss due to rheumatoid arthritis. *Occup Med (Lond).* 2006;56(1):18-27.

40. Goldman L, Ausiello D, eds. *Cecil Medicine.* 23rd ed. Philadelphia, PA: Saunders Elsevier; 2008.

41. Hakkinen A. Effectiveness and safety of strength training in rheumatoid arthritis. *Curr Opin Rheumatol.* 2004;16:132-137.

42. Roubenoff R, Roubenoff RA, Cannon JG, et al. Rheumatoid cachexia: cytokine-driven hypermetabolism accompanying reduced body cell mass in chronic inflammation. *J Clin Invest.* 1994;93:2379-2386.

43. Arnett FC, Edworthy SM, Bloch DA, et al. The American Rheumatism Association 1987 revised criteria for the classification of rheumatoid arthritis. *Arthritis Rheum.* 1988;31:315-324.

44. American College of Rheumatology. Criteria for the classification of systemic sclerosis (scleroderma). *MedicalCRITERIA.com.* http://www.medicalcriteria.com/criteria/reu_scleroderma.htm. Accessed February, 26, 2012.

45. Lupus Foundation of America. What is lupus? http://www.lupus.org/webmodules/webarticlesnet/templates/new_learnunderstanding.aspx?articleid=2232&zoneid=523. Accessed February 26, 2012.

46. The Henry Spink Foundation. Scleroderma fact sheet. http://www.henryspink.org/scleroderma.htm. Accessed February 26.2012.

47. Komocsi A, Vorobcsuk A, Faludi R, et al. The impact of cardiopulmonary manifestations on the mortality of SSc: a systematic review and meta-analysis of observational studies. *Rheumatology (Oxford).* 2010;51(6):1027-1036.

48. Centers for Disease Control and Prevention. Gout. http://www.cdc.gov/arthritis/basics/gout.htm. Accessed October 13, 2012.

49. U.S. National Library of Medicine. PubMed Health. Gout. http://www.ncbi.nlm.nih.gov/pubmedhealth/PMH0001459. Accessed October 13, 2012.

50. Dagfinrud H, Kvien TK, Hagen KB. Physiotherapy interventions for ankylosing spondylitis. *Cochrane Database Syst Rev.* 2004;4:CD002822.

51. Ottawa Panel. Ottawa Panel evidence-based clinical practice guidelines for therapeutic exercises in the management of rheumatoid arthritis in adults. *Phys Ther.* 2004;84(10):934-972.

52. de Jong Z, Vliet Vlieland TPM. Safety of exercise in patients with rheumatoid arthritis. *Curr Opin Rheum.* 2005;17(2):177-182.

53. Van den Ende CHM, Vliet Vlieland TP, Munneke M, Hazes JM. WITHDRAWN: Dynamic exercise therapy for treating rheumatoid arthritis. *Cochrane Database Syst Rev.* 2008;1:CD000322.

54. Häkkinen A, Mälkiä E, Häkkinen K, et al. Effects of detraining on neuromuscular function in patients with inflammatory arthritis. *Br J Rheumatol.* 1997;36(10):1075-1081.

55. Munneke M, de Jong Z, Zwinderman AH, et al. Effect of a high-intensity weight-bearing exercise program on radiologic damage progression of the large joints in subgroups of patients with rheumatoid arthritis. *Arthritis Rheum.* 2005;53(3):410-417.

56. Oldfield V, Felson DT. Exercise therapy and orthotic devices in rheumatoid arthritis; evidence-based review. *Curr Opin Rheumatol.* 2008;20(3):353-359.

57. Cairns AP, McVeigh JG. A systematic review of the effects of dynamic exercise in rheumatoid arthritis. *Rheumatol Int.* 2009;30(2):147-158.

58. Hurkmans E, van der Giesen FJ, Vliet Vlieland TP, Schoones J, Van den Ende EC. Dynamic exercise programs (aerobic capacity and/or muscle strength training) in patients with rheumatoid arthritis. *Cochrane Database Syst Rev.* 2009;4:CD006853.

59. Baillet A, Zeboulon N, Gossec L, et al. Efficacy of cardiorespiratory aerobic exercise in rheumatoid arthritis: meta-analysis of randomized controlled trials. *Arthritis Care Res.* 2010;62(7):984-992.

60. Scarvell J, Elkins MR. Aerobic exercise is beneficial for people with rheumatoid arthritis. *Br J Sports Med.* 2011;45(12):1008-1009.

61. Van den Ende CH, Breedveld FC, le Cessie S, et al. Effect of intensive exercise on patients with active rheumatoid arthritis: a randomized clinical trial. *Ann Rheum Dis.* 2000;59(8):615-621.

62. Strombeck B, Jacobsson LTH. The role of exercise in the rehabilitation of patients with systemic lupus erythematosus and patients with primary Sjögren's syndrome. *Curr Opin Rheumatol.* 2007;19:197-203.

63. Ammer K. Physiotherapy in seronegative spondylarthropathies. A systematic review. *Eur J Phys Med Rehabil.* 1997;7:114-119.

64. Elyan M, Kahn MA. Does physical therapy still have a place in the treatment of ankylosing spondylitis? *Curr Opin Rheumatol.* 2008;20(3):282-286.

65. Kraag G, Stokes B, Groh J, Helewa A, Goldsmith CH. The effects of comprehensive home physiotherapy and supervision on patients with ankylosing spondylitis: an 8-month followup. *J Rheumatol.* 1994;21(2):261-263.

66. Fernández-de-las-Peñas C, Alonso-Blanco C, Alguacil-Diego IM, Miangolarra-Page JC. One-year follow-up of two exercise interventions for the management of patients with ankylosing spondylitis: a randomized controlled trial. *Am J Phys Med Rehabil.* 2006;85:559-567.

67. Ince G, Sarpel T, Durgun B, Erdogan S. Effects of a multimodal exercise program for people with ankylosing spondylitis. *Phys Ther.* 2006;86(7):924-935.

68. WebMD. Rheumatoid arthritis progression. http://www.webmd.com/rheumatoid-arthritis/guide/ra-progression. Reviewed by David Zelman February 7, 2012. Accessed February 26, 2012.

69. Hansen M, Florescu A, Stoltenberg M, et al. Bone loss in rheumatoid arthritis influence of disease activity, duration of the disease, functional capacity and corticosteroid treatment. *Scand J Rheumatol.* 1996;25(6):367-376.

70. Haugeberg G, Ørstavik RE, Uhlig T, Falch JA, Halse JI, Kvien TK. Bone loss in patients with rheumatoid arthritis: results from a population-based cohort of 366 patients followed up for two years. *Arthritis Rheum.* 2002;46(7):1720-1728.

71. Huusko TM, Korpela M, Karppi P, Kautiainen H, Sulkava R. Threefold increased risk of hip fractures with rheumatoid arthritis in central Finland. *Ann Rheum Dis.* 2001;60:521-522.

72. Kroger H, Honkanen R, Saarikoski S, Alhava E. Decreased axial bone mineral density in perimenopausal women with rheumatoid arthritis—a population based study. *Ann Rheum Dis.* 1994;53:18-23.

73. Sambrook PN, Eisman JA, Champion GD, Yeates MG, Pocock NA, Eberl S. Determinants of axial bone loss in rheumatoid arthritis. *Arthritis Rheum.* 1987;30(7):721-728.

74. Bacon PA, Townend JN. Nails in the coffin: increasing evidence for the role of rheumatic disease in the cardiovascular mortality of rheumatoid arthritis. *Arthritis Rheum.* 2001;44:2707-2710.

75. del Rincón ID, Williams K, Stern MP, Freeman GL, Escalante A. High incidence of cardiovascular events in a rheumatoid arthritis cohort not explained by traditional cardiac risk factors. *Arthritis Rheum.* 2001;44(12):2737-2745.

76. Turesson C, Matteson EL. Cardiovascular risk factors, fitness and physical activity in rheumatic diseases. *Curr Opin Rheumatol.* 2007;19:190-196.

77. Dryer SJ, Boden SD. Natural history of rheumatoid arthritis of the cervical spine. *Clin Orthop Rel Res.* 1999;366:98-106.

CASE STUDY 11-1

Susan L. Edmond, PT, DSc, OCS

EXAMINATION

History

Current Condition/Chief Complaint

Ms. Icon was a 43-year-old female who had referred herself to physical therapy for treatment of diffuse musculoskeletal pain and limitations in functional activities secondary to fibromyalgia. Ms. Icon recently experienced an exacerbation of pain, primarily in her shoulders and neck. Ms. Icon also reported systemic fatigue. Ms. Icon's goal was to experience less pain and fatigue with her current activity level.

Clinician Comment *Fibromyalgia is a chronic condition that is characterized by dull constant pain in multiple muscles, ligaments and tendons located on both sides of the body, above and below the waist. Other symptoms include systemic fatigue and an inability to think clearly. This latter symptom is commonly called* brain fog. *Fibromyalgia is characterized by a lack of stage 4, restorative sleep. It is believed that this contributes to the fatigue and brain fog associated with this condition.[1] An estimated 2% of the population of the United States is affected by fibromyalgia. The cause or causes of fibromyalgia are unknown; however, risk factors include female sex, increasing age, a family history of fibromyalgia, sleep disorders and rheumatic disease.*

Social History/Environment

Ms. Icon lived with her husband and 2 children aged 10 and 15 years. English was her primary language. She was employed as a 2nd grade public school teacher. Her husband sustained a spinal cord injury 20 years ago, and has been a wheelchair user since then. Ms. Icon was therefore responsible for most housekeeping activities.

Ms. Icon lived in a one-story house in a residential neighborhood. In the past, she had enjoyed taking walks on dirt paths near her home, but states that she has not done so in a while due to schedule constraints.

Social/Health Habits

Nonsmoker, social drinker

Medical/Surgical History

Ms. Icon reported that she began experiencing insidious onset of dull, constant multiple joint pain above and below the waist and systemic fatigue 15 years ago, approximately 3 months after giving birth to her first child. She first attributed these symptoms to the increase in activities associated with caring for an infant, but sought medical attention about 2 months after the onset of symptoms when they did not subside. When first evaluated for these symptoms, her general practitioner told her that there was "nothing physically wrong with her." When Ms. Icon continued to seek a medical diagnosis and treatment, she was referred to a psychologist for counseling. Counseling did not reveal a psychological cause for her physical pain or fatigue, nor did it produce a change in her symptoms. Ms. Icon then became discouraged and decided not to pursue additional medical or psychological management.

Five years later, Ms. Icon experienced an exacerbation of symptoms, and returned to her general practitioner. He referred Ms. Icon to a rheumatologist, who diagnosed her with fibromyalgia. At that time, she was told that there was no effective treatment for fibromyalgia.

Otherwise, medical history was significant for 2 normal (vaginal) deliveries.

Clinician Comment *Ms. Icon's diagnosis was based in part on her report of constant bilateral multiple joint pain and systemic fatigue. Atypical of fibromyalgia, she did not report difficulty with cognition.*

Reported Functional Status

Ms. Icon reported that she was able to perform all necessary ADL including instrumental ADL. Specifically, she was able to teach her 2nd grade class, but reports that she was extremely fatigued by the end of the day. She was able to shop for her family and perform housecleaning activities, but reported an increase in pain and fatigue afterward, especially when she tried to perform too many activities in a short period of time. Pain was located primarily in her neck and both shoulders and to a lesser extent in her low back and knees. All symptoms diminished following 2 to 3 hours of rest.

Medications

Over the counter ibuprofen as needed.

Other Clinical Tests

No other medical tests were performed.

Clinician Comment *Since Ms. Icon had referred herself to physical therapy, it was especially important to consider whether to "treat," "refer and treat," or "refer." Ms. Icon presented with signs and symptoms of insidious onset of neck and bilateral shoulder pain consistent with a known diagnosis of fibromyalgia. Even though she was experiencing an exacerbation of symptoms, she had been diagnosed with fibromyalgia prior to beginning physical therapy. The subjective report was consistent with the signs and symptoms associated with this medical diagnosis. Based on the information provided at this point in the examination, there were no "red flags."*

The appropriate course of action was, therefore, to continue with the examination with the intent to "treat"; nevertheless, it was important to recognize that new medications to manage fibromyalgia had been developed since she last saw a physician for her condition. Ms. Icon might, therefore, benefit from a referral to a physician for pharmacological management.

Systems Review

Cardiovascular/Pulmonary

Seated, resting:
Heart rate: 73 bpm
Blood pressure: 120/85 mm Hg
Respiration rate: 12 breaths per minute

Integumentary

No discolorations or breaks in the integument were observed.

Musculoskeletal

Strength and AROM grossly assessed in the upper extremities and lower extremities and the spine: All were within functional limits, except for moderate limitations in bilateral shoulder elevation and neck lateral movements.
Height: 5'4"
Weight: 138 pounds (BMI 23.7)

Neuromuscular

No impairments in balance, gait, locomotion, transfers or transitions were observed.

Communication, Affect, Cognition, Language and Learning Style

Ms. Icon was alert and oriented to person, place and time. She engaged in conversation easily, followed all commands, and demonstrated motivation to adhere to a home program.

Clinician Comment *The systems review was unremarkable. This case was an example of a patient with a systemic condition. As such, it is likely that Ms. Icon had multiple impairments throughout her musculoskeletal system, however a complete musculoskeletal examination was not reasonable. In this case, the patient reported functional limitations primarily affecting 2 domains: systemic fatigue and pain in the neck and shoulders. While a screening examination of the entire musculoskeletal system was performed, the physical examination focused on these 2 concerns.*

Her pain and posture needed further examination. Tests and measures for her neck and shoulder range of motion, joint integrity and mobility, and muscle performance needed to be included. Finally, her aerobic capacity/endurance needed to be established.

Tests and Measures

Pain

She described her pain as a diffuse ache located in her neck and both glenohumeral joints. Any activity increased symptoms, including carrying packages and housework. Symptoms returned to baseline within 2 to 3 hours. Rest decreased symptoms. Pain at rest was reported to be a 2 on a visual analog scale, and increased to a 6 with activities of daily living, especially any movements into shoulder elevation such as reaching for objects on top shelves.

Pain was reproduced with palpation of the cervical paraspinals, upper trapezeii, scalenes, and sternocleidomastoid muscles. Pressure algometry revealed tenderness in 13 of 18 tender points.

In addition, during the palpation examination, no edema or effusion was noted in neck or shoulders. Bilateral spasms were palpable and were accompanied by reproduction of pain in cervical paraspinals, upper trapezeii, scalenes, and sternocleidomastoid muscles.

Clinician Comment *Fibromyalgia is characterized by the presence of tender points—specific anatomical locations where slight pressure causes pain. Eighteen tender points have been identified. The presence of pain with pressure on at least 11 of these 18 tender points using a pressure algometer is indicative of fibromyalgia. These 18 tender points are the back of the head, between the scapulae, the top of the shoulders, the front sides of the neck, the upper chest, the lateral elbow area, the upper hips, the sides of the hips, and the inner knees.[2] Ms. Icon met this criterion for diagnosing fibromyalgia syndrome.*

Posture

Patient demonstrates slight forward head.

Range of Motion (Including Muscle Length)

Neck Passive Range of Motion

Forward Bending	0 to 35	
	Firm end feel	
	Pain with overpressure*	
Backward Bending	WNL	
	LEFT	**RIGHT**
Side Bending	0 to 30	0 to 30
	Firm end feel	Firm end feel
	Pain with overpressure*	Pain with overpressure*
Rotation	0 to 50	0 to 50
	Firm end feel	Firm end feel
	Pain with overpressure*	Pain with overpressure*

*"Pain" is described by the patient as a stretching sensation.

Shoulder Passive Range of Motion

	LEFT	**RIGHT**
Flexion	0 to 150	0 to 155
	Firm end feel	Firm end feel
	Pain with resistance**	Pain with resistance**
Extension	WNL	WNL
Abduction	0 to 130	0 to 135
	Firm end feel	Firm end feel
	Pain with resistance**	Pain with resistance**
Lateral Rotation	0 to 60	0 to 60
	Firm end feel	Firm end feel
	Pain with overpressure*	Pain with overpressure*
Medial Rotation	WNL	WNL
Horizontal Adduction	WNL	WNL

*"Pain" is described by the patient as a stretching sensation.
**"Pain" is described by the patient as a sharp.

Special Tests

Shoulders

- Shoulder painful arc: Negative bilaterally within available range
- Apley scratch test: Decreased lateral rotation bilaterally

Clinician Comment *Ms Icon showed decreased passive range of motion in her neck for the ranges of forward bending, and bilateral side bending and rotation. Her shoulders had a range of motion deficit for passive range of motion in flexion, abduction and lateral rotation.*

Joint Integrity and Mobility

Cervical Spine

Occiput–C2 distraction: hypomobile, pain free
C2–T2 P-A Glides: WNL, pain free

Glenohumeral Joints

	LEFT	RIGHT
Distraction	Hypomobile, pain free	Hypomobile, pain free
Anterior Glide	Hypomobile, painful	Hypomobile, painful
Posterior Glide	Hypomobile, painful	Hypomobile, painful
Inferior Glide	Hypomobile, painful	Hypomobile, painful
Acromioclavicular Joints	WNL	WNL
Sternoclavicular Joints	WNL	WNL
Scapulothoracic Joints	WNL	WNL

Special Tests

Neck
- Vertebral artery test: Negative bilaterally
- Alar ligament test: Negative bilaterally

Shoulder
- Anterior apprehension test: Negative bilaterally
- Load and shift maneuver: Negative bilaterally
- Sulcus test: Negative bilaterally
- Hawkins test: Negative bilaterally
- Crank test: Negative bilaterally

Clinician Comment *On passive intervertebral movement testing, Ms. Icon shows decreased motion at her suboccipital joints. She also shows a decrease in all glenohumeral accessory joint motions.*

Muscle Performance (Including Strength, Power, and Endurance)

Manual Muscle Testing Neck

	LEFT	RIGHT
Capital Extension	N	N
Cervical Extension	N	N
Combined Neck Extension	N	N
Capital Flexion	N	N
Cervical Flexion	N	N
Cervical Rotation	N	N

N = Normal, 5/5.

Manual Muscle Testing Shoulders

	LEFT	RIGHT
Scapular Musculature	N	N
Flexion	G	G
Extension	N	N
Abduction	G	G
Horizontal Abduction	N	N
Horizontal Adduction	N	N
Lateral Rotation	G	G
Medial Rotation	N	N

N = Normal, 5/5; G = Good, 4/5.

Resisted Isometric Testing Neck

Forward Bending	Strong, pain free	
Backward Bending	Strong, painful	
	LEFT	**RIGHT**
Side Bending	Strong, painful	Strong, painful
Rotation	Strong, painful	Strong, painful

Resisted Isometric Testing Shoulders

	LEFT	RIGHT
Flexion	Strong, pain free	Strong, pain free
Extension	Strong, pain free	Strong, pain free
Abduction	Strong, pain free	Strong, pain free
Adduction	Strong, pain free	Strong, pain free
Lateral Rotation	Strong, pain free	Strong, pain free
Medial Rotation	Strong, pain free	Strong, pain free
Horizontal Abduction	Strong, pain free	Strong, pain free
Horizontal Adduction	Strong, pain free	Strong, pain free

Special Tests

Shoulder/Scapula
- Drop arm test: Negative bilaterally
- Supraspinatus test: Negative bilaterally
- Yergason's test: Negative bilaterally
- Speed's test: Negative bilaterally
- Lateral scapular slide test: Increased scapular movement bilaterally

Clinician Comment *Ms. Icon showed decreased strength in bilateral shoulder flexion, abduction and lateral rotation.*

Cranial and Peripheral Nerve Integrity

- Upper Quarter Myotomal Screen: WNL

Special Tests

- Slump Test: Negative
- Spurling's test: Negative bilaterally

Sensory Integrity

- WNL bilateral upper extremities

Reflex Integrity

- WNL Biceps, Brachioradialis and Triceps reflexes

Aerobic Capacity/Endurance

- 6-Minute Walk Test: 430 meters. Patient reported mild fatigue after testing.

Clinician Comment *Tests of endurance are commonly used to quantify impairments in patients with several types of conditions, including cardiac and pulmonary disease, neuromuscular disorders and arthritis. To date, no tests of endurance have been validated on patients with fibromyalgia. The 6-Minute Walk Test was used because it is a functional test that quantifies limitations in endurance, and because data on healthy subjects are available for comparison. Ms. Icon should have been able to walk 618 meters during the 6-Minute Walk Test.[3] Her performance is approximately 70% of this expected value and indicates decreased walking tolerance.*

The physical examination revealed signs and symptoms consistent with musculoskeletal pain. No "red flags" had been identified. There was therefore no need for referral. If symptoms did not subside with physical therapy management, or if, upon questioning, the patient expressed interest in being evaluated for pharmacological treatment, then a referral to a physician would be indicated.

This patient appeared to have symptoms consistent with fibromyalgia (tender points with associated pain and fatigue), but also had impairments that were consistent with localized musculoskeletal pain. Specifically, Ms. Icon had decreased range of motion and accessory motion, and decreased strength in the glenohumeral joint, which is consistent with adhesive capsulitis. She also had tenderness, spasm and decreased range of motion in her cervical paraspinal muscles. These latter findings, in conjunction with pain with resisted isometric testing, are indicative of cervical pain of muscular origin. These 2 musculoskeletal disorders could have arisen as a result of the fibromyalgia. Conversely, they could have developed independent of her primary diagnosis, possibly in part because of Ms. Icon's impaired posture.

Based on the patient's diagnosis, reported symptomatology, and tissue irritability, the therapist determined that the patient should be able to tolerate a moderately vigorous physical therapy program.

EVALUATION

Diagnosis

Practice Pattern

Ms. Icon was a 43-year-old female second grade teacher with a known medical diagnosis of fibromyalgia. Symptoms had been present for 15 years. At the time of her initial examination, she reported fatigue with activities of daily living and a recent increase neck and bilateral shoulder pain. Symptoms could have been attributable directly to fibromyalgia; however this patient also demonstrated decreased range of motion and accessory motion, and strength in both shoulders, which is also consistent with mild adhesive capsulitis. She also presented with tenderness, spasm and decreased range of motion in her cervical paraspinal muscles, consistent with a muscle strain. Symptoms of fibromyalgia with resultant decrease in activity level and impaired posture were likely causes of neck pain and shoulder adhesive capsulitis. Suboccipital joint hypomobility likely contributed to impaired posture.

These findings placed her in the musculoskeletal practice pattern of the following:

- Pattern B: Impaired posture
- Pattern D: Impaired joint mobility, motor function, muscle performance and range of motion associated with connective tissue dysfunction
- Pattern E: Impaired joint mobility, motor function, muscle performance and range of motion associated with localized inflammation

International Classification of Functioning, Disability, and Health Model

See ICF Model on p 460.

Prognosis

Prognosis was good for reducing the signs and symptoms of fibromyalgia and musculoskeletal symptoms in the neck and shoulder. Given the patient's physical findings, lack of comorbidities and excellent motivation, it was anticipated that she would benefit from physical therapy.

Plan of Care

Intervention

- Patient education regarding correct posture and strategies to maintain correct posture with activities of daily living.
- Patient education regarding pacing oneself with daily activities
- Home exercise instruction: stretching, strengthening and aerobic exercises
- Passive range of motion to neck and bilateral shoulders

ICF Model of Disablement for Ms. Icon

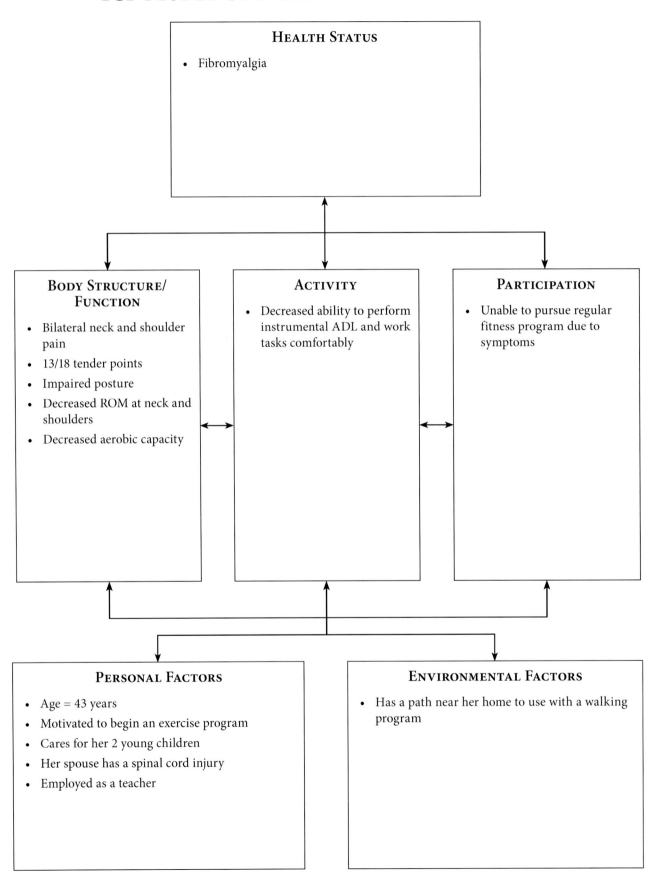

Health Status

- Fibromyalgia

Body Structure/ Function

- Bilateral neck and shoulder pain
- 13/18 tender points
- Impaired posture
- Decreased ROM at neck and shoulders
- Decreased aerobic capacity

Activity

- Decreased ability to perform instrumental ADL and work tasks comfortably

Participation

- Unable to pursue regular fitness program due to symptoms

Personal Factors

- Age = 43 years
- Motivated to begin an exercise program
- Cares for her 2 young children
- Her spouse has a spinal cord injury
- Employed as a teacher

Environmental Factors

- Has a path near her home to use with a walking program

- Bilateral shoulder strengthening exercises
- Joint mobilization/manipulation to upper cervical spine and bilateral glenohumeral joints.
- Soft tissue mobilization to affected cervical musculature

Clinician Comment *The physical therapist hypothesized that by addressing all of the patient's impairments in conjunction with a program for managing fibromyalgia, the patient's pain would diminish and she would experience an improvement in her functional levels. This hypothesis was corroborated by a critical review stating that the best evidence supports treating patients with adhesive capsulitis with stretching and stretching exercises, and with joint mobilization/manipulation[4]; and a different critical review in which the authors supported managing patients with nonspecific neck pain with exercise and manual therapy.[5]*

Treatment of fibromyalgia consists of instruction in techniques to get adequate sleep, reduce stress, and pace oneself with daily activities. Exercise is also an integral component of a treatment plan for fibromyalgia.[1,6]

Several recent critical reviews have addressed the efficacy of exercise in the treatment of fibromyalgia. There is strong evidence supporting the implementation of an aerobic exercise program to manage symptoms and improve physical function,[7-10] as well as for performing strengthening exercise to achieve these same objectives.[8-10] The evidence suggests that aerobic exercises are superior to resistance exercises, when both are performed at moderate to high intensity levels,[10] although optimal outcomes are likely achieved when different types of exercises are included in an exercise program.[9]

Proposed Frequency and Duration of Physical Therapy Visits

This patient was scheduled for physical therapy 3 times per week for 3 weeks, and then 2 times per week for 3 weeks for a total of 15 visits. The expected time frame to meet all goals was therefore 6 weeks.

Anticipated Goals

1. Patient to demonstrate good understanding of self-management of fibromyalgia (1 week).

2. Patient to demonstrate correct posture and awareness of mechanisms to maintain appropriate posture with daily activities (2 weeks).

3. Patient to be independent with a home exercise program and demonstrate knowledge of appropriate progression of exercise program following discharge from physical therapy (3 weeks).

4. Patient to experience a decrease in neck and bilateral shoulder pain to a 1 on a 1-10 visual analog scale at rest, and a 4 with activity on a visual analog scale (3 weeks).

5. Neck and bilateral shoulder range of motion to be WNL (4 weeks).

6. Neck and bilateral shoulder accessory motion to be WNL (4 weeks).

7. Bilateral shoulder strength to be WNL (5 weeks).

8. Patient to experience a decrease in neck and bilateral shoulder pain to a 0 on a 1 to 10 visual analog scale at rest, and a 2 with activity on a visual analog scale (5 weeks).

9. Patient to walk 618 meters during the 6-Minute Walk Test (6 weeks).

10. Patient to experience no fatigue with current activity level (6 weeks).

Expected Outcome (6 weeks)

1. Patient will report minimal pain and fatigue and report unrestricted ADL, instrumental ADL, and work tasks.

2. Patient to be independent managing her fibromyalgia symptoms.

Discharge Plan

Patient to continue with home exercise program and self-measures. Patient to return to physical therapy if symptoms return or if other symptoms attributable to fibromyalgia arise.

INTERVENTION

Coordination, Communication, and Documentation

Document all aspects of Ms. Icon's physical therapy care in her outpatient physical therapy record. Provide patient with written instructions describing each of her home exercises.

Patient-/Client-Related Instruction

Instruct in home exercise program. Provide patient education regarding correct posture and benefits of maintaining correct posture with activities of daily living. Provide patient education regarding need to pace self with activities, and to the need to continue with home exercise program once discharged from physical therapy.

Procedural Interventions

Therapeutic Exercise

Aerobic Capacity/Endurance Conditioning or Reconditioning

Mode
Walking on a dirt pathway near her home (home exercise).
Intensity
During each walk, the patient maintains a heart rate of 70% of her maximum heart rate (which is approximately 110 beats per minute). As the patient becomes more conditioned, she should be able to walk greater distances while maintaining 70% of her maximum heart rate.

Duration

Begin with 10 minutes and gradually increase to 30 minutes.

Frequency

Begin with 3 times per day, but as duration increases, decrease frequency to 2 then 1 time per day.

Description of the Intervention

Before beginning the walking exercise, the patient spends 5 minutes gradually increasing her walking speed. She spends 5 minutes gradually decreasing her walking speed after ending her walking exercise.

Progression for Duration

- Week 1 and 2: The patient walks for 10 minutes.

- Week 3 and 4: The patient walks for 20 minutes during 1 walk and for 10 minutes during the 2nd walk.

- Week 5 and 6, and after discharge: The patient walks for 30 minutes.

Progression for Frequency:

- Week 1 and 2: The patient walks 3 times per day: once in the morning, once in the afternoon, and once in the evening.

- Week 3 and 4: The patient walks 2 times per day: once in the morning and once in the evening.

- Week 5 and 6, and after discharge: The patient walks 1 time per day.

Flexibility Exercises

Mode

Active/passive movements for neck (home exercise).

Intensity

The patient moves her neck until she feels a stretch in her neck muscles.

Duration

Initially, the patient holds the stretch for 15 seconds. Over the course of approximately 1 week, the patient increases the hold time to 30 seconds.

Frequency

The patient performs this exercise 5 times, 3 times per day.

Description of the Intervention

The patient positions herself on her back with her head on a pillow that is shallower (scooped out) in the center than at the edges. The patient rolls her head to the left side until she feels a stretch in her neck muscles, and holds this position. The patient repeats this exercise on the right side.

Mode

Active/passive movements for neck (home exercise)

Intensity

The patient moves her neck until she feels a stretch in her neck muscles.

Duration

Initially, the patient holds the stretch for 15 seconds. Over the course of approximately 1 week, the patient increases the hold time to 30 seconds.

Frequency

The patient performs this exercise 5 times, 3 times per day.

Description of the Intervention

The patient grasps the back and sides of her lower neck with both hands. While holding the lower part of her neck still, the patient bends her head forward slightly.

Mode

Active/passive movements, shoulder reaching (home exercise)

Intensity

The patient moves her arms until she feels a stretch in her shoulder.

Duration

The patient initially holds the stretch for 15 seconds. Over the course of approximately 1 week, the patient increases the hold time to 30 seconds.

Frequency

The patient performs this exercise 5 times, 3 times per day.

Description of the Intervention

The patient positions herself on her back holding onto a dowel with her arms by her side and her palms facing upward shoulder-width apart. With her elbows straight, the patient moves the dowel up in front of her and then tries to keep moving it over her head until she feels a stretch in her shoulders. The patient holds this position. Afterward, the patient moves the dowel as high in front of her as she can, and then moves it down toward her left side until she feels a stretch in her shoulder. The patient holds this position. The patient repeats this exercise on the right side. Finally, the patient brings her arms back down to her side, still holding onto the dowel. She then bends her elbows to 90 degrees, and holding her elbows by her side, moves her hands out away from her trunk to the left. The patient holds this position. The patient repeats this exercise on the right side.

Strengthening Exercise

Mode

Resistive movements of the shoulder

Intensity

The patient repeats this exercise until she feels fatigue in her shoulder muscles or until the exercise becomes fairly difficult to perform, whichever happens first, up to 3 sets of 10 repetitions.

Duration

About 5 minutes.

Frequency

Once a day.

Description of the intervention

The patient stands with her back against the wall with arms at her side, holding a 5-pound weight with her left hand. The patient slowly brings her arm up and forward, and back down to her side. The patient repeats this exercise on the right side.

Mode

Resisted movements of the shoulder.

Intensity

The patient repeats this exercise until she feels fatigue in her shoulder muscles or until the exercise becomes fairly difficult to perform, whichever happens first, up to 3 sets of 10 repetitions.

Duration

About 5 minutes.

Frequency

Once a day.

Description of the Intervention

The patient stands with her back against the wall with her arms at her side, holding a 5-pound weight with her left hand. The patient slowly brings her arm up and out to the side, and back down to her side, keeping her palms up. The patient repeats this exercise on the right side.

Mode

Resisted movements of the shoulder

Intensity

The patient repeats this exercise until she feels fatigue in her shoulder muscles or until the exercise becomes fairly difficult to perform, whichever happens first, up to 3 sets of 10 repetitions.

Duration

About 5 minutes.

Frequency

Once a day.

Description of the Intervention

The patient lies on her stomach on a bed with her left arm out to the side, elbow bent to 90 degrees, and forearm off the bed, fingers pointing toward the floor, holding a 5-pound weight with her left hand. The patient slowly brings her hand up and toward her head, keeping her elbow bent to 90 degrees and her upper arm on the bed. The patient repeats this exercise on the right side.

Mode

Active movements, scapular stabilization

Intensity

The patient performs the exercise until she feels her arm getting tired or the exercise becomes noticeably more difficult to perform.

Duration

About 5 minutes.

Frequency

Once a day.

Description of the Intervention

The patient is instructed to perform this exercise only if she feels as though she will not lose her balance. The patient places a small theraball on a low table and stands next to the table. The patient bends forward and positions her left hand on the top of the theraball, her elbow slightly bent, and her trunk over the ball, putting weight on the ball. Next, the patient moves her trunk to the left and right, and forward and backward, while balancing with her hand on the theraball. The patient repeats this exercise on the right side.

Manual Therapy Techniques, Including Mobilization/Manipulation

Administer grades III and IV joint mobilization distraction techniques to suboccipital joints and grades III, IV and V mobilization / manipulation distraction, anterior, posterior and inferior glides to bilateral glenohumeral joints.

Administer soft tissue mobilization techniques to bilateral cervical paraspinals, upper trapezeii, scalenes and sternocleidomastoid musculature.

> **Clinician Comment** *For this patient, all exercises should be performed on a daily basis. This patient will therefore be instructed to perform all exercises at home. The therapist will review the exercises during physical therapy visits, and ensure that the patient is performing them correctly. By instructing the patient in home exercises, vs having her perform them in the clinic, the patient can maximize the effect of the exercise program and better utilize clinic time for patient instruction and manual techniques.*

REEXAMINATION

Ms. Icon was reevaluated after 4 weeks of treatment.

Subjective

The patient reported that she had been adhering to her home exercise program.

Objective

Posture

WNL

Pain

She stated that the interventions were effective in reducing pain to a 1 at rest and a 4 with her usual activities. No pain was reported with palpation of the cervical paraspinals, upper trapezeii, scalenes, and sternocleidomastoid muscles. Pressure algometry revealed tenderness in 5 of 18 tender points. No spasm in cervical area to palpation.

Range of Motion

Neck PROM was WNL for all movements, no pain with overpressure.

Shoulder Passive Range of Motion

	LEFT	RIGHT
Flexion	0 to 170	0 to 165
	Firm end feel	Firm end feel
	Pain with overpressure	Pain with overpressure
Extension	WNL	WNL
Abduction	0 to 150	0 to 150
	Firm end feel	Firm end feel
	Pain with overpressure	Pain with overpressure
Lateral Rotation	0 to 70	0 to 70
	Firm end feel	Firm end feel

	LEFT	RIGHT
Lateral Rotation	No pain with overpressure	No pain with overpressure
Medial Rotation	WNL	WNL
Horizontal Adduction	WNL	WNL

Joint Integrity and Mobility

Cervical Spine: WNL

Glenohumeral Joints

	LEFT	RIGHT
Distraction	Hypomobile, pain free	Hypomobile, pain free
Anterior Glide	Hypomobile, pain free	Hypomobile, pain free
Posterior Glide	Hypomobile, pain free	Hypomobile, pain free
Inferior Glide	Hypomobile, pain free	Hypomobile, pain free

Muscle Performance

- Manual Muscle Testing Neck: WNL

Manual Muscle Testing Shoulder

	LEFT	RIGHT
Flexion	G	G
Extension	N	N
Abduction	G	G
Horizontal Abduction	N	N
Horizontal Adduction	N	N
Lateral Rotation	G	G
Medial Rotation	N	N
N = Normal, 5/5; G = Good, 4/5.		

Resisted Isometric Testing Neck

Forward Bending	Strong, pain free	
Backward Bending	Strong, pain free	
	LEFT	**RIGHT**
Side Bending	Strong, pain free	Strong, pain free
Rotation	Strong, pain free	Strong, pain free

Special Tests

- Lateral Scapular Slide Test: WNL

Aerobic Capacity/Endurance

6-Minute Walk Test: 550 meters; patient reported mild fatigue after testing.

Assessment

Patient was independent with home exercises, and demonstrated good understanding of correct posture and self-measures. Patient demonstrated improvement in all impairments, and has subsequently experienced a decrease in pain and fatigue with functional activities. Goals related to neck and posture impairments have been met. Patient experienced improvements in shoulder range of motion and strength, but still requires additional therapy to address residual impairments. Fibromyalgia symptoms of pain and fatigue improved as well, but patient would benefit from additional physical therapy to continue to address these areas.

Plan

Discontinue interventions to cervical spine.

Continue physical therapy 2 times per week for an additional 2 weeks. Address residual shoulder impairments (strength, range of motion and accessory motion), and reinforce independence with continuing Ms. Icon's home program once discharged.

OUTCOMES

Ms. Icon attended 3 more visits, but cancelled her final session. Her husband had become ill, and she needed to care for him. She reported that she was "doing fine." No final reevaluation was performed.

REFERENCES

1. Mayo Clinic. Diseases and conditions: fibromyalgia. http://www.mayoclinic.org/diseases-conditions/fibromyalgia/basics/definition/con-20019243. Accessed February 2009.
2. Wolfe F, Smythe HA, Yunus MB, et al. The American College of Rheumatology 1990 Criteria for the classification of fibromyalgia: report of the multicenter criteria committee. *Arthritis Rheum.* 1990;33:160-172.
3. Enright PL, Sherrill DL. Reference equations for the six-minute walk in healthy adults. *Am J Respir Crit Care.* 1998;158:1384-1387.
4. Kelley MJ, McClure PW, Leggin BG. Frozen shoulder: evidence and a proposed model guiding rehabilitation. *J Orthop Sports Phys Ther.* 2009;39:135-148.
5. Hurwitz EL, Carragee EJ, van der Velde G, et al. Treatment of neck pain: noninvasive interventions: results of the Bone and Joint Decade 2000-2010 Task Force on Neck Pain and its Associated Disorders. *Spine.* 2008;35:S123-S152.
6. Clauw DJ. Fibromalgia: a clinical review. *JAMA.* 2014;311:1547-1555.
7. Brosseau L, Wells GA, Tugwell P, et al. Ottawa panel evidence-based clinical practice guidelines for aerobic fitness exercises in the management of fibromyalgia: part 1. *Phys Ther.* 2008;88:857-871.
8. Brosseau L, Wells GA, Tugwell P, et al. Ottawa panel evidence-based clinical practice guidelines for strengthening exercises in the management of fibromyalgia: part 2. *Phys Ther.* 2008;88:873-885.
9. Busch AJ, Webber SC, Brachaniec M, et al. Exercise therapy for fibromyalgia. *Curr Pain Headache Rep.* 2011;15:358-367.
10. Busch AJ, Webber SC, Richards RS, et al. Resistance exercise training for fibromyalgia. *Cochrane Database of Syst Rev.* 2013;12:CD010884.

12

Individuals With Motor Control and Motor Function Disorders

Lisa Brown, PT, DPT, NCS

CHAPTER OBJECTIVES

- Identify major components in the central nervous system and summarize the role each plays toward the production of human movement beginning at the premotor area.

- List the pathways by which sensory information from the body's periphery influence, modify or coordinate motor responses.

- Identify the 3 most frequent problems that reduce functional capacity in individuals with neuromuscular disorders.

- Contrast deficits produced from a lesion at the premotor cortex versus the motor cortex.

- Outline the possible motor control deficits that can occur with a lesion in the cerebellum.

- Describe the variations from normal movement characteristic of a sensory system dysfunction.

- Answer the question: How is deconditioning just as possible in patients with nonprogressive neuromuscular disorders as those with progressive disorders?

- Discuss how spasticity could change over time independent of underlying central control of movement deficits.

- Describe the effect that the autonomic nervous system can have on the response to exercise or exercise tolerance.

- List the general factors to be considered when prescribing exercise for an individual with neuromuscular disorders.

- Compare and contrast the treatment considerations versus exercise benefit for programs based on walking, treadmill walking, bicycle ergometry or arm crank ergometry for patients with neuromuscular disorders.

- Contrast the benefits with the detriments of adaptive and assistive devices use during exercise sessions.

- Discuss the change in energy requirements to be considered during exercise for patients post-stroke, post-spinal cord injury, and with traumatic brain injury.

- Identify the physiologic factors that contribute to the distinct complaints of weakness, fatigue, and deconditioning in patients with multiple sclerosis.

- Compare and contrast the exercise guidelines for patients with amyotrophic lateral sclerosis and those with Guillain-Barré syndrome.

CHAPTER OUTLINE

- Normal Movement
  - Supplemental and Premotor Cortex
  - Cerebral Cortex
  - Basal Ganglia and Diencephalon
  - Cerebellum
  - Brainstem
  - Spinal Cord
  - Peripheral Nervous System
  - Sensory System
  - Conclusion

Coglianese D, ed. *Clinical Exercise Pathophysiology for Physical Therapy: Examination, Testing, and Exercise Prescription for Movement-Related Disorders (pp 465-532).*
© 2015 Taylor & Francis Group.

The light turns red and the crossing sign appears. You have less than 12 seconds to cross a busy road before the traffic emerges again. For an individual with a healthy neuromuscular system this may seem like an easy task, but what if the individual has a history of a stroke with hemiplegia? What systems are affected that may affect their ability to cross this busy street in a safe and efficient manner? This chapter will briefly review the physiology of normal motor function, and examine the physiology of abnormal motor function within a variety of neurological diagnosis. The impact on movement and exercise prescription for these specialized populations will be presented. Now let's see if we can figure out how to help this individual cross the street.

Movement arises from the interaction of the individual, the task at hand, and the environment. How the individual presented above moves next needs to take into consideration the constraints of the task at hand, the environment around him, and the limitations posed on the individual by the neuromuscular disorder. When we consider the individual there are 3 main factors that control movement. First, movement is driven by cognition, broadly defined as attention, planning, problem solving, motivation, and emotion. Second, perception is the integration of sensory information from the environment and body systems to interpret and regulate movement. Lastly, action is the motor output that is produced by the individual to accomplish the task (Figure 12-1).[1] The understanding of motor control in its entire complexity is beyond the scope of this chapter. Designing an exercise program for individuals with neurologic deficits can be challenging because of the complex and varied patterns of not only neurological, but also physiological and musculoskeletal limitations, that affect our patients. We will focus our discussion primarily on the systems that influence movement at the level of the individual.

Normal Movement

The process underlying human movement is a complex coordination of neurological systems. The multiple systems involved each has a primary purpose, and also overlap and provide redundancy in the system that becomes important when we talk about injury and recovery. This section will provide a general overview of the primary systems involved in the production of human movement.

The nervous system can be divided into 2 primary systems: the central nervous system (CNS) and the peripheral nervous system (PNS). The CNS consists of the brain and spinal cord, while the PNS contains cranial and spinal nerves that extend outside of the brain and spinal cord.[2] For organizational purposes, we will start at the top of the CNS.

Supplemental and Premotor Cortex

The supplemental and premotor cortex regions are responsible for higher order motor planning with projections to the motor cortex.[2] The parietal and premotor areas are primarily involved in the identification of targets in space, choosing the action plan necessary to complete the intended task, and then programming the movement. Premotor areas transmit output information to the motor cortex that then continues on to the brainstem, and spinal cord via the corticospinal and corticobulbar tracts.[1,3]

Cerebral Cortex

The cerebral cortex is considered the highest level within the complex motor control system of the CNS. The cerebral cortex can act hierarchically affecting levels below it, and in parallel with other systems when acting independently on spinal motor neurons. There are multiple areas and pathways in the cerebral cortex that determine strategies for movement.[3] The primary motor cortex lies in the frontal lobe and controls movement on the contralateral side of the body. The primary somatosensory cortex is in the parietal lobe and controls sensation on the contralateral side of the body. These sensory and motor areas are topographically organized and known as the motor and sensory homunculus or "little man" so that motor function for the foot is represented adjacent to the motor area for the leg.[2]

Basal Ganglia and Diencephalon

The basal ganglia (BG) is located at the base of the cerebral cortex. The BG receives information from the cerebral cortex, and sends information back to the motor cortex through the thalamus. The primary functions of the BG include higher level cognitive aspects of motor control such as the planning of motor strategies.

The diencephalon is the next caudal structure and is made up of the thalamus and the hypothalamus. The thalamus is considered a relay center used to process information from multiple input pathways from the spinal cord, cerebellum,

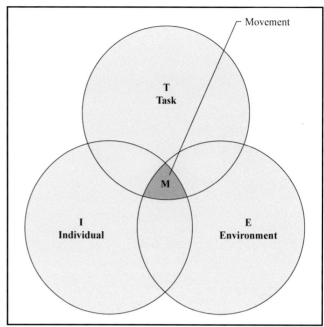

Figure 12-1. Movement emerges from the interactions between the individual, the task, and the environment. (Adapted from Shumway-Cook A. *Motor Control: Translating Research Into Clinical Practice.* 4th ed., North American Edition, Lippincott Williams & Wilkins).

brainstem, and cortex.[1] The hypothalamus is important in the control of autonomic, neuroendocrine, and limbic circuits (Figure 12-2).[2]

Cerebellum

The cerebellum is connected to the brainstem by tracts known as "peduncles." It receives inputs from the brainstem, spinal cord, and cerebral cortex, and produces outputs to the brainstem. The function of the cerebellum is simply the modulation of the motor output of the corticospinal and descending motor tracts with sensory signals.[1,2]

Brainstem

The brainstem is the next level of neural processing. The brainstem is composed of the midbrain, pons, and medulla and contains many of the cranial nerves.[2] The brainstem contains ascending and descending pathways transmitting sensory and motor information, with all descending motor pathways originating in the brainstem with the exception of the corticospinal tract. It receives sensory information from the skin and muscles of the head and neck, and vestibular and visual systems. The brainstem contains nuclei controlling motor output to the neck, face, and eyes, and are vital for postural control and locomotion.[1]

Spinal Cord

The spinal cord is the level involved in the initial reception and processing of information from the muscles, joints, and skin. The spinal cord consists of central gray matter

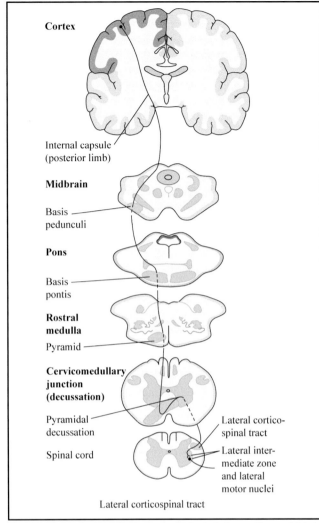

Figure 12-2. Corticospinal tract. (Adapted from Blumenfeld H. *Neuroanatomy Through Clinical Cases.* 2nd ed. Sinauer Associates Inc.)

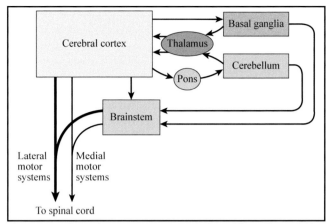

Figure 12-3. General motor organization. (Adapted from Blumenfeld H. *Neuroanatomy Through Clinical Cases.* 2nd ed. Sinauer Associates Inc).

surrounded by white matter that contains the ascending and descending pathways. The dorsal (posterior) horn of the spinal cord contains mainly sensory neurons while the ventral (anterior) horn contains mainly motor neurons. Lower motor neurons controlling the arms and legs reside in the ventral horn.[2] Both reflexive and voluntary control of posture and movement is controlled through motor neurons (Figure 12-3).[1]

Peripheral Nervous System

The PNS includes motor and sensory components of cranial and spinal nerves, and peripheral aspects of the autonomic nervous system. Axons in the peripheral nervous system extend from cell bodies originating in the brainstem, spinal cord, or dorsal root ganglia. The motor system, also termed lower motor neuron (LMN), includes alpha motor neurons located in the anterior horn cells of the brainstem and spinal cord, axons that arise from the anterior horn cells and form the spinal, peripheral, and cranial nerves, the

motor endplate of the axon, and the muscle fibers innervated by the motor nerve axon. Schwann cells protect axons in the PNS by creating myelin with large-diameter axons, and by providing support to small diameter axons. Approximately 25% of peripheral nerve fibers are myelinated, which speeds the rate of action potential conduction.[3]

Sensory System

The skin, muscles, and joints contain receptors that transmit sensory information via afferent axons to the spinal cord. The afferent fibers then travel in the spinal column and ascend to the brainstem. Fibers that run along the posterior or dorsal column of the spinal cord synapse on the dorsal column nuclei in the medulla to cross over to the contralateral hemisphere of the brain. These fibers then continue to ascend and synapse in the thalamus before finally ending in the primary sensory motor cortex. Dorsal column sensory neurons carry information about proprioception, vibration sense, kinesthetic sense, and light touch. This provides sensory input from joints and muscles contributing to motor and postural control. Sensory neurons that carry information about pain, temperature sense, and crude touch enter the spinal cord and immediately synapse in the gray matter of the spinal cord to cross over and ascend in the anterolateral white matter via the spinothalamic tract. The sensory neurons synapse next in the thalamus before continuing to the primary somatosensory cortex. Descending somatosensory output modulates activity of the skeletal muscles.[2,3]

Visual and vestibular systems also provide key information necessary for postural control and locomotion. The visual system allows object identification to determine movement and visual proprioceptive information about where the body is in space. Sensory information from the visual system is processed from the image detection on the retina, through the optic nerve to the optic chiasm where information travels through the optic tract. The optic tract forms synapses on neurons in several regions that, in turn, project to the visual cortex. The vestibular system provides sensory information about the position and motion detection of the head in space. This information contributes to the coordination of motor responses and gaze stabilization to maintain postural stability. The peripheral vestibular system consists of sensory receptors that transmit information via the eighth cranial nerve. The central vestibular system consists of 4 vestibular nuclei located in the medulla.[2]

Conclusion

There are several parallel pathways and feedback loops that connect all of these systems to produce and control movement. The corticospinal tract is a key motor pathway that begins in the primary motor cortex and descends through the brainstem, crossing over at the junction between the medulla and the spinal cord, to reach the spinal cord and control movement. Lesions occurring above this cross-over junction will produce weakness on the opposite side of the body, while lesions below this junction in the spinal cord cause weakness on the same, or ipsilateral side.

Upper motor neurons (UMN) project from the cortex to the brainstem or spinal cord and then form synapses on LMNs located in the brainstem motor nuclei and anterior horns of the spinal cord. LMN cranial nerves in the brainstem, and anterior spinal roots in the spinal cord then project out of the CNS to control muscle cells in the periphery.[2] Functional demands drive patterns of innervation that play a role in determining the characteristics of a muscle. Muscle fibers can be classified based on speed of shortening and morphological characteristics.[3] Type I muscle fibers, or slow oxidative slow-twitch muscle fibers, are fatigue-resistance fibers. Type II fibers can be further classified as either Type IIa or Type IIb. Type IIa fibers are referred to as fast oxidative fibers, are faster and bigger than Type I fibers, and are also fatigue resistant. Type IIb lack aerobic enzyme and fatigue easily.[3,4]

Muscle function can be defined in terms of strength, speed, and fatigue resistance. While the typical ratio of slow-twitch muscle fibers to fast is 50% to 50%, the characteristics can depend on the activity patterns to which the muscle is subjected. The ability of a muscle to produce force is determined by the descending motor control of the UMN system, the number of motor units recruited, the order of motor unit recruitment, type of muscle fibers available for innervation, and the amount of tension placed on the muscle.[4]

NEUROLOGICAL IMPAIRMENTS AFFECTING MOTOR CONTROL

Noted earlier in the chapter, "normal" movement is driven by the interaction of the individual with the environment while completing a specific task. Altered, or "abnormal" movements at the level of the individual can be influenced by pathology affecting the action, perception, or cognitive systems. For example, a neurological injury such as a stroke has a direct effect on the individual at the level of the motor cortex. Weakness (action), neglect (perception), or attention to task (cognition) can all affect the way the individual now moves post-stroke. This can pose a challenge to the performance of daily tasks, such as effectively crossing the street.

Despite the variability for potential lesion location and severity, the 3 most frequent problems that reduce functional capacity in individuals with neuromuscular disorders (NMDs) are altered motor function, fatigue, and difficulty exercising, and accessing activity all contributing to a sedentary and unhealthy lifestyle.[5]

Premotor Cortex

A lesion at the level of the associated or limbic cortices does not tend to produce profound motor deficits, but can alter the volitional or motivational control of movement.[2]

Motor Cortex

An insult to the motor cortex and UMNs of the corticospinal tract can result in impairments along the descending motor pathways. Abnormal central motor function causes a distortion in the central motor excitatory drive. This may in turn impair the ability to recruit and modulate motor neurons, decreasing force production. This irregular activation promotes abnormal movement patterns, or synergies, during functional tasks such as walking.[1] Individuals with more significant damage to the corticospinal tract show increased activation in premotor and supplemental motor cortices of the affected hemisphere during functional tasks.[6] These changes in pattern of brain activation appear to correlate with a decrease in functional outcomes. As motor recovery and function improve, there is a reduction in abnormal activation patterns.[6]

Subcortical

At the sub-cortical level the cerebellum and basal ganglia affect the coordination of motor output. A lesion at either of these structures will affect the timing of a movement resulting in either delayed initiation or termination, and the ability to grade and scale force produced. Pathology in the cerebellum can affect the accuracy of movement (dysmetria), and tends to be more prominent when multiple joints are involved across a larger trajectory at a faster speed (such as walking across the street) versus single-joint movements performed over a smaller range at a slower speed.[1] The ability to coordinate eye and head movements, postural sway, and the timing of equilibrium responses may also be affected. Loss of input from the cerebellum is thought to cause hypotonia or asthenia (generalized weakness).[3] Pathology in the basal ganglia can result in impaired timing of movements and movements that are either too small (hypokinetic/bradykinetic) or too large (hyperkinetic).[1]

Spinal Cord/Lower Motor Neuron

A lesion at the level of the LMN from the anterior horn of the spinal cord to the peripheral nerve will cause muscle weakness and atrophy. Lesions at the neuromuscular junction, and subsequent alterations in the mechanical properties of the muscles and joints themselves can further contribute to motor weakness.[2]

Peripheral Nervous System

Disorders arising from the PNS are broadly classified as either neuropathies when the lesion is confined to the nerve, or myopathies, when the pathology occurs in the muscle. A lesion of the sensory function will either follow a peripheral nerve distribution or a dermatomal pattern when the spinal nerve or dorsal root ganglion is affected. The most common symptoms of a peripheral sensory lesion are tingling, prickling, burning, or paresthesias. When motor function is involved, paralysis or paresis will occur in muscles innervated by the nerve distal to the lesion. Weakness will occur in a myotomal pattern, affecting all muscles innervated by that spinal level. Typically symptoms of peripheral nerve motor impairments would be weakness, muscle cramping, fasciculations, and hypotonicity. Deep tendon reflexes (DTRs) will also be diminished. In the autonomic nervous system preganglionic nerve fibers are myelinated. In the presence of demyelination or axonal degeneration, abnormalities in vascular control and sweating will occur.[3]

Sensory System Dysfunction

Disorders affecting the sensory system pathways can have a profound impact on movement and motor control. Disruption of sensory function in the dorsal column pathways will result in difficult maintaining postural control during voluntary and involuntary functional tasks. The lack of joint and motor position feedback can cause movements that are ataxic, uncoordinated, and inefficient. Impairments in the visual system that can affect mobility are visual fields cuts that may contribute to tripping and falls. Impairments of the vestibular system may cause deficits in gaze stabilization, postural control, and balance especially in complex environments and during dynamic activities.[1]

KEY IMPAIRMENTS AFFECTING MOVEMENT AND EXERCISE CAPACITY

Motor weakness is one of the most common and consistent consequences both of UMN and LMN lesions. Weakness can be caused by a lesion at any level in the neuromuscular system and is commonly classified by the severity and location of the distribution. The term "paresis" is used to describe a mild to moderate, or partial weakness, while "plegia" denotes a more severe or total loss of movement. Paralysis is another term used when there is no motor function present. The term *hemi* describes weakness on one side of the body, "para" describes weakness in the lower limbs, while the terms "tetra" or "quad" describe weakness noted in all 4 limbs.[1,2] For example, our patient who has had a cortical stroke with mild to moderate weakness on the right side of the body may be described as having "hemiplegia." Weakness from UMN and LMN lesions can also lead to secondary neuromuscular impairments affecting exercise participation, including muscle disuse atrophy, cardiovascular deconditioning, and contractions.[1] Specific muscle groups such as hip flexors and plantar-flexors have been noted to have a direct impact on gait speed when weak, which may in turn contribute to an increase in disability.[7,8] Therefore, a thorough understanding of the function of the motor system in the presence of a neurological deficit is a critical element throughout the course of care.

Aerobic Deconditioning

Reduced exercise performance and fitness can occur with muscle or neurological injury, loss of muscle tissue size and quality, or deconditioning. Individuals with both progressive as well as stable neuromuscular disorders tend to have some aspect of all of these deficits from either the pathology itself or as a result of disuse from a more sedentary lifestyle affecting overall mobility.[5] Individuals with NMD tend to live a more sedentary lifestyle and often present with a decreased amount of resting energy expenditure compared to able-bodied individuals. During even basic activities of daily living (ADL), however, movements are less efficient and there is an increased energy cost of physical activity, especially in more demanding tasks such as walking.[9] Secondary effects include cardiopulmonary compromise in the presence of NMD including a reduction in max and peak volume of oxygen consumed (VO_2), pulmonary ventilation, work rate or capacity, and endurance, which places an increased risk for hypertension (HTN), cardiovascular disease (CVD), and diabetes mellitus (DM).[10] Most aerobic interventions studied in slowly or rapidly progressing disorders demonstrate the potential for a positive response to aerobic exercise training. Short-term cardiovascular adaptations can be made with sub-maximal training similar to able-bodied individuals.[9,10] The severity of risk and impact of cardiovascular deconditioning varies depending on the neurological diagnosis and is discussed in more detail later in this chapter.

Abnormal Tone and Spasticity

Changes in muscle tone occur as a consequence of a UMN or LMN lesion. Muscle tone is defined as the muscles resistance to passive stretch.[1] Everyone has a certain amount of muscle tone. The spectrum of muscle tone ranges from low, or hypotonic, to high, or hypertonic (Figure 12-4). On one end of the spectrum, hypotonicity is defined as a reduction in the stiffness of a muscle to lengthening.[1] Hypotonicity is typically associated with lesions in the cerebellum and is

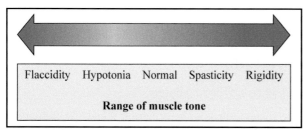

Figure 12-4. Range of muscle tone. (Adapted from Shumway-Cook A. *Motor Control: Translating Research Into Clinical Practice*. 4th ed., North American Edition, Lippincott Williams & Wilkins.)

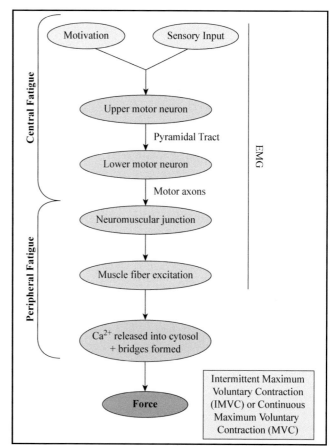

Figure 12-5. Fatigue. (Adapted from Lou J, Weiss MD, Carter GT. Assessment and management of fatigue in neuromuscular disease. *Am J Hosp Palliat Care*. 2010;27(2):145-157.)

thought to be due to a decrease in input from the cerebellum to the motor cortex.[3] The high end of "hypertonicity" is classified as either spasticity or rigidity. Levels of hypertonicity are caused by a lesion of the corticospinal pathways contributing to an amplified amount of alpha motor neuron excitability that results in an increase in resting muscle tone, and an elevated level of excitatory afferent input elicited by a quick muscle stretch.[1]

Spasticity is further defined as a velocity-dependent reflex response to muscle stretch. The role of spasticity in functional movements has been debated and the thought process has evolved. The evidence suggests that there is not a causal relationship between the level of spasticity an individual presents with and central control of movement.[11-13] The presence of spasticity changes the physical property of the muscle over time. An increase in muscle fiber size variability and extracellular matrix material may present clinically with an increase in muscle stiffness. This may alter the resting alignment of the affecting limb, placing it in a shortened position and at increased risk for developing contractures.[1] This may contribute to inefficient gait patterns and deconditioning.

Fatigue

Fatigue is a universal complaint among individuals with neuromuscular disorders and is a complex multidimensional impairment with both physiological and psychological aspects. More than 60% of individuals with neurological disorders suffer from fatigue, often described as sleepiness, weakness, exercise intolerance, or exhaustion.[14-19] It influences movement and performance in ADL, as well as overall health and quality of life. Physiologic fatigue can result from pathology that affects motor neuron pathways responsible for the force-producing capability of a muscle or for the perceived effort of the task.[14,15] Fatigue can be characterized by the amount of a time a muscle can sustain a certain force (endurance), or by the amount of decline in force or power output over a period of time.[20] Fatigue can be brought on by physical activity or stress and may stem from central or peripheral mechanisms. The term "central fatigue" refers to fatigue that arises from the loss of voluntary activation of muscles during activity or exercise due to a disruption in input from anywhere along the central nervous system, such as a lesion in the motor cortex in multiple sclerosis (MS).[14] A muscle receiving sub-optimal input from the CNS, known as

central activation failure (CAF), will not be able to develop its maximal force capacity.[14] Peripheral fatigue develops when there is muscle weakness or sensory loss from disorders of the LMN units, or from morphological changes at the level of the muscle.[15,20] Peripheral muscle fatigability is described as the failure to sustain the force of a muscle contraction over time.[15] This declining force during contraction is mainly attributed to changing intracellular ion levels negatively affecting contractile forces (Figure 12-5). Severity of motor fatigue is measured by the percentage of decline in force production.[14] In individuals with neurological disorders, even the sense of "normal" fatigue can be amplified by the pathological changes that occur throughout the motor systems.[15] Fatigue can vary depending on the task performed, the type of muscle power utilized (voluntary versus electrical stimulation, isometric versus dynamic, sustain versus intermittent, high versus low forces), and the contractile properties of the muscles.[20] How each individual perceives and responds to fatigue can also have an influence. Subjective complaints can be influenced by motivation, coping mechanisms, overall well-being, and social circumstances.[15]

In addition to motor dysfunction, other factors that may contribute to fatigue in individuals with neuromuscular disorders that need to be considered are reduced respiratory and cardiac function, chronic pain, sleep disorders, depression, malnutrition, and dehydration. Hypoventilation is more prominent in supine positions so may be first noted as complaints of morning somnolence, headaches, restlessness, and fatigue.[21] Pulmonary function tests including forced vital capacity (FVC) reflect both inspiratory and expiratory muscle strength and may be important to monitor in supine as well as seated positions for the most accurate assessment of respiratory function in individuals with NMD.

Autonomic Nervous System

Autonomic nervous system dysfunction can be present with most neurological pathologies and must be taken into consideration when developing an exercise prescription. The autonomic nervous system is a component of the PNS that controls autonomic functions such as heart rate (HR), sweating, smooth muscle contraction in the walls of blood vessels and bronchi, sex organs, and the pupils.[2] The efferent autonomic pathways are divided into the sympathetic and parasympathetic pathways. The sympathetic division stems from the spinal levels T1 through L2 and controls the "fight or flight" response. When stimulated, the neurotransmitter norepinephrine is released, increasing HR, blood pressure (BP), pupil size, and bronchodilation. The parasympathetic division stems from parasympathetic ganglion in the cranial nerves and at S2 to S4. When stimulated, acetylcholine is released to produce the opposite effect, decreasing HR and BP. Neurons in the cerebral cortex, basal forebrain, hypothalamus, midbrain, pons, and medulla contribute to autonomic control, along with afferent sensory information from the periphery.[2,3] Response to exercise or exercise tolerance can be blunted in the presence of autonomic dysfunction, including the use of HR as a measure of response or perceived exertion. Abnormal autonomic responses can be mild to severe depending on the contributing pathology.

Conclusion

When considering an exercise prescription for an individual with NMD, you must take into consideration the specific diagnosis, the subsequent limitations that affect movement, the rate of the disease progression, and the amount of clinical involvement to estimate the best potential for response to treatment.[22,23] For example, in a disease like amyotrophic lateral sclerosis (ALS) that is characterized by a rapid progression, the goal may be to slow or stabilize the disease, while in slowly progressing diseases such as Parkinson's disease (PD), there is evidence, which we will explore further, that there is the potential for positive and significant gains in strength and aerobic capacity.

PATIENT/CLIENT MANAGEMENT

The patient/client management process established by the American Physical Therapy Association (APTA) is described in the *Guide to Physical Therapy Practice*. The 5 key elements include examination, evaluation, diagnosis, prognosis, and intervention, are designed to maximize outcomes.[24]

Examination

Patient/Client History

The history includes information about the individual's current and past medical history. This information is gathered from the patients/clients themselves, caregivers, members of the health care team, and the medical record. The information obtained can also include items like general demographics, social history, occupation, growth and development, living environment, functional status, and activity levels, family history, medications, and social habits. The patient/client history should also contain a review of relevant laboratory and diagnostic tests results.[24] This information can be used to identify potential health risks and comorbidities of the individual to help determine the health restorative and preventive needs of the patients/clients and their implications for response to physical therapy intervention.[1]

Systems Review

The systems review is a brief overview of the general health of the patient/client. Key elements of the systems review include a brief appraisal of the cardiopulmonary, integumentary, musculoskeletal, and neuromuscular systems. It is also a point to determine the communication style, cognition, language, and learning style of the patient/client.[24]

The cardiopulmonary system requires particular attention when working with individuals with neuromuscular disorders. Various cortical as well as spinal cord injuries (SCIs) above the level of T6 can be associated with dysfunction of the autonomic nervous system.[25,26] In particular, regulation of sweating, HR, and BP may be impaired when there is pathology along the neuromuscular system. This may present itself clinically as bradycardia, diaphoresis, supine and orthostatic hypotension, and in severe cases can cause cardiac arrest.[3]

Resting HR, orthostatic BP, resting respiratory rate, and arterial saturation with pulse oximeter are all baseline measures that should be included prior to the initiation of testing.

Tests and Measures

The next step in the examination process is driven by the information gathered in the history and systems review. The physical therapist chooses relevant tests and measures to determine the underlying impairments contributing to the individual's functional limitations that are affecting his or her activity and participation levels. The key elements related to mobility and the ability to participate in exercise are discussed below in more detail.

Aerobic Capacity and Endurance

Maximal exercise testing is considered the gold standard for assessing aerobic capacity. Many individuals with neuromuscular disease with deficits in gait and balance, or

TABLE 12-1. BASELINE RANGES ESTABLISHED IN INDIVIDUALS WITH A HISTORY OF STROKE, MULTIPLE SCLEROSIS, TRAUMATIC BRAIN INJURY, AND PARKINSON'S DISEASE

PATIENT POPULATION	MEAN WALKING DISTANCE (M) ± SD
Sub-acute stroke[244]	215.8 ± 91.6 m
Chronic stroke[245,246]	384 to 398, 378.3 ± 123.1 m
Parkinson's diseases H&Y[5-3,247,248]	391.6 to 394.1 ± 98.4 to 99.9 m
Multiple sclerosis EDSS 2.0 to 6.5[35]	368.6 to 393.8 m
Chronic TBI[33]	403 to 417 ± 105 to 106 m
H&Y: Hoehn and Yahr Staging Scale; EDSS: Expanded Disability Status Scale; SD: standard deviation; m: meters.	

who suffer from pain or extreme fatigue, may not be able to participate in accurate maximal exercise assessment. Sub-maximal exercise testing can overcome many of these obstacles and is an effective assessment of aerobic capacity and performance.[27] Individuals who do require cardiovascular monitoring, are prescribed anti-anginal medication, or are considered to be at hemodynamic risk should be tested in a setting with trained medical personnel present or cleared by their physician for sub-maximal testing. Contraindications to exercise testing include labile angina, angina at rest, and frequent premature periventricular contractions (PVCs) at rest.[27]

Measures of exercise response that can easily be examined in all clinical settings includes HR, BP, respiratory rate (RR), rating of perceived exertion (RPE), arterial saturation using a pulse oximeter, breathlessness, and ratings of fatigue and pain. The Borg scale is one of the most common and considered the best tools used to rate levels of perceived exertion.[28]

There are a variety of sub-maximal exercise tests that can be performed in a clinical setting and are appropriate for individuals with neuromuscular disorders. Factors to consider when selecting an appropriate testing measure include consideration of the individual's primary and secondary pathology, mobility, the use of assistive devices for balance or gait, cognitive status, and level of independence.[27] Individuals should be familiarized with the testing equipment and provided at least one practice attempt to improve the validity of the test results. A typical protocol for exercise testing includes a low-load warm-up period, a progressive uninterrupted exercise with increased loads at consistent time intervals, followed by a recovery period.[29] Adequate rest should be allowed between practice and test attempts, and verbal encouragement should be standardized.

Submaximal exercise testing can be symptom limited, or have predetermined end points often defined by peak HR of 120 beats per minutes (bpm) or 70% of predicted HR_{max}. A peak metabolic equivalent (MET) level of 5 may also be used as an endpoint.[29]

Pay special attention to medications the individual may be taking and their effects on exercise response, mobility, and fatigue. For example, beta blockers suppress normal HR and BP response to exercise, while individuals with PD take medications to improve mobility and often need to time activity around their medication schedule.

Treadmill testing is the most common option for individuals who are ambulatory and have only minor impairments in balance. Treadmills with front and side rails should be used for safety, but subjects should be encouraged to minimize use of the upper extremities (UEs) during testing. Ramping treadmill protocols start at a slow comfortable pace until a comfortable walking speed is achieved. At fixed intervals the speed or grade is gradually increased over a period of 6 to 12 minutes. Treadmill testing is the preferred method of testing when possible since it is easier to achieve VO_{2max} walking a treadmill than seated on a cycle or at an arm ergometer.[30,31]

Cycle ergometer testing can be used for individuals with impaired balance or ambulation preventing effective participation in a timed walk test. Testing with a cycle ergometer requires decreased energy cost compared to treadmill testing. The UEs require less motion or stability, making it easier to obtain an accurate BP. For individuals with hemiparesis, foot straps can be used to secure the weaker extremity. Work intensity is adjusted by changes in resistance and/or pedaling rate and typically calculated in watts or kilopond meters per minute (kpm/min^{-1}).[29,30] A disadvantage to cycle ergometer testing is that quadriceps muscles often fatigue before the individual reaches maximum oxygen uptake.

Arm ergometry testing is the least effective method of assessment for aerobic capacity, but can be used as an option for individuals who are nonambulatory or have less than minimal use of their lower extremities (LEs). Protocols for arm ergometer testing require that the individual is seated in an upright position with the fulcrum of the handle adjusted to shoulder height. Cycle speed should be maintained at 60 to 70 revolutions/minute with a work increase of 10W at each 2-minute stage.[29] BPs can be monitored mechanically at slower speeds, but are often less accurate at higher speeds. An option can be to test the individual intermittently with 1-minute rest breaks between stages to assess BP.

The 6-Minute Walk Test (6MWT) is a commonly used measure of endurance and functional mobility outside of the home for ambulatory individuals with NMDs (Table 12-1).[32] The 6MWT is a reliable and valid measure utilized across

Modified Ashworth Scale for Grading Spasticity

Grade	Description
0	No increase in muscle tone
1	Slight increase in muscle tone, manifested by a catch and release or by minimal resistance at the end of the range of motion when the affected part(s) is moved in flexion or extension
1+	Slight increase in muscle tone, manifested by a catch, followed by minimal resistance throughout the remainder (less than half) of the ROM
2	More marked increase in muscle tone through most of the ROM, but affected part(s) easily moved
3	Considerable increase in muscle tone, passive movement difficult
4	Affected part(s) rigid in flexion or extension

Figure 12-6. Modified Ashworth Scale. (Reprinted from *Phys Ther.* 1987;67(2):206-207, with permission of the American Physical Therapy Association. Copyright © 1987 American Physical Therapy Association.)

diagnostic groups.[33-38] Timed walking tests can be utilized safely when maximal exercise testing is contraindicated.[27] Results correspond to functional ADL and can be used to detect change in functional ability following intervention.[27] Improvements in walking distance can be attributed to improvements in cardiac output, in mechanics of ventilation, or in muscular conditioning.[38]

Motor Function and Performance

The assessment of muscle strength impairment and endurance can be challenging depending on the ability of the patient to isolate movement for the most accurate assessment. Examination methods of strength need to be practical in terms of time, training, and equipment needed to be feasible in a clinical setting.

When a patient is able to isolate movement, the primary measure of muscle strength used in the clinical setting is manual muscle testing (MMT). MMT is a reliable measure of muscle strength, but is less discriminatory than hand-held dynamometry in grades > 3/5.[39]

The second most common method of strength assessment in a clinical setting is HHD. The standard devices are portable, easy to use, relatively inexpensive, and considered a valid and reliable measure of muscle strength especially when testing muscles that are naturally or pathologically weak.[39] The ability to accurately quantify muscle strength in presence of a neurological impairment can be challenging, but has been documented in several studies using HHD.[39-43]

LE motor strength and endurance assessment can be initiated during observation of a functional task. The 5 or 10 times Sit to Stand Test is a simple and practical test of function and endurance that correlates well with LE manual and dynametric strength measures.[44,45] A cut-off score of 12 seconds appears to discriminate between healthy and hemiparetic individuals.[45]

When abnormal movement patterns or synergies are present, a subjective descriptive analysis of resting alignment or start position of the limb, the ability of the patient to fractionate movements at each joint in gravity or gravity minimized positions, and the patterns of movement that emerge is often used as an initial measure of mobility. While impairment level assessment tools such as the Fugl-Meyer Lower Extremity Assessment (FM-LE) can be utilized to objectively quantify movement patterns, correlation to complex motor behaviors such as walking are not as predictive as measures of LE strength.[46]

Measures of motor performance can provide more significant information related to functional limitation such as gait. The upright motor control test (UMCT) is a measure of paretic LE motor control. The 2 major sections of the test are the flexion control test and the extension control test. The flexion control test is used to assess flexion control of the nonweightbearing extremity for purposes such as advancement of the limb in the swing phase of gait. The extension control test evaluates LE extension control of a single weight-bearing extremity with application for single-limb stance potential in gait. Muscle groups are graded as strong (actively completing a full motion within a given time frame), moderate (actively completing a partial to full motion within a given time), weak (only partial to no motion is noted over the allotted amount of time), or unable to perform.[47] UMCT scores are significantly associated with measures of gait speed and can be predictive of later walking outcomes.[48]

Tone/Spasticity

The evaluation of muscle tone in the presence of a neurological insult is performed to identify the lesion location and to differentiate the role of muscle stiffness and contracture as it relates to a functional problem.[49] The most utilized measurement scale for assessment of hypertonicity in the clinical setting is the modified Ashworth Scale (MAS). The MAS is an ordinal scale ranging from 0 (no change in muscle tone), to 4 (rigidity; Figure 12-6). The MAS is currently the clinical standard for assessment of spasticity that does not require instrumentation, but consistent training to necessary to maintain reliability. Limitations of the MAS are the weak correlation to functional limitations, and the lack of procedural standardization.[50,51]

The Tardieu Scale has been suggested as an alternative to the MAS as it assesses and compares the response of passive stretch at both slow and fast speeds. Tardieu also included the importance of maintaining a constant position of the limb segment proximal to the muscle group being tested. The scale has been further developed to include parameters to define the strength and duration of the stretch reflex, the angle at which the stretch reflex is activated, and the speed necessary to trigger the stretch reflex. Reliability and validity are not well defined at this point.[52]

Fatigue

The effects of fatigue can be assessed in a clinical setting either subjectively or objectively. Subjective fatigue of the individual should be assessed using a questionnaire or other source of patient-reported outcome measure. The Fatigue Severity Scale (FSS) is a commonly used assessment tool across neurologic diagnosis, especially in individuals with MS and PD.[18,53-55] The 9 item scale measures fatigue and the severity of its impact of daily activities and participation, and can clarify the relationship between fatigue and depressive symptoms.[56] The self-administered questionnaire asks participants to rate their fatigue on a 7-point scale when answering statements such as, "My motivation is lower when I am fatigued," and "Fatigue interferes with my work, family, or social life." The FSS has high validity, reliability, and internal consistency.[53,56]

Another common subjective measure is the single-item visual analog scale (VAS). Subjective reports of fatigue tend to be more practical for clinical use, are widely available, and easier for the patient to understand and participate in. The main limitations are that the assessment relies on the individual's interpretation of fatigue and may not correlate with severity of physical fatigue measured in an exercise protocol.[21]

Sensory Integrity

A thorough examination of the sensory system is necessary when considering an exercise program in the presence of a neurological deficit. Sensory impairments within the somatosensory, visual or vestibular systems can have a profound impact on mobility, postural control, and locomotion. Critical components of a somatosensory examination should include items for discriminative touch, proprioception, pain, and temperature. A comprehensive visual exam should include information on visual acuity, visual fields, depth perception, and oculomotor control. Vestibular function examination can include tests of gaze stabilization, postural control, balance, and dizziness.[1] While deficits in sensation may not be a primary predictor of gait speed potential, it is certainly a contributing factor.[7,8] Sensation related to fall risk and injury potential needs to be considered when establishing the mode of intervention that may provide the maximal aerobic and strengthening benefits.

Orthotic and Prosthetic Devices

LE orthotic devices are frequently prescribed to individuals with neurological disorders. They are indicated in the presence of weakness or abnormal muscle tone to improve alignment, positioning, and provide stability during functional activities such as transfers, standing, and gait. The most common types of LE orthotics utilized are ankle-foot orthotics (AFO) and knee-ankle foot orthotics (KAFO). The use of neuroprosthetics is a developing field. While a discussion of the complexities of LE bracing components is beyond the scope of this chapter, we will address the implications for gait quality and efficiency as it relates to aerobic capacity and training.

Abnormal gait patterns that arise because of motor neuron lesions contribute to an increased risk for falls, and an increase in energy expenditure during slow gait speeds.[49] Individuals who use an AFO demonstrate improvements—an increase in step length gait velocity and cadence, a decrease in double limb stance time, and more symmetrical single-limb stance times and step lengths—that all contribute to improved efficiency of gait.[57] Individuals wearing an articulating AFO or posterior leaf spring (PLS) demonstrate even more significant improvements in step length and gait velocity compared to those who use a solid AFO.[58] The use of neuroprosthetics for foot drop are an increasingly popular option despite the expense and limited coverage by insurance companies. Commercial neuroprosthetics are used primarily in individuals with hemiparesis to activate ankle dorsiflexion in swing. Correction of this component of gait allows an increase in gait velocity and overall function and participation levels.[59] A thorough team-based examination performed in a brace clinic that includes a physical therapist can assist when determining the most appropriate bracing options for each patient.

Adaptive and Assistive Devices

Assistive devices such as a single-point cane or walker are frequently used to improve the safety of walking when a significant gait disorder or history of falls in noted. While these devices can improve safety, balance, and gait economy, they can also interfere with postural responses in a fall and place increased strength and metabolic demands on the individual.[60-62] This high amount of variability in the effectiveness of an assistive device demonstrates the importance of a skilled assessment by a physical therapist to establish the needs and goals of each patient.

Safety is always of the highest priority. Since difficulty with gait is consistent among individuals with NMDs, it is important that we take into account the changes in efficiency that are noted when prescribing an assistive device. A single-point cane is often recommended with mild gait deviations and minimal risk for falls are noted. Gianfrancesco et al measured individuals with MS walking with and without a cane at self-selected and fast walking speeds. When a cane was introduced, subjects showed significantly improved gait symmetry and variability at self-selected walking speeds, and improved velocity at faster walking speeds compared to gait without a device.[63] The least-supportive devices like a single-point cane may improve gait parameters including velocity better than other more supportive devices[64] in the absence of a balance disorder of fall risk. There is little scientific evidence for the support of assistive devices for improvements in gait or balance with individuals with PD.[65]

In general, walkers and wheeled walkers are indicated for individuals with moderate to severe disability.[66] While the intension is to improve safety and decrease fall risk, these devices significantly alter gait parameters such as step length and velocity. This translates to a decrease in gait speed with increased energy demands demonstrated by a higher VO_2.[67] This is most likely due to the increased economy of walking with these types of devices that can contribute to fatigue and decreased activity tolerance. Careful assessment of the most appropriate device is necessary to maximize safety, activity tolerance, and participation.

Evaluation/Diagnosis/Prognosis

Once all the necessary data are collected in the examination, the physical therapist formulates a clinical judgment. The results of the tests and measures performed influence the evaluation process along with an appreciation for the loss of function, social considerations, and overall health and physical function.

Intervention

A well-rounded exercise program will include both aerobic and strengthening components. Fatigue also plays a prominent role in neurological disorders and should be considered when designing an intervention plan.

Strength training refers to exercises that improve the force-generating capacity of the muscle.[3] The ability to improve muscle strength and the capacity to which the improvement can occur is discussed is further detail within the diagnostic groups. There is a better understanding that strength training does not increase abnormal tone or exacerbate synergistic movement patterns, and is strongly advocated for individuals with neurological pathology.[1,11]

Cardiovascular fitness and participation in exercise is an important and necessary lifestyle behavior for individuals with neurological disorders who are more prone to sedentary lifestyles and the development of cardiovascular and pulmonary disorders. Aerobic and endurance training focus on improvements of aerobic capacity, and the duration that a person can maintain a certain activity.[68] A regular exercise routine decreases the risk of secondary risk factors that occur with a sedentary lifestyle and disability, and can improve of maintain functional abilities.

Fatigue contributes to a more sedentary lifestyle that can affect general fitness and well-being of individuals with NMDs. Fatigue is treatable and can often be at least partially reversible. Management of fatigue is an important component of patient care and can be achieved through a variety of recognized treatment options. Symptomatic treatment of the underlying disease is important to control the physiologic component of fatigue. Medications and cognitive behavioral therapy have also shown a positive response by providing coping strategies and decreasing fatigue levels.

A regular aerobic or resistance exercise routine even at low intensities can prevent deconditioning and muscle wasting, improve efficiency of movement, and decrease fatigue across many neurological diagnosis.[15,21]

DIAGNOSTIC-SPECIFIC RESPONSE TO EXERCISE

Introduction

Dysfunction of the adult nervous system can be caused by traumatic, slowly or rapidly progressing degenerative disorders. The pattern of neuronal loss can be distinctive to the disease and produce a range of impairments affecting function and ADL. The ability to adequately prescribe an exercise intervention depends on our knowledge of the underlying pathology, risk for primary and secondary impairments, and potential for recovery or disease progression. This section will attempt to outline this information for the most common disorders of the neuromuscular system.

Traumatic Injury

A traumatic injury to the neuromuscular system can be described as an initial insult to the nervous system followed by a period of recovery of function.

Stroke

Pathology

Stroke remains one of the third leading causes of death in the United States behind heart disease, and is a leading cause of disability.[69,70] The average incidence is about 114 per 100,000, with approximately 4 million stroke survivors alive in the United States.[3] Risk factors for ischemic strokes include HTN, atrial fibrillation, DM, age, and smoking.[70] The term "stroke" refers to hemorrhagic events and ischemic infarcts to the brain. Ischemic strokes make up about 87% of all stroke types and occur when there is inadequate blood supply to the brain. Ischemic strokes occur in either small vessels, resulting in more focal deficits, or large vessels that typically involve multisystem impairments. A blockage of the blood vessel can be caused by either an embolus or narrowing of the vessel known as stenosis.

Residual impairments post-stroke are due to injury or death of the brain tissue supplied by that vessel. A stroke in the middle cerebral artery (MCA) may present with contralateral weakness in the UE greater than the LE, contralateral sensory and vision loss, and language or visual spatial disorders. A stroke affecting the region supplied by the anterior cerebral artery (ACA) may present with contralateral weakness in the LE greater than the UE, contralateral sensory loss, abulia, and aphasia when the left hemisphere is involved. The most common deficits consistent with a stroke involving the posterior cerebral artery (PCA) include homonymous hemianopsia, memory loss, visual hallucinations, topographic disorientation, and sensory loss. Small-vessel lacunar infarcts often present with pure motor hemiplegia or hemisensory loss, or dysarthria. Border zone infarction presents with deficits in more proximal body structures such as the shoulder and hips, rather than distal body structures likes the hands and feet. Strokes that occur in the brainstem may present with impairments in cranial nerve function, oculomotor deficits, and ipsilateral ataxia, bilateral hemiparesis, and hemisensory loss.[2,3,71]

Hemorrhagic strokes make up the remaining 13% and occur when a cerebral blood vessel ruptures, resulting in bleeding into the brain tissue.[72] The largest risk factor is high BP. These types of strokes occur in a younger population and are more fatal, with approximately 38% dying within the first 30 days, but there is better recovery potential for those who survive.[70,72] Symptom presentation depends on the mechanism of the stroke, and the region of the brain that is affected. There may also be the indirect territories affected around the region of the stroke, or from nerve fibers that pass through the region of the stroke.[72] The most common locations affected by hemorrhages are the putamen (50%), thalamus (15%), pons (10), cerebellum (10%), and the lobar (15%). According to the American Heart Association, the primary impairments observed after stroke are weakness or numbness in 50% of patients, and impaired ability to walk without a device or assistance in 30%.[70]

Many risk factors for stroke are shared with coronary artery disease and are modifiable. These include HTN, DM, high cholesterol, obesity, cigarette smoking, and cardiac disease.[2,73]

Impairments Contributing to Decreased Mobility

Stroke is the leading cause of long-term disability in the United States.[70] While individuals post-stroke may present with a variety of deficits, motor function impairments such as weakness and discoordination are the most prominent that contribute to disability.[74] Damage to the primary motor cortex after a stroke affects central motor activation causing a loss of force production and excessive muscular cocontraction.[75] After stroke there is often an increased activation of the secondary motor areas but these projections have less excitatory effect.[6] This decreased ability to produce a consistent and coordinated force then results in further weakness due to a reduction in the number of recruitable motor units, a decreased amount of lean muscle mass in the paretic limb, a 20% to 25% increase in intramuscular fat in the hemiparetic limb compared to the nonparetic limb, a loss of Type I muscle fibers, and a diminished capacity for oxidative metabolism in the paretic limb.[74,76-78] Muscle weakness and atrophy with an increased prevalence of fast-twitch muscle fibers on the contralateral limb are strong predictors of gait deficit severity.[75] These central and peripheral impairments to motor function produce a grossly inefficient hemiparetic gait pattern with greater oxygen consumption necessary to sustain self-selected walking speeds, contributing to aerobic deconditioning.[79,80]

An alteration in tone may cause an increased stiffness in the muscle with subsequent connective tissue changes such as contractures.[11] Loss of range of motion (ROM), especially at the ankle and hip, can contribute to a decrease in gait speed and efficiency.[81]

A consistent goal among stroke survivors is to return to home and community activities through walking. Yet, ambulatory activities are reported well below that of healthy but sedentary age-matched peers.[82] Functional gait speed in stroke can be classified using the following self-selected gait speed parameters[83,84]:

- Physiologic: 0.1 m/s
- Household ambulation: < 0.4 m/s
- Limited community ambulation: 0.4 to 0/8 m/s
- Community ambulation: > 0.8 m/s

The energy requirements of a hemiparetic gait pattern have been reported to be as much as 55% to 100% more than age-matched controls.[74] Regardless of age, stroke survivors often present with a higher metabolic cost of walking demonstrated by dramatically lower peak VO_2 than their age-matched healthy peers, and commonly have a limited fitness reserve related to their poor walking economy.[85-87] This can contribute to feelings of fatigue that have been reported in up to 97% of individuals who have suffered a stroke, regardless of neurological recovery.[14]

With the increased effort necessary for gait and a compounding sense of fatigue, a decreased level of activity can be a natural progression.

Regardless of age, cardiovascular fitness affected by gait performance is markedly impaired within 4 to 6 weeks post-stroke.[76] The high-energy cost of walking also decreases participation in ADL, leading to a spiral of continued progression of weakness, muscle atrophy, impaired cardiovascular fitness, and eventual disability.[76]

While most treatment and recovery occurs in the first few weeks and months after stroke, many patients are left with residuals deficits that limit activity. There is a high prevalence of extreme sedentary lifestyles after stroke contributing to deconditioning, and recurrent stroke. The prevalence of cardiac disease in stroke survivors has been reported to be as high as 75%.[73,74,88] Recurrent strokes account for up to 25% of all new strokes annually.[3] Baseline aerobic capacity is often lower than in age-matched peers, and reduced activity levels may then contribute to an increased energy cost of movement, with further deconditioning leading to an increased risk for cardiovascular disease and recurrent stroke.[79]

Considering the prominence of cardiac disease, risk for recurrent stroke, and the strong association between strength, fitness levels, and gait speed to activity and participation, the evaluation and intervention of muscle weakness, aerobic capacity, and gait should be high priorities throughout the rehabilitation process.[89]

Intervention

The design of an intervention program for a person with a stroke is multifaceted. There is the primary drive for functional recovery, the basic principles of which include repetitive skilled training to promote reorganization of movement representations within the motor cortex.[90] Walking capacity post-stroke is directly correlated to paretic leg strength and cardiovascular fitness.[91] Understanding the factors that contribute most to mobility help up when designing an exercise program.

Improvements in muscle strength can be made in stroke by 10% to 75%. The main target of a resistance program is to affect peripheral contributions to motor weakness at the level of the muscle. An increase in the volume of muscle fibers and increases in the rate of torque development and motor unit discharge can increase the strength of a hemiparetic muscle.[90] Improvements in strength of key LE muscle groups contribute to improved gait quality, speed, and efficiency on the 6MWT.[89] Strength of knee flexors and extensors alone can predict home vs. community walking ability, while hip flexion and soleus muscle strengths have been associated with faster gait speeds.[81,83] The principle of strength training is the same for stroke as for able-bodied individuals. The American College of Sports Medicine (ACSM) recommendations for strengthening in stroke include lifting a load that allows 8 to 12 repetitions through the available ROM before fatigue performed 2 to 3 times per week with rest in between for recovery. The key element that is often overlooked is to increase the intensity through increased resistance as the ability to generate force improves.[92] Strength training alone has not been shown to alter the organization of the cortical motor map, but when combined with task-specific practice has been shown to improve function.[90] It was thought at one time that strengthening in the presence of spasticity or hypertonia would cause a further increase in muscle tone. We understand now that this is not the case, and that strengthening is a safe an effective intervention in the presence of abnormal muscle tone.[13] Strengthening can also provide the element necessary to tolerate and achieve the high intensity needed for aerobic conditioning or skill acquisition during repetitive task practice.[90]

Aerobic exercise should be an important component of stroke rehabilitation given the significant adverse health consequences of deconditioning, and the increased risk of recurrent stroke that is associated with physical inactivity.[70] The trend in current clinical practice, however, shows that the levels of cardiovascular stress induced in current rehabilitation programs is not at a high enough level to induce an aerobic training effect.[93] This is an important point to consider as training workload is considered more predictive of treatment response than age, previous fitness levels, or lesion location.[79]

Pang et al studied 480 subjects with mild to moderate stroke who participated in an aerobic exercise program for 20 to 40 minutes, 3 to 5 days per week while working at an intensity of 50% to 80% of their HR reserve with significant improvements in peak VO_2 and peak workload.[94] Aerobic conditioning in stroke can also improve independence in ambulation and increase walking speeds and endurance.[86,95] An increase in gait speed by as little as 0.16m/s is more likely to produce a meaningful improvement in level of disability.[96] As a preventive measure it has been shown to decrease systolic BP, and the risk of recurrent stroke.[79,89] Many studies follow exercise protocols recommended by ACSM. The ACSM suggests an aerobic exercise frequency of 3 to 5 times per week, for 20 to 30 minutes per session, at an intensity of 55% to 90% HR_{max}. For someone just starting an aerobic program an appropriate intensity would be to work at 40% to 50% HR_{max} and to then build up to as close to 90% HR_{max} as tolerated.[29] Duration can start with a few minutes and build intermittently. Fitness training is safe and feasible and can be most effective post-stroke when performed for >30 minutes 3 times per week while maintaining a HR >70% age-adjusted HR_{max} (220 – age %)[7] as the ultimate goal.[95] The most benefits are seen when training is provided for >12 weeks.

Walking at a fast walking speed, and treadmill walking with or without a harness, are considered the most effective modes of cardiovascular training.[89,90,97-99] Aerobic training with a treadmill improves cardiovascular fitness, gait speed, and tolerance, and may produce sub-cortical reorganization in acute and chronic stroke survivors.[80,88] For more severely deconditioned individuals post-stroke, exercise with short bouts of 2 to 3 minutes of treadmill walking followed by rest breaks appears to have positive benefits.[97] Home- or clinic-based task-specific walking programs also resulted in improvements in walking speed and endurance that were sustained several months after the intervention was completed.[99,100]

For individuals who do not have the balance necessary for treadmill walking or are unable to achieve speeds that would produce a cardiovascular benefit during overground walking, an arm-leg ergometer, recumbent bike, or arm bike may also be able to provide a cardiovascular benefit, but to a lesser degree. Cycle ergometry appears to be the most common method of aerobic training for individuals post stroke.[94] Hemiparetic limbs may also be comfortably secured to arm and leg pedals to better participate in the reciprocal movement, and have demonstrated potential for improved sub-maximal effort when involved in the training protocol.[79]

Programs focusing on a combination of aerobic training and strengthening are more beneficial for improving the efficiency of gait than strengthening programs alone.[90,101] Combining the 2 training modalities significantly improves VO_2 peak, walking economy, and exercise tolerance.[86] Exercise and plasticity response depend on the dose of stimulus delivered, the specificity of the mode of intervention provided, and the context of the task being practiced. Combining these primary elements of exercise for individuals with stroke can provide functional and health benefits that can improve activity and social participation.

Spinal Cord Injury

Pathology

SCI is a relatively rare but catastrophic and expensive event with an incidence of approximately 40 cases per million in the United States or 10,000 to 12,000 new cases annually. There are an estimated 232,000 to 316,000 people currently living with SCI.[3,102] From health care costs to lost wages, the estimated cost of management of SCI is approximately $4 billion annually.[103] The average age at the time of

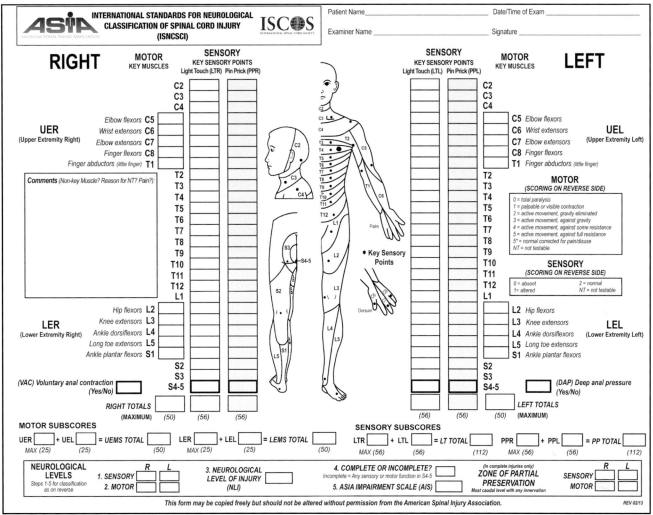

Figure 12-7. International Standards for Neurologic Classification of Spinal Cord Injury. From http://www.asia-spinalinjury.org/elearning/ASIA_ISCOS_high.pdf.

injury is 40.7 years with more than 80% of cases being male. Approximately 35% to 40% of SCIs are caused by a motor vehicle accident (MVA), while greater than 20% are related to falls, and 15% are related to acts of violence such as gunshot wounds. Less than 10% of SCIs are sports related such as while diving or playing contact sports. Other causes of SCI can be infection, tumor, thrombosis, or spinal degeneration. The incidence of SCI has decreased over the years with the implementation of preventive safety strategies such as seatbelt and drunk driving laws.[3,102,104]

The American Spinal Injury Association Impairment Scale (ASIA) is an impairment level scale used when grading injury severity in SCI. Motor and sensory function are identified at certain spinal levels and lesions are classified as either complete or incomplete. Complete lesions are defined as having no sensory or motor function below the level of the lesion including the lowest sacral segment. Incomplete lesions implies some sensory and motor function below the level of the lesion including the lowest sacral segments.[105] ASIA classification can change over time, and can be used when determining prognosis[102] (Figure 12-7; ASIA Scale).

The mechanism of injury can determine the type and severity of the injury. Most traumatic SCIs are caused by compression or displacement of the spinal cord due to excessive flexion, extension or rotational forces. Incomplete lesions typically fall into 5 categories:

1. Anterior cord syndrome is the most common pattern and is typically caused by an excessive flexion injury, MS, or anterior spinal artery infarct that disrupts the anterolateral pathways. Loss of pain and temperature sensation can be noted with damage to the spinothalamic tract, and bilateral loss of motor function is present with corticospinal tract injury.[2,3] Proprioception is typically spared.[105]

2. Posterior cord syndrome is a rare extension injury seen more in the elderly population. Patients will present clinically with a loss of proprioception often causing a wide base of support during gait. Motor function and pain and temperature sensation are intact. Larger lesions may encroach the corticospinal tracts, causing weakness.[2,105]

3. Central cord syndrome is often caused by degenerative narrowing of the spinal canal, tumor, or hyperextension

injury of the cervical spine. Clinical presentation depends on the size of the lesion. Smaller lesions may include the spinothalamic tracts with loss of pain and temperature sensation. Larger central cord lesions may present with anterior horn cells and corticospinal tract damage.[2] UEs are more affected than lower extremities.[3]

4. Brown-Séquard syndrome is most commonly caused by a stab or gunshot wound, and results in deficits on only one side of the spinal cord. Damage to the lateral corticospinal and posterior spinothalamic tracts will cause weakness, loss of proprioception, kinesthesia, and vibration on the ipsilateral side of the lesion. Loss of pain and temperature is noted slightly below the level of the lesion on the contralateral side of the lesion due to damage of the anterolateral fibers.[2]

5. Conus medullaris and conus equina syndrome are the result of damage to the base of the spinal cord and can present clinically with weakness, loss of sensation, and reflexive bladder.[3]

Patients with a SCI are further classified by level of injury and categorized as either having paraplegia if the injury affects the thoracic and lumbar regions only, or tetraplegia if the injury is in the cervical region with all 4 limbs, and trunk including respiratory muscles are involved. There is an approximately equal incidence of injuries that result in either paraplegia or tetraplegia,[3] with trend toward a decrease in rates of motor complete (ASIA A or B) injury.[106]

People with SCI have a close to normal life expectancy. Because of a more sedentary lifestyle, however, CVD becomes the leading cause of death ahead of respiratory disease, renal conditions, DM, and smoking in people who survive a traumatic SCI greater than 1 year.[107] The prevalence of asymptomatic and symptomatic CVD in SCI can be as high as 50% compared to 5% to 10% in able-bodied, age-matched peers.[25] Risk factors for CVD in SCI include lipid disorders, metabolic syndrome, obesity, physical inactivity, accelerated aging, and DM.[25,108,109] Other risks for CVD can be caused by the low BP and stroke volume in individuals with tetraplegia causing left ventricular hypertrophy, as well as a decreased volume and circulatory dysregulation in the LEs.[109,110] The risk for CVD is accelerated in this population and corresponds to the level of the injury, with a 16% increased risk for individuals with tetraplegia, a 70% increase risk for individuals with paraplegia, and a 44% increased risk for individuals with complete injuries.[25] Many studies have also observed a direct association between level of injury and peak oxygen uptake and the level of peak work obtained during physical activity, so that the higher the injury level the more blunted the response to physical activity.[110]

Impairments Affecting Mobility

While SCI is a devastating injury with a variable presentation, the most prominent deficit affecting mobility and participation in exercise is the loss of motor function. Motor function can be impaired from damage to the long corticospinal tracts that carry information from the motor cortex to the spinal cord, and damage to anterior horn cells, and spinal nerves that transmit information to the muscles.[3] Weakness can be a product of the SCI itself as well as muscle structure and contractile properties changes that occur because of deconditioning. Within 1 month of injury, muscle fibers below the level of the lesion are smaller, have less contractile property, and produce lower peak contractile forces. Muscle fibers begin to transform toward the fast-type phenotype and fatigue more rapidly.[109,110] These factors contribute to a decline in motor function, which then exacerbates muscle wasting and deconditioning, further impairing the daily energy expenditure in SCI.[25] Muscle weakness or paralysis can be extensive enough that voluntary exercise may be ineffective, or even impossible. Other effects of SCI that can restrict participation in exercise or are a cause of prolonged immobility are autonomic dysreflexia, fatigue, respiratory, and cardiovascular complications.

Autonomic dysreflexia (AD) can occur in spinal cord lesions above the level of T6. AD is associated with an elevated risk of CVD due to abnormal BP, HR variability, and a blunted HR response to aerobic exercise.[25] Individuals with autonomic dysfunction are at severe risk for both supine and orthostatic hypotension.[3] Symptoms of AD include headaches, HTN, bradycardia, diaphoresis, anxiety, and piloerection and can be caused by noxious stimulation such as bowel or bladder distention, tactile stimulation, or elevated BP during activity or exercise.[3] Signs for AD should be monitored carefully because when uncontrolled it can cause stroke, seizures, intracerebral hemorrhage or cardiac insult.[102] Considerations for exercise and the use of HR measures as a gauge of intensity may not be accurate in SCI because of AD.[111] AD in individuals with paraplegia presents as a lower HR complexity at rest and with exercise, and an exaggerated HR response during physical activity.[110,112] Individuals with tetraplegia may not be able to sufficiently activate the sympathetic nervous system to provide enough central circulatory support during increased activity levels. This will contribute to peak HR levels that will typically max out at about 120 beats per minute.[113] Deconditioning due to skeletal muscle paralysis will also contribute to altered autonomic cardiovascular modulation.[114]

Daily energy expenditure is lower in SCI because of lack of motor function, but also because of lack of opportunity and accessibility to physical activity. While individuals with paraplegia seemingly have more options for exercise, and the ability to achieve peak VO$_2$, they are only marginally more fit than individuals with tetraplegia.[110] Metabolic and skeletal muscle abnormalities due to deconditioning can be partially reversible in SCI through endurance training.[25] Considering the dramatic decline in activity levels of most individuals post-SCI, and the significant increased risk of CVD, initiation of a cardiovascular fitness program is appropriate even in the acute stages of recovery with maintenance a priority.

Cardiovascular fitness testing can be performed safely with most individuals with SCI. Exercise stress testing is an important first step to rule out CVD, provide an objective peak HR for the exercise prescription, and provide information on the baseline exercise tolerance of the individual.[115] Most sub-maximal fitness tests are conducted on a treadmill, with a cycle ergometer, or during overground walking but this may not be feasible for many individuals with SCI. The most common mode of exercise and cardiorespiratory testing in SCI is with an arm-crank ergometer.[110] The 6-Minute Arm Test (6MAT) is a sub-maximal arm ergometry test that is considered a reliable and inexpensive option for many clinic settings and can be performed on people with paraplegia and tetraplegia. Aerobic parameters used if signs of AD are not present are to work at 60% to 70% of age-predicted HR_{max}, or 11 to 15 on a Borg rating scale of perceived exertion.[116]

Consideration for the level of the injury needs to be made as physiologic responses to exercise are different from those without a SCI as discussed above, and risks of poorly designed programs are greater.[109]

Other tests that should be considered prior to implementing an exercise program are bone-mineral density testing to establish fracture risk, blood and glucose testing for baseline lipid and DM screening, and pulmonary function tests (PFT) to provide an objective baseline measure of ventilatory impairment, which inversely correlates to the level of the spinal cord lesion.[115]

Intervention

Major challenges to designing an endurance program for individuals with SCI is the reduced capacity to engage in large muscle endurance exercise because of LE weakness, a limited ability to stimulate and regulate the autonomic, cardiovascular systems, and temperature regulatory systems to support a high intensity of aerobic exercise. Secondary effects of the reduced activity levels that can further challenge activity is bone loss due to decreased exposure to weightbearing activities, skeletal and cardiac muscle atrophy, early-onset muscle fatigue, reduced lean mass, and an increase in fat percentages.[117] Individuals who rely of manual or power wheelchairs for mobility are at a higher risk for developing these secondary effects of deconditioning. Despite these limitations, with a well-designed program persons with SCI have the potential to benefit from exercise intervention to improve strength and aerobic capacity, and reduce the risk of health problems related to inactivity. Participation may need to include adaptive equipment or the use of electrical stimulation to achieve an aerobic benefit.

Individuals with tetraplegia have a 16% higher risk for developing cardiovascular illnesses compared to individuals with paraplegia.[25] More profound muscle weakness and loss of muscle mass combined with autonomic dysfunction contribute to the elevated risk. Initiation of a cardiovascular fitness routine early after injury may decrease this risk and reduce symptoms of orthostatic hypotension. Arm ergometry alone may be a challenge because of small muscle mass and easy peripheral fatigability. Tawashy et al presented positive effects of a UE circuit training program performed for a total of 30 minutes, 3 times per week, to minimize UE fatigue and boredom and to better facilitate improvements in aerobic capacity.[118] Exercise intensity cannot be predictably monitored with HR responses, so rating perceived exertion may be more accurate.

For individuals with paraplegia, options for training can be more accessible with the use of the UEs. Arm ergometry, wheelchair ergometry, and swimming are the most common modes of aerobic training, as they are accessible to those with residual or full UE muscle function. The magnitude of fitness achieved is typically inversely proportional to the level of the injury.[109] Individuals with tetraplegia can achieve the same gains in peak oxygen uptake using UE ergometry with assistance given to affix their hands to the device.[109] Hybrid training, or the use of an arm ergometer combined with functional electrical stimulation (FES) cycling at moderate and high intensity is a safe and feasible mode of cardiovascular training demonstrating superior improvements in VO_2 peak, stroke volume, LE muscle mass and strength compared to voluntary leg cycling or arm ergometry alone.[119-122] For individuals with long-standing muscle atrophy and deconditioning, strengthening of quadriceps muscles prior to the initiation of leg cycle FES enhances participation.

Electrically stimulated muscle contraction is utilized as a method of strengthening in SCI through indirect stimulation of the intact peripheral nerve. This method of exercise requires a functionally intact LMN system. There are several forms of electrically stimulated modes of exercise, including arm ergometry, leg cycling, leg exercise combined with UE exercise, lower body rowing, electrically stimulated standing, and bipedal ambulation with and without orthoses.[109] A systematic review performed by Nightingale et al on the benefits of FES gait revealed limited evidence for improvements in aerobic capacity or improvements in energy expenditure during gait, with stronger evidence supporting improvements in LE strength after training with FES.[123] While the current evidence is inconclusive, the trend is toward support of the intervention for multiple variables, with limitations primarily in the amount of available literature and the inconsistency in the methodology of assessment.

Jacobs and Nash et al used a circuit resistance training (CRT) program combining resistance exercise and high-speed, low-resistance arm ergometry with people with motor complete paraplegia. The purpose was to target both arm strength for UE injury prevention and cardiovascular endurance. After 12 to 16 weeks of 30- to 45-minute routines performed 3 times per week, the subjects demonstrated significant increases in peak VO_2, time to fatigue, and peak power output during arm testing, with no adverse effects.[124,125]

Recommended prescription guidelines for aerobic training are to work at an intensity of 40% to 80% of HR reserve, or 20 to 30 beats above resting HR, if stress test was not performed, for >30 minutes of continuous exercise. A frequency of 2 to 3 times per week is suggested with the most appropriate modality, which may include an arm or wheelchair ergometer, treadmill training, seated aerobics, swimming, electric stimulation leg cycle ergometry, or circuit resistance training.[115] In the presence of autonomic dysfunction in SCI, use of self-ratings of perceived exertion can be inconsistent when correlated with physiologic responses to exercise. This may not be a valid method of measuring exertion in the presence of tetraplegia more so than paraplegia.[126] Adapted sports-related activities are recommended to enhance participation. Exercise response during power wheelchair competition has the potential to reach or even surpass cardio-respiratory fitness training thresholds when performed for more than 30 minutes.[127] The mechanisms for improved aerobic capacity post-SCI are more likely due to improved muscle strength and oxygen perfusion than actual changes in cardiovascular response of HR, stroke volume, or cardiac output.[128]

Manual wheelchair users are more susceptible to chronic overuse injuries of the UEs due to the repetitive strain placed on them during daily mobility with a wheelchair. Resistance training should focus on UE and trunk muscles for joint protection, injury prevention, and promotion of improved mobility and function. Recommendations for resistance training are to work at an intensity of 50% to 80% one repetition maximum (1RPM), for 2 to 3 sets of 10 reps at least 2 times per week. Free weight, Nautilus equipment, and Therabands are all considered appropriate modalities.[115]

There are several unique risks in SCI that need to be considered prior to implementing an exercise program. As mentioned previously, autonomic dysfunction is common in lesions above the T6 spinal level, with more severe complication noted with complete SCIs. Symptoms of AD that need to monitored for are cardiac and circulatory dysfunction, clotting disorders, altered insulin metabolism, resting and exercise immunodysfunction, orthostatic hypotension, osteoporosis, joint deterioration, and thermal dysregulation at rest or with exercise.[109] Exercise in temperature-controlled environments, hydration throughout exercise routine, observing for signs of heat stress, bowel and bladder emptying prior to exercise, and careful observation of HR and BP responses to exercises are needed to decrease complications from autonomic dysfunction.

More than 50% of sublesional bone is lost within the first 6 months after an SCI, leaving the patient at an increased risk for fracture. Bone-mineral density testing should be considered, especially in individuals who have been nonweightbearing for extended periods of time.[109,115] Musculoskeletal-overuse injuries may be undetectable in areas where sensation or pain is diminished. Injuries may be detectable in the presence of swelling, increased spasticity or muscle spasms, warmth or erthema.[109] When using high-intensity electrical stimulation in the presence of sensory loss there is an increased risk of skin burns. Close monitoring of skin with frequent replacement of electrodes can decrease this risk.

Traumatic Brain Injury

Pathology

Traumatic or acquired brain injury (TBI) is defined as an injury to the head that disrupts the normal function of the brain. TBI is currently the leading cause of death and life-long disability in the United States. Each year approximately 1.7 million people sustain a TBI with approximately 50,000 deaths, 275,000 hospitalizations, and 80,000 to 90,000 people left with permanent disability. With approximately 5.3 million people currently living with disability caused by TBI, the estimated cost of direct and indirect medical costs combined with lost productivity is $60 billion. The groups most at risk are men, young children, adolescents, and the elderly. Falls and MVAs account for more than half of all TBIs, with assaults, sports-related injuries, and other occurrences accounting for the rest.[129,130]

TBIs can be categorized as either focal, which tend to be caused by a contact force, or diffuse, which tend to be caused by noncontact, acceleration-deceleration, or rotational forces. Primary damage is a direct result of the injury, while secondary brain damage occurs because of the body's reaction to the trauma. Secondary brain damage can continue for days to weeks after the initial injury and is influenced by medical management.[129]

Focal brain injuries typically result in cortical contusions or lacerations that are classified according to the location of the intracranial hemorrhage. Epidural hematoma (EDH) is typically formed when the middle meningeal artery ruptures between the dura and the skull. This is a rapidly expanding hemorrhage that forms a lens-shaped biconvex hematoma and can cause significant compression of the brain within hours of impact.[2] Subdural hematoma (SDH) can be chronic or acute and typically occurs after a shearing type injury that disrupts the bridging veins between the arachnoid and dura space. This venous injury forms a crescent-shaped hematoma and can takes days to weeks to present clinically depending on the age of the person and the velocity of the impact.[2,3]

Diffuse axonal injury (DAI) is a more widespread injury that indicates a more severe injury and accounts for 40% to 50% of hospital TBI admissions.[129] DAI is typically caused by acceleration-deceleration and rotational forces, and is the predominant reason for loss of consciousness post-TBI. The shearing injury of the axons impairs transport of protein from the cell body and causes swelling of the axon and axonal death. A secondary process of axonal injury occurs causing a loss of ion gradients across cell membranes. This metabolic cascade can cause cell death, or apoptosis, over a period of days, week, or even months after injury.[131] DAI can be seen throughout the brain regardless of the site of the initial injury, and is more often in midline structures including the parasagittal white matter of the cerebral cortex, corpus callosum, basal ganglia, brainstem, and cerebellum.[3]

The increase in volume in the intracranial space caused by either lesion type has secondary effects that can cause further brain damage. Normal intracranial pressure (ICP) in adults is less than 15 mm Hg.[2] Intracranial hemorrhage can cause an increase in blood volume or swelling of the brain, which can trigger an elevation in ICP. Severely elevated ICP can cause a decrease in blood flow with further brain ischemia, or a mass effect shifting brain tissue and causing herniation of brain tissue and compression of periventricular structures.[2,3]

TABLE 12-2. CLASSIFICATION OF TRAUMATIC BRAIN INJURY SEVERITY

CRITERIA	MILD	MODERATE	SEVERE
Structural imaging	Normal	Normal or abnormal	Normal or abnormal
Loss of Consciousness (LOC)	0 = 30 min	> 30 min and < 24 hours	> 24 hours
Alteration of consciousness/mental state (AOC)*	a moment up to 24 hours	> 24 hours. Severity based on other criteria	
Post-traumatic amnesia (PTA)	0 = 1 day	> 1 and < 7 days	> 7 days
Glasgow Coma Scale (best available score in first 24 hours)	13 to 15	9 to 12	< 9
Reprinted from Management of Concussion/mTBI Working Group. VA/DoD Clinical Practice Guideline for Management of Concussion/ Mild Traumatic Brain Injury. *J Rehabil Res Dev.* 2009;46(6):CP1-68.			

TBI is primarily classified as mild, moderate, or severe based on structural imaging, the duration of loss consciousness (LOC) and the Glasgow Coma Scale (GCS) (Table 12-2).[129] Impairments generally reflect both the focal and diffuse nature of the injury.

Impairments Affecting Mobility

After a TBI variable patterns of deficits are observed. Common impairments affecting mobility and participation in exercise include weakness, motor control abnormalities, altered cognition, and impaired balance.[49] Fatigue and poor sleep patterns are also prominent.[132] Spasticity does not appear to contribute to decreased economy of movement post-TBI.[12] Predictors of return to ambulation include the patient's ability to ambulate at admission to rehabilitation, and the duration of post-traumatic amnesia.[133]

Individuals following a TBI rapidly develop secondary sequelae related to the decreased level of mobility that comes with prolonged hospitalization. Mossberg et al studied the aerobic capacity of individuals post-TBI with minimal physical impairments and found that they presented with significantly lower peak responses for HR and VO$_2$, had impaired pulmonary efficiency, and overall decreased levels of cardiovascular fitness contributing to complaints of fatigue and decreased levels of participation.[134,135] TBI survivors are also 3 times more likely to die from circulatory conditions such as heart disease, stroke, and high BP as a consequence of a prolonged sedentary lifestyle. Despite these secondary complications, individuals with moderate to severe TBI provide consistent responses to maximal exercise testing, and can safely perform at sub-maximal and peak aerobic training.[30] Improvements in aerobic capacity are associated with improvements in aerobic efficiency.[136]

Fatigue has been reported as one of the most consistent impairments experienced by individuals who have suffered a TBI, with 50% to 80% reporting symptoms.[19,54] Complaints of fatigue are not necessarily correlated to injury severity or age at the time of the injury. Primary fatigue in TBI may be caused by impaired excitability of the motor cortex, and hypopituitarism.[19] Secondary fatigue may result from sleep

disorders, pain, depression, and deconditioning.[19,134,137] The greatest amount of fatigue is typically reported within the first 6 months of injury, with improvements noted between 6 and 12 months post-TBI.[19] After 12 months there is another trend of increased complaints of fatigue that are most likely due to the effects of deconditioning due to impairments in mobility.

Cycle ergometry, both upright and recumbent, are more commonly used during graded exercise modalities in the presence of balance and gait impairments. While both cycle and treadmill testing are reliable measures in TBI, treadmill testing is recommended when safe and feasible as it elicits a higher peak VO$_2$ and is more functional.[30,135] In the clinical setting submaximal testing such as the 6MWT are more accessible. The 6MWT is a reliable measure of gait speed and aerobic capacity in individuals with TBI.[33] Age-predicted HR$_{max}$ is a reliable measure of cardiovascular response and fitness in individuals with TBI, and can be utilized during the 6MWT as a measure of aerobic capacity.[135]

Intervention

Despite the variability in residual deficits in body structure and function post-TBI, many individuals consistently adopt a sedentary lifestyle confirmed by a decline of peak aerobic capacity to only 65% to 74% of their age-matched peers,[135,136] and a reduction in pulmonary function by 25% to 40%.[17] This trend toward deconditioning contributes to an increased risk of cardiovascular and cardiopulmonary disorders. Incorporating a lifelong program of aerobic training may play an important role overall physical capacity and in long-term mortality in TBI.[138]

Aerobic training in the presence of TBI has not been well documented, but the few studies to date demonstrate positive effects in physical endurance and metabolic capacity.[17] Mossberg et al followed 40 individuals with chronic TBI who participated in a standard physical therapy program with the addition of only 15 to 20 minutes of low-intensity aerobic exercise utilizing either a motorized treadmill, stair climber, recumbent or stationary bike. All participants demonstrated improvements in cardiorespiratory fitness with increased walking tolerance and decreased sub-maximal HR.[139] This finding supports the benefits of aerobic condition regardless of the modality used. While general fitness training has demonstrated consistent improvements in cardiovascular conditioning and exercise capacity, there is limited evidence translating into improvements in functional capacity.[137]

The evidence supporting the use of treadmill training with and without body weight support to promote neurological recovery is inconclusive in individuals with TBI.[140] This is most likely due to the very small samples sizes and extreme variability of impairments and deficit severity in TBI. When the primary purpose of treadmill training is to utilize it as a method of aerobic condition, response is more consistently favorable. Individuals who trained on a treadmill demonstrated greater VO_2 than those who trained on mechanical stairs or a bike ergometer. The need for more focused attention to task with a stationary bike or stair climber to maintain a high intensity may play a role in the varied responses. Stationary cycling and mechanical stair climbing tend to be more self-paced and exercise performance can be more consistently challenged using a treadmill.[141] Specific research has not been conducted to compare the effects of training with or without body weight support when balance safety is a concern and body weight support is available.

A combined aerobic and resistance program performed at an intensity of 60% to 80% age-adjusted HR_{max} for 25 minutes 2 to 3 days per week for 12 weeks demonstrated improvements in aerobic capacity, peak VO_2, peak power output, and respiratory efficiency.[141] Circuit training is thought to be particularly effective in the presence of TBI when attention and motivation are limited. Bhambhani et al used a protocol combining intermittent upper and lower body high-resistance, short-duration weight-lifting exercises with treadmill, cycle or arm ergometry. Subjects were encouraged to maintain an HR at or above 60% of their HR reserve, and at 12 weeks subjects presented improvements in peak power output, and peak VO_2.[31]

Individuals post-TBI with a higher number of residual symptoms and limited community integration are less likely to exercise, and also have higher levels of perceived disability and handicap. The design of an individualized and motivating program that meets the need of the person is associated with decreased impairment, elevated mood, and perceptions of better health.[138]

Degenerative Diseases

Degenerative diseases of the nervous system can affect gray matter, white matter, or both. Progression can be slow and over a period of decades with close to normal life expectancy, or rapid over a period of months to just a few years leading to death. The understanding of the pathology as well as the pattern of progression can be important when considering the goals of an exercise-based intervention. The following section will explore a variety of the most common disorders across the spectrum of disease progression.

Parkinson's Disease

PD is a slowly progressive neurodegenerative disease affecting as many as 1 to 1.5 million United States citizens. The average onset occurs in the fifth decade with an increasing incidence and prevalence as the population ages. Patients may notice initial subtle symptoms such as difficulty with writing, an asymmetrical resting tremor, or slowness of movements. The diagnosis is made by exclusion and assessment for cardinal clinical features that include resting tremor, muscular rigidity with a "cogwheeling" resistance to passive movement, bradykinesia, and loss of postural control. Diagnosis can often be confirmed by a positive response to levodopa or a dopamine antagonist.[142,143]

PD is caused by a degeneration of dopaminergic neurons in the substantia nigra pars compacta of the basal ganglia. The pattern of neuronal loss tends to be in the ventrolateral tier followed by the medial ventral tier, which is the opposite of normal aging.[144] Dopamine has both an excitatory and inhibitory effect on the thalamus.[2] This loss of dopamine has a net inhibitory effect on the thalamus, and is thought to play a key role in the slow movement and delayed initiation of movement seen in PD.[3,145] There is a suspected preclinical period of 5 to 15 years as symptoms typically do not present themselves until approximately 30% to 40% of dopaminergic neurons of the substantia nigra pars compacta and 70% to 80% of dopamine depletion in the striatum occurs.[142,146] While movement is not lost, depletion of dopamine in the striatum is thought to impair the learning of new movement sequences and causes a loss of reflexive or automatic movement.[3] Learning becomes extremely task specific, as does the ability to task shift as the dysfunction in the basal ganglia progresses.[20] Dopaminergic neurons that remain often contain characteristic cytoplasmic inclusions called *Lewy bodies* and can be found in all affected brainstem areas. Lewy body neuritis has been shown to correlate with the degree of cognitive impairments seen in patients with PD.[2,144] As this degeneration progresses, gait and balance disturbances become more prominent, leading to falls, a decline in mobility, and an increased risk of mortality.[146]

Disease staging is measured using the modified Hoehn and Yahr (H&Y) Staging Scale, which is a 7-point ordinal scale ranging from 1 (unilateral disease involvement) to 5 (wheelchair bound or bedridden unless aided). The H&Y scale has shown a high correlation in neuroimaging studies with dopaminergic loss, and with motor impairments, disability, and quality of life measures (Figure 12-8).[147]

Impairments Affecting Mobility

Bradykinesia is one of the most classic clinical features of PD that affects mobility. This hallmark sign of basal ganglia disorders refers to an overall slowness of movement and is a result of the excessive inhibition to the thalamus suppressing the motor cortical regions, and abnormal projections to brainstem locomotor areas contributing to posture and gait abnormalities.[3,145] Patients with bradykinesia also have difficulty planning, initiating, and executing tasks.[148] Bradykinesia is related clinically to decreases in muscle

Hoehn and Yahr scale	Modified Hoehn and Yahr scale
1: Unilateral involvement only usually with minimal or no functional disability	1.0: Unilateral involvement only
2: Bilateral or midline involvement without impairment of balance	1.5: Unilateral and axial involvement 2.0: Bilateral involvement without impairment of balance 2.5: Mild bilateral disease with recovery on pull test
3: Bilateral disease: mild to moderate disability with impaired postural reflexes, physically independent	3.0: Mild to moderate bilateral disease; some postural instability; physically independent
4: Severely disabling disease, still able to walk or stand unassisted	4.0: Severe disability; still able to walk or stand unassisted
5: Confinement to bed or wheelchair unless aided	5.0: Wheelchair bound or bedridden unless aided

Figure 12-8. Comparison between the original and modified Hoehn and Yahr scale. (Reprinted with permission from Goetz CG, Poewe W, Rascol O, et al. Movement Disorder Society Task Force report on the Hoehn and Yahr staging scale: status and recommendations. *Mov Disord.* 2004;19(9):1020-1028.)

activation acceleration rates presenting as decreased gait speed, and difficulty rising from a chair.[149]

Rigidity usually appears unilaterally in the initial stages of PD and can be felt in both agonist and antagonist muscles. It starts proximally in an upper limb and eventually spreads to all extremities and the trunk. One of the early signs of rigidity is loss of associated movements in one UE with decreased arm swing during gait that may affect gait speed. Axial rigidity limits rotation and extension of the trunk and spine, further limiting variability of movement during functional tasks such as walking.[3,148]

Bradykinesia and rigidity, among other symptoms related to PD, are thought to manifest themselves at a sub-clinical level for years prior to actually diagnosis and true functional decline.[142] While functional mobility may not be grossly affected in the pre- or even early stages of PD, research has shown that people with a diagnosis of mild to moderate PD present with significantly lower respiratory muscle strength and respiratory abnormalities even at rest.[150,151] In early diagnosis bradykinesia and rigidity have been found to affect gait, producing a decrease in stride length, impaired inter-limb coordination, and decreased cadence and velocity contributing to an increase in the energy cost of walking.[152,153] Walking economy has been found to be worse in individuals with even mild to moderate PD demonstrated by impairments in HR, minute ventilation, respiratory exchange rate, and RPEs during ambulation at speeds greater than 1.0 mph.[154] As the disease progresses individuals with PD experience a decline in walking, balance, and ADL that contribute to a progressive decline in participation.[144,145] Fatigue is also noted in PD and can be related to central activation failure from dopamine deficiency and abnormal levels of corticomotor excitability noted during exercise. Bradykinesia and rigidity may contribute to peripheral fatigue contributing to further aerobic deconditioning.

Autonomic dysfunction can affect the quality of life and participation levels of individuals with PD.[155] Symptoms of autonomic dysfunction are thought to be the result of damage to the postganglionic sympathetic efferences and loss of Lewy bodies in the peripheral sympathetic nervous system.[156] Symptoms can include orthostatic hypotension, lightheadedness, weakness, mental "clouding," syncope, or urinary and gastrointestinal dysfunction.[155,156] Triggers may be heat, some foods, alcohol, and exercise. Medications may also be a factor as amantadine and dopamine agonists can contribute to orthostatic hypotension.[156] If symptoms of AD are noted early in the disease process, consideration for a secondary cause, or other diagnosis such as multiple systems atrophy (MSA) should be made.[148,156]

Intervention

Despite neurological deficits in movement and respiratory function, individuals with mild to moderate PD who perform a regular exercise routine have the potential to achieve and maintain a normal aerobic capacity.[151] Exercise has also proven beneficial and effective for the improvement of physical functioning, health-related quality of life, strength, balance, and gait speed.[157] Regardless of H&Y stage, there is a significant correlation between subjects who exercise and their aerobic capacity. Sedentary individuals with PD produce lower VO_2 peak scores than those who exercise, further supporting the need for a regular cardiovascular routine in PD.[151] Considering the progressive nature of PD, and the relatively small window of effective medication management, participation in a well-designed exercise program is critical for minimizing disease-related and secondary impairments while maximizing quality of life. Under the direction of skilled a physical therapist, individuals with PD demonstrate improvements in walking economy, motor features of PD such as bradykinesia and rigidity, functional capacity, balance and flexibility.[157-162]

Increased compliance and long-term participation in an exercise routine was demonstrated with prescriptions that were based on current literature, were challenging and motivational, and provided a combination or variety of activities.[163] Since PD is a progressive disorder, lifelong participation is critical to maintaining the benefits.

Treadmill training has been demonstrated to improve gait speed and stride length in individuals with PD at H&Y stages 1 through 3.[164,165] Treadmill walking with and without body weight support can produce a faster and more stable gait pattern, including symmetrical step and stride lengths. These improvements were significantly more than just conventional gait training alone, and continued during overground gait for hours to even weeks after the intervention ceased.[166-168] Considering the decline in efficiency of walking and decrease in motor initiation in individuals with PD, conventional walking may be a less effective mode of exercise when attempting to produce a cardiovascular benefit.

A more symmetrical gait pattern can improve the economy of walking and allow individuals with PD to train within their age-predicted HR_{max} and improve cardiovascular fitness. When subjects participated in a graded exercise program on the treadmill up to 80% of the HR_{max}, they showed improvements in oxygen uptake, HR, and respiratory frequency.[169] Improvements in gait kinematics such as step length during and, for a period of time, after training on a treadmill are thought to be due to the proprioceptive information provided by the treadmill belt.[165] These improvements in step length also contribute to a more efficient gait pattern. Intensity of training has also been suggested to produce a normalized corticomotor excitability level (CEL) in early PD when training is performed at a high intensity[170] and has also shown to have an indirect benefit on measures of quality of life, motor impairments, and postural control, decreasing both fall risk and patient fear of falling.[171,172] Repetition in practice and specificity of training combined with a high-intensity practice condition have been demonstrated to facilitate motor learning, especially in those individuals with moderate to severe PD.[173] When considering that bradykinesia contributes to a slower gait velocity that can further enhance the secondary effects of cardiovascular deconditioning, high-intensity treadmill training may be the most task-specific and effective intervention for the improvement of aerobic capacity in PD as well as the improvement in bradykinesia and gait speed.

The estimate for maximum exercise capacity is lower for stationary cycling, but may be a more practical option for individuals with PD who have balance deficits and do not have access to a body weight-supported treadmill system.[174] There are initial data to suggest that forced exercise while cycling improves motor function in people with PD. Ridgel et al studied a small group of people with PD performing tandem biking with a partner who pedaled at a rate 30% higher than the subjects preferred rate and compared them to a group who pedaled alone at their preferred pedaling rate only. Subjects in both groups worked at 60% to 80% of their training HR_{max} and made significant improvements

in aerobic capacity. Only the forced exercise group made improvements in motor scores of the Unified Parkinson's Disease Rating Scale (UPDRS) including components for rigidity, bradykinesia, and tremors.[175] The mechanism of the motor improvements is not well understood, but the gains in aerobic fitness are further confirmed with moderate- to high-intensity exercise.

The amount of VO_2 obtained during exercise relies heavily on the individuals level of fitness combined with the muscle mass involved in the activity. Arm crank ergometry produces a VO_{2max} value less than cycling or treadmill walking in healthy younger populations. When considering a typically more sedentary population, people with PD do not seem to be able to produce a high enough intensity to achieve a cardiovascular benefit with UE exercise such as arm ergometer training.[174] It has been demonstrated in other populations with motor control disorders that combining leg and arm ergometry can produce a more effective cardiovascular benefit than cycling or arm bike alone.

Strength deficits are not often highlighted as a primary problem for individuals with PD. However, those with reported bradykinesia demonstrate decreased rates of force generation, and time to reach peak velocity when performing tasks such as sit to stand.[149,176] Individuals with mild to moderate PD have the potential to increase muscle strength and improve motor timing, similar to that of normal age-matched peers.[153] The addition of high-intensity eccentric resistance training has shown improvements in bradykinesia and gait speed that significantly exceed those of gains made with basic resistance training.[162] The primary muscle groups that should be considered when prescribing a strengthening exercise program include the LE muscles that are key for improvement of gait parameters and efficiency. Both free weights and Nautilus equipment are safe and effective during a recommended duration of strengthening 2 to 3 times per week. While effects can be seen in 8 to 12 weeks, the long-term benefits are best achieved with a consistent weekly routine.

Physical exercise in the form of aerobic and resistance training have several benefits for individuals with PD. Improvements in motor performance, symptoms related to PD, tolerance for daily activities, aerobic capacity, quality and longevity of life overwhelmingly supports the need for consistent exercise across the life span.[146] Key principles of exercise that also may promote neuroplasticity in PD include 1) intense activity maximizing synaptic activity, 2) complex activities promoting greater structural adaptations, 3) rewarding and stimulating activities promoting increased dopamine levels enhancing motor learning, 4) dopaminergic neurons responding both in a positive way to exercise, and a negative way to inactivity, and 5) early introduction of exercise, resulting in slowing of the disease process.[146,177]

Multiple Sclerosis

MS is a slow to moderately progressive degenerative disorder of the CNS. Prevalence is about 0.1% with about 350,000 to 400,000 people currently living with MS in the

United States. Peak age of onset is between 20 to 40 years, with a higher ratio of women to men affected.[2] The disease process is characterized by acute relapses, remissions, and chronic progression. Relapses are thought to occur with an acute inflammatory attack of T lymphocytes on oligodendroglial myelin, causing disruption of nerve conduction and a sudden change in clinical status. Discrete episodes of inflammatory response and demyelination occur insidiously, followed by a period of remission with full or partial symptom resolution thought to be due to remyelination.[2,178,179] Periods of chronic progression can occur at clinical and subclinical levels throughout the disease process. This is thought to be the result of incomplete remyelination leading to permanent axonal loss that appear as lesion sites on magnetic resonance imaging (MRI).[178] Destruction of axons is thought to be the essential cause of nonremitting disease progression and clinical disability in MS.[180] Diagnosis is confirmed based on the presence of clinical features, combined with white matter lesions found on MRI, or the presence of oligoclonal bands in the cerebrospinal fluid (CSF).[2] Immunomodulatory and immunosuppressant medications are used to partially ameliorate symptoms, decrease the number and frequency of relapses, and slow the progression of relapsing-remitting MS.[179]

Disease progression is routinely tracked in clinical practice using the Expanded Disability Status Scale (EDSS). This MS-specific scale rates the patient neurological status on an ordinal scale ranging from 0.0 (normal) to 10.0 (death). The scale combines pyramidal and functional measures to rate level of disability.[181,182]

Impairments Affecting Mobility

The clinical presentation of people with MS can be highly variable. Weakness and fatigue are the 2 most common deficits in body structure and function that have a negative impact on aerobic capacity, the ability to participate in exercise and aerobic conditioning activities, and overall levels of physical activity.[18,183] Autonomic dysfunction has been inconsistently noted with MS, but when present can also have detrimental effects.[184-186]

Weakness can be documented even in the early stages of the disease. The cortical demyelination that occurs during acute and chronic stages can lead to a decrease in motor unit firing rates, inadequate motor unit recruitment, and an increase in central motor conduction time.[2] This decrease in central, or cortically driven, activation produces impairments in the force and rate of voluntary muscle contraction.[187] There is also evidence of topographic changes in the cortical motor areas with deficits in conduction and excitation that correspond to changes in motor function. This suggests that there is also a process of neural plasticity that occurs with axonal damage in MS.[188] Peripheral weakness at the skeletal muscle and muscle fiber type appears to be similar to age-matched sedentary individuals without MS.[68] This indicates that changes in the quality of the muscle itself is most likely a response to deconditioning and immobility, and may potentially have a better response to strengthening. Increased body temperature has been shown to exacerbate

this process so many individuals with MS feel even weaker when they are warm.[2]

Weakness in the LE muscle groups can have a direct impact on walking speed,[189] which has shown to have an inverse correlation with EDSS level and deconditioning.[190] Respiratory muscle weakness, especially within the muscles responsible for inspiration, are found even in the early stages of MS. Weakness in these particular muscle groups can lead to an ineffective cough an impaired ability to adequately clear the airway, leading to a higher risk of respiratory complications and further aerobic deconditioning.[35,191]

Fatigue has a profound and global impact on individuals with MS and is reportedly the most common symptom present in up to 80% of individuals with MS.[18] Fatigue can be a primary impairment in people with MS because of dysfunction along the pathways of neural activation. Fatigue in MS can be related to hypometabolism in certain brain areas, or to the amount of diffuse axonal damage and brain atrophy.[14,192] This can be demonstrated by a compensatory increase in central motor drive exertion present during exercise, or delays in voluntary muscle activation. When activation of a muscle is incomplete, there is a greater perceived effort and level of fatigue compared to their healthy peers when performing the same activity.[18,193,194] Primary fatigue can also be associated with other side effects of MS including immune dysregulation, cortical hypofunction due to demyelination, and abnormal thyroid function. Fatigue can be considered a secondary impairment in response to sleep dysfunction, pain, depression, medication side effects, and physical deconditioning from reduced muscle performance.[18,192] Fatigue can be present in very early or late stages of MS[190] and is not necessarily associated with motor function changes or impairments in ambulation.[187] Fatigue can be directly correlated with a decline in respiratory muscle strength, endurance, depression, and a poor quality of life.[18,191,192]

Deconditioning from the above factors can have a profound impact on walking speed, walking endurance,[190] physical activity, participation,[183] and overall quality of life.[191] As the disease progresses deconditioning, cardiovascular, and pulmonary dysfunction tend to be more pronounced.[35,190,195] HR and BP responses appear to be blunted in many individuals with MS during graded exercise testing, possibly because of cardiovascular dysautonomia.[196,197] Autonomic dysfunction in MS is thought to be the result of a dysfunction of the central parasympathetic nervous system's HR responses.[195] This may impair perfusion to the brain and muscles causing early fatigue, HR response to exercise affecting performance, and attenuate sweating responses, causing increased susceptibility to heat stress.[196] An increased number of lesions found on MRI throughout the progression of MS, especially in the area of the midbrain, have been directly correlated to a decrease in cardiovascular function.[186,195]

There is evidence that individuals with MS can safely participate in physical activity in the form of strengthening exercise and aerobic conditioning at moderate to high intensities with reductions in MS symptoms, and improved function and quality of life.[55,191,193,198-202] Physical activity may also play an important role in modifying the progression of disability in MS.[199] While dose-response effects of exercise are variable in the current literature, both sub-maximal aerobic and strengthening programs even at low intensities can be effective, and are safe and well tolerated by people with MS.[196,203]

Strengthening in the form of progressive resistance exercise (PRE) is a safe and effect training tool in individuals with mild to moderate MS that has shown to improve muscle strength, decrease the perception of fatigue, and improve ambulation.[55,204-206] Despite the progressive nature of MS, PRE training has shown to induce improvements in force production with muscle hypertrophy similar to responses expected in subjects without MS.[206,207] Key principles of PRE are to perform a small number of repetitions with a high load until peripheral muscle fatigue is reached, to allow sufficient rest between exercise to allow for recovery, and to increase the load as the ability to generate force improves.[205] As a general guideline Petejan and White suggest selecting 1 to 2 exercise per major muscle groups, and exercising at 60% to 80% of a maximum voluntary contraction,[206,208] especially at the trunk and LEs. Exertion with temperature elevation may increase symptoms, so interval training and exercising in an air-conditioned environment may allow individuals with MS to tolerate increased exercise intensity.[196]

Strengthening can be performed using traditional free weights or Nautilus equipment. Cakt et al provided resistance using a cycle ergometer to target muscle groups and movements patterns associated with gait. This study applied the principle of PRE training by applying resistance during the pedaling action, and demonstrated significant improvements in duration of exercise tolerance, max workload, Timed Up & Go, Dynamic Gait Index, Functional Reach, FSS, Falls Efficacy Scale, and the Beck Depression Inventory compared to a home LE strengthening program and no exercise.[55] PRE has shown to significantly increase gait speed, endurance, and kinematics including increased step length, improved toe clearance, and decreased double limb support in individuals with moderate MD. Improvements in gait pattern allows for more efficient mobility and decreased levels of fatigue as well.[204,206,209]

In individuals with normal neuromuscular systems, high-resistance training through eccentric contractions produces an elevated muscle force at a low metabolic cost or level of perceived exertion. It is thought of as a more effective means of producing muscle hypertrophy and improvements in strength.[4,210] In individuals with MS, however, eccentric resistance exercise is less effective than standard concentric training methods, and typically not recommended.[211]

Mode of sub-maximal aerobic training for a person with MS needs to be individualized, taking into consideration underlying impairments or mobility restrictions that may affect the ability to participate at a high level. Program design needs to consider the individual person's goals, body, structure, and functional limitations secondary to MS, and level of disability. Cycling has often been considered a relevant training alternative for individuals who do not have access to or cannot tolerate training on a treadmill, or who may have impairments in postural control.[212] Walking and cycling have similar locomotor patterns with reciprocal flexion and extension movements at the hips, knees, and ankles and alternating muscle activation patterns.[55] Programs incorporating combined arm and leg ergometry have shown significant increases in maximal aerobic capacity, physical work capacity, strength, and quality of life in MS.[196] Petejan and White suggest parameters similar to those recommended by the ACSM for healthy individuals. Aerobic exercise 2 to 3 sessions per week for >20 minutes at 65% to 75% age adjusted HR_{max}, and resistance training starting at 2 sessions per week.[208]

Fatigue in MS has demonstrated inconsistent responses to medication management or exercise.[192] The sources or sources of fatigue, whether peripherally or centrally driven need to be clearly defined to design the most effective intervention. Treatment of comorbid conditions such as depression and sleep impairments can be necessary to alleviate fatigue. Fatigue has been shown to improve by up to 22% in individuals with MS who participate in a regular, sustained exercise routine.[15,212]

Pulmonary muscle strengthening and endurance training has demonstrated improvements in forced vital capacity, among other measures of pulmonary function, in individuals with mild to moderate MS.[35]

Adherence to an exercise program can be a major obstacle. Since MS is a progressive disease, compliance and consistency in a well-rounded program is imperative. Consideration of environmental and personal factors, along with exercise preferences is considered key in the promotion of exercise in individuals with MS.[196]

Amyotrophic Lateral Sclerosis

Pathology

ALS is a rare and rapidly progressive adult-onset degenerative disease of motor neurons with an incidence of 1.5 to 2.5 per 100,000.[213] Approximately 90% of cases occur sporadically while the remaining 10% may be from an inherited autosomal dysfunction.[3] Initial symptoms most often include weakness in the distal extremities with the presence both of UMN and LMN signs. "Amyotrophic" refers to symptoms of muscle weakness, atrophy, and fasciculations that are associated with LMN degeneration, while "lateral sclerosis" refers to the process of gliosis and scarring that occurs with degeneration of the lateral corticospinal tracts, brainstem, and cortex causing UMN signs such as hyperreflexia, Hoffman signs, Babinski, and clonus.[3,214] Bulbar signs including dysarthria and dysphagia, can be present in 20% to 25% of cases at the initial presentation and are caused by degeneration of corticobulbar fibers or the motor nuclei in the cranial nerves of the medulla.[2] Motor neurons of the oculomotor nuclei are spared with preserved control of oculomotor function.[3] The resulting muscle atrophy and weakness causes profound mobility limitations. Depending on initial clinical presentation, mean survival is 3 to 5 years.[215]

Disease progression through functional change is typically tracked using the ALS Functional Rating Scale (ALSFRS). This scale contains 10 functional items each rated on a 4-point ordinal scale from 0 (no movement or function) to 4 (normal function). Items that are measured include speech, swallowing, salivation, handwriting, cutting food, and handling utensils, dressing and hygiene, turning in bed, walking, climbing stairs, and breathing.[216]

Drug management of ALS relies primarily on one medication. Riluzole is currently the only medication that is approved for slowing the disease process of ALS and prolonging survival by anywhere from 2 to 24 months. The max benefit can be found when Riluzole is initiated earlier in the disease process before the onset of respiratory complications.[217] Aggressive multidisciplinary care and symptom management to maximize function and independence throughout the life span can support a longer life span and improved quality of life.[218]

Impairments Affecting Movement

Weakness is a primary symptom in ALS and stems not only from the disease process itself, but also from disuse. Peripheral denervation caused by degeneration of anterior horn cells leads to structural damage of the muscle fiber, affecting the ability of the muscle to produce a consistent and sustainable force. Axonal sprouting and reinnervation in the early stages of the disease allow partial innervation of surviving motor units.[219] Mitochondrial abnormalities in DNA impair the integrity of the muscle and further contribute to weakness.[220] Myelin loss appears in all areas of the spinal cord except in the posterior columns. This pattern of degeneration negatively affects force production capabilities, but allows the preservation of sensation.[3] As the disease progresses individuals with ALS will lose weight through the loss of lean muscle mass and a decrease in caloric intake, which is often exacerbated by bulbar muscle weakness and dysphagia.[221] These factors contribute to a spiral of further muscle weakness due to insufficient activity and loss of contractile proteins, even in the early stages of the diagnosis. Cramping with volitional movement, motor fasciculations, and complaints of stiffness are common. Other secondary effects of immobility that individuals with ALS are highly susceptible to are cardiovascular deconditioning contributing further to fatigue and respiratory complications.[222]

Deconditioning and a generalized feeling of fatigue are common complaints in individuals with ALS. Partially innervated motor units produce an inefficient muscle contraction with early fatigability.[219] This loss of force-producing capability in the PNS contributes to inefficient mobility and complaints of physiological fatigue. Deconditioning may also be secondary to hypoventilation and respiratory insufficiency.[223]

As a result of loss of UMN inhibition spasticity is a common and painful side effect. Combined with the progression of motor weakness, individuals with ALS are at risk for developing painful joint contractures.[224]

The diagnosis and management of respiratory function in individuals with ALS is a vital component of care as most deaths in ALS are due to respiratory failure.[217] Forced vital capacity and nocturnal oximetry are often used as measures of respiratory function, predictors of survival, and as markers for the initiation of external ventilatory or nutritional support.[217,223] Impairments in respiratory function can contribute to fatigue in individuals with ALS and are addressed with noninvasive positive pressure ventilation that may initially be introduced at night.[21]

Intervention

The rapid progression of ALS and nature of the motor neuron loss have caused controversy in the past as to whether exercise is appropriate in this population. The low incidence of ALS poses a challenge to researchers, but a handful of small but well-designed studies have shown that exercise can be physically and psychologically important for individuals with ALS. This is especially true in the early stages and middle stages of the disease process before significant muscle atrophy and deconditioning, take place.[222] Small-randomized controlled trials have shown small to moderate, but not statistically significant, gains in function following exercise.[220] Considering the aggressive progression of this disease, it can be important to note that even though the results did not show a significant gain, there also was not a decline in function, or adverse effects reported.

Strengthening at low to moderate resistance in the early to middle stages of the disease with aerobic conditioning at a sub-maximal level can be safe and effective.[222,225] It is widely accepted that strength training is most safe and beneficial with muscles that are unaffected, or are able to move throughout full range against gravity.[223] The implication of a 3/5 muscle grade is that there are an adequate amount of motor neurons available to tolerate resistance training without detrimental effects. Resistance training at a moderate intensity has been demonstrated to improve function as measured by the ALSFRS and quality of life without adverse effects.[226] Strengthening at a high intensity is not recommended as it may further damage mitochondria, increase extracellular and oxidative stress, and cause further damage to the muscle.[220] In the later stages of the disease, structured strengthening exercise may not be beneficial and may even be harmful as the performance of ADL alone may provide a training effect to excessively denervated muscles.[222] When muscle grades fall below a 3/5 strength or in the presence of spasticity, ROM exercises are an important addition to maintain efficient mobility and prevent painful contractures.

Aerobic conditioning is another important component of an exercise program in ALS at all stages because of the profound risk of respiratory complications that arise from the combination of muscle weakness, deconditioning, and secondary complications of dysphagia. Aerobic exercise can be performed safely also at submaximal levels at 50% to 60% of HR reserve, even in the presence of respiratory insufficiency and with the use of supplemental oxygen or with bilevel positive airway pressure support.[222,223] Intermittent breaks and rest periods are recommended to prevent overwork.

Mode of exercise has not been well studied in ALS to determine which activity may provide the most benefit. A small pilot study by Sanjak demonstrated improvements in gait speed, fatigue, and levels of perceived exertion in individuals with ALS following repetitive rhythmic treadmill walking with body weight support. Subjects were encouraged to train at a moderate intensity measured by a 20-point Borg scale, and were provided supplemental oxygen as needed to maintain oxygen saturations about 90%. Rest breaks were provided in between training period to avoid fatigue and overwork. Treadmill training with body weight support was a feasible method of aerobic conditioning, and measures of perceived exertion using a self-monitored Borg scale were reliable.[227] Other options for consideration are stationary bikes in the presence of balance impairments or trunk weakness, and swimming.

Individuals with ALS should be educated to not exercise to the point of fatigue or exhaustion. Energy should be preserved for patient safety and ADL. Symptoms of overwork should be monitored and avoided. These include muscle cramps, pain, muscle fasciculations, or extreme fatigue with an inability to perform ADL after exercise. With careful consideration and monitoring of program intensity, therapeutic exercise can reduce the rate of muscle weakness progression, decrease fatigue, improve quality of life, and can be safely initiated at most stages of the disease.[222,228]

Guillain-Barré Syndrome

Pathology

Guillain-Barré syndrome (GBS) is a rapidly progressing demyelinating disorder of the PNS that is typically preceded by an infectious event such as upper respiratory or gastrointestinal tract illness.[16] There are several clinical variants, but GBS usually refers to acute demyelinating inflammatory polyneuropathy. The incidence of GBS in the United States is approximately 1 to 3 per 100,000 and it typically affects otherwise healthy adults in their fifth to eighth decades.[16] Symptoms are caused by an autoimmune attack of the PNS affecting Schwann cells, resulting in demyelination.[229] Primary clinical symptoms include a rapid progression of symmetrical weakness in the arms and legs, and areflexia. Other common features include paresthesias with or without loss of sensation, pain, autonomic dysreflexia, cranial nerve involvement, and a high concentration of protein found in the CSF >1 week after onset of initial symptoms. Symptoms progress and then peak over a period of 1 to 4 weeks with as many as 21% to 30% requiring mechanical ventilator support because of respiratory muscle weakness.[16,26,230] This is followed by a plateau phase that can last for days to weeks. The longer it takes a patient to reach this plateau phase or "nadir," the longer the acute stay and the poorer the functional outcome.[16] The process of remyelination and recovery can vary. Patients with less severe disease can gradually recover muscle strength within 2 to 4 weeks after plateau and close to 80% recover ambulation by 6 months. Of these patients, 50%

may show residual neurological deficits such as dysesthesia, foot drop, and intrinsic muscle wasting, and 7% to 15% of these patients have enough residual deficits to present with a decrease in function. As many as 20% of patients who require ventilator support remain nonambulatory at 6 months and are considered the most severe.[16,231] Total recovery time can take up to 2 years with less than a quarter of patients noting continued activity and participation deficits.[232]

Impairments Affecting Mobility

The most common residual deficit in GBS affecting functional recovery is muscle weakness.[233] Forsberg et al reported that at 2 weeks 100% of patients present with submaximal muscle strength grades. At 1 year 62%, and at 2 years 55% of patients still present with submaximal muscle grades.[26] Adequate force production of a muscle depends on effective depolarization of alpha motor neurons in the PNS. Demyelination in the PNS in GBS affects depolarization by disrupting the propagation of an action potential, slowing the conduction velocity. This can cause dyssynchrony of the conduction, conduction block or may even result in complete axonal loss.[229] This produces a decrease in the quality and quantity of motor units recruited to generate or sustain muscle forces adequate enough for ADL. Muscles that are only partially innervated have the potential for overwork and are easily fatigued.[229,230]

A significant increase in muscle strength can be seen in the first 6 months, with up to 95% of strength expected to be "fully recovered" by 18 months. This rapid rate of motor return makes accurate and consistent measurement of muscle strength a critical element of the rehabilitation process not only to determine a patient's functional status, but to monitor the progress of recovery, establish a prognosis, and determine appropriate interventions.[234] Accepted principles of strength training in GBS include 3 main parameters:

1. Recognize and avoid overworking of a muscle. There is weak evidence in the polio literature that stress of a partially innervated motor unit can cause further permanent damage to the motor unit with subsequent decline in strength.[235] This theory remains controversial, but the basic concept remains in place for people with GBS. Symptoms of overwork are a delayed onset of muscle soreness 1 to 5 days after exercise with a reduction in the maximum force a patient can produce. If a patient demonstrates signs of overwork, rest is advised until baseline strength levels return, and then strengthening can be resumed at a lower intensity.

2. Avoid eccentric contractions.

3. Avoid strengthening until the muscle has achieved antigravity strength.[229]

Once the disease process has reached at least the plateau phase and the patient has achieved anti-gravity strength, strengthening recommendations are to perform short bouts of non-fatiguing exercise.[236] Resistance and program intensity can safely be increased if no adverse effects such as a decline in muscle weakness are noted.[237]

Fatigue remains the most persistent and disabling residual symptom of GBS and can be found in 38% to 86% of patients well beyond the 18-month point in their recovery.[15,16,234] Fatigue is often worse in older patients and females, and can be independent of any residual neurological deficits.[15] In the acute stage of GBS, fatigue can be described as primarily peripheral in origin. Demyelination disrupting nerve conduction will present as fatigability characterized by failure of a muscle to sustain the force of a muscle contraction over time.[15] Fatigue, however, is prominent throughout the recovery process, can be independent of the severity of muscle weakness, and often continues for many years, leading researchers to believe there is a combined central and peripheral component.[16] Garssen et al found signs of peripheral fatigability and central activation failure. The components of central fatigue are not as well understood, but it is hypothesized that this may be due to lack of or exhaustion of motor neurons in the motor cortex, or lack of patient motivation.[238] The effects of exercise on fatigue are not well studied and inconclusive, but overall the evidence demonstrates that exercise can be effective in patients who are neurologically recovered but complain of severe fatigue.[16,239,240]

The final consideration when implementing an exercise program for patients with GBS is to monitor diligently for signs of autonomic dysfunction, especially in the acute stage. Autonomic dysfunction is reported in approximately 70% of patients at 2 weeks, 50% of patients at 2 months, less than 20% of patients at 6 months to 1 year, and less than 10% of patients at 2 years after initial onset of symptoms.[26,184] Those patients who required mechanical ventilator support were more likely to demonstrate symptoms of autonomic dysfunction, and tended to have longer acute care hospital stays.[230] Uncontrolled HR and BP pressure are the most common symptoms and may be unreliable when used as a measure of exercise tolerance.[184] RPEs using a Borg measure may be more appropriate,[241] although accuracy, safety, and reliability have not been careful studied in this population.

SUMMARY

Accessible fitness programs and adaptive sports programs are needed to support lifelong fitness and participation. The best way to choose the correct intervention is to understand the problem we are attempting to address. Exercise programs designed for all individuals, including those with neurological disorders, need to be goal directed and performed at a high intensity to improve motor function and endurance to achieve a high level of activity and participation. When incorporating concepts of motor learning to encourage recovery of function along with improvements in exercise capacity, 3 key factors need to be considered. These include the individual's skill level, the conditions of the exercise being practiced or performed, and the feedback frequency.[173] A well-designed exercise program includes the 4 main components of exercise prescription specifying exercise mode, intensity, duration, and frequency. While many of the diagnostic groups discussed may tolerate parameters outlines by the ACSM, a thorough understanding of the pathology, implications for mobility, exercise potential, and risk factors involved unique to each person and diagnosis will promote the best performance and hopefully lifelong participation.

REFERENCES

1. Shumway-Cook A. *Motor Control: Translating Research Into Clinical Practice.* 4th ed, North American Edition. Philadelphia, PA: Lippincott Williams & Wilkins; 2011.
2. Blumenfeld H. *Neuroanatomy Through Clinical Cases.* 2nd ed. Sunderland, MA: Sinauer Associates Inc; 2010.
3. Goodman CC, Fuller K. *Pathology: Implications for the Physical Therapist.* 3rd ed. St. Louis, MO: Saunders Elsevier; 2008.
4. Clamann HP. Motor unit recruitment and the gradation of muscle force. *Phys Ther.* 1993;73(12):830-843.
5. McDonald CM. Physical activity, health impairments, and disability in neuromuscular disease. *Am J Phys Med Rehabil.* 2002;81(11 Suppl):S108-S120.
6. Kokotilo KJ, Eng JJ, Boyd LA. Reorganization of brain function during force production after stroke: a systematic review of the literature. *J Neurol Phys Ther.* 2009;33(1):45-54.
7. Kluding P, Gajewski B. Lower-extremity strength differences predict activity limitations in people with chronic stroke. *Phys Ther.* 2009;89(1):73-81.
8. Nadeau S, Arsenault AB, Gravel D, Bourbonnais D. Analysis of the clinical factors determining natural and maximal gait speeds in adults with a stroke. *Am J Phys Med Rehabil.* 1999;78(2):123-130.
9. McCrory MA, Kim HR, Wright NC, Lovelady CA, Aitkens S, Kilmer DD. Energy expenditure, physical activity, and body composition of ambulatory adults with hereditary neuromuscular disease. *Am J Clin Nutr.* 1998;67(6):1162-1169.
10. Kilmer DD. Response to aerobic exercise training in humans with neuromuscular disease. *Am J Phys Med Rehabil.* 2002;81(11 Suppl):S148-S150.
11. Giuliani CA. The relationship of spasticity to movement and considerations for therapeutic interventions. *Neurology Report.* 1997;21(3):78-84.
12. Dawes H, Bateman A, Culpan J, et al. The effect of increasing effort on movement economy during incremental cycling exercise in individuals early after acquired brain injury. *Clin Rehabil.* 2003;17(5):528-534.
13. Taylor NF, Dodd KJ, Shields N, Bruder A. Therapeutic exercise in physiotherapy practice is beneficial: a summary of systematic reviews 2002-2005. *Aust J Physiother.* 2007;53(1):7-16.
14. Zwarts MJ, Bleijenberg G, van Engelen BG. Clinical neurophysiology of fatigue. *Clin Neurophysiol.* 2008;119(1):2-10.
15. de Vries JM, Hagemans ML, Bussmann JB, van der Ploeg AT, van Doorn PA. Fatigue in neuromuscular disorders: focus on Guillain-Barré syndrome and Pompe disease. *Cell Mol Life Sci.* 2010;67(5):701-713.
16. van Doorn PA, Ruts L, Jacobs BC. Clinical features, pathogenesis, and treatment of Guillain-Barré syndrome. *Lancet Neurol.* 2008;7(10):939-950.
17. Mossberg KA, Amonette WE, Masel BE. Endurance training and cardiorespiratory conditioning after traumatic brain injury. *J Head Trauma Rehabil.* 2010;25(3):173-183.
18. MacAllister WS, Krupp LB. Multiple sclerosis-related fatigue. *Phys Med Rehabil Clin N Am.* 2005;16(2):483-502.
19. Bushnik T, Englander J, Wright J. Patterns of fatigue and its correlates over the first 2 years after traumatic brain injury. *J Head Trauma Rehabil.* 2008;23(1):25-32.
20. Allman BL, Rice CL. Neuromuscular fatigue and aging: Central and peripheral factors. *Muscle Nerve.* 2002;25(6):785-796.

21. Lou J, Weiss MD, Carter GT. Assessment and management of fatigue in neuromuscular disease. *Am J Hosp Palliat Care.* 2010;27(2):145-157.

22. Krivickas LS. Exercise in neuromuscular disease. *J Clin Neuromuscul Dis.* 2003;5(1):29-39.

23. Abresch RT, Han JJ, Carter GT. Rehabilitation management of neuromuscular disease: the role of exercise training. *J Clin Neuromuscul Dis.* 2009;11(1):7-21.

24. American Physical Therapy Association. *Guide to Physical Therapist Practice.* 2nd ed. Alexandria, VA: Author; 2003.

25. Myers J, Lee M, Kiratli J. Cardiovascular disease in spinal cord injury: an overview of prevalence, risk, evaluation, and management. *Am J Phys Med Rehabil.* 2007;86(2):142-152.

26. Forsberg A, Press R, Einarsson U, et al. Impairment in Guillain-Barré syndrome during the first 2 years after onset: a prospective study. *J Neurol Sci.* 2004;227(1):131-138.

27. Noonan V, Dean E. Submaximal exercise testing: clinical application and interpretation. *Phys Ther.* 2000;80(8):782-807.

28. Borg GA. Psychophysical bases of perceived exertion. *Med Sci Sports Exerc.* 1982;14(5):377-381.

29. American College of Sports Medicine. *ACSM's Resource Manual for Guidelines for Exercise Testing and Prescription.* 6th ed. Philadelphia, PA: Lippincott Williams & Wilkins; 2010.

30. Mossberg KA, Greene BP. Reliability of graded exercise testing after traumatic brain injury: submaximal and peak responses. *Am J Phys Med Rehabil.* 2005;84(7):492-500.

31. Bhambhani Y, Rowland G, Farag M. Effects of circuit training on body composition and peak cardiorespiratory responses in patients with moderate to severe traumatic brain injury. *Arch Phys Med Rehabil.* 2005;86(2):268-276.

32. Graham JE, Ostir GV, Fisher SR, Ottenbacher KJ. Assessing walking speed in clinical research: a systematic review. *J Eval Clin Pract.* 2008;14(4):552-562.

33. Mossberg KA. Reliability of a timed walk test in persons with acquired brain injury. *Am J Phys Med Rehabil.* 2003;82(5):385-390.

34. Eng JJ, Dawson AS, Chu KS. Submaximal exercise in persons with stroke: Test-retest reliability and concurrent validity with maximal oxygen consumption. *Arch Phys Med Rehabil.* 2004;85(1):113-118.

35. Fry DK, Pfalzer LA, Chokshi AR, Wagner MT, Jackson ES. Randomized control trial of effects of a 10-week inspiratory muscle training program on measures of pulmonary function in persons with multiple sclerosis. *J Neurol Phys Ther.* 2007;31(4):162-172.

36. van Loo MA, Moseley AM, Bosman JM, de Bie RA, Hassett L. Interrater reliability and concurrent validity of walking speed measurement after traumatic brain injury. *Clin Rehabil.* 2003;17(7):775-779.

37. Jackson AB, Carnel CT, Ditunno JF, et al. Outcome measures for gait and ambulation in the spinal cord injury population. *J Spinal Cord Med.* 2008;31(5):487-499.

38. Kosak M, Smith T. Comparison of the 2-, 6-, and 12-minute walk tests in patients with stroke. *J Rehabil Res Dev.* 2005;42(1):103-107.

39. Murphy MA, Roberts-Warrior D. A review of motor performance measures and treatment interventions for patients with stroke. *Top Geriatr Rehabil.* 2003;19(1):3-42.

40. Bohannon RW, Smith MB. Assessment of strength deficits in eight paretic upper extremity muscle groups of stroke patients with hemiplegia. *Phys Ther.* 1987;67(4):522-525.

41. Larson CA, Tezak WD, Malley MS, Thornton W. Assessment of postural muscle strength in sitting: Reliability of measures obtained with hand-held dynamometry in individuals with spinal cord injury. *J Neurol Phys Ther.* 2010;34(1):24-31.

42. Lu Y, Lin J, Hsiao S, Liu MF, Chen SM, Lue YJ. The relative and absolute reliability of leg muscle strength testing by a handheld dynamometer. *J Strength Cond Res.* 2011;25(4):1065-1071.

43. Morris SL, Dodd KJ, Morris ME. Reliability of dynamometry to quantify isometric strength following traumatic brain injury. *Brain Inj.* 2008;22(13-14):1030-1037.

44. Csuka M, McCarty DJ. Simple method for measurement of lower extremity muscle strength. *Am J Med.* 1985;78(1):77-81.

45. Mong Y, Teo TW, Ng SS. 5-repetition sit-to-stand test in subjects with chronic stroke: reliability and validity. *Arch Phys Med Rehabil.* 2010;91(3):407-413.

46. Bowden MG, Clark DJ, Kautz SA. Evaluation of abnormal synergy patterns poststroke: relationship of the Fugl-Meyer Assessment to hemiparetic locomotion. *Neurorehabil Neural Repair.* 2010;24(4):328-337.

47. Hislop HJ, Montgomery J. *Daniels and Worthingham's Muscle Testing: Techniques of Manual Examination.* 8th ed. St. Louis, MO: Elsevier Saunders; 2007.

48. Mercer VS, Chang S, Anderson M, Aull D, Macklin S, Rogers A. Relationship between clinical measures of paretic lower extremity motor control at 1 month and gait speed at 6 months post stroke. *J Neurol Phys Ther.* 2006;30(4):197.

49. Esquenazi A. Evaluation and management of spastic gait in patients with traumatic brain injury. *J Head Trauma Rehabil.* 2004;19(2):109-118.

50. Brashear A, Zafonte R, Corcoran M, et al. Inter- and intrarater reliability of the Ashworth Scale and the Disability Assessment Scale in patients with upper-limb poststroke spasticity. *Arch Phys Med Rehabil.* 2002;83(10):1349-1354.

51. Gregson JM, Leathley M, Moore AP, Sharma AK, Smith TL, Watkins CL. Reliability of the Tone Assessment Scale and the modified Ashworth scale as clinical tools for assessing poststroke spasticity. *Arch Phys Med Rehabil.* 1999;80(9):1013-1016.

52. Haugh AB, Pandyan AD, Johnson GR. A systematic review of the Tardieu Scale for the measurement of spasticity. *Disabil Rehabil.* 2006;28(15):899-907.

53. Herlofson K, Larsen JP. Measuring fatigue in patients with Parkinson's disease? The fatigue severity scale. *Eur J Neurol.* 2002;9(6):595-600.

54. Levine J, Greenwald BD. Fatigue in Parkinson disease, stroke, and traumatic brain injury. *Phys Med Rehabil Clin N Am.* 2009;20(2):347-361.

55. Cakt BD, Nacir B, Genc H, et al. Cycling progressive resistance training for people with multiple sclerosis: a randomized controlled study. *Am J Phys Med Rehabil.* 2010;89(6):446-457.

56. Krupp LB, LaRocca NG, Muir-Nash J, Steinberg AD. The fatigue severity scale. Application to patients with multiple sclerosis and systemic lupus erythematosus. *Arch Neurol.* 1989;46(10):1121-1123.

57. Esquenazi A, Ofluoglu D, Hirai B, Kim S. The effect of an ankle-foot orthosis on temporal spatial parameters and asymmetry of gait in hemiparetic patients. *PM R.* 2009;1(11):1014-1018.

58. Lewallen J, Miedaner J, Amyx S, Sherman J. Effect of three styles of custom ankle foot orthoses on the gait of stroke patients while walking on level and inclined surfaces. *J Prosthet Orthot.* 2010;22(2):78-83.

59. Laufer Y, Hausdorff JM, Ring H. Effects of a foot drop neuroprosthesis on functional abilities, social participation, and gait velocity. *Am J Phys Med Rehabil.* 2009;88(1):14-20.

60. Bateni H, Heung E, Zettel J, McLlroy WE, Maki BE. Can use of walkers or canes impede lateral compensatory stepping movements? *Gait Posture.* 2004;20(1):74-83.

61. Bateni H, Maki BE. Assistive devices for balance and mobility: benefits, demands, and adverse consequences. *Arch Phys Med Rehabil.* 2005;86(1):134-145.

62. Bateni H, Zecevic A, McIlroy WE, Maki BE. Resolving conflicts in task demands during balance recovery: does holding an object inhibit compensatory grasping? *Exp Brain Res.* 2004;157(1):49-58.

63. Gianfrancesco MA, Triche EW, Fawcett JA, Labas MP, Patterson TS, Lo AC. Speed- and cane-related alterations in gait parameters in individuals with multiple sclerosis. *Gait Posture.* 2011;33(1):140-142.

64. Holden MK, Gill KM, Magliozzi MR. Gait assessment for neurologically impaired patients. Standards for outcome assessment. *Phys Ther.* 1986;66(10):1530-1539.

65. Constantinescu R, Leonard C, Deeley C, Kurlan R. Assistive devices for gait in Parkinson's disease. *Parkinsonism Relat Disord.* 2007;13(3):133-138.

66. Souza A, Kelleher A, Cooper R, Cooper RA, Iezzoni LI, Collins DM. Multiple sclerosis and mobility-related assistive technology: systematic review of literature. *J Rehabil Res Dev.* 2010;47(3):213-223.

67. Protas EJ, Raines ML, Tissier S. Comparison of spatiotemporal and energy cost of the use of 3 different walkers and unassisted walking in older adults. *Arch Phys Med Rehabil.* 2007;88(6):768-773.

68. Carroll CC, Gallagher PM, Seidle ME, Trappe SW. Skeletal muscle characteristics of people with multiple sclerosis. *Arch Phys Med Rehabil.* 2005;86(2):224-229.

69. Roger VL, Go AS, Lloyd-Jones DM, et al. Heart disease and stroke statistics—2011 update: a report from the American Heart Association. *Circulation.* 2011;123(4):e18-e209.

70. Lloyd-Jones D, Adams RJ, Brown TM, et al. Executive summary: heart disease and stroke statistics—2010 update: a report from the American Heart Association. *Circulation.* 2010;121(7):948-954.

71. Jørgensen HS, Nakayama H, Raaschou HO, Olsen TS. Intracerebral hemorrhage versus infarction: stroke severity, risk factors, and prognosis. *Ann Neurol.* 1995;38(1):45-50.

72. Collins C. Pathophysiology and classification of stroke. *Nurs Stand.* 2007;21(28):35-39.

73. Gordon NF, Gulanick M, Costa F, et al. American Heart Association Council on Clinical Cardiology, Subcommittee on Exercise, Cardiac Rehabilitation, and Prevention; the Council on Cardiovascular Nursing; the Council on Nutrition, Physical Activity, and Metabolism; and the Stroke Council. *Circulation.* 2004;109(16):2031-2041.

74. Ivey FM, Macko RF, Ryan AS, Hafer-Macko CE. Cardiovascular health and fitness after stroke. *Top Stroke Rehabil.* 2005;12(1):1-16.

75. Hafer-Macko CE, Ryan AS, Ivey FM, Macko RF. Skeletal muscle changes after hemiparetic stroke and potential beneficial effects of exercise intervention strategies. *J Rehabil Res Dev.* 2008;45(2):261-272.

76. Kelly JO, Kilbreath SL, Davis GM, Zeman B, Raymond J. Cardiorespiratory fitness and walking ability in subacute stroke patients. *Arch Phys Med Rehabil.* 2003;84(12):1780-1785.

77. Ivey FM, Hafer-Macko CE, Macko RF. Task-oriented treadmill exercise training in chronic hemiparetic stroke. *J Rehabil Res Dev.* 2008;45(2):249-259.

78. Ryan AS, Dobrovolny CL, Smith GV, Silver KH, Macko RF. Hemiparetic muscle atrophy and increased intramuscular fat in stroke patients. *Arch Phys Med Rehabil.* 2002;83(12):1703-1707.

79. Potempa K, Lopez M, Braun LT, Szidon JP, Fogg L, Tincknell T. Physiological outcomes of aerobic exercise training in hemiparetic stroke patients. *Stroke.* 1995;26(1):101-105.

80. Luft A, Macko R, Forrester L, Goldberg A, Hanley DF. Post-stroke exercise rehabilitation: what we know about retraining the motor system and how it may apply to retraining the heart. *Cleve Clin J Med.* 2008;75(Suppl 2):S83-S86.

81. Mulroy SJ, Klassen T, Gronley JK, Eberly VJ, Brown DA, Sullivan KJ. Gait parameters associated with responsiveness to treadmill training with body-weight support after stroke: an exploratory study. *Phys Ther.* 2010;90(2):209-223.

82. Michael KM, Allen JK, Macko RF. Reduced ambulatory activity after stroke: the role of balance, gait, and cardiovascular fitness. *Arch Phys Med Rehabil.* 2005;86(8):1552-1556.

83. Perry J, Garrett M, Gronley JK, Mulroy SJ. Classification of walking handicap in the stroke population. *Stroke.* 1995;26(6):982-989.

84. Bowden MG, Balasubramanian CK, Behrman AL, Kautz SA. Validation of a speed-based classification system using quantitative measures of walking performance poststroke. *Neurorehabil Neural Repair.* 2008;22(6):672-675.

85. Ivey FM, Hafer-Macko CE, Macko RF. Exercise training for cardiometabolic adaptation after stroke. *J Cardiopulm Rehabil Prev.* 2008;28(1):2-11.

86. Saunders DH, Greig CA, Mead GE, Young A. Physical fitness training for stroke patients. *Cochrane Database Syst Rev.* 2009(4):003316.

87. Platts MM, Rafferty D, Paul L. Metabolic cost of over ground gait in younger stroke patients and healthy controls. *Med Sci Sports Exerc.* 2006;38(6):1041-1046.

88. MacKay-Lyons MJ, Howlett J. Exercise capacity and cardiovascular adaptations to aerobic training early after stroke. *Top Stroke Rehabil.* 2005;12(1):31-44.

89. Jørgensen JR, Bech-Pedersen DT, Zeeman P, Sørensen J, Andersen LL, Schönberger M. Effect of intensive outpatient physical training on gait performance and cardiovascular health in people with hemiparesis after stroke. *Phys Ther.* 2010;90(4):527-537.

90. Dobkin BH. Training and exercise to drive poststroke recovery. *Nat Clin Pract Neurol.* 2008;4(2):76-85.

91. Patterson SL, Forrester LW, Rodgers MM, et al. Determinants of walking function after stroke: Differences by deficit severity. *Arch Phys Med Rehabil.* 2007;88(1):115-119.

92. American College of Sports Medicine. *ACSM's Guidelines for Exercise Testing and Prescription.* 8th ed. Lippincott Williams & Wilkins; 2009:400.

93. MacKay-Lyons MJ, Makrides L. Cardiovascular stress during a contemporary stroke rehabilitation program: is the intensity adequate to induce a training effect? *Arch Phys Med Rehabil.* 2002;83(10):1378-1383.

94. Pang MY, Eng JJ, Dawson AS, Gylfadóttir S. The use of aerobic exercise training in improving aerobic capacity in individuals with stroke: a meta-analysis. *Clin Rehabil.* 2006;20(2):97-111.

95. Pang MY, Eng JJ. Determinants of improvement in walking capacity among individuals with chronic stroke following a multidimensional exercise program. *J Rehabil Med.* 2008;40(4):284-290.

96. Tilson JK, Sullivan KJ, Cen S, et al. Meaningful gait speed improvement during the first 60 days poststroke: minimal clinically important difference. *Phys Ther.* 2010;90(2):196-208.

97. Macko RF, Ivey FM, Forrester LW, et al. Treadmill exercise rehabilitation improves ambulatory function and cardiovascular fitness in patients with chronic stroke: a randomized, controlled trial. *Stroke.* 2005;36(10):2206-2211.

98. Ivey FM, Hafer-Macko CE, Macko RF. Exercise training for cardiometabolic adaptation after stroke. *J Cardiopulm Rehabil Prev.* 2008;28(1):2-11.

99. Sullivan KJ. Brown DA. Klassen T, et al. Effects of task-specific locomotor and strength training in adults who were ambulatory after stroke: results of the STEPS randomized clinical trial. *Phys Ther.* 2007;87(12):1580-1602.

100. Duncan PW, Sullivan KJ, Behrman AL, et al. Body-weight-supported treadmill rehabilitation after stroke. *N Engl J Med.* 2011;364(21):2026-2036.

101. van de Port IG, Wood-Dauphinee S, Lindeman E, Kwakkel G. Effects of exercise training programs on walking competency after stroke: a systematic review. *Am J Phys Med Rehabil.* 2007;86(11):935-951.

102. LiVecchi MA. Spinal cord injury. *Continuum (Minneap Minn).* 2011;17(3 Neurorehabilitation):568-583.

103. Sekhon LH, Fehlings MG. Epidemiology, demographics, and pathophysiology of acute spinal cord injury. *Spine (Phila Pa 1976).* 2001;26(24 Suppl):S2-S12.

104. Ho CH, Wuermser LA, Priebe MM, Chiodo AE, Scelza WM, Kirshblum SC. Spinal cord injury medicine. 1. Epidemiology and classification. *Arch Phys Med Rehabil.* 2007;88(3 Suppl 1):S49-S54.

105. Maynard FM Jr, Bracken MB, Creasey G, et al. International Standards for Neurological and Functional Classification of Spinal Cord Injury. American Spinal Injury Association. *Spinal Cord.* 1997;35(5):266-274.

106. Kattail D, Furlan JC, Fehlings MG. Epidemiology and clinical outcomes of acute spine trauma and spinal cord injury: experience from a specialized spine trauma center in Canada in comparison with a large national registry. *J Trauma.* 2009;67(5):936-943.

107. Garshick E, Kelley A, Cohen SA, et al. A prospective assessment of mortality in chronic spinal cord injury. *Spinal Cord.* 2005;43(7):408-416.

108. Groah SL, Nash MS, Ward EA, et al. Cardiometabolic risk in community-dwelling persons with chronic spinal cord injury. *J Cardiopulm Rehabil Prev.* 2011;31(2):73-80.

109. Nash MS. Exercise as a health-promoting activity following spinal cord injury. *J Neurol Phys Ther.* 2005;29(2):87-103.

110. Jacobs PL, Nash MS. Exercise recommendations for individuals with spinal cord injury. *Sports Med.* 2004;34(11):727-751.

111. Hayes AM, Myers JN, Ho M, Lee MY, Perkash I, Kiratli BJ. Heart rate as a predictor of energy expenditure in people with spinal cord injury. *J Rehabil Res Dev.* 2005;42(5):617-624.

112. Agiovlasitis SH, Heffernan KS, Jae SY, et al. Effects of paraplegia on cardiac autonomic regulation during static exercise. *Am J Phys Med Rehabil.* 2010;89(10):817-823.

113. Figoni SF. Exercise responses and quadriplegia. *Med Sci Sports Exerc.* 1993;25(4):433-441.

114. Wecht JM, Marsico R, Weir JP, Spungen AM, Bauman WA, De Meersman RE. Autonomic recovery from peak arm exercise in fit and unfit individuals with paraplegia. *Med Sci Sports Exerc.* 2006;38(7):1223-1228.

115. Myslinski MJ. Evidence-based exercise prescription for individuals with spinal cord injury. *J Neurol Phys Ther.* 2005;29(2):104-106.

116. Hol AT, Eng JJ, Miller WC, Sproule S, Krassioukov AV. Reliability and validity of the six-minute arm test for the evaluation of cardiovascular fitness in people with spinal cord injury. *Arch Phys Med Rehabil.* 2007;88(4):489-495.

117. Westcott WL, Rosa S. Spinal cord injury. *Strength Cond J.* 2010;32(6):16-18.

118. Tawashy AE, Eng JJ, Krassioukov AV, Miller WC, Sproule S. Aerobic exercise during early rehabilitation for cervical spinal cord injury. *Phys Ther.* 2010;90(3):427-437.

119. Brurok B, Helgerud J, Karlsen T, Leivseth G, Hoff J. Effect of aerobic high-intensity hybrid training on stroke volume and peak oxygen consumption in men with spinal cord injury. *Am J Phys Med Rehabil.* 2011;90(5):407-414.

120. Raymond J, Davis GM, Fahey A, Climstein M, Sutton JR. Oxygen uptake and heart rate responses during arm vs combined arm/electrically stimulated leg exercise in people with paraplegia. *Spinal Cord.* 1997;35(10):680-685.

121. Raymond J, Davis GM, van der Plas M. Cardiovascular responses during submaximal electrical stimulation-induced leg cycling in individuals with paraplegia. *Clin Physiol Funct Imaging.* 2002;22(2):92-98.

122. Raymond J, Davis GM, Climstein M, Sutton JR. Cardiorespiratory responses to arm cranking and electrical stimulation leg cycling in people with paraplegia. *Med Sci Sports Exerc.* 1999;31(6):822-828.

123. Nightingale EJ, Raymond J, Middleton JW, Crosbie J, Davis GM. Benefits of FES gait in a spinal cord injured population. *Spinal Cord.* 2007;45(10):646-657.

124. Jacobs PL, Nash MS, Rusinowski JW. Circuit training provides cardiorespiratory and strength benefits in persons with paraplegia. *Med Sci Sports Exerc.* 2001;33(5):711-717.

125. Nash MS, van de Ven I, van Elk N, Johnson BM. Effects of circuit resistance training on fitness attributes and upper-extremity pain in middle-aged men with paraplegia. *Arch Phys Med Rehabil.* 2007;88(1):70-75.

126. Lewis JE, Nash MS, Hamm LF, Martins SC, Groah SL. The relationship between perceived exertion and physiologic indicators of stress during graded arm exercise in persons with spinal cord injuries. *Arch Phys Med Rehabil.* 2007;88(9):1205-1211.

127. Barfield JP, Malone LA, Collins JM, Ruble SB. Disability type influences heart rate response during power wheelchair sport. *Med Sci Sports Exerc.* 2005;37(5):718-723.

128. American College of Sports Medicine. *ACSM's Resources for Clinical Exercise Physiology: Musculoskeletal, Neuromuscular, Neoplastic, Immunologic and Hematologic Conditions.* 2nd ed. Baltimore, MD: Lippincott Williams & Wilkins; 2010.

129. Greenwald BD, Burnett DM, Miller MA. Congenital and acquired brain injury. 1. Brain injury: epidemiology and pathophysiology. *Arch Phys Med Rehabil.* 2003;84(3 Suppl 1):S3-S7.

130. Centers for Disease Control. Traumatic brain injury. http://www.cdc.gov/TraumaticBrainInjury/index.html. Accessed June 12, 2014.

131. Dombovy ML. Traumatic brain injury. *Continuum (Minneap Minn).* 2011;17(3 Neurorehabilitation):584-605.

132. Mossberg KA, Amonette WE, Masel BE. Endurance training and cardiorespiratory conditioning after traumatic brain injury. *J Head Trauma Rehabil.* 2010;25(3):173-183.

133. Katz DI, White DK, Alexander MP, Klein RB. Recovery of ambulation after traumatic brain injury. *Arch Phys Med Rehabil.* 2004;85(6):865-869.

134. Mossberg KA, Ayala D, Baker T, Heard J, Masel B. Aerobic capacity after traumatic brain injury: comparison with a nondisabled cohort. *Arch Phys Med Rehabil.* 2007;88(3):315-320.

135. Bhambhani Y, Rowland G, Farag M. Reliability of peak cardiorespiratory responses in patients with moderate to severe traumatic brain injury. *Arch Phys Med Rehabil.* 2003;84(11):1629-1636..

136. Jankowski LW, Sullivan SJ. Aerobic and neuromuscular training: effect on the capacity, efficiency, and fatigability of patients with traumatic brain injuries. *Arch Phys Med Rehabil.* 1990;71(7):500-504.

137. Bateman A, Culpan FJ, Pickering AD, Powell JH, Scott OM, Greenwood RJ. The effect of aerobic training on rehabilitation outcomes after recent severe brain injury: a randomized controlled evaluation. *Arch Phys Med Rehabil.* 2001;82(2):174-182.

138. Gordon WA, Sliwinski M, Echo J, McLoughlin M, Sheerer MS, Meili TE. The benefits of exercise in individuals with traumatic brain injury: a retrospective study. *J Head Trauma Rehabil.* 1998;13(4):58-67.

139. Mossberg KA, Kuna S, Masel B. Ambulatory efficiency in persons with acquired brain injury after a rehabilitation intervention. *Brain Inj.* 2002;16(9):789-797.

140. Brown TH, Mount J, Rouland BL, Kautz KA, Barnes RM, Kim J. Body weight-supported treadmill training versus conventional gait training for people with chronic traumatic brain injury. *J Head Trauma Rehabil.* 2005;20(5):402-415.

141. Hunter M, Tomberlin J, Kirkikis C, Kuna ST. Progressive exercise testing in closed head-injured subjects: comparison of exercise apparatus in assessment of a physical conditioning program. *Phys Ther.* 1990;70(6):363-371.

142. Ng DC. Parkinson's disease. Diagnosis and treatment. *West J Med.* 1996;165(4):234-240.

143. Rao SS, Hofmann LA, Shakil A. Parkinson's disease: diagnosis and treatment. *Am Fam Physician.* 2006;74(12):2046-2054.

144. Lang AE, Lozano AM. Parkinson's disease. First of two parts. *N Engl J Med.* 1998;339(15):1044-1053.

145. Lang AE, Lozano AM. Parkinson's disease. Second of two parts. *N Engl J Med.* 1998;339(16):1130-1143.

146. Archer T, Fredriksson A, Johansson B. Exercise alleviates Parkinsonism: clinical and laboratory evidence. *Acta Neurol Scand.* 2011;123(2):73-84.

147. Goetz CG, Poewe W, Rascol O, et al. Movement disorder society task force report on the Hoehn and Yahr staging scale: status and recommendations. *Mov Disord.* 2004;19(9):1020-1028.

148. Jankovic J. Parkinson's disease: clinical features and diagnosis. *J Neurol Neurosurg Psychiatry.* 2008;79(4):368-376.

149. Bishop M, Brunt D, Pathare N, Ko M, Marjama-Lyons J. Changes in distal muscle timing may contribute to slowness during sit to stand in Parkinsons disease. *Clin Biomech (Bristol, Avon).* 2005;20(1):112-117.

150. Haas BM, Trew M, Castle PC. Effects of respiratory muscle weakness on daily living function, quality of life, activity levels, and exercise capacity in mild to moderate Parkinson's disease. *Am J Phys Med Rehabil.* 2004;83(8):601-607.

151. Canning CG, Alison JA, Allen NE, Groeller H. Parkinson's disease: an investigation of exercise capacity, respiratory function, and gait. *Arch Phys Med Rehabil.* 1997;78(2):199-207.

152. Winogrodzka A, Wagenaar RC, Booij J, Wolters EC. Rigidity and bradykinesia reduce interlimb coordination in Parkinsonian gait. *Arch Phys Med Rehabil.* 2005;86(2):183-189.

153. Scandalis TA, Bosak A, Berliner JC, Helman LL, Wells MR. Resistance training and gait function in patients with Parkinson's disease. *Am J Phys Med Rehabil.* 2001;80(1):38-43.

154. Christiansen CL, Schenkman ML, McFann K, Wolfe P, Kohrt WM. Walking economy in people with Parkinson's disease. *Mov Disord.* 2009;24(10):1481-1487.

155. Gallagher DA, Lees AJ, Schrag A. What are the most important nonmotor symptoms in patients with Parkinson's disease and are we missing them? *Mov Disord.* 2010;25(15):2493-2500.

156. Ziemssen T, Reichmann H. Cardiovascular autonomic dysfunction in Parkinson's disease. *J Neurol Sci.* 2010;289(1-2):74-80.

157. Goodwin VA, Richards SH, Taylor RS, Taylor AH, Campbell JL. The effectiveness of exercise interventions for people with Parkinson's disease: a systematic review and meta-analysis. *Mov Disord.* 2008;23(5):631-640.

158. Schenkman M, Hall D, Kumar R, Kohrt WM. Endurance exercise training to improve economy of movement of people with Parkinson disease: three case reports. *Phys Ther.* 2008;88(1):63-76.

159. de Goede CJ, Keus SH, Kwakkel G, Wagenaar RC. The effects of physical therapy in Parkinson's disease: a research synthesis. *Arch Phys Med Rehabil.* 2001;82(4):509-515.

160. Ellis T, de Goede CJ, Feldman RG, Wolters EC, Kwakkel G, Wagenaar RC. Efficacy of a physical therapy program in patients with Parkinson's disease: a randomized controlled trial. *Arch Phys Med Rehabil.* 2005;86(4):626-632.

161. Müller T, Muhlack S. Effect of exercise on reactivity and motor behaviour in patients with Parkinson's disease. *J Neurol Neurosurg Psychiatry.* 2010;81(7):747-753.

162. Dibble LE, Hale TF, Marcus RL, Gerber JP, LaStavo PC. High intensity eccentric resistance training decreases bradykinesia and improves quality of life in persons with Parkinson's disease: a preliminary study. *Parkinsonism Relat Disord.* 2009;15(10):752-757.

163. Ene H, McRae C, Schenkman M. Attitudes toward exercise following participation in an exercise intervention study. *J Neurol Phys Ther.* 2011;35(1):34-40.

164. Mehrholz J, Friis R, Kugler J, Twork S, Storch A, Pohl M. Treadmill training for patients with Parkinson's disease. *Cochrane Database Syst Rev.* 2010;(1):CD007830.

165. Bello O, Sanchez JA, Fernandez-del-Olmo M. Treadmill walking in Parkinson's disease patients: adaptation and generalization effect. *Mov Disord.* 2008;23(9):1243-1249.

166. Herman T, Giladi N, Hausdorff JM. Treadmill training for the treatment of gait disturbances in people with Parkinson's disease: a mini-review. *J Neural Transm.* 2009;116(3):307-318.

167. Miyai I, Fujimoto Y, Ueda Y, et al. Treadmill training with body weight support: its effect on Parkinson's disease. *Arch Phys Med Rehabil.* 2000;81(7):849-852.

168. Pohl M, Rockstroh G, Rückriem S, Mrass G, Mehrholz J. Immediate effects of speed-dependent treadmill training on gait parameters in early Parkinson's disease. *Arch Phys Med Rehabil.* 2003;84(12):1760-1766.

169. Pelosin E, Faelli E, Lofrano F, et al. Effects of treadmill training on walking economy in Parkinson's disease: a pilot study. *Neurol Sci.* 2009;30(6):499-504.

170. Fisher BE, Wu AD, Salem GJ, et al. The effect of exercise training in improving motor performance and corticomotor excitability in people with early Parkinson's disease. *Arch Phys Med Rehabil.* 2008;89(7):1221-1229.

171. Cakit BD, Saracoglu M, Genc H, Erdem HR, Inan L. The effects of incremental speed-dependent treadmill training on postural instability and fear of falling in Parkinson's disease. *Clin Rehabil.* 2007;21(8):698-705.

172. Herman T, Giladi N, Gruendlinger L, Hausdorff JM. Six weeks of intensive treadmill training improves gait and quality of life in patients with Parkinson's disease: a pilot study. *Arch Phys Med Rehabil.* 2007;88(9):1154-1158.

173. Onla-or S, Winstein CJ. Determining the optimal challenge point for motor skill learning in adults with moderately severe Parkinson's disease. *Neurorehabil Neural Repair.* 2008;22(4):385-395.

174. Protas EJ, Stanley RK, Jankovic J, MacNeill B. Cardiovascular and metabolic responses to upper- and lower-extremity exercise in men with idiopathic Parkinson's disease. *Phys Ther.* 1996;76(1):34-40.

175. Ridgel AL, Vitek JL, Alberts JL. Forced, not voluntary, exercise improves motor function in Parkinson's disease patients. *Neurorehabil Neural Repair.* 2009;23(6):600-608.

176. Stelmach GE, Teasdale N, Phillips J, Worringham CJ. Force production characteristics in Parkinson's disease. *Exp Brain Res.* 1989;76(1):165-172.

177. Fox CM, Ramig LO, Ciucci MR, Sapir S, McFarland DH, Farley BG. The science and practice of LSVT/LOUD: neural plasticity-principled approach to treating individuals with Parkinson disease and other neurological disorders. *Semin Speech Lang.* 2006;27(4):283-299.

178. Lucchinetti CF, Parisi J, Bruck W. The pathology of multiple sclerosis. *Neurol Clin.* 2005;23(1):77-105.

179. Brück W. The pathology of multiple sclerosis is the result of focal inflammatory demyelination with axonal damage. *J Neurol.* 2005;252(Suppl 5):3-9.

180. Brück W. Clinical implications of neuropathological findings in multiple sclerosis. *J Neurol.* 2005;252(Suppl 3):10-14.

181. Kurtzke JF. Rating neurologic impairment in multiple sclerosis: an expanded disability status scale (EDSS). *Neurology.* 1983;33(11):1444-1452.

182. Freeman J, Morris M, Davidson M, Dodd K. Outcome measures to quantify the effects of physical therapy for people with multiple sclerosis. *J Neurol Phys Ther.* 2002;26(3):139-144.

183. Motl RW, Snook EM, Schapiro RT. Symptoms and physical activity behavior in individuals with multiple sclerosis. *Res Nurs Health.* 2008;31(5):466-475.

184. Flachenecker P. Autonomic dysfunction in Guillain-Barré syndrome and multiple sclerosis. *J Neurol.* 2007;254(Suppl 2):II96-II101.

185. Kanjwal K, Karabin B, Kanjwal Y, Grubb BP. Autonomic dysfunction presenting as postural orthostatic tachycardia syndrome in patients with multiple sclerosis. *Int J Med Sci.* 2010;7:62-67.

186. Saari A, Tolonen U, Pääkkö E, et al. Cardiovascular autonomic dysfunction correlates with brain MRI lesion load in MS. *Clin Neurophysiol.* 2004;115(6):1473-1478.

187. Ng AV, Miller RG, Gelinas D, Kent-Braun JA. Functional relationships of central and peripheral muscle alterations in multiple sclerosis. *Muscle Nerve.* 2004;29(6):843-852.

188. Thickbroom GW, Byrnes ML, Archer SA, Kermode AG, Mastaglia FL. Corticomotor organisation and motor function in multiple sclerosis. *J Neurol.* 2005;252(7):765-771.

189. Benedetti MG, Piperno R, Simoncini L, Bonato P, Tonini A, Giannini S. Gait abnormalities in minimally impaired multiple sclerosis patients. *Mult Scler.* 1999;5(5):363-368.

190. Chetta A, Rampello A, Marangio E, et al. Cardiorespiratory response to walk in multiple sclerosis patients. *Respir Med.* 2004;98(6):522-529.

191. Koseoglu BF, Gokkaya NK, Ergun U, Inan L, Yesiltepe E. Cardiopulmonary and metabolic functions, aerobic capacity, fatigue and quality of life in patients with multiple sclerosis. *Acta Neurol Scand.* 2006;114(4):261-267.

192. Cantor F. Central and peripheral fatigue: exemplified by multiple sclerosis and myasthenia gravis. *PM R.* 2010;2(5):399-405.

193. Thickbroom GW, Sacco P, Kermode AG, et al. Central motor drive and perception of effort during fatigue in multiple sclerosis. *J Neurol.* 2006;253(8):1048-1053.

194. Andreasen AK, Jakobsen J, Petersen T, Andersen H. Fatigued patients with multiple sclerosis have impaired central muscle activation. *Mult Scler.* 2009;15(7):818-827.

195. Acevedo AR, Nava C, Arriada N, Violante A, Corona T. Cardiovascular dysfunction in multiple sclerosis. *Acta Neurol Scand.* 2000;101(2):85-88.

196. Heesen C, Romberg A, Gold S, Schulz KH. Physical exercise in multiple sclerosis: supportive care or a putative disease-modifying treatment. *Expert Rev Neurother.* 2006;6(3):347-355.

197. Hale LA, Nukada H, Du Plessis LJ, Peebles KC. Clinical screening of autonomic dysfunction in multiple sclerosis. *Physiother Res Int.* 2009;14(1):42-55.

198. Dalgas U, Stenager E, Ingemann-Hansen T. Multiple sclerosis and physical exercise: recommendations for the application of resistance-, endurance- and combined training. *Mult Scler.* 2008;14(1):35-53.

199. Motl RW, McAuley E. Longitudinal analysis of physical activity and symptoms as predictors of change in functional limitations and disability in multiple sclerosis. *Rehabil Psychol.* 2009;54(2):204-210.

200. Petajan JH, Gappmaier E, White AT, Spencer MK, Mino L, Hicks RW. Impact of aerobic training on fitness and quality of life in multiple sclerosis. *Ann Neurol.* 1996;39(4):432-441.

201. Romberg A, Virtanen A, Ruutiainen J, et al. Effects of a 6-month exercise program on patients with multiple sclerosis: a randomized study. *Neurology.* 2004;63(11):2034-2038.

202. Thickbroom GW, Sacco P, Faulkner DL, Kermode AG, Mataglia FL. Enhanced corticomotor excitability with dynamic fatiguing exercise of the lower limb in multiple sclerosis. *J Neurol.* 2008;255(7):1001-1005.

203. Sabapathy NM, Minahan CL, Turner GT, Broadley SA. Comparing endurance- and resistance-exercise training in people with multiple sclerosis: a randomized pilot study. *Clin Rehabil.* 2011;25(1):14-24.

204. Dalgas U, Stenager E, Jakobsen J, et al. Resistance training improves muscle strength and functional capacity in multiple sclerosis. *Neurology.* 2009;73(18):1478-1484.

205. Dodd KJ, Taylor NF, Denisenko S, Prasad D. A qualitative analysis of a progressive resistance exercise programme for people with multiple sclerosis. *Disabil Rehabil.* 2006;28(18):1127-1134.

206. Taylor NF, Dodd KJ, Prasad D, Denisenko S. Progressive resistance exercise for people with multiple sclerosis. *Disabil Rehabil.* 2006;28(18):1119-1126.

207. Dalgas U, Stenager E, Jakobsen J, Petersen T, Overgaard K, Ingemann-Hansen T. Muscle fiber size increases following resistance training in multiple sclerosis. *Mult Scler.* 2010;16(11):1367-1376.

208. Petajan JH, White AT. Recommendations for physical activity in patients with multiple sclerosis. *Sports Med.* 1999;27(3):179-191.

209. Gutierrez GM, Chow JW, Tillman MD, McCoy SC, Castellano V, White LJ. Resistance training improves gait kinematics in persons with multiple sclerosis. *Arch Phys Med Rehabil.* 2005;86(9):1824-1829.

210. Clarkson PM, Hubal MJ. Exercise-induced muscle damage in humans. *Am J Phys Med Rehabil.* 2002;81(11 Suppl):S52-S69.

211. Hayes HA, Gappmaier EPT, LaStayo PC. Effects of high-intensity resistance training on strength, mobility, balance, and fatigue in individuals with multiple sclerosis: a randomized controlled trial. *J Neurol Phys Ther.* 2011;35(1):2-10.

212. Rampello A, Franceschini M, Piepoli M, et al. Effect of aerobic training on walking capacity and maximal exercise tolerance in patients with multiple sclerosis: a randomized crossover controlled study. *Phys Ther.* 2007;87(5):545-555.

213. Logroscino G, Traynor BJ, Hardiman O, et al. Descriptive epidemiology of amyotrophic lateral sclerosis: New evidence and unsolved issues. *J Neurol Neurosurg Psychiatry.* 2008;79(1):6-11.

214. Rowland LP, Shneider NA. Amyotrophic lateral sclerosis. *N Engl J Med.* 2001;344(22):1688-1700.

215. Rowland GJ, Farag M, Bhambhani Y, et al. Relationship between peak aerobic power and cerebral hemodynamics in patients with traumatic brain injury. *Med Sci Sports Exerc.* 2002;34(5 Suppl 1):S56.

216. The Amyotrophic Lateral Sclerosis Functional Rating Scale. Assessment of activities of daily living in patients with amyotrophic lateral sclerosis. The ALS CNTF treatment study (ACTS) phase I-II Study Group. *Arch Neurol.* 1996;53(2):141-147.

217. Miller RG, Jackson CE, Kasarskis EJ, et al. Practice parameter update: the care of the patient with amyotrophic lateral sclerosis: drug, nutritional, and respiratory therapies (an evidence-based review): report of the Quality Standards Subcommittee of the American Academy Of Neurology. *Neurology.* 2009;73(15):1218-1226.

218. Miller RG, Jackson CE, Kasarskis EJ, et al. Practice parameter update: the care of the patient with amyotrophic lateral sclerosis: multidisciplinary care, symptom management, and cognitive/behavioral impairment (an evidence-based review): report of the Quality Standards Subcommittee of the American Academy of Neurology. *Neurology.* 2009;73(15):1227-1233.

219. Sharma KR, Miller RG. Electrical and mechanical properties of skeletal muscle underlying increased fatigue in patients with amyotrophic lateral sclerosis. *Muscle Nerve.* 1996;19(11):1391-1400.

220. Lui AJ, Byl NN. A systematic review of the effect of moderate intensity exercise on function and disease progression in amyotrophic lateral sclerosis. *J Neurol Phys Ther.* 2009;33(2):68-87.

221. Dupuis L, Pradat PF, Ludolph AC, Loeffler JP. Energy metabolism in amyotrophic lateral sclerosis. *Lancet Neurol.* 2011;10(1):75-82.

222. Dalbello-Haas V, Florence JM, Krivickas LS. Therapeutic exercise for people with amyotrophic lateral sclerosis or motor neuron disease. *Cochrane Database Syst Rev.* 2008;(2):005229.

223. Pinto AC, Alves M, Nogueira A, et al. Can amyotrophic lateral sclerosis patients with respiratory insufficiency exercise? *J Neurol Sci.* 1999;169(1-2):69-75.

224. Ashworth NL, Satkunam LE, Deforge D. Treatment for spasticity in amyotrophic lateral sclerosis/motor neuron disease. *Cochrane Database Syst Rev.* 2006;(1):004156.

225. Bohannon RW. Results of resistance exercise on a patient with amyotrophic lateral sclerosis. A case report. *Phys Ther.* 1983;63(6):965-968.

226. Bello-Haas VD, Florence JM, Kloos AD, et al. A randomized controlled trial of resistance exercise in individuals with ALS. *Neurology.* 2007;68(23):2003-2007.

227. Sanjak M, Bravver E, Bockenek WL, et al. Supported treadmill ambulation for amyotrophic lateral sclerosis: A pilot study. *Arch Phys Med Rehabil.* 2010;91(12):1920-1929.

228. Dal Bello-Haas V, Kloos AD, Mitsumoto H. Physical therapy for a patient through six stages of amyotrophic lateral sclerosis. *Phys Ther.* 1998;78(12):1312-1324.

229. Bassile CC. Guillain-Barré syndrome and exercise guidelines. *J Neurol Phys Ther.* 1996;20(2):31-36.

230. Meythaler JM, DeVivo MJ, Braswell WC. Rehabilitation outcomes of patients who have developed Guillain-Barré syndrome. *Am J Phys Med Rehabil.* 1997;76(5):411-419.

231. Fletcher DD, Lawn ND, Wolter TD, Wijdicks EF. Long-term outcome in patients with Guillain-Barré syndrome requiring mechanical ventilation. *Neurology.* 2000;54(12):2311-2315.

232. Forsberg A, Press R, Einarsson U, de Pedro-Cuesta J, Holmqvist LW. Disability and health-related quality of life in Guillain-Barré syndrome during the first two years after onset: a prospective study. *Clin Rehabil.* 2005;19(8):900-909.

233. Merkies IS, Schmitz PI, van der Meché FG, Samijn JP, van Doorn PA. Connecting impairment, disability, and handicap in immune mediated polyneuropathies. *J Neurol Neurosurg Psychiatry.* 2003;74(1):99-104.

234. El Mhandi L, Calmels P, Camdessanché JP, Gautheron V, Féasson L. Muscle strength recovery in treated Guillain-Barré syndrome: a prospective study for the first 18 months after onset. *Am J Phys Med Rehabil.* 2007;86(9):716-724.

235. Agre JC. The role of exercise in the patient with post-polio syndrome. *Ann N Y Acad Sci.* 1995;753:321-334.

236. Ropper AH. The Guillain-Barré syndrome. *N Engl J Med.* 1992;326(17):1130-1136.

237. Bensman A. Strenuous exercise may impair muscle function in Guillain-Barré patients. *JAMA.* 1970;214:468-469.

238. Garssen MP, Schillings ML, Van Doorn PA, Van Engelen BG, Zwarts MJ. Contribution of central and peripheral factors to residual fatigue in Guillain-Barré syndrome. *Muscle Nerve.* 2007;36(1):93-99.

239. Garssen MP, Bussmann JB, Schmitz PI, et al. Physical training and fatigue, fitness, and quality of life in Guillain-Barré syndrome and CIDP. *Neurology.* 2004;63(12):2393-2395.

240. Bussmann JB, Garssen MP, van Doorn PA, Stam JH. Analysing the favourable effects of physical exercise: Relationships between physical fitness, fatigue and functioning in Guillain-Barré syndrome and chronic inflammatory demyelinating polyneuropathy. *J Rehabil Med.* 2007;39(2):121-125.

241. Meythaler JM. Rehabilitation of Guillain-Barré syndrome. *Arch Phys Med Rehabil.* 1997;78(8):872-879.

CASE STUDY 12-1

Laura Klassen, DipPT, BPT, MSc

EXAMINATION

History

Current Condition/Chief Complaint

Mr. Julep, a 70-year-old White male, was diagnosed with a right side, lacunar stroke of thrombotic etiology, resulting in hemiparesis.

> **Clinician Comment** *The most common cause of ischemic stroke is thrombosis, which causes partial to complete arterial stenosis.[1] Lacunar cerebral vascular accidents occur in small perforating branches of the middle cerebral artery supplying blood to the diencephalon and ventral pons.[2] They typically result in localized lesions and a set of limited clinical signs and symptoms, as described by Brown in Chapter 12. Although usually smaller in size than the lesions caused by cortical strokes, subcortical lesions can have substantial impact on motor control. Axons from the primary, secondary, and supplementary motor cortices all converge in the corona radiata, before passing through the compact internal capsule.[3]*
>
> *Lacunar strokes are generally associated with better functional outcomes[4] and greater likelihood of discharge home[5] than other types of ischemic strokes. They are also generally associated with low rates of recurrence.[6] However, there are a variety of other personal contextual factors influencing rehabilitation outcomes and risks for recurrence.*
>
> *Mr. Julep's age and gender are personal contextual factors influencing stroke outcomes.[7] At 70 years of age, Mr. Julep is just slightly younger than the mean age for White males at time of stroke.[8] Increasing age has been associated with poorer functional recovery from stroke.[9,10] It has also been associated with decreased likelihood of return home.[5,11] Poor outcomes are particularly true in the very old[12] and those with severe strokes.[13] Increases in the number and severity of comorbidities that occur with aging may play a role in the association between age and rehabilitation outcomes.[5,11]*
>
> *When considered independently of other prognostic variables, age has been reported to have limited effect on functional outcomes[14] and discharge destination.[15] Therefore, age should not, in isolation, influence decisions regarding access to rehabilitation or intervention planning.*
>
> *Mr. Julep's gender weighs in his favor when considering stroke outcomes. Men are less likely to have in-hospital complications following stroke,[16] are more likely to achieve greater functional recovery[5] and are more likely to be discharged home.[8,11,15] Sociological factors may play a role in such findings.*

History of Current Complaint

Mr. Julep was admitted to an acute care hospital after developing rapid onset of a left lower facial droop, paresis of left arm and leg, dysarthria, and dysphagia. He was incontinent at time of admission. He was treated with alteplase (ie, tissue plasminogen activator [tPA]).

Mr. Julep received physical therapy care (30 minutes/day for 5 days) while in the acute care facility. He was transferred from acute care to a rehabilitation facility 8 days after his initial admission. He underwent a full interdisciplinary rehabilitation assessment during his first days there. The results of the physical therapy portion of that assessment are presented in the sections that follow.

> **Clinician Comment** *Incontinence had resolved in the acute post-stroke period, and dysarthria and dysphagia were resolving by time of admission to our rehabilitation facility. Therefore, these impairments were not expected to detrimentally influence rehabilitation outcomes or discharge destination.*
>
> *Those receiving tPA for acute treatment of stroke have been reported to have a 30% higher likelihood of minimal or no disability at 3 months' postintervention.[17] Although Mr. Julep is unlikely to present with minimal disability as a final outcome of his stroke, having received optimal acute treatment may have influenced the outcomes achieved.*
>
> *Earlier rehabilitation intervention is associated with better recovery of function.[5] Shorter intervals between stroke onset and admission to a rehabilitation facility have been reported to increase the likelihood of being discharged home; by a factor of 2, if the interval is 7 days or less.[11] Mr. Julep was admitted to a rehabilitation facility a short 8 days after his stroke. In the interim, he received early physical therapy intervention in the acute care facility, Therefore, the time between stroke onset and commencement of rehabilitation intervention was minimal.*

Social History/Environment

Mr. Julep was a retired farmer, who lived with his wife in a single-story house. His wife was in good health. He had 2 grown children. His daughter, son-in-law, and 2 grandchildren lived in the basement suite of his home. The house had 3 steps (no hand rail) at front entrance. Mr. Julep's hobbies included fishing, gardening, and watching sports on television.

Clinician Comment *Mr. Julep's wife attended many of his physical therapy assessment and treatment sessions, demonstrating interest and support for her spouse. His daughter and grandchildren also attended some treatment sessions.*

Patients with high levels of social support experience more rapid and extensive recovery of function following stroke.[18,19] Those living with another individual are also much more likely to be discharged home.[5,11,15,20] In one large epidemiological analysis, those living with a family member or friend were 4 times more likely to be discharged home than those who lived alone prior to the stroke.[11] This positive discharge outcome is likely associated with assistance that another person is able to provide with activities of daily living (ADL) and instrumental ADL (IADL).

Social/Health Habits

Mr. Julep smoked for 50 years, smoking 1 to 2 packs/day. He quit 5 years ago.

He was physically active while farming, but has lived an inactive lifestyle since retiring. He had never followed a regular exercise or fitness program and had not engaged in physically vigorous leisure activities since early adulthood. Mr. Julep reported that he typically walked approximately 0.5 km/day prior to his stroke.

Clinician Comment *Regular physical exercise/activity is a health strategy known to reduce risk of first stroke[21,22] and recurrence of stroke.[23] Conversely, infrequent physical activity prior to first stroke is a significant prognostic factor for institutionalization at 5 years.[24] Assisting Mr. Julep to become more physically active during his rehabilitation stay and to stay active in the long term was a priority in intervention planning.*

Mr. Julep's inactivity for a number of years had, no doubt, led to his physically deconditioned state and had likely had a negative impact on his cardiovascular, pulmonary, and musculoskeletal systems. Further deconditioning may have occurred during his acute hospital stay. Although Mr. Julep's deconditioned state was a modifiable health risk factor, it would be important to keep in mind that physical exercise had not been a regular part of Mr. Julep's life. Compliance with a regular exercise program, given limited past experience, may be challenging.[25]

It was fortunate that Mr. Julep had ceased smoking 5 years ago, as this might reduce the likelihood of recurrence of stroke.[26]

Medical/Surgical History

Mr. Julep presented with Type 2 diabetes mellitus. Blood sugar levels had fluctuated during the acute care stay and continued to do so until midway through his inpatient rehabilitation stay. As a result of diabetes, he presented with mild retinopathy.

Mr. Julep was diagnosed and successfully treated for prostate cancer in 1991.

Clinician Comment *Diabetes causes damage to the linings of arteries, leading to development, over time, of cardiovascular disease and risk for stroke.[27] Mortality following stroke is higher in those with diabetes.[28] Stroke outcomes are similar in those survivors with and without diabetes, but those with diabetes can be expected to take longer to achieve the same level of function.[28] As examination proceeds, further indications of arterial disease may be revealed, and other signs and symptoms associated with diabetes may be found.*

Medications

Mr. Julep was taking ticlopidine (250 mg, twice a day), an antiplatelet aggregate. He was also taking insulin humulin daily (100u/mL-NDH vial, 100u/mL regular vial). He required acetaminophen (325 mg, PRN) for back pain.

Relevant Clinical Tests

An initial computed tomography (CT) scan, performed immediately after hospital admission, ruled out a hemorrhagic stroke etiology. A follow-up CT scan, performed using a contrast medium, demonstrated a localized ischemic lesion in the posterior limb of the internal capsule on the right side. A carotid Doppler ultrasound test conducted on the fourth day of his acute hospital stay found significant stenosis, with minimal plaque formation, in the region of the right carotid bulb, just beyond the carotid bifurcation.

An initial electrocardiogram (EKG) demonstrated nonspecific ST and T wave changes. Repeat testing conducted just prior to transfer to the rehabilitation facility reported the same results. An initial chest X-ray showed no lung anomaly, but did make note of degenerative joint disease of the thoracic spine. A barium swallow test, conducted on the same day as the Doppler ultrasound, found a slight delay in the swallowing mechanism, a normal cough reflex, and a tendency to aspirate when attempting to swallow thin fluids. A pureed diet was recommended at that time.

Clinician Comment *The corticospinal and corticobulbar tracts travel from the primary motor cortex through the posterior limb of the internal capsule to lower motor neurons innervating the trunk and extremities (corticospinal) and the head and neck (corticobulbar). Secondary motor efferent fibers from the premotor and supplementary motor cortices pass through the genu and anterior limb of the internal capsule, respectively, on their way to the reticulospinal, rubrospinal and vestibulospinal nuclei in the brainstem.[3] Mr. Julep's presentation of hemiparesis was indicative of corticospinal tract damage, and his initial* *presentation of dysphagia and dysarthria were indicative of corticobulbar tract damage. In general, individuals with small, incomplete lesions of the corticospinal tract are expected to recover isolated movement of the arm and leg. Those with complete lesions of the corticospinal tract, but with preservation of supplementary and premotor efferents, may only recover movement that is dependent on abnormal, stereotyped synergies.[3] Assessment of extremity motor control in Mr. Julep's case would likely require evaluation of both isolated and synergistic movement.*

Severe stenosis of the right carotid artery placed Mr. Julep at significant risk of stroke recurrence.[29]

EKG testing assists in determining presence of cardiac ischemia. The ST segment and T wave are produced by ventricular repolarization.[30] Although the changes reported were nonspecific, they may be representative of early coronary artery disease. This possibility needed to be kept in mind when choosing tests and measures and planning physical interventions.

Reported Functional Status

Mr. Julep was right-hand dominant. Prior to the stroke, he was independent in all ADL and IADL activities. He assisted his wife in providing care to his grandchildren when his daughter and son-in-law were working and was the primary person responsible for finances, vehicle maintenance, and yard maintenance. He assisted his son-in-law during peak farm seasons of crop seeding and harvesting.

During the initial examination, Mr. Julep reported that since the stroke, he required some assistance and supervision to ensure safety with most activities, including walking. He was observed to walk for short distances using a front-wheeled walker. He was observed to use his right arm and leg to maneuver the wheelchair. Mr. Julep reported dressing independently if clothes were laid out for him, but he needed assistance with bathing and toileting. He reported that most activities required more effort and time than they had before the stroke and that he tired easily.

Mr. Julep reported that he now managed a regular diet, although he did choke occasionally when drinking fluids.

Clinician Comment *Mr. Julep reported that he tired easily during physical activity. General physical deconditioning, possible left ventricular dysfunction (EKG), diabetes, and decreased motor control may all have contributed to his complaint.*

Those with stroke typically demonstrate substantially decreased peak oxygen (O_2) consumption during submaximal exercise and as much as double the energy costs associated with walking, compared to age- and gender-matched individuals without stroke.[8] Decreased O_2 availability and increased energy costs of moving may both be contributing to his sense of increased effort in performing ADL.

In summary, Mr. Julep presented with a lacunar, motor stroke for which he received tPA as part of optimal, immediate medical stroke management. He was slightly younger than the average stroke patient and had a strong social support system. However, he had lived an inactive lifestyle for the past 5 years and presented with the comorbid conditions of Type 2 diabetes and carotid artery disease. EKG results suggested possible initial signs of coronary artery disease, as well.

Mr. Julep's admission to a rehabilitation facility meant that he was considered a good candidate for rehabilitation intervention. A systems review was required to guide selection of most appropriate tests and measures for physical therapy assessment purposes.

Systems Review

Cardiovascular/Pulmonary

Seated resting values for vital signs were as follows: heart rate (HR) of 84 beats per minute (bpm), blood pressure (BP) of 150/90 mm Hg, respiratory rate of 16, and arterial O_2 saturation of 90%. Lower extremities were cool to touch and mottled in appearance, beginning below the knees bilaterally. Mild edema was noted in the left hand, foot, and ankle. There were no signs or symptoms of deep vein thrombosis.

Mr. Julep demonstrated a strong and nonproductive cough on request. Chest expansion felt slightly decreased on left (hemiplegic) side as compared to right to manual palpation. He denied shortness of breath when completing physical activities, despite finding most activities tiring.

Clinical Comments *Impaired circulatory status in bilateral lower extremities was most likely related to the diagnosis of Type 2 diabetes. Edema was likely the result of decreased voluntary movement and dependent position of distal segments of the arm and leg. Impaired chest expansion on the left side may have been related to a combination of decreased trunk motor control on the affected side and sitting posture, which saw him side-flexed on the left, with center of body mass (COM) displaced to the right.*

Cardiorespiratory fitness can be defined as the ability to perform prolonged physical activity. It is dependent on the capacity of circulatory, respiratory, and muscular systems to supply and use O_2 during physical activity.[31]

Cardiorespiratory fitness has been measured to be ~50% of that of age-matched controls in those with stroke[32] and to decrease quickly following stroke.[33] When decreased fitness is combined with very high rates of energy expenditure (as previously discussed), it was not surprising that Mr. Julep was experiencing fatigue and an increased sense of effort when performing functional mobility tasks. Post-stroke fatigue was found in 39% of participants in a 2001 Swedish study.[34]

Integumentary

Mr. Julep presented with mild trophic skin changes in both lower extremities below the knees and with thickened toenails. A scab, measuring 1 cm in diameter, was present on the left medial malleolus. The area surrounding it was reddened. Mr. Julep reported that this abrasion had been present for some time. No other skin lesions were noted.

Clinical Comments *The skin and nail issues identified were most likely related to Mr. Julep's diagnosis of Type 2 diabetes.*

Musculoskeletal

Mr. Julep was 69 inches in height; weighed 190 pounds and had a body mass index (BMI) of 28.06, which placed him in the overweight category.[35]

Mr. Julep reported intermittent low and mid back pain of moderate intensity (6/10 on VAS numeric rating scale). He was observed to sit in a kyphotic posture with forward chin poke.

Mr. Julep did not present with subluxation of the left shoulder and did not complain of pain at rest or during passive movement of the shoulder. He did, however, present with some limitations in joint ranges of motion (ROMs) and muscle flexibility for trunk and left extremities that were noted as needing additional assessment during the scan.

Clinician Comment *Although Mr. Julep was not obese, being overweight makes diabetes management more problematic.[28]*

Absence of shoulder pain is a positive indicator as regards potential use of the hemiplegic arm in daily activities.[36] A more detailed assessment of shoulder ROMs is important to determination of the risk for development of shoulder pain.[36]

Given the presence of degenerative joint changes in the thoracic spine, it is likely that there are degenerative joint changes in the lumbar and cervical spines as well. More detailed assessment of trunk mobility/ROM will be important, as trunk and pelvic mobility are important to many locomotor activities.

Neuromuscular

Transfers

General observation during performance of transfers and moving between sitting and lying confirmed that Mr. Julep presented both with paresis and dependence on abnormal synergies for movement of the left arm and leg. The left leg was observed to bear Mr. Julep's entire body weight very briefly without assistance during a full standing transfer. Mr. Julep was observed to use the left leg to lift the left wheelchair pedal in preparation for transfers.

Balance

Mr. Julep was able to safely maintain quiet sitting over the edge of a hospital bed with feet dangling. However, when reaching forward beyond arm span in this position, he required supervision.

Mr. Julep was able to stand independently for short periods, but required close supervision. He required verbal cues to maintain left hip and knee extension. Ankle postural motor strategy responses in response to postural sway were noted to be deficient on the left side.

Locomotion

Mr. Julep walked slowly with a front-wheeled walker for short distances only, requiring supervision and minimal assist to correct the path of the walker.

Clinical Comments *Use of a walker promotes safety (Brown, Chapter 12) and symmetry. It also encourages upper extremity weightbearing, with elbow extension, wrist extension, and palmar grasp, increasing functional use of the upper extremity. However, a walker alters gait characteristics, and may not be the type of walking aide best suited for long-term use in Mr. Julep's case.*

Sensory and Perceptual Integrity

Mr. Julep wore glasses for decreased acuity both in far and near vision. He demonstrated no evidence of a visual field defect or visual neglect. He denied any loss of normal sensation in his left arm, but did indicate that his feet felt numb and that it did not hurt when he accidentally banged his left foot and ankle against the wheelchair footrest.

Clinical Comments *Although Mr. Julep appeared to present with a motor stroke, tactile sensory impairments due to involvement of thalamocortical sensory afferent fibers that travel in the posterior limb of the internal capsule[3] or due to peripheral neuropathy in the lower extremities were possibilities, making it important to assess somatic sensation.*

Communication, Affect, Cognition, Language, and Learning Style

Mr. Julep's dysarthria had resolved sufficiently by the time of admission to the rehabilitation facility, so that his communication was no longer affected by it. However, communication was hampered by a long-standing hearing impairment that required the use of a hearing aid in the left ear.

Mr. Julep was always pleasant and cooperative. However, he demonstrated little variation in emotional responses, resulting in an affect that could be described as flattened. He was alert and consistently oriented to person, place, and time. He demonstrated the ability to sustain attention, but had some difficulty in selectively attending when in a busy environment, especially if tired because of poor sleep the night before. His short-term memory appeared to be impaired, as evidenced by incomplete recall of events in physical therapy sessions from 1 day to the next. Mr. Julep did not spontaneously engage in problem solving regarding performance of mobility activities, but would participate if prompted and guided.

> **Clinician Comment** *Mr. Julep's hearing impairment was expected to make verbal instruction less effective than demonstration during treatment sessions.*
>
> *Hinkle found that age, cognitive status, and initial function accounted for 42% of the variance in functional recovery at 3 months following motor strokes.[9] Assessment of Mr. Julep's cognition was warranted. It should be noted that cognitive dysfunction may not be due only to Mr. Julep's recent stroke.[15]*
>
> *During the systems review Mr. Julep showed deficits in ROM and sensory integrity. He was observed to demonstrate clinical signs of paresis/weakness, as well as dependence on synergy for movement in the left arm and leg. Both his muscle performance and muscle function needed to be examined.*
>
> *Mr. Julep's aerobic capacity needed to be measured in addition to his ability with self-care and home management tasks. Examining his ADL and IADL status would also be part of the occupational therapy assessment.*
>
> *The rate of depression following stroke is reported to range from 18% to 68%.[37-39] Depression is one of a number of factors that can contribute to the fatigue experienced by individuals with neurologic disorders (Brown, Chapter 12). Depression has been linked to lower levels of independence following stroke.[40] Upon reflection, assessment for depression by clinical psychologist was likely warranted, but was not completed. The Beck Depression Inventory would have been an appropriate tool.[7]*

Tests and Measures

Cognitive Status

Concerns about cognitive status arose during the Systems Review. Cognitive status was assessed using the Mini-Mental State Examination (MMSE). This measure includes 11 questions with a total score that can range from 0 to 30. Mr. Julep's score was 25/30.

> **Clinician Comment** *The MMSE[TM] is reported to have good reliability, the ability to differentiate among diagnostic groups, and the ability to differentiate those with disorders from those without.[41] Mr. Julep's score is indicative of mild cognitive impairment.[4]*

> *A mild impairment is not considered a major factor in predicting rehabilitation outcomes.[5,9] It does, however, warrant consideration when choosing teaching methods used in the rehabilitation program.*

Posture

Mr. Julep's posture was observed both in sitting and standing. When observed in the sagittal plane, he presented with a "slouched" sitting posture, demonstrating chin poke, increased thoracic kyphosis, slightly reversed lumbar lordosis, and a posterior pelvic tilt. In the frontal plane, his trunk was noted to be slightly side flexed to the left and the left shoulder to be 1 inch lower than the right. Mr. Julep stood in a forward lean posture. Slight winging of left scapula was observed. He stood more asymmetrically than he sat, with his left hip and knee semi-flexed and with his COM shifted diagonally to the right and forward over his base of support (BOS). His left shoulder was more than 1 inch lower than the right and trunk side flexion on the left was increased. Mr. Julep was able to correct both sitting and standing postural asymmetry with manual contact guidance and cueing. In sitting, he demonstrated limited correction of abnormalities seen in sagittal plane, particularly at pelvis and lumbar spine despite cueing and manual contact assistance.

> **Clinician Comment** *Observational assessment of posture provides a simple, but holistic, first picture of the musculoskeletal system and the effects of neurological impairments. Postural asymmetry appears to be due to nonstructural limitations, as these could be corrected with effort and light manual cues. Abnormal thoracic kyphosis and lumbar lordosis may be structural in nature, thus limiting attempts at correction. However, tight hamstring muscles may be contributing to posterior pelvic tilt. A position of posterior pelvic tilt increases both lumbar lordosis and thoracic kyphosis. Assessment of trunk mobility, hip extension ROM, and hamstrings muscle extensibility will assist in determining whether improvements in pelvic and trunk posture might be achieved through treatment. Poor vertical alignment increases the energy expended to counteract the forces of gravity in upright postures.[42]*

Range of Motion (Including Muscle Lengths)

Limitations in joint ROMs and muscle lengths were assessed using a combination of goniometry and visual comparison between left and right sides of the body. Mr. Julep was found to have slight limitation in neck side flexion to the right, limited trunk side flexion ranges of 20 degrees to the left and 15 degrees to the right, combined neck and trunk rotation ranges of 75 degrees to the left and 65 degrees to the right, and lumbar extension ROM to just slightly beyond neutral.

Passive hip extension ranges of motion were limited to 5 degrees on the right and 0 degrees on the left. Passive straight leg raise (SLR) was determined to be 45 degrees on the left and 60 degrees on the right. Ankle dorsiflexion, measured with knees flexed, were 5 degrees on the left and 10 degrees on the right. With knees extended, dorsiflexion ranges were 0 degrees on the left and 5 degrees on the right.

Left shoulder flexion was limited to 130 degrees, abduction to 120 degrees, and external rotation to 60 degrees. There was a capsular joint end feel at the limits of passive ranges of motion. Left forearm supination was limited to 75 degrees. Left thumb flexion, extension, abduction and opposition were all limited by 1/4 range.

Using the modified Ashworth Scale to evaluate resistance to passive movement, Mr. Julep generally presented with grade 1 to 1+ spasticity in the typical decorticate distribution for the left arm and leg, as well as left trunk side flexors. However, left ankle plantar flexors were graded as 2, and unsustained clonus was elicited from the left ankle plantar flexors.

Clinician Comment *Limitations that could potentially affect performance of mobility tasks and left upper extremity function were targeted for assessment. Limited spinal mobility may affect gait and bed mobility activities.[42] Limited hip extension ROM may contribute to shortened step lengths, as a trailing limb position is not possible to achieve without excessive forward trunk lean.[42] Limited hamstrings muscle extensibility (as measured using SLR) may contribute to posterior pelvic tilt and slouched sitting posture.[42] Limited ankle dorsiflexion ROM and plantar flexor muscle extensibility (as evidenced by greater limitation in dorsiflexion ROM when tested with knee extended) will likely hinder performance of sit-to-stand[43] and gait,[42] as well as the ability to use ankle strategies effectively to control postural sway and balance in standing.[42]*

Mr. Julep may be developing a capsular pattern of restriction for the left shoulder that could lead to development of shoulder pain in the future.[36] Precautions in handling the left upper extremity as well as encouraging functional range active-assisted movement at the shoulder are required to ensure that this does not occur. The modified Ashworth Scale demonstrates good interrater and intrarater reliability in individuals with acute stroke.[44]

Mr. Julep presented with mild spasticity that would be unlikely to limit performance of mobility tasks and ADL, perhaps with the exception of the left ankle plantar flexors.

Sensory and Perceptual Integrity

Mr. Julep did not present with either homonymous hemianopia or visual extinction on testing. There was no evidence of impairment in light touch sensation for the left lower half of the face or any extremities, although Mr. Julep did describe light touch as feeling less distinct for his left arm and leg. There was no tactile extinction for the left arm or leg. The ability to distinguish between sharp and dull sensory stimuli was intact for the upper extremities, but moderately severe and patchy impairment was found for areas below the knees bilaterally. There was no impairment in joint position sense (ie, proprioception) for either the left arm or leg.

Clinician Comment *Intact proprioception in the left arm and leg may enhance possibilities for motor recovery. Individuals with lacunar strokes, presenting without severe sensory deficits, have demonstrated a trend toward more frequent recovery of isolated upper extremity movement.[3]*

The patchy distribution of impairment in sharp/dull sensation for the distal lower extremities is more likely associated with diabetic peripheral neuropathy than with the subcortical lesion. This impairment increases the risk of injury to the shins, ankles, and feet caused by trauma, such as banging feet/ankles on wheelchair foot pedals.

Muscle Performance (Including Strength, Power, and Endurance)

The Motricity Index (MI) was used to evaluate extremity strength. Mr. Julep's summed arm and leg scores were 59/100 and 69/100, respectively. Scores for individual test items were as follows: pinch grip 26 (able to hold a 2.5 cm cube against a weak pull), elbow flexion 19 (movement through full range against gravity, but not against resistance), shoulder abduction 14 (movement present, but not full range/not against gravity), ankle dorsiflexion 19 (movement full range against gravity, but not against resistance), knee extension 25 (movement full range against resistance, but weaker than other side), and hip flexion 25 (movement against gravity, but weaker than other side).

Clinician Comment *The Motricity Index was developed specifically for use in evaluating hemiplegic arm and leg strength.[45,46] Six test items, representative of movement at each limb segment, are evaluated, using a 5-level, weighted rating scale that is based on the Medical Research Council (MRC) manual muscle testing scale. All movements are tested in sitting, taking approximately 5 minutes to complete.*

The Motricity Index is reported to have good interrater reliability scores for arm and leg.[45,47] The validity of this tool has been determined through correlations with dynamometer strength scores[48] and with grip strength scores.[49]

Mr. Julep demonstrated greater recovery distally than proximally in the upper extremity. Having some ability to grasp and release with the left hand suggests a reasonable prognosis for left arm function.[49] Ability to grasp and release could be expected to increase the frequency with which Mr. Julep would attempt to use the arm for reaching, thus forcing increased attempted movement at shoulder and elbow. A systematic review of motor recovery after stroke found that patients with small lacunar strokes showed relatively good motor recovery.[50]

5 Times Sit to Stand Test

Lower extremity muscle endurance was evaluated using the 5 Times Sit to Stand Test described by Brown in Chapter 12. Mr. Julep completed the test in 20.6 seconds.

Clinician Comment *The intrarater, interrater and test-retest reliabilities of this measure, when used with a stroke population, were reported to be excellent if raters viewed video clips of test methods prior to use.[51] Mr. Julep's score was above the mean, but within the computed standard deviation for scores reported for individuals with stroke.[51]*

Motor Function (Motor Control and Learning)

Mr. Julep was observed to use his left arm to support some body weight when rising from sitting to standing and when walking with the walker. The arm was also observed to perform assistive functions such as holding the wheelchair seat belt buckle, as well as simple grasp and manipulate functions, such as applying the left wheelchair brake. However, Mr. Julep was not observed to use this arm effectively when moving between side lying and sitting or for propelling his wheelchair, instead demonstrating a weak associated reaction in the pattern of the abnormal flexion synergy during performance of these tasks.

The Chedoke-McMaster Stroke Assessment: Impairment Inventory: Stage of Recovery of Arm and Leg was used to assess motor control as it pertained to the ability to isolate (ie, fractionate) movement and recruit muscles in a variety of combinations, as opposed to 2 stereotypical patterns.[36]

The left arm and hand presented with stages 3/7 and 4/7, respectively. The left leg and foot presented with stages 5/7 and 4/7, respectively. Stage 3/7 indicated that willed movement in the patterns of the flexion and extension synergies was possible. Stages 4 and 5 indicated progressive improvement in the ability to recruit muscles in more complex movement patterns and to isolate movement. Although Mr. Julep was able to dorsiflex, then plantar flex, his foot through full range with the knee flexed in sitting, he was not able to dorsiflex the ankle through full available range with the knee held in an extended position.

Clinician Comment *The Chedoke-McMaster Stroke Assessment Impairment Inventory: Stage of Recovery of Arm and Leg has good-excellent intrarater and interrater reliability (intraclass correlation coefficient [ICC] = 0.93 to 0.98; 0.85 to 0.97, respectively), and test-retest reliability (ICC = 0.84 to 0.92).[36] The inventory uses a 7-point scale, corresponding to Brunnstrom's stages of motor recovery following stroke to score motor performance.*

Although an impairment tool that evaluates stage of recovery from dependence of abnormal synergies for limb movement may not be as predictive of future functional outcomes as a measure of strength (see Chapter 12 for discussion), it does provide information important to the retraining of extremity motor control by providing a progression framework for increasing fractionation (ie, isolating movement to 1 joint or limb segment) and recruiting muscles to more complex functional synergies including ability to recruit muscles from opposing flexion and extension synergies at adjacent joints. For example, active ankle dorsiflexion from the flexion synergy combined with knee extension from the extension synergy are required to produce an effective ankle postural motor strategy response to posterior displacement of the COM in standing.[42] Ability to recruit this more complex muscle synergy would be represented by Stage 5 recovery of the foot, which Mr. Julep had not yet reached.

Gait, Locomotion, Balance

Gait

The following asymmetries in spatial and temporal gait characteristics and gait deviations were observed:

- Decreased step lengths bilaterally, right step length shorter than left
- Decreased single limb support time on left leg as compared to right
- Excessive forward trunk lean during left stance phase
- Excessive contralateral pelvic drop during left stance phase
- Decreased hip extension during terminal stance, left more limited than right
- Excessive left knee flexion during loading and rapid left knee extension from mid-stance to terminal stance
- Decreased left knee extension with foot flat at initial contact
- Absence of left heel off in terminal stance

Clinician Comment *Asymmetries in step lengths and single limb support times are common following stroke.[52] Asymmetries, as well as the gait deviations observed, can most likely be attributed to Mr. Julep's presentation of muscle weakness, dependence on abnormal synergies, and limitations in joint ROM and muscle extensibility.[42] Impaired balance also likely contributed to asymmetry in single limb support time.*

Locomotion

Performance of locomotor and ambulatory activities was evaluated using 3 standardized measures: the Chedoke-McMaster Stroke Assessment: Disability Inventory, the Modified Emory Ambulation Profile, and the 10 meter walk test.

Chedoke-McMaster Stroke Assessment: Disability Inventory

This inventory includes a gross motor function index composed of 10 items and a walking index composed of 5 items. Each item is rated using the same 1 to 7 point scale that is used with the Functional Independence Measure (FIM).[42]

Results of testing were as follows:

1. Bed mobility: Supine to side lying on strong side: 5/7 (supervision required; cueing required for left arm participation)

2. Bed mobility: Supine to side lying on weaker side: 6/7 (modified independence)

3. Bed mobility: Side lying to long sitting through strong side: 5/7 (supervision, cueing)

4. Bed mobility: Side lying to sitting on side of bed through strong side: 4/7 (minimal assistance at trunk and left arm)

5. Bed mobility: Side lying to sitting on side of bed through weaker side: 4/7 (minimal assistance at trunk and left arm)

6. Remain standing for 30 seconds: 5/7 (supervision, cueing)

7. Transfer to and from bed toward strong side: 5/7 (cueing to achieve optimal starting position for sit to stand and to complete turn before attempting to sit down)

8. Transfer to and from bed toward weaker side: 4/7 (minimal assistance to maintain balance, cueing to achieve optimal starting position for sit to stand, cueing for left arm participation and cueing to complete turn before sitting down)

9. Transfer up and down from floor to chair: 3/7 (moderate assistance)

10. Transfer up and down from floor to standing: 3/7

11. Walk indoors, 25 meters (m): 4/7 (minimal contact assistance to correct path of front-wheeled walker, as walker gradually deviates to the left)

12. Walk outdoors, over rough ground, ramps, and curbs, 150 m: 1/7 (unable to walk 150 m, requires moderate assistance to manage a ramp, curb, and a short distance over rough ground).

13. Walk outdoors several blocks, 900 m: 1/7 (unable to walk for this distance)

14. Walk up and down stairs: 4/7 (railing on right, 2 feet/step, leading with the right when ascending and with the left when descending, minimal assistance).

15. Age appropriate walking distance for 2 minutes (2-point bonus if able to walk more than 84 m). Score = 0/2

Mr. Julep's total score was 54/100. All activities required more time to complete than what would be considered reasonable.

Sit to Stand

Although sit-to-stand is not an item on the Chedoke-McMaster disability inventory, it was decided to assess this activity in more detail. Mr. Julep was able to perform sit-to-stand with supervision from a regular height surface using his arms to assist. In preparation for rising, Mr. Julep's feet were often asymmetrical with left positioned forward of the right. He demonstrated decreased and asymmetrical forward displacement of COM during flexion momentum and momentum transfer, with diagonal displacement to the right. He typically demonstrated incomplete extension of left hip and knee during the extension phase of rising to standing. When rising from a lower than a standard height surface, he required minimal contact assistance.

Car Transfers

Although transfer to/from a car is not an item on the disability inventory, this task was assessed. Mr. Julep required moderate assistance with the task

Clinician Comment *Interrater and test-retest reliability of the Chedoke-McMaster Stroke Assessment Disability Inventory, are reported to be excellent,[42] and the validity of the inventory has been extensively studied.[42,53] The minimal clinically important difference (MCID) for the Disability Inventory has been reported as 7 to 8 points.[54]*

Modified Emory Ambulation Profile

The Modified Emory Ambulation Profile Scale is used to evaluate the ability to walk under varying task and environmental conditions. The time required to complete each of 5 tasks is multiplied by an assistive device factor ranging from 1 (no assistance) to 6 (ankle-foot orthotics (AFO) and walker or quad cane required). As Mr. Julep used a walker, his time scores were multiplied by a factor of 4.

Results of testing were as follows:

1. Walk on floor: 23.5 sec × 4 = 94

2. Walk on carpet: 29 sec × 4 = 116

3. Timed Up & Go: 64.4 sec × 4 = 257.6

4. Obstacles: over a series of 2 bricks and around a trash bin: 75.5 sec × 4 = 302

5. Stairs (4 steps): 65.7 × 4: (railing substituted for walker) = 262.8

Summed score = 1032.4

Clinician Comment

Clinician Comment *The modified Emory Ambulation Profile has excellent interrater[55] and test-retest[56] reliability for summed scores. Profile scores have been found to correlate with those of timed walking tests.[56,57]*

Mr. Julep walked slightly slower on carpet than on firm flooring and demonstrated difficulty with foot clearance on this semi-compliant surface. There is carpeting in most rooms of his house. Managing obstacles and turns, as would be required for safe household ambulation, were substantial challenges.

Walking Velocity

Measured over the middle 5 meters of a 10-meter walkway. Mr. Julep's walking velocity was 0.31 m/sec.

Clinician Comment *Test-retest reliability of walking velocity scores for individuals with stroke has been reported to be excellent for those requiring physical assistance to ambulate and to be good for those able to walk without physical assistance.[58] Minimal detectable change scores (90% confidence intervals) have been reported to range from 0.05 to 0.08 m/sec.[59]*

Based on his measured walking velocity, Mr. Julep would be classified, at present, as a household ambulator. A velocity of 0.4 m/sec would be required to be classified as limited community ambulator.[31,60] Using a walker as an ambulatory aid is an impediment to improvement in walking velocity.

Balance

The Berg Balance Scale (BBS) was used to evaluate Mr. Julep's ability to maintain balance under a variety of task conditions. His total score at admission to the rehabilitation program was 34/56.

Clinician Comment *The internal consistency, interrater reliability, intrarater reliability, and test-retest reliability of the BBS have been reported as excellent when used with stroke populations.[61] Moderate to excellent sensitivity of BBS scores have also reported, but with evidence of floor and ceiling effects.[61] The minimal detectable change (MDC) score for the BBS has been estimated to be 5.8 and 6.9 points, respectively, at 90% and 95% confidence intervals for individuals receiving rehabilitation following stroke when assessed by 2 different raters.[62] For those requiring an ambulation assistive device, an MDC of 7 points would be appropriate to be 90% confident that genuine change had occurred.[62] BBS scores should be used with caution for predicting fall risk for individuals with chronic stroke, particularly when a walking aid is being used.[63] The same caution would likely apply to those with more acute stroke.*

Excellent correlations with the Barthel Index, Functional Independence Measure, and gait speed have been reported, and scores have been found to be predictive of disability level at 90 days post-stroke.[61] Those stroke patients scoring >20 on admission and >40 on discharge have been reported to be more likely to be discharged home.[64]

Sitting

While sitting over the side of his hospital bed, Mr. Julep required minimal contact assistance to remain stable when reaching down to his feet. Other sitting activities were performed without risk to his safety. For this reason, dressing his lower body was performed sitting in the wheelchair. Left upper extremity protective reactions were observed but appeared insufficient to prevent loss of balance in response to large amplitude displacements of the COM. Equilibrium reaction responses in sitting appeared decreased in amplitude for trunk and left extremities.

Mr. Julep was able to reach 6 to 8 inches beyond arm span safely in lateral and forward directions when feet were resting on the floor. When sitting on a hospital bed with feet dangling, Mr. Julep could reach forward a distance of 5 inches, but required supervision to ensure safety when doing so.

Standing

Postural motor strategies were observed during postural sway in quiet standing and during completion of test items from the BBS. Ankle strategy responses demonstrated decreased dorsiflexor and plantar flexor muscle activity on the left. Hip strategies demonstrated decreased excursions of forward/backward displacement of the pelvis. Left knee wobble was observed intermittently, and the knee assumed a position of semi-flexion frequently during testing. Stepping postural motor strategies were not evaluated during the initial assessment due to patient apprehension, but were identified as items for future assessment.

Aerobic Capacity and Physical Endurance

Clinician Comment *Independent sitting balance has been identified as an important predictor of discharge home,[15] and of rehabilitative outcomes.[65,66]*

6-Minute Walk Test

The 6-Minute Walk Test (6MWT) was used to evaluate aerobic capacity and physical endurance under submaximal test conditions. The distance walked with front-wheeled walker in 6 minutes was 120.6 meters. Rate of perceived exertion (RPE), as measured using the Borg scale,[67] was 13/20 (somewhat hard). HR was 102 bpm and BP was 165/100 mm Hg immediately following completion of the test.

Clinician Comment *Although maximal exercise testing is considered the gold standard for assessment of aerobic capacity, this method was not feasible within the rehabilitation facility for the reasons identified in Chapter 12. Mr. Julep was cleared for submaximal exercise testing by his physical medicine specialist. To reduce the possibility of an adverse cardiac event during testing, a conservative predetermined end point of 70% of predicted HR maximum $[(220 - age) \times 0.7] = 105$ bpm was chosen for testing. Lighter intensity exercise has been suggested for those with suspected coronary artery disease who have not undergone an exercise EKG.[7]*

The 6MWT test has demonstrated excellent test-retest reliability as well as criterion validity and sensitivity to change in a stroke population.[68]

Mr. Julep's 6MWT distance score was substantially lower than the established baseline value for subacute stroke indicated in Box 12-1 of Chapter 12 (215.8 ± 91.6 meters). This comparatively poorer score may be related to Mr. Julep's use of a walker in combination with his deconditioned state. An MDC of 54.1 meters has been reported for the 6MWT.[68] Given Mr. Julep's low initial score, this value might not be a realistic benchmark of true change if he continued to use a walker for ambulation.

It is common for individuals with stroke who are undergoing rehabilitation to achieve lower workloads, lower HRs and lower BP responses than expected norms with sub-maximal exercise testing.[69] O_2 uptake at submaximal workloads is greater than in healthy individuals, but peak O_2 uptake is lower.[8] MacKay and Makrides[70] found that peak O_2 uptake at 26 days following stroke was lower than that required to meet the physiologic demands for daily living.

Fatigue Severity Scale

Fatigue was measured using the Fatigue Severity Scale (FSS). Mr. Julep's averaged FSS score was 5.4/7.

Clinician Comment *Fatigue is a common complaint in individuals who have experienced stroke,[71,72] is among the worst symptoms of stroke for approximately 40% of stroke clients,[73,74] and has been found to persist as a complaint for at least 2 years post-stroke.[72] Fatigue is also a common symptom of diabetes. Although findings of fatigue frequently overlap with findings of depression in those with recent stroke, fatigue may be present in the absence of depression.[72] Fatigue, independent of depression, has been found to be a significant factor associated with health-related quality of life.[75]*

The FSS, as discussed in Chapter 12, is a 9-item self-report questionnaire. This scale has been used to measure fatigue in stroke populations,[72,75] demonstrating excellent internal consistency for the stroke group [C = 0.95] and good test-retest reliability [rho = 0.88] within a normal subset of study participants in a recent study.[72] An MDC_{95} for FSS scores in a stroke population has been reported to be 0.15.[72]

Mr. Julep's score was substantially higher than the average of 3.9 ± 1.84 reported by Valko et al[72] for individuals with chronic stroke, and the cut-off score for normal-range fatigue of 4 that was suggested by Van de Port et al.[75]

Self-Care and Home Management, Including Activities of Daily Living and Instrumental Activities of Daily Living

Functional Independence Measure

Overall functional status and care giver burden was quantified using the Functional Independence Measure (FIM). At time of admission to our rehabilitation facility, Mr. Julep's total FIM score was 98/126, his motor sub-score was 70/91 and his social-cognitive sub-score was 28/35. Scores for individual items were as follows: self-care: feeding (6), grooming (6), bathing (5), dressing upper body (5), dressing lower body (5), toileting (5), bladder management (7), bowel management (6), transfers to bed, chair, wheelchair (6), transfer to toilet (5), transfer to tub or shower (4), walking or using wheelchair (4; can't walk 150 feet), stairs (5), comprehension (6), expression (6), social interaction (6), problem solving (5), memory (5).

Clinician Comment *The FIM scores each of 13 items on a 7-point ordinal scale ranging from independent (7) to dependent (1).[12,76] Test items are typically grouped into 2 main sub-scores (motor, social-cognitive) and 6 minor sub-scores (self-care, continence, transfers, locomotion, communication, and social cognition).[16] The total maximum score that can be achieved is 126.*

FIM scores on admission have been found to be strongly associated with functional recovery during inpatient rehabilitation,[77] as well as with discharge destination.[11,16] The Canadian Institute for Health Information[11] has developed a conceptual framework for modeling the likelihood of being discharged home based on factors commonly referenced in the stroke literature. They reported that a high motor function score on the FIM (51 to 91) was the strongest predictor of discharge home, increasing the likelihood of this discharge destination by a factor of 6. They also reported that those with high FIM social-cognitive subscale scores (30 to 35) were 2.5 times more likely to be discharged home than those with low scores (5 to 20). The scores that Mr. Julep obtained on the FIM strongly suggest that he will be able to return home upon discharge.

EVALUATION

Diagnosis

Practice Pattern

Mr. Julep was classified into Pattern 5D: Impaired Motor Function and Sensory Integrity Associated with Non Progressive Disorders of the Central Nervous System—Acquired in Adolescence or Adulthood.

International Classification of Functioning, Disability and Health Model

See ICF model on p 508.

Prognosis

Predictions about functional recovery and discharge destination are influenced by stroke characteristics, medical management of stroke, presentation of impairments and activity limitations caused by the stroke, comorbidities, and personal and environmental contextual factors. All of these variables, as they relate to Mr. Julep, have been discussed (see Examination and Tests and Measures sections).To summarize, factors with positive influences on functional outcomes and discharge destination include: lacunar stroke, early intervention with tPA, male gender, strong social support, short interval between stroke onset and commencement of rehabilitation services, minimal cognitive impairment, early return of motor function, and good sitting balance. Factors with negative influences on outcomes include: comorbidities of Type 2 diabetes and carotid vascular disease, an inactive lifestyle prior to stroke, and high BMI.

Clinician Comment *Considering all of these variables enhances the clinician's ability to determine appropriate treatment goals and expectations, which are the foundations for intervention planning. It was predicted that Mr. Julep would return to live with his wife and family, and would achieve independence in household ambulation and ADL activities. It was also predicted that limited community ambulation would be possible, with supervision. It was also predicted that Mr. Julep would be able to participate in modified forms of his leisure activities of gardening and fishing.*

Plan of Care

Prevention

Primary prevention of stroke recurrence and effective management of Type 2 diabetes were considered critical to Mr. Julep's future health and were addressed by a comprehensive interdisciplinary intervention plan. As part of this plan, the physical therapist was responsible for education regarding the possible benefits of regular aerobic exercise. Benefits that were discussed included improved physical activity tolerance, possible reduction of fatigue, management of risk for stroke recurrence, as well as management of weight and blood sugar levels. The physical therapist was also responsible for counseling regarding ongoing participation in physical activity.

Clinician Comment *Exercise improves insulin sensitivity and assists in normalizing plasma glucose levels by increasing carbohydrate metabolism, thus reducing plasma glucose levels.*

Intervention

Mr. Julep required an intensive program of task-specific training in bed mobility, sit-to-stand, transfers, walking under varying task and environmental conditions, as well as upper extremity support (ie, weightbearing), reach and grasp activities, ADL and IADL activities. Occupational therapy (OT) team members were tasked with addressing ADL and IADL training and worked in conjunction with physical therapy on upper extremity function. Motor-learning principles were employed during practice to enhance performance, as well as retention and transfer of improved performance. Because of hearing loss and mild cognitive impairment, frequent demonstration, repetitive teaching methods, written instructions, and diagrams were required for practice of mobility tasks.

In addition to task-specific training, Mr. Julep required a program of strengthening, stretching, and flexibility exercises for trunk and left extremities, a standing balance retraining program, and an aerobic exercise training program. In this case description, strength training, gait training and aerobic training were emphasized.

Precautions that were considered when planning and implementing physical therapy interventions included monitoring HR and BP, as well as observing for signs of low blood sugar levels. Individuals with Type 2 diabetes who take insulin may develop hypoglycemia during/following exercise, but the risk of this occurring is much less than it is in those with Type 1 diabetes. Symptoms of hypoglycemia may occur hours after completing exercise. Carbohydrates were made available during and after exercise, and hydration during exercise was encouraged.

Diabetic neuropathy affecting sensation in bilateral lower extremities warranted education and diligent care during exercise and task-specific training. Because of the presence of back pain and degenerative joint changes, choice of body positioning for strengthening and stretching exercises had to be considered, and frequent feedback regarding comfort needed to be elicited.

ICF Model of Disablement for Mr. Julep

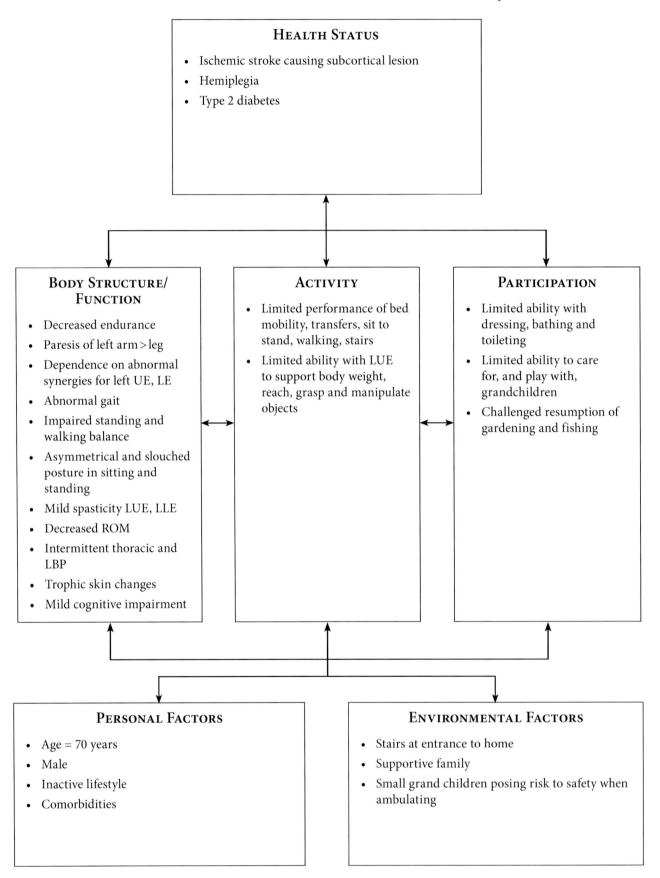

Proposed Frequency and Duration of Physical Therapy Treatment Sessions

Two, 50-minute sessions/day, 5 days per week were planned for the remaining 4 weeks of inpatient physical therapy rehabilitation. Inpatient programming was planned so Mr. Julep would spend approximately 50% of each treatment session on activities in standing by the beginning of week 2 of the remaining 4 weeks of inpatient program Strength training occurred 3 times per wk. Stretching and mobility exercises, balance training, and task-specific training were completed daily. Physical endurance training was completed 2 times per week using overground walking initially, and progressing to include both overground walking and treadmill walking. Appropriate use of upper extremity for weightbearing, reaching, grasping, and manipulating were encouraged during all treatment sessions.

> **Clinician Comment** *Current best practice recommendations for stroke care suggest a minimum of 1 hour of direct therapy from each relevant core therapy.*[78]

Anticipated Goals

Mr. Julep and his wife participated in goal setting with each team member. Involvement of individual and family in goal setting and treatment planning increases the patient's adherence to therapy.[79]

Physical therapy goals agreed on were as follows:

1. Bed mobility: Independent supine to side lying to left/right in hospital bed (1 week).
2. Bed mobility: Independent lie-to-sit in hospital bed (1 week).
3. Independent sit-to-stand to/from hospital bed (1 week).
4. Independent sit-to-stand from standard height chair without arms (1 week).
5. Independent sit-to-stand from toilet (1 week).
6. Independent transfers to/from wheel chair (1 week).
7. Independent wheelchair propulsion using upper extremities (1 week).
8. Independent sit-to-stand from sofa height, compliant surface (2 weeks)
9. Transfer to/from car with supervision (3 weeks).
10. Independent ambulation with walker in rehabilitation facility (3 weeks).
11. Walk with single point cane and supervision (3 weeks).
12. Walk for a continuous distance of ≥300 meters with single-point cane (4 weeks).
13. Transfer up from floor to standing and/or sitting with minimal contact assistance of 1 (4 weeks).
14. Ascend/descend a set of 5 stairs independently using railing on right (4 weeks).

Expected Outcomes

1. Walk independently using a single-point cane indoors (8 weeks).
2. Walk with supervision using a single-point cane outdoors (8 weeks).
3. Walk for a distance of ≥500 meters before resting (8 weeks).
4. Cast fishing rod with right arm when standing on a semi-compliant surface with supervision (8 weeks).
5. Hoe a 1-meter square patch of garden with supervision (8 weeks).

Discharge Plan

Mr. Julep was to be discharged home to live with his wife and family, with a plan to attend outpatient programming, 2 times per week, for 1 month. He would have a predischarge needs assessment 2 weeks prior to discharge, which would include a home visit attended by physical therapy and OT rehabilitation team members. He was to spend a weekend at home 1 week prior to being discharged.

Follow-up reviews with members of the rehabilitation team were planned for 3 months, 6 months, and 12 months following discharge from the outpatient service.

INTERVENTION

Coordination, Communication, and Documentation

Coordination of the components of the rehabilitation intervention program was achieved through weekly team meetings of which Mr. Julep and his wife were part. The initial physical therapy assessment and plan of care were both documented in the heath record. Communication regarding progress being made toward treatment goals occurred at team meetings and through weekly documented progress reports. Reexamination occurred at discharge, and at the completion of outpatient programming.

Patient-/Client-Related Instructions

Mr. Julep and his family received information about the proposed plan for inpatient care and the discharge plan. They were provided information by various team members about prevention of stroke recurrence and management of Type 2 diabetes. Team members discussed the information with Mr. Julep and his family and answered any questions arising from discussions. Support was provided by the team for Mr. Julep's family.

In collaboration with the physical therapist, the OT provided Mr. Julep, his wife, and his daughter written instructions and diagrams of upper extremity reach and grasp activities on a table-top surface that could be practiced outside of formal treatment sessions. Physical therapy was responsible for teaching the wife and daughter how to assist with safe ambulation. The patient and his family were also provided written instructions and diagrams for completion of bed mobility tasks, sit to stand, transfers to/from wheelchair, and lower extremity stretching exercises that Mr. Julep was to perform independently at least once each day.

Mr. Julep was encouraged by OT and physical therapy to use his left arm for ADL and IADL such a brushing his hair, turning on light switches, and holding a juice cup in his left hand while using the right hand to remove the lid. He was also encouraged to use the left arm to assist with wheelchair propulsion. He was provided with a daily diary in which he recorded use of the left arm.

Mr. Julep, his wife and daughter received instruction in monitoring HR while walking. They also received instruction in monitoring RPE.

Clinician Comment *Setting expectations early in the rehabilitation process for some independent practice and practice supervised by family was implemented to increases the total amount of intervention time per week. Augmented task practice and exercise has been demonstrated to have a small, favorable effect on performance of daily activities.[80,81]*

Providing practical training to family care providers has been found to decrease both burden and anxiety that these family members experience upon discharge to home.[82]

Encouraging Mr. Julep to use both arms for wheelchair propulsion was intended to provide another opportunity for Mr. Julep to use his left arm in a functional context.

Procedural Interventions

Therapeutic Exercise

Flexibility Exercises

Mode
Active movement, use of transition positions, passive stretching
Duration
10 to 15 minutes
Frequency
Daily
Description of Intervention
- Trunk side flexion
  - Position: Elbow support side lying on each side (part of the task of moving from side lying ↔ sitting)
  - Activity: Active trunk shortening on uppermost side causing lengthening on lowermost side by drawing uppermost side ear to shoulder and shoulder to hip while extending elbows to achieve side sitting.

- Trunk extension
  - Position: Prone lying, elbows bent, palms down, hands positioned just ahead of shoulders
  - Activity: partial pushup with pelvis remaining on treatment mat (part of task of moving from floor ↔ sitting or standing).
  - Note: Discontinue if back pain worsens
- Trunk rotation
  - Position: crook lying with arms outstretched in 90-degree horizontal abduction, palms turned up
  - Activity: shoulder horizontal adduction, neck and trunk flexion with rotation to reach left outstretched arm across body to touch palm to palm of outstretched right arm (similar to movement components of an upper body flexion strategy for rolling supine to side lying).
- Hip extension: both left and right legs
  - Position 1: half kneeling with one foot forward, side of body in contact with treatment mat, hand on treatment mat for support/stability
  - Activity 1: forward weight shift with hip extension
  - Position 2: forward lunge standing
  - Activity 2: forward weight shift with bilateral knee semi-flexion
- Hamstrings stretch: both left and right legs
  - Position: sitting with heel resting on foot stool; palms stacked and resting on same knee
  - Activity: Hinge forward from hips to bring nose forward over knees while keeping knee straight and maintaining a straight trunk posture
- Calf stretch: both left and right legs
  - Position: sitting with heel resting on foot stool; belt positioned around forefoot, ends grasped in hands
  - Activity: Draw toes toward knee by pulling on belt while keeping knee straight.
  - Progress to calf stretch in forward lunge position with hands support on wall.

Hamstrings and calf stretches in sitting position were designated for additional independent practice on a daily basis.

Clinician Comment *A number of the treatment positions and exercises described above challenge muscle strength, muscle endurance and balance, in addition to addressing flexibility issues. Several positions used were relevant to transitioning from one position to another, thus were set in a purposeful context. For example, half kneeling is an important transition position used to move from the floor to either sitting or standing. Forester and Young have reported that approximately 75% of individuals* *with stroke fall in the 6-month period following discharge from the hospital.[83] Therefore, learning how to transition from the floor to sitting and/or standing is an important activity.*

The hip flexor stretches performed in half kneeling and forward lunge standing both require the thigh to move posterior in relation to the pelvis, resulting in a trailing limb position. Achievement of a trailing limb position and increased hip extension angle in terminal stance has been associated with higher walking velocity.[59]

Muscle Strength, Power and Endurance Training: Trunk and Lower Extremities

Mode
Gravity + body weight-resisted exercise, gravity + elastic-resisted exercise.

Duration
~50 to 60 minutes

Frequency
3 times per week

Intensity
The amount of resistance used and/or the number of exercise repetitions were revisited at the beginning of each week.

Progression
The method of progression varied slightly for each exercise. Most activities commenced with 2 sets of 8 repetitions, progressing to 3 sets of 12. Exercises performed in standing commenced with back to wall and with bilateral hand support on table positioned in front, with progression to standing away from the wall with unilateral, left hand support. All strengthening exercises performed in standing commenced with core abdominal muscle "setting."

Description of Intervention
Abdominal strengthening commenced with trunk curls with rotation in crook lying, progressing to backward lean trunk curls with rotation in sitting. Hip and knee extensors were strengthened using a combination of wall squats and task specific sit-to-stand practice. As a progression for both wall squats and sit-to-stand, a staggered position with right foot ahead of left was used to increase required force output from the left lower extremity. As a progression for sit-to-stand practice, the height of the sitting surface was progressively lowered. Hip abductors were strengthened in standing using lateral stepping to both left and right with elastic resistance. Strength and endurance of hip flexors was targeted using repetitive alternating stool step touches in standing. Knee curls was performed against elastic resistance in sitting. Mr. Julep was instructed to pull his foot back along the floor until the tips of the toes were directly under the knee (as per optimal foot starting position for sit-to-stand). Plantar flexors were strengthened using bilateral heel raises in standing, progressing to unilateral, left heel raise with right leg positioned forward on a step stool and to practice of "push-off" in walk standing. Bilateral toe raises were initially performed

in sitting, with progression to performance in standing in conjunction with practice of backward postural sway.

Clinician Comment *To the extent possible, strengthening exercises were performed within functional contexts. To challenge standing balance and endurance, as well as to increase the weightbearing, support function of the left upper extremity, it was decided to conduct a significant portion of the strengthening exercise program in standing with left hand positioned forward on a table top. Wall support behind the patient was used initially to provide a tactile postural reference and to provide additional external support.*

From observation of gait characteristics and gait deviations, it appeared that Mr. Julep had difficulty supporting his body weight and sustaining forward progression during left leg stance. Strengthening of hip and knee extensors was targeted to assist in reducing the excessive knee flexion and forward trunk lean observed during stance. Strengthening of hip extensors as well as ankle plantar flexors was intended to increase the production of horizontal forces needed to propel the COM forward and create a trailing limb position during left-leg stance.[42] Strengthening of hip abductors was intended to enhance control of mediolateral stability and reduce contralateral pelvic drop during left leg stance.[42]

There is evidence in the descriptive literature of associations between strength of hemiparetic muscle groups and functional ambulation outcomes. Nadeau et al found a significant relationship between hip flexor strength and natural (ie, customary) walking velocity.[84] At maximal walking velocity, significant relationships were found for both hip flexor and ankle plantar flexor strength. Kim and Eng found high correlations for plantar flexor strength with both gait velocity and stair climbing.[85] They found moderate correlations for hip flexor and knee flexor strength with both gait velocity and stair climbing.

There is also evidence of associations between strength and the activity of sit-to-stand. Strength of knee flexors of both affected and unaffected legs has demonstrated moderate to good correlations with 5 rep sit-to-stand (STS) scores,[51] and strength of knee extensors of both leg has demonstrated moderate correlations with independent performance of STS.[86]

There is ample evidence supporting improvements in muscle strength with progressive resisted exercise training in individuals with stroke. However, the evidence for increases in strength translating to improved functional outcomes is mixed.

Two noncontrolled studies have suggested translation of strength gains to functional outcomes. Weiss et al found improvements in lower extremity strength, gait and balance following a high intensity lower extremity strength training program.[87] Jorgensen et al reported improvements in walking speed using a program that combined high intensity, body weight-supported treadmill training, progressive resistance strength training and aerobic exercise.[88] *As 3 different interventions were delivered simultaneously, it is not possible to determine the extent to which each contributed to improved walking speed.*

A 2009 Cochrane review that included 4 trials of resistance training and 9 trials using a mix of aerobic and resistance training found insufficient evidence for the beneficial effects of strength training on walking speed or walking tolerance.[89]

A 2008 review including both randomized controlled trials (RCTs) and noncontrolled studies, a mix of acute, subacute, and chronic stroke populations, and interventions of either high-intensity resistance training alone or in combination with aerobic training, found that 9 of 11 studies reported an improvement in gait speed.[90] *The average change in speed computed for all studies was 0.13 m/s. The average effect size for improved gait speed was 1.5, which is considered to be a substantial effect. Gains in lower extremity strength were associated with improvements in activity limitations (particularly ambulation, but also stair climb in one study and chair rise in another study), and improved participation in 2 studies.*[90]

Earlier RCTs found strong evidence for increased strength, but limited, inconclusive, or conflicting evidence for improved functional performance.[91-93]

In summary, although relationships between strength and functional outcomes have been reported, the evidence from RCTs and systematic reviews for increased strength translating to improved functional outcomes is limited. With this in mind, careful consideration must be given to the amount of treatment time spent performing strength training that is not task specific or does not challenge other impairments while achieving the purpose of strength training.

Balance, Coordination and Agility Training

Mode(s)

Balance in quiet standing was challenged by: changing the size and/or shape of the BOS (eg, stand with feet together, tandem stand); changing/reducing sensory feedback (eg, eyes closed, stand on foam) and by combining these changes.

Dynamic standing balance was challenged in a variety of ways:

- Using standing positions for most strengthening exercises.

- Practicing ankle, hip and stepping postural motor strategies using internally and externally generated displacing forces of varying directions, amplitudes and velocities.

Balance and agility were challenged using an obstacle course that required changing direction, turning, stepping around and over obstacles, and stepping backward while walking, as well as by walking in environments with moving obstacles. Balance was also challenged by progressing to dual task activities (eg, walking while carrying a grocery bag, while holding a grandchild's hand).

Intensity

Timely progressions in difficulty of balance requirements

Duration

10 to 15 minutes of balance-specific training.

Frequency

4 to 5 times per week.

Clinician Comment *Balance training was included as part of Mr. Julep's intervention plan for the purposes of reducing risk of falls, improving safety and performance of activities occurring in standing positions, and facilitating progression to a single-point cane for ambulation.*

There is some evidence of a relationship between balance and functional outcomes. For example, balance has been found to be significantly related to self-selected and maximal walking velocities.[84] *There is also evidence of beneficial effects of balance training in acute stroke. Hammer et al found improvements in balance with physical therapy interventions, reporting that interventions performed at least twice per week were required to achieve improvements.*[94] *In a 2010 systematic review, Lubetzky-Vilnai and Kartin reported moderate evidence for improved balance performance for individualized training programs in the acute stage (0 to 6 months) of stroke for those with moderately severe stroke, with the results of 5 studies categorized at level III evidence and 6 at level IV.*[95] *The authors noted that most studies included other treatment methods in addition to balance training, making it difficult to determine the extent of the specific effects of balance training.*

Van de Port et al has suggested that specific balance training interventions were required, noting that gait-specific training without balance training did not result in measurable improvements in balance in the study conducted.[96]

Gait and Locomotion Training

Increasing both velocity and endurance were emphasized in Mr. Julep's gait training program.

Modes

Both treadmill and overground training were used.

Duration

The amount of time spent walking progressed to an average of 30 minutes per day over the course of inpatient rehabilitation. This average included aerobic training activities 2 days per week.

Frequency

Daily

Description of Intervention

Partial body weight support of 25% was used for the first week of treadmill training only. Intermittent verbal cues and assistance were provided to increase ankle dorsiflexion in swing and at initial contact, knee extension at initial contact, as well as left hip extension and left ankle plantarflexion in terminal stance when walking on the treadmill. Treadmill speed was progressively increased (see aerobic exercise training for more details).

Overground training included progression to single-point cane, use of a walking grid to enhance gait symmetry, obstacle course work, practice in avoiding moving obstacles, walking outdoors on uneven surfaces, and dual-task practice.

Clinician Comment *The ability to walk is an important factor in determining discharge destination after stroke[97] and is typically identified by patients as the goal of highest priority. Walking performance is affected by motor control, cardiorespiratory fitness, dynamic balance and, possibly, muscle strength.[98] All were addressed in the development and delivery of Mr. Julep's treatment plan.*

The amount of gait training and the methods of training used addressed a number of the principles of experience-dependent neural plasticity described by Kleim and Jones (2008), including: use it and improve it, specificity, repetition matters, intensity matters, and salience matters.[99]

One of the advantages of including treadmill training as part of a gait training program is the ability to "force" increases in gait velocity in a safe environment. Although partial body weight support increases safety, there are concerns that it also reduces the work of treadmill walking. To ensure that work load was sufficient to increase aerobic fitness, partial body weight support was discontinued after the first week of treadmill training.

In a recently published study, body-weight support treadmill training, whether instituted 2 or 6 months following stroke, did not result in better walking outcomes at 1 year post-stroke than a progressive home exercise program managed by a physical therapist.[100] At this point, it is not known if earlier introduction of treadmill walking, as occurred in Mr. Julep's case, using minimal body weight support, would produce superior outcomes than other forms of gait training in the longer term.

Aerobic Capacity/Endurance Conditioning or Reconditioning

Mode

Both fast overground walking and treadmill walking were used for aerobic training. A temporary dorsiflexion assist device, fashioned using a tensor bandage,[101] was used during initial aerobic training sessions on the treadmill to prevent toe drag. Interval training was used initially. Walking velocity and distance were recorded at each training session. Warm up and cool down for each training session involved walking at customary (ie, natural) walking velocity.

Safety: A training bout was to be discontinued if HR exceeded 110 bpm, systolic BP exceeded 220 mm Hg or diastolic BP exceeded 115. HR, BP, and level of perceived exertion were monitored during endurance training.

Intensity

Warm-up and cool down were performed at an RPE of 9 to 10/20.

Training commenced with an RPE of 11 to 12/20, progressing to an RPE of 13 over the course of inpatient rehabilitation. Walking overground progressed to ≥1.5 km/hour. Walking on the treadmill commenced at a velocity of ~1.5 km/hr and progressed to ≥2 km/hour.

Duration

A duration of 16 minutes was used initially (6 min walk overground, rest/stretch, 5 min walk on treadmill, rest/review activity diary, 5 min walk on treadmill), progressing to a total of 30 minutes at time to discharge to outpatient program.

Frequency

2 times per week.

Clinician Comment *As indicated in Chapter 12, fast walking over ground and treadmill walking are considered the most effective methods of aerobic training post-stroke. Both are task specific and have been found to also improve walking performance.[89,102] The repetitive nature and task specificity inherent in the methods of endurance training chosen were expected to facilitate activity-dependent neural plasticity (see previous discussion about gait training).*

The goal of endurance training is to improve aerobic fitness in the hopes of reducing the energy cost of ADL,[7] thereby increasing levels of activity and social participation. Specific inclusion of endurance training in a rehabilitation program is needed because other components of the rehabilitation program may not be sufficiently intense to cause an aerobic training effect.[70]

There is evidence of improved peak O_2 consumption and peak workload with aerobic training regardless of stage of stroke[102] and regardless of significant comorbidity.[103] There is also evidence of decreased submaximal energy expenditure in chronic stroke populations with endurance training.[104] A Cochrane systematic review found sufficient evidence to support the inclusion of cardio-respiratory training involving walking in post-stroke rehabilitation.[89]

Other benefits of endurance training that have been reported in stroke populations include: reduced risk of future cardiovascular events,[103,105] improved management of diabetes by enhancing glucose regulation,[106] reduced body weight, and improved body composition.[103]

Maintaining a regular endurance training program after discharge from rehabilitation care will be needed to achieve/maintain optimal effects.[7] As stated in Chapter 12, the greatest benefits are achieved with programs lasting longer than 12 weeks. It will be important to encourage Mr. Julep to maintain aerobic training using overground walking after discharge from rehabilitation programming.

Because Mr. Julep had not undergone a graded exercise test with EKG monitoring, and because he might have been at risk for exertion-related adverse cardiac complications related to coronary artery disease, it was decided to commence with lighter-intensity exercise with gradual progression. Mr. Julep was educated as to symptoms of cardiac distress and the need to stop if these occurred. A guideline of ~75% of predicted heart rate maximum [(220 − age) × 0.75] was chosen as the HR at which a training bout would be discontinued. The upper limit for systolic BP was set below the values of 250 mm Hg recommended for termination of graded exercise testing in stroke populations.[7]

Choosing an initial target velocity for overground aerobic training was based on Mr. Julep's velocity score on the 10-meter walk test. Goal velocities for both training methods were chosen based on functional gait classifications (see Chapter 12). Sullivan et al suggest training at faster velocities on a treadmill improves walking more than training at slower velocities.[107] In that study, average training velocity was ~2 mph, which is approximately 3 km/hr. Overground walking velocity was expected to change substantially when Mr. Julep began using a single-point cane instead of a walker. It was anticipated that he would be able to walk faster on the treadmill than when walking over ground with the walker or when walking with the cane.

Functional Training for Home, Community and Leisure Reintegration Including Instrumental Activities of Daily Living

Task-specific skill training in physical therapy sessions included practice of gait activities (already discussed), as well as bed mobility, sit-to-stand, transfers (horizontal and vertical), and management of stairs. The objectives of task-specific skill training involving these mobility tasks were to improve both efficiency and independence. ADL were addressed in OT treatment sessions.

Motor learning principles were applied, including random order of task practice, delayed feedback, intermittent feedback, and a focus on knowledge of results. Transfer of learning was addressed with practice under environmental conditions that would be encountered at home. For example, STS was practiced from progressively lower height sitting surfaces and compliant sitting surfaces to simulate stand-up from a sofa. STS was also practiced while holding objects of various weights and sizes.

Practice of lying ↔ sitting commenced with a force control strategy.[42] Practice progressed to an asymmetrical momentum strategy for rising to sitting, coming up over the left side, as this is the side on which he would get out of bed at home.

Initial practice of STS emphasized repositioning on sitting surface and foot positioning for optimal starting position. It included part practice of the flexion-momentum phase, (emphasizing symmetrical horizontal transfer of the COM),

part practice of flexion-momentum combined with momentum transfer, both of which were followed immediately by whole practice of the task.

Practice of vertical transfers began with a floor ↔ sitting transfer, using side sitting, 4-point kneeling, 2-point kneeling and half kneeling (with right leg forward) as transition positions. Practice was performed with Mr. Julep's right side next to chair/bed. Practice progressed to floor ↔ standing transfers.

Clinician Comment *A force control strategy[42] for lie-to-sit was used initially, as it was possible to complete independently despite poor/fair abdominal muscle strength. Practice from both left and right side lying was included. During practice, use of the left upper extremity to assist in supporting and moving the axial body, and trunk side flexion were facilitated as needed and were emphasized in instruction that proceeded practice. Performance was progressed to an asymmetrical momentum strategy[101] in order to reduce the time required to complete the task of rising to sitting.*

Prescription, Application of Devices and Equipment

Mr. Julep progressed from walking with a front-wheeled walker to walking with a single-point cane.

Clinician Comment *A walker enhances safety when walking, as it provides a substantial increase to the size of the base of support. However, it increases metabolic demands, interferes with postural motor stepping strategies used to regain balance, decreases step lengths, and decreases walking velocity (Brown, Chapter 12). In addition, it is cumbersome Using a cane allows for less limitation in community ambulation activities.*

REEXAMINATION (4 WEEKS)

Mr. Julep's progress was monitored regularly and reported in health record progress notes. Full reexaminations occurred at 4 weeks (discharge from inpatient programming), and again at 8 weeks (discharge from outpatient programming). Reassessment reports were documented separately from progress notes in the health record.

Subjective

Mr. Julep reported that he was using his left arm more when dressing, grooming, and eating. He reported feeling safe walking with the front-wheeled walker and that he was walking the distance from his room to the dining room by himself without stopping to rest. However, he did not yet feel safe walking alone with a single-point cane. Mr. Julep reported feeling less tired than when he was first admitted to the rehabilitation program.

He was very excited about returning home to live.

Objective

Cognitive Status

Mr. Julep's MMSE score was unchanged at time of reexamination (25/30).

Pain/Posture

Mr. Julep rated his back pain as 4 to 5/10 on the Visual Analog Scale (VAS). Less postural asymmetry was observed in sitting and standing. He was able to achieve a neutral lumbar lordosis and pelvic tilt position in sitting with verbal cueing. A very slight forward trunk lean was observed in standing, but Mr. Julep is now able to maintain hip and knee at 0 degrees when standing.

Range of Motion (Including Muscle Lengths)

Trunk side flexion range of motion had increased to 25 degrees to the left and 20 degrees to the right. Combined neck and trunk rotation had increased slightly to the right and was 75 degrees to both left and right sides at time of reexamination.

Hip extension range of motion had increased to 5 degrees on the left. SLR had increased to 60 degrees bilaterally. Ankle dorsiflexion on the left, with knee extended, had increased to 0 degrees.

Left shoulder ROM for external rotation had increased to 70 degrees, left forearm supination remained at 75 degrees, and left thumb range of motion had improved, although ranges were still slightly less than those for the right thumb.

Upon reexamination, spasticity was found to have generally decreased to grade 1, except for the left ankle plantar flexors, which remained at grade 2. Unsustained clonus at left ankle continued to be demonstrated.

Sensory and Perceptual Integrity

Mr. Julep now describes light touch as feeling the same on left and right extremities.

Muscle Performance

Motricity Index scores had improved slightly: upper extremity 70/100, lower extremity 75/100. Individual items scores that had changed included: elbow flexion of 25, shoulder abduction of 19, and ankle dorsiflexion of 25.

5 Timed STS: The time to complete the test improved to 16.9 sec from the initial time of 20.6 sec.

Clinician Comment *In order to achieve a full score for any item on the Motricity Index, normal power (ie, equal to the strength of the nonhemiplegic extremity segment) is required. Although there were indications of improved strength for all extremity segments tested, the Motricity Index did not capture all of these. It may have been beneficial to use a hand-held dynamometer (as suggested by Brown, Chapter 12) for testing movements included in the Motricity Index. A dynamometer would have generated ratio level data, which may have indicated improvements in strength that were not captured by the Motricity Index. However, there would be some question as to whether small gains in force production would have been clinically significant.*

Motor Function (Motor Control and Motor Learning)

Chedoke-McMaster Stroke Assessment Impairment Inventory: Stage of Recovery of Arm and Leg: On reassessment, the left arm and hand presented with stages 4 and 5 of recovery respectively, and the left leg and foot presented with stages 6 and 5 respectively, all demonstrating improvement by 1 stage.

Gait, Locomotion and Balance

Chedoke-McMaster Stroke Assessment: Disability Inventory

Mr. Julep's total score increased from 54/100 on initial assessment to 75/100, a change that was greater than the reported MCID for this measure (see Tests and Measures Section).

Modified Emory Ambulation Profile

At time of discharge, Mr. Julep used a single-point cane, rather than a walker when completing the tasks included in the mEAP. Close supervision was required during performance of the obstacles task.

1. Walk on floor: $20.2 \times 2 = 40.4$
2. Walk on carpet: $25.6 \times 2 = 51.2$
3. Timed Up & Go: $46.6 \times 2 = 93.2$
4. Obstacles: $65.5 \times 2 = 131$
5. Stairs: $58.1 \times 2 = 116.2$

Summed score = 432. This score was substantially lower than the initial summed score of 1032.4. Much of the reduction could be attributed to the change in type of assistive walking device.

Customary Walking Velocity

Measured while walking with a single-point cane was 0.56 m/sec, a substantial improvement over his initial walking velocity with the walker of 0.31 m/sec.

Clinician Comment *Brown (Chapter 12) suggested that an increase of 0.16 m/sec likely produces a meaningful improvement in participation. With this change in walking velocity, Mr. Julep is more likely to engage in walking in the community.*

BBG

Mr. Julep's score improved to 42/56 from the initial score of 34/56.

Postural Motor Stepping Strategies

When externally generated displacing forces (of sufficient amplitude to elicit stepping postural motor strategies) were applied in a controlled environment, Mr. Julep demonstrated sufficient response time and amplitude of responses with the right leg to regain balance. However, when forced to step with the left leg instead, responses were insufficient to regain balance in lateral and posterior directions.

Aerobic Capacity

6MWT distance at time of discharge was 252 m, as compared to 120.6 m at admission. The change in score exceeded the MDC of 54.1 m (see Tests and Measures Section).

Mr. Julep's FSS score at time of discharge was 5.2, as compared to 5.4 at time of admission which is greater than the MDC reported for this measure (reported in Tests and Measures Section).

Clinician Comment *As training effects are believed to take 8 to 12 weeks to achieve maximum benefit, a good portion of the improvement in distance walked may be attributed to the change from a walker to a cane and, possibly, to improvements in motor control and balance.*

Self-Care and Home Management, Including Activities of Daily Living and Instrumental Activities of Daily Living

Mr. Julep's total FIM score at time of discharge was 106. His motor sub-score had increased by 8 points to 78/91. His social-cognitive sub-score had not changed.

Assessment

Improvements in primary and secondary impairments were achieved. In addition, gains were made in the performance of mobility tasks, including ambulation. Edema of left hand had resolved, but there was still mild edema of the left foot and ankle. There had been no change in the size of the abrasion on the left ankle. Blood sugar levels were stable and well controlled at time of discharge from inpatient rehabilitation. Mr. Julep lost 6 pounds during his inpatient rehabilitation stay.

Of the 7 goals anticipated to be met within 1 week, all were met except for independent STS from toilet, which was met within 2 weeks. Independent STS from sofa was achieved in 3 weeks, rather than in 2 weeks. Independent ambulation with the walker, supervised transfers to/from car, and supervised walking with a single-point cane were achieved in the suggested 3-week time frame. Transfer up from floor to sitting with minimal contact assistance was achieved in 4 weeks, but transfer up to standing directly from the floor continued to require moderate assistance at

4 weeks. Walking a continuous distance of ≥ 300 meters with a single-point cane was not achieved at 4 weeks, but ascending/descending stairs independently using a railing was.

Task-specific training, along with improvements in balance, motor control (particularly the lower extremity), and flexibility contributed to accomplishing treatment goals that were achieved.

Discharge

Mr. Julep was successfully discharged home to live with his wife and family. He attended 2, 60-minute outpatient treatment sessions for 4 weeks, missing only 1 session due to a cold.

Mr. Julep was provided with a 30- to 45-minute home program of stretching and strengthening exercises. These were reviewed with Mr. Julep and his wife. This program was to be completed 3 times each week, on the weekdays on which he was not attending outpatient programming. An exercise diary was provided in which Mr. Julep could record the number of times/week the exercises were completed and the number of repetitions and sets completed. Mr. Julep was instructed to walk indoors/outdoors for 20 to 30 minutes 2 times each week. He was asked to record his RPE for each walk completed, along with the date, in the exercise diary. He was also encouraged to attend the stroke group exercise program that ran 2 days per week at a public recreation facility.

It was planned that Mr. Julep would walk on the treadmill for 25 to 30 minutes during each outpatient visit. The remainder of his outpatient treatment time would be spent in review/revision of strength training and flexibility exercises as necessary, progression of balance and gait training activities, as well as continued practice of rising from the floor to standing.

OUTCOME (END OF OUTPATIENT PROGRAM, 8 WEEKS)

On reexamination at 8 weeks, Mr. Julep had improved his Motricity Index score for shoulder abduction to 25 and his Chedoke-McMaster Inventory stage of recovery for the arm to 5. His STS time decreased to 15.8 sec. His BBS score increased to 45/56. When forced to step with the left leg in response to large displacements of his COM, his postural motor stepping strategy was sufficient to regain balance in a lateral direction, but not in a posterior direction. His Chedoke-McMaster Stroke Assessment: Disability Inventory score had increased to 80/100 and his customary walking velocity (with single-point cane) had increased to .6 m/sec.

Mr. Julep met the goal of walking for a continuous distance of 300 meters at 5 weeks and 500 meters at 8 weeks. He was walking independently with a straight cane indoors by 8 weeks, and outdoors with supervision by 8 weeks. He was able to maintain his balance when casting a fishing rod with the right arm and when hoeing a small garden patch at 8 weeks, but required supervision for both activities because of decreased balance confidence.

REFERENCES

1. Caro JJ, Migliaccio-Walle K, Sshak KJ, Proskorovsky I, O'Brien JA. The time course of subsequent hospitalizations and associated costs in survivors of an ischemic stroke. *BMC Health Serv Res.* 2006;6(1):99.

2. Blumenfeld H. *Neuroanatomy Through Clinical Cases.* Sunderland, MA: Sinauer Associates Inc; 2002.

3. Shelton F and Reding M. Effect of lesion location on upper limb recovery after stroke. *Stroke.* 2001;32:107-112.

4. Samuelsson M, Soderfeldt B, Olsson GB. Functional outcome in patients with lacunar infarcts. *Stroke.* 1996;27: 842-846.

5. Massucci M, Perdon L, Agosti M, et al. Prognostic factors of activity limitation and discharge destination after stroke rehabilitation. *Am J Phys Med Rehabil.* 2006;85:963-970.

6. Murat Sumer M, Erturk O. Ischemic stroke subtypes: risk factors, functional outcomes and recurrence. *Neurol Sci.* 2002;22:449-454.

7. Gordon NF, Gulanick M, Costa F, et al. Physical Activity and Exercise Recommendations for stroke survivors An American Heart Association scientific statement from the Council on Clinical Cardiology, Subcommittee on Exercise, Cardiac Rehabilitation, and Prevention; the Council on Cardiovascular Nursing; the Council on Nutrition, Physical Activity and Metabolism; and the Stroke Council. *Circulation.* 2004;109(16):2031-2041.

8. Holroyd-Lecuc JM, Kapral MK, Austin PC, Tu JV. Sex differences and similarities in the management and outcome of stroke patients. *Stroke.* 2000;31:1833-1837.

9. Hinkle JL. Variables explaining functional recovery following motor stroke. *J Neurosci Nurse.* 2006;38(1):6-12.

10. Weimer C, Ziegler A, Konig IR, Diener HC. Predicting functional outcome and survival after acute ischemic stroke. *J Neurol.* 2002;249:888-895.

11. Canadian Institute for Health Information. Factors predicting discharge home from inpatient rehabilitation after stroke. *Analysis in Brief.* May 5, 2009. https://secure.cihi.ca/free_products/aib_nrs_stroke_e.pdf. Accessed December 28 2011.

12. Paolucci S, Antonucci G, Troisi E, et al. Aging and stroke rehabilitation: a case-comparison study. *Cerebrovasc Dis.* 2003;15:98-105.

13. Black-Schaffer RM and Winston C. Age and functional outcome after stroke. *Top Stroke Rehabil.* 2004;11:23-32.

14. Bagg S, Pombo AP, Hopman W. Effect of age on functional outcomes after stroke rehabilitation. *Stroke.* 2002;33:179-185.

15. Frank M, Conzelmann M, Engelter S. Prediction of discharge destination after neurological rehabilitation in stroke patients. *Eur Neurol.* 2010;63:227-233.

16. Roquer J, Capello AR, Gomis M. Sex difference in first-ever acute stroke. *Stroke.* 2003;34;1581-1585.

17. National Institute of Neurological Disorders and Stroke rt-PA Stroke Study Group. Tissue plasminogen activator for acute ischemic stroke. *N Engl J Med.* 1995;333(24):1581-1587.

18. Glass TA, Matchar DB, Belyea M, Feussner JR. Impact of social support on outcome of first stroke. *Stroke.* 1993;24:64-70.

19. Ricci S, Celani MG, La Rosa F, et al. SEPIVAC: a community-based study of stroke incidence in Umbria, Italy. *J Neurol Neurosurg Psychiatr.* 1991;54:695-698.

20. Nguyen T-A, Page A, Aggarwal A, Henke P. Social determinants of discharge destination for patients after stroke with low admission FIM instrument scores. *Arch Phys Med Rehabil.* 2007;88:740-744.

21. Willey JZ, Moon YP, Paik MC, Boden-Albala B, Sacco RL, Elkind MSV. Physical activity and risk of ischemic stroke in the Northern Manhattan Study. *Neurology.* 2009;73:1774-1779.

22. Goldstein LB, Adam JR, Becker K, et al. Primary prevention of ischemic stroke: a statement for healthcare professionals from the Stroke Council of the American heart Association. *Stroke.* 2001;32:280-299.

23. Sacco RL, Benjamin EJ, Broderick JP, et al. American Heart Association Prevention Conference. IV. Prevention and Rehabilitation of Stroke. Risk Factors. *Stroke.* 1997;28(7):1507-1517.

24. Hankey GJ, Jamrozik K, Broadhurst RJ, Forbes S, Anderson CS. Long-term disability after first-ever stroke and related prognostic factors in the Perth Community Stroke Study, 1989-1990. *Stroke.* 2002;33(4):1034-1040.

25. Iverson, MD, Fossel AH, Ayers K, Palmsten A, Wang HW, Daltroy LH. Predictors of exercise behavior in patients with rheumatoid arthritis 6 months following a visit with their rheumatologist. *Phys Ther.* 2004;84(8):706-716.

26. Bak S, Sindrup SH, Alslev T, Kristensen O, Gaist D. Cessation of smoking after first-ever stroke: a follow-up study. *Stroke.* 2002;33:2263-2269.

27. American Heart Association. http://www.americanheart.org/print_presenter.jhtml;jsessionid=T10XXRLIKKOGGCQFCXPSCZQ?identifier=4756. Accessed January 8, 2012.

28. Jorgensen HS, Nakayama H, Raaschou HO, Olsen TS. Stroke in patients with diabetes. The Copenhagen Stroke Study. *Stroke.* 1994;25:1977-1984.

29. Rothwell PM, Warlow CP. Prediction of benefit from carotid endarterectomy in individual patients: a risk-modelling study. *Lancet.* 1999;353:2105-2110.

30. Ganong WF. *Review of Medical Physiology.* 23rd ed. New York: Lange Medical Books/McGraw-Hill; 2005.

31. Bowden MG, Balasubramanian CK, Behrman AL, Kautz SA. Validation of a speed-based classification system using quantitative measures of walking performance post stroke. *Neurorehabil Neural Repair.* 2008;22(6):672-675.

32. Ivey FM, Macko RF, Ryan AS, Hafer-Macko CE. Cardiovascular health and fitness after stroke. *Top Stroke Rehabil.* 2005;12(1)1-16.

33. MacKay-Lyons MJ, Howlett J. Exercise capacity and cardiovascular adaptations to aerobic training early after stroke. *Top Stroke Rehabil.* 2005;12(1):31-44.

34. Glader EL, Stegmayr B, Asplund K. Poststroke fatigue: a 2-year follow-up study of stroke patients in Sweden. *Stroke.* 2001;33:1327-1333.

35. National Heart Lung and Blood Institute: Obesity Education. Calculate your body mass index. http://www.nhlbisupport.com/bmi. Accessed January 12, 2012.

36. Gowland C, Van Hullenar S, Torresin W, et al. *Chedoke-McMaster Stroke Assessment: Development, Validation and Administration Manual.* Hamilton: Chedoke-Mcmaster Hospitals and McMaster University; 1995.

37. Aben I, Demollet J, Lousberg R, Verhey F, Wojceichowski F, Honig A. Personality and vulnerability to depression in stroke patients. *Stroke.* 2002;33:2391-2395.

38. Gresham GE, Staton WB. Rehabilitation of the stroke survivor. In: Barnett HJM, Morh JP, Stein BM, et al, eds. *Stroke: Pathophysiology, Diagnosis and Management.* 3rd ed. New York: Churchill Livingstone; 1998:1389-1399.

39. Kronenberg G, Katchanoy J, Endres M. Post-stroke depression: clinical aspects, epidemiology, therapy and pathophysiology [article in German]. *Nervenarzt.* 2006;77(10):1179-1182, 1184-1185.

40. Parikh RM, Robinson KG, Lipsey JR, Starkstein SE, Fedoroff JP, Price TR. The impact of poststroke depression on recovery in activities of daily living over a 2-year follow-up. *Arch Neurol.* 1990;47:785-789.

41. Folstein MF, Folstein SE, McHugh PR. Mini-Mental State: a practical method for grading the cognitive status of patients for the clinician. *J Psychiatr Res.* 1975;12(3):189-198.

42. Shumway-Cook A, Woollacott MH. *Motor Control Translating Research into Clinical Practice.* Philadelphia, PA: Lippincott Williams & Wilkins; 2007.

43. Carr J, Shepherd R. *Neurological Rehabilitation Optimizing Motor Performance.* Oxford: Butterworth-Heinemann; 1998.

44. Gregson JM, Leatheley M, Moore AP, Sharma AK, Smith TL, Watkins CL. Reliability of the Tone Assessment Scale and the modified Ashworth scale as clinical tools for assessing poststroke spasticity. *Arch Phys Med Rehabil.* 1999;80(9):1013-1016.

45. Collin C and Wade D. Assessing motor impairment after stroke: a pilot reliability study. *J Neurol Neurosurg Psychiatry.* 1990;53(7):576-579.

46. Demeurrise G, Demol O, Robage E. Motor evaluation of vascular hemiplegia. *Euro Neurol.* 1980;19:382-389.

47. Collen F, Wade D, Bradshaw C. Mobility after stroke: reliability of measures of impairment and disability. *Int Disab Stud.* 1990;12:6-9.

48. Cameron D and Bohannon RW. Criterion validity of lower extremity Motricity Index scores. *Clin Rehabil.* 2000;14:208-211.

49. Sunderland A, Tinson DJ, Bradley EL, Langton Hewer R. Arm function after stroke: an evaluation of grip strength as a measure of recovery and a prognostic indicator. *J Neurol Neurosurg Psychiatry.* 1989;52:1267-1272.

50. Hendricks HT, van Limbeek J, Geurts A, Zwarts MJ. Motor recovery after stroke: a systematic review of the literature. *Arch Phys Med Rehabil.* 2002;83:1629-1637.

51. Mong Y, Teo TW, Ng SS. 5-repetition sit-to-stand test in subjects with chronic stroke: reliability and validity. *Arch Phys Med Rehabil.* 2010;91(3):407-413.

52. Hsu AL, Tang PF, Jan MH. Analysis of impairments influencing gait velocity and asymmetry of hemiplegic patients after mild to moderate stroke. *Arch Phys Med Rehabil.* 2003;84:1185-1193.

53. Huijbregts MP, Gowland C, Gruber R. Measuring clinically-important change with the activity inventory of the Chedoke-McMaster Stroke Assessment. *Physiother Can.* 2000;52:295-304.

54. Gowland C, Stratford P, Ward M, Moreland J, Torresin W, Van Hullenaar S. Measuring physical impairment and disability with the Chedoke-McMaster Stroke Assessment. *Stroke.* 1993;24:58-63.

55. Baer HR, Wolf SL. Modified Emory Ambulation Profile: an outcome measure for the rehabilitation of post stroke gait dysfunction. *Stroke.* 2001;32:973-979.

56. Liaw LJ, Hsieh C, Lo SK, Lee S, Huang MH, Lin JH. Psychometric properties of the modified Emory functional ambulation profile for stroke patients. *Clin Rehabil.* 2006;20(5):429-437.

57. Wolf SL, Catlin PA, Gage K, Gurucharri K, Robertson R, Stephen K. Establishing the reliability and validity of measurements of walking time using the Emory Functional Ambulation Profile. *Phys Ther.* 1999;79(12):1122-1133.

58. Fulk GD and Echternach JL. 2008. Test-retest reliability and minimal detectable change of gait speed in individuals undergoing rehabilitation after stroke. *J Neurol Phys Ther.* 2008;332:8-13.

59. Mulroy SJ, Klassen T, Gronley JK, Eberly VJ, Brown DA, Sullivan KT. Gait parameters associated with responsiveness to treadmill training with body-weight support after stroke: an exploratory study. *Phys Ther.* 2010;90(2):209-223.

60. Perry J, Garrett M, Gronley JK, Mulroy S. Classification of walking handicap in the stroke population. *Stroke.* 1995;26:982-989.

61. Blum L, Korner-Bitensky N. Usefulness of the Berg Balance Scale in stroke rehabilitation: a systematic review. *Phys Ther.* 2008;88:559-566.

62. Stevenson TJ. Detecting change in patients with stroke using the Berg Balance Scale. *Aust J Physiother.* 2001;47(1):29-38.

63. Harris JE, Eng JJ, Marigold DS, Tokuno CD, Louis CL. Relationship of balance and mobility to fall incidence in people with chronic stroke. *Phys Ther.* 2005;85:150-158.

64. Wee JY, Wong H, Palepu A. Validation of the Berg Balance Scale as a predictor of length of stay and discharge destination in stroke rehabilitation setting. *Arch Phys Med Rehabil.* 2003;84:731-735.

65. Kwakkel G, Wagenaar RC, Kollen BJ, Lankhorst GJ. Predicting disability in stroke—a critical review of the literature. *Age Ageing.* 1996;25:479-489.

66. Brauer SG, Bew PG, Kuys SS, Lynch MR, Morrison G. Prediction of discharge destination after stroke using the motor assessment scale on admission: a prospective multi-site study. *Arch Phys Med Rehabil.* 2008;89(6):1061-1065.

67. Borg GA. Psychological basis for physical exertion. *Med Sci Sports.* 1982;14:377.

68. Fulk GD, Echternach JL, Nof L, O'Sullivan S. Clinometric properties of the six-minute walk test in individuals undergoing rehabilitation post stroke. *Physiother Theory Pract.* 2008;24(3):195-204.

69. Monga TN, Deforge DA, Williams J, Wolfe LA. Cardiovascular responses to acute exercise in patients with cerbrovascular accidents. *Arch Phys Med Rehabil.* 1988;69(11):937-940.

70. MacKay MJ, Makrides L. Exercise capacity early after stroke. *Arch Phys Med Rehabil.* 2002;83:1697-1702.

71. DeGroot MH, Phillips SJ, Eskes GA. Fatigue associated with stroke and other neurologic conditions: implications for stroke rehabilitation. *Arch Phys Med Rehabil.* 2003;84(11):1714-1720.

72. Valko PO, Bassetti CL, Bloch KE, Held U, Baumann CR. Validation of the Fatigue Severity Scale in a Swiss cohort. *Sleep.* 2008;31(11):1601-1607.

73. Ingles JL, Eskes GA, Phillips SJ. Fatigue after stroke. *Arch Phys Med Rehabil.* 1999;80:173-178.

74. Glader EL, Stegmayr B, Asplund D. Poststroke fatigue: a 2-year follow-up study of stroke patients in Sweden. *Stroke.* 2001;33:1327-1333.

75. Van de Port IGL, Kwakkel G, Schepers VPM, Heinemans CTI. Is fatigue an independent factor associated with activities of daily living, instrumental activities of daily living and health-related quality of life in chronic stroke? *Cerebrovasc Dis.* 2007;23:40-45.

76. Hamilton BB, Laughlin JA, Fiedler RC, Granger CV. Interrater reliability of the 7-level Functional Independence Measure (FIM). *Scand J Rehabil Med.* 1995;27:253-256.

77. Alexander M. Stroke rehabilitation outcome: a potential use of predictive variables to establish levels of care. *Stroke.* 1994;25(1):128-134.

78. Lindsay P, Bayley M, Hellings C, Hill M, Woodbury E, Phillips S. Canadian Best Practice Recommendations for Stroke Care (updated 2008). *CMAJ.* 2008;179(12):S1-S25.

79. Evans RL, Bishop DS, Matlock AL, et al. Family interaction and treatment adherence after stroke. *Arch Phys Med Rehabil.* 1987;68:513-517.

80. Teasell RW, Kalra L. What's new in stroke rehabilitation: Back to basics. *Stroke.* 2005;36:215-217.

81. Kwakkel G, van Peppen R, Wagenaar RC, et al. Effects of augmented exercise therapy time after stroke: a meta-analysis. *Stroke.* 2004;35:2529-2539.

82. Kalra L, Evans A, Perez I, et al. Training carers of stroke patients: randomized controlled trail. *BMJ.* 2004;328:1099-1204.

83. Forester A, Young J. Incidence and consequences of falls due to stroke: a systematic inquiry. *BMJ.* 1995;311:83-86.

84. Nadeau S, Arsenaault AB, Gravel D, Bourbonnais D. Analysis of clinical factors determining natural and maximal gait speeds in adults with stroke. *Am J Phys Med Rehabil.* 1999;78(2):123-130.

85. Kim CM, Eng JJ. The relationship of lower extremity muscle torque with locomotor performance in persons with stroke. *Phys Ther.* 2003;83:49-57.

86. Eriksrud O, Bohannon RW. Relationship of knee extension force to independence in sit-to-stand performance in patients receiving acute rehabilitation. *Phys Ther.* 2003;83(6):544-551.

87. Weiss A, Suzuki T, Bean J, Fielding RA. High intensity strength training improves strength and functional performance after stroke. *Am J Phys Med Rehabil.* 2000;79:369-376.

88. Jorgensen JR, Bech-Pedersen DT, Zeeman P, Sorensen J, Andersen LL, Schonberger M. Effects of intensive outpatient physical training on gait performance and cardiovascular health in people with hemiparesis after stroke. *Phys Ther.* 2010;90(4):527-537.

89. Saunders DH, Greig CA, Mead GE, Young A. Physical fitness training for stroke patients. *Cochrane Database Syst Rev.* 2009(4):CD003316.

90. Pak S, Patten C. Strengthening to promote functional recovery poststroke: an evidence-based review. *Top Stroke Rehabil.* 2008;14(3):177-1999.

91. Van Peppen R, Kwakkel G, Wood-Dauphinee S, Hendricks H, Van der Wees P, Dekker J. The impact of physical therapy on functional outcomes after stroke: what's the evidence? *Clin Rehabil.* 2004;18:833-862.

92. Eng JJ. Strength training in individuals with stroke. *Physiother Can.* 2004;56:189-201.

93. Morris SL, Dodd KJ, Morris ME. Outcomes of progressive resistance strength training following stroke: a systematic review. *Clin Rehabil*. 2004;18:27-39.

94. Hammer A, Nilsagard Y, Wallquist M. Balance training in stroke patients—a systematic review of randomized, controlled trials. *Adv Physiother*. 2008;10(4):163-172.

95. Lubetzky-Vilnai A, Kartin D. The effects of balance training on balance performance in individuals poststroke: a systematic review. *J Neurol Phys Ther*. 2010;34(3):127-137.

96. Van de Port IG, Wood-Dauphinee S, Lideman E. Kwakkel G. Effects of exercise training programs on walking competency after stroke: a systematic review. *Am J Phys Med Rehabil*. 2007;86(11):935-951.

97. De Quervain JA, Simon SR, Leurgans S, Pease WS, McAlister FA. Gait pattern in the early recovery period after stroke. *J Bone Joint Surg*. 1996;78:1506-1514.

98. Bowden MG, Embry AE, Gregory CM. Physical therapy adjuvants to promote optimization of walking recovery after stroke. *Stroke Res Treat*. 2011;2011:601416.

99. Kleim JA, Jones TA. Principles of experience-dependent neural plasticity: Implications for rehabilitation after brain damage. *J Speech Lang Hear Res*. 2008;51(1):S225-S239.

100. Duncan PW, Sullivan KJ, Behrman A, et al. Body-weight-supported treadmill rehabilitation after stroke. *N Engl J Med*. 2011;364:2026-2036.

101. Davies PM. *Steps to Follow: A Guide to the Treatment of Adult Hemiplegia*. Berlin: Springer-Verlag; 1985.

102. Pang MYC, Eng JJ, Dawson AS, Gylfadóttir S. The use of aerobic exercise training in improving aerobic capacity in individuals with stroke: a meta-analysis. *Clin Rehabil*. 2006;20(2):97-111.

103. Rimmer JH, Rauworth AE, Wang EC, Nicola TL, Hill B. A preliminary study to examine the effects of aerobic and therapeutic (nonaerobic) exercises on cardiorespiratory fitness and coronary risk reduction in stroke survivors. *Arch Phys Med Rehabil*. 2009;90(3):407-412.

104. Macko RF, DeSouza CA, Tretter LD, et al. Treadmill aerobic exercise training reduces the energy expenditure and cardiovascular demands of hemiparetic gait in chronic stroke patients: a preliminary report. *Stroke*. 1997;82:879-884.

105. Hambrecht R, Wolf A, Gielen S, et al. Effect of exercise on coronary endothelial function in patients with coronary artery disease. *N Engl J Med*. 2000;342(7):454-460.

106. Franklin BA, Sanders W. Reducing the risk of heart disease and stroke. *Phys Sportsmed*. 2000;28(10):19-26.

107. Sullivan KJ, Brown DA, Klassen T, et al. Effects of task-specific locomotor and strength training in adults who were ambulatory after stroke: results of the STEPS randomized clinical trial. *Phys Ther*. 2007;87(12):1580-1602.

CASE STUDY 12-2

Vanina Dal Bello-Haas, PT, PhD

EXAMINATION

History

Current Condition/Chief Complaint

Mrs. Jelly was a 59-year-old White woman with a diagnosis of bulbar-onset amyotrophic lateral sclerosis (ALS). Mrs. Jelly was experiencing neck pain.

Clinician Comment *Although muscle weakness is the cardinal impairment in ALS, the type and severity of impairments, activity limitations, and participation restrictions that manifest will vary. The differences in presentation depends on the localization and extent of motor neuron loss, the degree and combination of lower motor neuron (LMN) and upper motor neuron (UMN) loss, pattern of onset and progression, body region(s) affected, and stage of the disease. Typically at disease onset, signs or symptoms are asymmetrical and focal. Progression of the disease leads to increasing numbers and severity of impairments, and signs and symptoms progress in a contiguous manner. This means signs and symptoms spread from one focal region (eg, bulbar in the case of Mrs. Jelly) to an anatomically adjacent area (eg, cervical in the case of Mrs. Jelly).*

Bulbar-onset ALS is seen in 20% to 25% of cases. The term bulbar-onset *indicates involvement of motor nuclei of the cranial nerves IX, X, XI, XII or degeneration of the corticobulbar tract, resulting in muscle weakness and wasting of the tongue, pharynx, larynx, and soft palate. Bulbar-onset ALS occurs more frequently in middle-aged women, and initial symptoms include difficulty chewing, swallowing, and speaking.*[1,2]

History of Current Complaint

About 1 month prior to her initial physical therapy appointment, Mrs. Jelly noticed that the back of her neck and her upper shoulders were quite sore by the end of a work day. Mrs. Jelly reported the pain was present throughout the day, but she tried to ignore it. By the end of the day, however, the pain ("aching pain") was quite severe. Mrs. Jelly also noticed that her head "felt heavy" by the end of the day. Mrs. Jelly often had difficulty finding a comfortable position for sleeping. She reported that she woke frequently during the night, and often woke up with a headache.

Clinician Comment *People with ALS typically develop cervical extensor muscle weakness, initially. Early symptoms of cervical weakness includes neck stiffness, heaviness, and fatigue with holding the head up or difficulties in keeping the head upright with unexpected movements (eg, in an accelerating car).*[3,4]

Although the poor sleep and early morning headaches may be related to neck pain, respiratory muscles may also be weak. Early signs and symptoms of respiratory muscle weakness include fatigue, dyspnea on exertion, difficulty sleeping in supine, frequent awakening at night, excessive daytime sleepiness, and morning headaches due to hypoxia.[5] *People with ALS may not complain of respiratory symptoms initially, because they tend to decrease their overall level of physical activity due to fatigue or increasing muscle weakness.*

Social History/Environment

Mrs. Jelly lived in a condominium with her husband of 30 years. Mr. Jelly had a stroke affecting his left side 5 years prior, was independent in activities of daily living (ADL) and instrumental ADL (IADL), but used a motorized wheelchair for mobility. Mr. Jelly did not work. The Jellys had 3 adult children: 2 who lived in a different state and a third who lived in Asia. Mrs. Jelly reported that she had a strong support network of friends and coworkers.

Employment/Work (Job/School/Play)

Mrs. Jelly was an administrative assistant at a local university. Mrs. Jelly was very concerned about her ability to continue to work because of increasing difficulty she was experiencing with her speech. In particular, Mrs. Jelly was concerned about losing her health benefits.

Clinician Comment *The financial realities of living with ALS and trying to navigate the health care and reimbursement systems can be daunting and overwhelming. Individuals should be referred to a social worker as early as possible. The usual 24-month waiting period for Medicare was eliminated for Social Security Disability Insurance (SSDI) recipients disabled by ALS as a result of extensive lobbying of Congress by The ALS Association (ALSA).*

Social/Health Habits

Mrs. Jelly was a nonsmoker and drank alcohol only on social occasions. Mrs. Jelly walked daily during her lunch hour with a colleague—she aimed to walk 30 to 45 minutes per day, 5 days per week. Mrs. Jelly reported that she "greatly treasures the daily walks," as this was an opportunity for her to chat with her colleague about personal and work issues. Mrs. Jelly was finding that on some days her walks were taking her longer to complete and that sometimes she had to stop because of leg cramps.

Clinician Comment *The etiology of muscle cramping is not well understood. Muscle cramps are thought to be related to hyperexcitability of motor axons, and in people with ALS, cramps occur in uncommon sites such as the tongue, jaw, neck, abdomen, as well as in more typical sites.[3]*

Family History

Mrs. Jelly's family history was negative for ALS. Her parents both died of natural causes in their late 80s. Mrs. Jelly had 2 younger brothers, one aged 38 and the other aged 45. She had a maternal cousin who was diagnosed with multiple sclerosis (MS) at the age of 45.

Clinician Comment *More than 90% of cases of ALS are classified as sporadic (ie, no clear family history), and the cause of sporadic ALS is unknown. The remaining 5% to 10% are classified as familial ALS (FALS), which is transmitted as an autosomal dominant disease.[6,7] About 15% to 20% of people with FALS (ie, about 1% of all patients with ALS) have a mutation in the gene encoding an enzyme called copper-zinc superoxide dismutase.[8]*

Medical/Surgical History

Mrs. Jelly was diagnosed with bulbar-onset ALS 11 months prior to the initial physical therapy appointment. About 6 months prior to her diagnosis, Mrs. Jelly noticed that she was having difficulty pronouncing certain words. She also noted that she began to choke when drinking coffee or water. This progressed to difficulty chewing and swallowing. On physical exam, tongue fasciculations and a brisk jaw reflex were noted. Diagnostic tests ruled out any other conditions that may have accounted for signs and symptoms. An electromyography (EMG) determined active denervation of the left hand and chronic denervation of the thorax. Mrs. Jelly was diagnosed with clinically probable ALS with laboratory support. Mrs. Jelly had no other medical problems. Past surgical history included a tonsillectomy at age 10.

Clinician Comment *ALS diagnosis is one of exclusion, eg, neuroimaging and clinical laboratory studies are performed and other all other diagnoses that might be the cause of signs and symptoms must be excluded. The El Escorial criteria, widely accepted criteria used for the diagnosis of ALS for clinical practice, therapeutic trials, and other research purposes, classifies ALS into "clinically definite," "clinically probable," "clinically probable with laboratory support," and "possible" categories.[9] More information can be found online at http://www.alsa.org/assets/pdfs/fyi/criteria_for_diagnosis.pdf.*

A criticism of the El Escorial criteria is that they favor clinical signs over electrodiagnostic findings, reducing sensitivity. Recently developed Awaji-shima criteria[10] allow for electrophysiological evidence of LMN to be considered as equivalent to clinical signs. This makes the category of "clinically probable ALS with laboratory-support" redundant since all categories of the Awaji-shima criteria include evidence from electrodiagnostic findings.

The Awaji-shima criteria[10] are as follows:

(i)   Clinically definite ALS: clinical or electrophysiological evidence of LMN and UMN signs in the bulbar region and at least 2 spinal regions, or the presence of LMN and UMN in 3 spinal regions.

(ii) Clinically probable ALS: clinical or electrophysiological evidence of LMN and UMN in at least 2 regions,

> with some UMN signs necessarily rostral to the LMN signs.
>
> (iii) *Clinically possible ALS: clinical or electrophysiological signs of LMN and UMN signs in 1 region; or UMN signs are found alone in 2 or more regions; or LMN signs are found rostral to UMN signs.*

Reported Functional Status

Prior to the diagnosis of ALS, Mrs. Jelly was very active. As noted previously, she walked daily. Mrs. Jelly had been very active in several volunteer organizations, including participating in overseas missions, but was no longer involved because she was embarrassed about her speech and fatigued by the end of most work days. At the time of the initial physical therapy appointment, Mrs. Jelly did not need any assistance for ADL or IADL. Depending on the day, however, she noted that having to complete additional activities in the evening could be fatiguing. She also noted that she was slower in completing tasks.

Medications

Mrs. Jelly was taking Rilutek (riluzole). In addition, she took calcium with vitamin D, vitamin E, vitamin C, and coenzyme Q10(CoQ10). Mrs. Jelly reported no allergies.

> **Clinician Comment** *There is no cure for ALS, and clinical trials of medications for reducing mortality and treating symptoms of ALS are ongoing.*
>
> *Rilutek is the only Food and Drug Administration (FDA)-approved medication to treat ALS. Riluzole is a glutamate inhibitor. Studies have found that the drug delays disease progression modestly, extending survival for about 2 to 4 months. Although usually well tolerated, adverse effects include asthenia, nausea, vomiting, dizziness, liver toxicity, and neutropenia.[11,12]*
>
> *Medical management of ALS is symptomatic and there are many medications and interventions that are used to treat symptoms. Practice guidelines for the management of ALS[13,14] have been published and can be found online at http://www.neurology.org/content/73/15/1218.full.html.*
>
> *As Mrs. Jelly is postmenopausal, calcium with vitamin D is being taken to prevent bone loss.*
>
> *The oxidative stress/free-radical damage hypothesis contributes to the theory that "high-dose" antioxidants may be beneficial for people with ALS. To date, there is no evidence of beneficial effects in humans. CoQ10 is a component of the respiratory chain of mitochondria. Normally, CoQ10 acts both as an electron carrier and as a potent antioxidant.[15]*
>
> *Mrs. Jelly's interview revealed that she had neck pain, progressive speech difficulties and muscle weakness, symptoms of respiratory muscle weakness, fatigue, and concerns about*

the progression of her ALS. Based on the physical therapy interview, the other health care professionals who should be involved with her care, in addition to her neurologist, include: a speech-language pathologist, a registered dietician, a social worker, an occupational therapist. The roles for each of these practitioners will be presented in more detail in the plan of care.

Systems Review

Cardiovascular/Pulmonary

- Heart rate (HR) = 88
- Blood pressure (BP) = 129/70
- Respiratory rate (RR)= 18
- Oxygen saturation was 92% on room air
- No accessory muscle use evident in sitting

Musculoskeletal

Fasciculations were noted in the neck musculature, upper chest, and left hand. Slight atrophy of the left anatomical snuff area was noted.

> **Clinician Comment** *Fasciculations are common in individuals with ALS, although they are rarely an initial symptom. The etiology of fasciculations remains unclear and is thought to be related to hyperexcitability of motor axons.[3]*

Anthropometrics

- Height = 167.6 cm (5 feet, 6 inches)
- Weight = 52.3 kg (115 pounds)
- Body mass index (BMI) = 18.6

> **Clinician Comment** *As nutrition status has been identified as a prognostic factor for survival and disease complications,[16] careful attention to nutrition and hydration is required.*
>
> *People with bulbar muscle weakness will have difficulty chewing, swallowing, and manipulating food inside the mouth or moving food into the esophagus. They may take in less than optimal fluid and caloric needs, which results in weight loss. Although, some weight loss can be expected due to loss of muscle mass as the disease progresses, excessive weight loss is more indicative of inadequate nutritional intake. Laboratory blood counts and chemistries would confirm signs of dehydration and undernourishment. BMI confirms a registered dietician should be involved in overall management of Mrs. Jelly.*

Integumentary

- Skin integrity = No integumentary abnormalities were noted.

Clinician Comment *Skin integrity is usually not compromised in people with ALS, even in the late stage of the disease, because sensation is normally preserved. However, skin inspection should be performed regularly, especially when the patient becomes immobile. Pay particular attention to contact points between the body and assistive, adaptive, orthotic, protective and supportive devices, mobility devices, and resting and sleeping surfaces.*

Musculoskeletal

- Gross symmetry/posture: Overall, Mrs. Jelly's sitting posture was slumped throughout the interview. Mrs. Jelly occasionally rested her chin on her fist. When prompted, Mrs. Jelly was able to correct her posture.

- Gross range of motion (ROM)/strength: Cervical spine ROM was within normal limits (WNL). Mrs. Jelly lacked some eccentric control when moving the head into full flexion.

  - Lower and upper extremity ROM and gross muscle strength was WNL. Strength testing of quadriceps muscles brought on muscle cramping bilaterally.

  - Mrs. Jelly was able to perform sit-to-stand with arms folded with no difficulty.

  - Mrs. Jelly was able to walk a distance of 5 meters on her tip-toes and on her heels.

Neuromuscular

No impairments were noted in locomotion, transfers, or transitions. No gait abnormalities were noted during locomotion.

Communication, Affect, Cognition, Language, and Learning Style:

Mrs. Jelly slurred her words and occasionally had to repeat herself to be understood. She had a flat affective. Mrs. Jelly answered questions appropriately and could follow 3-step commands. She reported she preferred to have information presented to her in both written and verbal formats to ensure she "doesn't miss anything."

Clinician Comment *Mrs. Jelly presents with a flat affect. It was not clear whether the flat affect was due to cognitive changes or, perhaps, depression. She could, however, answer questions appropriately and could follow 3-step commands.*

Although once considered separate cognitive impairments, symptoms ranging from mild deficits to severe frontotemporal dementia (FTD) are now considered part of the

ALS disease spectrum. ALS-associated FTD signs include: cognitive decline, executive functioning impairments, difficulties with planning, organization and concept abstraction, and personality and behavior changes. Individuals with ALS, without FTD, can have difficulties with verbal fluency, language comprehension, memory, abstract reasoning, and generalized impairments in intellectual function.[17-19] People with bulbar-onset ALS are more likely to have cognitive impairments than patients with limb-onset disease.[20] Clinicians should screen for cognitive impairments. No ALS-specific cognitive test or measure exists. The Mini-Mental State Examination (MMSE)[21] has been used in clinical studies; however, it may not be sensitive enough to identify frontotemporal function impairments. If dementia or cognitive impairments are suspected, executive function, language comprehension, memory, and abstract reasoning should be examined and referrals to appropriate health care professionals may be warranted (eg, neuropsychologist).[22]

Living with ALS, a devastating disease with no cure, and experiencing loss after loss as the disease progresses can result in psychological impairments, such as depression or anxiety. Depression can interfere with sleep, cause fatigue, and greatly affect a person's quality of life, as well as alter one's ability to cope with, and adapt to, the progressive changes and losses of the disease. Clinicians should screen for depression and make the appropriate referral for further assessment and management, eg, psychologist (psychological counseling), psychiatrist or neurologist (medications).

Mrs. Jelly's systems review indicated low BMI, which was likely an indicator of progressive dysphagia. She reported cervical pain. Altered posture was observed throughout the interview. Based on the findings from the systems review, screening for depression and further assessment of muscle strength, especially hand strength, were warranted.

Tests and Measures

Pain

Mrs. Jelly rated her neck pain as 8 to 9/10 (at its worst) using the 10-point visual analog scale (VAS), and described it as "aching." The pain is 4/10 in the morning upon waking and progresses to 8 to 9/10 by the end of the day.

Posture

Mrs. Jelly held her head forward, both the standing and seated position. Bilateral shoulder girdles were held in a protracted position. She had a moderate increase in thoracic kyphosis. With verbal cues to correct her posture, Mrs. Jelly was able to hold herself more erect and could maintain this position for short periods of time.

Clinician Comment *The clinical assessment of posture in people with ALS is largely subjective and descriptive in nature.*

Muscle Performance (Including Strength, Power and Endurance)

MUSCLE GROUP	GRADE
Cervical flexion	4/5
Cervical extension	3+/5
Cervical right rotation	4+/5
Cervical left rotation	4+/5
Cervical right side flexion	4+/5
Cervical left side flexion	4+/5

	RIGHT* (POUNDS)	RIGHT (POUNDS)	AGE/GENDER RANGE MEAN (SD)[1]	LEFT (POUNDS)	LEFT (POUNDS) AGE/GENDER MEAN (SD)[23]
Grip (Jamar dynamometer)	55.5	33 to 86 57.3 (12.5)		32	31 to 76 47.3 (11.9)
Tip pinch (pinch gauge)	11	9 to 16 11.7 (1.7)		7.5	8 to 13 10.4 (1.4)
Lateral (key) pinch (pinch gauge)	14.5	11 to 21 15.7 (2.5)		10.5	12 to 19 14.7 (2.2)
Palmar pinch (pinch gauge)	15.5	11 to 26 16.0 (3.1)		10.5	11 to 21 15.4 (3.0)

*Dominant side.

Clinician Comment *Specific deficits in muscle strength can be measured with manual muscle testing (MMT), isokinetic muscle strength testing, or hand-held dynamometry. In clinical practice, MMT or hand-held dynamometry is preferred due to efficiency. As the disease progresses, the physical therapist must weigh the emotional and physical costs of repeated formal muscle testing against the benefits of what this information provides in the greater context of the individual's overall evaluation and management plan. Specifically, it can be clearly evident muscles when are wasted and limbs cannot be moved against gravity.*

Compared to a female aged 55 to 59, Mrs. Jelly's left grip and pinch strength was below the mean, or below, or close to, the lower end of the range. She was not complaining, however, of activity limitations (eg, dressing) or participation restrictions (eg, work). Although premorbid grip and pinch values were not available, the wasting in the anatomic snuff and the EMG findings suggested that it was likely that the findings in her left hand findings were due to ALS.

Tone and Reflexes

Using the Modified Ashworth spasticity scores, Mrs. Jelly showed 1+ for both upper extremities. She had a clonic jaw reflex, hyperreflexia in both upper extremities, hyporeflexia in both lower extremities, and a positive right Babinski reflex.

Clinician Comment *The Modified Ashworth Scale[23] is used clinically to assess resistance to passive movement and reflects only an aspect of spasticity. Psychometric properties have not been tested in ALS populations. Limited reliability and lack of sensitivity exist with lower grades (eg, 1, 1+, and 2).[24,25] Deep tendon and pathological reflex testing also assist in determining UMN and LMN involvement.*

Respiratory Function

Auscultation: normal breath sounds throughout; no adventitious sounds

Cough: strong; effective for secretion clearance

Diaphragmatic excursion: 4 cm

Forced vital capacity (FVC) was assessed using a hand-held spirometer. Mrs. Jelly had slight difficulty maintaining a tight lip seal on the apparatus due to orofacial weakness:

FVC = 95% predicted (sitting)

FVC = 93% predicted (lying)

Clinician Comment *Supine FVC may be a better indicator of diaphragm weakness than erect FVC. Monitoring of FVC or VC is important—although there is no firm evidence, current practice guidelines suggest that for optimal safety and efficacy the percutaneous endoscopic gastrostomy (PEG) procedure should be offered to the patient and completed before the individual's FVC/VC falls below 50% of predicted.[25]*

Although Mrs. Jelly had difficulty finding a comfortable position for sleeping, woke frequently during the night, and often woke with a headache, her FVC in sitting was WNL. Her FVC in lying did not vary much from her FVC in sitting.

Fatigue

Mrs. Jelly rated her fatigue as 8/10 at its worst, which generally occurred by the end of her work day.

Clinician Comment *Fatigue is very common in individuals with ALS. As motor neurons die, the remaining neurons are overburdened. Weakened muscles must work at a higher percentage of their maximal strength to perform the same activity, which also hastens muscle fatigue.[26] Fatigue may also be related to sleep disturbances, respiratory impairments, hypoxia, and depression. No ALS-specific measures exist; the Fatigue Severity Scale[27] has been used in clinical trials.*

Functional Status

Mrs. Jelly rated herself at 90% using the Schwab and England Activities of Daily Living Scale; 90% corresponds to "completely independent; able to do all chores with some degree of slowness, difficulty, and impairment; may take twice as long as usual; beginning to be aware of difficulty."

Clinician Comment *The Schwab and England Activities of Daily Living Scale[28] is an 11-point global measure of functioning that asks the rater to report ADL function from 100% (normal) to 0% (vegetative functions only). The scale has been used to examine function in individuals with ALS, has been found to have excellent test-retest reliability, to correlate well with qualitative and quantitative changes in function, and to be sensitive to changes over time.*

Disease-Specific Measures

The ALS Functional Rating Scale-Revised was used to assess Mrs. Jelly's function and her scores appear next.

AMYOTROPHIC LATERAL SCLEROSIS FUNCTIONAL RATING SCALE-REVISED SCORES

ITEM	SCORE	DESCRIPTOR
Speech	3	Detectable speech disturbance
Salivation	3	Slight but definite excess of saliva in mouth; may have nighttime drooling
Swallowing	3	Early eating problems—occasional choking
Handwriting (pre-ALS dominant hand)	4	Normal
Cutting food and handling utensils (patients without gastrostomy)	3	Somewhat slow and clumsy, but no help needed
Dressing and hygiene	3	Independent and complete self-care with effort or decreased efficiency
Turning in bed; adjusting bed clothes	3	Somewhat slow and clumsy, but no help needed
Walking	4	Normal
Climbing stairs	4	Normal

AMYOTROPHIC LATERAL SCLEROSIS FUNCTIONAL RATING SCALE-REVISED SCORES

ITEM	SCORE	DESCRIPTOR
Dyspnea	4	Normal
Orthopnea	4	Normal
Respiratory insufficiency	4	Normal

Clinician Comment *The ALSFRS-R[29] examines the functional status of patients with ALS. The patient is asked to rate his or her function using a scale from 4 (normal function) to 0 (unable to attempt the task). The ALSFRS-R was expanded from the original 10-point scale to include additional respiratory items, and has been found to have internal consistency, construct validity, and to have retained the properties of the original scale. Telephone administration of the ALSFRS-R has also been found to be reliable.[30]*

Mrs. Jelly's ALSFRS-R scores indicated she had bulbar function and some ADL impairments, likely due to the left hand weakness.

Psychosocial Function

With the Beck's Depression Inventory (BDI), Mrs. Jelly's score was 19, which was indicative of borderline clinical depression.

Clinician Comment *The BDI[31] consists of 21 items. Each item is a list of 4 statements arranged in increasing severity about a particular symptom of depression. The BDI has been used in ALS clinical studies.*

EVALUATION

Diagnosis

Practice Pattern

The Preferred Practice Pattern that best applied to Mrs. Jelly's case was Neuromuscular Practice Pattern 5E: Impaired motor function and sensory integrity associated with progressive disorders of the central nervous system (CNS).

Clinician Comment *Depending on the stage of the disease and the resultant impairments, activity limitations and participation restrictions, several practice patterns may apply.*

International Classification of Functioning, Disability and Health Model of Disability

See ICF model on p 526.

Prognosis

With respect to neck pain, Mrs. Jelly's prognosis was good. It was expected that her neck pain could be relieved, at least in the shorter-term, with modifications to work environment, use of a cervical collar, and rest.

Clinician Comment *It is imperative that the physical therapist have a solid understanding of the nature and course of ALS in order make effective decisions regarding the prognosis (eg, what impairments, limitations, restrictions can be restored; what impairments, limitations, restrictions require compensatory strategies; and what impairments, limitations, restrictions cannot be affected by physical therapy interventions at all).*

With regard to the plan of care, management of people with ALS is complex because of the progressive and devastating nature of the disease, and the progressive number and severity of impairments, activity limitations, participation restrictions, and accompanying psychosocial issues that manifest. Future impairments, activity limitations, and participation restrictions need to be considered and management needs to be planned for accordingly.

Care requires a comprehensive and multidisciplinary approach. It is clear that Mrs. Jelly would benefit from other health care professionals' assessments and management, even though she was in the earlier stages of ALS. Specialized centers or clinics that meet rigorous standards set by the ALSA and the Muscular Dystrophy Association (MDA) are considered to be the most advantageous for the management of individuals with ALS. Research has found that patients attending a multi-disciplinary clinic lived longer than those in the general neurology cohort.[32]

The assessment a physical therapist would complete and area of assessment foci would be determined by the physical therapy setting, eg, whether the physical therapist is a member of a multi-disciplinary clinic and what other health care professionals are part of the team.

Plan of Care

Interventions

Interventions identified for Mrs. Jelly included the following:

- Patient-/client-related instruction regarding her current impairments, activity limitations and participation restrictions, the plan of care (also provided in written format), the discharge plan, and the reevaluation plan.

- Patient-/client-related instruction regarding energy conservation, sleep health and positioning, physical activity, and exercise log.
- A soft cervical collar to wear at work and during recreational walking.
- A work environment assessment and recommendations.
- A flexibility and strengthening exercise program.
- A revised recreational walking program.
- Referrals to other health care professionals (eg, Mrs. Jelly's neurologist, a speech language pathologist, a registered dietician, a psychologist, and an occupational therapist).

Clinician Comment *Based on Mrs. Jelly's history and presentation, the focus of physical therapy intervention for Mrs. Jelly was largely compensatory and preventive. Compensatory interventions were directed toward modifying activities, tasks or the environment to minimize limitations and restrictions (eg, cervical collar, energy conservation, work environment changes). Preventive intervention was directed toward minimizing potential impairments (eg, secondary effects of immobility).*

Proposed Frequency and Duration of Physical Therapy Visits

Mrs. Jelly would be scheduled for 4 physical therapy sessions initially with 3 sessions planned for interventions and education and 1 for reassessment. It was anticipated that as the disease progressed, Mrs. Jelly would benefit from additional physical therapy visits.

Anticipated Goals

1. Mrs. Jelly would demonstrate understanding of, and adhere to, use of the cervical collar (Visit #1).
2. Mrs. Jelly would demonstrate understanding of, and adhere to, use of daily energy conservation techniques, sleep health, and positioning (Visit #1).
3. Mrs. Jelly would demonstrate understanding of, and ability to use, the Borg CR-10 Rate of Perceived Exertion (RPE) scale[33] and a physical activity and exercise log to monitor exercise and activity effort (Visit #1).
4. Mrs. Jelly would demonstrate understanding of the rationale for and independence with a revised walking program and flexibility and strengthening exercise program (Visit #2).
5. Mrs. Jelly would have a good understanding of, and adhere to, work environment modifications to decrease muscle strain and fatigue (Visit #4).
6. Mrs. Jelly's cervical pain would decrease from 8/10 to 3/10 on the pain VAS (Visit #4).

ICF Model of Disablement for Mrs. Jelly

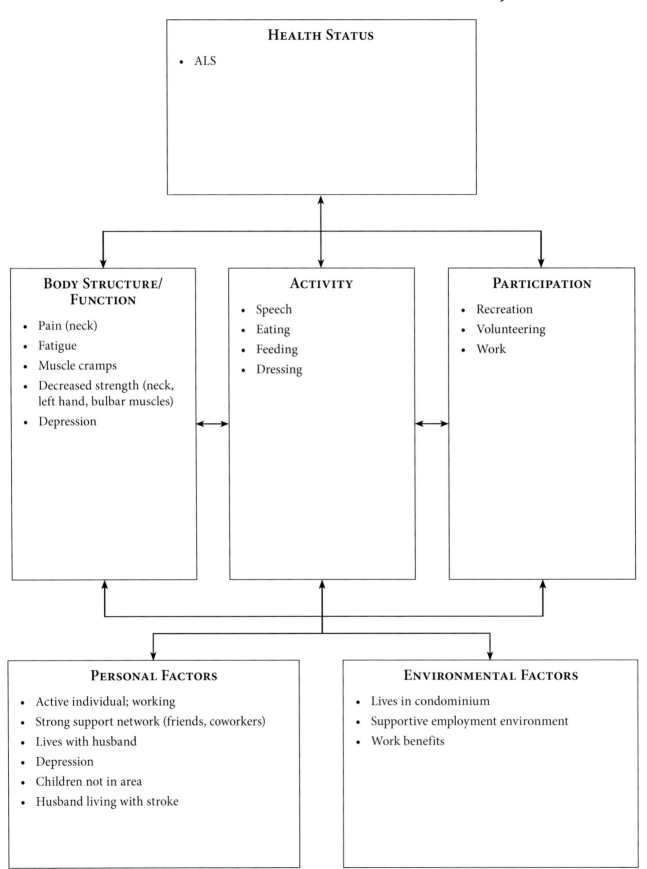

Expected Outcomes (by Reassessment Visit 4 to Occur 2 Weeks After Visit 3)

1. Mrs. Jelly would report minimal (1 to 2/10) to no cervical pain during work activities.

2. Mrs. Jelly would demonstrate excellent understanding and 100% adherence with energy conservation techniques, sleep health, and positioning, use of cervical collar, revised recreational walking program, flexibility and strengthening exercise program, use of RPE, and completion of the physical activity and exercise log.

3. Mrs. Jelly would demonstrate excellent understanding and 100% adherence with work environment modifications.

Discharge Plan

It was anticipated that Mrs. Jelly would be ready for discharge from physical therapy to her own care when she achieved the established anticipated goals and expected outcomes. The plan of care, including the discharge plan, was discussed with Mrs. Jelly who reported she was in agreement.

INTERVENTION

Coordination, Communication, and Documentation

Coordinated and ongoing dialogue with members of the multi-disciplinary team regarding current status, care, and plans for the future was essential. Ongoing communication with patient, family, referral sources, and other caregivers regarding progress toward goals would be pursued. Documentation would include all aspects of care, including initial examination/evaluation, daily treatment notes, telephone conversations, progress reports, reexaminations, and discharge summary.

Patient-/Client-Related Instructions

- Mrs. Jelly was informed about the plan of care, frequency of visits, and discharge plan.

- Mrs. Jelly received written and verbal information about energy conservation, sleep health and positioning, use of the cervical collar, use of the RPE, revised walking program, flexibility and strengthening exercise program (with figures), and physical activity and exercise log.

- Mrs. Jelly received written and verbal information about work environment modifications.

- Mrs. Jelly was provided the websites for ALSA and the MDA.

Clinician Comment *ALSA and MDA are national voluntary organizations that provide many functions and programs for people with ALS and their families and caregivers (eg, written and video educational materials, local education programs, patient and caregiver support groups, equipment loan programs, respite programs, transportation programs, advocacy programs, and ALS awareness programs).*

Printed educational materials can be downloaded and given to Mrs. Jelly.

Procedural Interventions

Prescription, Application, and, as Appropriate, Fabrication of Devices and Equipment (Assistive, Adaptive, Orthotic, Protective, Supportive, and Prosthetic)

Supportive Device

Mrs. Jelly was provided with a soft foam collar and instructed regarding use during work, prolonged sitting, and during recreational walking.

Clinician Comment *For mild to moderate cervical weakness, a soft foam collar is recommended. Soft collars are comfortable and usually well tolerated by patients, but wear-induced compressibility requires they be replaced frequently. For moderate to severe weakness, a semi-rigid or rigid collar is prescribed. These collars provide very firm support, but can be very warm, may cause discomfort at points of body contact, and, may feel confining. Although a soft collar is appropriate based on the assessment and has been prescribed, if Mrs. Jelly was agreeable, a semi-rigid collar could also be prescribed for the longer term—as the disease progresses, the cervical weakness will progress and a semi-rigid collar will be needed.*

Functional Training in Work (Job/School/Play), Community, and Leisure Integration or Reintegration, Including Instrumental Activities of Daily Living, Work Hardening, and Work Conditioning

Work Environment Recommendations

The following alterations to Mrs. Jelly's work station were recommended:

- Computer tabletop articulating forearm troughs to relieve muscle strain and weight of the limbs when working on the computer.

- Elevation of the computer screen to allow viewing at eye level and to avoid cervical muscle fatigue

- Full-back computer chair with head support.
- Ergonomic keyboard to reduce fatigue.

Energy Conservation

Mrs. Jelly was provided with written and verbal instruction about energy conservation, planning her daily and weekly activities, pacing activities to avoid increased fatigue.

Clinician Comment *Both the MDA and the ALSA websites have resource materials related to energy conservation—see http://www.als-mda.org/publications/everydaylifeals/ch2/ or http://web.alsa.org/site/DocServer/FYI_Minimizing_Fatigue.pdf?docID=29218.*

Physical Activity and Exercise Log

Mrs. Jelly was provided with a physical activity and exercise log to use until her reassessment visit. Written and verbal instruction regarding use of the log was provided.

Clinician Comment *A physical activity and exercise log that the physical therapist can review is an important component to include in the overall management plan for people with ALS, in particular when prescribing exercise. The patient should be educated in self-monitoring. The log should collect data about the activity or exercise, the level of exertion, the level of fatigue during and after, and "side effects" (eg, signs of overuse, which include: the inability to perform daily activities following exercise because of exhaustion or pain; a reduction in maximum muscle force that gradually recovers; or increased or excessive muscle cramping, soreness, fatigue, or fasciculations).*

Therapeutic Exercise Prescription

Flexibility Exercise Program Consisting of Stretching and Active Range of Motion Exercises

Mode

Upper extremity (UE), lower extremity (L/E), hands—Active ROM and stretching exercises

Intensity

ROM exercises—no greater than moderate effort

Stretching exercises—maintain stretch below discomfort point

Duration

20-second hold for each stretching exercise

10 to 15 minutes total each session

Frequency

5 repetitions of each exercise; 2 sessions per day (eg, U/E exercises [first session] and LE exercises [second session]).

Clinician Comment *An individualized flexibility exercise program composed of ROM and stretching exercises and targeting major muscles and joints is considered standard care for people with ALS. This type of exercise program is appropriate for Mrs. Jelly and is implemented for preventive purposes (eg, prevent contractures and maintain ROM). In addition, Mrs. Jelly is experiencing cramping with walking, so should be engaging in stretching exercises.*

Strengthening Exercise Program for Right Hand

Mode

Soft ball or Eggerciser

Intensity

Not greater than moderate effort

Duration

2 set of 8 repetitions of each exercise

Frequency

3 times per week

Clinician Comment *How advisable was it for Mrs. Jelly to be engaged in strengthening exercises and, if so, which muscles should be targeted?*

When designing a strengthening exercise program for a person with ALS, the physical therapist must take into consideration the stage of the disease, how quickly the disease is progressing (fast versus slow), the nature and severity of impairments (eg, respiratory function, cognitive impairments, fatigue), psychosocial and financial issues, and patient goals. Prescribing exercise, in particular strengthening (or aerobic) modes, is not a simple and straightforward process.

Reduced activity, particularly if prolonged, reduces function of the neuromuscular system, in addition to other systems. Strength loss through inactivity and disuse can significantly debilitate individuals with ALS, making them highly susceptible to deconditioning, and muscle and joint tightness leading to contractures and pain. Thus, a balance between overuse fatigue and disuse atrophy needs to be struck when prescribing strengthening (and aerobic) exercise.

The effects of exercise programs have not been extensively studied and are not well understood, despite the high incidence of muscle weakness in people with ALS. A Cochrane review of exercise for people with ALS identified only 2 studies that met the methodological quality inclusion criteria, indicating a dearth of randomized and well-controlled research. The 2 included studies were too small to determine to what extent exercise is of benefit for people with ALS. However, the mean difference in the primary outcome, function as measured by the ALS Functional Rating Scale, was statistically significant for the exercise group, and adverse effects, such as increased muscle cramping, muscle soreness or fatigue, were not reported by the investigators.[34]

Research indicates highly repetitive or heavy resistance exercise can cause prolonged loss of muscle strength in weakened, denervated muscle.[35] In individuals with other neuromuscular diseases,[36,37] research has found that overuse weakness does not occur in muscles with a Manual Muscle Test (MMT) grade of 3 or greater; moderate resistance exercises can increase strength in muscles with a MMT grade of 3 or greater; strength gains are proportional to initial muscle strength; and heavy eccentric exercise should be avoided. Exercise may produce functional benefits; however, the extent of psychological benefits have yet to be confirmed.

Mrs. Jelly had cervical extensor weakness and left hand weakness. Based on the findings and "complete picture," compensatory versus restorative interventions were more appropriate to address this weakness. Although a general strengthening program could be prescribed to maximize strength in nonaffected or mildly affected muscles in order to delay time to when function becomes impaired, because of fatigue, in Mrs. Jelly's case, it was better to focus on a revised walking program and active ROM exercises rather than specific UE and LE strengthening. Mrs. Jelly was right-hand dominant. Since prescribing strengthening exercises was an appropriate option to consider to increase or maintain her strength for functional purposes, this exercise would not have been excessively fatiguing.

Aerobic Capacity/Endurance Conditioning or Reconditioning

Mode
Walking program
Intensity
Self-selected pace
RPE = 3 on Borg CR-10 RPE
Duration
10 minutes per session
Frequency
2 times per day: once at noon and once after work

Clinician Comment *In the case of Mrs. Jelly, walking was an enjoyable and social activity and one of the few activities she had been continuing. Mrs. Jelly was also exhibiting signs and symptoms of depression. Thus, rather than completely eliminating walking as an activity, it was preferable to make the activity a safer one for her status. Initial first steps included: decreasing the strain and cervical muscle fatigue in order to decrease overall fatigue; implementing energy conservation strategies so that energy was conversed for the walking program; and, modifying the*

exercise program (eg, shorter sessions, RPE = 3, moderate). Signs and symptoms of overwork and fatigue could then be monitored, and the plan and walking program reassessed.

For people with ALS, exercise program goals include: maximizing functional capacity of the innervated muscle fibers; preventing or minimizing the effects of disuse atrophy; preventing limitations in ROM and muscle length; and maximizing aerobic capacity, endurance, and functional level for as long as possible.

Both the physical therapist and Mrs. Jelly need to recognize and accept that people with ALS will become weaker and more functionally limited despite any type or amount of exercise. Although modest improvements may occur at the onset of an exercise training program, the severity as well as the number of impairments will increase. Overall function will inevitably decrease over time.

People with ALS should be advised to exercise for several brief periods throughout the day, with sufficient rest in between. If signs of overuse occur (see physical activity and exercise log), exercises should be stopped until symptoms resolve, and further evaluation is conducted.

In people with ALS, the safe range for therapeutic exercise narrows, and the degree to which the range narrows is dependent on the extent of disease involvement and the rate of disease progression. A weak or denervated muscle is more susceptible to overwork damage because it is already functioning close to its maximal limits. ADL alone may cause impaired muscles to act as though in training and exercise that would improve normal muscles may actually cause overwork damage in impaired muscles. The remaining motor units will respond to training, and these motor units must work harder to handle a given amount of exercise stress.[38]

Special attention must be paid to developing an exercise program, in particular resistance or endurance, for people with ALS. Exercise programs should be at moderate to low intensities and should be carefully monitored. Exercise programs must be at a level that will minimize disuse atrophy, but be cautious enough to avoid fatigue and overwork, as both may be detrimental.[39] Thus, the physical therapist needs to continuously balance exercise "underwork" and exercise "overwork" and adjust the program (eg, type of exercise or activity, intensity) accordingly based on the individual's response to exercise, and other disease-specific factors (eg, respiratory impairments) in order to prevent excessive fatigue and potential overwork damage. People with ALS should be advised not to carry out any activities to the point of extreme fatigue, and should keep track of symptoms of overuse (see physical activity and exercise log). Once exercise becomes so tiring or is so difficult that it prevents the individual from completing daily activities, it is no longer appropriate.

REEXAMINATION

The first reexamination of Mrs. Jelly took place as planned, 2 weeks after Visit #3.

Subjective

Mrs. Jelly reported that she was wearing her cervical collar as directed. She reported that she no longer had severe neck pain. She was utilizing her energy-conversation strategies and was dividing up her exercise sessions throughout the day. She was participating in her walking program and reported no problems with her exercises or walking program. She reported that she did not experience any signs or symptoms of overwork postexercising.

Mrs. Jelly had successfully negotiated with her supervisor to have 2 20-minute rest periods during the work day, one mid-morning and one mid-afternoon. Mrs. Jelly reported that end-of-work-day fatigue was not as much of an issue anymore. She was even considering resuming 1 volunteer activity per week.

Mrs. Jelly reported that her neurologist had prescribed Celexa (citalopram) for her depressive symptoms. She had been taking the medication for a week at the time of the reassessment. She reported she "hasn't noticed much difference yet." Mrs. Jelly reported that she had appointments booked to see a speech language pathologist and registered dietician in the next 2 weeks. Her neurologist had provided information about a PEG and Mrs. Jelly was "thinking about this option."

Clinician Comment *When pervasive, depressive symptoms need to be treated aggressively with psychopharmacological medications. If left untreated psychosocial impairments can adversely affect an individual's ability to adapt, cope, and participate in the plan of care. Unfortunately, antidepressant medications usually take several weeks (up to 6 weeks) to work, and some clients may need to trial different medications to find one that is effective. Psychological well-being has been found to be an important prognostic factor. Individuals with psychological well-being were found to have significantly longer survival times compared to those with psychological distress. Mortality rates were 6.8 times greater in those experiencing psychological distress.[40] These findings were confirmed in a later study that found degree of physical disability, disease progression, and survival could be predicted by the patient's psychological status.[41]*

A PEG, a type of gastrostomy tube inserted via endoscopic surgery that creates a permanent opening into the stomach for the introduction of food, is useful for stabilizing body weight/mass. Although there is no firm evidence, for optimal safety and efficacy the PEG procedure should be offered to the patient and completed before the individual's FVC/VC falls below 50% of predicted.[25] Studies have found PEG insertion may prolong survival and survival was greatest for patients with a VC greater than 50% predicted at the time of the procedure.[42,43] It is important for physical therapists to be aware that a PEG does not prevent the risk of aspiration.[44,45]

Objective

Pain

Mrs. Jelly reported her neck pain was 0 to 1/10 in the morning upon waking and 2/10 by the end of some work days (VAS).

Posture

No changes noted.

Clinician Comment *No changes expected.*

Muscle Performance

Examination not completed.

Clinician Comment *The reexamination visit took place 2 weeks after the initial visits. Mrs. Jelly was not complaining of any new signs or symptoms, nor was she reported any signs or symptoms of overwork. Significant changes in muscle strength were not expected at this point in time. If Mrs. Jelly had new complaints of additional signs and symptoms or limitations or restrictions, reassessment of muscle strength would have been warranted.*

Functional Training in Work (Job/School/Play), Community, and Leisure Integration or Reintegration, Including Instrumental Activities of Daily Living, Work Hardening, and Work Conditioning

Mrs. Jelly had implemented the work environment recommendations as well as the energy conservation instructions identified for her. Mrs. Jelly's physical activity and exercise log were reviewed. Her verbal report of the lack of signs and symptoms of overwork was confirmed in her log entries.

Assessment

Mrs. Jelly implemented the recommendations and was managing well at the time of reassessment. As her disease progressed in the future, Mrs. Jelly would benefit from physical therapy to address any additional impairments, activity limitations, and participation restrictions that would appear.

Plan

Mrs. Jelly will be reevaluated in 3 months.

OUTCOMES

Discharge

Mrs. Jelly planned to continue with her program independently and would contact physical therapy before her next appointment, as needed.

Clinician Comment *Think about what might be next for Mrs. Jelly. It was likely that in 3 months, bulbar impairments would have progressed, her FVC might be decreased, L hand weakness would have progressed, and new impairments and activity limitations (UE > LE because of the contiguous nature of ALS) might be present. Additional compensatory interventions would likely need to be implemented and eventually "exercise" would be composed, more so, of functional performance activities.*

In terms of overall prognosis for Mrs. Jelly, people with bulbar-onset ALS have a poorer prognosis than those with limb-onset ALS. Five-year survival rates were reported to be 9% and 16% for those with bulbar-onset ALS, compared to 37% and 44% for limb-onset.[46,47] Fifty percent survival probability after initial symptom onset is slightly greater than 3 years, unless mechanical ventilation is used to sustain breathing.[1] In most individuals, death occurs within 3 to 5 years after diagnosis and usually results from respiratory failure.[48]

Think about you, as the physical therapist involved in Mrs. Jelly's care. Is there a role for you as a physical therapist as the disease progresses? What is the role?

REFERENCES

1. Haverkamp LJ, Appel V, Appel SH. Natural history of amyotrophic lateral sclerosis in a database population: validation of a scoring system and a model for survival prediction. *Brain.* 1995;118:707.
2. Brooks BR. The natural history of amyotrophic lateral sclerosis. In: Williams AC, ed. *Motor Neurone Disease.* London: Chapman and Hall; 1994:121.
3. Swash M. Clinical features and diagnosis of amyotrophic lateral sclerosis. In: Brown R Jr, Meininger V, Swash M, eds. *Amyotrophic Lateral Sclerosis.* London: Martin Dunitz Ltd; 2000:3.
4. Mitsumoto H, Chad DA, Pioro EK: Clinical features: signs and symptoms. In: Mitsumoto, H, Chad DA, Pioro EK, eds. *Amyotrophic Lateral Sclerosis.* Philadelphia, PA: F.A. Davis; 1998:47.
5. Rochester DF, Esau SA. Assessment of ventilatory function in patients with neuromuscular disease. *Clin Chest Med.* 1994;15(4):751-763.
6. Norris F, Shepherd R, Denys E, et al. Onset, natural history and outcome in idiopathic adult motor neuron disease. *J Neurol Sci.* 1993;118(1):48-55.
7. Strong MJ, Hudson AJ, Alvord WG. Familial amyotrophic lateral sclerosis, 1850-1989: a statistical analysis of the world literature. *Can J Neurol Sci.* 1991;18(1):45-58.
8. Rosen DR. Mutations in Cu/Zn superoxide dismutase gene are associated with familial amyotrophic lateral sclerosis. *Nature.* 1993;364(6435):362.
9. Brooks BR, Miller RG, Swash M, et al. El Escorial revisited: revised criteria for the diagnosis of amyotrophic lateral sclerosis. *Amyotroph Lateral Scler Other Motor Neuron Disord.* 2000;1(5):293-293.
10. de Carvalho M, Dengler R, Eisen A, et al. Electrodiagnosis criteria for diagnosis of ALS. Consensus of an International Symposium sponsored by IFCN. December 3-5, 2006, Awiji-shima, Japan.
11. Lacomblez L, Bensimon G, Leigh PN, Guillet P, Meininger V. Dose-ranging study of riluzole in amyotrophic lateral sclerosis. Amyotrophic Lateral Sclerosis/Riluzole Study Group II. *Lancet.* 1996;347(9013):1425-1431.
12. Bensimon G, Lacomblez L, Meininger V. A controlled trial of riluzole in amyotrophic lateral sclerosis. ALS/Riluzole Study Group. *N Engl J Med.* 1994;330(9):585-591.
13. Mathiowetz V, Kashman N, Volland G, Weber K, Dowe M, Rogers S. Grip and pinch strength: normative data for adults. *Arch Phys Med Rehabil.* 1984;66(2):69-74.
14. Pandyan AD, Johnson GR, Price CI, Curless RH, Barnes MP, Rodgers H. A review of the properties and limitations of the Ashworth and Modified Ashworth scales as measurements of spasticity. *Clin Rehabil.* 1999;13(5):373-383.
15. Beal MF. Aging, energy, and oxidative stress in neurodegenerative diseases. *Ann Neurol.* 1995;38:357.
16. Desport JC, Preux PM, Truong TC, Vallat JM, Sautereau D, Couratier P. Nutritional status is a prognostic factor for survival in ALS patients. *Neurology.* 1999;53(5):1059-1063.
17. Wilson CM, Grace GM, Munoz DG, He BP, Strong MJ. Cognitive impairment in sporadic ALS: a pathologic continuum underlying a multisystem disorder. *Neurology.* 2001;57(4):651-657.
18. Strong MJ, Grace GM, Orange JB, Leeper HA, Menon RS, Aere C. A prospective study of cognitive impairment in ALS. *Neurology.* 1999;53(8):1665-1670.
19. Abrahams S, Leigh PN, Harvey A, Vythelingum GN, Grisé D, Goldstein LH. Verbal fluency and executive dysfunction in amyotrophic lateral sclerosis (ALS). *Neuropsychologia.* 2000;38(6):734-747.
20. Abrahams S, Goldstein LH, Al-Chalabi A, et al. Relation between cognitive dysfunction and pseudobulbar palsy in amyotrophic lateral sclerosis. *J Neurol Neurosurg Psychiatry.* 1997;62(5):464-472.
21. Folstein MF, Folstein SE, McHugh PR. "Mini-mental state". A practical method for grading the cognitive state of patients for the clinician. *J Psychiatr Res.* 1975;12(3):189-198.
22. Miller RG, Jackson CE, Kasarskis EJ, et al. Practice Parameter update: the care of the patient with amyotrophic lateral sclerosis: multidisciplinary care, symptom management, and cognitive/behavioral impairment (an evidence-based review): report of the Quality Standards Subcommittee of the American Academy of Neurology. *Neurology.* 2009;73(15):1227-1233.
23. Bohannon RW, Smith MB. Interrater reliability of a modified Ashworth scale of muscle spasticity. *Phys Ther.* 1987;67(2):206-207.
24. Pandyan AD, Price CM, Barnes MP, Johnson GR. A biomechanical investigation into the validity of the Modified Ashworth scale as a measure of elbow spasticity. *Clin Rehabil.* 2003;17(3):290-293.
25. 25. Miller RG, Jackson CE, Kasarskis EJ, et al. Practice Parameter update: the care of the patient with amyotrophic lateral sclerosis: drug, nutritional, and respiratory therapies (an evidence-based review): report of the Quality Standards Subcommittee of the American Academy of Neurology. *Neurology.* 2009;73(15):1218-1226.
26. Kilmer DD. The role of exercise in neuromuscular disease. *Phys Med Rehabil Clin N Am.* 1998;9(1):115-125, vi.
27. Krupp LB, LaRocca NG, Muir-Nash J, Steinberg AD. The fatigue severity scale. Application to patients with multiple sclerosis and systemic lupus erythematosus. *Arch Neurol.* 1989;46(10):1121-1123.
28. Schwab R, England A. Projection technique for evaluating surgery in Parkinson's disease. In: Gillingham J, Donaldson I, eds. *Third Symposium on Parkinson's Disease.* Edinburgh, Scotland: Livingstone; 1969.

29. Cedarbaum JM, Stambler N, Malta E, et al. The ALSFRS-R: a revised ALS functional rating scale that incorporates assessments of respiratory function. *J Neurol Sci.* 1999;169(1-2):13-21.

30. Kaufmann P, Levy G, Montes J, et al. Excellent inter-rater, intra-rater, and telephone-administered reliability of the ALSFRS-R in a multicenter clinical trial. *Amyotroph Lateral Scler.* 2007;8(1):42-46.

31. Beck AT, Ward CH, Mendelson M, Mock J, Erbaugh J. An inventory for measuring depression. *Arch Gen Psych.* 1961;4:561-571.

32. Traynor BJ, Alexander M, Corr B, Frost E, Hardiman O. Effect of a multidisciplinary amyotrophic lateral sclerosis (ALS) clinic on ALS survival: a population based study, 1996-2000. *J Neurol Neurosurg Psychiatry.* 2003;74(9):1258-1261.

33. Borg G. *Borg's Perceived Exertion and Pain Scales.* Champaign, IL: Human Kinetics; 1998.

34. Dalbello-Haas V, Florence JM, Krivickas LS. Therapeutic exercise for people with amyotrophic lateral sclerosis or motor neuron disease. Cochrane Database Syst Rev. 2008;2:CD005229.

35. McCartney N, Moroz D, Garner SH, McComas AJ. The effects of strength training in patients with selected neuromuscular disorders. *Med Sci Sports Exerc.* 1988;20(4):362-368.

36. Kilmer DD, McCrory MA, Wright NC, Aitkens SG, Bernauer EM. The effect of a high resistance exercise program in slowly progressive neuromuscular disease. *Arch Phys Med Rehabil.* 1994;75(5):560-563.

37. Aitkens SG, McCrory MA, Kilmer DD, Bernauer EM. Moderate resistance exercise program: its effect in slowly progressive neuromuscular disease. *Arch Phys Med Rehabil.* 1993;74(7):711-715.

38. Coble NO, Maloney FP. Effects of exercise in neuromuscular disease. In: Maloney FP, Burks JS, Ringel SP, eds. *Interdisciplinary Rehabilitation of Multiple Sclerosis and Neuromuscular Disorders.* New York: Lippincott; 1985:228.

39. Ribchester RR. Activity-dependent and independent synaptic interactions during reinnervation of partially denervated rat muscle. *J Physiol.* 1988;401:53-75.

40. McDonald ER, Wiedenfeld SA, Hillel A, Carpenter CL, Walter RA. Survival in amyotrophic lateral sclerosis: the role of psychological factors. *Arch Neurol.* 1994;51(1):17-23.

41. Johnston M, Earll A, Giles M, McClenahan R, Stevens D, Morrison V. Mood as a predictor of disability and survival in patients diagnosed with ALS/MND. *Br J Health Psych.* 1999;4(2):127-136.

42. Mathus-Vliegen LM, Louwerse LS, Merkus MP, Tytgat GN, Vianney de Jong JM. Percutaneous endoscopic gastrostomy in patients with amyotrophic lateral sclerosis and impaired pulmonary function. *Gastrointest Endosc.* 1994;40(4):463,-469.

43. Mazzini L, Corrà T, Zaccala M, Mora G, Del Piano M, Galante M. Percutaneous endoscopic gastrostomy and enteral nutrition in amyotrophic lateral sclerosis. *Neurology.* 1995;242(10):695-698.

44. Jarnagin WR, Duh QY, Mulvihill SJ, Ridge JA, Schrock TR, Way LW. The efficacy and limitations of percutaneous endoscopic gastrostomy. *Arch Surg.* 1992;127(3):261-264.

45. Kadakia SC, Sullivan HO, Starnes E. Percutaneous endoscopic gastrostomy or jejunostomy and the incidence of aspiration in 79 patients. *Am J Surg.* 1992;164(2):114-118.

46. Rosen AD. Amyotrophic lateral sclerosis. Clinical features and prognosis. *Arch Neurol.* 1978;35(10):638-642.

47. Tysnes OB, Vollset SE, Larsen JP, Aarli JA. Prognostic factors and survival in amyotrophic lateral sclerosis. *Neuroepidemiology.* 1994;13(5):226-235.

48. Ringel SP, Murphy JR, Alderson MK, et al. The natural history of amyotrophic lateral sclerosis. *Neurology.* 1993;43(7):1316-1322.

Individuals With Multi-System Disorders

Melanie A. Gillar, PT, DPT, MA

CHAPTER OBJECTIVES

- List the most common risk factors for cancer and discuss which could be prevented through behavioral changes.

- Identify the differences between benign neoplasms and malignant neoplasms.

- Discuss cell differentiation and the difference between well-differentiated cells and cancer cells.

- Describe how radiation therapy, chemotherapy, and immunotherapy work to treat cancer.

- Summarize the potential benefits of exercise in individuals with cancer.

- Summarize exercise prescription and testing for individuals with cancer.

- Name the 3 main types of diabetes and explain how they are similar and/or different.

- Identify and describe the 3 tests most commonly used to diagnose diabetes.

- List the risk factors for diabetes that can be modified and those that cannot.

- Discuss abnormal insulin metabolism in individuals with diabetes.

- Identify exercise prescription guidelines for individuals with diabetes.

- List the major characteristics of fracture blisters.

- Contrast and compare acute compartment syndrome and chronic compartment syndrome.

- Describe complex regional pain syndrome (CRPS) and distinguish between CRPS I and CRPS II.

- Identify the signs and symptoms of fat embolism syndrome.

CHAPTER OUTLINE

- Cancer
  - Epidemiology
  - Pathology/Pathophysiology
  - Physical Therapy Management
    - Exercise and Cancer
    - Exercise Testing and Prescription
    - General Considerations
- Diabetes Mellitus
  - Prediabetes
  - Diagnosis: Diabetes, Prediabetes, and Gestational Diabetes
  - Epidemiology
  - Associated Morbidity/Mortality
  - Associated Costs
  - Pathology/Pathophysiology
    - Insulin Metabolism
    - Type 1 Diabetes
    - Type 2 Diabetes
    - Gestational Diabetes Mellitus

Coglianese D, ed. *Clinical Exercise Pathophysiology for Physical Therapy: Examination, Testing, and Exercise Prescription for Movement-Related Disorders* (pp 533-574).
© 2015 Taylor & Francis Group.

Advances in science, medicine, and rehabilitation in the latter part of the 20th century have produced large numbers of citizens who survive into their 70s, 80s, and 90s. This phenomenon is often referred to as the "graying of America." Concurrently there have been aggressive advances in managing both acute and chronic disease and the development of life-sustaining technologies in critical care and trauma that support the recovery and maintenance of life. The result is that many Americans are successfully living and functioning with multi-system disorders. Many, if not most of these individuals, are unwilling to merely survive, but wish to thrive in their remaining years. Physical therapists often manage the care of these individuals with multi-system disorders to address the functional limitations associated with the movement-related impairments that compromise an individual's ability to participate and thrive.

Physical therapists who practice in acute or chronic care settings, in a school system, in rehabilitation facilities, in home health or in the outpatient environment will all receive referrals for patients and clients with multi-system disorders. Often they will elicit the history, signs, symptoms, and associated information that would identify these people when interviewing someone who has been referred for what appears to be a "simple" musculoskeletal injury. It is not uncommon for a physical therapist to learn during a patient interview that the patient has a history of cancer, heart disease, hypertension or diabetes in addition to the presenting complaints from a sprain or strain. The possibility of new disease development, disease progression or disease recurrence exists with any patient. Physical therapists can recognize that possibility and address all such issues by attending to details during the examination. The challenge of rehabilitation in

this population is to provide the interventional support that allows patients to achieve successful outcomes and remain functional despite the existence of advanced chronic disease, severe trauma, and multi-system disorders. This chapter will consider the physiology of abnormal cell development that affects normal structure and function in patients with cancer, diabetes, and musculoskeletal trauma, some of the more common multi-system disorders that occur in patients who are referred to physical therapists for the management of their movement related impairments. Each section in this chapter initiates discussion with the epidemiology and pathology/pathophysiology of these multi-system disorders and then examines how the patient/client management model described in the *Guide to Physical Therapist Practice* can and should be applied to management of these patient populations.

CANCER

The term *cancer* does not describe a single disease but refers to more than 100 different diseases.[1,2] This group of diseases is characterized by uncontrolled growth and spread of abnormal cells.[2-4] Cancer can originate in almost any part of the body and behaves differently depending on its organ of origin.[1-3] When cancer cells spread and travel to another part of the body, this is referred to as metastasis. Regardless of where a cancer may spread, it is always named for the body organ of origin and takes its characteristics with it to the new site.[2,3] For example, metastatic breast cancer in the lungs will continue to behave like breast cancer and if viewed under a microscope will continue to look like a cancer that originated in the breast.[2]

Just as cancer is not a single disease, there is more than one cause of cancer. Causative agents are usually divided into 2 categories, external or environmental (tobacco, chemicals, radiation, and infectious organisms) and internal or genetic (inherited mutations, hormones, immune conditions, and mutations that occur from metabolism).[4,5] The American Cancer Society (ACS) estimates that 5% of all cancers are genetic while the rest are related to other factors, the result of damage (mutations) to genes that occur over a lifetime.[4] It is thought that most cancers develop as a result of multiple environmental, viral, and genetic agents working together or repeated exposure to a single carcinogenic (cancer-producing) agent.[1,5]

According to the ACS all cancers caused by cigarette smoking and heavy use of alcohol could be prevented completely.[4] Research suggests that about one-third of the cancer deaths that were expected to occur in 2009 were related to nutrition, physical inactivity, and overweight or obesity and therefore could have been prevented (Box 13-1).[6] Some cancers are related to infectious agents, such as hepatitis B virus, human papillomavirus, human immunodeficiency virus, *Helicobacter pylori*, and others and could be prevented through behavioral changes, vaccines or antibiotics. In 2009 it was expected that more than 1 million skin cancers would be diagnosed. These cancers could have been prevented by appropriate protection from sun exposure.

Epidemiology

Cancer is second only to heart disease as a cause of death in the United States.[7] In fact, 1 in every 4 deaths in the United States is due to cancer.[4,8] However, when deaths are aggregated by age, starting in 1999 statistics demonstrated that cancer surpassed heart disease as the leading cause of death for people under the age of 85.[8,9] In 2009, the ACS estimated that there would be a total of 1,479,350 new cancer cases and an expected 562,340 deaths from cancer in the United States. This translates to more than 1500 deaths each day from cancer (Table 13-1).[4,8]

Anyone can develop cancer. The risk of developing cancer increases as we age. Approximately 77% of all cancers are diagnosed at age 55 and older.[4] In the United States, the lifetime risk for men of all races developing cancer is a little less than 1 in 2 while for women of all races the risk is a little more than 1 in 3.[4,8,10] The National Cancer Institute (NCI) estimates that as of January 2005, there were ~11.1 million Americans alive who had a history of cancer.[4] Some of these individuals were cancer free while others had continued evidence of their disease and may have been undergoing treatment.

In early stages, most cancers are asymptomatic. Cancer is most often detected or diagnosed after a tumor can be felt or when other symptoms develop. These symptoms may develop because the cancer has grown large enough to impinge on nearby organs, blood vessels, and nerves. Unexplained weight loss, fever, fatigue, pain, and changes in the skin are some of the nonspecific signs and symptoms of cancer. However, there are many other conditions that may cause these symptoms as well. Other signs and symptoms may be more indicative of cancer. These include changes in bowel habits or bladder function, sores that do not heal, unusual bleeding or discharge, thickening or a lump in the breast or other body part, indigestion or difficulty swallowing, change in a wart or mole, a nagging cough or hoarseness. Other cancers, however, develop in places where there may be no symptoms until the cancer has grown quite large. Pancreatic cancer is an example of this type of cancer. By the time there are signs and symptoms, the cancer has usually reached an advanced stage.[11] The earlier a cancer is diagnosed, the more likely it is that treatment will be successful and that the cancer can be cured. When a physical therapist is interviewing an individual over the age of 50 who presents with the nonspecific signs and symptoms of cancer, or, those signs and symptoms that are more indicative of cancer, they should consider the possibility of cancer.

The ACS, the Centers for Disease Control and Prevention (CDC), the NCI, and the North American Association of Central Cancer Registries (NAACCR) collaborated to produce an annual report to the nation on the current status of cancer in the United States, issuing their first report in 1998. That first report documented a sustained decline in cancer

Box 13-1. Most Common Risk Factors for Cancer

- Age
- Certain hormones
- Tobacco
- Heredity
- Sunlight
- Alcohol
- Ionizing radiation
- Nutrition
- Certain chemicals and other substances
- Physical inactivity
- Some viruses and bacteria
- Overweight

Adapted from National Cancer Institute. October 4, 2006. www.cancer.gov/cancertopics/wyntk/overview/page4. Accessed May 14, 2010.

death rates for the first time since national record keeping was begun in the 1930s.[12] Since then, subsequent reports have confirmed this finding and provided updates. In their report published in 2010, death rates declined for the 3 most common cancers in men (lung, prostate, and colorectal cancers) and for 2 of the 3 leading cancers in women (breast and colorectal cancer; Box 13-2).[13] The 2009 statistics further delineated the decline in death rates by 2.0% per year from 2001 and 2005 in men and by 1.6% per year in women from 2002 and 2005.[8] (This compares with declines of 1.5% in men from 1993 to 2001 and 0.8% per year in women from 1994 to 2002.)

The 5-year relative survival rate for all cases of cancers diagnosed between 1996 and 2004 is 66%.[4] Survival rates vary greatly depending on the type of cancer and stage at diagnosis. The 5-year relative survival rate represents the percentage of cancer patients who are living 5 years after diagnosis relative to persons without cancer regardless of whether they are disease free, have relapsed or are currently undergoing treatment. It is important to remember that 5-year relative survival rates are most useful for monitoring progress in the early detection and treatment of cancer and they do not represent the proportion of people who are cured permanently since cancer deaths can occur beyond 5 years after diagnosis.

The overall costs for cancer are considerable. The National Institutes of Health (NIH) estimates that in the year 2008, a total of $228.1 billion was spent on cancer; $93.2 billion went to direct medical costs (total of all health expenditures), $18.8 billion for indirect morbidity costs (lost productivity due to illness) and $116.1 billion for indirect mortality costs (lost productivity due to premature death).[4]

TABLE 13-1. NEW CANCER CASES AND DEATHS BY SELECT CANCER SITES AND SEX: 2014 UNITED STATES ESTIMATES

ESTIMATED NEW CASES		ESTIMATED DEATHS	
Male	*Female*	*Male*	*Female*
Prostate 233,000 (27%)	Breast 232,670 (29%)	Lung and bronchus 86,930 (28%)	Lung and bronchus 72,330 (26%)
Lung and bronchus 116,000 (14%)	Lung and bronchus 108,210 (13%)	Prostate 29,480 (10%)	Breast 40,000 (15%)
Colon and rectum 71,830 (8%)	Colon and rectum 65,000 (8%)	Colon and rectum 26,270 (8%)	Colon and rectum 24,040 (9%)
Urinary bladder 56,390 (7%)	Uterine corpus 52,630 (6%)	Pancreas 20,170 (7%)	Pancreas 19,420 (7%)
Melanoma of the skin 43,890 (5%)	Thyroid 47,790 (6%)	Liver and intrahepatic bile duct 15,870 (5%)	Ovary 14,270 (5%)
Kidney and renal pelvis 39,140 (5%)	Non-Hodgkin's lymphoma 32,530 (4%)	Leukemia 14,040 (5%)	Leukemia 10,050 (4%)
Non-Hodgkin's lymphoma 38,270 (4%)	Melanoma of the skin 32,210 (4%)	Esophagus 12,450 (4%)	Uterine corpus 8,590 (3%)
Leukemia 30,100 (4%)	Kidney and renal pelvis 24,780 (3%)	Urinary bladder 11,170 (4%)	Non-Hodgkin's lymphoma 8,590 (3%)
Oral cavity and pharynx 30,220 (4%)	Ovary 21,980 (3%)	Non-Hodgkin's lymphoma 10,470 (3%)	Liver and intrahepatic bile duct 7,130 (3%)
Pancreas 23,530 (3%)	Pancreas 22,890 (3%)	Kidney and renal pelvis 8,900 (3%)	Brain and other nervous system 6,230 (2%)
All other sites 167,850	All other sites 169,630	All other sites 83,160	All other sites 65,130
All sites 855,220 (100%)	All sites 810,320 (100%)	All sites 310,010 (100%)	All sites 275,710 (100%)

*Excludes basal and squamous cell skin cancers and in situ carcinoma except urinary bladder.
Percentages may not total 100% due to rounding
Reprinted with permission from the American Cancer Society. Cancer Facts & Figures 2014. Atlanta, GA: American Cancer Society; 2014.

Pathology/Pathophysiology

Normal, healthy cells grow, divide, and die in an orderly fashion. Cancer cells continue to grow and divide to form new abnormal cells.[3] A neoplasm (often referred to as a tumor) is the abnormal mass of tissue that results from the failure of cells to divide normally and die within the expected time frame. Neoplasms can be benign or malignant. Benign neoplasms have the same cell type as the parent cell, but grow at an abnormal rate.[14] They do not metastasize nor do they invade the surrounding tissue.[14,15] They are usually encapsulated.[1] Benign neoplasms cause problems when they grow large enough to compress other organs and interfere with

vital functions.[1,14] Alternatively, malignant neoplasms have the tendency to grow rapidly and spread widely. Malignant neoplasms extensively infiltrate and invade the surrounding tissue.[1] With their rapid rate of growth, malignant neoplasms tend to compress blood vessels and outgrow their blood supply with resultant tissue ischemia and necrosis.

Cells divide and bear offspring during a process called cell proliferation. Cell proliferation is normally regulated so that the number of cells that are actively dividing equals the number of cells dying or being shed. Cell differentiation is defined as the process whereby cells are transformed into different and more specialized cell types. Cell differentiation determines the structure, function, and life span of a cell.

BOX 13-2. TOP 15 CANCER SITES IN MEN AND WOMEN

MALE	FEMALE
• Prostate	• Breast
• Lung and fronchus	• Lung and bronchus
• Colon and rectum	• Colon and rectum
• Urinary bladder	• Corpus and uterus, not otherwise specified (NOS)
• Melanoma of the skin	• Melanoma of the skin
• Non-Hodgkin's lymphoma	• Non-Hodgkin's lymphoma
• Kidney and renal pelvis	• Thyroid
• Leukemia	• Ovary
• Oral cavity and pharynx	• Pancreas
• Pancreas	• Leukemia
• Stomach	• Kidney and renal pelvis
• Liver and intrahepatic bile duct	• Urinary bladder
• Esophagus	• Cervix uteri
• Brain and other nervous system	• Oral cavity and pharynx
• Myeloma	• Brain and other nervous system

Adapted from Edwards BK, Ward E, Kohler BA, et al. Annual report to the nation on the status of cancer, 1975-2006, featuring colorectal cancer trends and impact of interventions (risk factors, screening, and treatment) to reduce future rates. *Cancer.* 2010,116(3):544-573.

Well-differentiated cells are no longer able to divide and bear offspring. Cancer cells fail to undergo normal cell proliferation and differentiation processes. Because cancer cells lack cell differentiation, they do not function properly nor do they die in the same time frame as normal cells. Altered cell differentiation also results in changes in cell characteristics and cell function that distinguishes cancer cells from fully differentiated normal cells. The inability of cancer cells to differentiate prevents cancer cells from performing their normal functions and results in a variety of tissue changes including pain, cachexia, decreased immunity, anemia, leukopenia, and thrombocytopenia.[14] Because tumor cells take the place of normally functioning parenchymal tissue, the initial symptoms of cancer usually reflect the site of involvement. Lung cancer, for example, usually presents with impaired respiratory function.[1]

Metastasis is the term used to describe the development of a secondary cancer in a location distant from the location of the primary cancer. With metastasis, cancer cells travel to other areas of the body via the blood or lymphatic systems. The most common sites for cancer metastases are the lungs, bone, liver, and brain.[15] With spread via the circulatory system, the blood-borne cancer cells typically follow the venous flow that drains the site of the neoplasm.[1] The lymphatic channels empty into the venous system as well, so even with spread via the lymphatic channels, cancer cells that survive may eventually gain access to the circulatory system. Not all people with metastatic cancer have symptoms. When there are symptoms, the type and frequency of the symptoms depend on the size and location of the metastasis.[15] For example, cancer that has metastasized to the bone frequently causes pain and may result in bone fractures, while cancer that metastasizes to the brain may cause a variety of symptoms that include seizures, headaches, and dizziness.

According to the ACS, there are 3 major types of treatment for cancer: surgery, radiation therapy (RT), and chemotherapy.[16] Surgery is the oldest form of cancer treatment and can be used in combination with other treatments. Surgery and radiation are used to treat localized cancers while chemotherapy is particularly helpful when used to treat cancer that is widespread or has metastasized. Another form of cancer treatment is immunotherapy. It is relatively new compared to the 3 main forms of cancer treatment and still plays a fairly small role in treating most cancers.[17]

RT is the use of ionizing radiation to kill cancer cells and to shrink tumors. Radiation may come from an external source (external-beam RT) or it can be delivered by radioactive material placed in the body, near the cancer cells (internal RT, implant therapy or brachytherapy). RT works by injuring or destroying cells in the area being treated by damaging their genetic material. This makes it impossible for cancer cells to continue to grow and divide.[18] RT damages both cancer cells and healthy cells though most normal, healthy cells recover from the effects of radiation and resume normal function.

It is well known that RT, especially external-beam RT, causes significant long-term or chronic changes to the connective tissue.[5] Though changes such as fibrosis, atrophy, and contraction of tissue can occur to any irradiated area, this is especially true of collagen. Edema, decreased range of motion (ROM), and impaired function are some of the impairments associated with fibrosis of connective tissue. Radiation also has a fibrotic effect on the circulatory and lymphatic systems. This is typically seen as a loss of elasticity and contractility of the irradiated vessels that transport the blood, lymph, and waste products from the area being treated. This may result in lymphedema or decreased vascularity of some of the tissues.

Chemotherapy uses drugs to destroy cancer cells. A combination of drugs has been found to be more effective than treatment with one drug alone. These drugs destroy cancer cells by preventing them from growing or multiplying. Chemotherapy can also harm normal, healthy cells, especially those that divide quickly.[19] The side effects from chemotherapy are a result of this damage to healthy cells. Fortunately, healthy cells usually repair themselves after chemotherapy.

Chemotherapy drugs can be classified as either cell cycle specific or cell cycle nonspecific.[1] Drugs are classified as cell cycle specific when they exert their action during a specific phase of the cell cycle. Methotrexate, an antimetabolite agent, works by interfering with DNA synthesis thus interrupting the S phase of the cell cycle. In contrast, cell cycle-nonspecific agents exert their effect during all phases of the cell cycle. Cytoxan (cyclophosphamide), an alkylating agent,[5] acts by disrupting DNA when cells are in their resting state and when they are dividing.[1] Cell cycle-specific and cell cycle-nonspecific chemotherapy drugs are often combined to treat cancer since they differ in their mechanisms of action.

Immunotherapy, also referred to as biologic therapy or biotherapy, uses the body's immune system to fight diseases, including cancer.[17] It may be used alone but is most often used as an adjuvant to enhance the effects of the primary therapy. The 2 main types of immunotherapy are active immunotherapies and passive immunotherapies.[20] Active immunotherapies act by stimulating the body's own immune system to fight the disease. Passive immunotherapies use components of the immune system (such as antibodies) made in the lab to start the attack on the disease. At present, monoclonal antibodies (passive immunotherapies) are the most widely used form of cancer immunotherapy.[20,21] Two commonly used monoclonal antibodies are Herceptin (trastuzumab) and Rituxan (rituximab).[5,21] Herceptin is used to treat metastatic breast cancer in patients whose tumors produce excess amounts of human epidermal growth factor receptor 2 (HER-2) protein. Rituxan is used in the treatment of non-Hodgkin's lymphoma.

Fatigue is the most common side effect reported by patients undergoing cancer treatments and can be a side effect of surgery, RT, and chemotherapy. It has been reported that ~90% of cancer patients experience cancer-related fatigue (CRF) during RT or chemotherapy.[22] The National Comprehensive Cancer Center (NCCN) Fatigue Guidelines Committee developed the most commonly used definition of CRF. They defined CRF as "an unusual, persistent, subjective sense of tiredness related to cancer or cancer treatment that interferes with usual functioning."[23] The etiology of CRF is poorly understood and the relative contributions of the disease itself, the treatment modalities, and comorbid conditions remain unclear.[24] The current thinking is that the etiology of CRF likely involves the dysregulation of a number of interrelated physiological, biochemical, and psychological systems.[23,24] CRF is different from the fatigue experienced after the flu, exercise or other exertion. It has both subjective and objective components and may include symptoms such as physical weakness or tiredness, depression, impaired cognitive function, and impaired ability to sustain social relationships.[23] A recently published review in the Cochrane Database of Systematic Reviews evaluated the effect of exercise on CRF.[25] Twenty-eight studies were included in this review. The results of the review suggest that exercise can be helpful in reducing fatigue both during and after treatment for cancer. However, there was insufficient evidence to determine the best type or intensity of exercise for reducing the fatigue associated with cancer. This clearly presents an opportunity for management by physical therapists as well as for further research to determine the most effective exercise parameters (best type of exercise [aerobic versus resistance], mode, frequency, intensity, and duration of exercise) to assist in the management of CRF. Other impairments that are common in cancer patients and managed by physical therapists include impaired cardiorespiratory endurance, lymphedema, pain, muscle weakness, and neuropathy.

Physical Therapy Management

Exercise and Cancer

There has been an abundance of research on the benefits of exercise in the general population. In comparison, research on the benefits of exercise in individuals with cancer is still in its infancy. The traditional recommendations for individuals with cancer included rest and limiting physical activity. Though that still may be the case if movement causes severe pain, rapid heart rate or shortness of breath, beginning in the late 1980s research demonstrated that moderate intensity aerobic exercise training was of benefit to individuals with cancer throughout the various stages of treatment, recovery, remission, and palliative care.[14,26] This research concluded that not only did exercise improve physiological performance measures, but there were also psychological benefits including enhanced quality of life (QOL). Some of the possible benefits of exercise may include[27]:

- Improved balance, lower risk of falls and fractures

- Prevention of muscle atrophy due to inactivity

- Reduced risk of heart disease

- Reduced risk of osteoporosis

- Improved blood flow to the legs and decreased risk of blood clots

- Decreased nausea
- Fewer symptoms of fatigue
- Improved flexibility and strength
- Improved self-esteem
- Enhanced self-confidence and independence
- Lower risk of anxiety and depression
- Better weight control

Though the ideal level of exercise for individuals with cancer has not yet been determined, an effective exercise program should be customized for the individual's current level of fitness/functioning and include activities directed at improving aerobic conditioning, muscular strength, and flexibility.

Exercise Testing and Prescription

For individuals with cancer, whether they are currently undergoing active treatment or have had cancer in the past, it is absolutely essential that a complete history, systems review, and examination (including functional exercise testing) be performed prior to beginning any exercise program. When managing individuals with cancer the focus is on identifying signs and symptoms that would indicate the cancer itself and/or the cancer treatments have had an impact on cardiorespiratory function, muscular performance, the integumentary system, sensory integrity, and functional abilities.

Exercise testing prior to beginning an exercise program is essential in this population. An exercise test will assess whether it is safe for an individual with cancer to begin an exercise program and provide the data that will allow for the design of an individualized exercise prescription.[14] The exercise test performed in this population is typically a submaximal test. These submaximal exercise tests can be field tests, clinical tests or the more formal graded exercise test. Field tests provide information on a subject's fitness category and include the 6- and 12-Minute Walk Tests, the Cooper 1.5 Mile Walk Test, the Rockport Fitness Test, and the 12-Minute Run Test. Clinical exercise tests such as the Timed Up & Go Test, the Modified Shuttle Walk, and the Bag and Carry Test provide additional information on coordination, balance, and motor planning. Submaximal graded exercise tests appropriate for individuals with cancer include the Modified Bruce Treadmill Test, the Astrand-Rhyming Cycle Ergometer Test as well as the Single Stage Submaximal Walking Test. Graded exercise testing provides good predictive information on the individual's maximal oxygen (O_2) consumption and level of fitness. As always, the history and systems review will direct the selection of the appropriate exercise test for each individual. Graded exercise tests are appropriate for individuals with a complex medical history or when there is a need to assess potential risk factors associated with performing exercise. The American College of Sports Medicine (ACSM) recommends examination of the cardiovascular system with a graded exercise test with 12-lead electrocardiogram (EKG) in individuals with any of the following:

- Known cardiac, pulmonary or metabolic disease
- Two or more of the risk factors for cardiac disease such as elevated cholesterol levels, smoking, hypertension or diabetes mellitus
- One or more of the following signs/symptoms of cardiac disease such as dizziness, chest pain, irregular heart rates or rhythms, or shortness of breath
- Chemotherapy agents that are toxic to the heart or lung such as doxorubicin hydrochloride (Adriamycin) or bleomycin sulfate (Blenoxane)
- RT that may have caused pulmonary fibrosis, pneumonitis or pericarditis

As discussed earlier in this section, research has found that moderate-intensity aerobic exercise training was beneficial to individuals with cancer. Moderate exercise is defined as activity that takes as much effort as a brisk walk.[28] Two of the methods for determining training heart rate (HR) for aerobic exercise training are the heart rate reserve (HRR) also known as the Karvonen method and the maximum heart rate (HR_{max}). These methods can be difficult to use in this population since individuals with cancer may have inappropriate HR responses to exercise and large physiologic changes on a day-to-day basis from the disease, their treatments or changes in medications.[14] Alternative methods for determining exercise intensity in this population include HR response based on O_2 consumption or metabolic equivalent (MET) levels and Borg's Rating of Perceived Exertion Scale (RPE). Drouin and Pfalzer[14] have suggested 3 intensities of exercise training for individuals with cancer (Table 13-2). The high- and moderate-intensity aerobic exercise training should be preceded by a 5- to 10-minute warm-up period[27] and followed by a 5- to 10-minute cool-down period.[14,27]

The generalized weakness and deconditioning associated with cancer treatments can be more debilitating than the disease itself and not every person with cancer will be able to participate in moderate intensity aerobic exercise training. Though 30 minutes per day of exercise training is optimal, this may not be possible for severely deconditioned individuals. Research has demonstrated that cardiorespiratory fitness gains are similar when physical activity is divided into 3 10-minute sessions and would be an option for getting these individuals started on an aerobic exercise training program.[28] Individuals who are confined to bed or who are ambulating less than 50% of the time[5] and those who fatigue with mild exertion may benefit from low levels of physical activity such as ROM exercises and gentle resistance exercises until their tolerance for activity improves.[5,14]

The goal of exercise in individuals recovering from cancer treatments or in remission is to return them to their prior level of function both physically and psychologically. For this population participation in aerobic exercise training can lead to improved fitness, physical work capacity, and cardiovascular response to exercise. They typically begin with moderate intensity exercise training and then progress to increased levels of training.[14]

TABLE 13-2. SUGGESTED INTENSITIES OF EXERCISE TRAINING FOR INDIVIDUALS WITH CANCER

	EXERCISE PRESCRIPTION	
High-intensity training (to promote fitness)	30 to 45 minutes, 3 to 5 days per week 70 to 90% of HR_{max} (60% to 85% HRR)	RPE 14 to 16
Moderate-intensity training (to promote health)	Accumulate 30 minutes most days per week 50% to 70% HR_{max} (40% to 60% HRR)	RPE 11 to 13
Low-intensity training (activity to maintain function and prevent deconditioning)	3 to 5 minutes of activity that is well tolerated several times per day or below 50% of HR_{max}	Gradually increase exercise duration and intensity

RPE: rate of perceived exertion; HRR: heart rate reserve; HR_{max}: maximum heart rate.

Adapted from Drouin J, Pfalzer, L. Cancer and Exercise. *National Center on Physical Activity and Disability (NCPAD)*. March 5, 2009. http://www.ncpad.org/disability/fact_sheet.php?sheet=195. Accessed May 14, 2010.

General Considerations

There are certain precautions and contra-indications specific to cancer patients[14,27]:

- Monitoring vital signs during exercise is essential in the immunosuppressed population. Cancer patients should be watched closely for signs of cardiopulmonary compromise including dyspnea, pallor, diaphoresis, and fatigue during exercise. Patients should be instructed to monitor their pulse rate, respiratory rate, and BP when exercising on their own.

- The RPE should not exceed 11 (light) to 13 (somewhat hard) for moderate-intensity training or submaximal testing.

- Patients should be advised not to exercise within 2 hours of chemotherapy or RT. Increased circulatory response resulting from exercise may have a potentially negative impact on the patient.

- In the presence of anemia, adjustments may need to be made in exercise intensity and duration because of increases in pulse and respiratory rates from hypoxia, which may lead to fatigue with minimal exertion. Interval exercise with frequent, short sessions throughout the day may be more appropriate in the presence of anemia.

- Hematological values (hematocrit, hemoglobin, white blood cells, and platelets) must be monitored in patients undergoing active treatment to determine if exercise may be initiated.

- In patients with compromised skeletal integrity, non-weightbearing activities such as cycling, rowing, and swimming may be a better choice. However, water activities may not always be appropriate for the immunosuppressed population. In the presence of impaired sensation, a stationary bicycle would be a better choice to lessen the risk of falls.

- In patients who have had severe bouts of vomiting or diarrhea, there may be an electrolyte imbalance and they should have their electrolytes checked prior to initiating exercise.

- If patients still have a catheter in place, resistance training that use muscles in the area of the catheter should be avoided.

- Patients should be advised to contact their physician if they experience any of the following abnormal responses including fever; extreme or unusual fatigue; unusual muscular weakness; irregular heartbeat; palpitations; chest pain; leg pain or cramps; unusual joint pain; unusual bruising or nosebleeds; sudden onset of nausea during exercise; rapid weight loss; severe diarrhea or vomiting; disorientation; confusion; dizziness; light-headedness; blurred vision; fainting; pallor; night pain or pain not associated with any injury.

Finally, it is important to remember that in this population exercise is something that individuals can do to exert some control over their care and their body. It's something they can do for themselves, not something that is done to or for them.

Management by physical therapists of this population is directed toward identifying the multi-system impact of cancer as it affects the musculoskeletal, neuromuscular, cardiovascular, and pulmonary systems to produce impairments that affect movement and functional performance. Physical therapy interventions are directed toward prescribing treatment programs and interventions to reduce or alleviate impairments and functional limitations.

DIABETES MELLITUS

Diabetes mellitus (DM) is a group of metabolic diseases marked by hyperglycemia (high levels of blood glucose) and the development of long-term macrovascular, microvascular, and neuropathic complications. It is a disorder of carbohydrate, protein, and fat metabolism that results from an imbalance of insulin availability and insulin need.[1] There are 3 main types of diabetes, Type 1 diabetes, Type 2 diabetes

TABLE 13-3. PLASMA GLUCOSE LEVELS			
TEST	**NORMAL**	**PREDIABETES (IMPAIRED GLUCOSE TOLERANCE)**	**DIABETES**
Fasting Plasma Glucose Test (FPG)	< 100 mg/dl (5.6 mmol/l)	100 to 125 mg/dl (5.6 to 6.9 mmol/l)	≥ 126 mg/dl (7.0 mmol/l)*
Oral Glucose Tolerance Test (OGTT)	< 140 mg/dl (7.8 mmol/l)	140 to 199 mg/dl (7.8 to 11.0 mmol/l)	≥ 200 mg/dl (11.1 mmol/l)*

*Positive test results on any of these 3 tests should be confirmed with a second test on a different day.
Adapted from Porth CM. *Essentials of Pathophysiology: Concepts of Altered Health States.* 2nd ed. Philadelphia, PA: Lippincott Williams & Wilkins; 2007; American Diabetes Association. Diagnosis and classification of diabetes mellitus. *Diabetes Care.* 2010;33:S62-S69.

and gestational diabetes mellitus (GDM). In addition, there are other types of diabetes that result from specific genetic conditions, surgery, medications, infections, pancreatic disease, and other illnesses. These types of diabetes account for 1% to 5% of all cases diagnosed.[29]

Prediabetes

Prediabetes is a condition in which blood glucose levels are elevated, but are not high enough to be classified as diabetes. Please refer to Table 13-3 Plasma Glucose Levels.[1,30] Individuals with prediabetes have impaired fasting glucose (IFG) or impaired glucose tolerance (IGT) or sometimes both and are at increased risk for developing Type 2 diabetes, heart disease, and stroke.[29] IFG and IGT are associated with metabolic syndrome. Metabolic syndrome is defined as a collection of risk factors that include obesity (especially abdominal or visceral obesity), dyslipidemia of the high-triglyceride and/or low-high-density lipoprotein (HDL) type and hypertension in addition to insulin resistance or glucose intolerance. Elevated levels of insulin and glucose are linked to damage to the lining of coronary and other arteries, which is a key step in the development of heart disease, stroke, and peripheral vascular disease (macrovascular complications).[30-32] Having prediabetes does not have to mean that the development of Type 2 diabetes is inevitable. Studies have shown that individuals with prediabetes who lose weight and increase their physical activity can prevent or delay diabetes[29,33] and even return their blood glucose levels back to normal.[29]

Diagnosis: Diabetes, Prediabetes, and Gestational Diabetes

The Fasting Plasma Glucose Test (FPG), the Oral Glucose Tolerance Test (OGTT), and the Random Plasma Glucose Test are the 3 tests most commonly used to diagnose diabetes.[33] The FPG is the preferred test to diagnose diabetes. It is convenient and is most reliable when done in the morning. It measures blood glucose levels after at least 8 hours without eating. It will, however, miss some diabetes or prediabetes that can be found with the OGTT. Studies have demonstrated that the OGTT is more sensitive than the FPG test for

diagnosing prediabetes, but it is less convenient to administer. It measures blood glucose levels after at least 8 hours without eating and 2 hours after drinking a beverage containing 75 grams of glucose dissolved in water.[29,33] Both the FPG and OGTT are used to detect diabetes and prediabetes, but the Random Plasma Glucose Test, also known as the casual plasma glucose test, in combination with symptom assessment (increased urination, increased thirst, unexplained weight loss) is used solely to diagnose diabetes.[33] It measures blood glucose levels without regard to when an individual last ate. Positive tests results on any of these 3 tests should be confirmed by repeating either the FPG or OGTT on a different day (Table 13-4). Gestational diabetes is diagnosed using the OGTT and based on plasma glucose values. When testing for gestational diabetes, it is preferable to use 100 grams of glucose in liquid for the test. Blood glucose levels are checked 4 times during the test. Blood glucose levels that are above normal on at least 2 of these tests indicate that the woman has gestational diabetes. It is also important to note that in 2009 an international expert committee recommended the use of the hemoglobin A1C assay for the diagnosis of diabetes.[34] The committee determined that an A1C value of 6.5% or greater should be used for the diagnosis of diabetes. The committee's findings were referred to practice groups for review of the implications and for further recommendations.

Epidemiology

In 2008 United States Statistic reports, ~1.6 million new cases of diabetes were diagnosed in people aged 20 years and older in 2007.[29] It is estimated that 23.6 million people or 7.8% of the United States population, have diabetes. Of those 23.6 million people, 17.9 million have been diagnosed with diabetes and 5.7 million have yet to be diagnosed. There are approximately 186,300 people aged 20 and younger who have diabetes (Type 1 or Type 2). This corresponds to 0.2% of all people in this age group. Although Type 2 diabetes is still rare in this age group, it is being diagnosed more frequently in children and adolescents of American Indian, African American, Hispanic/Latino American, and Asian/Pacific Islander descent. For Americans living in the United States who are age 20 years and older, 23.5 million or 10.7% of all people in this age group have diabetes. For Americans age

TABLE 13-4. HOW DIABETES AND PREDIABETES ARE DIAGNOSED

TEST	TEST DESCRIPTION	DIAGNOSIS
Fasting Plasma Glucose Test (FPG)	The FPG is the preferred test to diagnose diabetes. It is convenient and is most reliable when done in the morning. It measures blood glucose levels after at least 8 hours without eating.*	Diabetes or pre-diabetes
Oral Glucose Tolerance Test (OGTT)	The OGTT is more sensitive than the FPG test for diagnosing prediabetes, but it is less convenient to administer. It measures blood glucose levels after at least 8 hours without eating and 2 hours after drinking a beverage containing glucose.*	Diabetes or pre-diabetes
Random Plasma Glucose Test	This test along with an assessment of symptoms is used only to diagnose diabetes. It measures blood glucose levels without regard to when an individual last ate.*	Diabetes
*Positive test results on any of these 3 tests should be confirmed with a second test on a different day. Adapted from National Institute for Diabetes and Digestive and Kidney Diseases. Diagnosis of diabetes. NIH Publication No. 09-4642, October 2008.		

60 years or older, 12.2 million or 23.1% of all people in this age group have diabetes.

Associated Morbidity/Mortality

Diabetes is the sixth leading cause of death in the United States and the fifth leading cause of death by disease.[7] Diabetes, however, is likely to be underreported as a cause of death. Studies have reported that only 35% to 40% of those individuals with a history of diabetes had diabetes listed anywhere on their death certificate and only 10% to 15% had it listed on their death certificate as the underlying cause of death.[29] For example, coronary heart disease, stroke, and end-stage renal disease are all complications of diabetes that may be listed as the cause of death while the diagnosis of diabetes goes unlisted. It is estimated that the overall risk for death among individuals with diabetes is approximately twice that of individuals without diabetes of a similar age.

Associated Costs

The overall costs for diabetes are substantial. In 2007, the total cost (direct and indirect) for diabetes was estimated at $174 billion; $116 billion went to direct medical costs and $58 billion for indirect costs (disability, work loss, premature mortality).[29,35]

Pathology/Pathophysiology

Insulin Metabolism

The body uses glucose, fatty acids, and other substrates as the source of fuel to provide for the body's energy needs.[1] Insulin and glucagon control the body's energy metabolism. It is insulin, however, that has the effect of lowering the blood glucose level. It lowers blood glucose levels by increasing the transport of glucose into body cells and by decreasing the production and release of glucose into the bloodstream by the liver. An individual with uncontrolled diabetes is unable to transport glucose into either fat or muscle cells and glucose continues to accumulate in the blood.[1,5] The result is fuel deprivation and essential starvation of the body's cells and an increase in the breakdown of fat and protein.[1] The kidneys attempt to compensate for the imbalance in blood glucose accumulation and restore normal levels by excreting the excess glucose in the urine. Excess glucose in the urine acts as an osmotic diuretic, which causes the excretion of an increased amount of water as well.[5]

When glucose is not available to serve as fuel for the cell, the body relies on fat stores for energy.[5] Fat cell breakdown and mobilization results in the formation of breakdown products known as ketones. Ketones accumulate in the blood and are excreted via the kidneys and lungs. Ketones produce hydrogen ions. The production of hydrogen ions by the ketones increases the acidity of blood and interferes with acid-base balance. Accumulation of hydrogen ions can cause the blood pH to fall and can result in metabolic acidosis. When the renal threshold for ketone metabolism is exceeded, the overflow ketones appear in the urine as acetone (ketonuria). Excretion of a large amount of glucose and ketones increases osmotic diuresis, resulting in fluid and electrolyte loss via the kidneys. Critical electrolyte loss that occurs when potassium and sodium are excreted in the urine can produce severe dehydration, electrolyte deficiency, and worsening acidosis. Additionally, when fats are metabolized as the primary source of energy, there may be an increase in the circulating lipid level to 5 times the normal amount. This significant elevation of blood lipids can contribute to the development of atherosclerosis and its resultant cardiovascular complications.

Insulin is also required for the transport of amino acids (the building blocks of proteins) into cells.[5] Under normal circumstances, proteins are continually being broken down and rebuilt. In the absence of insulin to transport amino acids into the cells, the balance between building and breakdown is altered and there is an increase in protein catabolism. The loss of protein that results from protein catabolism interferes with the inflammatory response process and the tissue's ability to repair itself.

Another metabolic role for insulin relates to its effect on the smooth muscle tone in arterial walls. Insulin is a directly acting arterial vasodilator.[36] It relaxes arterial wall muscles thus increasing blood flow. In the absence of adequate insulin, blood flow, especially in the microvascular system, is reduced because of contraction of the arterial wall muscles.

During exercise there can be as much as a 20-fold increase in whole body O_2 consumption depending on the intensity and duration of activity. It is thought that even greater increases may occur in the working muscles.[37] To meet the energy requirement of increased O_2 consumption, skeletal muscles increase the utilization of glycogen and triglyceride fuel stores as well as relying on free fatty acids resulting from the breakdown of triglycerides in adipose tissue and glucose released from the liver. Blood glucose levels are remarkably well maintained during exercise with hypoglycemia rarely occurring in nondiabetic individuals. This is possible because of hormonally mediated metabolic adjustments that occur during exercise.[5,37] Hepatic glucose production is triggered by a decrease in plasma insulin and the presence of glucagon during exercise.[37] During periods of prolonged exercise, increases in plasma glucagon and catecholamines provide the necessary glucose for use by muscles and other body tissues.[5,37]

Insulin-deficient patients with Type 1 diabetes aren't able to make these hormonal adjustments during exercise.[5,37] Because insulin-deficient individuals routinely have a low circulating insulin level, the active cells essentially sense impending starvation or lack of fuel, which triggers the release of an excessive amount of glucagon and catecholamines. Release of these hormones stimulates a further increase in glucose mobilization, which significantly increases the already high circulating levels of glucose and ketones, compounding the problem. This may precipitate ketoacidosis if the hyperglycemia and ketosis are at a sufficiently high level and/or if the individual is dehydrated. When high levels of insulin are present in these same individuals as a result of insulin administration, this can ease or even prevent the increased mobilization of glucose and other substrates that are induced by exercise, and hypoglycemia may result.[37] Though this is possible in individuals with Type 2 diabetes who take insulin or sulfonylurea therapy, it tends to be less of a problem in this group. In this population, exercise is thought to improve insulin sensitivity and assist in bringing elevated plasma glucose levels into the normal range.[5,37]

Type 1 Diabetes

Type 1 diabetes was previously known as insulin-dependent DM or juvenile-onset diabetes. In Type 1 diabetes, the beta cells of the pancreas have been destroyed by the body's immune system. The beta cells are the only cells that produce insulin, the hormone that regulates blood glucose. Type 1 has been further subdivided into Type 1a and Type 1b.[1] Type 1a, immune-mediated diabetes, is characterized by autoimmune destruction of beta cells. Type 1b, idiopathic diabetes,

is used to describe those cases of beta cell destruction where no evidence of autoimmunity is present. What differentiates Type 1a from Type 1b is the presence of islet autoantibodies.[38] Only a very small percentage of individuals with Type 1 diabetes have Type 1b and most are usually of African or Asian descent.[1].

It is estimated that Type 1 diabetes accounts for 5% to 10% of all diagnosed cases of diabetes[29] and of those, 95% have Type 1a diabetes.[1] Type 1 diabetes is usually diagnosed in children and young adults, although onset can occur at any age (Table 13-5). The onset of Type 1 diabetes is often sudden. In addition to the common symptoms, nausea, vomiting or stomach pains often accompany the abrupt onset of Type 1 diabetes.[39] The risk factors for Type 1 diabetes are less clear than those for Type 2 or GDM, but autoimmune, genetic, and environmental factors are involved in developing Type 1 diabetes (Table 13-6).[29]

Type 2 Diabetes

Type 2 diabetes was previously known as noninsulin-dependent DM or adult-onset diabetes, though it can occur at any age, even during childhood. Ninety percent to 95% of all diagnosed cases of diabetes are Type 2.[29,30] This type of diabetes usually begins as insulin resistance. In insulin resistance, the muscle, liver, and fat cells do not utilize insulin properly. Initially the pancreas is able to keep up with the additional demand by producing more insulin. In time, however, the pancreas gradually loses the ability to produce sufficient insulin in response to the demand placed on it by meals. Development of Type 2 diabetes is associated with advancing age, obesity, family history of diabetes, history of GDM, impaired glucose metabolism, physical inactivity, and race/ethnicity. The risk factors for Type 2 diabetes that cannot be modified are age, previous history of GDM, family history, and race/ethnicity. Type 2 diabetes usually develops more insidiously than Type 1 diabetes, and many individuals with Type 2 diabetes have no signs or symptoms. Or, symptoms may be so mild that they are ignored. The symptoms of Type 2 diabetes (see Table 13-5) include increased urination, increased thirst, fatigue, blurred vision, and frequent infections and sores that are slow to heal. At times the diagnosis of diabetes is not made until someone seeks treatment for a complication of diabetes such as blurred vision (microvascular complication) or heart disease (macrovascular complication).

Gestational Diabetes Mellitus

GDM is a form of glucose intolerance that is first diagnosed during pregnancy. It is thought to be caused by the hormones of pregnancy that block the action of the mother's insulin, making it difficult for insulin to do its job of controlling blood sugar or by insufficient production of insulin to meet the demands of pregnancy. GDM develops when the pancreas is unable to produce sufficient insulin to keep blood glucose levels within an acceptable range. GDM occurs more frequently among African Americans, Hispanic/Latino Americans, and American Indians.[29] Asian Americans and

TABLE 13-5. SIGNS AND SYMPTOMS OF DIABETES

SIGN/SYMPTOM	TYPE 1	TYPE 2	GESTATIONAL DIABETES MELLITUS (GDM)
Polyuria (excessive urination)	Yes	Yes	Yes, though most pregnant women have to urinate more frequently.
Polydipsia (excessive thirst)	Yes	Yes	Yes
Polyphagia (excessive hunger)	Yes	Is usually not present in people with Type 2 diabetes.	Yes, though most pregnant women feel hungrier.
Unexpected weight loss	Yes	Yes, but more common in Type 1. Many people with Type 2 have problems with obesity.	
Blurred vision	Yes	Yes. This is frequently a symptom that prompts an individual to seek medical treatment.	Yes
Numbness or tingling in hands or feet	Yes	Yes. This is frequently a symptom that prompts an individual to seek medical treatment.	
Fatigue	Yes	Yes. This is frequently a symptom that prompts an individual to seek medical treatment.	
Very dry skin	Yes	Yes	
Sores that are slow to heal	Yes	Yes	
Frequent infections	Yes	Yes. This is frequently a symptom that prompts an individual to seek medical treatment.	
Often asymptomatic		Yes	Yes. Many women are surprised to learn that they have GDM since they frequently have no symptoms.

Adapted from Porth CM. *Essentials of Pathophysiology: Concepts of Altered Health States.* 2nd ed. Philadelphia, PA: Lippincott Williams & Wilkins; 2007; Goodman CC, Boissonnault WG, Fuller KS. *Pathology: Implications for the Physical Therapist.* 2nd ed. Philadelphia, PA: Saunders; 2003; Centers for Disease Control and Prevention. Basics about diabetes. March 12, 2010. http://www.cdc.gov/diabetes/consumer/learn.htm#. Accessed May 29, 2010; BC HealthGuide. Gestational diabetes. February 10, 2010. http://www.bchealthguide.org/kbase/topic/special/hw197466/sec5.htm. Accessed May 29, 2010.

Pacific Islanders are also at greater risk for developing GDM.[40] Obese women and women with a family history of diabetes are also at greater risk for developing GDM[29] as are women who have had GDM during an earlier pregnancy or who have given birth to at least one baby weighing more than 9 pounds.[40] Frequently, there are no symptoms and women are surprised to learn that they have GDM. When they do have symptoms they may include increased thirst, increased urination, increased hunger, and blurred vision.[41] GDM requires treatment to normalize maternal blood glucose levels to avoid complications in the unborn child. Five percent to 10% of women with GDM are found to have Type 2 diabetes after pregnancy.[29] In addition, women who have had GDM have a 40% to 60% chance of developing diabetes in the next 5 to 10 years.

Complications

Diabetes is associated with significant complications. These complications can be divided into acute and chronic complications. The acute complications of diabetes include diabetic ketoacidosis and hyperosmolar (nonketotic) coma. Uncontrolled diabetes often leads to biochemical imbalances that can cause these life-threatening events. In addition to the acute complications listed above, the CDC in its 2007 National Diabetes Fact Sheet[29] reported specific complications of diabetes in the United States (Table 13-7).

Physical Therapy Management

At present, there is no known cure for diabetes. Management is directed at regulation of blood glucose levels and usually includes a combination of dietary management,

TABLE 13-6. RISK FACTORS FOR TYPE 1, TYPE 2, AND GESTATIONAL DIABETES MELLITUS

Type 1 diabetes mellitus risk factors	• The risk factors for Type 1 DM are less clear than those for Type 2 DM or GDM, but autoimmune, genetic, and environmental factors are involved in developing Type 1 diabetes.
Type 2 diabetes mellitus risk factors	• Family history of diabetes (parent, brother, or sister) • Physical inactivity • Race/ethnicity: African American, Alaska Native, American Indian, Asian American, Hispanic/Latino American, or Pacific Islander • Overweight or obese • Older age (45 years or older) • History of GDM or delivery of at least one baby weighing more than 9 pounds • Hypertension (greater than or equal to 140/90 mm Hg in adults) or being treated for high blood pressure • HDL cholesterol < 35 mg/dL and/or triglyceride level > 250 mg/dL • Previous history of impaired glucose tolerance (IGT) or impaired fasting glucose (IFG) • Polycystic ovary syndrome (PCOS) • Acanthosis nigricans, a condition characterized by a dark, velvety rash around the neck or armpits • History of cardiovascular disease
Gestational diabetes mellitus risk factors	• Family history of diabetes (parent, brother, or sister) • Race/ethnicity: African American, Hispanic/Latino American, American Indian, Asian American, or Pacific Islander • Age (25 or older) • Obesity • History of GDM or delivery of at least one baby weighing more than 9 pounds • Diagnosis of prediabetes

DM: diabetes mellitus; HDL: high-density lipoprotein.

Adapted from Centers for Disease Control and Prevention. National diabetes fact sheet: general information and national estimates on diabetes in the United States, 2007. Atlanta, GA: U.S. Department of Health and Human Services, Centers for Disease Control and Prevention, 2008. http://www.cdc.gov/diabetes/pubs/pdf/ndfs_2007.pdf; National Institute for Diabetes and Digestive and Kidney Diseases. Diagnosis of diabetes. NIH Publication No. 09-4642, October 2008; National Institute of Diabetes and Digestive and Kidney Diseases. What I need to know about gestational diabetes. NIH Publication No. 06-5129, April 2006.

exercise, and antidiabetic drugs with the goal of keeping blood glucose, lipid, and BP at normal levels. Education is an essential component in the management of diabetes. Individuals with diabetes must understand the relationship among food intake, exercise, medication, and blood glucose.

Dietary Management

Individuals with Type 1 diabetes require insulin supplementation. The amount of insulin required to maintain blood sugar is variable and is determined by food intake and physical activity. Patients with Type 1 diabetes are encouraged to eat consistent amounts and types of food at specific and routine times. Blood glucose levels are closely monitored. This is performed daily with home monitoring devices and several times per year with the A1C laboratory test. Results of this test reflect average blood glucose over a 2- to 3-month period.

Type 2 diabetes is most frequently managed with proper nutrition and exercise, sometimes in conjunction with oral medication. Insulin may be required when adequate control of blood glucose levels cannot be achieved with oral medications. Weight loss, if indicated, is also an important management tool.

Managing Medications With Exercise

The benefits of exercise are well known. For individuals with Type 2 diabetes, the benefits of a regular exercise program include an increase in carbohydrate metabolism, which results in lower plasma glucose levels,[5] better weight control, decreased body fat, increased HDL,[5] decreased triglycerides,[5]

TABLE 13-7. COMPLICATIONS OF DIABETES

Heart disease and stroke	In 2004, heart disease was listed on 68% of diabetes-related death certificates and stroke was listed on 16% of diabetes-related death certificates in individuals aged 65 years and older. Adults with diabetes die of heart disease 2 to 4 times more frequently than adults without heart disease, and their risk for stroke is 2 to 4 times higher.
Hypertension	In 2003 to 2004, 75% of adults with self-reported diabetes had blood pressure readings greater than or equal to 130/80 mm Hg or took prescription medications to control hypertension.
Blindness	Among adults aged 20 to 74 years of age, diabetes is the leading cause of new cases of blindness. Diabetic retinopathy results in 12,000 to 24,000 new cases of blindness each year.
Kidney disease	Diabetes is the leading cause of kidney failure. In 2005, diabetes accounted for 44% of the new cases of kidney failure.
Nervous system disease	It is estimated that 60% to 70% of individuals with diabetes have mild to severe forms of nervous system involvement including impaired sensation or pain in the hands or feet, slowed digestion of food in the stomach, carpal tunnel syndrome and erectile dysfunction. Close to 30% of individuals with diabetes aged 40 years or older have impaired sensation in their feet. Severe diabetic neuropathy is a major contributing factor to lower extremity amputations.
Amputations	More than 60% of nontraumatic lower limb amputations occur in individuals with diabetes. In 2004, ~71,000 nontraumatic lower-limb amputations were performed in individuals with diabetes.
Dental disease	Periodontal disease is more common in people with diabetes than in the general population with almost one-third having severe periodontal disease. Young adults with diabetes have approximately twice the risk of periodontal disease compared to those without diabetes.
Complications of pregnancy	When diabetes is poorly controlled before conception and during the first trimester of pregnancy there is the risk of major birth defects in 5% to 10% of these pregnancies as well as the possibility of spontaneous abortions in 15% to 20% of these pregnancies.
Other complications	Individuals with diabetes have also been found to be more susceptible to other illnesses and once they become ill, frequently have poorer prognoses. Individuals with diabetes aged 60 years or older are 2 to 3 times more likely to report an inability to walk one-quarter mile, climb stairs, do housework or use a mobility aid when compared with individuals in their same age group without diabetes.

Adapted from Centers for Disease Control and Prevention. National diabetes fact sheet: general information and national estimates on diabetes in the Unites States, 2007. Atlanta, GA: U.S. Department of Health and Human Services, Centers for Disease Control and Prevention, 2008. http://www.cdc.gov/diabetes/pubs/pdf/ndfs_2007.pdf.

and an improvement in insulin sensitivity.[5,37] It has also been found to be beneficial in preventing the complications associated with Type 2 diabetes. In individuals with insulin-dependent diabetes, the benefits of exercise must be weighed with the increased risk of hypoglycemia.[1,5,37] In some individuals, the symptoms of hypoglycemia may occur hours after completing their exercise. They need to be aware that this is a possibility and that they may need to adjust their diabetes medication dose, their carbohydrate intake, or both.[1,5] This is something the physical therapist must consider when prescribing and administering exercise programs in individuals with altered insulin metabolism.

Physical Therapy/Exercise Testing and Prescription

For an individual with the pathologic diagnosis of either Type 1 or Type 2 diabetes, it is essential that a complete history, systems review, and examination, (including functional exercise testing), be performed prior to beginning any exercise program. The history should focus on eliciting any signs or symptoms that indicate that the DM has had an impact on the cardiovascular system, eyes, kidneys, feet, and/or nervous system. Impairment of any of these could have a deleterious effect on movement-related functions. The examination should screen for the presence of macrovascular, microvascular or neuropathic complications of DM that could significantly affect and alter the performance of exercise such as heart disease, peripheral vascular disease, retinopathy, nephropathy, peripheral neuropathy, and autonomic neuropathy. Examination of the cardiovascular system with a graded exercise test with EKG may be indicated if the individual is at risk for underlying cardiovascular disease (CVD) based on any of the following criteria[37,42]:

- Initiating exercise >60% HR_{max} or > brisk walking
- Age >35

- Age > 25 years and
  - Type 2 diabetes of > 10 years' duration
  - Type 1 diabetes of > 15 years' duration
- Additional risk factors for coronary artery disease (CAD), eg, BP > 140/90, smoking, dyslipidemia or family history of premature CAD
- Presence of any complications of diabetes (eg, retinopathy, nephropathy, peripheral neuropathy)
- Peripheral vascular disease
- Autonomic neuropathy

Individuals with known CAD require a diagnostic evaluation to assess for an ischemic response to exercise, identify the ischemic threshold, and to test for the predisposition to arrhythmia during exercise.[37] This diagnostic evaluation specifically focuses on evaluation of left ventricular function at rest and during exercise. Resting tachycardia (HR > 100 beats per minute), orthostasis, failure of the heart rate to increase during exercise or undesirable exercise-induced elevation of blood pressure may be indicative of autonomic neuropathy.[37,42]

Caution must be taken before proceeding with an exercise program in individuals with some specific complications of diabetes including retinopathy, peripheral neuropathy, autonomic neuropathy, and nephropathy.[43] In individuals with proliferative or severe nonproliferative diabetic retinopathy, vigorous aerobic or resistance exercise may be contraindicated because of the risk of triggering vitreous hemorrhage or retinal detachment. In the presence of impaired pain sensation of the extremities there is obviously increased risk of skin breakdown and infection as well as Charcot joint destruction. Therefore, it may be prudent to encourage activities that do not involve weightbearing such as swimming or bicycling. In individuals with autonomic neuropathy there can be an increased risk of exercise-induced injury as a result of decreased cardiac responsiveness to exercise (blunting of BP and HR response to exercise),[42,43] postural hypotension, impaired thermoregulation resulting from impaired skin blood flow and sweating, impaired night vision, and impaired thirst with an increased risk of dehydration and gastroparesis with unpredictable food delivery.[37,43] There is a strong association between autonomic neuropathy and CVD in individuals with diabetes.[43] It is recommended that individuals with diabetic autonomic neuropathy undergo cardiac investigation prior to increasing their physical activity beyond their usual level of activity. In addition, these individuals are also at risk for silent ischemia (dyspnea, diaphoresis, orthostasis) and must be closely monitored during exercise.[42] There can also be an increase in urinary protein excretion with physical activity.[43] This increase is in proportion to the acute increase in BP. Microalbuminuria and proteinuria are associated with an increased risk of CVD in individuals with a history of these conditions. In previously sedentary individuals with diabetic nephropathy, it is important to perform an exercise EKG stress test before they begin an exercise program that will be significantly more demanding than their usual level of activity.

In individuals with Type 1 diabetes, vigorous activity is avoided in the presence of hyperglycemia and ketosis.[43] In individuals with Type 2 diabetes, it has not been deemed necessary to postpone exercise solely based on blood glucose levels > 300 mg/dl, particularly in a postprandial state provided the individual feels well, is adequately hydrated, and there is no evidence of ketosis. As previously discussed, hypoglycemia is a possibility in individuals with Type 1 diabetes.[1,5,37] Consequently, there is a need to adjust diabetes medication dosing and potentially carbohydrate intake to balance the metabolic response to exercise.[1,5] Postexercise hypoglycemia is also a possibility in individuals with Type 2 diabetes who take insulin or sulfonylurea therapy, though it tends to be less of a problem in this group.[37]

In 1996 the United States Surgeon General's report recommended that all people participate in aerobic activity of moderate intensity for at least 30 minutes on most, if not all, days of the week.[28,43] Currently, the recommended frequency of aerobic training for this population is 4 to 7 days per week, or every other day.[42,43] General recommendations of this type assume a lack of movement-related impairment and are generally prescribed using a generic formula intended to address the general population. For example, exercise intensity for an aerobic training program can be calculated using Karvonen's formula (HR reserve): $[(HR_{peak} - HR_{rest}) \times (40\%$ to $70\%)] + HRrest$,[42] which assumes that an exercise test has been performed that documented the resting and peak exercise HR and that there were no untoward responses in HR, BP, or other signs and symptoms of a pathologic response. The duration and frequency of this aerobic training prescription can then be set at 20 to 30 minutes, preceded by a 5- to 10-minute warm-up period, and followed by a 5- to 10-minute cool-down period, and performed 3 to 5 times per week.[37,42,43] These general guidelines are a reasonable starting point for patients with a history of diabetes; however, the essential individual changes in prescription will be made as a result of the actual exercise test findings. Exercise testing, (as described in Chapter 6 and discussed in Chapter 7), is appropriate and necessary in this population. Given the abnormalities associated with glucose mobilization and cellular uptake, careful monitoring of blood sugar and insulin levels is essential to prescribing a safe and effective level of exercise for these patients.

To improve glycemic control, assist with weight maintenance, and reduce the risk of CVD, the American Diabetes Association (ADA) recommends at least 150 min/week of moderate intensity aerobic training (40% to 60% of maximum O_2 consumption (VO_{2max}) or 50% to 70% of HR_{max}) and/or at least 90 min/week of vigorous aerobic exercise (> 60% of VO_{2max} or > 70% of HR_{max}.[43] The duration of aerobic training should be 20 to 30 minutes with an additional 5- to 10-minute warm-up and cool down.[42] Blood glucose monitoring is an essential part of the aerobic training program for the individual with diabetes (Table 13-8).[42] Though hypoglycemia is the most common problem for diabetics who exercise, hyperglycemia is also a risk, especially for those individuals with Type 1 diabetes who are not

TABLE 13-8. MONITORING AND MANAGING BLOOD GLUCOSE LEVELS BEFORE AND DURING EXERCISE

BLOOD GLUCOSE	WHAT TO DO	COMMENTS
< 70 mg/dL	Hypoglycemia. Do not exercise.	Ingest carbohydrates
70 to 100 mg/dL	Snack	15 g of carbohydrates every hour of moderately intense activity
100 to 300 mg/dL	Proceed with exercise program	
> 300 mg/dL and on oral meds	Try 10 to 15 minutes of activity	If BG rises: stop If BG drops: continue, rechecking every 10 to 15 minutes
> 300 mg/dL and on insulin	Should be checked for ketones (via urine dip stick or Precision Xtra® glucose meter)	If (+) ketones: avoid activity If (–) ketones: participate with close blood glucose monitoring

Adapted from American Physical Therapy Association. Physical fitness and type 2 diabetes. September 13, 2007. http://www.apta.org/AM/Template.cfm?Section=PFSP_Pocket_Guides&Template=/MembersOnly.cfm&ContentID=44367. Accessed May 29, 2010.

in glycemic control.[44] Carbohydrate intake and or insulin injections/infusion should be adjusted prior to beginning to exercise based on blood glucose levels and exercise intensity to prevent hypoglycemia. In order to avoid the risk of hypoglycemia associated with exercise, injecting insulin into exercising limbs should be avoided. Abdominal site injections are recommended. Increased consumption of carbohydrates may be necessary when exercising late in the evening to minimize the risk of nocturnal hypoglycemia. In addition, carbohydrates should be readily available during and after exercise.[37]

Studies have also shown resistance training to have beneficial effects in individuals with Type 2 diabetes.[43] The strength training prescription for these individuals is prescribed in response to examination and exercise testing that documents deficiencies that are either generalized or specific. Functional exercise testing such as a timed stair climb or the Timed Up & Go assessment can be extremely useful to elicit deficits and establish a baseline level of performance. Exercise prescription can be made using the overload principle and having the subject train at 50% to 60% of maximum, or, in severely limited patients, an intermittent training program performing the limited task has also been shown to be beneficial. The current recommendations for specific resistance training of muscle groups or activities that are limited are use of an 8 to 10 repetition max beginning with one set and progressing to 3 sets.[42,43] Exercises should include 8 to 10 of the major muscle groups involved and be performed 2 to 3 days per week.

General Considerations

There are several other important considerations in individuals with diabetes. The proper footwear and socks are essential to minimize trauma to the feet. The footwear should fit properly and have adequate cushioning and support to prevent blisters. The socks should be made of an absorbent material to keep the feet dry. Individuals must be taught to closely monitor their feet for blisters, redness or other signs potential injury.[37] It is essential that they be well hydrated since dehydration can affect blood glucose levels. They should be encouraged to consume adequate fluids (eg, 17 ounces of fluid 2 hours before exercise) and to continue to drink during exercise. Adequate precautions should be taken when exercising in extremely hot or cold environments.

Management by physical therapists of this population is directed toward identifying the multi-system impact of diabetes as it affects the musculoskeletal, neuromuscular, cardiovascular, and pulmonary systems to produce impairments that affect movement and functional performance. Physical therapy interventions are directed toward prescribing treatment programs and interventions to reduce or alleviate impairments and functional limitations.

MUSCULOSKELETAL TRAUMA

The musculoskeletal system accounts for nearly 70% of body mass and is subject to a wide array of injuries.[1] Musculoskeletal injuries result from a variety of physical and mechanical forces and include blunt tissue trauma (hematomas, lacerations, and contusions), disruption of tendons and ligaments (sprains, strains, and dislocations) and fractures of the bony structures. Factors such as age, environment or activity also play a role and can place an individual at greater risk for injury. For example, high-speed motor vehicle accidents (MVA) are a common cause of musculoskeletal trauma in adults younger than 45 years of age with the greatest risk in the 16- to 19-year-old age range.[1,45] Childhood injuries are most often the result of falls, bicycle-related injuries, and sports injuries.[1] The most frequent cause of injuries in individuals 65 years of age and older is falls.[46] Falls are also the most frequent cause of injury and death and the most common cause of nonfatal injuries and hospital admissions for trauma in this population.[46,47] Each year approximately 35% to 40% of adults 65 and older experience at least one fall.[46] Falls are also the most common cause of fractures and traumatic brain injuries in this age group.[47]

Complications of Musculoskeletal Trauma

The complications associated with musculoskeletal trauma include impaired bone healing (malunion or nonunion), fracture blisters, compartment syndrome, complex regional pain syndrome, and fat embolism syndrome. Please refer to Chapter X for information on impaired bone healing.

Fracture Blisters

Fracture blisters are defined as skin bullae and blisters that represent areas of epidermal necrosis with separation of the epidermis from the underlying dermis by edema fluid.[1] The blisters can be either filled with clear fluid or blood.[48] They are most frequently associated with severe injuries such as those resulting from an MVA or a fall from a significant height, but can also occur after excessive joint manipulation, dependent positioning, heat application or from peripheral vascular disease.[1] Fracture blisters most frequently occur at the tibia, ankle, and elbow or areas where there is little soft tissue between the skin and the bone. It is thought that a major factor in the development of fracture blisters is injury to the dermal-epidermal junction caused by excessive shearing of the skin during the mechanism of fracture.[48] Fracture blisters are associated with a higher incidence of complications, they delay surgical management, and there is an increased risk of infection, particularly in individuals with DM.

Compartment Syndrome

Compartment syndrome (CS) occurs when the tissue pressure (interstitial pressure) within an enclosed space (eg, abdominal and limb compartments) is greater than the perfusion pressure,[1,49] resulting in compromised blood flow and muscle and nerve damage. In this chapter, the discussion will be limited to a discussion of limb compartment syndrome as an illustration of how this pathology can produce significant impairment issues that need to be addressed by physical therapy management.

Fascia is the inelastic membrane that surrounds and separates groups of muscles from one another in the upper and lower extremities. The area inside this enclosed space is referred to as a compartment. Each compartment includes muscle tissue, nerves, and blood vessels. CS can occur whenever increased tissue pressure in a compartment restricts the blood flow to the muscles and nerves within that compartment. If left untreated, the outcome will be tissue ischemia with subsequent necrosis and nerve damage with resultant functional impairment. Data suggest that the ischemic threshold for normal muscle is reached when pressure within the compartment increases to 20 mm Hg below the diastolic pressure or 30 mm Hg below the mean arterial pressure.[50]

Compartment syndrome can occur when there is an increase in the compartment's volume due to trauma, swelling, vascular injury, and bleeding or venous obstruction, a decrease in the size of the compartment that is associated with constrictive dressings, casts, closure of fascial defects or burns, or, a combination of the 2.[1,49,50] One of the most significant causes of CS is the bleeding and edema associated with fractures and bone surgery.[1] Contusions and soft tissues are also frequently associated with CS.

There are 2 types of CS, acute and chronic. Acute CS is usually associated with a traumatic event such as a fracture or crush injury. The hallmark symptom of acute CS is severe pain that is out of proportion to the injury or physical findings, and does not respond to traditional control methods such as elevation and pain medication.[1,51,52] Sensory changes such as numbness, tingling and loss of sensation, diminished reflexes, and motor impairment are indications of nerve compression. Symptoms usually begin within hours of the injury, but can be delayed up to 64 hours after injury.[1,51] Muscle necrosis can occur in as little as 4 to 8 hours, making it extremely important that individuals at risk for CS are identified and appropriate treatment is initiated.[1,52]

Conservative management consists of decreasing the compartmental pressures and may include splitting a cast or removal of restrictive dressings.[1,52] These measures are frequently sufficient to reduce much of the underlying pressure and relieve many of the symptoms. Elevation of the extremity to the level of the heart will often reduce the edema. Elevation beyond this is contraindicated because it will decrease arterial blood flow and narrow the arteriovenous pressure gradient, which will worsen the ischemia.[52] When conservative measures fail, a fasciotomy is indicated to decompress the compartment, normalize compartment pressures, and restore blood flow to the affected tissues. Rhabdomyolysis and subsequent renal failure are the most severe life-threatening complications of CS.[51,52]

Chronic CS also known as chronic exertional compartment syndrome is an overuse injury of the lower extremity. It is typically seen in athletes such as long-distance runners, basketball players, skiers, and soccer players.[52] It most frequently involves the anterior and lateral compartments.[51] Usually an individual is pain free at rest. Chronic CS typically presents as exercise-induced pain that dissipates quickly when the exercise is stopped. The exact mechanism of injury is not fully understood. It is thought that the stress of hard-surface exercise leads to edema, increasing the compartment volume with a resultant increase in intramuscular pressure that then leads to tissue ischemia and pain.[1,51] It is not the medical emergency that acute CS is and usually responds to conservative management consisting of rest from the aggravating activity. As in the management of any overuse syndrome, ice and elevation may assist with the recovery as well as the use of nonsteroidal anti-inflammatory medications. For obvious reasons, compression would be contraindicated. If conservative management fails, a fasciotomy may be indicated.

TABLE 13-9. SYMPTOMS OF COMPLEX REGIONAL PAIN SYNDROME

In addition to the cardinal symptom of CRPS, pain that is out of proportion to the severity of the injury, which worsens rather than improves over time, may spread to the entire extremity, and may be exacerbated by emotional stress. Other symptoms of CRPS include:

SENSORY	Hyperesthesia—Increased sensitivity
	Allodynia—Perception of pain resulting from a stimulus that would not ordinarily cause pain
VASOMOTOR	Temperature asymmetry and/or skin color changes and/or skin color asymmetry
SUDOMOTOR	Sweating changes and/or sweating asymmetry
EDEMA	Swelling and stiffness in affected joints
MOTOR	Impaired range of motion and/or motor dysfunction (weakness, tremor, dystonia)
TROPHIC	Changes in hair, nail and skin growth patterns and nutritional status

Adapted from National Institute of Neurological Disorders and Stroke. Complex regional pain syndrome fact sheet. May 19, 2010. Parrillo SJ. Complex regional pain syndrome. March 23, 2010. http://www.emedicine.com/emerg/topic497.htm#section~clinical Accessed May 29, 2010; Harden RN, Stanton-Hicks M, Wilson PR. Proposed new diagnostic criteria for complex regional pain syndrome. *Pain Med*. 2007;8:326-331.

Complex Regional Pain Syndrome

Complex Regional Pain Syndrome (CRPS) is a chronic pain condition. CRPS presents as pain that is out of proportion to the severity of the injury that gets worse rather than better over time. It is thought to be the result of dysfunction in the central or peripheral nervous systems.[53] CRPS has been further divided into CRPS I and CRPS II. CRPS I (previously known as *reflex sympathetic dystrophy*) is most frequently triggered by tissue trauma or immobilization,[54] while CRPS II (also known as *causalgia*) is associated with a nerve injury.[5,53,54] In the United States, the incidence of CRPS after fractures and contusions is 10% to 30% while the incidence after peripheral nerve injuries is 1% to 15%.[54] It affects persons of all ages though most experts agree that it is most commonly seen in women.

The cardinal symptom of CRPS is intense, burning pain that is out of proportion to the severity of the injury. In addition, other symptoms can include the presence of edema, abnormal sensory, motor, sudomotor, vasomotor, and/or trophic findings.[55] These include increased skin sensitivity, changes in nail and hair growth patterns, changes in skin temperature, color and texture, swelling and stiffness in affected joints, and motor impairment (Table 13-9).[53-55] Though the symptoms of CRPS vary in severity and duration, they may all contribute to movement-related impairments and functional limitations. Since there is no specific diagnostic test for CRPS, it is diagnosed primarily based on the history and clinical examination.[5] Consequently, physical therapists are well positioned to identify the development of these signs and symptoms and can be instrumental in ensuring that these issues are accurately diagnosed early in the course of development. Diagnostic testing is used to either rule out other diagnoses[53] or may be used to evaluate secondary changes that may assist in establishing a diagnosis.[5]

The cause of CRPS remains poorly understood. Most researchers agree that CRPS is a neurologic disorder affecting the central and peripheral nervous systems.[53] One of the most recent hypotheses suggests that pain receptors in the involved extremity become responsive to the group of nervous system messengers collectively known as catecholamines. In animal studies, norepinephrine (a catecholamine released by sympathetic nerves) acquires the ability to activate pain pathways following tissue or nerve injury. Another hypothesis suggests that the immune response is triggered in postinjury CRPS (CRPS II), which then leads to the typical inflammatory symptoms of warmth, redness, and edema in the involved extremity. Thus CRPS may result from a disruption in the healing process. It is most likely that CRPS is the result of multiple causes that produce similar symptoms.

There is no known cure for CRPS. Treatment is directed at relief of the painful symptoms associated with CRPS. Treatment interventions include physical therapy, psychotherapy, sympathetic nerve blocks, medication, surgical sympathectomy, spinal cord stimulation, and intrathecal drug pumps.[53] It has been suggested that early diagnosis and treatment may help in limiting the disorder, but there has been insufficient evidence to date from clinical studies to support this.

Fat Embolism Syndrome

Fat Embolism Syndrome (FES) is a collection of clinical signs and symptoms that result when fat droplets are released into the small blood vessels of the lungs and other organs after long-bone[1,56-58] or pelvic[58,59] fractures. It is thought that the fat emboli are released from the bone marrow or adipose tissue at the fracture site into the venous system through torn veins.[1] FES is also associated with trauma other than fractures as well as nontraumatic surgical conditions (eg, liposuction, cardiopulmonary bypass, joint replacement) and medical conditions (eg, acute pancreatitis, DM, sickle cell crisis).[1,57-59]

It is important to note that fat embolization and FES are not synonymous. Fat embolization involves the presence of fat droplets in the systemic circulation.[1,55] Fat embolization after long-bone trauma is a common occurrence yet the actual incidence of the clinical syndrome known as FES is low.[56-59] The incidence of FES has been estimated at 3% to 4% with 90% of all cases linked to blunt trauma.[58] Fat embolization is usually asymptomatic and nonlife-threatening whereas FES can be fatal. The main signs and symptoms of FES are respiratory distress, cerebral dysfunction, and petechial rash.[58] The petechial rash typically develops within 24 to 36 hours while respiratory distress is usually seen anywhere from 12 to 72 hours after injury. Respiratory dysfunction varies in severity from mild (dyspnea, tachypnea) to severe, where the signs and symptoms may appear indistinguishable from adult respiratory distress syndrome (ARDS).[58,59] Cerebral dysfunction initially manifests as subtle changes in behavior and signs of disorientation,[1] develops after the onset of respiratory system dysfunction[59] and is thought to result from emboli in the cerebral circulation as well as respiratory depression.[1] This may progress to agitated delirium, seizures or focal defects.[1,59] The diagnosis of FES is made based on clinical signs and symptoms since laboratory and radiographic findings are nonspecific and can be inconsistent.[56,59,60]

Medical management is prophylactic or supportive, directed at management to ensure adequate oxygenation and ventilation, hemodynamic stability, hydration, prophylaxis of deep vein thrombosis, and stress-related gastrointestinal bleeding, as well as nutrition.[58,60] Studies suggest that early stabilization of long-bone fractures reduce recurrent fat embolism and FES,[58,60] and reduce the incidence of ARDS 5-fold.[58] The mortality rate for FES is 10% to 20%, with older individuals with comorbidities and/or decreased physiologic reserves having worse outcomes.

At present the underlying pathophysiology for FES is unclear.[1,56] There are currently 2 theories (the mechanical theory and the biochemical theory) that explain how fat emboli result in FES.[55,58] The mechanical theory hypothesizes that when fat droplets are released into the venous circulation, the larger particles become lodged in and block pulmonary capillaries while the smaller particles are able to pass through the lung capillaries and enter the systemic circulation.[1,58] The droplets deposited in the pulmonary capillaries then travel through the arteriovenous shunts to the brain. Microvascular lodging of these droplets produce local ischemia and inflammation that result in the release of inflammatory mediators, platelet aggregation, and vasoactive amines.[58] The biochemical theory proposes that hormonal changes resulting from trauma and/or sepsis trigger a systemic release of free fatty acids as chylomicrons. Acute-phase reactants, such as C-reactive proteins, then cause chylomicrons to coalesce and create the physiologic reactions described in the mechanical theory. This second theory helps to explain the presence of FES in nontraumatic situations.

Evaluation and Management of Musculoskeletal Trauma

History

Issues to focus on while interviewing and taking a history from patients who have sustained musculoskeletal trauma would include the mechanism of injury, date of onset and course of events, recent hospitalization, any surgical procedures as a result of the injury, preexisting medical conditions as well as any other health-related conditions that might affect the current injury. If during this phase of the examination the patient reports he or she had surgery to "relieve the pressure" in one or more limbs, this may indicate that the patient developed CS as a complication of the injury. This would then direct the clinician to inspect the skin for fasciotomy scars during the systems review. Another example would be the geriatric patient who sustained a femur fracture and reports that he or she spent time in the intensive care unit (ICU) on a ventilator. This might lead the clinician to suspect that the patient had developed ARDS as a complication of FES.

Systems Review

During the systems review the physical therapist should pay particular attention to the presence of edema, the skin integrity, the skin color, presence of scar formation, gross symmetry of the limbs, gross ROM, gross strength, balance, locomotion and transfers, and transitions. In a patient who has sustained a fracture, the presence of skin bullae or blisters may indicate that the patient had developed fracture blisters as a complication of their fracture. Another example of a finding during the systems review is the presence of shiny, glossy skin over the area of injury with excessive rubor, warmth to the touch, and the inability of the patient to tolerate even light touch. This may indicate the presence of CRPS. This would then direct the clinician to select appropriate tests in the integumentary integrity, pain, and sensory integrity categories to provide them with additional information. It might also direct the clinician to refer the patient back to their physician for further evaluation of the possibility of CRPS and, if confirmed, the medical management of this complication of musculoskeletal trauma.

Tests and Measures

As always, the findings from the history and systems review will direct the selection of tests and measures for each individual. The following categories of tests and measures would most likely be considered in patients who have sustained musculoskeletal trauma:

Aerobic capacity and endurance; anthropometric characteristics; assistive and adaptive devices; cranial and peripheral nerve integrity; gait, locomotion and balance; integumentary integrity; joint integrity and mobility; motor function (motor control and motor learning); muscle performance (including strength, power and endurance); orthotic; protective and supportive devices; pain; posture; ROM including muscle length; self-care and home management (including activities of daily living [ADL] and instrumental ADL [IADL]); and sensory integrity.

Physical therapists are in the forefront of providing treatment interventions to individuals who have sustained musculoskeletal trauma as well as the sequelae of the complications of musculoskeletal trauma. Physical therapists manage the impairments and functional limitations associated with these complications that are identified during the evaluation process. The most commonly identified impairments and functional limitations in this population include pain; impaired joint mobility, motor function and ROM; impaired motor performance and impaired gait, locomotion, and balance.

REFERENCES

1. Porth CM. *Essentials of Pathophysiology: Concepts of Altered Health States.* 2nd ed. Philadelphia, PA: Lippincott Williams & Wilkins; 2007.
2. SEERs (Surveillance Epidemiology and End Results) Training Web Site. http://training.seer.cancer.gov/disease/cancer/. Accessed May 14, 2010.
3. American Cancer Society. February 24, 2009. http://www.cancer.org/docroot/CRI/content/CRI_2_4_1x_What_Is_Cancer.asp?rnav=cri. Accessed May 14, 2010.
4. American Cancer Society. Cancer Facts & Figures 2009. Atlanta: American Cancer Society; 2009.
5. Goodman CC, Boissonnault WG, Fuller KS. *Pathology: Implications for the Physical Therapist.* 2nd ed. Philadelphia, PA: Saunders; 2003.
6. National Cancer Institute. October 4, 2006. http://www.cancer.gov/cancertopics/wyntk/overview/page4#top. Accessed May 14, 2010.
7. Leading Causes of Death. National Center for Health Statistics. December 31, 2009. http://www.cdc.gov/nchs/fastats/lcod.htm. Accessed May 14, 2010.
8. Jemal A, Siegel R, Ward E, Hao Y, Xu J, Thun MJ. Cancer statistics, 2009. *CA Cancer J Clin.* 2009;59(4):225-249.
9. Jemal A, Siegel R, Ward E, et al. Cancer statistics, 2006. *CA Cancer J Clin.* 2006;56(2):106-130.
10. Horner MJ, Ries LAG, Krapcho M, et al. *SEER Cancer Statistics Review 1975-2006.* Bethesda, MD: National Cancer Institute; 2009.
11. American Cancer Society. Revised January 6, 2010. http://www.cancer.org/docroot/CRI/content/CRI_2_4_3X_What_are_the_signs_and_symptoms_of_cancer.asp?rnav=cri. Accessed May 14, 2010.
12. Jemal A, Clegg LX, Ward E, et al. Annual report to the nation on the status of cancer, 1975-2001, with a special feature regarding survival. *Cancer.* 2004;101(1):3-27.
13. Edwards BK, Ward E, Kohler BA, et al. Annual report to the nation on the status of cancer, 1975-2006, featuring colorectal cancer trends and impact of interventions (risk factors, screening, and treatment) to reduce future rates. *Cancer.* 2010,116(3):544-573.
14. Drouin J, Pfalzer, L. Cancer and exercise. National Center on Physical Activity and Disability (NCPAD). March 5, 2009. http://www.ncpad.org/disability/fact_sheet.php?sheet=195. Accessed May 14, 2010.
15. National Cancer Institute. September 1, 2004. http://www.cancer.gov/cancertopics/factsheet/Sites-Types/metastatic. Accessed May 14, 2010.
16. American Cancer Society. February 24, 2009. http://www.cancer.org/docroot/CRI/content/CRI_2_4_4X_How_Is_Cancer_Treated.asp?rnav=cri. Accessed May 15, 2010.
17. American Cancer Society. August 25, 2009. http://www.cancer.org/docroot/ETO/content/ETO_1_4X_What_Is_Immunotherapy.asp?sitearea=ETO. Accessed May 16, 2010.
18. National Cancer Institute. August 25, 2004. http://www.cancer.gov/cancertopics/factsheet/Therapy/radiation. Accessed May 15, 2010.
19. National Cancer Institute. June 29, 2007. http://www.cancer.gov/cancertopics/chemotherapy-and-you/page2. Accessed May 15, 2010.
20. American Cancer Society. August 25, 2009. http://www.cancer.org/docroot/ETO/content/ETO_1_4X_Types_of_Immunotherapy.asp?sitearea=ETO. Accessed May 15, 2010.
21. American Cancer Society. August 25, 2009. http://www.cancer.org/docroot/ETO/content/ETO_1_4X_Monoclonal_Antibody_Therapy_Passive_Immunotherapy.asp?sitearea=ETO&viewmode=print&. Accessed May 16, 2010.
22. American Cancer Society. October 8, 2008. http://www.cancer.org/docroot/MIT/content/MIT_2_3X_Cancer-Related_Fatigue_Plagues_Many_Patients.asp?sitearea=MIT. Accessed May 15, 2010.
23. Morrow GR. Cancer-related fatigue: causes, consequences, and management. *Oncologist.* 2007;12(Suppl 1):1-3.
24. Ryan JL, Carroll JK, Ryan EP, Mustian KM, Fiscella K, Morrow GR. Mechanisms of cancer-related fatigue. *Oncologist.* 2007;12 (Suppl 1):22-34.
25. Cramp F, Daniel J. Exercise for the management of cancer-related fatigue in adults. *Cochrane Database Syst Rev.* 2008;2:CD006145.
26. Young-McCaughan S. Exercise in the rehabilitation from cancer: *Medsurg Nurs.* 2006;15(6): 384-387.
27. American Cancer Society. June 4, 2008. http://www.cancer.org/docroot/MIT/content/MIT_2_3x_physical_activity_and_the_cancer_patient.asp?sitearea=MIT. Accessed May 15, 2010.
28. Centers for Disease Control and Prevention. 1996 Surgeon general's report on physical activity and health. S/N 017-023-00196-5. http://www.cdc.gov/nccdphp/sgr/sgr.htm. Accessed July 29, 2008.
29. Centers for Disease Control and Prevention. National diabetes fact sheet: general information and national estimates on diabetes in the United States, 2007. Atlanta, GA: U.S. Department of Health and Human Services, Centers for Disease Control and Prevention; 2008.
30. American Diabetes Association. Diagnosis and classification of diabetes mellitus. *Diabetes Care.* 2010;33:S62-S69.
31. American Heart Association. http://www.americanheart.org/print_presenter.jhtml;jsessionid=T1oXXRLIKKOGGCQFCXPSCZQ?identifier=4756. Accessed May 25, 2010.
32. The Cleveland Clinic Health Information Center. February 9, 2007. http://www.clevelandclinic.org/health/health-info/docs/3000/3057.asp?index=10783. Accessed May 25, 2010.
33. National Institute for Diabetes and Digestive and Kidney Diseases. Diagnosis of diabetes. NIH Publication No. 09-4642, October 2008.
34. American Diabetes Association. International expert committee report on the role of the A1C assay in the diagnosis of diabetes. *Diabetes Care.* 2009;32:1327-1334.
35. American Diabetes Association. Economic costs of diabetes in the U.S. in 2007. *Diabetes Care.* 2008;31(3):596-615.
36. Connell JM. Role of insulin in regulation of vascular endothelial function. Presented at Society of Endocrinology AM, London, UK. Endocrine Abstracts 2001; 2: SP8.
37. American Diabetes Association. Physical activity/exercise and diabetes. *Diabetes Care.* 2004;27(Suppl 1):S58-S62.
38. Winter WE, Harris N, Schatz D. Immunological markers in the diagnosis and prediction of autoimmune type 1a diabetes. *Clinical Diabetes.* 2002;20(4):183-191.
39. Centers for Disease Control and Prevention. Basics about diabetes. March 12, 2010. http://www.cdc.gov/diabetes/consumer/learn.htm#. Accessed May 29, 2010.
40. National Institute of Diabetes and Digestive and Kidney Diseases. What I need to know about gestational diabetes. NIH Publication No. 06-5129, April 2006.
41. BC HealthGuide. Gestational diabetes. February 10, 2010. http://www.bchealthguide.org/kbase/topic/special/hw197466/sec5.htm. Accessed May 29, 2010.
42. American Physical Therapy Association. Physical fitness and type 2 diabetes. September 13, 2007. http://www.apta.org/AM/Template.cfm?Section=PFSP_Pocket_Guides&Template=/MembersOnly.cfm&ContentID=44367. Accessed May 29, 2010.

43. Sigal RJ, Kenny GP, Wasserman DH, Castaneda-Sceppa C, White RD. Physical activity/exercise and type 2 diabetes: a consensus statement from the American Diabetes Association. *Diabetes Care.* 2006;29(6):1433-1438.

44. Whaley MH, Brubaker PH, Otto RM, eds. *ACSM's Guidelines for Exercise Testing and Prescription.* 7th ed. Philadephia, PA: Lippincott Williams & Wilkins; 2006.

45. Centers for Disease Control and Prevention. Teen drivers: Fact sheet. April 26, 2010. http://www.cdc.gov/MotorVehicleSafety/Teen_Drivers/teendrivers_factsheet.html. Accessed May 29, 2010.

46. Centers for Disease Control and Prevention. Injury among older adults. October 9, 2007. http://www.cdc.gov/ncipc/olderadults.htm. Accessed May 29, 2010.

47. Centers for Disease Control and Prevention. Falls among older adults: an overview. October 6, 2009. http://www.cdc.gov/ncipc/factsheets/adultfalls.htm. Accessed May 29, 2010.

48. Strauss EJ, Petrucelli G, Bong M, Koval KJ, Egol KA. Blisters associated with lower-extremity fracture: results of a prospective treatment protocol. *J Orthop Trauma.* 2006;20(9):618-622.

49. Weinmann M. Compartment syndrome. *Emerg Med Serv.* 2003;32:36.

50. Olson SA, Glasgow RR. Acute compartment syndrome in lower extremity musculoskeletal trauma. *J Am Acad Orthop Surg.* 2005;13:436-444.

51. Swain R, Ross D. Lower extremity compartment syndrome. *Postgrad Med.* 1999;3:159-162,165,168.

52. Wallace S, Goodman S, Smith DG: Compartment syndrome, lower extremity. February 9, 2009. http://www.emedicine.com/orthoped/topic596.htm. Accessed May 29, 2010.

53. National Institute of Neurological Disorders and Stroke. Complex regional pain syndrome fact sheet. May 19, 2010. http://www.ninds.nih.gov/disorders/reflex_sympathetic_dystrophy/detail_reflex_sympathetic_dystrophy.htm. Accessed May 29, 2010.

54. Parrillo SJ. Complex regional pain syndrome. March 23, 2010. http://www.emedicine.com/emerg/topic497.htm#section~clinical. Accessed May 29, 2010.

55. Harden RN, Stanton-Hicks M, Wilson PR. Proposed new diagnostic criteria for complex regional pain syndrome. *Pain Med.* 2007;8:326-331.

56. Parisi DM, Koval K, Egol K. Fat embolism syndrome. *Am J Orthop.* 2002;31:507-512.

57. Mellor A, Soni N. Fat embolism. *Anaethesia.* 2001;56:145-154.

58. Kirkland L. Fat embolism. August 4, 2009. http://www.emedicine.com/med/topic652.htm. Accessed May 29, 2010.

59. Georgopoulos D, Bouros D: Fat embolism syndrome: clinical examination is still the preferable diagnostic method. *Chest.* 2003;123:982-983.

60. Habashi NM, Andrews PL, Scalea TM. Therapeutic aspects of fat embolism syndrome. *Injury.* 2006;37(Suppl 4): S68-S73.

CASE STUDY 13-1

Melanie A. Gillar, PT, DPT, MA

EXAMINATION

History

Current Condition/Chief Complaint

Dr. Lacrosse was a 92-year-old White male referred to home physical therapy after he sustained a left pubic ramus fracture from a fall in his home. Dr. Lacrosse was having difficulty with locomotion and hip movements secondary to the pain in his groin. He hoped to return to being able to walk without pain.

History of Current Complaint

Dr. Lacrosse was a medical school graduate whose primary language was English. He fell while chasing a mouse in his living room. He remembered turning quickly and then falling. Dr. Lacrosse landed on his left side and hit his head. There was no loss of consciousness, but he was unable to get up. His wife called 911 and he was taken by ambulance to the emergency department (ED) with chief complaint of left hip and groin pain. Plain films in the ED were negative for a hip or pelvic fracture. Dr. Lacrosse was admitted for further workup. A subsequent computed tomography (CT) scan revealed a left pubic ramus fracture. He was discharged to home 3 days after his admission and referred to a certified home health agency (CHHA) for home health care services including physical therapy.

Social History/Environment

Dr. Lacrosse was a retired psychiatrist who had worked in both an academic medical center and as a consultant to the New York Police Department (NYPD). He was married and lived with his wife, who was ~20 years younger, in a high-rise apartment building with a doorman at the entrance. Mrs. Lacrosse was currently undergoing radiation therapy (RT) status post (s/p) lumpectomy for breast cancer. Mrs. Lacrosse was very supportive and would be able to assist her husband with activities of daily living (ADL) and manage all instrumental ADL (IADL) during his recovery period. There were no steps to enter the building, but there were 2 steps without railings to access the apartment's terrace. Dr. Lacrosse had bilateral hearing aids and wore glasses to read. He was discharged to home with a raised toilet seat and standard folding walker.

Social/Health Habits

Dr. Lacrosse never smoked and he denied alcohol use. He spent his leisure time reading and enjoyed sculpting in the "studio" he had in his apartment. He did not participate in any regular exercise other than walking.

Medical/Surgical History

Dr. Lacrosse's past medical history was as follows: hypertension (20 years prior), cardiac arrhythmia (24 years prior), prostate cancer (20 prior, in remission), s/p bilateral hernia repairs and osteoarthritis (OA) in both feet. His hypertension and cardiac arrhythmia were well managed on a medication regimen of digoxin, Cozaar (losartan potassium), and amiloride hydrochloride.

Reported Functional Status

Prior to hospitalization, Dr. Lacrosse was completely independent with all ADL and participated in IADL, but shared responsibility for them with his wife who was primarily responsible for household chores. He was able to ambulate independently indoors and outdoors without an assistive device. At the time of the physical therapy evaluation, Dr. Lacrosse required assistance with locomotion and self-care. He was not able to participate in IADL.

Medications

Cozaar (losartan potassium) 25 mg daily (QD), digoxin 0.125 mg QD, amiloride hydrochloride 5 mg twice a day (BID), Colace (docusate) 100 mg 3 times per day (TID). The patient refused pain medications because he did not want to take a chance that they would cause some gastrointestinal (GI) disturbance. Medications prior to hospitalization were the same except for the addition of the Colace.

Other Clinical Tests

During the previous year, Dr. Lacrosse had blood tests and an electrocardiogram (EKG).

Clinician Comment *The interview provides the clinician with the opportunity to gather a wealth of information about patients beyond the presenting complaint. It allows the clinician to listen to how they present and express themselves and what their concerns are and to observe their thought processes. How they listen and interpret information may give important information about their hearing and cognition. If there appears to be impaired memory, do they acknowledge it when they are asked about it or do they seem to be unaware of the problem? Asking them specific questions during the past medical history (PMH), eg, such as "Do you have a history of heart disease, diabetes, cancer, etc"? may trigger the sharing of a diagnosis they have failed to mention that may have a bearing on how their case is managed. What is their perception of their limitations and what are their goals? A patient's answer to this question provides the clinician with important information that will be useful later when developing and implementing the plan of care. If the patient understands that the plan of care recommended will address his or her concerns (as well as additional concerns identified by the clinician), this can often be the key to compliance with the prescribed regimen. In the home, having a family member or caregiver present during the interview can be extremely helpful. In this case, having the patient's wife present during the interview provided verification of the accuracy of the patient's report as to both the events preceding the fall and his prior functional status.*

Pelvic fractures are rare injuries when compared to fractures in other body regions. They comprise 3% to 8% of all skeletal injuries.[1] The pelvic ring is defined as the continuous osseous cage formed by the paired innominate bones, which are composed of the ilium, ischium, and pubis, and the sacrum, including the relatively rigid articulations at the sacroiliac joints and the symphysis pubis. Stable pelvic fractures are ones that do not disrupt any joint articulations.[2] Dr. Lacrosse sustained a pubic ramus fracture, which is considered a stable fracture and one that is treated symptomatically.[3]

Fractures of the pubic rami occur commonly in the elderly,[4,5] and there is evidence that their incidence is increasing.[4] In a study by Hill et al,[4] the overall incidence of a fracture of a pubic ramus in the general population during the study period was 6.9/100,000/year while the incidence in patients over 60 years of age was 25.6/100,000/year. Alost and Waldrop[5] in their study found that 56% of the pelvic fractures in the patients studied were pubic rami fractures.

There is evidence in the available literature that the majority of the pelvic fractures seen in the elderly are caused by low-energy/moderate trauma, usually in the form of a fall from standing height.[1,3] In a study by Hill et al,[4] 87.4% of the fractures was a result of a simple fall with 55.7% a result of a fall at home. Since Dr. Lacrosse's fall was from a standing height and occurred at home, it would fit into this category.

A study by Alost and Waldrop[5] suggests that though the mechanism of injury in most geriatric patients is usually a fall, a less severe mechanism of injury than that seen in younger patients who most often sustain pelvic fractures as a result of a motor vehicle accident, there is a significantly greater mortality associated with pelvic fractures in geriatric patients. Exacerbation of preexisting cardiovascular disease was thought to be the cause of the increased mortality seen in this population. Dr. Lacrosse had a history of both hypertension and cardiac arrhythmia, but fortunately for him, there was no evidence of an exacerbation of his underlying cardiovascular disease during his hospital course, at the time of my initial visit or during the course of his home care services.

There are surprisingly few articles available on stable or closed pelvic fractures and several studies noted this. The vast majority of the available literature on all aspects of pelvic fractures and their management deal with those fractures that are a result of high-energy or blunt trauma, most frequently motor vehicle accidents. These fractures and their management are very different because they are associated with many potentially life-threatening injuries.[5]

There was, however, a study by Koval et al[6] published in 1997 that evaluated the outcome of elderly patients who sustain pubic rami fractures. Of note was that the demographics reported in their study was similar to that reported for elderly patients who sustain femoral neck fractures or intertrochanteric hip fractures. In addition, prefracture dependency, general health status, and ambulatory status were also found to be similar between those groups of patients. Of particular interest for this case study was that Dr. Lacrosse fit the patient profile for the patients in their study. He too was community dwelling and ambulatory prior to sustaining a pubic ramus fracture. Ninety-five percent of the patients who sustained an acute pubic ramus fracture required hospitalization for pain control and physical therapy. In Dr. Lacrosse's case he was admitted for further work-up because of his severe pain and negative radiographs. Once he had further imaging studies (CT scan) and the diagnosis of pubic ramus fracture was made, Dr. Lacrosse was referred for physical therapy that consisted primarily of gait training and then he was discharged to home for further management. Seventeen percent of the patients studied had additional imaging studies before the diagnosis of pubic ramus fracture was made. There was, however, a significant difference between Dr. Lacrosse's length of stay and the average length of stay (LOS) of the patients in the study. His LOS was 4 days, which was considerably less than their average length of stay of 14 days.

Several studies have suggested that underlying osteoporosis may be a risk factor for pelvic fractures,[3] though there has been little direct evidence to support that fractures of the pelvis sustained in low-energy trauma are associated with osteoporosis.[2] This is an area for further study. There is, however, available literature describing the risk factors for falls in the elderly. An article by Palmer[7] provides a comprehensive summary of these risk factors. According to Palmer, accidental falls such as the one Dr. Lacrosse experienced are not random occurrences, but they are predictable and preventable. Falls occur in 50% of community-dwelling persons over the age of 80. After every fall, an elderly patient is at increased risk of hospitalization, nursing home placement, and death. Risk factors that have been identified as predictive of falls in the elderly include the following:

- *Sedative use*
- *Cognitive impairment*
- *Abnormalities of gait and balance*
- *Disability of the lower extremities*
- *Difficulty performing tandem gait*
- *Small calf circumference*
- *Impaired vision*
- *Low body mass index*
- *Incontinence*
- *Depression*

Based on the information gathered during the history, Dr. Lacrosse's only risk factor was impaired vision. However, chasing a mouse and turning quickly were clearly not usual activities for Dr. Lacrosse and had to have been a major contributing factor for his fall.

Systems Review

Cardiovascular/Pulmonary

Seated resting values: heart rate (HR): 66 irregular; blood pressure (BP): 150/93 (According to patient and his wife this was within his normal range.) Respiratory rate (RR): 14; Edema: None present

Integumentary

There was a healing scab at the crown of patient's head and ecchymotic areas at the left hip and elbow. No other areas of skin breakdown were noted.

Musculoskeletal

Gross range of motion (ROM) was intact. Gross muscle strength of both upper extremities and of both ankles and knees was intact. All hip motions elicited pain and therefore gross muscle strength of the hips was not assessed. Dr. Lacrosse exhibited a forward head, kyphotic posture. Height: 5 feet, 7 inches; weight: 135 pounds; body mass index (BMI): 21.1.

Neuromuscular

Gait

Impaired. Patient required supervision and verbal cueing for sequencing of the walker and his lower extremities. The patient was weightbearing as tolerated (WBAT) left lower extremity (LE) and was able to ambulate ~40 feet with a standard walker.

Locomotion

Impaired ability to transition sit to supine secondary to pain and impaired ability to perform bathtub transfers for showering.

Balance

No impairment noted.

Motor Function

Intact.

Communication, Affect, Cognition, Language, and Learning Style

Dr. Lacrosse was alert and oriented to person, place, and time. He was an accurate historian and his communication was appropriate. Even with his bilateral hearing aids, his hearing was impaired. It was important to speak clearly and slowly to him in order for him to hear what was said without repetition. As a result, he learned best through demonstration.

Dr. Lacrosse would benefit from education regarding safety, use of appropriate assistive device(s), ADL, and an exercise program.

Clinician Comment *The Guide to Physical Therapist Practice (Guide)[8] describes the systems review as a brief or limited examination of the cardiovascular/pulmonary, integumentary, musculoskeletal, and neuromuscular systems as well as the communication ability, affect, cognition, language, and learning style of the patient. The systems review consists of a minimum mandatory set of tests that have been selected for each of the systems based on their reliability and validity as screens for potential pathology, impairment, functional limitation, and disability related to the movement system. The information gathered during the systems review in combination with the history helps to identify patient/client needs and to generate diagnostic hypotheses that need to be further investigated with additional tests and measures. The systems review also* *assists the physical therapist to identify potential problems that may require consultation with or referral to another provider.*

Though Dr. Lacrosse was already at home, this was still the acute phase of his recovery and rehabilitation (Injury occurred December 28 and initial home physical therapy visit was January 3). The acuteness of his injury was an important consideration when performing the systems review as well as later when choosing the procedural interventions. In the case of pelvic fractures, the limiting factor during "physical" testing was pain since pain is the hallmark of pelvic fractures. This was the reasoning behind the decision to perform only gross ROM and muscle strength tests.

The information gathered during Dr. Lacrosse's systems review, in combination with the information from his history, identified needs that would direct the physical therapy interventions to address his impairments (pain with functional movements and activities) and functional limitations (inability to transition sit to supine without assistance for his lower extremities, his inability to ambulate without an assistive device and his inability to perform self-care in the usual manner). It also identified the need for additional tests and measures in the following categories:

- *Environmental, Home, and Work (Job/School/Play) Barriers*
- *Pain*
- *Self-Care and Home Management (Including ADL and IADL)*

In addition, it identified an elevated BP despite an existing medication regimen. According to the guidelines published in The Seventh Report of the Joint National Committee on Prevention, Detection, Evaluation and Treatment of High Blood Pressure,[9] most patients with hypertension will require 2 or more antihypertensive medications to achieve a BP < 140/90. Dr. Lacrosse had a history of hypertension and was taking Cozaar, an angiotensin receptor blocker that is used in the treatment of hypertension (causes relaxation of the smooth vascular muscle) at the recommended dosage and amiloride hydrochloride, which is a potassium-sparing diuretic, also at the recommended dosage.[10]

At the time of initial visit his BP was 150/93 and on subsequent visits his BP remained within this range (140 to 150 for systolic and 85 to 95 for his diastolic). According to both the patient and his wife, this was a normal BP reading for him. Dr. Lacrosse reported that he and his physician feel that his current medication regimen was keeping his BP under good control and there was no need to modify his medication regimen. Follow-up with his physician confirmed this.

Tests and Measures

Clinician Comment *The tests and measures utilized were incorporated into the required initial physical therapy visit form utilized by the CHHA.*

Environmental, Home and Work (Job/School/Play) Barriers

Home safety assessment performed to evaluate home safety and identify any current barriers that required remediation. None were identified.

Clinician Comment *This can be accomplished with checklists or questionnaires of current and potential barriers. A "Home Safety Assessment" checklist that is answered, "Yes," "No" or "Not Applicable" was used to identify any safety issues in Dr. Lacrosse's apartment. There was also an area to identify what action(s) was taken if anything was found to be unsafe or inadequate. The checklist included the following items:*

- *Are the rooms cluttered?*
- *Is the lighting adequate?*
- *If throw rugs are present, are they properly secured?*
- *Are there skid-resistant mats in risk areas of the bathroom?*
- *If there are stairs, are they unobstructed and do they have nonslip surfaces and handrails?*
- *Is there any durable medical equipment (DME) safety equipment such as tub seat or grab bars present?*
- *Does the patient have adequate sensory capabilities regarding water temperature?*
- *Are electrical appliances away from the tub/shower?*
- *Are the electrical and telephone cords safely positioned?*
- *If there is DME equipment, is it appropriate, in good condition, and is the patient using it appropriately?*
- *Are there any obstructions near the stove or oven?*
- *Is the patient able to access emergency assistance?*

There was also an area to identify if anything unsafe or unusual was found in the home. If anything unsafe or unusual was identified there was an area to describe what was found and when other members of the health care team were informed. The home safety assessment performed in Dr. Lacrosse's apartment did not identify any safety issues or barriers that required remediation.

Pain

The pain assessment performed included the use of a numeric rating scale, which revealed that Dr. Lacrosse's pain was 8/10. The pain was localized to his groin. The pain was triggered by any hip movement and when getting in and out of bed.

> **Clinician Comment** *The pain assessment used included not only a numeric rating scale (NRS), but questions regarding the frequency of pain, type of pain, location of pain, precipitating factors, signs/symptoms of pain, as well as any control measures. There was also an area to include any recommendations. The numeric rating scale is a 0 to 10 intensity scale where zero indicates that there is no pain and 10 is the worst pain imaginable. The pain assessment performed revealed that Dr. Lacrosse's pain was 8/10, was localized to his groin, and was triggered by any hip movement and when getting in and out of bed. This pain report was consistent with the pain patterns reported by patients with pelvic fractures. Further research supports the use of an NRS both in cognitively impaired and cognitively intact older adults.[11,12] The NRS, when combined with additional questions about frequency of pain, type of pain, etc, allows the clinician to gather the necessary information to choose appropriate procedural interventions to manage a patient's pain and/or make appropriate recommendations about pain control to a patient's physician. In addition, this combination scale can be used to monitor a patient's response to physical therapy interventions and/or pain medication.*

Self-Care and Home Management (Including Activities of Daily Living and Instrumental Activities of Daily Living)

Information gained through interview and observation identified that Dr. Lacrosse required assistance for lower extremity dressing and to sponge bathe. A raised toilet seat allowed him to be independent performing toilet transfers.

> **Clinician Comment** *The Guide[8] defines self-care management as the ability to perform ADL such as bed mobility, transfers, dressing, grooming, bathing, eating, and toileting. Home management is defined as the ability to perform the more complex IADL such as maintaining a home, shopping, and performing household chores.*
>
> *There are many ways to gather the data for this category. As previously indicated, the initial physical therapy visit used a form required by the CHHA. This was a very comprehensive form. An entire area of the form was devoted to "Functional Assessment," which included the patient's prior level of function, all aspects of bed mobility, transfers, shower/tub transfers, how the patient toilets, whether he is able to feed, dress, bathe or groom himself as well as IADL information, including managing in the kitchen, shopping, and housework. One of the advantage of working with a patient in the home is that if through interview or report a deficit is identified in any of the aforementioned areas, it is easy to ask for a demonstration and then to figure out how best to remediate the problem. In the case of Dr. Lacrosse, the data were gathered for this category through interview and observation. It was able to be determined that Dr. Lacrosse had been independent with all ADL prior to hospitalization and participated in IADL but shared responsibility for them with his wife, who was primarily responsible for household chores. At the time of the initial visit Dr. Lacrosse required assistance for LE dressing and to sponge bathe. A raised toilet seat allowed him to be independent performing toilet transfers.*
>
> *It's important to complete the interview portion of the initial visit prior to beginning the systems review and tests and measures because if a patient states that he or she is unable to perform a specific task or activity, the therapist can test the ability to perform that task and ask for a demonstration during the exam. A common example is when the patient reports that he or she is unable to perform LE dressing activities such as donning and doffing pants. More often than not these same patients have adequate ROM and muscle performance to be able to perform the activity. When asked to demonstrate why they are unable to put on their pants, it is frequently observed that they are used to doing this activity standing and have never considered that it could be done in sitting or even supine. In the case of Dr. Lacrosse, his pain with all hip motions would explain his report that he required assistance with LE dressing and to sponge bathe. In addition, his pain with all hip motions, coupled with his need for a walker to ambulate, would correlate with his difficulty transferring into and out of his tub for showering thus necessitating the need to sponge bathe.*

EVALUATION

Diagnosis

Practice Pattern

Based on the above history, systems review, and tests and measures, this patient is classified into Musculoskeletal Pattern 4G: Impaired Joint Mobility, Muscle Performance, and Range of Motion Associated with Fracture

International Classification of Functioning, Disability and Health Model

See ICF model on p 558.

ICF Model of Disablement for Dr. Lacrosse

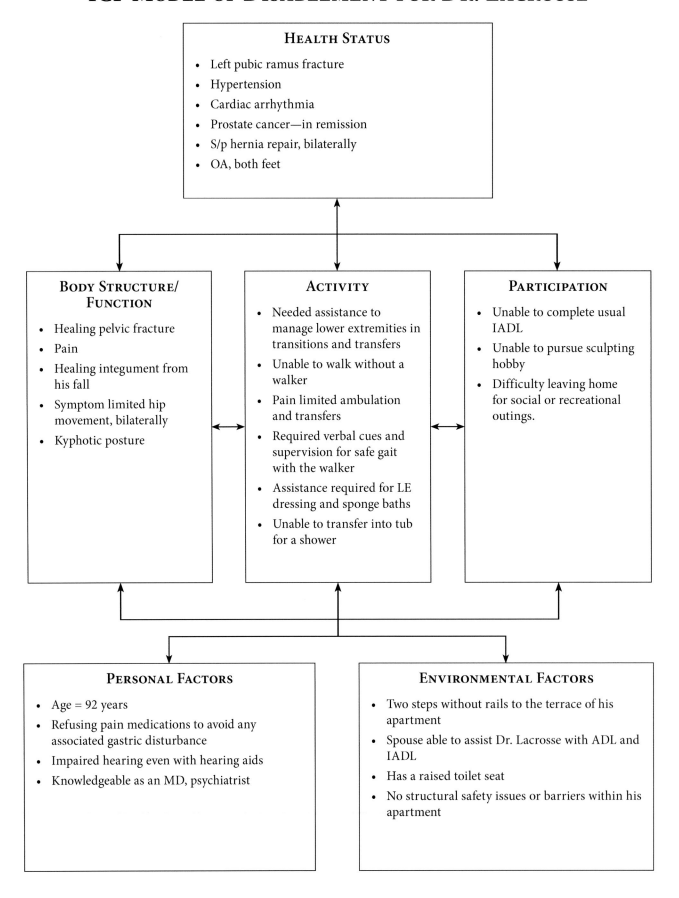

Health Status

- Left pubic ramus fracture
- Hypertension
- Cardiac arrhythmia
- Prostate cancer—in remission
- S/p hernia repair, bilaterally
- OA, both feet

Body Structure/ Function

- Healing pelvic fracture
- Pain
- Healing integument from his fall
- Symptom limited hip movement, bilaterally
- Kyphotic posture

Activity

- Needed assistance to manage lower extremities in transitions and transfers
- Unable to walk without a walker
- Pain limited ambulation and transfers
- Required verbal cues and supervision for safe gait with the walker
- Assistance required for LE dressing and sponge baths
- Unable to transfer into tub for a shower

Participation

- Unable to complete usual IADL
- Unable to pursue sculpting hobby
- Difficulty leaving home for social or recreational outings.

Personal Factors

- Age = 92 years
- Refusing pain medications to avoid any associated gastric disturbance
- Impaired hearing even with hearing aids
- Knowledgeable as an MD, psychiatrist

Environmental Factors

- Two steps without rails to the terrace of his apartment
- Spouse able to assist Dr. Lacrosse with ADL and IADL
- Has a raised toilet seat
- No structural safety issues or barriers within his apartment

Prognosis

This 92-year-old male was in good health and independent prior to his fall. His hospitalization course was brief and at the time of initial visit, 6 days after his fall, he was already able to ambulate 40 feet in his apartment with a walker with supervision and verbal cueing for sequencing of the walker and his LEs. Though he was unwilling to take any pain medications, he was willing to do whatever was asked of him despite the pain. It was anticipated that over the course of 3 to 6 months, beyond the 4 weeks of anticipated physical therapy, Dr. Lacrosse would make a complete or near complete recovery.

Plan of Care

Interventions

- Patient-/client-related instruction regarding his current condition, the plan of care, and the discharge plan.

- Endurance reconditioning program will consist of an in-home, timed walking prescription based on his current functional walk test (maximum of 40 feet with assistive device).

- Patient will be instructed in his prescribed home exercise program (HEP) that had been written out (his preferred learning style). Frequency of performance equals 2 to 3 times daily for a 15- to 20-minute session equaling a total duration of ~40 minutes.

- Gait training will progress from use of a walker to use of a straight cane on level surfaces and stairs.

- Patient education will include instruction regarding safety with an assistive device.

- Bed mobility training will incorporate the use of upper extremities and sliding movement techniques to strengthen arms/trunk and minimize hip pain.

- As pain with hip movements decreases, will begin LE dressing instruction and initiate tub transfer training for showering.

Proposed Frequency and Duration of Physical Therapy Visits

Over the course of 4 weeks, Dr. Lacrosse will be seen for 10 visits; 3 times per week for 2 weeks and then 2 times per week for 2 weeks.

Anticipated Goals

1. Patient to have sufficient decrease in pain with hip movements so that he is independent transitioning from sit to supine (2 to 3 weeks), independent performing LE dressing (2 to 3 weeks), and independent with tub transfers for showering (4 weeks).

2. Patient to be able to ambulate independently indoors with a straight cane on all level surfaces in his apartment (3 weeks) and independent with a straight cane on stairs so that he is able to negotiate the 2 steps to his terrace (4 weeks).

3. Patient's endurance capacity will increase to allow for independent mobility (with straight cane), within the apartment (3 weeks), and able to walk outside of his living area to the front of his building and access curb side transportation (4 weeks).

Expected Outcomes

Over the 3 to 6 months following the completion of physical therapy, it could be anticipated that the patient would resume participation in IADL and he will be able to ambulate outdoors with a straight cane on all surfaces, weather permitting.

Discharge Plan

Patient will be ready for discharge from home health physical therapy to his own care when he has achieved the anticipated goals listed above. The plan of care including the discharge plan was discussed with the patient, who was in agreement.

INTERVENTIONS

Patient-/Client-Related Instruction

Dr. Lacrosse received instruction about his plan of care and discharge plan as previously discussed. In addition, he was educated about his current condition, what to expect in terms of pain, progression to a cane, etc, as well as explanations for the procedural interventions chosen and why they would benefit him. He received instructions about safety issues when ambulating with an assistive device, including placement of the device, how to make sure the walker was "locked" in the open position, etc. Dr. Lacrosse was also instructed in a HEP and provided with a written copy of his HEP.

Procedural Interventions

Therapeutic Exercise Prescription

Aerobic Capacity/Endurance Conditioning or Reconditioning:

Mode
Walking program
Intensity
RPE < 11, symptoms < 3 to 4/10
Duration
One to 5 minutes to cover 5 to 50 feet
Frequency
One time every waking hour until total feet walked for the day is 300 to 500 feet

Dr. Lacrosse was instructed in a walking program that consisted of ambulating short distances, (5- to 10-foot segment minimums) for a minimum of 30 feet for every hour that he was awake. He was instructed that the distance he walked each time could be short with rests in between, but it was essential that he walked every hour for a total of 300 to 500 feet per day.

Clinician Comment *An hourly ambulation schedule can be prescribed for patients with instructions to total their distance walked over the course of the day. This is an effective tool for reconditioning patients after hospitalization as the duration and frequency of walking is within their control and they can easily add the distances and track their progress. The frequency and intensity of walking prescriptions are not as important as the total duration of walking in cases of severe impairment (ability to walk less than 500 feet in 6 minutes). Once the patient is able to complete a total of 500 feet without pain or loss of balance, it is possible to add in the component of "intensity" to the exercise prescription by combining the distance to be walked with a specific time frame. There is research to support the efficacy of intermittent training in improving aerobic conditioning,[13] and there are studies to support the efficacy of a walking program in improving walk endurance capacity.[14]*

Strength, Power, and Endurance Training

Mode
Isometric and against gravity, strengthening exercises.

Intensity
Slow movements through entire ROM, as able, and avoid undue fatigue.

Duration
Fifteen to 20 minutes (for entire routine of identified exercises).

Frequency
10 repetitions, 2 to 3 times per day.

An HEP was developed for Dr. Lacrosse consisting of active exercise in supine and sitting as well as isometric exercises in supine.

- Gluteal sets in supine with 5-second hold both LEs.
- Quad sets in supine with 5-second hold both LEs.
- Ankle pumps in supine to be performed simultaneously with both ankles. Dr. Lacrosse was instructed to perform each repetition slowly to achieve maximal ROM.
- Heel slides in supine alternating legs. Dr. Lacrosse was instructed to perform each repetition slowly to maximize ROM and minimize pain on affected side.
- Marching in place sitting in a straight back chair to be performed slowly to achieve maximal ROM.
- Knee extension in sitting in straight back chair to be performed slowly and with 5-second hold, alternating legs.

Gait and Locomotion Training

Gait training—Progress from walker to straight cane (including stair climbing).

Functional Training in Self-Care and Home Management

Activities of Daily Living Training
Bed mobility and transfer training; LE dressing

Prescription, Application, and, as Appropriate, Fabrication of Devices and Equipment (Assistive, Adaptive, Orthotic, Protective, Supportive, and Prosthetic)

Assistive Device
Prescribe an adjustable straight cane when the patient was ready to progress to gait training with a cane.

Clinician Comment *There is next to nothing published in the literature about physical therapy interventions after pelvic fracture. Koval et al[6] in their article discuss that "physical therapy was started when symptoms allowed and consisted of unrestricted weight-bearing ambulation using a walker. Patients progressed to using a cane as tolerated." That's true, but what about the other interventions? The demographics reported in their study were similar to those reported for elderly patients who sustain femoral neck fractures or intertrochanteric hip fractures. In addition, prefracture dependency, general health status and ambulatory status were also found to be similar between these 2 groups of patients. Dr. Lacrosse fit the patient profile for the patients in their study. A search of the literature was then completed to identify recommended physical therapy interventions after hip fracture.*

Many studies discussed patients receiving "physical therapy" and there was general agreement that physical therapy interventions are indicated after hip fracture, but few discussed exactly what specific physical therapy interventions were utilized. Naglie et al[15] studied elderly patients (at least 70 years old) status postsurgical repair of a hip fracture that were randomly assigned to receive either postoperative interdisciplinary care or usual care during their hospitalization. Interdisciplinary care included routine assessment and care by an internist-geriatrician, physical therapist, occupational therapist, social worker, and clinical nurse specialist. In addition, interdisciplinary rounds were held twice weekly to set goals for the patients and monitor their progress. The physical therapy interventions included early mobilization full weightbearing on the operative leg and twice-daily physical therapy sessions. This is an example of physical therapy interventions that were provided but specific details about what those interventions were are not indicated. However, the study looked at outcomes at 3 and 6 months and whether there was a decline from baseline in terms of ambulation, chair or bed transfers, and place of residence. It could be postulated from this that interventions included gait and transfer training as well as functional training in self-care.

Kauffman et al[16] in their 1987 article were a bit more specific in discussing the physical therapy interventions after hip fracture. They acknowledged that the physical therapy was individualized to the patient and fracture type. In addition, they described the standard physical therapy interventions after hip fracture as ROM, strengthening exercises, and gait training.

Tinetti et al[17] in their study looked at whether a home-based systematic multicomponent rehabilitation strategy (SMR) resulted in better outcomes relative to usual care (UC). They discussed that the usual components of home care physical therapy after hip fracture included various combinations of muscle strength conditioning, ambulation, transfer, and balance training. They also contend that though home health aides may provide some assistance with ADL, most patients after hip fracture receive limited retraining in self-care either from an occupational therapist or rehabilitation nurse. For the purpose of their study, the physical therapy component of the SMR strategy was designed to identify and remediate impairments in upper extremity and LE strength, balance, transfers, gait, and bed mobility. The interventions for gait, transfers, and bed mobility included instruction in safer, more effective techniques, the provision of and training in the use of assistive devices, as well as environmental modifications. Patients were also instructed in individualized HEPs that they were to do daily on their own.

The UC physical therapy interventions consisted of gait training and transfer training, as well as strengthening and ROM exercises. The specific interventions and duration of the physical therapy were left up to the discretion of the physical therapist. Their conclusion was that the SMR program was no more effective in promoting recovery than the usual home-based rehabilitation. They conclude by saying: "The challenge that remains is to determine the composition and duration of rehabilitation and home services that ensures optimal functional recovery most efficiently in older persons who fracture a hip."

More recently Mangione and Palombaro[18] in their case report noted that exercise is the least-examined factor affecting outcome in patients' status post-hip fracture. They listed the general categories of physical therapy interventions provided in this population as including active-assistive, active, and resistance exercises as well as transfer and gait training, instructions on weightbearing limitations and precautions, and moist heat. They too pointed out the lack of complete exercise prescriptions that include the frequency, intensity, and duration for patients after hip fracture. They designed a program based on the overload and specificity principles for the subject with good results. It would be difficult to generalize the results of this type of exercise prescription for Dr. Lacrosse because he was seen in the period immediately postfracture. His fracture had not fully healed whereas their subject was seen 1 year after surgery for repair of her hip fracture.

Intuitively it makes sense to provide physical therapy interventions to address the limited ROM and pain with functional movements and activities that are 2 of the common impairments associated with hip and pelvic fractures. It is also fairly clear from the limited available literature that transfers and gait training are appropriate physical therapy interventions for this population. It is less clear from the literature that functional training in self-care is a routine part of physical therapy interventions. In Dr. Lacrosse's geographic area and in the home health setting, LE dressing instruction, recommendations for bathing/showering options, etc, are a routine part of the physical therapy interventions provided to patients who have sustained pelvic and hip fractures. What is not clear from the review of the literature is which exercises are most appropriate in the weeks immediately following a fracture. It makes good sense to instruct patients in exercises such as ankle pumps and circles as well as other active ROM exercises to improve circulation, to prevent blood clots and maintain available ROM. Starting patients on mild strengthening exercises such as gluteal sets and quad sets would also seem to make good sense. However, the question that remains unanswered is the specificity of exercise that is most effective in facilitating return to function after hip or pelvic fractures, particularly in the elderly.

REEXAMINATION

Objective

Observation of gait and assessment of pain was ongoing and permitted patient to be progressed to gait training with straight cane, including stair climbing, LE dressing instruction, bed mobility, and tub transfer training at the appropriate time. Observed the patient's response to exercise every visit and modified his HEP accordingly.

OUTCOMES

Discharge

Dr. Lacrosse was seen for a total of 10 physical therapy visits over the course of 4 weeks. At that point he had achieved his anticipated goals and was discharged from home health physical therapy to his own care. No further physical therapy intervention was indicated. At the time of discharge, he no longer had pain with hip movements and was independent transitioning sit to supine, performing LE dressing, and transferring into and out of the tub for showering. In addition, he was independent ambulating with a straight cane indoors on all level surfaces in his apartment and was able to negotiate the 2 steps to his terrace. He was instructed to continue performing his HEP once daily and encouraged to do as much walking as possible.

Clinician Comment *In their study, Koval et al[6] found that there were 38 patients for whom 1-year minimum follow-up was available (range 12 to 70 months). At this follow-up, 35 of the 38 patients (92%) were living at home and 32 of the 38 patients (84%) had no or only mild complaints of hip/groin pain. Thirty-five patients (92%) had returned to their prefracture ambulatory status and 36 of 38 patients (95%) had returned to their prefracture ability in performing ADL. Their conclusion was that patients with pubic ramus fractures have a good prognosis with regard to long-term pain relief and functional outcome.*

At 4-year follow-up, Dr. Lacrosse was still living at home with his wife, had no complaints of hip or groin pain, was independent performing his ADL, had resumed participation in IADL, and was back to sculpting. The only significant difference was in his ambulation status. He now required a cane to ambulate on all surfaces indoors and did not go outdoors unless accompanied by his wife.

REFERENCES

1. Morris RO, Sonibare A, Green DJ, Masad T. Closed pelvic fractures: characteristics and outcomes in older patients admitted to medical and geriatric wards. *Postgrad Med J.* 2000;76:646-650.
2. McKinnis LN. *Fundamentals of Orthopedic Radiology.* Philadelphia, PA: F. A. Davis Company, 1997.
3. Melton LJ 3rd, Sampson JM, Borrey BF, Ilstrup DM: Epidemiologic features of pelvic fractures. *Clin Orthop.* 1981;155:43-47.
4. Hill RMF, Robinson CM, Keating JF. Fractures of the pubic rami: epidemiology and five-year survival. *J Bone Joint Surg Br.* 2001;83-B:1141-1144.
5. Alost T, Waldrop RD. Profile of geriatric pelvic fractures presenting to the emergency department. *Am J Emerg Med.* 1997;15:576-578.
6. Koval KJ, Aharonoff GB, Schwartz MC, et al. Pubic rami fracture: a benign pelvic injury? *J Orthop Trauma.* 1997;11(1):7-9.
7. Palmer R. Falls in the elderly: predictable and preventable. *Cleve Clin J Med.* 2001;68(4):303-306.
8. American Physical Therapy Association. *Guide to Physical Therapist Practice.* 2nd ed. 2001;81:9-744.
9. Chobanian AV, Bakris GL, Black HR, et al. Seventh report of the Joint National Committee on Prevention, Detection, Evaluation, and Treatment of High Blood Pressure. *Hypertension.* 2003;42(6):1206-1252.
10. Holland N, Adams MP. *Core Concepts in Pharmacology.* Upper Saddle River, NJ: Prentice Hall; 2003.
11. Ware LJ, Epps CD, Herr K, Packard A. Evaluation of the Revised Faces Pain Scale, Verbal Descriptor Scale, Numeric Rating Scale and Iowa Pain Thermometer in older minority adults. *Pain Manag Nurs.* 2006;7(3):117-125.
12. Bergh I, Sjöström B, Odén A, Steen B. An application of pain rating scales in geriatric patients. *Aging (Milano).* 2000;12(5):380-387.
13. Christensen EH, Hedman R, Saltin B: Intermittent and continuous running. *Acta Physiol Scand.* 1960;50:269-286.
14. MacRae PG, Asplund LA, Schnell JF, Ouslander JG, Abrahamse A, Morris C. A walking program for nursing home residents: effects on walk endurance, physical activity, mobility, and quality of life. *J Am Geriatr Soc.* 1996;44(2):175-180.
15. Naglie G, Tansey C, Kirkland JL, et al. Interdisciplinary inpatient care for elderly people with hip fracture: a randomized controlled trial. *CMAJ.* 2002;167(1):25-32.
16. Kauffman TL, Albright L. Wagner C. Rehabilitation outcomes after hip fracture in persons 90 years and older. *Arch Phys Med Rehabil.* 1987;68:369-371.
17. Tinetti ME, Baker DI, Gottschalk M, et al. Home-based mulitcomponent rehabilitation program for older persons after hip fracture: a randomized trial. *Arch Phys Med Rehabil.* 1999;80(8):916-922.
18. Mangione KK, Palombaro KM. Exercise prescription for a patient 3 months after hip fracture. *Phys Ther.* 2005;85:676-687.

CASE STUDY 13-2

*Melanie A. Gillar, PT, DPT, MA
and Nancy Gage, PT, DPT*

EXAMINATION

History

Current Condition/Chief Complaint

Ms. Ledger was a 66-year-old White woman who was referred to physical therapy to assist with right upper extremity mobility. Three weeks prior to the initial physical therapy appointment she had undergone a right modified mastectomy and axillary lymph node dissection. Ms. Ledger was scheduled to begin radiation therapy (RT) in 3 weeks.

Ms. Ledger reported pain associated with her recovery from her recent surgery that resulted in significant limitations in her mobility and function. She reported difficulty finding a comfortable position for sleeping. In addition, she needed to be able to comfortably maintain a position of prolonged right shoulder flexion/abduction to allow for the initial mapping for RT and subsequent treatments.

History of Current Complaint

Ms. Ledger was diagnosed with breast cancer 9 months prior to the initial physical therapy appointment, A routine mammogram showed an area of increased density in her right medial breast. A follow-up mammogram and ultrasound performed 1 week later showed a suggestion of a spiculated density measuring 2.0 to 2.5 cm. She underwent an ultrasound-guided core biopsy 10 days after the follow-up mammogram and ultrasound. The biopsies were positive for a Stage 2/3 infiltrating carcinoma in all cores. The tumor was Estrogen Receptor/Progesterone Receptor (ER/PR) positive and HER-2 negative. She began a course of neoadjuvant chemotherapy, Femara (letrozole), prior to her surgery.

Clinician Comment *Breast cancers can vary tremendously in terms of severity and long-term prognosis. It is the staging of the disease that determines the seriousness. The American Joint Committee on Cancer uses the TNM classification system.[1,2] Staging is the system used to identify the extent of the tumor (T), spread to lymph nodes (N), and metastases (M) when first diagnosed. These* *categories are further broken down with a suffix indicating the degree of involvement.*

T (Primary tumor)	(x, 0, is, 1 to 4) size or direct extent of primary tumor
T x	Primary tumor cannot be evaluated
T0	No evidence of primary tumor
T is	Carcinoma in situ (LCIS, DCIS or Paget's disease of the nipple
T1, T2, T3, T4	Size and/or extent of the primary tumor
N (Lymph nodes)	(x, 0, 1 to 3) amount of spread to regional lymph nodes
N x	Regional nodes cannot be evaluated
N0	No regional lymph node involvement
N1, N2, N3	Number and/or extent of spread to regional lymph nodes
M (Metastasis)	(x, 0, 1) presence or absence of metastasis
M x	No distant metastasis can be evaluated
M0	No distant metastasis present
M1	Metastasis is present
LCIS: lobular carcinoma in situ; DCIS: ductal carcinoma in situ.	

These criteria may be then translated into a more simple classification of staging.

Stage	Definition
Stage 0	Carcinoma in situ (present only in the layer of cells in which it began).
Stage 1, 2, 3	The higher the number, the more extensive the disease: larger tumor size, and/or spread to nearby lymph nodes and/or organs adjacent to the primary tumor.
Stage 4	The cancer has spread to another organ.
Data from American Cancer Society. Breast Cancer Facts and Figures 2007-2008. Atlanta: American Cancer Society Inc.; and National Cancer Institute. September 25, 2008. http:// www.cancer.gov/cancertopics/pdq/treatment/breast/ HealthProfessional/page1. Accessed October 28, 2008.	

Breast cancer can be treated in a variety of ways including surgery, (RT), chemotherapy, and hormonal therapy. The first step in treatment is the removal of the cancer. Also important in the initial treatment planning is testing of the tumor itself. The estrogen receptor assay is a lab test performed to see whether estrogen receptors are present. Is the tumor estrogen receptor positive (ER+), and likely to respond to hormonal therapy? Or is the tumor estrogen receptor negative (ER–), and therefore unlikely to respond to hormone therapy? Another common test is the HER2/ neu genetic test. Cancers that have this gene tend to be very aggressive and may respond to Herceptin as part of an adjuvant chemotherapy treatment plan.[3]

Neoadjuvant chemotherapy is administered prior to surgery with the intent of reducing tumor size to make surgery more manageable and less extensive. A major benefit to neoadjuvant chemotherapy is the potential to increase breast conservation and possibly eliminate the need for a mastectomy. Preoperative chemotherapy allows for an in situ assessment of the tumor behavior during chemotherapy and to determine effectiveness of different cytotoxic drugs avoiding the unnecessary administration of medications to which the cancer is resistant.[4]

Social History/Environment

Ms. Ledger was an active 66-year-old woman. She was divorced and lived alone in a single-family 2-story home with her 3 dogs. She had 4 grown children, 2 of whom lived out of state. All were very supportive. She also had a strong support network of friends and coworkers.

Employment/Work (Job/School/Play)

Ms. Ledger was a third-grade teacher. She had taken the school year off to accommodate medical appointments and treatments. She hoped to return in the fall for at least 1 more year of teaching prior to her retirement. She expressed concern about her ability to perform at her previous work level.

Social/Health Habits

Ms. Ledger was a nonsmoker and she reported only rare use of alcohol.

Family History

Ms. Ledger's family history was significant for 2 maternal aunts with breast cancer; one diagnosed at the age of 40 and the other at the age of 90. Her mother died of dementia and her father died of chronic obstructive pulmonary disease (COPD). She had one sister who was alive and well.

Medical/Surgical History

Ms. Ledger's past medical history was significant for hypercholesterolemia, endometriosis, asthma, and degenerative disc disease. There was a question of a recent episode of pneumonia. She reported that she had taken estrogen for 20 years. Past surgical history included a hysterectomy, bilateral salpingo-oophorectomy secondary to endometriosis, an appendectomy, tonsillectomy, right ankle reconstruction, and a caesarean section. As mentioned earlier, Ms. Ledger had surgery 3 weeks prior to the initial physical therapy appointment.

Clinician Comment *Ms. Ledger underwent a modified radical mastectomy as well as axillary lymph node dissection (ALND). A modified radical mastectomy removes the breast, skin, nipple areola, and some axillary lymph nodes but spares the pectoralis muscles. An ALND is the surgical resection and histological examination of the first 2 layers of lymph nodes in the axilla. Level 3 nodes may also be removed.*

Reported Functional Status

Prior to the diagnosis of breast cancer, Ms. Ledger was very active. She walked her 3 dogs a distance of ~1 mile each day and gardened in the spring and summer. She reported a decline in her energy level that she believed was related to both her chemotherapy as well as her recent surgery. She needed assistance for all but light housework and activities of daily living (ADL). She was unable to perform any yard work and she was not able to handle her dogs on a leash. Her goal was to return to work as a third-grade teacher at the beginning of the next school year, 5 months away. She wanted to work in her garden.

Medications

Ms. Ledger was taking Femara, Zometa (zoledronic acid), calcium with vitamin D, Lipitor (atorvastatin), Flovent (fluticasone), albuterol, and Klonopin (clonazepam). She was allergic to penicillin, sulfa drugs, tetracycline, and bees.

Clinician Comment *Femara, an aromatase inhibitor, is an anti-estrogen drug that is Food and Drug Administration (FDA) approved and typically used for the adjuvant treatment of postmenopausal women with hormone receptor-positive, early-stage breast cancer.*

Femara is also approved for the extended adjuvant treatment of early-stage breast cancer in postmenopausal women who are within 3 months of completing 5 years of tamoxifen therapy. And finally, as in the case of Ms. Ledger, Femara is approved for the treatment of estrogen receptor-positive or unknown breast cancer that has metastasized.[5]

Zometa is a member of the group of medications known as bisphosphonates *that are used to treat hypercalcemia in the blood associated with a malignancy. The primary pharmacologic action of zoledronic acid is the inhibition of bone resorption.[5]*

Calcium with vitamin D is a dietary supplement taken to prevent bone loss.[5]

Lipitor is a cholesterol-lowering medication that blocks the production of cholesterol in the body.[5] Atorvastatin reduces low-density lipoprotein (LDL) cholesterol and total cholesterol in the blood. Atorvastatin is used to treat high cholesterol and to lower the risk of stroke, heart attack, or other heart complications.

Flovent is a corticosteroid that is used in the maintenance treatment of asthma.[5] When used regularly, it prevents the wheezing and shortness of breath seen in asthma, bronchitis, and some types of emphysema. It works directly in the lungs to make breathing easier by reducing the swelling and inflammation of the airways. It is not indicated for an acute asthma attack.

Albuterol is taken as needed for the treatment of acute episodes of bronchospasm or the prevention of the symptoms of asthma.[5]

Klonopin is indicated for the treatment of panic disorders, characterized by the occurrence of unexpected panic attacks and the associated concern of experiencing additional attacks.[5] It is in a class of drugs known as benzodiazepines.

Other Clinical Tests

A chest computed tomography (CT) scan, brain magnetic resonance imaging (MRI) scan, thoracic spine MRI, positron emission tomography (PET) staging, and bone density exam were performed within the month following the breast core biopsies. The test results appear below.

Computed Tomography Scan

- No significant mediastinal adenopathy identified. Previously identified structure appeared simply to represent a pericardial recess.

- Persistent small bilateral pleural effusions similar to exam 6 months earlier.

- Multifocal small sclerotic lesions had developed in the thoracic spine consistent with sclerotic metastatic disease. In addition, there appeared to be small lytic lesions on the anterior aspect of T7 and T8.

Brain Magnetic Resonance Imaging

- No evidence of intracranial metastatic disease. Questionable metastatic disease involving skull and proximal cervical spine.

- No evidence of acute infarction or acute or chronic intracranial hemorrhage or significant atrophy. Minimal periventricular signal white matter abnormality was nonspecific.

Magnetic Resonance Imaging Thoracic Spine

- Innumerable sclerotic foci scattered throughout the cervical, thoracic, and the proximal lumbar spine and the margin of this study. These findings were thought to be consistent with metastatic disease. There was no evidence of a pathological fracture or a bony expansion. There was no evidence of central canal or foraminal narrowing.

- There were chronic-appearing degenerative and/or post-traumatic changes in the cervical spine and the cord may be contacted at multiple levels. There was little or no impingement associated with this. This might be better evaluated with a dedicated cervical MRI if clinically indicated.

- There were disc osteophyte complexes and/or small disc protrusions as described above, but no cord contact or impingement is identified.
- Bilateral pleural effusions.

Positron Emission Tomography Staging

- Diffuse metastatic disease in the spine and pelvis.
- Moderate pleural effusions and left renal calcifications.

Bone Density Exam

"All regions are much, much better than average for age, with no sign of evolving osteoporosis or osteopenia. Excellent bone mineral density (BMD)."

Clinician Comment *The results of the MRI of the thoracic spine and the PET staging revealed that Ms. Ledger had metastatic disease, which would indicate that she had Stage 4 breast cancer (cancer that had spread to another organ) and not Stage 2/3 as originally thought.*

Nothing appeared in the interview that would contraindicate Ms. Ledger's participation in physical therapy. The system review would further evaluate her status as well as assist in the selection of indicated tests and measurements.

Systems Review

Cardiovascular/Pulmonary

- Heart rate (HR) = 82
- Blood pressure (BP) = 149/89
- Respiratory rate (RR) = 14
- Oxygen saturation was 99% on room air
- Edema: There was no edema noted in the distal extremities including Ms. Ledger's right arm, forearm, and hand.

Clinician Comment *Lymphedema is an accumulation of the protein-rich lymphatic fluid in the interstitial tissue that causes swelling, most often in the arm(s) and/or leg(s) and occasionally in other parts of the body.[6] Lymphedema can develop when lymphatic vessels are missing or impaired (primary), or when lymph vessels are damaged or lymph nodes removed or damaged (secondary), as in the case of surgical or radiotherapeutic interventions. It has been reported that approximately 25% of patients will develop lymphedema after breast cancer surgery and that can increase to 38% if the patient receives RT.[7] Onset of lymphedema is often slow and subtle, beginning with a heavy or full sensation in the limb before*

progressing to full blown swelling. Lymphedema onset is usually within the first 2 or 3 years following treatment, but may occur as many as 30 years later.

Integumentary

- Skin integrity: The skin was dry and flaky with some peeling skin in the area around the mastectomy scar.
- Presence of scar formation: Mastectomy scar was a healed 8-inch incision, extending from the lateral chest wall in line with the axilla at the level of the fifth and sixth ribs to the sternum. Axillary lymph node dissection scar was well healed but with adhesions throughout.

Musculoskeletal

- Gross symmetry/posture—Overall, Ms. Ledger's posture was slumped and asymmetric throughout the interview. When prompted, she attempted to correct her spine and shoulder girdle posture but was only partially successful.
- Gross ROM/strength—Both lower extremities, left upper extremity, and cervical spine were without impairments in gross mobility and strength. The entire right upper extremity was limited and painful with movement. The patient was reluctant to perform any right shoulder motions secondary to fear and pain.
- Height = 5 feet, 4 inches
- Weight = 166 pounds
- Body mass index (BMI) = 28.5

Neuromuscular

No impairments noted in balance, locomotion, transfers or transitions.

Communication, Affect, Cognition, Language, and Learning Style:

Ms. Ledger was a pleasant, cooperative woman. She was alert, oriented, and eager to "get moving." She and her daughter asked many very appropriate questions specific to physical therapy as well as her overall plan of care. She was appropriately concerned with moving her right upper extremity and fearful of increasing her pain.

She stated that "as a teacher she preferred to understand what was being done and why." She also reported doing best with slow, clear explanations in "layman's" terms. Ms. Ledger had no barriers to learning. All educational needs would be addressed verbally in the clinic and she would be given written instructions as well.

Clinician Comment *Ms. Ledger's interview revealed that she had pain, restrictions in self-care and home management tasks and concerns about whether she had adequate right upper extremity mobility for the planned RT sessions. The systems review confirmed the limitations in right upper extremity ROM and strength as well* *as noted impaired posture and integument characteristics, namely, decreased scar mobility. Because of her extensive axillary surgery and planned RT, Ms. Ledger was at high risk for developing lymphedema. Anthropometric measures of baseline girth and volume were indicated to be taken of her upper extremities, as well, in the tests and measures portion of the examination.*

Tests and Measures

Pain

Ms. Ledger rated her pain as 8/10 using the 10-point Numeric Rating Scale.

Clinician Comment *There are numerous, well documented ways to assess pain. Three that have been found to be valid and reliable are:*

- *The Visual Analog Scale (VAS), which is a 10-cm line on which the patient marks the spot he or she feels corresponds to the level of pain. One endpoint on the line is labeled "no pain" and the other endpoint is labeled "worst pain possible."*
- *The Numeric Rating Scale (NRS) uses a 0 to 10 intensity scale, where zero indicates that there is no pain and 10 is the worst pain imaginable.*
- *The Verbal Rating Scale (VRS) asks patients to choose a word that best describes their pain.[8]*

Self-Care and Home Management (Including Activities of Daily Living and Instrumental Activities of Daily Living)

Ms. Ledger was not able to sleep on her right side because of pain. She reported difficulty dressing. She had not been able to resume driving. The Shoulder Pain and Disability Index (SPADI) was used to establish Ms. Ledger's baseline. Her initial score was 97.8.

Clinician Comment *The SPADI is a 13-item, 2-part questionnaire in which the patient rates his or her pain and level of difficulty with basic daily activities.[9] A higher score is associated with a higher degree of functional limitations. The score is calculated by adding the scores from both parts of the questionnaire, dividing that number by the highest score possible, and then multiplying by 100. The highest score possible is 130 if all the questions are answered. If an item is deemed not applicable, no score is calculated for that item. The SPADI has been found to be reliable and valid in measuring disability in community based patients reporting shoulder pain due to musculoskeletal pathology. The SPADI is available at http://www.workcover.com/worker/reference-library/forms under Documents A – Z.*

Integument

Pliability—The scar was thick and restricted laterally with decreased mobility and adhesions throughout.

Axillary web syndrome/lymphatic cording—There was significant and diffuse cording present throughout the right upper arm, axilla, lateral chest wall, and abdomen.

Clinician Comment *A formal or standardized scar-rating tool was not used to assess Ms. Ledger's soft tissue changes but there are several scar rating tools available that are both valid and reliable. The Vancouver Scar Scale was developed to assess burn scars and is the most widely used scar-rating scale.[10] It has been shown to be a valid, reliable, and feasible tool to objectively evaluate scars after breast cancer surgery. It looks at 4 parameters related to wound maturation, appearance, and function of healed skin. It also assesses pliability, pigmentation, vascularity, and scar height independently. The scar is assigned points for each of these categories and the sum is tallied for the final score. The maximum score is 13 and the lower the score, the "better" the scar. Inter-rater reliability was significant with Spearman's correlation coefficient of 0.66 for the overall score (all p values < 0.001).*

It is estimated that 90% of patients treated with RT for breast cancer will develop some degree of radiation-induced dermatitis.[11] Early effects are those that occur within 90 days of initiation of radiation and include: dryness, epilation, pigment changes, and erythema. Dry and moist desquamation may also develop. Late effects, occurring more than 90 days after completion of RT, may include: atrophy, fibrosis characterized by progressive induration, edema, and thickening of the dermis. Pigmentation changes, telangiectasias, and dermal necrosis can also occur several months after RT has been completed. Physical therapy is crucial during this phase to educate the patient in skin care, prevent postural changes, and maintain joint integrity. Measurement of these changes has tended to be very subjective.

One tool that has been preliminarily investigated for reliability and validity is the Skin Toxicity Assessment Tool (STAT).[12] This tool looks at not only the physical description of the skin, but also asks for patient subjective comments. In addition, there is a section for treatment recommendation. The STAT has been found to have an inter-observer level of agreement for eliciting subjective complaints of 72% to 92% (95% confidence interval (CI) = 63% to 96%; k = 0.33 to 0.68). The inter-observer agreement when scoring skin reactions ranged from 65% to 97.5% (k = 0.46 to 0.81). There is a significant correlation between objective and subjective toxicity scores (p < 0.05).

Lymphatic cording is thought to occur from lymphatic disruption following breast or axillary surgery.[13] Lymphatic cording in the upper quarter is characterized by axillary pain radiating down the upper extremity/chest wall, decreased shoulder ROM, and a palpable or visible web of subcutaneous tissues, especially with upper extremity abduction.[14] Previously named axillary web syndrome because it was first described in the axilla, lymphatic cording more accurately describes the condition as symptoms can extend beyond the axilla, including the chest wall and abdomen. The condition is thought to be a result of lymphovenous injury secondary to positioning in surgery, lymphovenous stasis, or hypercoagulability caused by surgery.[13,14] Another theory suggests that cording may be a result of thrombosed lymphatics and a variant of Mondor's disease.[14] The severity of cording is described as mild, mild-moderate, moderate, moderate to severe, or severe.[14,15] Review of the literature yielded limited information and no studies related to the reliability of this classification system.

Posture

Ms. Ledger held her right upper extremity in a guarded "sling" position in both the standing and seated position. Her right shoulder was elevated and internally rotated. Her scapula was protracted and there was a moderate increase in thoracic kyphosis with an increased flattening of her cervical lordosis. With verbal cues to correct her posture, Ms. Ledger sat a little more erect but did not change her shoulder girdle position.

Clinician Comment *The clinical assessment of posture is largely subjective and descriptive in nature. The plumb line is inexpensive and commonly used for clinical assessment of posture. It establishes a line of reference that coincides with the midline of the body in anterior, posterior, and lateral views.[16] Kendall and McCreary[16] use this plumb line to describe a "standard posture." The visual assessment of posture may have only fair intrarater reliability and poor interrater reliability.[17]*

Range of Motion (Including Muscle Length)

With Ms. Ledger positioned in supine, ROM measures were recorded for her bilateral upper extremities. Cervical spine measures were subjectively assessed with Ms. Ledger seated.

MOTION	RIGHT (Passive Only)	LEFT (Active)	LEFT (Passive)
Shoulder flexion	150 degrees	175 degrees	180 degrees
Shoulder abduction	141 degrees	170 degrees	180 degrees
Shoulder internal rotation	70 degrees	70 degrees	70 degrees

MOTION	RIGHT (Passive Only)	LEFT (Active)	LEFT (Passive)
Shoulder external rotation *Painful/ apprehensive	60 degrees	85 degrees	90 degrees
Shoulder extension	25 degrees	50 degrees	60 degrees
Elbow extension	–10 degrees	0 degrees	0 degrees
Elbow flexion	135 degrees	135 degrees	135 degrees
CERVICAL RANGE OF MOTION			
Forward bend	Full		
Backward bend	Full		
Side bend right	¾		
Side bend left	½		
Rotation right	¾		
Rotation left	½		

Clinician Comment *Goniometric shoulder measurements have high intrarater reliability when taken either in sitting or in supine.[18,19] There is a decreased reliability when taken in one position and then another.[18] It is therefore important to remain consistent in the positioning and in the documentation of the positioning.*

Chen et al[20] identify visual estimation (VE) as a quick and easy way to measure cervical range of motion, but report errors have been estimated to be as great as differences of 5 degrees and 45 degrees. They go on to state that it is too unreliable and its use should be discouraged. They recommend single inclinometry as it has been proven reliable for all active motions but clarify it is most reliable when performed by the same therapist using the same procedure. Youdas et al[21] have also discouraged the use of VE, citing the use of a goniometer or a cervical ROM instrument that was found to have good to high intrarater reliability. Although VE is used as a means for measuring spinal ROM, it may not be the better choice.

Muscle Performance (Including Strength, Power, and Endurance)

MUSCLE GROUP	RIGHT	LEFT
Shoulder flexion	2-/5	4+/5
Shoulder abduction	2-/5	4+/5
Shoulder internal rotation	3/5	5/5

MUSCLE GROUP	RIGHT	LEFT
Shoulder external rotation	2/5	4+/5
Shoulder extension	3+/5	5/5
Elbow extension	3+/5	5/5
Elbow flexion	3+/5	5/5
Middle trapezius	2/5	3+/5
Middle deltoid	2/5	3+/5
Rhomboids	2/5	3/5

Clinician Comment *A literature review performed by Cuthbert and Goodheart[22] found the Manual Muscle Test (MMT) to be a useful clinical tool, but because of the many factors contributing to decreased muscle performance, additional research is required to establish its validity. Other studies, however, have shown the MMT to highly correlate to the hand-held dynamometer, whose reliability has been established.[23] In a study conducted by Bohannon,[24] he concluded that his results "cast doubt in the suitability of MMT as a screening tool for muscle impairment." Though MMT is a commonly used and convenient test, additional research is needed. Hand-held dynamometry might have been the better choice.*

Anthropometric Measures

Upper Limb Volume for Baseline Lymphedema Assessment

Circumferential measurements:

	RIGHT UPPER EXTREMITY*	LEFT UPPER EXTREMITY
MCP	16.6 cm	17 cm
Ulna styloid (US)	15.1	15.2
5 cm above US	17.1	18.4
10 cm	20.7	21.0
15 cm	24.3	24.2
20 cm	25.5	26.2
25 cm	25.4	25.8
30 cm	29.5	29.5
35 cm	31.5	31.0
40 cm	32.8	30.8
Total volume	1837.6 ml	1823.3 ml
Difference	0.07% (patient is right (R) handed)	

MCP: metacarpophalangeal joints.

Clinician Comment *Lymphedema limb assessment can be performed a number of ways: water displacement, tape measure, Perometer (Pero-System), or bioimpedence.[25-28]*

With the factors of cost and convenience considered, a tape measure, with circumferential measurements at 5 cm intervals and subsequent volume calculations, was used.

The volume of a truncated cone is calculated as follows:

$$V = h\ (C1^2 + C1C2 + C^2)/12\pi$$

V is the volume of the segment and C (1) and C (2) are the circumferences at the end of each segment, and h is the distance between them (segment length).

Circumferential girth measurements are a reliable, valid, and fairly easy way to measure for presence of limb edema.[25] Water displacement, although messy and time consuming, is an effective and reliable measurement tool for limb volume.[25,26] Because of the relative ease, convenience and no cost, circumferential girth measurements were used to establish baseline limb volume. The results of these measurements, a 0.07% difference in the right upper extremity in a right-handed individual, indicated that at baseline there is no significant difference between the 2 upper extremities.

EVALUATION

Diagnosis

Practice Pattern

Ms. Ledger fit into several of the Preferred Practice Patterns.

Musculoskeletal Practice Patterns

4B Impaired Posture

4D Impaired Joint Mobility, Motor Function, Muscle Performance, and Range of Motion Associated With Connective Tissue Dysfunction

Integumentary Practice Pattern

7A Primary Prevention/Risk Reduction for Integumentary Disorders

International Classification of Functioning, Disability, and Health Model of Disability

See ICF Model on p 569.

Prognosis

Ms. Ledger had an excellent physical therapy prognosis. It was expected that she would achieve and maintain the ROM required for RT. It was anticipated that she would return to all ADL and light household activities upon completion of RT. Her goal of returning to work as a school teacher in 5 months depended on her response to the medical treatment of her cancer.

ICF Model of Disablement for Ms. Ledger

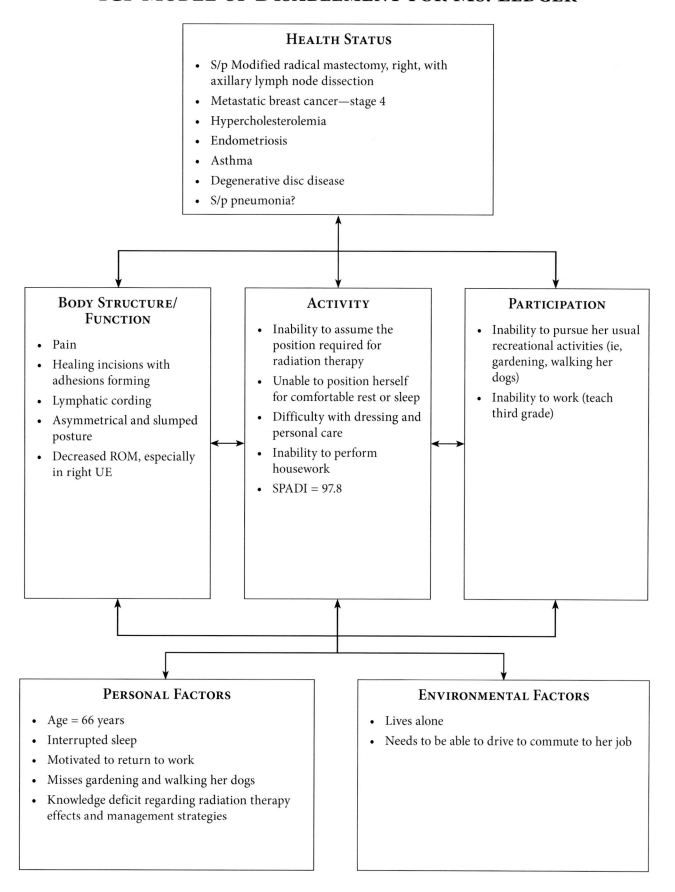

Health Status

- S/p Modified radical mastectomy, right, with axillary lymph node dissection
- Metastatic breast cancer—stage 4
- Hypercholesterolemia
- Endometriosis
- Asthma
- Degenerative disc disease
- S/p pneumonia?

Body Structure/ Function

- Pain
- Healing incisions with adhesions forming
- Lymphatic cording
- Asymmetrical and slumped posture
- Decreased ROM, especially in right UE

Activity

- Inability to assume the position required for radiation therapy
- Unable to position herself for comfortable rest or sleep
- Difficulty with dressing and personal care
- Inability to perform housework
- SPADI = 97.8

Participation

- Inability to pursue her usual recreational activities (ie, gardening, walking her dogs)
- Inability to work (teach third grade)

Personal Factors

- Age = 66 years
- Interrupted sleep
- Motivated to return to work
- Misses gardening and walking her dogs
- Knowledge deficit regarding radiation therapy effects and management strategies

Environmental Factors

- Lives alone
- Needs to be able to drive to commute to her job

Plan of Care

Interventions

Interventions planned for Ms. Ledger included:

- Patient-/client-related instruction regarding her current condition, the plan of care, and the discharge plan.

- Patient education on skin care and lymphedema-prevention guidelines. She would also be instructed to include use of Aquaphor (Eucerin) and daily moisturizing to minimize skin changes before and during RT.

- Manual therapy techniques consisting of: soft tissue mobilization to normalize tissue density of the cervical, shoulder and scapular muscles, scar mobilization and skin tractioning for cording release.

- Scapula and glenohumeral joint mobilization to allow for RT positioning.

- Wand exercises for shoulder flexion, abduction, and extension beginning in supine and progressing to standing. Later the exercises would progress to strengthening with 1- to 2-pound cuff weight or TheraBand.

- An endurance reconditioning program would begin once other interventions were underway and she showed that she could meet a functional walk standard of 500 feet. It was anticipated that she would have a program with timed walking prescription.

- Patient would be instructed in her prescribed home exercise program (HEP), which would be provided in a written form also.

Proposed Frequency and Duration of Physical Therapy Visits

Ms. Ledger would be scheduled for 3 physical therapy sessions per week for 3 weeks in preparation for RT. It was also anticipated that she will need an additional 6 to 8 visits over the course of her RT.

Anticipated Goals

1. Ms. Ledger would have a good understanding of, and comply with, lymphedema precautions and skin care (1 week).

2. Ms. Ledger would tolerate mobilization techniques to mobilize her scar and decrease lymphatic cording (2 to 3 weeks).

3. She would demonstrate independence with an initial HEP (2 to 3 weeks).

4. Her right shoulder flexion would increase to 165 degrees and abduction to 150 degrees to allow for positioning during RT (3 weeks).

5. Ms. Ledger's pain would decrease from 8/10 to 4/10 on the NRS (6 weeks).

6. The mobility of her mastectomy scar would normalize and lymphatic cording would be eliminated or, at least, reduced (8 weeks).

7. Ms. Ledger's right shoulder ROM would be her optimum and tolerant of overpressure at end ranges (10 weeks).

8. All upper extremity MMT show greater than 3+/5 strength, at least (12 weeks).

9. She would be independent in a full home program of mobility, strengthening, and postural correction exercises in addition to a walking program (16 weeks).

Expected Outcomes (16 weeks)

1. Ms. Ledger would resume her previous level of ADL and IADL tasks.

2. She will have an excellent understanding and 100% compliance with lymphedema guidelines/precautions to allow safe return to all previous activities.

3. She would estimate that she would be able to return to, at least, 85% to 90% of her work tasks.

Discharge Plan

The patient would be ready for discharge from physical therapy to her own care when she achieved the anticipated goals and expected outcomes listed above. The plan of care, including the discharge plan, has been discussed with the patient, who was in agreement.

INTERVENTION

Coordination, Communication, and Documentation

Coordinated dialogue with both medical and radiation oncologists, as well as her surgeon, to clarify the required movement for radiation field mapping and treatment would be undertaken, and thereafter as needed. Ongoing communication with patient, family, referral sources, and other caregivers regarding progress toward goals would be pursued. Documentation would include all aspects of care, including initial examination/evaluation, daily treatment notes, telephone conversations, progress reports, reexaminations, and discharge summary.

Patient-/Client-Related Instructions

The patient and her family were informed regarding the plan of care, frequency of visits, and discharge plan as previously discussed.

Ms. Ledger received written and verbal information pertaining to lymphedema prevention guidelines. She was also given information on how to access the National Lymphedema Network (NLN). Lymphedema guidelines are published on the website (http://www.lymphnet.org). Side effects and adverse effects that may occur during and after the delivery of RT, such as fatigue, skin changes, sensation changes, and breast swelling will also be covered throughout the course of therapy. Additional information was also provided on current conservative treatment options, should she develop lymphedema.[6,7]

Skin care, precautions, and preparation for radiation therapy would be reviewed. An integumentary protection technique consisting of skin preparation with Aquaphor daily before RT begins and then continued following the delivery of RT would be reviewed with Ms. Ledger.

A written postural HEP would be initiated along with general activity guidelines, including an endurance reconditioning program.

> **Clinician Comment** *The lymphedema guidelines from the NLN focus on 5 key areas: skin care, activity/lifestyle, avoidance of limb constriction, compression garments, and temperature extremes. Printed educational materials adapted from the NLN guidelines were available to give to Ms. Ledger.*

Procedural Interventions

Manual Therapy Techniques (Including Mobilization/Manipulation)

Ms. Ledger would be seen for scar management and release of lymphatic cording. The manual therapy techniques utilized would include: soft tissue mobilization to normalize tissue density of the cervical, shoulder and scapular muscles, scar mobilization, and skin tractioning for cording release.

> **Clinician Comment** *Although Moskovitz et al[29] suggest that lymphatic cording is self-resolving in a 3-month period, Wyrick et al[13] found a much shorter resolution time with physical therapy intervention. A 3.6-week time frame was the average for acute-onset and only the "late-onset" cases required longer interventions of up to 10 weeks.*

Therapeutic Exercise Prescription

Body Mechanics and Postural Stabilization; Flexibility Exercises

Mode
Active and against gravity, flexibility, and postural exercises.

Intensity
Slow movements through entire ROM, as able, and avoid undue fatigue.

Duration
10 to 15 minutes (for entire routine of identified exercises).

Frequency
10 repetitions, 2 to 3 times per day.

Ms. Ledger would be shown and given an opportunity to practice the exercise program. As her proficiency with the exercises improves, the program will become a HEP to address postural corrections and right shoulder and scapular mobility.

- Cervical side bend and rotation stretching—In sitting, the patient would be instructed to perform gentle stretches to the point of moderate tension only, with a 20-second hold.
- Postural corrections—In sitting, the patient would be instructed in scapula retraction and depression along with gentle chin tuck to restore normal postural alignment, with a 10-second hold.
- Wall walking for shoulder flexion to be performed bilaterally to maintain symmetry and prevent substitution, with a 20-second hold.

Ms. Ledger would be instructed to perform each repetition slowly to achieve maximal benefit.

> **Clinician Comment** *In people with cancer, exercise and physical activity have been shown to improve fitness, reduce fatigue, and modestly reduce weight and body fat. There is also a strong correlation between strenuous exercise and quality of life.[30]*

Aerobic Capacity/Endurance Conditioning or Reconditioning

Mode
Walking program.

Intensity
RPE < 11.

Duration
3 to 5 minutes to cover 250 feet.

Frequency
Once every waking hour until total feet walked for the day is 2000 to 2500 feet.

Ms. Ledger would be instructed in a walking program that would consist of ambulating a minimum of 250 feet for every hour that she was awake. She would be instructed that the distance she walked each time could be short with rests in between, but that it was essential that she walked every hour for a total distance each day of 2000 to 2500 feet.

> **Clinician Comment** *An hourly ambulation schedule with instructions for the patient to total their distance walked over the course of the day is an effective tool for reconditioning patients after hospitalization as the duration and frequency of walking is within their control and they can easily add the distances and track their progress. The frequency and intensity of walking prescriptions are not as important as the total duration of walking when the patient is severely impaired (ability to walk less than*

500 feet in 6 minutes). Once the patient is able to complete a total of 500 feet without shortness of breath or significant fatigue, it is possible to add in the component of "intensity" to the exercise prescription by combining the distance to be walked within a specific time frame. There is research to support the efficacy of intermittent training in improving aerobic conditioning[31] and there are studies to support the efficacy of a walking program in improving walk endurance capacity.[32]

Functional Training in Self-Care and Home Management

Energy Conservation Techniques

Ms. Ledger would receive assistance, as needed, to help her plan her daily and weekly activities but also guidelines for pacing the activities to avoid increased fatigue.

Instrumental Activities of Daily Living Training

Ms. Ledger would have the opportunity to seek advice on how to organize her kitchen to make meal preparation easier.

Injury Prevention or Reduction

Ms. Ledger would have the opportunity to practice simulated IADL tasks—including those requiring forward bending, squatting or lifting—to ensure she was using correct body mechanics.

Prescription, Application, and, as Appropriate, Fabrication of Devices and Equipment (Assistive, Adaptive, Orthotic, Protective, Supportive, and Prosthetic)

Supportive/Prosthetic Device

Ms. Ledger would be referred to a qualified vendor for prosthetic devices and mastectomy bras. If she began to show lymphedema signs in her right upper extremity, her physician would be notified and assistance provided to acquire appropriate compression garments as appropriate.

REEXAMINATION

The first reexamination took place 3 weeks after the initial physical therapy appointment and on the day of anticipated radiation field mapping. Results were as follows:

Subjective

"I feel so much better. I'm anxious to begin radiation."

Objective

Pain

Ms. Ledger reported her pain had improved from 8/10 to a 2/10 on VAS.

Self-Care and Home Management

Ms. Ledger reported she was able to sleep on her right side. She was performing light household chores and she was able to reach overhead with very little pain (eg, she could empty the dishwasher and reach to put plates on the second shelf). Her SPADI score had improved to 11.6.

Integumentary System

Scar/skin integrity—The skin in the area of mastectomy scar was smooth and well moisturized. The scar was well healed and pink. There was good mobility of the scar medially; adhesions persisted at the lateral end of the scar.

The lymphatic cording was reduced from severe to moderate with elimination of the cording in the abdomen inferior to the mastectomy scar. Cording was also reduced in the antecubital area, but persisted in the upper arm, lateral chest wall, and the axilla.

Posture

Ms. Ledger self-corrected her posture during treatment sessions. Her posture was symmetrical with only trace protraction in right shoulder girdle.

Range of Motion

MOTION	RIGHT (ACTIVE)	LEFT (ACTIVE)
Shoulder flexion	165 degrees (was 150 degrees)	175 degrees
Shoulder abduction	165 degrees (was 141 degrees)	170 degrees
Shoulder internal rotation	90 degrees	90 degrees
Shoulder external rotation	90 degrees (was 60 degrees and extremely painful/apprehensive)	85 degrees
Shoulder extension	25 degrees	50 degrees
Elbow extension	0 degrees (was –10 degrees)	0 degrees
Elbow flexion	135 degrees	135 degrees

She was also able to achieve and maintain the overhead position of shoulder flexion/abduction required for RT without pain.

Muscle Performance

MUSCLE GROUP	RIGHT	LEFT
Shoulder flexion	3/5 (was 2/5)	4+/5
Shoulder abduction	3/5 (was 2/5)	4+/5
Shoulder internal rotation	4/5 (was 3/5)	5/5
Shoulder external rotation	4/5 (was 2/5)	4+/5
Shoulder extension	4+/5 (was 3+/5)	5/5
Elbow extension	4+/5 (was 3+/5)	5/5
Elbow flexion	4+/5 (was 3+/5)	5/5
Middle trapezius	3/5 (was 2/5)	3+/5
Middle deltoid	3/5 (was 2/5)	3+/5
Rhomboids	3-/5 (was 2/5)	3/5

Work, Community, and Leisure Reintegration

Ms. Ledger had not returned to work and would remain at home the rest of the summer. She had not yet returned to her leisure activities secondary to fatigue as well as a busy schedule of medical appointments. Her surgeon had not yet cleared her to walk her dogs.

Assessment

Ms. Ledger made excellent progress with her program. She increased the passive and active ROM of her shoulder and reported decreased pain. She was starting to resume self-care and home management activities. She was able to achieve and maintain the overhead position required for RT. She would continue to benefit from physical therapy to further increase her ROM.

Plan

The frequency of treatment sessions was reduced to 2 times per week for 3 weeks and then 1 time per week for 3 weeks to span the projected course of her RT. It was anticipated that she may then need 2 to 4 visits over the remaining 4 to 6 weeks to complete the treatment plan. Treatment sessions would continue to work on glenohumeral and scapula mobilization and progress to shoulder and scapula stabilizer strengthening. Continue to provide education and support regarding skin care changes with RT. Continued monitoring and education regarding skin care would also be indicated as she progressed toward returning to her previous level of activity.

OUTCOMES

Discharge

Ms. Ledger continued to receive physical therapy throughout her course of RT. She received a total of 21 physical therapy treatments. She had achieved all the anticipated goals and reached the desired functional outcomes listed below:

- Her skin had healed, and she was fit for and received a breast prosthesis.

- She was compliant with skin care and prevention guidelines for lymphedema.

- She was dressing without assistance, performing all ADL, self-care activities, and sleeping well.

- She was independent in her HEP and had an excellent understanding of activity progression.

- She was in the process of organizing her classroom and decorating her bulletin boards without limitations in preparation to begin her final year as a third-grade teacher.

Her only stated restriction was with reaching in extreme overhead positions with her right upper extremity.

Clinician Comment *Other self-report shoulder assessment tools include the Disabilities of the Arm, Shoulder and Hand (DASH), the American Shoulder and Elbow Surgeons standardized shoulder form (ASES), the Simple Shoulder Test (SST) and the University of California at Los Angeles (UCLA) Shoulder Score. These have all been found to have good reliability, validity, and responsiveness and while there is a high correlation among the scores, the tools are not equivalent in their assessment of function.*[33] *Because the diagnosis of breast cancer and its subsequent treatment, including surgery, chemotherapy, and RT is more complex than a simple shoulder disability, in retrospect, the SPADI is most appropriate for the short-term measurement of functional outcome.*

A long-term quality of life survey such as the Quality of Life in Adult Cancer Survivors (QLACS) may also have been useful in this case.[34] *The QLACS has 47 items and 12 domains: 7 generic and 5 cancer specific. The generic domains are physical pain, negative feelings, positive feelings, cognitive problems, sexual problems, social avoidance, and fatigue. The cancer-specific domains are financial problems resulting from cancer, distress about the family, distress about reoccurrence, appearance concerns, and benefits of cancer. In a study by Avis et al,*[34] *the QLACS was evaluated for test-retest reliability, concurrent and retrospective validity, and responsiveness. The results of that study showed good test-retest reliability and high internal consistency. The generic domain summary showed consistency with other health-related quality of life (HRQL) tools. The cancer-specific domains exhibited divergent validity with generic HRQL but not cancer specific. The QLACS showed a satisfactory predictive validity for factors previously shown to correlate with HRQL. Although lengthy, this tool may have been useful in determining the overall outcome status for Ms. Ledger.*

REFERENCES

1. American Cancer Society. Breast Cancer Facts and Figures 2007-2008. Atlanta, GA: American Cancer Society Inc. http://www.cancer.org/research/cancerfactsfigures/breastcancerfactsfigures/breast-cancer-facts--figures-2007-2008. Accessed June 2, 2014.
2. National Cancer Institute. September 25, 2008. http://www.cancer.gov/cancertopics/pdq/treatment/breast/HealthProfessional/page1. Accessed October 28, 2008.
3. Seidman AW, Fornier MN, Esteva FJ, et al. Weekly trastuzumab and paclitaxel therapy for metastatic breast cancer with analysis of efficacy by HER2 immunophenotype and gene amplification. *J Clin Oncol.* 2001;19(10):2587-2595.
4. Mieog JS, van der Hage JA, van de Velde CJ. Neoadjuvant chemotherapy for operable breast cancer. *Br J Surg.* 2007;94(10):1189-1200.
5. RxList. The Internet Drug Index. http://www.rxlist.com. Accessed June 2, 2014.
6. Moseley AL, Carati CJ, Pillar NB. A systematic review of common conservative therapies for arm lymphoedema secondary to breast cancer treatment. *Ann Oncol.* 2007;18:639-646.
7. Bicego D, Brown K, Ruddick M, Storey D, Wong C, Harris SR. Exercise for women with or at risk for breast cancer-related lymphedema. *Phys Ther.* 2006;86(10):1398-1405.
8. Paice JA, Cohen FL. Validity of a verbally administered numeric rating scale to measure cancer pain intensity. *Cancer Nurs.* 1997;20(2):88-93.
9. MacDermid J, Solomon P, Prkachin K. The Shoulder Pain and Disability Index demonstrates factor, construct and longitudinal validity. *BMC Musculoskelet Disord.* 2006;7:12.
10. Truong P, Abnousi F, Yong C, et al. Standardized assessment of breast cancer surgical scars integrating the Vancouver Scar Scale, Short-Form Mcgill Pain Questionnaire, and patients' perspectives. *Plast Reconstr Surg.* 2005;116(5):1291-1299.
11. Harper JL, Franklin LE, Jenrette JM, Aquero EG. Skin toxicity during breast irradiation: pathophysiology and management. *South Med J.* 2004;97(10):989-993.
12. Berthelet E, Truong P, Musso K, et al. Preliminary reliability and validity testing of a new Skin Toxicity Assessment Tool (STAT) in breast cancer patients undergoing radiotherapy. *Am J Clin Oncol.* 2004;27(6):626-631.
13. Wyrick SL, Waltke LJ, Ng AV. Physical therapy may promote resolution of lymphatic cording in breast cancer survivors. *Rehab Oncol.* 2006;24:29-34.
14. Kepics JM. Physical therapy treatment of axillary web syndrome. *Rehab Oncol.* 2004;22:21-22.
15. Severied K, Simpson J, Templeton B, York R, Hummel-Berry K, Leiserowitz A. Lymphatic cording among patients with breast cancer or melanoma referred to physical therapy. *Rehab Oncol.* 2007;25:8-13.
16. Griegel-Morris P, Larson K, Mueller-Klaus K, Oatis CA. Incidence of common postural abnormalities in the cervical, shoulder, and thoracic regions and their association with pain in two age groups of healthy subjects. *Phys Ther.* 1992;72(6):425-431.
17. Fedorak C, Ashworth N, Marshall JB, Paull H. Reliability of the visual assessment of cervical and lumbar lordosis: how good are we? *Spine (Phila Pa 1976).* 2003;28(16):1857-1859.
18. Sabari JS, Maltzev I, Lubarsky D, Liszkay E, Homel P. Goniometric assessment of shoulder range of motion: comparison of testing in supine and sitting positions. *Arch Phys Med Rehabil.* 1998;79(6):647-651.
19. Riddle DL, Rothstein JM, Lamb RL. Goniometric reliability in the clinical setting: shoulder measurements. *Phys Ther.* 1987;67:668-673.
20. Chen J, Solinger AB, Poncet JF, Lantz CA. Meta-analysis of normative cervical motion. *Spine (Phila Pa 1976).* 1999;24(15):1571-1578.
21. Youdas JW, Carey JR, Garrett TR. Reliability of cervical spine range of motion—a comparison of three methods. *Phys Ther.* 1991;71(2):98-104.
22. Cuthbert SC, Goodheart GJ Jr. On the reliability and validity of manual muscle testing: a literature review. *Chiropr Osteopat.* 2007;15:4.
23. Bohannon RW. Measuring knee extensor muscle strength. *Am J Phys Med Rehabil.* 2001;80:13-18.
24. Bohannon RW. Manual muscle testing: does it meet the standards of an adequate screening test? *Clin Rehabil.* 2005;19:662-667.
25. Taylor R, Jayasinghe UW, Koelmeyer L, Ung O, Boyages J. Reliability and validity of arm volume measurements for assessment of lymphedema. *Phys Ther.* 2006;86(2):205-214.
26. Sander AP, Hajer NM, Hemenway K, Miller AC. Upper-extremity volume measurements in women with lymphedema: a comparison of measurements obtained via water displacement with geometrically determined volume. *Phys Ther.* 2002;82(12):1201-1212.
27. Warren AG, Brorsun H, Borud LJ, Slavin SA. Lymphedema: a comprehensive review. *Ann Plas Surg.* 2007;59(4):464-472.
28. Cornish BH, Ward LC, Thomas BJ, Bunce IH. Quantification of lymphoedema using multi-frequency bioimpedance. *Appl Radiat Isot.* 1998;49(5-6):651-652.
29. Moskovitz AH, Anderson BO, Yeong RS, Byrd DR, Lawton TJ, Moe RE. Axillary web syndrome after axillary dissection. *Am J Surg.* 2001;181(5):434-439.
30. Valenti M, Porzio G, Aielli F, et al. Physical exercise and the quality of life in breast cancer survivors. *Int J Med Sci.* 2008;5(1):24-28.
31. Christensen EH, Hedman R, Saltin B: Intermittent and continuous running. *Acta Physiol Scand.* 1960;50:269-286.
32. MacRae PG, Asplund LA, Schnell JF, Ouslander JG, Abrahamse A, Morris C. A walking program for nursing home residents: effects on walk endurance, physical activity, mobility, and quality of life. *J Am Geriatr Soc.* 1996;44(2):175-180.
33. McClure P, Michener L. Measures of adult shoulder function: The American Shoulder and Elbow Surgeons Standardized Shoulder Form Patient Self-Report Section (ASES), Disabilities of the Arm, Shoulder, and Hand (DASH), Shoulder Disability Questionnaire, Shoulder Pain and Disability Index (SPADI), and Simple Shoulder Test. *Arthritis Care Res.* 2003;49(S5):S50-S58.
34. Avis NE, Ip E, Foley KL. Evaluation of the Quality of Life in Adult Cancer Survivors (QLACS) scale for long-term cancer survivors in a sample of breast cancer survivors. *Health Qual Life Outcomes.* 2006;4:92.

Financial Disclosures

Dr. Joanell A. Bohmert has no financial or proprietary interest in the materials presented herein.

Dr. Lisa Brown has no financial or proprietary interest in the materials presented herein.

Cheryl L. Brunelle has no financial or proprietary interest in the materials presented herein.

Dr. LeeAnne Carrothers has no financial or proprietary interest in the materials presented herein.

Dr. David Chapman has no financial or proprietary interest in the materials presented herein.

Dr. Cynthia Coffin-Zadai has not disclosed any relevant financial information.

Dr. Debra Coglianese has no financial or proprietary interest in the materials presented herein.

Kathleen Coultes has no financial or proprietary interest in the materials presented herein.

Dr. Vanina Dal Bello-Haas has no financial or proprietary interest in the materials presented herein.

Dr. Skye Donovan has no financial or proprietary interest in the materials presented herein.

Dr. Susan L. Edmond has no financial or proprietary interest in the materials presented herein.

Dr. Nancy Gage has no financial or proprietary interest in the materials presented herein.

Dr. Paul D. Gaspar has no financial or proprietary interest in the materials presented herein.

Dr. Melanie A. Gillar has no financial or proprietary interest in the materials presented herein.

Laura Klassen has no financial or proprietary interest in the materials presented herein.

Dr. Kerri Lang has no financial or proprietary interest in the materials presented herein.

Dr. Daniel Malone receives royalties from SLACK Incorporated for his work, *Physical Therapy in Acute Care*.

Dr. Mary Jane Myslinski has no financial or proprietary interest in the materials presented herein.

Dr. Lola Sicard Rosenbaum has no financial or proprietary interest in the materials presented herein.

Dr. Brian D. Roy has no financial or proprietary interest in the materials presented herein.

Dr. Robert M. Snow has no financial or proprietary interest in the materials presented herein.

Dr. Alison L. Squadrito has no financial or proprietary interest in the materials presented herein.

Dr. Jane L. Wetzel has no financial or proprietary interest in the materials presented herein.

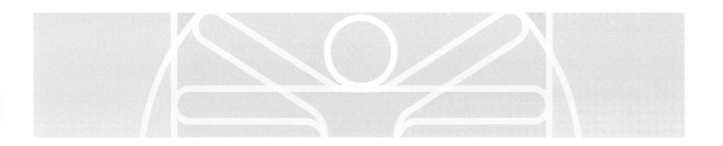

Index

Printed in the United States
by Baker & Taylor Publisher Services